# The Comprehensive Treatment of the Aging Spine

**Minimally Invasive and Advanced Techniques**

# The Comprehensive Treatment of the Aging Spine

## Minimally Invasive and Advanced Techniques

**Edition: 1**

**James Joseph Yue, MD**
Associate Professor
Yale University School of Medicine
Department of Orthopaedic Surgery and
 Rehabilitation
New Haven, Connecticut

**Richard D. Guyer, MD**
President, Texas Back Institute
Plano, Texas
Associate Clinical Professor
Department of Orthopedics
University of Texas, Southwestern Medical
 School
Dallas, Texas

**J. Patrick Johnson, MD, FACS**
Neurosurgeon, Spine Specialist
Director of Education, Spine Fellowship and
 Academic Programs
Co-Director, Spine Stem Cell Research Program
Director, California Association of Neurological
 Surgeons
Los Angeles, California

**Larry T. Khoo, MD**
Director of Minimally Invasive Neurological
 Spinal Surgery
Los Angeles Spine Clinic
Los Angeles, California

**Stephen H. Hochschuler, MD**
Chairman, Texas Back Institute Holdings
Paradise Valley, Arizona

**SAUNDERS**

ELSEVIER

MT

# ELSEVIER
SAUNDERS

1600 John F. Kennedy Blvd.
Ste 1800
Philadelphia, PA 19103-2899

ISBN: 978-1-4377-0373-3

THE COMPREHENSIVE TREATMENT OF THE AGING SPINE
MINIMALLY INVASIVE AND ADVANCED TECHNIQUES

---

Notice

Knowledge and best practice in this field are constantly changing. As new research and experience broaden our understanding, changes in research methods, professional practices, or medical treatment may become necessary.

Practitioners and researchers must always rely on their own experience and knowledge in evaluating and using any information, methods, compounds, or experiments described herein. In using such information or methods they should be mindful of their own safety and the safety of others, including parties for whom they have a professional responsibility.

With respect to any drug or pharmaceutical products identified, readers are advised to check the most current information provided (i) on procedures featured or (ii) by the manufacturer of each product to be administered, to verify the recommended dose or formula, the method and duration of administration, and contraindications. It is the responsibility of practitioners, relying on their own experience and knowledge of their patients, to make diagnoses, to determine dosages and the best treatment for each individual patient, and to take all appropriate safety precautions.

To the fullest extent of the law, neither the Publisher nor the authors, contributors, or editors, assume any liability for any injury and/or damage to persons or property as a matter of products liability, negligence or otherwise, or from any use or operation of any methods, products, instructions, or ideas contained in the material herein.

---

**Library of Congress Cataloging-in-Publication Data**

The comprehensive treatment of the aging spine : minimally invasive and advanced techniques / [edited by] James Joseph Yue ... [et al.]. — 1st ed.
    p. ; cm.
  Includes bibliographical references.
  ISBN 978-1-4377-0373-3
  1. Spine—Diseases—Treatment. I. Yue, James J.
  [DNLM: 1. Spinal Diseases—diagnosis. 2. Spinal Diseases—therapy. 3. Aged. 4. Aging—physiology. 5. Physical Therapy Modalities. 6. Spine—surgery. WE 725 C7378 2011]
  RD768.C645 2011
  617.4'71--dc22                                                      2010001778

*Acquisitions Editor:* Adrianne Brigido
*Developmental Editor:* Anne Snyder
*Publishing Services Manager:* Debbie Vogel/Anitha Raj
*Project Manager:* Sruthi Viswam/Kiruthiga Kasthuri
*Design Direction:* Ellen Zanolle

Printed in the United States of America

Last digit is the print number:  9  8  7  6  5  4  3  2  1

6/20/11

*To my mother, Mary Jude, for her endless wisdom and encouragement and eternal motivaton.*

*James J. Yue*

*I dedicate this book to my wonderful wife, Shelly, whose inspiration and love has sustained me through my career and taught me how to live life to its fullest. I also dedicate this endeavor to the thousands of patients who will hopefully benefit from the advances discussed in this book.*

*Richard D. Guyer*

*I dedicate the efforts of this book to all my family, friends, mentors, and patients, who have taught me to be the best surgeon possible; and to my fellows and residents, whom I have taught to be a better surgeon than me.*

*J. Patrick Johnson*

*This book is dedicated to all whom endeavor to ease the pain and suffering of spinal disease. From therapist to surgeon and from master to student, I pray that these pages will not only guide you in the labors of today, but also to the discoveries of tomorrow. I give humble thanks to the devotion of my residents and fellows, both past and present, without whom this volume and all other academia would not be possible. And at the end, I am the most grateful to Kristine, Miya and Taka, whose boundless love and understanding is the beacon that lights my way every single day.*

*Larry T. Khoo*

*I would like to dedicate this book to Ralph Rashsbaum, MD, without whose friendship and guidance for more than forty years, The Texas Back Institute would not have existed.*

*Stephen H. Hochschuler*

# Contributors

**Khalid M. Abbed, MD**
Assistant Professor of Neurosurgery
Chief, Yale Spine Institute
Director, Minimally Invasive Spine Surgery
Director, Oncologic, Spine Surgery, Neurosurgery
Yale School of Medicine
New Haven, CT, USA

**Kathleen Abbott, MD, RPT**
Interventional Physiatrist
Pioneer Spine and Sports Physicians, P.C.
Glastonbury, CT, USA

**Nduka Amankulor, MD**
Resident
Department of Neurosurgery
Yale University School of Medicine
New Haven, CT, USA

**Carmina F. Angeles, MD, PhD**
Clinical Instructor/Spine Fellow
Neurosurgery
Stanford University Medical Center
Stanford, CA, USA

**Ali Araghi, DO**
Assistant Clinical Professor
Texas Back Institute
Phoenix, AZ, USA

**Rajesh G. Arakal, MD**
Orthopaedic Spine Surgeon
Texas Back Institute
Plano, TX, USA

**Sean Armin, MD**
Neurosurgeon
Riverside Neurosurgical Associates
Riverside, CA, USA

**Farbod Asgarzadie, MD**
Department of Neurosurgery
Loma Linda University Medical Center
Loma Linda, CA, USA

**Darwono A. Bambang, MD, PhD**
Division of Orthopaedic and Spine
Gading-Pluit Hospital Senior Lecturer
Orthopedic Department
Faculty of Medicine, Taruma Negara University
Jakarta Utara, Indonesia

**Jose Carlos Sauri Barraza**
Department of Orthopaedics
Centro Médico ABC
Mexico City, Mexico

**John A. Bendo, MD**
Director, Spine Services
New York University Hospital for Joint Diseases
Assistant Professor of Orthopedic Surgery
New York University School of Medicine
New York, NY, USA

**Edward C. Benzel, MD**
Chairman, Department of Neurosurgery
Neurological Institute
Cleveland Clinic
Cleveland, OH, USA

**Jason A. Berkley, DO**
Staff Physician, Department of Nanology
Neurology/Interventional Spine Pain Management
Institute for Spinal Disorders
Cedars Sinai Medical Center
Los Angeles, CA, USA

**Rudolf Bertagnoli, MD**
Chairman
First European Center for Spine Arthroplasty and
Associated Non Fusion Technologies
St. Elisabeth Krankenhaus Straubing, KKH
Bogen, Germany

**Obeneba Boachie-Adjei, MD**
Weill Medical College of Cornell University
Professor of Orthopaedic Surgery
Hospital for Special Surgery
Attending Orthopaedics Surgeon
Chief of Scoliosis Service
New York Presbyterian Hospital
Attending Orthopaedics Surgeon
Memorial Sloan-Kettering Cancer Center
Associate Attending Surgeon
New York, NY, USA

**Alan C. Breen, DC, PhD, MIPEM**
Professor of Musculoskeletal Health Care
Institute for Musculoskeletal Research and Clinical Implementation
Anglo-European College of Chiropractic
Bournemouth, Dorset, UK

**Courtney W. Brown, MD**
Assistant Clinical Professor
Department of Orthopedics
University of Colorado
Denver, CO, USA

**Chunbo Cai, MD, MPH**
Spine Clinic
Department of Physical Medicine
Kaiser Permanente Medical Center
San Francisco, CA, USA

**Charles S. Carrier**
Clinical Research Coordinator
Orthopaedic Spine Service
Massachusetts General Hospital
Boston, MA, USA

**Thomas J. Cesarz, MD**
Instructor
Orthopaedics
University of Rochester Medical Center
Rochester, NY, USA

**Boyle C. Cheng, PhD**
Assistant Professor
University of Pittsburgh
Co-Director
Spine Research Laboratory
Pittsburgh, PA, USA

**Kenneth M.C. Cheung, MBBS, MD, FRCS, FHKCOS, FHKAM(Orth)**
Clinical Professor
Department of Orthoapedics and Traumatology
University of Hong Kong
Pokfulam, Hong Kong

**Etevaldo Coutinho, MD**
Instituto de Patologia da Coluna
São Paulo, Brazil

**Reginald J. Davis, MD, FACS**
Chief of Neurosurgery
Greater Baltimore Medical Center
Towson, MD, USA

**Adam K. Deitz**
CEO
Ortho Kinematics, Inc.
Austin, TX, USA

**Perry Dhaliwal, MD**
Department of Clinical Neurosciences
Division of Neurosurgery
University of Calgary
Calgary, Alberta, Canada

**Rob D. Dickerman, DO, PhD**
Neurological and Spine Surgeon
North Texas Neurosurgical Associates
Adjunct Professor of Neurosurgery
University of North Texas Health Science Center
Fort Worth, Texas;
Professor
Texas Back Institute
Plano, TX, USA

**David A. Essig, MD**
Department of Orthopaedic Surgery
Yale University School of Medicine
New Haven, CT, USA

**Alice Fann, MD**
Atlanata VA Medical Center
Department of Rehabiliation Medicine
Emory University School of Medicine
Decatur, GA, USA

**Michael Fehlings, MD, PhD**
Neurosurgeon
Toronto Western Hospital
Toronto, Ontario, Canada

**Lisa Ferrara, PhD**
President
OrthoKinetic Technologies, LLC and OrthoKinetic Testing Technologies, LLC
Southport, NC, USA

**Richard G. Fessler, MD, PhD**
Professor
Department of Neurosurgery
Northwestern University Feinberg School of Medicine
Chicago, IL, USA

**Zair Fishkin, MD, PhD**
Attending Surgeon
Department of Orthopaedic Surgery
Buffalo General Hospital
Buffalo, NY , USA

**Amy Folta, PharmD**

**Kai-Ming Gregory Fu, MD, PhD**
Spine Fellow
Neurological Surgery
University of Virginia
Charlottesville, VA, USA

**Shu Man Fu, MD, PhD, MACR**
Professor of Medicine and Microbiology
Margaret M. Trolinger Professor of Rheumatology
Division of Clinical Rheumatology and Center for Immunity, Inflammation, and Regenerative Medicine
University of Virginia School of Medicine
Charlottesville, VA, USA

**Anand A. Gandhi, MD**
Interventional Pain Management
Laser Spine Institute
Scottsdale, AZ, USA

**Elizabeth Gardner, PhD**
Resident
Department of Orthopaedic Surgery
Yale New Haven Hospital
New Haven, CT, USA

**Steven R. Garfin, MD**
Professor and Chair
Department of Orthopaedics
University of California, San Diego
San Diego, CA, USA

**Hitesh Garg, MBBS, MS(Orth)**
Fellowship in Spine Surgery
Yale University School of Medicine, USA
Associate Consultant
Spine Surgery
Artemis Health Institute
Gurgaon, Haryana, India

**Avrom Gart, MD**
Assistant Clinical Professor
Physical Medicine and Rehabilitation
UCLA, Medical Center
Medical Director
Spine Center
Cedars-Sinai Medical center
Los Angeles, CA, USA

**Samer Ghostine, MD**
Department of Neurosurgery
Loma Linda University Medical Center
Loma Linda, CA, USA

**Brian P. Gladnick, BA**
Weill Cornell Medical College
New York, NY, USA

**Ziya L. Gokaslan, MD, FACS**
Department of Neurosurgery
The Johns Hopkins Hospital
Baltimore, MD, USA

**Jeffrey A. Goldstein, MD**
Director of Spine Service
New York University Hospital for Joint Diseases
New York, NY, USA

**Oren N. Gottfried, MD**
Assistant Professor
Department of Neurosurgery
Duke University Medical Center
Durham, NC, USA

**Grahame C. D. Gould, MD**
Resident Physician
Neurosurgery
Yale New Haven Hospital
New Haven, Connecticut, USA

**Jonathan N. Grauer, MD**
Associate Professor
Department of Orthopaedics and Rehabilitation
Yale University School of Medicine
New Haven, CT, USA

**Richard D. Guyer, MD**
President, Texas Back Institute
Plano, Texas;
Associate Clinical Professor
Department of Orthopedics
University of Texas, Southwestern Medical School
Dallas, TX, USA

**Eric B. Harris, MD**
Director, Multidisciplinary Spine Center
Director of Orthopaedic Spine Surgery
Department of Orthopaedics
Naval Medical Center San Diego
San Diego, CA, USA

**Christopher C. Harrod, MD**
Resident
Harvard Combined Orthopaedic Residency Program
Boston, MA, USA

**Paul F. Heini, MD**
Associate Professor
University of Bern
Bern, Switzerland

**Shawn F. Hermenau, MD**
Spine Fellow
Orthopaedic Surgery
Yale University School of Medicine
New Haven, CT, USA

**Stephen H. Hochschuler, MD**
Chairman
Texas Back Institute Holdings
Paradise Valley, AZ, USA

**Daniel J. Hoh, MD**
Assistant Professor
Department of Neurosurgery
University of Florida
Gainesville, FL;
Department of Neurological Surgery
Keck School of Medicine
University of Southern California
Los Angeles, CA, USA

**Wei Huang, MD, PhD**
Assistant Professor
Rehabilitation Medicine
Emory University
Atlanta, GA, USA

**R. John Hurlbert, MD, PhD, FRCSC, FACS**
Associate Professor
Department of Clinical Neurosciences
University of Calgary
Calgary, Alberta, Canada

**J. Patrick Johnson, MD, FACS**
Neurosurgeon, Spine Specialist
Director of Education, Spine Fellowship and Academic Programs
Co-Director, Spine Stem Cell Research Program
Director, California Association of Neurological Surgeons
Los Angeles, CA, USA

**Jaro Karppinen, PhD, MD**
Professor
Physical and Rehabilitation Medicine
Institute of Clinical Sciences
University of Oulu
Oulu, Finland

**Tony M. Keaveny, PhD**
Professor
Departments of Mechanical Engineering and Bioengineering
University of California
Berkeley, CA, USA

**Larry T. Khoo, MD**
Los Angeles Spine Clinic
Los Angeles, CA, USA

**Choll W. Kim, MD**
Associate Clinical Professor
Department of Orthopaedic Surgery
University of California San Diego
Spine Institute of San Diego
Center for Minimally Invasive Spine Surgery at Alvarado Hospital
Executive Director, Society for Minimally Invasive Spine Surgery
San Diego, CA, USA

**Terrence Kim, MD**
Orthopaedic Surgeon
Cedars Sinai Spine Center
Los Angeles, CA, USA

**Woo-Kyung Kim, MD, PhD**
Professor and Chair of Neurosurgery
Gachon University
Gil Medical Center
Spine Center
Incheon, South Korea

**Joseph M. Lane, MD**
Professor of Orthopaedic Surgery
Assistant Dean, Medical Students
Weill Cornell Medical College
Orthopaedics
Hospital for Special Surgery
Chief, Metabolic Bone Disease Service
Hospital for Special Surgery
New York, NY , USA

**Jared T. Lee, MD**
Resident
Harvard Combined Orthopaedic Residency Program
Boston, MA, USA

**Robert E. Lieberson, MD, FACS**
Clinical Assistant Professor
Department of Neurosurgery
Stanford University Medical Center
Stanford, CA, USA

**Lonnie E. Loutzenhiser, MD**
Orthopaedic Spine Surgeon
Panorama Orthopedics & Spine Center
Golden, CO, USA

**Malary Mani, BS**
University of Washington
Seattle, Washington, WA

**Satyajit Marawar, MD**
Spine Fellow
Upstate University Hospital
Syracuse, NY, USA

**Jason Marchetti, MD**
Medical Director of Inpatient Rehabilitation
Mayhill Hospital
Denton, TX, USA

**H. Michael Mayer, MD, PHD**
Professor of Neurosurgery
Paracelsus Medical School
Salzburg, Austria;
Medical Director and Chairman
Schön-Klink München Harlaching
Munich, Germany

**Vivek Arjun Mehta, BS**
Medical Student
Department of Neurosurgery
The Johns Hopkins Hospital
Baltimore, MD, USA

**Fiona E. Mellor, BSc (Hons)**
Research Radiographer
Institute for Musculoskeletal Research and Clinical Implementation
Anglo-European College of Chiropractic
Bournemouth, Dorset, UK

**Christopher Meredith, MD**
Desert Institute for Spine Care
Phoenix, AZ, USA

**Vincent J. Miele, MD**
Neurosurgical Spine Fellow
Cleveland Clinic
Cleveland, OH , USA

**Jack Miletic, MD**
Interventional Spine/Pain Management
Institute for Spinal Disorders
Cedars Sinai Medical Center
Los Angeles, CA, USA

**Christopher P. Miller, BA**
Department of Orthopaedics and Rehabilitation
Yale University School of Medicine
New Haven, CT, USA

**Florence Pik Sze Mok, MSc, PDD, GC, BSc**
PhD Candidate
Orthopaedic & Traumatology
Li Ka Shing Faculty of Medicine
The University of Hong Kong
Hong Kong

**Joseph M. Morreale, MD**
Spine Surgeon
Center for Spinal Disorders
Thornton, CO, USA

**Kieran Murphy, MB, FRCPC, FSIR**
Professor and Vice Chair
Department of Medical Imaging
University of Toronto
Toronto, Ontario, Canada

**Frank John Ninivaggi, MD, FAPA**
Assistant Clinical Professor
Yale Child Study Center
Yale University School of Medicine
Associate Attending Physician
Yale-New Haven Hospital
New Haven, CT, USA

**Donna D. Ohnmeiss, Dr.Med.**
President
Texas Back Institute Research Foundation
Plano, TX, USA

**Chukwuka Okafor, MD, MBA**
Orthopaedic Surgery
Bartow Regional Medical Center
Lakeland, FL, USA

**Wayne J. Olan, MD**
Clinical Professor Radiology and Neurosurgery
The George Washington University Medical Center
Washington, DC;
Director
Neuroradiology/ MRI
Suburban Hospital
Bethesda, MD, USA

**Leonardo Oliveira, BSc**
Masters Degree (in course)
Radiology
Universidade Federal de São Paulo
São Paulo, Brazil

**Manohar Panjabi, PhD**
Professor Emeritus
Orthopaedics and Rehabilitation
Yale University School of Medicine
New Haven, CT, USA

**Jon Park, MD**
Director, Comprehensive Spine Neurosurgery
Director, Spine Research Laboratory and Fellowship Program
Stanford, CA, USA

**Scott L. Parker, BS**
Medical Student
Department of Neurosurgery
The Johns Hopkins University School of Medicine
Baltimore, MD, USA

**Rajeev K. Patel, MD**
Associate Professor
University of Rochester Spine Center
Rochester, NY, USA

**Robert Pflugmacher, MD**
Associate Professor
Department of Orthopaedic and Trauma Surgery
University of Bonn
Bonn, Germany

**Frank M. Phillips, MD**
Professor, Spine Fellowship
Co-Director, Orthopaedic Surgery
Head, Section of Minimally Invasive Spinal Surgery
Rush University Medical Center
Chicago, IL, USA

**Luiz Pimenta, MD, PhD**
Associate Professor
Neurosurgery Universidade Federal de São Paulo
São Paulo, Brazil;
Assistant Professor
University of California San Diego
San Diego, CA, USA

**Colin S. Poon, MD, PhD, FRCPC**
Assistant Professor of Radiology
Director of Head and Neck Imaging;
Director of Neuroradiology Fellowship
Department of Radiology
University of Chicago
Chicago, IL, USA

**Ann Prewett, PhD**
President and CEO
Replication Medical, Inc.
Cranbury, NJ, USA

**Kamshad Raiszadeh, MD**
Spine Institute of San Diego
Center for Minimally Invasive Spine Surgery at Alvarado Hospital
San Diego, CA, USA

**Amar D. Rajadhyaksha, MD**
New York University Hospital for Joint Diseases
Department of Orthopaedic Surgery
Division of Spine Surgery
New York, NY, USA

**Kiran F. Rajneesh, MD, MS**
Research Fellow
Department of Neurological Surgery
University of California, Irvine
Orange, CA, USA

**Ravi Ramachandran, MD**
Resident Physician
Department of Orthopaedics and Rehabilitation
Yale University School of Medicine
New Haven, CT, USA

**Luis M. Rosales**
Assistant Professor
School of Medicine
Universidad Nacional Autonoma de Mexico
Mexico City, DF, Mexico

**Hajeer Sabet, MD, MS**
Spine Surgery Fellow
Department of Orthopaedic Surgery
Rush University
Chicago, IL, USA

**Barton L. Sachs, MD, MBA, CPE**
Professor of Orthopaedics
Executive Assistant Director of Neurosciences and
Musculoskeletal Services
Medical University of South Carolina
Charleston, SC, USA

**Nelson S. Saldua, MD**
Staff Spine Surgeon
Department of Orthopaedic Surgery
Naval Medical Center San Diego
San Diego, CA, USA

**Dino Samartzis, DSc, PhD (C ), MSc, FRIPH, MACE, Dip EBHC**
Research Assistant Professor
Department of Orthopaedics and Traumatology
University of Hong Kong
Pokfulam, Hong Kong

**Srinath Samudrala, MD**
Neurosurgeon
Cedars-Sinai Institute for Spinal Disorders
Los Angeles, CA, USA

**Harvinder S. Sandhu, MD**
Associate Professor of Orthopedic Surgery
Weill Medical College of Cornell University;
Associate Attending Orthopaedic Surgeon
Hospital for Special Surgery
Assistant Scientist
Hospital for Special Surgery
New York, NY, USA

**Karl D. Schultz, Jr. MD, FRCS**
Practicing Neurosurgeon
Northeast Georgia Medical Center
Gainesville, GA, USA

**Stephen Scibelli, MD**
Neurosurgeon
Cedars-Sinai Institute for Spinal Disorders
Los Angeles, California

**Christopher I. Shaffrey, MD**
Harrison Distinguished Professor
Neurological and Orthopaedic Surgery
University of Virginia
Charlottesville, VA, USA

**Jessica Shellock, MD**
Orthopedic Spine Surgeon
Texas Back Institute
Plano, TX, USA

**Ali Shirzadi, MD**
Senior Resident
Neurological Surgery Residency Program
Department of Neurosurgery
Cedars-Sinai, Los Angeles, CA

**Josef B. Simon, MD**
Division of Neurosurgery
New England Baptist Hospital
Boston, MA, USA

**Kern Singh, MD**
Assistant Professor
Orthopaedic Surgery
Rush University Medical Center
Chicago, IL, USA

**Zachary A. Smith, MD**
Department of Neurosurgery
UCLA Medical Center
Los Angeles, CA, USA

**David Speach, MD**
Associate Professor
Orthopaedics and Rehabilitation
University of Rochester School of Medicine
Rochester, NY, USA

**Sathish Subbaiah, MD**
Assistant Professor
Neurosurgery
Mount Sinai School of Medicine
New York, NY, USA

**Deydre Smyth Teyhen, PT, PhD, OCS**
Associate Professor, Doctoral Program in Physical Therapy
U.S. Army-Baylor University Doctoral Program in Physical Therapy
Fort Sam Houston, TX, USA

**Gordon Sze, MD**
Professor of Radiology
Section Chief of Neuroradiology
Yale University School of Medicine
New Haven, CT, USA

**G. Ty Thaiyananthan, MD**
Assistant Clinical Professor of Neurosurgery
Department of Neurological Surgery
University of California, Irvine
Irvine, CA, USA

**William Thoman, MD**
Northwestern University
Chicago, IL, USA

**Eeric Truumees, MD**
Adjunct Faculty
Bioengineering Center
Wayne State University
Detroit, MI, USA

**Aasis Unnanuntana, MD**
Fellow
Orthopaedic Surgery
Hospital for Special Surgery
New York, NY, USA

**Alexander R. Vaccaro, MD, PhD**
Professor of Orthopaedics and Neurosurgery
Co-Director
Thomas Jefferson University/Rothman Institute
Philadelphia, PA, USA

**Sumeet Vadera, MD**
Neurosurgery Resident
Cleveland Clinic
Department of Neurological Surgery
Cleveland, OH, USA

**Shoshanna Vaynman, PhD**
The Spine Institute Foundation
Los Angeles, CA, USA

**Michael Y. Wang, MD, FACS**
Associate Professor
Departments of Neurological Surgery and Rehabilitation Medicine
University of Miami Miller School of Medicine
Miami, FL, USA

**Peter G. Whang, MD**
Assistant Professor
Department of Orthopaedics and Rehabilitation
Yale University School of Medicine
New Haven, CT, USA

**Andrew P. White, MD**
Instructor in Orthopaedic Surgery
Harvard Medical School
Spinal Surgeon
Beth Israel Deaconess Medical Center
Boston, MA, USA

**Timothy F. Witham, MD, FACS**
Assistant Professor of Neurosurgery
Director, The Johns Hopkins Bayview Spine Center
Johns Hopkins University School of Medicine
Baltimore, MD, USA

**Kirkham B. Wood, MD**
Chief, Orthopaedic Spine Service
Department of Orthopaedic Surgery
Massachusetts General Hospital
Boston, MA, USA

**Eric J. Woodard, MD**
Division of Neurosurgery
New England Baptist Hospital
Boston, MA, USA

**Kamal R.M. Woods, MD**
Department of Neurosurgery
Loma Linda University Medical Center
Loma Linda, CA, USA

**Kris Wai-ning Wong, PhD**
Senior Lecturer
Discipline of Applied Science
Hong Kong Institute of Vocational Education
Hong Kong

**Huilin Yang**
Professor
Department of Orthopedics
Suzhou University Hospital
Suzhou, China

**Weibin Yang, MD, MBA**
Physical Medicine and Rehabilitation Service
VA North Texas Health Care System
University of Texas Southwestern Medical School
Dallas, TX, USA

**Anthony T. Yeung, MD**
Desert Institute for Spine Care
Phoenix, AZ, USA

**Christopher A. Yeung, MD**
Desert Institute for Spine Care
Phoenix, AZ, USA

**Philip S. Yuan, MD**
Memorial Orthopedic Surgical Group
Long Beach, CA, USA

**James Joseph Yue, MD**
Associate Professor
Yale School of Medicine
Department of Orthopaedic Surgery and Rehabilitation
New Haven, CT, USA

**Navid Zenooz, MD**
Musculoskeletal Radiology Fellow
Yale University School of Medicine
New Haven, CT, USA

**Yinggang Zheng, MD**
Desert Institute for Spine Care
Phoenix, AZ, USA

**Linqiu Zhou, MD**
Department of Rehabilitation Medicine
Jefferson Medical College
Thomas Jefferson University
Philadelphia, PA, USA

**Dewei Zou, MD**
China PLA Postgraduate Medical School
Orthopedic
Surgical Division
Beijing, China

# Preface

The treatment of spinal disorders is often challenging and demanding for both patient and clinician. These challenges and demands are often amplified in the elderly patient. The concepts and methods presented in *The Comprehensive Treatment of the Aging Spine: Minimally Invasive and Advanced Techniques* are aimed at assisting the clinician in approaching the complexities of the aging spine. Osteoporosis, diabetes, cardiovascular and cerebral vascular disease, poor nutrition, and other co-morbidities often mandate a collective decision making process. In addition, the fundamentals of spinal anatomy, spinal embryology, biomechanics, biochemistry of spinal implants, and radiologic changes that occur in the aging spine are delineated for the clinician. Knowledge of non-operative/conservative treatment modalities such as land and aquatic therapy, acupuncture, injections, medication, and yoga therapies is a prerequisite to the initial management of the aging spine, especially in the presence of such co-morbidities.

If non-operative care does not sufficiently remedy the patient's symptoms, operative intervention may be necessary. An emphasis on decision making and operative options for differing pathologies such as spinal stenosis, spondylolisthesis, scoliosis, cervical myelopathy, osteoporotic fractures and fixation, and spinal tumors are presented. Each chapter underscores the relevant pathology, surgical technique, outcomes, and complications that can occur in the operative treatment of the aging spine.

New developments and emerging technologies are introduced to the clinician. The use of cyberknife therapy, nanotechnologies, endoscopic, and ozone therapies are reviewed. Innovative approaches such as the lateral approach to the spine (Extreme Lateral [XLIF] and Guided Lateral [GLIF]) are reviewed and described. Lastly, the economic impact of the aging spine is reviewed in terms of the cost benefit of caring for spinal disorders in the aging population.

# Contents

# PART 1

# Introduction to the Aging Spine

# 1

# Embryology of the Spine

*Zair Fishkin and John A. Bendo*

## KEY POINTS

- Gastrulation is the beginning of organogenesis and the time when the embryo is most susceptible to internal and external insults that may lead to congenital defects.

- Congenital spinal defects are often associated with abnormalities of the cardiac and renal systems because both these organ systems arise out of embryonic mesoderm precursors and develop at the same time as the spine.

- Failure of the cranial and caudal neural pores to close in the first 25 to 27 days post gestation results in anencephaly and spina bifida, respectively.

- Segmental shift of adjacent somites during embryogenesis may lead to defects of formation.

- Defects of segmentation may result from hemimetamer hypoplasia, osseous metaplasia of the intervertebral disc, or a bony bar in the posterior elements. The resulting deformity depends on the location of the congenital defect and remaining active growth centers.

## INTRODUCTION

Although a thorough understanding of mammalian embryology may not be required for the spine clinician, a fundamental grasp of the concepts of organogenesis, especially pertaining to the spine and central nervous system, may provide insight to the pathoanatomy and pathophysiology of common ailments affecting the spine. The following chapter is a summary of the key points that drive embryogenesis and result in common orthopedic diseases of the spine.

## GASTRULATION

The intrauterine process by which the human form develops can be divided into two phases, the embryonic period and the fetal period. The embryonic period lasts from conception to approximately 52 days post gestation. It is a vital period for organogenesis, occurring at a time when the embryo is most prone to external and internal teratogenic insults. The next 7 months encompass the fetal period, a time for tissue specialization and growth.

Immediately following fertilization, the zygote undergoes rapid cell division. Approximately 16 cells make up a ball-like structure called the morula. By the eighth day of gestation, the morula develops two fluid-filled cavities, the primitive yolk sac and the amniotic cyst. The cysts are separated by a double-layer disc of cells. Of these two cell layers, the epiblast lies adjacent to the amniotic sac; it will eventually give rise to all three germ layers during gastrulation, the process by which a two-layer disc becomes a three-layer disc.

Gastrulation begins in the third week of gestation and gives rise to three distinct germ layers, the ectoderm, the mesoderm, and the endoderm. The initial phase of gastrulation begins with formation of the primitive streak, which is sometimes named the primitive groove (Figure 1-1). This midline thickening of the germinal disc terminates in the primitive node. Under control of embryonic growth factors, cells of the epiblast layer migrate inward to form the mesoderm and the endoderm through the process of invagination. Cells migrating farthest from the epiderm and closest to the yolk sac become the endoderm. The remaining epiblast cells will eventually differentiate into

the ectoderm (Figure 1-2). The migrating cells that are sandwiched between the endoderm and ectoderm layers will become the mesoderm. Control of these migrations is maintained through various cell-signaling pathways that also contribute to establishment of the body axes in all planes. The signaling pathways, or organizer genes, are secreted by the primitive streak and mesoderm. The cranial direction of the embryonic disc is established by a specialized area of cells, referred to as the anterior visceral endoderm, that expresses genes required for formation of the head and cerebrum. The dorsal-ventral axis is regulated by growth factors in the TGF-β family including bone morphogenic protein-4, fibroblast growth factor, and the sonic hedgehog gene.

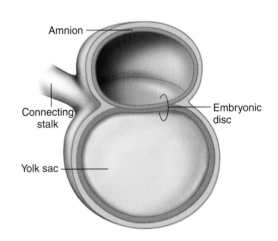

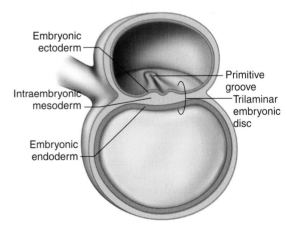

■ **FIGURE 1-1** **Top:** Approximately 8 to 12 days after gestation, the embryo contains two fluid-filled cavities, the primitive yolk sac and amnion, which are separated by the embryonic disc, a double layer of cells containing the epiblast. **Bottom:** Beginning in the third week following gestation, a primitive streak or groove forms in the epiblast. This thickening marks the beginning of gastrulation, the process by which the two-layer disc becomes three layers: ectoderm, mesoderm, and endoderm.

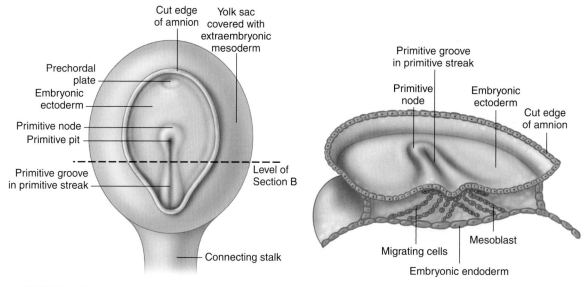

**■ FIGURE 1-2**   During the process of invagination, cell migration begins in the primitive streak and progresses in a predictable pattern. The deepest cells form the endoderm, while the cells staying superficial form the ectoderm. Cells migrating between the two layers will be the precursors to the mesoderm layer.

Control of sidedness is regulated by fibroblast growth factor-8, Nodal, and Lefty-2, all of which are secreted on the left side of the germinal disc. An additional protein, Lefty-1, is secreted to prevent migration of the left sided growth factors across the midline.[1]

At the cranial end of the primitive streak is a specialized collection of cells, the primitive node. Cells migrating cranially into the primitive node will eventually form the prechordal plate, while those migrating more posterior will fuse with cells in the hypoblastic layer to form the notochordal process. By day 16 or 17 of gestation, the lateral edges of the endoderm continue to invaginate; the two edges will eventually meet and pinch off the notochordal process, forming the definitive notochord. This is the earliest beginning of the bony vertebrae and the remainder of the skeleton. Cell migration continues for approximately 7 days, at which point the primitive streak begins to close in a cranial to caudal direction.

## SOMITE PERIOD

The presence of the notochord induces proliferation of the mesoderm. At approximately 17 days of gestation the mesoderm thickens into two masses, each located directly adjacent to the notochord. This initial layer, termed the paraxial mesoderm, continues to spread laterally to eventually differentiate into three distinct areas, paraxial mesoderm, intermediate mesoderm, and lateral mesoderm. During the somite period, lasting from approximately 19 to 30 days post fertilization, the paraxial mesoderm will develop into segmental bulbs of tissue on either side of the notochord (Figure 1-3). The first pair of somites will appear adjacent to the notochord, and they will continue to develop in a cranial to caudal direction until a total of 42 to 44 pairs of somites appear by the end of the fifth week of gestation. The first 24 somite segments are responsible for the cervical, thoracic, and lumbar spine. Somites 25 through 29 contribute to formation of the sacrum, while pairs 30 through 35 are responsible for coccyx formation. The rest of the 42 to 44 somite pairs disappear through a process of regression, which occurs at approximately 6 weeks of gestation.

The somites continue to differentiate into two distinct tissues. Ventromedial cells develop into the sclerotome, while dorsolateral cells develop into the dermatomyotome. The latter cells will eventually give rise to the integument system and dorsal musculature of the body, while the sclerotome will migrate to surround the notochord and give rise to the vertebral column. Regulation of sclerotome formation is controlled by proteins coded by the sonic hedgehog gene, which is expressed by cells of the notochord. This process of sclerotome migration will begin by the fourth week of gestation. Each sclerotome will be divided by an intersegmental vessel and a loose area

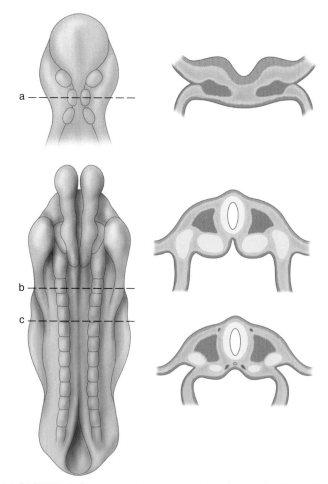

**■ FIGURE 1-3**   Human embryo at approximately 3 weeks of gestation; the embryo is approximately 1.5 to 2.5 mm in length at this point of development. Note that the cranial portion is wider than the caudal portion, with open neuropores at both ends. Ten pairs of somites have formed at this point in development. Cross-sectional electron micrographs show the neural tube with sclerotome and dermatomyotome cell masses on both sides of the midline. *(Reprinted from Müller, O'Rahilly: J Anat 203: 297–315, 2003.)*

of intersegmental mesenchyme. In addition, a pair of myotomes and accompanying segmental nerves will be associated with each sclerotome.

As the process of differentiation continues, each sclerotome will divide into a cranial region of relatively loosely packed cells and a caudal portion of rapidly proliferating and densely packed cells. At this point in spinal development, classic embryology texts describe a phenomenon by which the pace of proliferation is so great that the caudal part of the one sclerotome begins to overgrow into the cranial portion of the adjacent sclerotome and thereby fusing to create a single mass of tissue destined to become the precartilaginous vertebral body. Parke (The Spine, 1999) suggests that this theory of "resegmentation" may not be accurate, and provides compelling evidence toward an alternate route of vertebral body formation. In his summary of the recent evidence, Parke outlines a pathway of spinal development which begins with a uniform layer of axial mesenchyme surrounding the notochord. The sclerotomal organization is still maintained with an intersegmental vessel, a nerve, and a peripheral layer of dermatomyotome associated with each segment. However, the uniform mesenchyme undergoes a period of differentiation by which densities develop within the loose tissues. These dense regions will develop into the intervertebral discs and eventually pinch off the notochord which will be trapped within the dense tissue to become the nucleus pulposus.[2] The loose tissues between the discs form the cartilaginous centrum, which is the precursor of the vertebral bodies. The caudal portion of the centrum undergoes rapid proliferation, and cells migrate peripherally to surround the neural tube, forming the membranous neural arches which will serve to protect the neural elements. In total, each bony vertebral segment will consist of five ossification centers, one centrum, two neural arches, and two costal elements.

Ossification of the vertebral bodies occurs around the ninth week of gestation and begins at the thoracolumbar junction. Ossification then proceeds in both cranial and caudal directions, with the caudal segments demonstrating a quicker rate of ossification compared with the cranial segments. Ossification of the posterior arches begins at approximately the same time but begins in the cervical vertebrae and proceeds in a caudal direction. As the two neural arch centers approach midline, they begin to fuse, forming the lamina and spinous process. Fusion of the neural arches first occurs in the lumbar segments during the first year of life and proceeds cranially. Fusion is not completed until ages of 5 to 8 years. The costal ossification centers have a variable role in vertebral body formation. In the cervical spine, these centers have a minimal contribution and may contribute to part of the foramen transversarium. In the thoracic spine, these ossification centers are the precursors of the ribs. In the lumbosacral spine, the costal ossification centers are responsible for formation of the transverse processes and the anterolateral portion of the sacrum.[2]

## UPPER CERVICAL SPINE

The upper cervical spine must provide stable support for the cranial vault, and must also position the head and its sensory organs in space. This region has uniquely adapted to the evolutionary requirement of each species. In humans, this area is well suited to support a large cranium while providing approximately ± 80 degrees of lateral rotation and ± 45 degrees of flexion/extension.

A detailed anatomic study of cervical spine anatomy was presented by O'Rahilly and Meyer in a serial time reconstruction of human embryos ranging from 8 to approximately 16 weeks of gestation.[3] It is generally believed that the most cranial 4 or 5 pairs of somites are responsible for the occipital-atlas complex. Development of this junction is regulated by growth factors derived from the notochord as it crosses into the cranium. The notochord travels through the middle or slightly anterior portion of each centrum, and up through the future dens at the level of the axis. It then makes an anterior directed turn to enter the skull just above the level of the dens. At this time, each centrum is divided by a thickening of the notochord that will develop into the nucleus pulposus. The true boundary between the spine and cranium is not fully understood, with some authors suggesting that the atlas is a standalone accessory cranial bone with the true head-neck boundary being between the C1 and C2 articulation.

O'Rahilly and Meyer describe the centrum of the axis as being composed of three axial columns which they termed X, Y, and Z. The first and most cranial column, X, will develop an articulation with the anterior tubercle of C1, forming the atlanto-dens joint space.[4] By approximately 9 weeks of gestation, the X column, or future dens, is already bounded posteriorly by the transverse ligament and anchored into the occipital condyles by the alar ligamentous complex. Columns Y and Z are separated by the remnants of an intervertebral disc that may persist well into birth. Although it is generally accepted that column Z will form the centrum of the axis, the fate of column Y remains uncertain. Some believe that it is incorporated into the axis centrum, while other embryologists believe, based on reptilian studies, that it is incorporated into the centrum of the atlas. Calcifications in the three columns are readily visible by the time the embryo reached a length of 120 mm; however, fusion will not take place until 6 to 8 years of age. In some instances, the tip of the dens may calcify independently without fusion to the remaining axis; this is termed os odontoideum.

## NEURAL DEVELOPMENT

The neural elements likewise form during gastrulation. Under control of growth factors secreted by the prechordal plate, the ectoderm begins to thicken at the cranial end to form the neural plate and the lateral edges of the germinal disc fold to form the neural crests. This process is primary neurulation. As previously discussed, the neural crests meet in the midline to form the neural tube. The tube has two open ends, the cranial and caudal neuropores, both of which communicate with the amniotic cavity. This communication allows for prenatal detection of central nervous system markers in amniotic fluid if neural tube closure has failed to complete. There are likely multiple foci at which neural tube closure initiates and progresses both cranially and caudally in a zipperlike fashion. The cranial neuropore is generally first to close, and final closure is not complete until about 25 days post gestation.[1] The caudal neuropore closes approximately 2 days later. Failure of neuropore closure at the cranial end results in anencephaly, a deficiency of skull, scalp, and forebrain. Failure of caudal neuropore closure results in spina bifida. Once closure is completed, the neural tube must separate from the ectoderm. This process is termed dysjunction; premature separation during this step of neurulation may pull primitive mesenchyme tissues inside the developing neural tube, resulting in a lipomeningocele or lipomyelomeningocele.[5] Incomplete separation may lead to cutaneous sinuses that communicate with the spinal canal.

Thickenings in the neural tube give rise to the proencephalon (forebrain), mesencephalon (midbrain), and rhombencephalon (hindbrain). A cervical flexure will form connecting the rhombencephalon to the developing spine. The neural tube contains a lumen, the central canal of the spinal cord, which is in continuity with the cerebral ventricles. The neural tube wall consists of rapidly dividing neuroepithelial cells. These cells develop into neuroblasts and form a thick layer called the mantle. While in the mantle layer, the primitive neuroblast cells remain relatively apolar. Neuroblastic differentiation involves transformation of the apolar cells into a bipolar form, with elongation of one end to form the primitive axon and complex specialization of the other end to form the dendrites. At the completion of maturation, this cell will be the neuron. Axons of the neuron will protrude peripherally through the mantle layer and form the marginal layer of the spinal cord. The mantle layer, which contains the cell nuclei, does not undergo myelination and becomes the gray matter of the spinal cord. The axons in the marginal layer will get myelinated and become the white matter.

As the neuroblast proliferates, the spherical neural tube begins to thicken both ventrally and dorsally. The two areas of neuroblast are separated by the sulcus limitans, which prevents cell migration between the two layers. The ventral thickenings will form the basal plate which houses the motor horn cells. The dorsal thickenings will form the alar plate which contains the dorsal sensory neurons. The sympathetic chain is made up of neurons that accumulate in the "intermediate horn," a small thickening of cells that is found between the alar and basal plates at the level of the thoracic and upper lumbar spine. Neurons of the dorsal sensory horn become known as interneurons or associated neurons. These cells project axons that enter the marginal zone and extend proximally or distally to form communications between afferent and efferent neurons.

The spinal nerves begin to form in the fourth week after gestation. Each nerve is composed of a ventral motor root and a dorsal sensory root. Axons of the ventral motor horn cells project through the marginal zone and coalesce outside of the neural tube into the ventral motor root. These axons will continue to the motor endplates of the muscles formed from its respective sclerotome.

The dorsal sensory root begins its development from neural crest cells, which are of ectodermal origin. These cells migrate laterally during formation of the neural tube, forming the dorsal root ganglia, which contain the cell bodies. Axons project proximally and distally from the ganglia. The proximal axons make up the dorsal sensory roots and enter the neural tube on its dorsal surface into the dorsal horn to communicate with the sensory neurons. The distal axons join with the ventral motor fibers to compose the spinal nerve. They will terminate in the end organs to bring afferent feedback to the central nervous system.

## SACRUM AND CONUS MEDULLARIS DEVELOPMENT

Development of the neural structures in the caudal terminus of the spine deserves some special attention. At their respective most distal points, the neural tube and notochord coalesce into an undifferentiated cellular mass that will develop into the coccyx, sacrum, and fifth lumbar vertebrae. This process is the beginning of secondary neurulation. A single canal will form within this mass through a process called canalization. Debate exists in the literature as to whether this newly formed neural tube is initially continuous with the primary neural tube or whether the two coalesce at a later point in development. It is known that the chick embryo develops two distinct neural tubes that anastomose in the sacral region, while in a mouse embryo, the secondary neural tube forms as an extension of the primary neural tube. The pathway of secondary neurulation in humans is not yet elucidated; however, it is known that the distal portion of the tube and central canal will regress in a cephalic direction via a process called retrogressive differentiation. This will give rise to the conus medullaris and will leave behind a thin film of pia mater tissue called the filum terminale.[5] Nerve root compression may result when an abnormally thick filum terminale is present (usually greater than 2 mm in diameter).

As retrogressive differentiation continues, the position of the conus medullaris relative to the bony spine continues to change. The conus ascends from the level of the coccyx early in embryogenesis to rest at approximately the L2-3 disc space by the time of birth. Asymmetric rates of growth between the bony spine and the cord result in further caudal migration of the conus during the fetal period so that it comes to its final resting place at L1-2 by a few months after birth. Any final resting position of the cord at or below the L2-3 disc space would imply a tethered cord.

## ASSOCIATED ANOMALIES

While discussing spinal embryology, it is important to remember that spinal development is not an isolated event. Multiple organ systems are developing in parallel with the spine and often share the same germinal tissue source. Any internal or external insult to the developing embryo may affect other organ systems. The mesoderm is particularly involved in the genesis of several organs. Paraxial mesoderm, the precursor of the centrum and vertebral column, is also responsible for formation of the dermis, skeletal muscle, and the connective tissue of the head.[6] The intermediate and lateral mesoderm is responsible for formation of the urogenital, cardiac, and renal systems. In children with known congenital spinal defects, the incidence of associated anomalies has been reported as high as 30% to 60%.[7] The most common organ system to be affected is the genitourinary system. Mesoderm tissues that make up the spinal column also contribute to formation of the mesonephros. While it is the medial region of the mesoderm that forms the vertebrae, the ventrolateral region forms the genitourinary organs.[8] The cardiopulmonary system is also commonly involved in conjunction with a congenital spinal abnormality. These anomalies may be fatal and should be diagnosed and treated before their associated problems progress. Diagnosis of both congenital spinal defects and associated anomalies may be made on prenatal ultrasound examination.

The timing of insult during fetal development also affects the rate of associated anomalies. Tsou (1980) divided a group of 144 patients with congenital spinal anomalies into two groups: embryonic anomalies, defined as those that occurred in the first 56 days post fertilization, and fetal anomalies, defined as those that occurred from day 57 of gestation to birth.[9] They found that the rate of associated defects was 7% in the fetal group as compared with 35% in the embryonic group. Associated orthopedic anomalies included Klippel-Feil syndrome, acetabular dysplasia, clubfoot, congenital short leg, Sprengel deformity, coxa vara, radial clubhand, and thumb aplasia. Nonorthopedic associated anomalies included dextrocardia, hypospadia, microtia, lung aplasia, pulmonary arterial stenosis, imperforate anus, mandibular anomalies, cleft palate, and hemidiaphragm.[9]

## CONGENITAL SPINAL ANOMALIES

Normal spinal development involves coordination between cellular tissues and signaling pathways. Mesenchyme provides the cellular building blocks for the structural tissues of the spine while the notochord provides signaling molecules to organize normal development. Congenital spinal defects may be the result of defects in mesenchymal building blocks, genetic defects in the signaling pathways, or a combination of both. The most commonly used classification system for congenital spinal defects, however, is not based on the etiology of disease but rather on the radiographic morphology. Moe et al. proposed a classification system that breaks congenital spinal defects into three main groups: defects of formation, defects of segmentation, and complex defects of the neural tube.

### Defects of Formation

Defects of formation are defined as absence of any structural portion of the vertebral ring. The resultant deformity is a result of the anatomic structure that failed to form properly. The most common morphological result of a failure of formation is a hemivertebra or wedge vertebra. Classification of hemivertebra depends on the presence of growth plates on either side of the body. A fully segmented hemivertebra has growth plates on both sides and is separated by a disc from both the cranial and caudal adjacent vertebral body. A semisegmented hemivertebra only has one growth plate, and thus an intervertebral disc is only found adjacent to either the cranial or caudal segment. A nonsegmented hemivertebra has no active growth plates or discs to separate it from the body above or below. This is a stable situation with minimal potential for increasing deformity with growth. Another stable situation may occur when plasticity of both the cranial and caudal adjacent vertebral bodies allow the adjacent bodies to conform to the shape of a hemivertebra, thus keeping the pedicles in line with the rest of the spine. This stable situation, in which the hemivertebra is referred to as being incarcerated, does not result in a deformity and usually does not require treatment.

Although it is generally agreed that hemivertebrae are the result of the failure of formation, the exact pathophysiology has not yet been elucidated. It is helpful to separate failures of formation as those occurring during the embryonic period and those that occur in the fetal period. During the embryonic stage, most authors propose a theory of "segmental shift," which occurs during the sclerotomic pairing phase of embryogenesis.[9] As the somites join in the midline, it is assumed that each somite is in the same developmental phase as its counterpart across the midline. This development usually proceeds in a predictable pattern from a cranial to caudal direction. Asynchronous development of one somite in a hemimetameric pair may prevent normal midline fusion and result in a caudal shift of the column such that the two contralateral pairs are in a synchronous phase of development. This would leave an isolated out-of-phase hemivertebra without a cross-midline counterpart (Figure 1-4). This segmental shift theory is further supported by the presence of double-balanced hemivertebra where each of the asynchronous hemi-vertebra is found on one side of the midline. The most caudal hemivertebra is commonly found at the lumbosacral junction where there is no further room for compensation from the somite below. Another mechanism for hemivertebra formation may result from a physiologic insult to the somite precursor during the embryonic period. Although midline fusion occurs between corresponding somites, the injured hemimetameric pair may undergo growth retardation of variable severity. Mild growth retardation may result in a hypoplastic hemivertebra in which the growth plates are formed, but the rate of growth is not equal to the opposite side. More severe forms of sclerotome growth retardation may result in a failure of segmentation and will be discussed later.

Insults to the growing spine during the embryonic stage tend to globally affect the vertebral segment, including both posterior and anterior elements. Insults occurring during the fetal period tend to be more specific and only

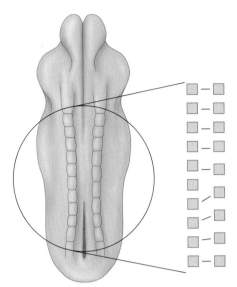

■ **FIGURE 1-4** Hemimetameric pairing: a defect of formation may occur when adjacent pairs of somites are out of developmental phase with their cross-midline counterpart. This results in a caudal shift of hemimetameric pairing. An isolated hemivertebra is left without a cross-midline counterpart. This hemivertebra may be balanced by another hemivertebra at the sacral end of the contralateral side, resulting in minimal overall deformity. *(Reprinted from Tsou PM et al: Clin Orthop Relat Res 152: 218, 1980.)*

affect a portion of the vertebra, the centrum being the area most commonly afflicted. Centrum hypoplasia and aplasia is described by Tsou as a spectrum of growth retardation that occurs from 2 to 7 months post fertilization during a period of normally rapid vertebral growth.[9] A vascular etiology for centrum aplasia and hypoplasia was proposed by Schmorl and Junghanns; however, this has not yet been proven. Identification of these failures of formation is clinically important as they may often result in structural deformity of the spine. Centrum aplasia and posterior hemicentrum have been shown to cause an isolated kyphotic deformity, while wedge vertebra, posterior corner hemivertebra, and a lateral hemicentrum more commonly cause a mixed kyphoscoliotic deformity.[6]

## Defects of Segmentation

Defects in segmentation occur when two or more adjacent vertebrae fail to fully separate resulting in a complete or partial loss of the growth plate. The extent and location of the defect largely determines the resultant deformity. One mechanism of segmentation failure involves a more advanced form of hemimetamer hypoplasia. As cells of the sclerotome undergo their migration, they first feed formation of the centrum, followed by the neural arches. A deficiency in the quantity of sclerotome would first manifest itself as a deficit in the neural arch formation, as they are last to receive the migrating cells. The resultant hypoplasia has a variable amount of penetrance. In the mildest form, only the lamina may be fused, followed by fusion of the facet joints. More severe forms involve fusion of the entire hemivertebra in which the adjacent level lamina, facet joints, and pedicles are fused into a single posterolateral bar.

Segmentation defects may also occur during formation of the intervertebral disc or the adjacent articulations. By the late embryonic period, mesodermal cells have migrated around the notochord and formed dense collections of tissues which will form the annulus fibrosus. In a more common form of segmentation defect, the anterior portion of the annulus undergoes first what Tsou describes as a cartilaginous transformation, followed by osseous metaplasia.[9] A bony bar forms between two or more adjacent vertebral bodies as ossification continues into childhood. This anterior tether may result in a severe kyphotic deformity that worsens with continued growth.

Posterior elements are also prone to failures of segmentation. The articulating facet joints form via condensation of mesenchymal tissues that extend in a superior and inferior direction away from the pedicle. Injury to the developing mesenchyme in the neural arches during the later portion of

the embryonic period may interrupt normal development of the apophyseal joints. A cartilaginous bridge forms between the superior and inferior articulating processes of two adjacent vertebral segments. This bridge undergoes ossification during early childhood and provides a posterior growth tether. Unilateral involvement would lead to a lordoscoliotic deformity and bilateral bars would lead to a pure lordotic deformity.

## Spina Bifida

Derived from the Latin term *bifidus*, spina bifida literally means a spine split in two. Although the severity of the disease may range from a benign incidental finding on x-ray to severe neurologic damage, the etiology remains the same, a failure of the embryonic vertebral arches to fuse. Causes for this lack of fusion are multifactorial. Mitchell (1997) suggested a weak genetic component by demonstrating an increased risk in siblings of affected children and even further increased risk with multiple affected siblings.[10] Environmental factors also play a role in the etiology of spina bifida. Mitchell correlated incidence with time of season, geographic location, ethnicity, race, socioeconomic status, maternal age and parity, and maternal nutritional status, specifically the dietary intake of folic acid and alcohol. Although the mechanism by which folic acid aids in neural tube closure is unknown, the role of folic acid as a substrate in DNA synthesis has been well described. An enzyme called methyl tetra hydroxy folate reductase (MTHFR) is involved in folate metabolism during DNA synthesis. Genetic alterations in this enzyme may lead to decreased enzymatic activity and increase the dietary folate requirements for proper DNA synthesis. As neural tube closure has been shown to begin early in the embryonic period, it is vital to begin folate supplementation as early as possible in the prenatal period and encourage dietary supplementation during family planning.

Spinal bifida occulta, one of the more benign forms of spinal bifida, results from a failure of fusion of the lamina. This relatively common finding has a reported incidence of 10% to 24% in the general population. The disease implies involvement of the posterior arches only and sparing of the cord and meninges from the pathology. Patients typically do not present with any neurological symptoms. Physical exam signs may include skin indentation and/or patches of irregular hair growth in the region of the lower lumbar spine. The most typical diagnosis is made an incidental finding on an x-ray of the lumbar spine. Rarely, associated defects may exist in conjunction with spina bidifa occulta. These may include a tethered cord, distortion of the cord by fibrous bands, syrinx, lipomyelomeningocele, a fatty filum terminale, or diastematomyelia. Collectively, these associated disorders are grouped into a term called occult spinal dystrophism.

Spina bifida cystica refers to a more severe form of spina bifida; it can be broken down into several subgroups based on the degree of the involved tissue layers.[6] The first group, spina bifida with meningocele, involves the meninges as well as the posterior arches. A cystic pouch is present within the meninges without involvement of the spinal cord or nerve roots. Patients are typically spared neurologically. Physical exam findings may be similar to those of spina bifida occulta, but also include subcutaneous lipomas and hemangiomas adjacent to the lesion. Spina bifida with myelomeningocele is the next most severe form of spina bifida. This disease results from failure of fusion in the posterior arches with involvement of the spinal cord and meninges. By definition, in spina bifida with myelomeningocele, the neural elements are not exposed to the external environment and are covered by a membranous cerebrospinal fluid–filled sac. This disease typically presents with neurological disorder based on the neurological level of the lesion. Associated anomalies include Arnold-Chiari malformation, hydrocephalus, scoliosis, and kyphosis. The most severe manifestation of spina bifida cystica is myeloschisis. In this severe presentation the neural elements are completely exposed. Neurologic injury is certain and infections are common.

## CONCLUSION

Clinicians treating spinal disorders may benefit from an understanding of the processes that drive spinal embryogenesis and the origin of common disorders affecting the spine. The process of embryogenesis is extremely complicated, but incredibly well synchronized. Multiple events happen in series and in parallel, all under the control of signaling pathways that are just now becoming understood. Spine development has been widely elucidated using human and animal data; however there remain many unknowns, especially on a molecular level. It is vital to remember that disorders of spinal development may not be isolated events; other organ systems are often affected. Awareness and early intervention may be required for optimal patient care.

## References

1. T.W. Sadler, Medical embryology, ninth ed., Lippincott Williams & Wilkins, Baltimore, 2004.
2. H.N. Herkowitz, S.R. Garfin, F.J. Eismont, G.R. Bell, Rothman-Simeone the spine, WB Saunders, Philadelphia, 1999.
3. R. O'Rahilly, D.B. Meyer, The timing and sequence of events in the development of the human vertebral column during the embryonic period proper, Anat. Embryol. (Berl) 157 (2) (1979) 167–176.
4. R. O'Rahilly, F. Muller, D.B. Meyer, The human vertebral column at the end of the embryonic period proper. 2. The occipitocervical region, J. Anat. 136 (1) (1983) 181–195.
5. J.D. Grimme, M. Castillo, Congenital anomalies of the spine, Neuroimaging Clin. N. Am. 17 (1) (2007) 1–16.
6. K.M. Kaplan, J.M. Spivak, J.A. Bendo, Embryology of the spine and associated congenital abnormalities, Spine J. 5 (5) (2005) 564–576.
7. D. Jaskwhich, et al., Congenital scoliosis, Curr. Opin. Pediatr. 12 (1) (2000) 61–66.
8. G.D. MacEwen, R.B. Winter, J.H. Hardy, Evaluation of kidney anomalies in congenital scoliosis, J. Bone Joint Surg. Am. 54 (7) (1972) 1451–1454.
9. P.M. Tsou, Embryology of congenital kyphosis, Clin. Orthop. Relat. Res. (128) (1977) 18–25.
10. L.E. Mitchell, Genetic epidemiology of birth defects: nonsyndromic cleft lip and neural tube defects, Epidemiol. Rev. 19 (1) (1997) 61–68.

# 2

# Applied Anatomy of the Normal and Aging Spine

*Rajesh G. Arakal, Malary Mani and Ravi Ramachandran*

**K E Y   P O I N T S**

- Cervical disc herniations most often affect the exiting root.
- Lumbar posterolateral herniations most often affect the root of the respective lower foramen.
- Acquired lateral recess stenosis is most often a result of hypertrophy of the superior articulating facet.
- Degenerative spondylolisthesis is most common at L4-5 and can entrap the L4 nerve root.
- Aging affects every aspect of the spine, from mineral density of the bones, to the physiology of the intervertebral discs, to the muscular scaffold around the spine.

"Chance favors the prepared mind." The spinal column consists of 33 vertebrae and is divided into seven cervical, twelve thoracic, and five lumbar vertebrae. The lumbar vertebrae articulate with the sacrum, which in turn articulates with the pelvis. Below the sacrum are the four or five irregular ossicles of the coccyx.

## THE VERTEBRAE

The articulations of the spine are based on synovial and fibrocartilaginous joints. The overall morphology of the vertebral column has a basic similarity, with the exception of the first two cervical vertebrae and the sacrum. A vertebra consists of a cylindrical ventral body of trabecularized cancellous bone and a dorsal vertebral arch that is much more cortical. From the cervical to the lumbar spine, there is a significant increase in the size of the vertebral bodies. An exception is the sixth cervical vertebra, which is usually shorter in height than the fifth and seventh vertebrae. In the thoracic spine, the vertebral body has facets for rib articulations. The posterior aspect of the vertebra starts with a posterior apex or spinous process. This process then flows into flat lamina that arch over the spinal canal and attach to the main body through a cylindrical pillar or pedicle. The transverse processes are found at the junction of the confluence of the laminae and pedicles and extend laterally. In the upper six cervical vertebrae, this component is part of the bony covering of the vertebral arteries. In the thoracic spine, the transverse process articulates with ribs. A mature and robust transverse process is found in the lumbar spine, with the remnant neural arch structure forming a mammillary process (Figure 2-1).

There are points of articulation between the individual vertebral segments between an inferior and ventral facing facet and a superior and dorsal facing facet. It is a diarthrodial, synovial joint. The shape of the facets is coronally oriented in the cervical spine, thus allowing for flexion-extension, lateral bending, and rotation. The facets are sagitally oriented in the lumbar spine and thus resist rotation, while allowing for

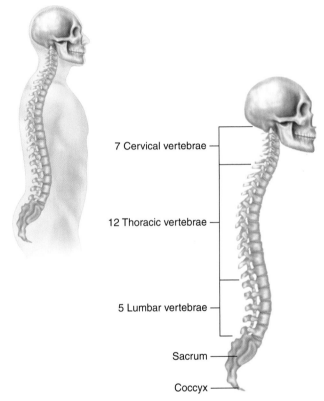

7 Cervical vertebrae

12 Thoracic vertebrae

5 Lumbar vertebrae

Sacrum

Coccyx

■ **FIGURE 2-1** The Vertebrae

some flexion and some translational motion.[1] Lateral to these joints are mamillary bony prominences upon which muscles can originate and insert.

The pedicles are the columns that connect the posterior elements to the anterior vertebral body. The transverse pedicle widths vary in size, but generally tend to larger dimension from the midthoracic to the lumbar spine, with a decrease of pedicle width from the lower cervical to the upper thoracic spine. Sagittal pedicle height increases from C3 to the thoracolumbar junction and then decreases from the upper lumbar region to the sacrum. The angles at which the pedicles articulate to the body also vary depending on the level. The windows formed between the pedicles transmit the nerves and vessels that correspond to that body segment.

The portion of the posterior arch most subject to stress by translational motion is the pars interarticularis, which lies between the superior and inferior articular facets of each mobile vertebra. Clinically, fracture of this elongated bony segment in the C2 vertebra results in the hangman's fracture; in the lower lumbar spine, it results in isthmic spondylolisthesis. The shear forces often result in ventral displacement of the superior articular facet, pedicle, and vertebral body and in maintenance of the attachments of the inferior articular facets and relationships to the lower vertebrae.[2] In cadaveric studies, the L5 pars region was particularly susceptible to fracture, given its smaller cross-sectional area of 15 mm[2] compared to the L1 and L3 vertebrae, which had over a fourfold increase.[3]

## Cervical Vertebrae

Forward flexion and rotation are largely attributed to the first two cervical vertebrae. The atlas is the first cervical vertebra. It is a bony ring with an anterior and posterior arch connected with relatively two large lateral masses. The superior articular facet of the lateral mass is sloped internally to accommodate the occipital condyles. The inferior portion is sloped externally to articulate with the axis. This inferior articulation allows for rotational freedom while limiting lateral shifts. The posterior arch of C1 is grooved laterally to fit the vertebral arteries as they ascend from the foramen transversarium of C1 to penetrate the posterior atlanto-occipital membrane within 20 to 15 mm lateral to the midline. It is recommended that one remain within 12 mm lateral to midline during dissection of the posterior aspect of the ring.[4] The anterior arch connects the two lateral masses, and the anterior tubercle in the most ventral portion is the site of attachment for the longus colli. The ventral side of the anterior arch has a synovial articulation with the odontoid process. The odontoid is restrained at this site with thick transverse atlantal ligaments that attach to the lateral masses (Figure 2-2).

The axis is the second cervical vertebra. The odontoid process, a remnant of the centrum of C1, projects from the body of C2 superiorly. This anatomy, unique to the cervical spine, allows for a strong rotational pivot with limitations on horizontal shear. Apical ligaments attach superiorly and alar ligaments attach laterally on the odontoid to the base of the skull at the basion. The basion is the anterior aspect of the foramen magnum. The superior aspects of the lateral masses are directed laterally and are convex to accommodate the atlas. The inferior articulations of the axis are similar to the remainder of the subaxial spine with a 45 degree sagittal orientation of the facets.

The cervical vertebrae are smaller in dimension than the lumbar vertebrae because they bear less weight than their lumbar counterparts. They are wider in the coronal plane in relation to the sagittal plane. The superior lateral edges of the vertebrae form the uncinate processes. The lateral processes have openings for the superior transit of the vertebral artery; these are called the foramen transversarium. During instrumentation of the lateral masses, it should be noted that as one descends from the upper cervical levels to C6, the foramen is more laterally positioned respective to the midpoint of the lateral mass. Anterior and posterior cervical musculature attach to their respective tubercles in the lateral portions of the transverse process. The seventh cervical vertebra is a transitional segment and has a long spinous process or vertebra prominens. The vertebral arteries usually enter the transverse foramen at C6 and omit the passage through the C7 foramen.

## Thoracic Vertebrae

The thoracic vertebrae are heart-shaped and have dual articulations for both ribs as well as for the superior and inferior vertebrae. The transverse diameter of the pedicles is smallest from T3 to T6. At T1, the transverse diameter

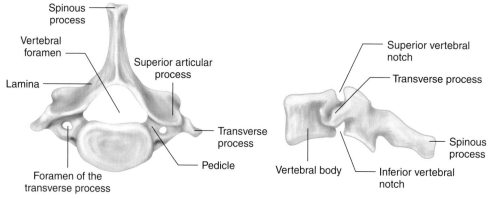

**■ FIGURE 2-2**   Cervical Vertebrae

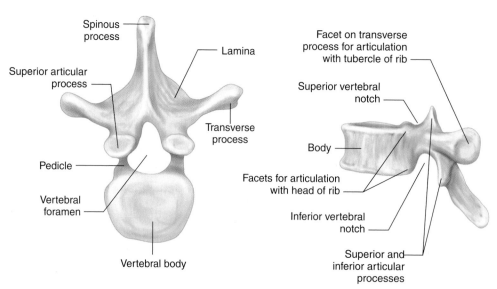

**■ FIGURE 2-3**   Thoracic Vertebrae

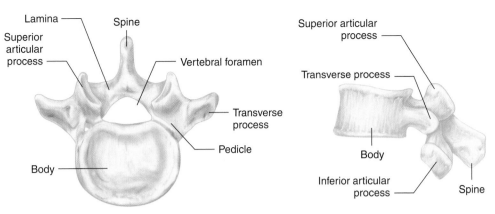

■ **FIGURE 2-4** Lumbar Vertebrae

is larger, with an average of 7.3 mm in men and 6.4 mm in women.[5] The first thoracic vertebra has a complete facet on the side of the body for the first rib head and an inferior demifacet for the second rib head. The ninth to twelfth vertebrae have costal articulations with their respective ribs. The last two ribs are smaller and do not attach to the sternum. The thoracic facets are rotated 20 degrees forward on the coronal plane and 60 degrees superiorly on the sagittal plane (Figure 2-3).

## Lumbosacral Spine

The lumbar vertebrae are much larger in overall relative proportion. The articular facets are concave and directed approximately 45 degrees medially on the coronal plane. The fourth transverse process tends to be smallest in comparison to the proximal lumbar segments. The fifth transverse process is the most robust (Figure 2-4).

The sacrum is the complex of five fused vertebra that articulates with the fifth lumbar vertebrae. There are both dorsal and ventral foramina. The ventral portion is relatively larger. The dorsal aspect of the sacrum is composed of ridges that are formed from the fusion of the spinous processes of the respective sacral vertebrae. At the superior margin, the articulation with the fifth lumbar vertebra is almost purely dorsal. This provides necessary restraint from a ventral translation at the lumbosacral junction.

The coccyx is the rudimentary remnant of the tail. It acts to provide attachment for the gluteus maximus and the pelvic diaphragm.

Loss of normal bone within the vertebrae is characteristic of osteoporosis. Primary osteoporosis affects the trabecular bone and is associated with vertebral compression fractures. This is most commonly seen in postmenopausal women, secondary to the sensitivity of the skeleton to estrogen loss.[6] Secondary osteoporosis affects the trabecular and cortical bone and is a result of aging and prolonged calcium deficiency.

## INTERVERTEBRAL DISC

The fibrocartilaginous nature of the disc provides mobility while maintaining relative structural orientation in the spine. The disc is most commonly divided into the outer annulus fibrosus and the inner nucleus pulposus. The annulus is a concentric mesh that surrounds the nucleus and resists tensile forces. The individual lamella can run obliquely or in a spiral manner in relation to the spinal column. Furthermore, there can be alterations in the direction of the fibers. On a sagittal section, the fibers are pointed slightly to the nucleus pulposus in its proximity, find a vertical orientation moving outward, and then finally bow out at its periphery. The fibers of the nucleus and inner lamellae are interposed into the cancellous bone of the vertebrae. The outer rings penetrate as Sharpey fibers with dense attachments into the vertebral periosteum and the anterior and posterior longitudinal ligaments (Figure 2-5).

The nucleus pulposus is usually confined within the annulus. It has a large number of fusiform cells in a heterogenous matrix. This allows for the ability of the disc material to bulge and recoil back with pressure. The fibers are not in any one orientation in histologic section and are the embryological remnant of the notochord.

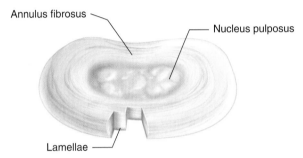

■ **FIGURE 2-5** Anatomy of the intervertebral disc

From the cervical to the lumbar spine, there are further variations at the disc level. There are uncovertebral "joints" that develop during the first decade; these are superior extensions of the uncinate processes with a corresponding slope from the superior vertebra. Anteriorly, the discs are wider in the cervical and lumbar spine, which results in cervical lordosis and a lumbar lordosis of 40 to 80 degrees. The thoracic kyphosis from 20 degrees to 50 degrees is mostly attributed to a disproportionately larger posterior vertebral body and smaller anterior height to contrast with a uniform disc height.

Disc degeneration with aging may be a component of the enzymatic activity resulting in an active breakdown of collagen, proteoglycans, and fibronectin. Proteoglycans are diminished with aging.[7] Aggrecan is degenerated by various enzymes including cathepsins, matrix metalloproteinases, and aggrecanases. Various mutations in genes can result in a genetic predisposition to disc degeneration, including defects of genes involving vitamin D receptor,[8] collagen IX,[9] collagen II, and aggrecan.

## LIGAMENTS

The dorsal lamina articulate with the adjacent segments through the ligamentum flavum, interspinous ligaments, supraspinous ligaments, and intertransverse ligaments. The ligamentum flavum attaches superiorly on the ventral side of the lamina, laterally on the base of the articulating facets, and inferiorly on the superior aspect of the lamina. With aging, the fibers may lose some of the material properties allowing for redundancy and laxity with extension. The ligamentum is a dual-layered structure that flows along both sides of the spine, with a central deficiency. The spinous processes are connected by the oblique interspinous ligaments. The supraspinous ligament connects the apices of the spinous processes. In the cervical spine, this structure is known as the ligamentum nuchae (Figure 2-6).

## Intraspinal Ligaments

The anterior longitudinal ligament drapes ventrally from the axis to the sacrum. Superficial layers span multiple segments with the deep layer spanning one spinal segment. In a similar fashion, the posterior longitudinal

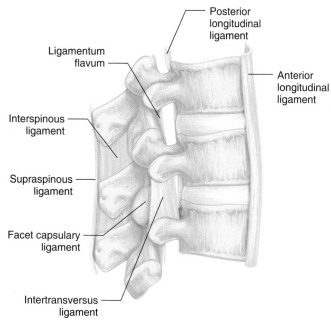

Posterior
longitudinal
ligament

Ligamentum
flavum

Anterior
longitudinal
ligament

Interspinous
ligament

Supraspinous
ligament

Facet capsulary
ligament

Intertransversus
ligament

■ **FIGURE 2-6**  Ligaments of the spine

ligament (PLL) has superficial and deep layers. The deep layer forms a dense central vertical strap with lateral attachments to the disc. Disc protrusions are likely more frequent posterolaterally, secondary to the stronger tether centrally. The peridural membrane is an additional layer between the PLL and the dura.[10]

## THE NERVE ROOTS

Due to the differential growth of the lower segments of the spine in relation to the more cranial segments, the dorsal and ventral roots converge to form the spinal nerve at a more oblique angle toward the intervertebral foramen more distally. In the cervical region, the root and the spinal nerve are at the same level as the disc and the intervertebral foramen. In the lumbar spine, the contributing roots for the nerve are descending to the next lower foramen. A posterolateral disc herniation will affect the nerve root of the respective lower foramen. The spinal nerves typically are in close proximity to the underside of the respective pedicle with narrower margins in the cervical and thoracic spine, and approximately 0.8 to 6.0 mm in the lumbar spine.[11] The lumbosacral root ganglia are usually in the intraforaminal region with variations medial and lateral to the foramina.

Anatomic variations can exist, with prevalence from 4% to 14% in various reports. Apart from anomalous levels of origin, there can be interconnections and divisions between nerves both intradural and extradural. Furthermore, the origins of the motor segments from within the ventral horn may allow for contributions to more than one nerve root. The description of the furcal nerve is most commonly applied to the cross-connection between the fourth and fifth lumbar nerve roots.[12] This is relevant because of the interconnections of the femoral and obturator nerves of the lumbar plexus to the lumbosacral trunk of the sacral plexus. Compression can result in mixed neurologic findings warranting careful investigation into the underlying pathology.

## THE INTERVERTEBRAL FORAMEN

The nerves traverse through the vertically elliptical window of the foramen. The borders of the foramen are defined anteriorly by the dorsal intervertebral disc and posterior longitudinal ligament. The posterior border is bounded by the ligamentum flavum and the facet capsule. Frequently, it is a sagittal narrowing that results in pathologic nerve compression. Furthermore, the nerves can be tethered by transforaminal ligaments with attachments to the capsule, pedicle, and disc.

## INNERVATION OF THE SPINE

Emanating from the dorsal root ganglion are rami communicantes that connect to the autonomic ganglion. Sinuvertebral nerves emanate from the rami communicantes close to the spinal nerve and enter back into the spinal canal to divide into branches than may innervate the posterior longitudinal ligament, and possibly, the dorsolateral aspects of the disc.[13] Branches may innervate more than one disc level, leading to the nonspecific locations of back pain. Afferent pain fibers are well documented within the histologic analysis of the sinuvertebral nerve. Meningeal fibers of these pain afferents to the ventral aspect of the dura may allow for explanations of back pain with dural distortion. There are intraspinal ligaments of Hoffman which normally tether the dura ventrally. Adhesions in the ventral aspect of the dura can also be acquired, resulting in a more anchored structure susceptible to external compression (Figure 2-7).

## NUTRITIONAL SUPPORT FOR THE VERTEBRA AND DISC

Paired segmental arteries branch posteriorly from the aorta to supply the second thoracic to the fifth lumbar vertebrae. These segmentals approach the middle of the vertebral artery and divide into dorsal and lateral branches. The dorsal branch courses lateral to the foramen, gives off the dominant spinal branch artery, and then supplies the posterior musculature. The spinal branch arteries off the dorsal artery are the major arterial supply to the vertebrae and the spinal canal. Segmentation off the dorsal branch vascularizes the posterior longitudinal ligament and dura, and enters in the center of the concavity of the dorsal vertebra. Anastomoses are common between fine branches from the left and right of each segment as well as from cranially and caudally. The lateral segmental branch has offshoots that penetrate the cortical body and the anterior longitudinal ligament.

An important variation is the contribution of segmental arteries in the lower thoracic or upper lumbar region to form a large radicular artery of Adamkiewicz, which joins the anterior spinal artery at the level of the conus medullaris.[14] Although the disc has no direct arterial supply, disc nutrition is dependent on the diffusion principles, size, and charge of particles. Specifically, the central aspect of the disc has a collective negative charge and is reliant on effective glucose transport from the vasculature of the endplates. Alterations of the precarious nutritional diffusion with age and pathologic processes can initiate a degenerative cascade.

## MUSCULAR ANATOMY

The muscles that are involved in spinal motion are the largest in the body. The strength of contraction is related to size, fiber type, and number but not limited to these factors. Other factors that may be pertinent to the competence of the muscular system with aging include the effect of neural stimulation, hormones, and conditioning. In the lumbar spine, the spinalis muscle goes between the spinous processes. The multifidi go upward and span two to four segments. The longissimus inserts into the tips of the spinous processes. The iliocostalis inserts into the ribs, and is the most lateral of the posterior lumbar spine intrinsic musculature. The psoas major acts anteriorly and is an important stabilizer in standing and sitting postures. As there are altered use patterns and conditioning with age, important stabilizers are affected, contributing to spinal deformity and altered motion (Figure 2-8).

## PATHOLOGIC CHANGES IN AGING

With aging, degenerative processes can result in the common pathologies of spinal stenosis, spondylolisthesis, spondylosis, diffuse idiopathic skeletal hyperostosis, and degenerative scoliosis. These changes will be discussed in greater detail in the following chapters. Anatomic changes in the normal joints and perineural structures result in slowly progressive narrowing and compression of the nerves. In the cervical spine, spinal stenosis can be both central and foraminal. Central compression can result in spondylotic myelopathy. Degenerative changes of the facet joints can result in joint laxity and instability. Such pathologic subluxation can give rise to degenerative spondylolisthesis. Arthritic changes can result in mechanical irritation and pain. The cluster of changes in the spinal complex can also result in a scoliotic collapse or adult degenerative scoliosis.

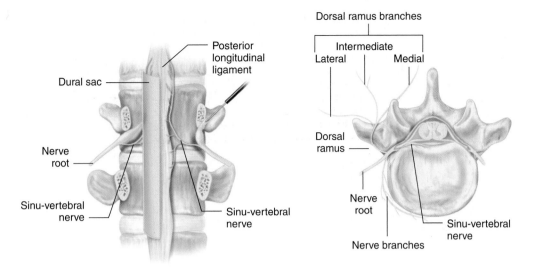

■ **FIGURE 2-7**    Innervation of the spine

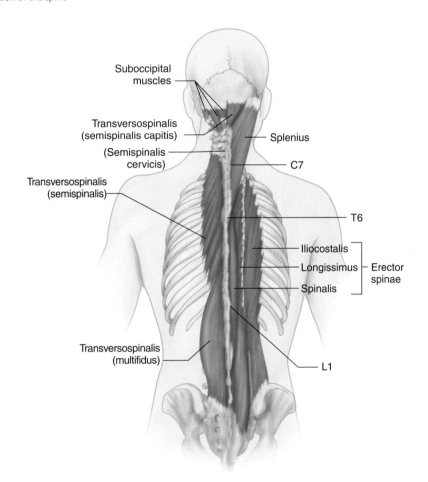

■ **FIGURE 2-8**    Posterior musculature of the spine

## Spinal Stenosis

Local pain and discomfort can result from pathologic changes in the caliber of the spinal canal both centrally and at the foraminal level. Direct mechanical compression of the dural sac and the nerve roots can result in pain and extremity weakness. Pain in the axial region can arise from pathologic changes to the sinuvertebral nerve and posterior primary ramus. Cervical stenosis is most commonly acquired or a result of degenerative spondylotic changes. As the intervertebral discs collapse, the annular bulge can narrow the canal. Furthermore, posterior buckling of the ligamentum flavum can contribute to cord compression. Osteophytes may form both centrally and foraminally, exacerbating the compression. In the lumbar spine, similarly, the stenosis may be both central and/or lateral. Lateral recess stenosis is usually the result of hypertrophy of the superior articulating facet. Foraminal stenosis can result from direct osteophytic growth, facet subluxation, or a vertical disc collapse. Degenerative synovial cysts can often result in compression and can mimic symptoms of spinal stenosis (Figure 2-9).

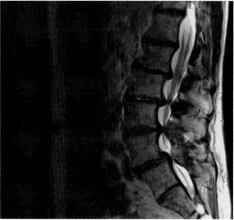

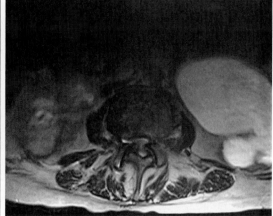

■ **FIGURE 2-9**   T2 MRI saggital and axial image of spinal stenosis

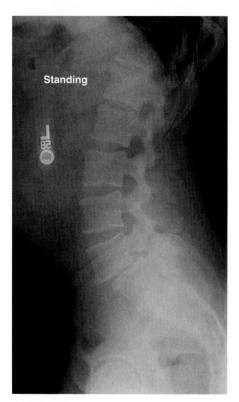

Standing

■ **FIGURE 2-10**   Lateral radiograph demonstrating anterolisthesis

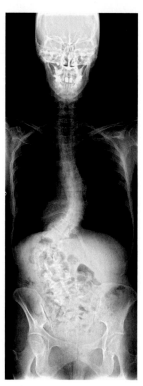

■ **FIGURE 2-11**   Scoliosis view of adult degenerative scoliosis

## Spondylolisthesis

Degenerative spondylolisthesis is most commonly a result of the pathologic degeneration of the facet joints. Asymmetry of this degeneration can result in a rotational deformity, along with translation. The L4-5 level is the most common level and can result in entrapment of the L4 root. The root can be caught between the inferior articulating facet of L4 and the body of L5 (Figure 2-10).

## Diffuse Idiopathic Skeletal Hyperostosis (DISH)

DISH predominantly affects middle-aged men and is characterized by prolific bone formation around the spine and in the extremities. Associated diseases are diabetes mellitus and gout. The most commonly affected area is the thoracolumbar spine. Often large spurs form on the anterolateral aspect of the vertebral body and flow into a contiguous bar. This is more common on the right side. The most common complaint is stiffness. The facet joints and sacroiliac joints are largely spared in this entity (Figure 2-12).

## Degenerative Scoliosis and Kyphosis

Scoliosis, as a subset in patients with no preexisting scoliosis at the time of skeletal maturity, can be a disease of the degenerative cascade, osteoporosis, trauma, and/or iatrogenic from prior surgical intervention. Although any curve has the potential for progression, large curves greater than 60 degrees tend to progress with greater probability. One of the greatest risk factors for kyphosis is osteoporosis and the ensuing compression fracture (Figure 2-11).

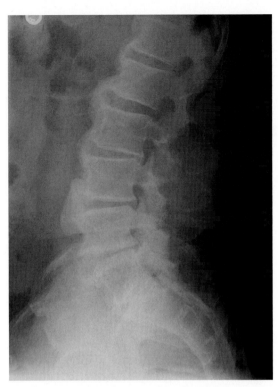

■ **FIGURE 2-12** Diffuse Idiopathic Skeletal Hyperostosis

## References

1. J.P.J. Van Schaik, H. Verbiest, et al., The orientation of the laminae and facet joints in the lower lumbar spine, Spine 10 (1985) 59–63.
2. W.R. Francis, J.W. Fielding, Traumatic spondylolisthesis of the axis, Orthop. Clin. North Am. 9 (1978) 1011–1027.
3. J.A. McColloch, E.E. Transfelt, Macnab's backache, Williams & Wilkins, Baltimore, 1997.
4. E.C. Benzel, Anatomic consideration of the C2 pedicle screw placement (letters to the editor), Spine 21 (1996) 2301–2301.
5. P.V. Scoles, A.E. Linton, B. Latimer, et al., Vertebral body and posterior element morphology: the normal spine in middle life, Spine 13 (1988) 1082–1086.
6. B.L. Riggs, L.J. Melton III, Evidence for two distinct syndromes of involutional osteoporosis, Am. J. Med. 75 (1983) 899–901.
7. G. Lyons, S.M. Eisenstein, M.B. Sweet, Biochemical changes in intervertebral disc degeneration, Biochim. Biophys. Acta 673 (1981) 443–453.
8. Y. Kawaguchi, M. Kanamori, H. Ishihara, et al., The association of lumbar disc disease with vitamin D receptor gene polymorphism, J. Bone Joint Surg. Am. 84 (2002) 2022–2028.
9. T. Kimura, K. Nakata, N. Tsumaki, et al., Progressive generation of the articular cartilage and intervertebral discs: an experimental study in transgenic mice bearing a type IX collagen mutation, Int. Orthop. 20 (1996) 177–181.
10. G. Dommissee, Morphological aspects of the lumbar spine and lumbosacral regions, Orthop. Clin. North Am. 6 (1975) 163–175.
11. N.A. Ebraheim, R. Xu, M. Darwich, et al., Anatomic relations between the lumbar pedicle and the adjacent neural structures, Spine 15 (1997) 2338–2341.
12. J.A. McCulloch, P.H. Young, Essentials of spinal microsurgery, Lippincott-Raven, Philadelphia, 1998.
13. M.D. Humzah, R.W. Soames, Human intervertebral disc: structure and function, Anat. Rec. 229 (1988) 337–356.
14. M.T. Milen, D.A. Bloom, J. Culligan, et al., Albert Adamkiewicz (1850-1921)—his artery and its significance for the retroperitoneal surgeon, World J. Urol. 17 (1999) 168–170.

# Histological Changes in the Aging Spine

3

*Kiran F. Rajneesh, G. Ty Thaiyananthan, David A. Essig, and Wolfgang Rauschning*

**K E Y   P O I N T S**

- The aging spine is predisposed to various disorders, with back pain being the primary complaint.
- Intervertebral disk degeneration is the commonest pathology in the aging spine.
- Osteoporosis of the vertebral bodies is a preventable cause of back pain.
- Facet joint degeneration can lead to painful facet joint syndrome.
- Back pain in older patients is amenable to treatment with a better understanding of the disease pathogenesis.

## INTRODUCTION

Back pain is one of the most common reasons for office visits to a physician. It accounts for 2% of all visits, surpassed only by routine examinations, diabetes, and hypertension.[1] Back pain is a condition that predominantly affects the older population. Increased survival rates, better health care outcomes, and improved economic status will increase the number of older people in our society. At present, persons older than 65 years constitute 13% of our population. In 30 years, they will constitute 30% of the United States population, and by the year 2050 they will makeup 60% of the population.[2] It is of paramount importance to recognize this trend of aging in the population and plan how best to fulfill the health needs of this growing part of our society.

Aging is a natural, inevitable, physiological change that leads to compromises in physical, mental, and functional abilities. At a cellular level, it represents decreased regeneration and repair, and increased catabolic changes that gradual deterioration in function. The spine, composed of the framework of vertebral columns and intervertebral disks encasing the spinal cord, is not insensitive to the onslaught of changes that occur during aging. The aging of the spinal cord results in decreased strength and agility and increased reflex times. However, the predominant effects of aging in the spine involve the mechanical components of the spine. Histologically, they can be classified as aging of the disks, the vertebral bodies, the facet joints, and the muscles and ligaments.

## INTERVERTEBRAL DISK

The intervertebral disks are remnants of the notochord and are interspersed between adjacent vertebral bodies of the spine except between the fused bodies of the sacrum and the coccyx. The intervertebral disks are composed of a circular ring of more resilient annulus fibrosus, which holds a central core of gelatinous material called the nucleus pulposus (Figure 3-1). Biochemically, both the annulus fibrosus and the nucleus pulposus contain proteoglycans in addition to water. The amount of water varies and is responsible for their varied characteristics and, consequently, their functions. The intervertebral disks derive their nutrition by diffusion across vertebral endplates. As the rate of permeability decreases with aging, the health of the disk is threatened.

The intervertebral disks are primarily shock absorbers and are resistant to compressive forces. During the process of aging, the daily wear and tear

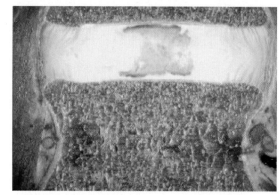

■ **FIGURE 3-1** Intervertebral disk. Outer annulus fibrosus surrounding inner nucleus pulposus. *(Courtesy of Wolfgang Rauschning, MD.)*

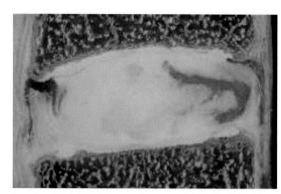

■ **FIGURE 3-2** Neovascularization at periphery of an annular tear. *(Courtesy of Wolfgang Rauschning, MD.)*

damage of years of mechanical stress compounded by decreased nutrition and water predispose the disks to degeneration. Associated with these local changes, systemic changes of aging such as decreased structural protein synthesis, impaired water metabolism, and decreased physical activity serve as additional insults to the fragile microenviroment of the aging disks.

The pathophysiology of disk degeneration involves a multitude of cellular and biochemical changes. Proteoglycans, responsible for the osmotic gradient and thus the hydration of the disk, are lost. There is overall fragmentation of type I and type II collagen within the disk, with an increase in the ratio of type I to type II collagen fibers. Furthermore, there is an increase in degradative enzymatic activity including cathepsins and matrix metalloproteinases (MMPs). As a result, there is a decrease in the biomechanical and load-sharing ability of the disk.

Due to decreased turgor and nutrition of the disks, radial and concentric fissures appear in the initial phases of degeneration. The normal avascular disks may develop microvascular capillaries at the periphery of the annulus fibrosus as a compensatory mechanism for decreased nutrition (Figure 3-2).

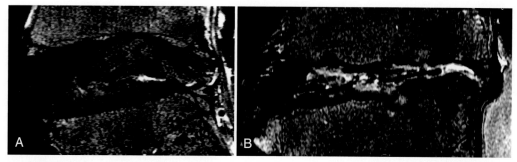

■ **FIGURE 3-3**    Degenerative changes on T2-weighted MRI. Note the decreased brightness of the intervertebral disk, the annular fissures, and the disk-space narrowing.

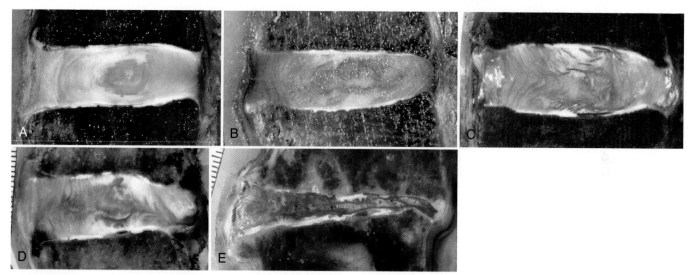

■ **FIGURE 3-4**    Cascade of disk degeneration. **A**, Healthy disk with an intact nucleus pulposus and annulus fibrosus. Weakening of or injury to the annulus coupled with loss of hydration and proteoglycans of the nucleus can lead to loss of disk height and subsequent endplate changes (**B-E**) *(Courtesy of Wolfgang Rauschning, MD.)*

However, this impaired neovascularization is detrimental, contributes to microedema, and exposes the disks to the body's immune cells for the first time in adult life. Also, there is dissection of the microstructural organization of the annulus fibrosus. The radial fissures eventually enlarge and follow the path of least resistance posterolaterally in relation to the vertebral bodies and overlying the intervertebral foramina. In the late stages of disk degeneration, the nucleus pulposus tracks out over the intervertebral foramina and can compress the exiting spinal nerve, potentially causing symptoms of radiculopathy.

Plain x-ray films show decreased intervertebral spaces, accompanied by deformed endplates and osteophyte formation. However, these are terminal changes and not helpful from an early diagnostic point of view. Magnetic resonance imaging (MRI) is regarded as the gold standard for early detection of disk degeneration. Disk desiccation (unhealthy disks are darker due to lesser water content), disk bulge due to deformed annulus fibrosus, and radial tears within the disk are early makers of disk degeneration[3] (Figures 3-3, 3-4). Novel imaging techniques such as MR spectroscopy to measure lactic acid within the disk (an early sign of disk degeneration), diffusion tensor imaging (DTI) for measuring water content within the disk, and functional MRI (fMRI) for task dependent signal intensity changes have been proposed and warrant further study.

## VERTEBRAL BODIES

The vertebral bodies are the primary support of the spinal cord and are osseous in nature. They differentiate from the segmental sclerotomes in embryological life and form the framework to support the spinal cord and its vascular supply. Vertebral bodies are composed of cancellous bone and are best adapted to resist compressive loads (Figure 3-5). However, this

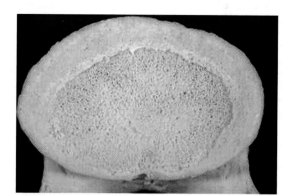

■ **FIGURE 3-5**    The vertebral body is composed of cancellous bone.

same property predisposes the cancellous bones to accelerated changes during aging. They are supplied by a rich network of vascular channels at low pressure, compared to cortical bones found elsewhere in the body which have haversian canals with high-pressure vascular channels. The increased vascularity in vertebral bodies, coupled with a low pressure system, increases their surface area ratio and sensitizes them to minute changes in hormones and other factors in the extracellular fluids. On a biochemical level, the cancellous bone is a lattice network composed of collagen and noncollagen proteins and calcium hydroxyapatite. The osteoid framework is laid down by osteoblasts and resorbed and restructured by osteoclasts, both of which are under the influence of parathyroid hormone (PTH) and calcitonin.

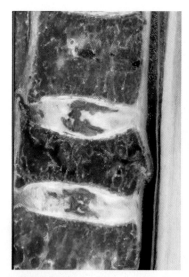

■ **FIGURE 3-6**   Compression fracture.

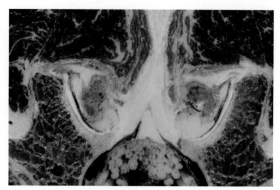

■ **FIGURE 3-7**   Facet joints are composed of synovial joints lined with synovium and articular cartilage. *(Courtesy of Wolfgang Rauschning, MD.)*

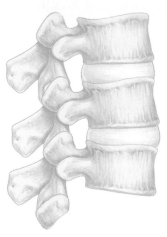

■ **FIGURE 3-8**   The three-column motion segment. 70% of the axial load is borne by the intervertebral disk, while up to 30% may be borne by the facet complex.

The bone density is maximal at 25 years of age and decreases with aging. Osteoporosis is characterized by decreased bone formation and mineralization as well as decreased bone density.[4] This effect is multifactorial in nature. During aging, there is a decrease in absorption and assimilation of nutrients including calcium and vitamin D. Decreased conversion of vitamin $D_2$ to vitamin $D_3$ in kidneys decreases the mineralized components of the bone.[5] There is also a general decline in production of various hormones influencing bone formation including PTH, estrogen, and glucocorticoids, which decrease osteoblastic activity. Furthermore, there is an increase in IL-6, TNF-$\alpha$, and other chemokines due to impaired immunity which increases osteoclastic activity. In addition, there is usually an overall decline in physical activity and exercise and decreased quality of diet in the elderly. All these factors together precipitate an osteopenic state.

Patients usually present with overwhelming back pain brought on after sudden physical activity, after lifting objects, or after coughing or bending. Plain radiographs show a decreased vertebral body height, decreased bone density (a 30% reduction in mineralization from baseline is required to visualize osteopenia on plain radiographs), and compression fractures (Figure 3-6). The bone density scan, also known as the dual energy x-ray absorptiometry (DEXA) scan, is an enhanced form of x-ray technology and the gold standard for imaging osteoporosis. The results of a DEXA scan are expressed as a T-score, which is an index of standard deviation. A T-score of less than −2.5 is significant for osteoporosis. Quantitative CT is an alternative imaging modality but requires high-resolution CT scanners and may not be available at all centers.[6] High-resolution MR imaging has been proposed and is focused on assessing bone structure directly rather than only assessing mineralization.[7]

## FACET JOINTS

Facet joints are the only true synovial joints within the vertebral column. The facet joint is located between two adjacent vertebral bodies with the upper facet facing downwards and medially and the lower facet facing upward and laterally. The facets articulate with a thin interspersed cartilage and are surrounded by a synovial sac and innervated by rich nerve endings (Figure 3-7). In a healthy young individual, the intervertebral disk is the anterior load-bearing structure and the facet is the posterior load-bearing structure. Hence facet joints are referred to as the three-joint complex, with two facets and the intervertebral disk (Figure 3-8). These joints allow flexion-extension and some torsion of the spine.[8] During aging, facet joint pathology is always secondary to disk degeneration. Increased load is subsequently transferred to the facet joints, which were designed for small load-bearing capacity. This increased load causes facet joint degeneration. The cartilage is the first structure to be affected, with resultant synovial inflammation, joint space narrowing, and osteophyte formation resulting in central or foraminal stenosis and spondylolisthesis (Figures 3-9, 3-10). The resulting inflammation causes irritation of the nociceptive nerve endings, causing back pain sometimes referred to as "facet joint syndrome."[9]

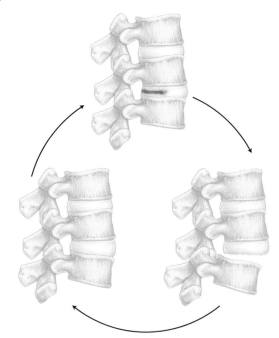

■ **FIGURE 3-9**   Degenerative cascade. Disk degeneration leading to increased facet loading and degeneration resulting in instability and spondylolisthesis.

On plain radiographs, sclerosis and osteophyte formation can be visualized in facet joints, demonstrating late stages of degeneration. MR imaging of the cartilage revealing focal erosions may be the earliest sign of facet

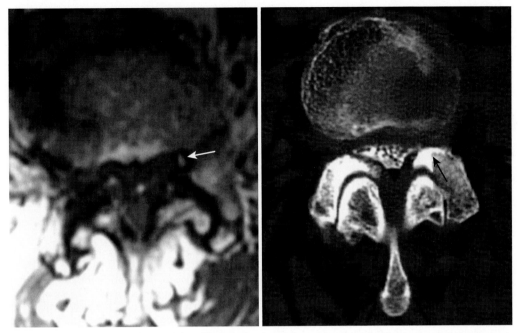

■ **FIGURE 3-10**    MRI and CT evidence of foraminal and central stenosis as a result of facet osteophyte development.

degeneration and may be amenable to rescue measures. Facet hypertrophy, apophyseal malalignment, and osteophyte formation may be recognized on CT scans.[10]

## MUSCLES AND LIGAMENTS

The intrinsic and extrinsic muscles, along with the ligaments, maintain the spine at optimal tension and maintain the normal physiological primary curvatures.[11] The ligamentum flavum connects adjacent vertebrae along the anterior edge of the lamina. It is primarily composed of elastin, and allows flexion and extension. The elastin content is responsible for the tensile strength of the ligamentum flavum. During aging, the muscles lose the ability to attain tetanic contractions, have decreased contractile force, and undergo atrophy. This atrophy is due to a decline in nutrition and hormonal status, in addition to decreased physical activity. Microscopically the muscles show decreased collagen fiber content and increased fatty infiltration. The ligamentum flavum has decreased elastin content and becomes lax and bulging, destabilizing the vertebral column.[12] These changes predispose the aging spine to disk degeneration, compression fractures, and spinal stenosis by altering the normal curvature and the normal tension within the spine.

Plain x-ray studies may show calcifications and altered curvatures of the spine. However, MR imaging may show atrophy of specific muscles, fatty infiltration. and impaired architecture of ligaments in aging.

## SUMMARY

Aging results in irreversible, permanent changes to the spinal column. The findings of disk, facet, vertebral body, and ligamentous pathology play an interrelated role in the aging spine. Thus, the management of these patients must take into account all of these interrelated elements. Future treatment challenges will not only center on treating end-stage disease, but also in preventing disease progression.

## References

1. B.I. Martin, R.A. Deyo, S.K. Mirza, et al., Expenditures and health status among adults with back and neck problems, Jama 299 (2008) 656–664.
2. V. Turkulov, N. Madle-Samardzija, O. Niciforovic-Surkovic, C. Gavrancic, [Demographic aspects of aging], Med Pregl 60 (2007) 247–250.
3. W. Johannessen, J.D. Auerbach, A.J. Wheaton, et al., Assessment of human disc degeneration and proteoglycan content using T1rho-weighted magnetic resonance imaging, Spine 31 (2006) 1253–1257.
4. Y.L. Lee, K.M. Yip, The osteoporotic spine, Clinical orthopaedics and related research (1996) 91–97.
5. T.L. Nickolas, M.B. Leonard, E. Shane, Chronic kidney disease and bone fracture: a growing concern, Kidney international, 2008.
6. H. Shi, W.C. Scarfe, A.G. Farman, Three-dimensional reconstruction of individual cervical vertebrae from cone-beam computed-tomography images, Am J Orthod Dentofacial Orthop 131 (2007) 426–432.
7. A. Zaia, R. Eleonori, P. Maponi, R. Rossi, R. Murri, MR imaging and osteoporosis: fractal lacunarity analysis of trabecular bone, IEEE Trans Inf Technol Biomed 10 (2006) 484–489.
8. A. Fujiwara, K. Tamai, M. Yamato, et al., The relationship between facet joint osteoarthritis and disc degeneration of the lumbar spine: an MRI study, Eur Spine J 8 (1999) 396–401.
9. P.P. Raj, Intervertebral disc: anatomy-physiology-pathophysiology-treatment, Pain Pract 8 (2008) 18–44.
10. M. Barry, P. Livesley, Facet joint hypertrophy: the cross-sectional area of the superior articular process of L4 and L5, Eur Spine J 6 (1997) 121–124.
11. M. Yamada, Y. Tohno, S. Tohno, et al., Age-related changes of elements and relationships among elements in human tendons and ligaments, Biological trace element research 98 (2004) 129–142.
12. H. Kosaka, K. Sairyo, A. Biyani, et al., Pathomechanism of loss of elasticity and hypertrophy of lumbar ligamentum flavum in elderly patients with lumbar spinal canal stenosis, Spine 32 (2007) 2805–2811.

# 4

# Natural History of the Degenerative Cascade

*Ali Araghi and Donna D. Ohnmeiss*

**KEY POINTS**

- For many years, the mechanics of the spine and how spinal tissues respond to the demands placed upon them has been studied, as well as the role of mechanical loading in impacting degeneration of spinal structures.
- The body of knowledge continues to grow, giving us greater insight into the complicated biochemistry of the intervertebral disc.
- Degeneration of the spinal segment is a very complex process, which is complicated by the high degree of interrelationship of the various spinal structures.
- The specific details of disc-related pain mechanisms resulting in a patient's clinical symptoms remain elusive.
- Along with disc degeneration, the posterior elements also degenerate, which may produce pain arising from the facet joints and, often, pain related to central or foraminal stenosis.

## NATURAL HISTORY OF THE DEGENERATIVE CASCADE

The degenerative process encompasses every element of the spine: the ligamentous structures, facet joints, intervertebral discs, endplates, and vertebral bodies. Changes occur in a sequential fashion on a multitude of levels, including the gross visual level, the radiographic level, the biomechanical level, and the biochemical level. Unfortunately, the changes seen in the normal aging spine are very similar to the changes seen in the pathologic and symptomatic spine. Hence, it becomes extremely difficult to differentiate the symptomatic conditions from the manifestations of a normal aging spine. It is only after understanding the normal changes associated with aging that we may be able to identify some of the pathologic changes.

The natural history of degenerative disc disease has been studied for many years. Lees and Turner, in 1963, followed 51 patients with cervical radiculopathy for 19 years and found that 25% had worsening of the symptoms, 45% had no recurrence, and 30% had what they classified as mild symptoms.[1] Nurick studied the nonsurgical treatment of 36 patients with cervical myelopathy over 20 years.[2] Sixty-six percent of the patients who presented with early symptoms did not progress, and approximately 66% of patients with moderate to severe symptoms did not progress either. The patients who progressed tended to be the younger patients.

## ANATOMY AND GENERAL MECHANISMS OF PAIN

In order to understand the degenerative cascade of the spine, it is of paramount importance to understand the normal function of the different structures and how they interrelate with each other. The facet joints are designed to bear approximately 10% to 30% of the load in the lumbar spine, depending on the patient's position. The articular cartilage that bears such loads is supported by the subchondral bone. The subchondral bone also serves to provide nutrition to the articular cartilage. The facet joints are diarthrodial synovial joints that have a capsule. The capsules together with the ligaments constrain joint motion. The medial and anterior capsule is formed by a lateral extension of the ligamentum flavum. The capsules and ligaments are innervated by primary articular branches from larger peripheral nerves and accessory articular nerves. Such nerves consist of both proprioceptive and nociceptive fibers. They are monitored by the central nervous system, and may perceive excessive joint motion (potentially due to instability or an injury) as a noxious stimulus and mediate a muscular reflex to counteract such excursions. Nociceptive free nerve endings and mechanoreceptors have been isolated in the human facet capsules and synovium. Such nerve endings may perceive chemical stimuli or mechanical stimuli such as instability, trauma, or capsular distention as noxious stimuli. Joint effusions, commonly seen on MRIs, may prevent such reflexes due to capsular distention, similar to a distended knee joint and absent patellar reflex. Substance P, a pain-related neuropeptide, has been identified in synovium. Higher concentrations have been found in arthritic joints. Additionally, capsular free nerve endings have been found to become sensitized in arthritic joints. This has caused otherwise dormant nerve endings to become reactive to motion that was perceived as normal in nonarthritic conditions.

The intervertebral disc is another significant component of the degenerative cascade. The sinuvertebral nerve innervates the posterior and posterolateral aspect of the intervertebral disc, as well as the posterior longitudinal ligament (PLL) and the ventral aspect of the thecal sac. The lateral and anterior aspect of the disc is innervated by the gray ramus communicans. These free nerve endings have been found primarily in the outer one third of the annulus, and have been found to be immunoreactive for painful neuropeptides. Some complex endings have been identified within the annulus as well. The considerable overlap of the descending and ascending nerve endings with branches of the sinuvertebral nerves of the adjacent one to two discs makes identifying the exact pain generator even more difficult when performing clinical diagnostic tests. Leakage of such neuropeptides out of the disc in the presence of annular tears, onto the nearby dorsal root ganglion (DRG), can cause irritation of the DRG and become another source of pain. The PLL fibers are closely intertwined with the posterior annulus. The PLL has been identified to contain a variety of free nerve endings. Hence any irritation of the posterior annulus and disc can cause irritation of these nerve endings. Such irritation can be mechanical secondary to pressure from a herniated disc, abnormal motion from instability, or mechanical incompetence of the annulus. Irritants can also be chemical such as low pH fluids, cytokines, or neuropeptides that can leak out from the disc via annular tears.

Cortical bone, bone marrow, and periosteum have been found to be innervated by nerves containing nociceptive neuropeptides such as calcitonin, gene-related peptides, and substance P. Periosteal elevation, such as in cases of infection, tumor, or hematoma, can be painful. Periosteal tears in cases such as fractures, inflammation, or subsidence (e.g., in osteoarthritic conditions) can cause pain. Vascular congestion from bone infarcts or sickle cell can cause the intramedullary nerve fibers to initiate a painful response.

Nociceptive nerve fibers have been identified in varying concentrations within the fibrous tissue of spondylolytic pars defects as well.

The spine is covered with muscles and tendons in which the main nociceptive nerve endings are unencapsulated. Pain may be mediated by chemical or mechanical conditions or both. The mechanonociceptive units may respond to disruption, stretch, or pressure. Direct injury can cause damage to the intrafascicular nerve fibers or cause a hematoma and edema, which can lead to a chemically mediated pathway. Such a pathway can begin by release of nociceptive sensitizing chemicals such as histamine, potassium, and bradykinin from the damaged tissues. This, in turn, can lead to altered vascular permeability and an influx of the inflammatory cells. It is through such neuropeptides that sensitization of the receptors occurs and, in combination with interstitial edema, this can cause primary muscular pain. At times, the mechanical effect of spasm of a major muscle group in and of itself can cause further trauma to the muscle, and potentiate the pain cascade.

## PATHOGENESIS OF LUMBAR DEGENERATION

During childhood and the first two decades of life, the spinal motion segments generally function in a physiologic manner and the disc maintains its hydrostatic properties. Hence, the disc maintains its height and its normal relationship with the facets, allowing the facets to experience normal loads and physiologic motion. The canal and the foramen are usually patent and the ligamentum flavum is only a few millimeters thick. Invagination of the disc into the endplates (Schmorl nodes) and some facet asymmetry may be seen, but are generally not symptomatic. In the next 20 years, however, degeneration does occur and annular tears occur that lead to disc bulging and protrusion, which can then cause loss of disc space height and loss of hydrostatic properties. This, in turn, will cause increased loads on the facets and initiate facet hypertrophy and neural encroachment. Such hypertrophy, when present in combination with loss of disc height, potentiates foraminal compromise. Ligamentum flavum hypertrophy occurs as well, which together with facet hypertrophy potentiates central canal compromise. Loss of disc height can certainly cause loss of stature in the elderly population.

## BIOCHEMICAL CHANGES

Numerous biochemical changes occur in the disc as a result of aging. The gelatinous nature of the disc degenerates into a more fibrotic state due to loss of water content. It is important to understand that a normal disc is composed of 80% water and 20% collagen and proteoglycans. The negatively charged glycosaminoglycans are what allows the nucleus to retain its water content and osmotic pressure. The actual cascade of nucleus degeneration occurs in the following order. First, there is loss of distinction between the nuclear and annular fibers and an increase in the collagen content of the disc, followed by the loss of the negative charges mentioned earlier and loss of water content, greatly reducing the proteoglycan aggregates. In fact, during the breakdown of the glycosaminoglycans, there is also a significant loss of chondroitin sulfate in comparison to keratin sulfate. The annulus degenerates by a decrease in cellularity and metabolic activity. The annulus is the only portion of the disc that in its healthy state has vascularity. This vascularity decreases with degeneration, which may hinder the healing process. Proteoglycan content decreases and large collagen fibrils appear. The large fibrils when present in a biomechanically vulnerable portion of the annulus may increase the likelihood of annular tears. Such tears generally occur due to a rotational force and occur in the posterolateral annulus. With annular disruption, changes take place within the disc itself. Vascularized granulation tissue forms along the margins of the annular ruptures and may pass as far as into the nucleus.[3] Unlike discs from asymptomatic subjects, among discs taken from back pain patients, nerve endings extended deep into the annulus and in some cases into the nucleus. Such nerves produced substance P.[4] These changes within the disc likely play a role in discogenic pain. Also, such changes may challenge disc regeneration as a pain-relieving intervention.

The cartilaginous endplate serves as a nutrition gradient for the healthy disc. Degeneration of the disc has been associated with a decrease in the diffusion capability across the endplate and sclerosis of the endplate, which in turn negatively affects the nutrition of the disc.[5] This is thought to at least have a negative impact on the biochemical medium within the disc, if it is

not the actual cause. These types of degenerative and nutritional changes within the disc will likely pose a significant challenge to disc regenerative therapies.

Kirkaldy-Willis et al. inspected 50 lumbar cadaveric specimens and also analyzed morphologic changes in 161 patients' lumbar spines intraoperatively.[6] It is such observations that have provided links between the different aspects of the degenerative cascade, leading to a better understanding of the transformation of a healthy level in the spine to a stenotic level with spondylolisthesis and instability.

## BIOMECHANICAL CHANGES

The theory of the three joint complex, and the interdependence of these elements, was recognized and described by Farfan and co-workers.[7] This interdependence and sequence of degeneration is outlined in Figure 4-1. Furthermore, the increased risk of the lower two levels for degeneration, secondary to their increased lordotic shape of the disc as well as their increased vulnerability to rotational injuries due to the exaggerated obliquity of their facet joints, was recognized. The two mechanisms of propagation of degeneration that were described consisted of a minor rotational injury causing facet injuries and annular tears and a repetitive compressive injury causing minor damage to the cartilage plate, which would serve as an early stimulus for progressive disc degeneration over time. Additionally, it was postulated that the abnormal stresses of a degenerated segment will affect the adjacent levels. The biochemical changes are accompanied and potentiated by biomechanical factors. The healthy disc has hydrostatic properties that allow the nucleus to convert axial compressive forces to tensile strain on the annular fibers as well as evenly share the load over the endplates. The oblique arrangement of the crossing collagen fibrils in the annulus allow it to convert the axial loads to tensile strains. In fact, the annulus is largely made of type I collagen which provides the tensile strength seen in tendons, whereas the nucleus is largely made of type II collagen. In the degenerative cascade, loss of hydrostatic properties occurs in the annulus and nucleus, and the osmotic pressure of the disc decreases, allowing an increase in creep by a factor of two. The disc loses its ability to imbibe water and to evenly distribute the loads that it is under. This is due to changes in the molecular meshwork of the proteoglycan collagens. Annular fissures occur, and, as a result of repetitive trauma, coalesce together and become radial tears. Radial tears render the disc even more incompetent. Such factors, particularly when potentiated by biochemical changes, cause resorption of disc material, and facilitate adjacent endplate sclerosis. Rarely may resorption lead to spontaneous fusion of the disc. Herniations are generally more likely in the earlier stages of degeneration when the intradiscal pressures are higher than in the more advanced stages. Offending osteophytes, however, are more likely in the more advanced stages of degeneration.

The medial and anterior facet joint capsules are made of approximately 80% elastin and 20% collagen. Degeneration starts by a synovial inflammatory response and fibrillation of the articular cartilage of the joint. This progresses to gross irregularity of the articular cartilage and formation of osteophytes. Eventually, one of the articular processes may fracture and become a loose body as well as contribute to capsular laxity, which will allow excessive motion of the joint and instability. The facet and disc changes cause mechanical incompetence of a motion segment and may lead to abnormal sagittal translation, further compromising the neural elements (Figure 4-2). Compensatory posturing is observed in the elderly with spinal stenosis as a forward flexed posture in an attempt to put the spine into flexion and increase the space available for the neural elements. This posturing will offload the degenerated facets and potentially decrease facet pain as well.

## THE THREE STAGES OF INSTABILITY

The theory of biomechanical degenerative instability was described by Kirkaldy-Willis and Farfan in 1982.[8] They defined instability as a clinical entity when the patient changes from mild symptoms to severe symptoms acutely with minimal activity or provocation. This was explained as abnormal joint deformation with stress, which produces a symptomatic reaction in the affected area, hence causing pain. The factors that affect such instability are primarily the increased motion of the joint and, secondarily, the physical changes that occur within the joint with repetitive trauma. They

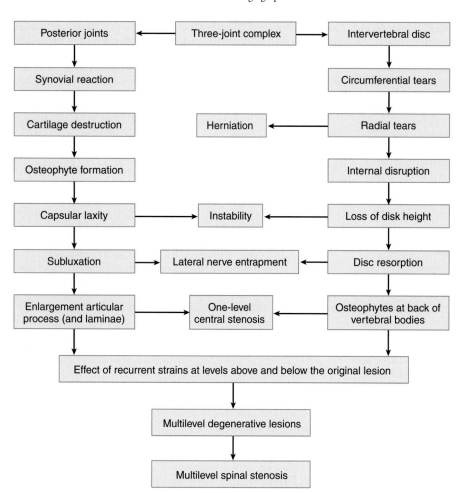

```
Posterior joints ← Three-joint complex → Intervertebral disc
        ↓                                          ↓
Synovial reaction                          Circumferential tears
        ↓                                          ↓
Cartilage destruction    Herniation ←       Radial tears
        ↓                                          ↓
Osteophyte formation                       Internal disruption
        ↓                                          ↓
Capsular laxity    →     Instability   ←    Loss of disk height
        ↓                                          ↓
Subluxation    →    Lateral nerve entrapment  ←  Disc resorption
        ↓                                          ↓
Enlargement articular    One-level    ←    Osteophytes at back of
process (and laminae)  central stenosis         vertebral bodies
        ↓
Effect of recurrent strains at levels above and below the original lesion
        ↓
Multilevel degenerative lesions
        ↓
Multilevel spinal stenosis
```

■ **FIGURE 4-1** Overview of the interrelation of disc and posterior element degeneration. *(From Kirkaldy-Willis WH, et al: Pathology and pathogenesis of lumbar spondylosis and stenosis, Spine 3:320, 1978.)*

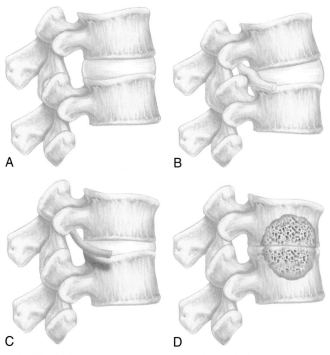

**A**    **B**

**C**    **D**

■ **FIGURE 4-2** As the spinal segment progresses from normal (**A**) to degenerative, positional changes may become more pronounced such as nerve root compression in extension (**B**), or patients leaning forward to increase the narrowed foramen (**C**). Eventually, the segment collapses and osteophytes form (**D**).

divided the clinical symptoms into three phases. First, a stage of temporary dysfunction, second, an unstable phase, and lastly, a stabilization phase. In the temporary dysfunction stage, the increased abnormal motion may actually manifest itself as decreased overall motion secondary to acute inflammation, muscle spasm, or guarding. The spinous processes may be held in midline or to one side secondary to spasm and hence limit lateral bending and rotation. Vertebral tilting and rotation are coupled in the spine and produce lateral bending. Abnormal excursion of the facets may be seen on lateral flexion and extension radiographs. Generally, significant abnormal shear or translation does not occur if there is a healthy disc present. In the second stage, the changes become more constant and long-lasting, yet the spine still has increased motion present. As stage two progresses the changes become more irreversible. Stage three is accompanied by advanced degeneration and loss of disc height as well as the presence of stabilizing osteophytes. This stage is generally more stable and less prone to instability. Some of the key clinical findings of each stage are summarized in Table 4-1.

In this context, injury is defined as any force that is too great for the joint to withstand. Such forces do not necessarily have to be from a significant traumatic episode or from lifting a heavy object, but simply from uncoordinated muscle activity supporting the patient's body weight. Injury can cause trauma to the articular surface and capsule of the facets, as well as to the endplates and disc annulus. . However, much larger external trauma is required for injury to the other ligamentous tissues and muscles. Facet joint articular surface injuries will start with fibrillation and progress to erosion and eburnation. Finally, subchondral fractures can lead to complete fractures and loose bodies as alluded to earlier in this chapter. By the same token, the synovial membrane will thicken through this inflammatory process and develop an effusion, which can become exudative and create fibrosis. If capsular tears occur, they may cause initial instability. Recovery with minor trauma is usually complete, though it can lead to a more prolonged vulnerable (unstable) phase.

With major traumatic episodes, the damage is different in that endplate fractures or detachment of peripheral annulus from the endplate can occur. This is especially likely if the segment is already in a more unstable phase. The body's reparative process consists of microvascular invasion and loss of normal annular and nuclear cells. This, in turn, will lead to loss of discheight. Such changes generally occur at the same time as when the facets begin to fragment, hypertrophy, and override. This, in combination with the thickening of the ligamentum flavum, will lead to central and foraminal stenosis. Repetitive injuries cause fibrosis and scar formation, but can also prolong the unstable phase. In cases of prolonged instability, the eventual loss of disc space height and formation of endplate osteophytes will stabilize the segment. Depending on the mode of impact of the forces, different parts of the spine will be injured and the reparative process will vary. Such variations are the determining factor for whether the reparative process will further destabilize the segment. Such instabilities may occur after multiple traumatic episodes or after only one.

The different modes of injury can induce episodic severe dysfunction by their interaction with the pathologic processes already present in the spine. The forces can be applied as direct axial compression. These forces are typically less damaging to the discs or facets when they are in their healthier phase, but further down the degenerative cascade, when there are more degenerative changes in the discs and annulus, the effects of such forces can become more damaging. Injury can also be directed in a torsional direction. Such injuries tend to put more stress on the facets and outer annular fibers. Facet injuries are even more pronounced in the lower

lumbar and lumbosacral spine where the facets are more coronally oriented and more prone to torsional injuries. Additionally, forces can cause a creep effect over time. Axial creep may cause bulging of the disc and loss of discheight, especially at the lumbosacral junction where the forces are applied at an angle. Also important to note is that the erect patient adds extension to the lumbosacral junction which further narrows the canal and foramen. Injuries occurring with the patient in a semi-prone position can cause the segment to experience further unilateral foraminal narrowing, which, along with preexisting axial creep, can cause dynamic foraminal nerve entrapment. Torsional creep will cause rotation of one vertebra on the other, which can cause bulging of the posterolateral corner of the annulus. This, along with the rotated posterior facet and lamina, can lead to lateral recess and foraminal narrowing.

## CLINICAL INSTABILITY AND DIAGNOSTIC IMAGING

Instability can be suspected based on symptoms of recurrent low back pain and sciatica without any neurologic deficit that starts with minimal trauma and is relieved by rest and bracing. Repetitive recurrence in a short period of time is typical. Another suspicious sign of instability is symptoms of pain, temporarily relieved by manipulation or mobilization of the spine, recurring with minimal activity. Pain on forward bending with a painful clunk on trunk extension is a sign of instability. Rotoscoliosis may be present as well. Most of such injuries occur in the lower lumbar region (L4-5 greater than L5-S1, in a 2:1 ratio). However, the presence of a deep-seated L5 within the pelvis (intercrestal line being at L4-5 disc or upper portion of L5 vertebral body) and elongated L5 transverse processes, protects the L5-S1 level and increases the chances of injury to the L4-5 level. Conversely, a high position of the L5 vertebral body (intercrestal line at lower portion of L5 vertebral body or the L5-S1 disc space) along with short L5 transverse processes increases the chances of L5-S1 injury.

Careful attention to x-rays can identify signs of instability, such as McNab traction spurs, which occur below the rims of the endplates, or the presence of gas in the disc space, sometimes referred to as Knutsson sign. Lateral flexion/extension x-rays can help identify instability by revealing a dynamic spondylolisthesis or retrolisthesis. Such malalignments can cause narrowing of the neural foramen, especially in the presence of decreased

| Phase | I Dysfunction | II Unstable | III Stabilization |
|---|---|---|---|
| Symptoms | Low back pain<br>Often localized<br>Sometimes referred<br>Movement painful | Those of dysfunction<br>Giving way of back: "catch"<br>Pain on coming to standing position after flexion | Less low back pain<br>Mainly leg pain |
| Signs | Local tenderness<br>Muscle contracted<br>Hypomobility<br>Extension painful<br>Seldom neurology<br>Abnormal decreased movement | Detection of abnormal movement (inspection, palpation)<br>Observation of "catch," sway, or shift when coming erect after flexion | Muscle tenderness<br>Stiffness<br>Reduced movement<br>Scoliosis<br>Some neurology |
| Radiological changes | Spinous processes malaligned<br>Irregular facets<br>Early disc changes | Anteroposterior:<br>Lateral shift<br>Rotation<br>Abnormal tilt<br>Malaligned spinous processes<br>Oblique:<br>Opening facets<br>Lateral:<br>Spondylolisthesis (in flexion)<br>Retrospondylolisthesis (in extension)<br>Abnormal opening of disc<br>Abnormal change in pedicle height<br>CT changes:<br>Disc bulging | Enlarged facets<br>Loss of disc height<br>Osteophytes<br>Small foramina<br>Reduced movement<br>Scoliosis |

**TABLE 4-1    Clinical observations seen in the Kirkaldy-Willis classification stages of spinal degeneration**

From Bertilson BC, et al: Inter-examiner reliability in the assessment of low back pain (LBP) using the Kirkaldy-Willis classification (KWC), Europ Spine J 2006:1696.

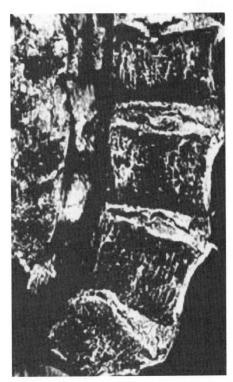

■ **FIGURE 4-3** Different stages of degeneration present in the same lumbar spine. *(From Kirkaldy-Willis WH, et al: Pathology and pathogenesis of lumbar spondylosis and stenosis, Spine 3:324, 1978.)*

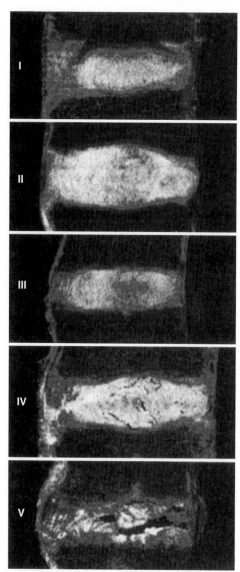

**■ FIGURE 4-4** Stages I through V of degeneration in the lumbar spine, based on the Thompson classification. *(From Thompson JP, et al: Preliminary evaluation of a scheme for grading the gross morphology of the human intervertebral disc, Spine 15:411-415, 1990.)*

discspace height. If flexion/extension radiographs demonstrate an exaggerated increase in posterior heights of the disc along with decreased anterior height of the disc of one level in comparison to the other levels, this may also be a sign of instability. This finding is sometimes referred to as "rockering." Less commonly evaluated radiographic modalities include anterior/posterior side bending films, which may demonstrate asymmetric tilting of the vertebral body, or decreased bending to one side (which stems from decreased tilt and rotation in a coupled fashion) with a paradoxical increase in disc height on the side to which the patient is bending. Exaggerated closure of the disc on the ipsilateral side as the bending can also occur. Lateral listhesis is due to abnormal rotation of the vertebral body during side bending, which is yet another sign of instability. Spinous process malalignment and pedicle asymmetry are important to be noted on the AP films as well. CT scanning a patient while rotated to the left and right side (with similar positioning to that of Judet views) can show gapping of the facet joint on the side opposite to the rotation of the vertebral body. This causes the superior articulating process to shift anteriorly and narrow the lateral recess on the ipsilateral side as the gapping. Such a finding can be consistent with dynamic nerve entrapment in the lateral recess.

## CONCLUSION

In summation, we have to compile the degenerative changes of each of the different parts of the spine, and apply them to the theory of the interrelated three-joint (tripod) complex. Injury to one part of the spine can cause abnormal motion and load transfers, and hence affect the other parts of the spine over time. Loss of disc height causes the posterior facets to sublux and the superior articular process of the level below to migrate upward and anteriorly, hence narrowing the lateral recess and possibly impinging on the traversing root. This is especially true when there is concomitant hypertrophy of the superior articular process. Depending on the amount of loss of disc height, the neural foramen can be narrowed as well and cause exiting root impingement. If the initial injury was asymmetric with respect to one facet joint, then that facet can degenerate, hypertrophy, stretch the capsule, and become more lax than the other side. In such a case scenario, a rotational deformity begins to occur which can simultaneously cause eccentric bulging of the disc due to its rotational instability, and cause unilateral lateral recess stenosis. Experimental work supports the concept that abnormal motion at one level causes nonphysiologic strains at the adjacent levels which can lead to multi-level involvement. This can explain why degeneration is typically seen in multiple adjacent levels of the spine in different stages of the cascade (Figure 4-3). Posterior element laxity and increased motion can exert additional forces on an already partially degenerated disc, render the segment incompetent to physiologic loads, and cause a degenerative spondylolisthesis. Certainly the reverse order of events can occur as well, possibly more often. When formulating a surgical treatment plan for a patient, it is of paramount importance to diagnose which of the stages of instability best fits the patient's spine at the time of treatment (Figure 4-4). Most stage I and early stage II will respond to conservative treatment. However, decompression alone for late stage II can lead to further instability and may be better accompanied by a fusion. Stage III, on the other hand, may best be treated with decompression alone without fusion.

## References

1. F. Lees, J.W. Turner, Natural history and prognosis of cervical spondylosis, BMJ 2 (1963) 1607–1610.
2. S. Nurick, The natural history and the results of surgical treatment of the spinal cord disorder associated with cervical spondylosis, Brain 95 (1972) 101–108.
3. B. Peng, J. Hao, S. Hou, et al., Possible pathogenesis of painful intervertebral disc degeneration, Spine 31 (2006) 560–566.
4. A.J. Freemont, T.E. Peacock, P. Goupille, et al., Nerve ingrowth into diseased intervertebral disc in chronic back pain, Lancet 350 (1997) 178–181.
5. J.P. Urban, S. Smith, J.C. Fairbank, Nutrition of the intervertebral disc, Spine 29 (2004) 2700–2709.
6. W.H. Kirkaldy-Willis, et al., Pathology and pathogenesis of spondylosis and stenosis, Spine 3 (1978) 319–328.
7. H.F. Farfan, Effects of torsion on the intervertebral disc lesions, Can J Surg 12 (1969) 336.
8. W.H. Kirkaldy-Willis, H.F. Farfan, Instability of the lumbar spine, Clin. Orthop. Relat. Res. 165 (1982) 110–123.

# 5

# History and Physical Examination of the Aging Spine

*Courtney W. Brown and Lonnie E. Loutzenhiser*

> **K E Y   P O I N T S**
>
> - Problems affecting the aging spine are a multifactorial degenerative process affecting both the soft tissues and bony structures.
> - These degenerative processes affect global balance, both sagittal and coronal, and produce neurological findings.
> - Any physical findings must correlate with radiographic studies.
> - Past history of surgery will influence the patient's findings.
> - Some apparent spinal problems may represent other pathology.

## INTRODUCTION

With the increasing longevity in our society, the aging spine has become a ubiquitous problem. Natural physiological aging affects both soft tissue and bony structures, leading to the degenerative process in the spine. Each individual patient's spinal problem has to be correlated and related to that individual's physiological history, which includes genetics; familial, environmental, and/or occupational problems; as well as the multiple comorbidities with which all of us must live. Perhaps it would be best to outline these various areas of influence to better understand how our histories affect our aging spines.

## PAST MEDICAL HISTORY

### Congenital/Familial/Genetic

Abnormal skeletal spine development may occur on a congenital, familial, or genetic basis. This may include various combinations of failure of formation or segmentation of the vertebrae leading to such problems as hemivertebrae, congenital fusions (Klippel-Feil), and congenital scoliosis. These abnormalities may lead to an abnormal stress and wear and tear to relatively normal adjacent levels of the spine, thus having a detrimental effect on these levels through ligamentous and disc degeneration. This may lead to a progressively painful or unstable spine.

Adolescent idiopathic scoliosis, which appears to be genetic in origin, has a totally different influence on the spine as we mature, and can range from a stable balanced spine to a progressive curve with neurological compression and/or global spinal imbalance. Usually, this develops as a slow, progressive vertebral body subluxation secondary to the disc degeneration in the scoliotic levels. This may not occur until later years and at that time, become symptomatic. Aside from spinal pain, as a lumbar curve increases, patients may complain of the rib cage sliding against the pelvis as they become shorter.

### Occupational/Environmental/Psychological

A patient's occupation has a significant impact on the speed and severity of degenerative problems that occur in the adult spine. Certainly, a day laborer who performs loaded twisting of the spine, thus creating annular shearing, is much more likely to have traumatic breakdown of the discs and ligamentous structures than someone with a sedentary occupation. Additionally, smoking decreases the blood supply and nutrition to the vertebral endplates and the intervertebral discs, therefore negatively affecting their healing capabilities. Psychological stress can negatively affect a spine problem and potentiate the pain response to the degeneration. Thus, the patient's pain threshold and psychological instability may produce increased symptoms through the combination of chronic pain, secondary gain, and subsequent depression. If the symptoms persist, symptom magnification may be a dominant factor. Thus, the physical disease of the spine may be overtaken by the patient's psyche. The possibility of alcohol abuse and malnutrition also needs to be considered.

### Comorbidities

Comorbidities, such as diabetes mellitus, cardiovascular disease, or renal disease, can produce neuropathic pain or neurological deficits. These may be extremely difficult to treat, either nonoperatively or operatively. Uncontrolled diabetes mellitus is well known to produce peripheral neuropathy leading to denervation, as well as pain. Cardiovascular disease, such as an aortic aneurysm or peripheral vascular disease, may cause vascular claudication mimicking spinal pathology. Additionally, patients may have a neurological disorder, such as Charcot-Marie-Tooth disease, that may affect the extremities as well as bowel and bladder function. Pulmonary pathology, such as a Pancoast tumor, may mimic the findings in patients with neck symptoms.

## HISTORY

### Origin of Pain

Pain can be described in multiple ways. The first should be the location and quality, as well as the severity of the pain. The pain must be described in terms of sharpness, dullness, burning, numbness, or throbbing. Is the pain intermittent or constant? Is it alternating in severity? The exacerbating or relieving factors should be noted. Is the pain improving or is it progressively getting worse? The pain may become better or worse with positioning. If worse, the etiology may be tumor or infection. Is the pain associated with any neurological symptoms? Any history of previous spinal procedures, as well as the result of those procedures, is crucially important to note and understand, as there may be some component of permanent damage as a result. The rating of pain from 1 to 10 may be misleading as patients who are repetitively questioned to quantify may become overly conditioned and magnify their response.

### Neurological History

History of weakness, falls, gait abnormalities, difficulty with fine motor movement, bowel or bladder dysfunction, and/or sexual dysfunction are all potential signs of myelopathy. This should be obtained in the initial history, which should also include questions about grip strength, dropping items such as coffee cups, or burning the fingers. Upper extremity weakness or pain needs to be noted, along with any associated radicular symptoms into the arms or legs.

## Past Surgical History

Any prior surgical history is important, as it may influence the spine. However, most important is the history of any prior spine procedures, their cause, what the procedure was, and what the results of the intervention were. Residual problems following the surgery become extremely important to document, and having copies of the medical record, including the operative notes, can be extremely important.

## PHYSICAL EXAMINATION

Physical examination should incorporate the patient's stature, habitus, ability to ambulate with or without assistive devices, and quality of gait, as well as the neurological status.

## Global Balance

This should include visible appreciation and palpation of a patient's spine, evaluating it for local or global kyphosis or hyperlordosis, whether it be in the cervical, thoracic, lumbar, or lumbosacral regions. Sagittal balance should be clinically appreciated and measured with a plumb bob. Positive sagittal balance is when the patient's head and neck are forward of his or her sacrum. Negative sagittal balance is when the head and neck are posterior to the sacrum. Coronal imbalance is a left or right deviation of the plumb bob from the C7 spinous process to the gluteal cleft.

## Gait

A patient's gait should be observed when walking outside the examining room. Patients who walk with a wide-based gait may have spinal stenosis. However, if they also walk with a positive sagittal balance (leaning forward), this can also be global imbalance secondary to previous spinal surgery, degenerative spondylolisthesis, spinal stenosis, or a preexisting spinal deformity. When walking, the patient's foot and knee position must be observed. If the legs are externally rotated, patients will commonly be out of global balance, and externally rotating the extremity or flexing the knees will allow them to stand more erect. If this occurs, the important part of evaluation is that of having the patient stand with feet in neutral position, knees straightened to normal position, and then observing their overall global posture. Commonly, these patients will suddenly lean into increased positive sagittal balance. Long x-rays, both AP and lateral, should be obtained with the lower extremities in this corrected position.

## Neurological

Neurological evaluation should include sensory and motor exams, as well as reflexes, of both the upper and lower extremities. Abdominal sensation and reflexes are also extremely important. Sensation, including light touch, pinprick, pressure, and proprioception, must be evaluated throughout the whole body. Individual muscle groups need to be examined for muscle strength, atrophy, or focal or global weakness. Dr. Stanley Hoppenfeld's book on orthopedic neuroanatomy is by far the best for quick visual understanding. His simplifying concept for individual extremity nerve evaluation is that the area of sensation and the underlying muscle and reflex are commonly innervated by the same nerve.

## Specific Cervical Neurological Levels

### C5 Neurological Findings

The motor exam of the C5 nerve root is best examined with the deltoid muscle, which is almost purely innervated by C5 (axillary nerve). The biceps can also be tested but is also innervated by a component of the C6 root.

The sensory distribution of the C5 nerve root is best tested over the deltoid muscle on the lateral aspect of the arm (axillary nerve).

The biceps reflex is the best test to assess C5 function. However, this also has a component of C6 as well.

### C6 Neurological Findings

There is no pure motor exam of the C6 nerve root, as there is cross innervation by the C5 and C7 nerve roots. The best muscles to test for evaluating the C6 nerve root are the biceps (also innervated by C5 via the musculocutaneous nerve) and the wrist extensors (extensor carpi radialis longus (ECRL) and extensor carpi radialis brevis (ECRB) innervated by C6 nerve and the extensor carpi ulnaris (ECU) innervated by C7, all via the radial nerve).

The sensory distribution of the C6 nerve root is best assessed over the lateral forearm, thumb, index finger, and radial half of the long finger (musculocutaneous nerve).

The reflex exam of the C6 nerve root can best be assessed with the brachial radialis reflex (purely C6) or with the biceps reflex (C5 component also).

### C7 Neurological Findings

There are multiple muscle groups used to test the function of the C7 nerve root. The triceps is purely innervated by the C7 root via the radial nerve. There are two major muscles in the wrist flexor group, the FCR and flexor carpi ulnaris (FCU). The flexor carpi radialis (FCR) is innervated by C7 via the median nerve and is the stronger of the two. The FCU is innervated by the C8 nerve via the ulnar nerve. Finger extensors are primarily innervated by the C7 nerve root. However, there is a component of C8 innervation also.

The most common area of C7 sensory innervation is the long finger. However, there can be some component of the C6 and C8 crossover.

The reflex exam of the C7 nerve root can be assessed with the triceps reflex.

### C8 Neurological Findings

C8 motor function is assessed by testing the strength of the finger flexors. There are two finger flexors, the flexor digitorum superficialis (FDS) and the flexor digitorum profundus (FDP). The FDS and the radial half of the FDP are innervated by the median nerve, while the ulnar half of the FDP is innervated by the ulnar nerve.

The best anatomical areas to assess sensory function of the C8 nerve root are the ulnar aspect of the forearm and the ring and small fingers.

There is no C8 reflex exam.

### T1 Neurological Findings

The motor function of the T1 nerve is best tested with the ring abductors (dorsal, interosseous, and abductor digiti quinti). The sensory area of the T1 nerve root is over the ulnar aspect of the proximal forearm and distal arm.

There is no deep tendon reflex to assess the T1 nerve root.

### Thoracic and Abdominal Neurological Findings

Thoracic neurological findings are primarily sensory and will correspond to an intercostal space. This may indicate a thoracic disc herniation. There are no reflexes for these sensory thoracic nerves.

Abdominal musculature contraction, sensation, and reflexes are evaluated by partial sit-ups, watching for a proximal or distal shift of the umbilicus. This shift may indicate intracanal pathology.

### T12 to L3 Neurological Findings

The motor exam of the T12 to L3 nerve roots is best examined with the iliopsoas muscle by testing hip flexion in a seated position.

The sensory distribution of the L1 nerve root is best tested just over and distal to the inguinal ligament anterior on the proximal thigh, the L2 obliquely just distal to L1 on the anterior mid thigh, and the L3 obliquely over the distal anterior thigh and patella.

There is no testable reflex for the T12 to L3 nerve roots.

### L2 to L4 Neurological Findings

The motor exam of the L2 to L4 nerve roots is best examined with the quadriceps muscle group and the hip adductor muscle group. The quadriceps muscle group, which is innervated by L2 to L4 nerve roots (femoral nerve), is tested with resisted knee extension in a sitting position, while the hip adductor group, also innervated by the L2 to L4 nerve groups, is tested with resisted hip adduction from an abducted position, either sitting or supine. The sensory distribution of the L2 and L3 nerve roots has been described above, and the sensory distribution and reflex exam of L4 will be described below.

## L4 Neurological Findings

The motor exam of the L4 nerve root is best examined with the tibialis anterior muscle, which is most purely innervated by L4 (deep peroneal nerve) and by resisted ankle dorsiflexion and inversion.

The sensory distribution of the L4 nerve root is best tested over the anteromedial lower leg.

The patellar reflex is the best test to assess L4 function. However, it has a component of L2 and L3 as well.

## L5 Neurological Findings

The motor exam of the L5 nerve root can be assessed with multiple muscle groups, including the extensor hallucis longus (EHL), the extensor digitorum longus (EDL), and the extensor digitorum brevis (EDB) – all innervated by the deep peroneal nerve – and the gluteus medius (superior gluteal nerve). The EHL is tested by resisted dorsiflexion of the great toe, while the EDL and the EDB are tested by resisted dorsiflexion of the remaining toes. The gluteus medius is tested by resisted abduction of the hip while lying in a lateral position.

The sensory distribution of the L5 nerve root is best tested over the lateral leg and the dorsal foot, most specifically the first dorsal web space on the foot.

The posterior tibialis reflex is the only way to test L5 reflex function. However, it is hard to elicit.

## S1 Neurological Findings

The motor exam of the S1 nerve root can be examined by the peroneus longus and brevis muscles (superficial peroneal nerve), the gastrocnemius muscle complex (tibial nerve), and the gluteus maximus (inferior gluteal nerve). The peronei are tested by resisted foot eversion in plantar flexion. The gastrocsoleus complex is tested with ankle plantar flexion. However, it is so strong that manual muscle testing is hard to perform. The best way to assess ankle plantar flexion is by asking the patient to toe walk and assess the toe walk, watching for weakness. The gluteus maximus is best tested with resisted hip extension in the prone position.

Sensory distribution of the S1 nerve root is best tested over the lateral and plantar aspect of the foot.

The Achilles reflex is the best test to assess S1 nerve root function.

## S2-4 Neurological Findings

The motor exam of the S2-4 nerve roots is difficult as the motor supply of the S2-4 nerve roots supply the bladder and the intrinsic muscles of the foot. Therefore, any toe deformities should be appreciated.

The sensory distribution of the S2-4 nerve roots supplies the anal sphincter.

## Vascular

The patient history and physical evaluation are extremely important in determining whether or not the patient may have vascular claudication or neurogenic claudication. Aortic aneurysm can simulate low back pain and is best appreciated by abdominal palpation with the hips and knees flexed, relaxing the abdominal muscles. Peripheral vascular disease can mimic neurological claudication. However, this should be eliminated by palpation of peripheral pulses and checking for hair distribution or stasis dermatitis.

## Summary

The following will be usual physical findings in multiple spinal diagnoses but must be correlated to their imaging studies:

1.  Spinal stenosis, central or foraminal

    A.  Loss of global balance
    B.  Neurogenic claudication (exam may be normal or have focal deficits)
    C.  Progressive wide-based gait

2.  Herniated nucleus pulposus

    A.  Cervical: radicular and/or myelopathic symptoms
    B.  Thoracic: radicular and/or myelopathic symptoms
    C.  Lumbar: radicular and/or motor and/or cauda equina symptoms

3.  Degenerative disc disease/degenerative spondylolisthesis

    A.  Cervical: radicular/local pain
    B.  Thoracic: radicular/local pain

4.  Spondylolisthesis

    A.  Stance
    B.  Hamstrings
    C.  Increased lumbar lordosis
    D.  Neurological symptoms can be static or dynamic.

5.  Adolescent idiopathic scoliosis/de novo scoliosis

    A.  Global imbalance, both sagittal and coronal
    B.  Rotational imbalance
    C.  Rib hump and lumbar prominence.
    D.  Leg length discrepancy/pelvic tilt/sacral obliquity

6.  Osteoporotic vertebral body fractures

    A.  Local tenderness
    B.  Percussive local pain
    C.  Kyphosis/sagittal imbalance
    D.  Neurological deficit: radicular or myelopathic

# The Role of Nutrition, Weight, and Exercise on the Aging Spine

*Kiran F. Rajneesh and G. Ty Thaiyananthan*

**KEY POINTS**

- Nonpharmacological treatment of back pain is an integral part of management in older patients.
- Nutritional balance of macronutrients and micronutrients is essential in the aging spine.
- Optimal exercise activities in older patients confer multiple benefits to the aging spine.
- Obesity in the elderly can accelerate the degeneration of the spine.
- Balanced nutrition, adequate exercise, and weight control in the elderly population can be achieved by better health education and represents primary prevention of back pain.

## INTRODUCTION

The aging spine is subject to multiple onslaughts of metabolic slowdown, mechanical wear and tear, and immunological compromise. The process of aging is irreversible, but its detrimental fallout can partly be compensated by conditioning. Nutrition, weight control, and exercise are factors that can counter excessive decompensation of the aging spine.

## NUTRITION

Elderly populations are predisposed to malnutrition due to a variety of causes. The physiological changes associated with aging are altered glucose regulation and impaired hormonal homeostasis. There is decreased absorption of macronutrients (carbohydrates, proteins, and fatty acids) as well as micronutrients.[1] The decreased absorption of micronutrients in the elderly population is significant for cobalamin, calcium, vitamin D, riboflavin, and niacin.

Calcium absorption declines in both sexes in the elderly, and is directly related to vitamin D metabolism. Cobalamin (vitamin $B_{12}$) absorption decreases in the elderly and predisposes them to subacute combined degeneration of the spinal cord.[2] Other vitamin B complexes may also have malabsorption, leading to neuropathies. The elderly have consistently lower levels of vitamin D. In a European study, vitamin D levels are lowest in winter in the elderly.[3] This tendency of decreased sun exposure and decreased capacity of the aging kidney to convert vitamin D to active form may reduce endogenous levels of vitamin D. Western diets only supply 25% to 50% of the vitamin D daily requirement; hence, supplementation in the elderly is crucial.

Other coexisting conditions in the elderly can also cause imbalances in nutrition. Extensive use of antibiotics can cause cobalamin deficiency. Other disorders such as Alzheimer disease may cause the patient to forget about having a meal. Parkinson disease and other movement disorders may prevent patients from feeding themselves adequately. Diabetes, hypertension, and other chronic conditions may directly, or indirectly, through the drugs used for treatment, cause anorexia in the elderly.

Anorexia and decreased food intake is prevalent in the elderly population.[4] Other than the previously noted causes of anorexia, elderly patients also suffer from psychological anorexia. It may originate from various life events such as loneliness, death of a spouse, lack of social life, estrangement from family, and loss of independence. It is important to recognize these major life events and provide the elderly population with counseling and support. Anorexia may also originate from the natural process of aging and changes within the central nervous centers for feeding and hydration. Although this change is inevitable and irreversible, it should not necessarily lead to undernourishment but merely readjust the food intake to the new levels. However, due to the complex interactions of aging, coexisting conditions, and life events occurring around aging, it may lead to malnutrition if not monitored.

The often neglected facet of malnutrition in the elderly population is the socioeconomic conditions that may hinder intake of well-balanced foods. Physicians and healthcare workers fail to take into account that most elderly people are not in control of their food intake. They may live at chronic care homes and group homes; thus they may only have access to standardized diets and have difficulty changing their diet to meet their specific health needs. Also, the elderly may not have a source of income to afford the diet or the dietary supplements we may recommend.

The elderly population is thus nutritionally vulnerable to deficiencies due to a combination of biological, social, and psychological causes. The nutritional deficiencies can affect various parts of the aging spine. Calcium and vitamin D imbalance affecting the vertebral column, vitamin B complexes such as B6 affecting the peripheral nerve conduction, decreased proteins causing paraspinal muscle atrophy, and vitamin B complex deficiency causing dorsal column symptoms illustrate a few examples. Thus it is important to anticipate these problems and actively monitor nutritional status in the elderly and supplement with easily available and affordable alternatives.

## OBESITY

Obesity in the elderly population is a growing problem. Obesity is defined as a body mass index (BMI) greater than 30 kg/m². A BMI between 25 to 29 kg/m² is classified as overweight. The prevalence of obesity in the general population in the United States for the year 2007 is between 25% and 29% in most states, as published by the Centers for Disease Control (CDC) in their annual report. A multicenter study in Europe called Survey in Europe on Nutrition and the Elderly: a Concerted Action (SENECA) published a report noting that 20% of the elderly population was obese.[1]

Traditionally, obesity is measured as an index of height and body weight. During aging, the elderly undergo height reduction due to muscle atrophy and bone resorption. On an average, an elderly patient undergoes a 1.5 to 2 cm height reduction over a span of 10 years. Thus, BMI may not be an accurate index of obesity in the elderly. Intra-abdominal fat content assessed by abdominal girth measurement may be a better index. However, there is no established standard protocol for it yet.

In the elderly population, the spinal column and its mechanical components over the years undergo wear and tear, metabolic slowdown, and impaired repair. These predispose the aging spine to disc degeneration, osteoporosis, and muscle atrophy. Obesity and overweight further assault the aging spine. The vertebral column is a weight-bearing column transmitting the weight of the head and the torso to the pelvis, and subsequently to the lower limbs.

Obesity increases the stress on the aging vertebral column by increasing the load-bearing capacity. This excessive load-bearing of the vertebral column predisposes the spinal cord to disc degeneration, facet joint syndrome, and hyperostosis.[5] Obesity also predisposes the elderly to nerve entrapment syndromes in the spine and in the limbs such as carpal tunnel syndrome.[6] Radicular back pain has a higher incidence in the elderly with obesity compared to healthy elderly people.[7] Also, back pain is more severe in obese patients compared to healthy elderly patients. The SF-36 (Short Form) physical component summary score and disease-specific measure and the Oswestry Disability Index are 1.5 times worse in obese elderly patients with spinal diseases as compared to controls.[7] Obesity also decreases the functional status of elderly patients and predisposes them to multisystem pathologies.

The 10-year trend of obesity published by the CDC conveys a message of a growing epidemic, with a 10% increase in prevalence across the country. It is important to not only recognize obesity but also to identify overweight elderly patients and provide health education to prevent their progression to obesity.

## EXERCISE

The aging process affects the spine extensively. The spinal cord may develop segmental degeneration or may undergo global degeneration. The disease processes affecting the aging spine may have variable rates of progression and intensity of affliction. Exercise or physical conditioning may help alleviate some of these conditions and may prevent onset of many more conditions.

Exercise or physical preconditioning is a process wherein the body is trained to attain optimal efficiency with maximal benefits and minimal discomfort. Physiologically, exercise fine tunes the underlying metabolic processes and cellular machinery by acting through specific stimuli.

During the process of aging, the spine undergoes wear and tear of its mechanical components and osteoporosis. (Refer "Histological Changes of Aging Spine." Chapter 3) Briefly, osteoporosis is a condition, prevalent in elderly patients, in which bone mass decreases in vertebrae. This decreased bone mass predisposes the elderly to pathological fractures on minor physical trauma. Osteoporosis is amenable to exercise.

Exercise prevents osteoporosis in the vertebral column and increases bone mass. The principle of exercise in osteoporosis is based on Wolff's law.[8] Wolff's law states that bone density and strength are a function of the direction and magnitude of mechanical stresses acting on that bone.[9] Weight-bearing exercises are performed in osteoporosis patients.[10] These include exercise like step training, where the patient spends 10 minutes of stepping up and down from a platform of about 6 to 8 inches in height. It is important to advise elderly patients to take adequate rest to prevent hypoxia. Also, elderly patients should be recommended to use good shock-bearing shoes and perform the exercise in a safe environment. The weight-bearing exercise facilitates osteoblastic activity and promotes increased bone mass.

Corrective exercises play a vital role in the aging spine. Corrective exercises attempt to restore normal architecture to the aging spine. In the kyphotic spines of estrogen-depleted elderly women, it may be useful to retrain the extensor muscles of the back.

For back pain, traction exercises may help relieve the pain and strengthen muscle tone. The exercises include pelvic tilts, knee to chest, lower back rotation, and hamstring stretch exercises. Low back pain may be alleviated by lumbar stabilization exercises aimed at stabilizing the spine and strengthening the muscles.

Aerobic exercises and swimming may contribute to healthy living by conditioning other organ systems but have no effect on the aging spine.[11]

## SUMMARY

Aging is an irreversible physiological process with many challenges. However, the spinal disorders associated with aging can be prevented by careful monitoring and maintenance of nutrition, weight management, and exercise regimen. These factors are amenable to modifications by patients and may alter or stop disease progression and improve the quality of life.

## References

1. W.A. van Staveren, L.C. de Groot, J. Burema, et al., Energy balance and health in SENECA participants. Survey in Europe on Nutrition and the Elderly, a Concerted Action, Proc. Nutr. Soc. 54 (1995) 617–629.
2. G.M. Hunter, R.E. Irvine, M.K. Bagnall, Medical and social problems of two elderly women, BMJ. 4 (1972) 224–225.
3. R.P. van der Wielen, M.R. Lowik, H. van den Berg, et al., Serum vitamin D concentrations among elderly people in Europe, Lancet 346 (1995) 207–210.
4. I.M. Chapman, C.G. MacIntosh, J.E. Morley, et al., The anorexia of ageing, Biogerontology 3 (2002) 67–71.
5. H. Julkunen, O.P. Heinonen, K. Pyorala, Hyperostosis of the spine in an adult population: its relation to hyperglycaemia and obesity, Ann. Rheum. Dis. 30 (1971) 605–612.
6. N. Lam, A. Thurston, Association of obesity, gender, age and occupation with carpal tunnel syndrome, Aust. N. Z. J. Surg. 68 (1998) 190–193.
7. J.C. Fanuele, W.A. Abdu, B. Hanscom, et al., Association between obesity and functional status in patients with spine disease, Spine 27 (2002) 306–312.
8. E.H. Burger, J. Klein-Nulen, Responses of bone cells to biomechanical forces in vitro, Adv. Dent. Res. 13 (1999) 93–98.
9. H.M. Frost, From Wolff's law to the Utah paradigm: insights about bone physiology and its clinical applications, Anat. Rec. 262 (2001) 398–419.
10. K. Elward, E.B. Larson, Benefits of exercise for older adults. A review of existing evidence and current recommendations for the general population, Clin. Geriatr. Med. 8 (1992) 35–50.
11. G.C. Gauchard, P. Gangloff, C. Jeandel, et al., Physical activity improves gaze and posture control in the elderly, Neurosci. Res. 45 (2003) 409–417.

# 7

# The Psychology of the Aging Spine, Treatment Options, and Ayurveda as a Novel Approach

*Frank John Ninivaggi*

**KEY POINTS**

- Aging denotes progressive chronological thresholds characterized by significant change.
- Physical changes like pain and fatigue herald limitations that require viable adaptations.
- Western "technomedicine" offers a range of proven medical and surgical interventions.
- Complementary and alternative medicine may offer additional therapeutic approaches.
- Ayurveda, Traditional Indian medicine, is a novel option recently available in the West.

## INTRODUCTION AND OVERVIEW

This chapter is a clinically-oriented discussion of the emotionally colored meanings that aging and declining physical status exert as life stressors in advancing years. Traditional Western and alternative Eastern medical perspectives, notably Ayurveda, are reviewed.

Older age brings numerous successes, healthy achievements, and pragmatic perspectives that enrich a meaningful life. Medical problems, however, challenge this. The aging spine, for example, typically becomes less agile; flexibility and the range of movements previously achieved with ease diminish. Pain and fatigue ensue. Activities of daily living become arduous. People notice these physical limitations in subtle and often disconcerting ways. The subliminal impact of age and physical changes is often insidious, and eventually adds to the burden that real physical limitations impose. As aging progresses and the recognition of progressive restrictions increases, quality-of-life challenges require action.

Aging is an inescapable process of metabolic and functional alterations, all of which have their sequelae. Resilience is more fragile; people take fewer risks and intentionally minimize change. Although everyone can expect the inevitable cast of aging, there is much variability in its effects. Genetic, environmental, traumatic, and lifestyle factors contribute to how health and disease interact. The way a person chooses to live can often influence genetic predispositions and ordinary wear and tear. Achieving and maintaining optimal health includes freedom from pain and its perception as suffering. Impairments in biopsychosocial functioning, especially related to musculoskeletal events, however, become a common challenge. A working knowledge of aging has pragmatic value. Screening for emerging disabilities affords the physician a valuable clinical perspective. When indicated, patients can be referred to specialists who conduct formal assessments of physical and mental function.

Wellness and healthy functioning are noticeably disturbed when decompensations in formerly healthy equilibriums occur. At this point, a physician may make a formal diagnosis. Disease and diagnosis, as such, do not denote "disability." These say little about their functional impact. Signs and symptoms do reflect that some "impairment" has occurred.[1] Measuring diminished functioning adds to quantifying decompensations from previous baselines. A brief discussion of these concepts follows.

For these reasons, good clinical care requires that perceived impairments be carefully assessed using standardized protocols performed by specialists. Imaging studies are also invaluable. Evaluations must be correlated with the performance of a specific task or the overall performance of a complex range of defined tasks, particularly when a demand for action is required. "Tasks" are complex physical or mental actions having an intended result, for example, reading a book or riding a bicycle. Complex tasks, for example, are those encountered in occupational performance or "work." These require the participation and coordination of multiple mental and physical systems. Other examples include time spent working at a computer, ability to lift items of a specific weight, walking, taking a shower, or driving a car. "Limitations" in these functions are ordinarily a reflection of an inability to intentionally accomplish these acts. These "impairments" denote derangements in the structure or function of organs or body parts and, to some extent, can be objectively measured. If, however, less defined syndromic symptoms are in excess of hard data measurements, estimated functional capacity can be ascertained by using clinical findings that have multidimensional consistency relative to typical reference populations. When a physician recommends that one or more behavioral tasks be curtailed because of "direct threat," namely, risk of injury or harm to self or others, a provider "restriction" has been imposed.

After a range of therapeutic interventions and rehabilitative efforts has occurred, a functional capacity test of physical abilities measures the patient's enduring impairments in ability to perform a defined task or tasks. Limitations in ability are called the "residual functional incapacity"; conversely, defined tasks that a patient is able to perform constitute the "residual functional capacity." Capacity here denotes real-time ability to perform a task successfully. This is an individual's current ability to work based on his or her capacity not only to tolerate symptoms but also to anticipate rewards and success.

The concept of "disability" is complex. It denotes an inability to perform or substantial limitations in major life activity spheres: personal, social, and occupational. Disabilities are due to limitations, especially impairments caused by medical and psychiatric conditions (including subjective pain reports) at the level of the whole person, not merely isolated parts or functions. From a functional perspective, "occupational disability" denotes current capacity insufficient to perform one or more material and substantial occupational duties currently demanded and accomplished previously. Last, the term "handicap" denotes an inability measured largely by the socially observable limitations it imposes. Handicap connotes the perception or assumption by an outside observer that the subject or patient suffers from a functional limitation or restriction. The term "handicap" implies that freedom to function in a social context has been lost. In this sense, people with handicaps can benefit from added supports. "Accommodations" that modify or reduce functional demands or barriers are given to them. Opportunities in social contexts, therefore, afford expanded freedom for more activities.

In this way, participation restrictions diminish. Intolerance to pain and fatigue are the most frequent reasons patients stop working and claim disability.

Striving for and maintaining a good quality of life or better is a fundamental value for everyone. This encompasses not only developing new strengths both mentally and physically, but also preserving current assets. Efforts in this direction prevent functional limitations and ameliorate disabilities. These include, for example, maintaining upright and stable posture, agile ambulation, and freedom from the limitations and burdens that pain imposes. Routine medical care and available specialized care afford opportunities to benefit from the advances that rational scientific medicine has to offer. The progressive globalization of diverse cultures, moreover, has introduced Eastern systems of wellness and healthcare not previously recognized or even available in the West. One of the inestimable benefits of this expanding diversification is the widening scope of health-enhancing treatment options. The cultural diversity and traditions of both physicians and patients make it wise for the contemporary healthcare provider to be cognizant of medical systems other than those typically regarded as conventional in Western terms. The prudent physician must always distinguish what is merely wishful thinking from what is yet unproven but within the context of realistic discovery and future confirmation.

Among these, Ayurveda – Traditional Indian Medicine – will be introduced both theoretically and as a range of interventions dealing with the management of aging and orthopedic problems. Ayurveda is a novel treatment option or adjunct among more traditional Western modalities. Given such choices, each person has opportunities to choose proactively, while realistically assessing his or her own specific needs and preferences in selecting healthcare. Different approaches may complement one another or be used integratively. In an available framework of rational and diverse treatment options, choices grounded in scientific evidence and trusted traditions may serve as a basis for good, well-rounded clinical care.[2,3]

## UNDERSTANDING THE PATIENT'S PERSPECTIVE

Adequately understanding how patients perceive their distress, and the problems involved in seeking help and choosing helpers, is fundamental to good care. The extent to which a provider appreciates and utilizes this understanding substantially contributes to patient compliance and better outcomes.

When a patient finally recognizes that signs and symptoms, especially pain, fatigue, and diminished functioning, are not transitory and may be progressively worsening, mixtures of distress, ambivalence, curiosity, and denial interact. Anxiety further blurs clear thinking and discrimination. For older patients, conscious fears about more permanent loss of functioning and subtle fears about reduced life span, even death, are present. Anxiety, fear, and inhibitions go hand-in-hand.

Older patients are acutely aware of changes in physical and psychological functioning. Identifying and adequately adapting to these degenerative changes is difficult, since even acclimating to the inevitable, ordinary changes met with in daily life can be trying. Patients often dread the efforts required to undergo a variety of tests, some of which are arduous and time-consuming, and others that are, in fact, painful (for example, discogram). A patient's insurance may not adequately cover some diagnostic procedures, or even some recommended surgery. This can present not only a financial burden but also an important psychological stressor to older patients whose incomes and earning capacities are limited.

Often, patients talk with family members and friends before deciding to consult a physician. Although many patients are now more knowledgeable about medical illnesses and treatments than in the past, especially because of media exposure and availability of internet data, the personal nature of the problem and its attendant emotional conflicts continue to exert significant cognitive dissonance and avoidance. It is not uncommon for patients to become clinically depressed secondary to the stress and diminished functioning resulting from orthopedic problems. Developing a stooped posture or various degrees of kyphosis, for example, affects one's physical appearance and adds to lowered self-esteem and withdrawal. Many become progressively isolated and remain homebound. In previous generations, the phrase "shut-in" described such confinement.

These considerations highlight the importance of the initial diagnostic process for the physician. Surgeons need to consider possible referral for further psychiatric assessment and treatment of anxiety and depression. The art and science of medicine, interviewing, and the physician-patient relationship intersect here. In contrast to problems in older patients, an often overlooked issue is the presentation of pain with or without orthopedic injury in the young adult. Behaviors with a high risk for orthopedic injury, such as motorcycle and race car driving, are more common in this population. Previous histories of substance abuse, even current malingering, must be high on one's clinical index of suspicion to help avoid wrong and puzzling diagnoses, and treatments that appear to fail or seem resistant.

Explicit and subtle factors contribute to a good interview. Attentiveness, composure, active listening, and sensitive responsiveness are fundamental. A recognition of the inevitable anxiety and cognitive strain under which a patient in distress labors should remind the physician to go slowly in questioning, speak clearly, and reiterate important diagnostic questions. Most patients, because of anxiety, have a difficult time hearing and understanding discussions with the doctor. Older patients, in addition, may be less receptive because of the aging process itself. People in pain show irritability and impatience. The physician's attentiveness to these and other features of the patient's presentation will facilitate a meaningful yield in accurately assessing signs, symptoms, and history. Listening attentively to what is said and what seems left out is important. Carefully assessing the extent of a patient's expectations for recovery from pain and limited functioning is important. Written materials outlined by the surgeon before, during, and after a surgical procedure are often useful. When tailored to the specific patient and his or her particular condition, they are seen as believable and help consolidate diagnostic and treatment information, and minimize misunderstanding and error. All aspects of patient-physician contact should facilitate the entire diagnostic and treatment process. Telephone inquiries, waiting rooms, and administrative and nursing personnel can set the stage for a productive interview and more accurate data collection. Tightly managed pre-op assessments also ensure better post-op compliance with rehabilitative recommendations such as adherence to physical therapy.

Last, orthopedic surgery teams tend to have multiple participants. With so many caregivers in the field, the wise chief surgeon intentionally takes the lead and orchestrates, within reason, the specific and overall flow of care, always keeping the needs of the individual patient in mind. Ideally, a designated contact person will be assigned to the patient throughout the process. Patients are aware of this. Compliance and better outcomes result.

## WESTERN PERSPECTIVES ON THE PSYCHOLOGY OF AGING

Aging denotes the effects of the passage of time on the body as well as its interpretation, as felt in emotional terms. Physical changes and attendant pathology are typically tangible and measureable. Emotional changes are much more subtle. These progressive changes are reflections of the continuing process of crossing "chronological thresholds." Each person's life is an autobiography of both change and continuity. A "considered" life has been looked at in a purposeful way. In the process, real opportunities open. One can choose to take an active role rather than merely being passive. Ongoing self-examination, self-exploration, and action are basic tools. Transformations of perspective, if purposely thought out, become essential for successfully traversing the inevitable changes that occur across the lifespan. Creative and lively attitudes bring rewarding results.

Why would a person want to be proactive? This chapter will make it clear that aiming for optimal health and biopsychosocial balance is essential to a sound lifestyle. The motivations for this are grounded in both biology and psychology. Biological survival means adapting to the constantly changing environment in as healthy a way possible. Psychological survival means creating conditions that strive for positive quality of life and result in meaningful satisfaction. Survival presumes intelligence, flexibility, and recognition of novel opportunities for success. This shores up functional viability on all levels, physical and psychological.

A new conceptual paradigm called the *biopsychospiritual* model[4] has recently been advanced. This enriched perspective recognizes the integral nature of body, mind, and spirit and includes such considerations as sacredness of life, refinement of consciousness, and the deepening fruitfulness that a proactive life may take over the lifespan. Profound respect for life and a renewed humane outlook underlie this approach. These considerations have pragmatic value. They can result in a sense of self-empowered creativeness that engenders the rational therapeutic optimism so essential to functional generativity across life's chronological thresholds and challenges.

The passage of time changes both body and mind, often in incompatible ways that can be confusing. The enrichments that adaptive intelligence brings over the years also enable people to more sharply sense their developing medical problems. Biological aging denotes the effects of internal physicochemical changes. Menopause and andropause are well known conditions. "Osteopause"—a decline in robust bone integrity—is also real. These include both decelerations in functioning and the impact of external aggressions such as trauma, disease, sun, wind, ionizing radiation, and extremes of temperature, to name just a few. Psychological aging is affected by perceptions of self and others: a sense of self and self-image, and earlier experiences with others. Viewing and identifying with how parents and grandparents age undeniably shapes one's self-image. How significant others physically change over time never goes unnoticed. Although our "biological clock" is out of our personal control, our "psychological clock" is, in fact, the timing we create for ourselves. Forced retirement, for example, solely owing to pain and health challenges, some of which may be treatable, repairable, or reversible, is a prime instance of biology colliding with psychology.

After young adulthood, at about age 30, a perceptible decline occurs in the physical self, the body. In middle adulthood, the 40s, one becomes more realistically able to assess both one's positive assets and those considered less desirable. After 50, noticeable declines in mental flexibility make it more of a challenge to implement change based on one's recognition of real and subtle limitations. At this time, the ill health of others seems to stand out. The death of a loved one or spouse is not uncommon. After 60, stark awareness of aging and some degree of chronic pain confront most people. This results in less energy, mobility, and stamina. One's memory tends to decline as well. Stressors become more frequent; adaptation to stressful life events is less resilient in advancing years. Dysphoria and clinical depression, at times, may add to the burden of aging. The National Center for Health Statistics in the United States shows that the suicide rate rises after age 65, especially for the Caucasian male population.

Anxiety accompanies tangible limitations of functioning in the course of aging. Anxiety, often felt as a low-grade sense of malaise, also tends to intensify with age. Irrational fears may develop. Pain and progressive functional limitations exacerbate feelings of harsh loneliness. Many older adults wish to remain in the workforce, and dread the occupational limitations that health challenges impose. Experts in work-related disability research have shown that the beneficial effects of work do outweigh the risks related to work. The far-reaching rewards associated with work are substantially greater than the harmful effects of a long-term lack of meaningful work. Aside from the financial advantages, work enhances self-esteem, structure, and social affiliation.

As aging and the concomitant suffering associated with pain increase, the problem of isolation becomes pronounced. Isolation is not only purely social. More important, the negative effects of isolation derive from subjectively interpreted feelings of withdrawal, disinterest, and anhedonia. These typically provoke subtle feelings of unconscious envy and conscious feelings of jealousy in complicated ways that further exacerbate mental equanimity. Such complex emotions elicit excessive anxiety, which tends to destabilize the mind. Less than optimal thinking processes, poorer decision-making skills, and a hypervigilant state marked by dysphoria result.

Various degrees of emotional contentment, to be sure, also accompany the aging process. The core of the biopsychosocial self has its base in the physical body. The conscious and unconscious sense of this awareness is termed "body image." Identity, confidence, and mental equanimity are stabilized to the extent that body image is ego-syntonic or pleasurably felt. Self-esteem strengthens. As the body and its functioning naturally decline, however, body image suffers. People then experience various degrees of emotional malaise, discomfort, and unhappiness.

The patient's physical appearance and perception of being fit, attractive, beautiful, or handsome are intimately involved in the aging process. The attendant decline in functioning makes this more poignantly felt. The aesthetic sense of beauty is based on innate biological and evolutionary programs along with individually-acquired learning. The roots of the perception

of attractiveness rest on the perception of symmetry, proportion, and novel complexity. Attractiveness results more from biological characteristics whereas beauty and self-confidence add emotional depth, the psychological dimension. As aging and illness occur, the physical body becomes less symmetrical. Female and male attractiveness appear to diminish. More rigidly fixed postures and their emotionally-laden facial expressions become etched in. Looking in the mirror is a distressing reminder. When others respond to the patient with disdain after noticing a less than attractive appearance, this distress is reinforced. These changes, moreover, signal that something should be done. The patient wonders what can be done to help or correct undesirable changes. Questions about how to repair the burgeoning deterioration that is perceived to be the source of distress come to the fore. The more that physical deterioration can be ameliorated, the more an individual's sense of being fit is strengthened.

Typically, the decade of the sixties introduces the inevitability of bodily aches and pains, less than optimal posture, and, perhaps, some degree of structural deformity. This stark confrontation with the reality of the physical side of the self spares few. The perception and interpretation of this painful recognition stimulate upset, ambivalence, and emotional discomfort. An individual's emotional response to pain is felt as suffering. The patient's description of pain is often inarticulate and requires the sensitive, explorative questioning of the physician. This again attests to the importance of diagnostic interviewing and establishing a positive therapeutic relationship.

Although natural decline over the course of chronological thresholds is inevitable, it is possible to manage these in ways that optimize overall health. This can restore a more harmonious physical appearance, a goal most patients eagerly desire. The upshot of this is a more confident mental attitude.

## WESTERN PERSPECTIVES ON MANAGING THE AGING PROCESS

People perceive and handle stressful life events situationally; moreover, stressors and their management change over time. The cumulative effects of stress and life's complexities add to existing anxieties and may exacerbate chronic physical ailments.

As aging progresses, emerging medical problems and the process of effectively dealing with them take on increased importance. In addition to the burdens that the possible development of heart disease, hypertension, and diabetes may have for patients, the aging spine can suffer a variety of structural and functional changes. With age, disks in the spine dehydrate and lose their function as shock absorbers. Adjoining bones and ligaments thicken and become less pliable. Disks may then pinch and put pressure on nearby nerve roots and spinal cord, causing pain and diminished functioning.

Age-related modeling of bone is associated with ligamentous laxity, facet hypertrophy, and an unstable spine. The clinical presentation of back pain, deformities, and shortened stature typically results from disk degeneration, vertebral wedging, and vertebral collapse. Back pain can have cervical, thoracic, or lumbar etiologies. Musculoskeletal problems include lumbar back sprains and strains, osteoarthritic degenerative disk disease, rheumatoid arthritis, spondylosis, ankylosing spondylitis, lumbar spinal stenosis, spondylolisthesis, and herniated disks. Osteoporosis can cause spinal compression fractures, kyphosis, and pain. Besides genetic factors, trauma, and aging, the combination of poor diet, less-than-optimal exercise, and smoking contributes to bone problems.

Western medicine offers a range of conservative medical and surgical interventions. Conservative therapies include dietary modification, exercise, and medications such as nonsteroidal antiinflammatories, analgesics (acetaminophen, aspirin), opioids to block pain impulses to the brain and modulate the perception of pain, muscle relaxants, tricyclic antidepressants, antiseizure medications, cortisone injections, and nerve blocks. In addition, physical therapy, chiropractic, and orthotics such as spinal bracing are employed. When these are not adequate to restore functioning, surgical interventions provide more options. Orthopedic implants are arguably a major innovation that can return patients to the workforce and ultimately cut healthcare costs on all levels.

Psychiatry offers help in its treatments to reduce anxiety, depression, and help modulate the impact of stress. Managing the mind through various types of psychotherapies helps enhance generativity. This, in turn, fosters health enthusiasm, productivity, a meaningful life, supportive relationships, and minimizes stagnation. Psychopharmacological interventions complement psychotherapies.

## EASTERN PERSPECTIVES ON MEDICINE AND PSYCHOLOGY

Western European and North American evidenced-based conventional medicine is called allopathic medicine. This "technomedicine" rests on tangible data. Standardized protocols objectively test its hypotheses and offer pragmatic clinical approaches. Building on its several thousand-year-old Greek and Latin foundations, it has become increasingly scientific over the last centuries. Its methodology and findings are objectively verifiable using statistically valid and reliable parameters. In contrast, Eastern medical systems originating in ancient India and China reputedly have their roots in traditions that span thousands of years, well into the pre-Christian era. Eastern medical systems are clinical, at times philosophical, and exceedingly subtle. They espouse axiomatic ontological hypotheses, some of which appear as untestable assertions. Their epistemological methodologies, however, are strong, although entirely empirical. This non-Western orientation is best viewed by Westerners in its own native métier for it to be grasped, understood, and not distorted by the truncating effects of partisan bias.

Traditional Chinese Medicine (TCM) and Indian medicine (Ayurveda) are the two most established medical systems in Eastern medical traditions. TCM and Acupuncture have been increasingly available in the West for the last 25 years. Ayurveda has only recently emerged in Western countries. This chapter introduces Ayurveda as a primary complementary and alternative treatment option.

Ayurveda is Traditional Indian Medicine (TIM). Its adherents regard it as originating roughly 6,000 years ago. Through the travels of its Hindu and Buddhist followers, it spread to Tibet, China, Japan, Korea, and other Far East regions between 1,500 and 2,000 years ago. Today, the clinical practice of Ayurveda retains many perspectives and methods rooted in its origins. In the last 25 years, it has been introduced in Europe and only recently in the United States. In terms of the translation of its age-old concepts into Western ideas and testable hypotheses, Ayurveda in America remains in its infancy. Modern scientific methodologies are only now being used to examine the safety and effectiveness of treatments that have been empirically used for thousands of years. Western training programs, especially those affiliated with large universities and medical schools, have only just begun offering standardized curricula. Contemporary Ayurveda is a medical system *in statu nascendi*, in the process of being born.

In modern-day India, tribal peoples called *adivasis* living in central and southern geographical areas (for example, Kerala) are believed by archaeologists to be descendants of Bhimbetkans, Indian aboriginals whose origins date back to the Mesolithic period, roughly circa 30,000 BC to 7,000 BC. These indigenous people, who make up about 8 % of the total population, are not generally integrated in mainstream Indian society. They practice what they call "tribal medicine," using single herb remedies, many of which are still referred to by idiosyncratic names. Current studies, however, demonstrate that these herbs correlate directly with the range of herbs used in standard Ayurvedic practice for the last several thousand years until now.

Ayurveda is preeminently a health and wellness system. Nevertheless, a wide variety of integrated propositions from biological, psychological, philosophical, and spiritual sources frame it as a foremost system of medical treatment. In many ways, it is a philosophy of medicine pragmatically applied. The roots of Ayurveda remain deeply planted in its cultural origins and may appear unfathomable, even fanciful, to Western thinkers. In terms of understandability, much less acceptance, it is hoped that Ayurveda's epistemological style with its ontological orientation (for example, the concept of the Five Great Gross Elements) will present an inviting challenge rather than evoke an automatic dismissal merely because of the apparent "foreignness" of such unfamiliar conceptualizations.

Medical science in Ayurveda begins with the individual. Each person is an integral whole composed of three principal dimensions: physical body, mental functioning, and a spiritual/consciousness base. This perspective is, in essence, a monistic one that eschews dualisms of all sorts. To understand the naturally integrated operation of these component dimensions, however, careful distinctions are made for heuristic purposes. Assessments

and treatments, therefore, are based on recognizing complex dynamic interactions among biological, psychological, social, environmental, and spiritual/consciousness factors. Mutative subtle energies believed to be essential forces on all these levels drive their organization into patterns experienced in the form of wellness and disease presentations discernable in terms specific to Ayurvedic theory.

## AYURVEDA: TRADITIONAL INDIAN MEDICINE

Introducing Ayurveda, with its almost 6,000 years of prehistory, history, and development, in a few paragraphs is a formidable task. In order not to misrepresent or oversimplify this complex edifice of ideas, the following schematic outline is presented. Only the outer edges of Ayurveda's *Weltanschauung* (German), *darshana* (Sanskrit), or worldview can be addressed in this brief primer.[4]

The history and development of Ayurveda reputedly spans 6,000 years, for most of which time, only an oral tradition existed. When the sacred scriptures of ancient India emerged in the Vedic period (circa 3,000 BC to 600 BC) in the four *Vedas – Rig, Sama, Yajur,* and *Atharva,* Ayurveda gradually became formally organized. Its three great fathers, in the respective foundational texts that bear their names, later codified it: *Charaka Samhita* (c. 1,000 BC), *Sushruta Samhita* (c. 660 BC and supplemented by Nagarjuna c. AD 100), and *Asthanga Sangraha of Vagbhata* (c. AD 7th century).[5,6,7]

The word "Ayurveda" derives from two Sanskrit terms, *ayus* meaning life or the course of living, and *veda* meaning knowledge, science, or wisdom. Ayurveda as the wisdom of life denotes an organized set of propositions that contain philosophical, ethical, cosmological, medical, and therapeutic principles aimed at generating, maintaining, optimizing, and restoring physical health and psychological well-being. This implies the absence of illness, disease, and suffering. The well-known system of yoga, in fact, originally came from the *Vedas* and later codifications arranged by the Indian sage, Patanjali (circa AD 100). Yoga practices differ in emphasis from Ayurveda but are an ancillary part of it. They complement Ayurvedic treatments.

As a medical and surgical system, Ayurveda has main subspecialties: internal medicine, surgery, otolaryngology, ophthalmology, obstetrics, gynecology, pediatrics, toxicology, psychiatry, anti-aging, rejuvenation, reproductive, and aphrodisiac medicine.

Each individual is considered an integral triune to the extent that active work is directed toward integration of bodily needs (*sharira*), refinement of psychological abilities (*manas*), and sensitivity to the consciousness-enhancing practices that stabilize these. Responsiveness to seasons and the changing environment (*kala parinama*) makes Ayurveda exceedingly aware of the inevitable imbalances and disease processes that present themselves and require attention at these times. I refer to this self-environment connectivity as "eco-concordance."

A strong ethical framework is an intrinsic part of Ayurveda. The standard of care aims for continuing improvement toward the recognition and treatment of mental and physical disorders. Not only does this add to good patient care but also to the refinement of diagnostic acumen and the effectiveness of treatment interventions. Saving life and easing suffering are axiomatic values. Ayurveda's three great texts make this explicit. Patient beneficence, protecting from harm together with actively promoting wellness, respect for all persons and individual self-direction, and fair and just socially responsible practices are the training standards of Ayurvedic practitioners. The Ayurvedic Oath (*Sisyopanayaniya* Ayurveda), in fact, may have preceded the Hippocratic Oath; both have striking correlations in their guidelines.

Ayurveda's conceptual models imply a complex and multitiered worldview. Key ideas often present as metaphors. These suggest overarching principles; what they actually refer to remains open to examination in terms of Western concepts of physics and physiology. Sanskrit names are included here in italics.

Fundamental Ayurvedic propositions include the following: the Five Great Gross Elements (*Pancha Mahabhutanis*) – Ether, Air, Fire, Water, and Earth; the biological *doshas* –*Vata, Pitta, Kapha; Agni* – how cells and tissues process molecules, the digestive and assimilative processes, metabolic rate, and cellular transport mechanisms; the seven bodily tissues (*sapta dhatus*) – plasma, blood, muscle, fat, bone, marrow and nerve tissue, and reproductive tissue; *Ojas* – immunity, stress modulation, and resistance to disease; *Prakruti* – an individual's "biopsychospiritual" constitutional type;

*Samprapti* – pathogenesis; *Vikruti* – specific disease syndromes in an individual; *Ahara* – diet; *Vihara* – lifestyle; *Dravyaguna Shastra* – pharmacognosy, pharmacology, materia medica, and therapeutics.

The Five Great Gross Elements are concepts that reside on the borders of philosophy, cosmology, and the material world of atoms and molecules. These five Elements – Ether, Air, Fire, Water, and Earth – are considered primary pentads, elemental substances composing matter in all its varied states of density. The Elements are the building blocks of tissues. As protosubstances, Elements carry strong metaphorical and emblematic connotations that imply a representation of physiological functioning when considered from the viewpoint of biological life. For example, each bodily tissue has a varied composition of Elements suggesting its character, especially useful as it relates to choosing specific therapeutic herbs of similar Elemental composition. Ginger (*Zingiber officinale*), for example, is thought to have a high Fire content and is used to stimulate digestive processes (*Agni*), which require such a "hot" (actively potent) energy to promote optimal functioning.

The three biological *doshas* – Vata, Pitta, and Kapha – are the backbone of Ayurveda. These *doshas* had traditionally been termed "humors" in historically Western medical systems such as those of ancient Greece and Rome, as travelers from the East influenced these developing medical systems. The original idea of a *dosha*, a biological and energetic substance, however, originated much earlier in ancient India. The work of Charaka, the internist, and subsequently the compilations of Sushruta, the surgeon, codified this. The word *dosha* literally means spoiling, fault, or darkener. This refers to the *dosha's* inherent ability to become vitiated or agitated. This disruption then alters the condition of tissues and the body's equilibrium. This action is, in fact, a positive homeostatic mechanism regulating the health of the body. There are only three *doshas*. In biological organisms, each operates as both a bioenergetic substance and a regulatory force. *Doshas* are biopsychological principles of organization both structurally and functionally, the least common organizational denominator of tissues and mind.

*Vata* connotes wind, movement, and flow. Its principal characteristic is propulsion. It is responsible for all motion in the body from cellular to tissue and musculoskeletal systems, acuity and coordination of the senses of perception, equilibrium of tissues, respiration, and nerve transmission. It is said to possess erratic, cold, dry, and clear qualities. *Vata* underlies the body's symmetry and proportion. When the proper flow of *Vata* through the body is impaired, pain is felt and distortions in form appear.

*Pitta* is described as the biological fire humor. Its etymological derivation is associated with digestion, heating, thermogenesis, and transformation. *Pitta's* chief action is digestion or transformation occurring through cellular, tissue, and organ levels to psychological, cognitive, and emotional spheres of mind (*Manas*). It is said to possess hot, flowing, and sharp qualities. The fundamental Ayurvedic conception of *Agni*, the energy of the digestive fire, is inextricably tied to the activity of its biological container, *Pitta dosha*.

*Kapha* is the biological water humor. Its chief characteristic is cohesion and binding. The word *Kapha* means phlegm and water flourishing, and suggests qualities of cohesiveness and firmness. *Kapha* maintains the stability of bodily tissues and imparts protection, structure, and denseness. It is said to possess heavy, dense, solid, and cold qualities, and the attribute of mass.

Each individual possesses a unique composition of all three *doshas*, each one contributing qualitative and quantitative uniqueness to that person. They are the overarching regulators of biopsychological functioning in health and disease.

*Agni*, a central Ayurvedic concept, refers to the way one's genetic constitution programs basic metabolic processes, the dynamics of anabolism and catabolism. Its centrality is only second to the conception of the *doshas*. *Agni* was described historically in various ways (for example, fire itself; the sun; and the divine force) as early as the *Rig-Veda* and *Atharva-Veda*. In ancient times, it was seen as the power behind all forms of transformation, the mediator between macrocosm and individual. As the primordial energetic dimension of *Pitta dosha*, *Agni* functions to control the rate and quality of all biological and mental dynamic processes. Thirteen subspecies of *Agni* are described in relation to their respective actions at cellular, tissue, and system levels. *Agni* as the heat element in processes of thermogenesis also aids the body's own infection control self-management.

In Ayurveda, *Agni* and the concept of digestion are interchangeable as functional ideas. *Agni*, however, far transcends the more circumscribed meaning that digestion denotes in Western physiology (for example, intraluminal hydrolysis of fats, proteins, and carbohydrates by enzymes and bile salts, digestion by brush border enzymes and uptake of end-products, and lymphatic transport of nutrients). Digestion in Ayurveda includes processes that transform raw, nonhuman substances (foods, herbs, sensory impressions, and so forth) by using material and psychological "digestive" mechanisms. *Vata*, *Pitta*, *Kapha*, and *Agni* handle these in order for those raw nutrients to become actively utilizable, assimilable, and form part of the biopsychological structure of the person. Clinically, the condition of one's *Agni* correlates with current health or disease. Optimizing *Agni* by diet, herbs, and lifestyle is fundamental to all treatments.

The physical body is composed of seven bodily tissues (*sapta dhatus*): plasma, blood, muscle, fat, bone, marrow and nerve tissue, and reproductive tissue. Each has micro-sized (subtle and invisible) and macro-sized (gross and visible) channels of circulation (*srotas*) that function to transport nutrients, wastes, and other substances both in their respective tissues and to other bodily tissues, organs, and systems. Plasma (*rasa*) as the total water content of the body, holds a special place since it is considered to pervade the entire body with essential nutrients and the moisture that sustains the fullness of vitality (*prinana*).

*Ojas* is the Sanskrit term referring to the bioenergetic bodily substance of immunity, strength, and vital energy reserves. It is the crucial Ayurvedic theory of the body's innate capacity for immune resistance to disease. In Traditional Chinese Medicine, the concept of *Yin* and *Jing* or "Life Essence" believed to reside in the kidneys compares with the Ayurvedic concept of *Ojas*. Some contemporary Ayurvedic researchers have suggested that the entire conceptualization of *Ojas* and its implications might correlate with the functioning of the hypothalamus in terms of the stress response, and with the energy of cellular mitochondria as the powerhouses of the cell. In Ayurveda's materia medica, for example, the herb ashwaganda (*Withania somnifera*) has been used for thousands of years as a powerful adaptogen, increasing resistance to cellular, physiological, and mental stress, restoring homeostasis, and enhancing stamina and mental performance. It is believed to contain and enhance the body's store of *Ojas*.

The Ayurvedic idea of individualized constitutional types or *prakruti* is a cornerstone of basic theory and practical therapeutics. The sine qua non of constructing individualized treatment plans rests on this. *Prakruti* denotes a person's unique biopsychological (anatomical, physiological, and psychological) template of predispositions, capacities, abilities, preferences, strengths, and vulnerabilities. It is a quotient of the endowment and interactions of each of the three *doshas* (*Vata*, *Pitta*, and *Kapha*) from birth onward. It is measured and determined solely on clinical grounds, and includes physical appearance, strength, quality of digestive processes, and psychological attributes. *Prakruti* does not essentially change throughout the lifetime. It is an important criterion for determining and recommending individualized diet and lifestyle choices.

*Vikruti* is the clinically observable imbalance of the *doshas* that pathological processes impose on the *prakruti*. Disease (*roga*) plays itself out within the field of the ill person (*vikruti*).

Disease etiology (*nidana*) is multifactorial. In addition to microbes (*krimi*), trauma (*pidaja*), genetic predispositions (*sahaja roga*), congenital (*garbhaja*), acquired (*jataja*), seasonal (*kalaja*), and inevitable, for example, aging (*swabhavaja*) influences, Ayurveda has traditionally espoused an agriculturally-oriented metaphor of "field and seed." The field is the *prakruti* – body, mind, and consciousness ground of strength. The seeds of illness are its genetic and acquired proneness to vulnerabilities. If *prakruti* and *Ojas* are balanced, the body and mind are less susceptible to disease. Whatever the precipitating causes of illness, the balance and integrity of *doshas* inevitably become disrupted, and, if left unchecked, lead to disease.

*Samprapti* denotes pathogenesis proper. When *Agni* or digestive and assimilative strength becomes impaired, an individual's *dosha* complement becomes unbalanced; for example, the level of *Pitta* is too low and the force of *Vata* too high. This leads to an abnormal buildup of toxic substances (*Ama*) in the body. They, along with congenital and acquired defective tissue and organ sites, launch the pathogenic process that gradually results in manifest disease. The six stages of *Samprapti* are the following:

1. *Sanchaya* or preclinical Stage 1 in which some *doshas* may abnormally begin to accumulate;
2. *Prakopa* or preclinical Stage 2 in which the *doshas* become aggravated and function in abnormal ways;

3. *Prasara* or preclinical Stage 3 in which the abnormal *doshas* are dislodged from their normal resting sites and begin spreading abnormally throughout the body;

4. *Stana-Samshraya* or clinical Stage 4 in which the abnormal *doshas* localize in an already defective tissue or organ; an aura of symptoms now becomes perceptible;

5. *Vyakti* or clinical Stage 5 during which the consolidated disease manifests in clear-cut signs and symptoms, and

6. *Bheda* or clinical Stage 6 in which the consolidated disease differentiates in specific ways along the lines of one's *dosha* quotient (*prakruti*) coupled with pathological tissue involvement. At this stage, complications arise.

Diagnostic methods in Ayurveda are essentially clinical. Diagnostic evaluation of the patient follows a tenfold process originally outlined by Charaka. Some of its features include assessing *prakruti*, *vikruti* with its pain and signs and symptoms of illness, tissue quality by inspection of morphology and functional status, body proportions, mental and emotional characteristics, digestive strength, energy level and stamina, and age-related abilities and limitations. An additional eightfold examination formulated in the 1500s also includes Ayurvedic pulse diagnosis.

Ayurveda has developed systems of nutrition as dietetics and specific food intake (*ahara*) over the course of thousands of years. It is a unique system incorporating the aforementioned theoretical elements and matching their analyses to recommendations for food options. An individual's *prakruti* and *vikruti* in the context of prevailing seasonal influences are taken into account. Foods function to maintain and enhance health, and, at specific times, act therapeutically. Ayurvedic therapy aims at balancing the *doshas* and restoring their optimal proportions for each *dosha's* single and coordinated efficiency. When *doshas* are properly aligned, *Agni's* operation optimizes and reinforces *dosha* stabilization.

Lifestyle and behavioral practices (*vihara*) are crucial features of Ayurveda's pursuit of wellness. Based on constitutional predispositions, strengths, weaknesses, and current needs at a specific age and in a specific season, recommendations for daily hygiene, exercise, development of mental faculties (for example, study, yoga postures, breath expansions/*pranayama*, and meditation), and suitable recreational activities are suggested. Guidelines for highly ethical standards (*sadvritta*) closely related to classical Western values and behaviors considered righteous and reasonable are included. Without requiring the ritualized constraints of a religion, Ayurveda incorporates the Hindu and Buddhist doctrine of *karma*, which ethically denotes accountability and taking personal responsibility for thoughts and actions. A proactive life by choice and adherence to medical guidelines includes a specific diet to maintain constitutional balance, appropriate responsiveness to the effects of time (for example, chronological age, diurnal variations, and seasons), and a suitable lifestyle. Besides the absence of disease and disability, wellness promotes functional integrity, strength, endurance, flexibility, and balance. Changes promoting wellness also presume newly-gained insights into motivations, attitudes, emotional dispositions, and behaviors. Moreover, a realization of belonging to the shared community of the one human family and the ultimate unity of all nature counters unrealistic feelings of isolation or narcissistically-based specialness.

*Dravyaguna Shastra* is Ayurveda's age-old science of medicine, a herbo-mineral pharmacopoeia. Herbal supplementation (*aushadha*) is used both prophylactically and as active treatment for disorders. About 700 herbs are recognized and used, although there are thousands more being employed in less standardized ways.

Modern research in the therapeutic effectiveness of Ayurvedic herbs has laid particular emphasis on the role of phytochemicals and natural antioxidants contained in these traditional herbal and spice substances. Phytochemicals are nonessential nutrients. The function of these micronutrients is protection against tissue damage and for disease prevention. Some of the proposed mechanisms for these effects include antioxidant activity, anti-inflammatory action, glutathione synthesis, effects on biotransformation enzymes involved in carcinogen metabolism, induction of cell cycle arrest and apoptosis, and inhibition of tumor invasion and angiogenesis.

Specific fractions of edible substances contain *phytochemicals*. These are flavonoids, isoflavones, allyl sulfides, catechins, anthocyanins, polyphenols, carotenoids, terpenes, and plant sterols. All phytonutrients are of plant origin – fruits, vegetables, herbs, and spices. They target unstable free radicals, known as reactive oxygen species (atoms, ions, or molecules with one or more unpaired electrons that bind to and destroy cellular components) both in general and specific ways to scavenge them and prevent pathogenic membrane disruption. This beneficial action is accomplished by neutralizing damaging ions and thereby reducing the oxidative stress that impairs endothelial cell integrity throughout the entire circulatory system. For example, phytonutrients make low density lipoproteins (LDL cholesterol) less likely to be oxidized by free radicals, become trapped in the intravascular lumen, attract calcium, and form plaques that narrow arterial patency and encourage blood clot formation. Additionally, antioxidant activity reduces excessive crosslinking of collagen molecules, thus strengthening connective tissue throughout the body and benefiting bone, ligaments, and joints. Another important mechanism of herbal treatments is the role of nitric oxide production by the endothelium to enhance vasodilation and arterial perfusion.

Lastly, Ayurveda's preeminent radical detoxification program – *Panchakarma* – is a five-step process that occurs over a period of several weeks and which must be closely supervised by a qualified practitioner. A few typically-used substances and modified treatment protocols will be discussed later in a consideration of orthopedic problems.

## AYURVEDIC PERSPECTIVES ON AGING

Normative fluctuations of *doshas* and specific *dosha* dominance are metrics used to denote epochs in the lifecycle. Older age becomes progressively noticeable in the later 50s and increasingly thereafter. This correlates with a predominance of *Vata dosha*. All of *Vata's* key qualities begin to affect the entire person: dryness, coldness, stiffness, rigidity, hardness, roughness, constriction/spasm versus looseness/hypermobility cycles, reduced tissue mass, and increased frailty. The body's harmonious symmetry and its proportions diminish. For example, intervertebral disks tend to become dehydrated and exert pressure on adjacent nerve roots. Stature and posture change. The aberrant flow of *Vata* in vitiated tissues and channels of circulation signals pain. This influences an individual's *Biopsychospiritual* makeup, and a general trend toward ungroundedness (unsteady gait, loss of confidence, and anxiety) becomes apparent. Cognition, although wiser from years of adaptive experience, may lack the swiftness, alacrity, and recall once present.

The appearance of aging is observed in face, body posture, and attitude. Older persons may look tired, downtrodden, burdened, dry, even sullen and angry. Much of this results from pain and the increasing constraints on previously enjoyed levels of functioning.

It is fair to add that an individual's past history of learning, achievements, and successes on material, emotional, and spiritual levels also has etched multiple contours of self-confidence and pragmatic memory. These inner resources along with social ties counter isolation and loneliness. They add to the satisfaction a favorable quality of life has engendered as aging proceeds.

## AYURVEDIC PERSPECTIVES ON MANAGING THE AGING PROCESS WITH RESPECT TO BONE

A comprehensive discussion of optimal age-management strategies and therapies unique to Ayurveda is beyond the scope of this chapter. Ayurvedic interventions always involve a multitiered approach that aims to modulate the deterioration associated with aging by enhancing the competence of repair mechanisms. A strong emphasis on *Vata* modulation and normalization through diet, seasonal, and lifestyle recommendations is the basis of all treatments. Included are specific prescriptions for physical exercise (*vyayama*), oil massage, gentle yoga stretches for musculoskeletal flexibility, and herbal adjuncts. The entire field of *Rasayanas* or rejuvenation medicine affords an untapped treasure trove awaiting examination by Western research. Because Ayurveda is profoundly holistic, all the aforementioned are components of an intense, one-to-one therapeutic relationship with a practitioner who acts as physician, coach, and, at times, psychotherapist. In this way, anxiety, fear, and depression, at times the deepest unconscious sources of pain and suffering, are addressed and managed.

Bone (*asthi*) is considered one of the seven major tissues composing the material substance of the physical body (*sharira*). Bone, its membranous coverings (*purishadhara kala*), articular joints (*sandhi*), cartilage (*tarunashti*), and channels of circulation (*asthivaha srotas*) are major components of the skeletal system. It is primarily derived from three of the Five Great Gross Elements or principles of organization of matter: Earth and Water (*Kapha* dimension) and Air (*Vata* dimension). The Sanskrit term *asthi* means to stand and endure. A major function of bone is support (*dharana*); bone also acts to protect vital organs and contributes to the shape and form of the body. Vagbhata (c. AD 700) asserts that bone tissue nourishes nerve and marrow tissue (*majja dhatu*) in critical ways. In terms of *doshas*, the substance of bone is essentially of *Kapha* origin. Two subspecies of *Kapha* are dominant: *Avalambaka Kapha*, centered in the thorax and vertebral column, and *Shleshaka Kapha*, situated in joint fluids and apposing structures such as disks and articular surfaces.

Bone, moreover, is one of the body's largest containers of *Vata dosha*, particularly *Vyana Vata* (pulsatile, rhythmic expansion and contraction) and *Apana Vata* (downward, eliminative action). Periosteal coverings are considered the membranes (*purishadhara kala*) containing and contributing to the nourishment of bone.

The principal repository of *Vata* in the entire body resides in the large intestine or colon. The colon's own membranes share a functional tie and the same name with all osseous membranes. This important correlation links the health and pathology of the colon with the health and pathology of the skeletal system. Its implications for treatment are profound. Western science regards the colon as having several important functions including resorption of water, electrolytes, and minerals back into the body, further digestion of various kinds of sugars and fiber, production of vitamins, especially vitamin K (needed for blood clotting and bone nutrition), and storage of indigestible foodstuff as stool for eventual elimination. Ayurvedic theory asserts that *Prana Vata* carries *Prana*, the primary life force. The Indian concept of *Prana* is equivalent to the Chinese concept of *Qi/Chi*. *Prana Vata* and minerals in foods and herbs rich in *Prana* are absorbed through the *purishadhara kala* membrane of the colon to directly supply bone tissue all over the body. In addition, Ayurveda regards the marrow internal to bone to be closely associated with nervous system functioning. This connection underscores the experience of pain associated with dysfunctions of bone and bone marrow.

Ayurveda's three foundational texts, *Charaka Samhita*, *Sushruta Samhita*, and *Asthanga Sangraha* of Vagbhata describe pain syndromes related to bone. In addition, a later work, Madhava Nidana (c. AD 650–950)[8] introduced the conceptualization of *amavata*. This toxic *Vata* condition has much in common with rheumatoid arthritis, and is marked by inflammation and edema.

The etiological field that sets the stage for the development of bone pathology and pain has general and specific triggers. Included are dietary practices that lead to impaired *Agni* and weakened digestive processes (for example, cold foods, and heavy foods, such as meat and cheeses, in excess), and *Vata* aggravating diets (for example, cold, dry foods, lack of sufficient oil in diet, excess of raw vegetables, use of traditionally incompatible food combinations: milk and fish, milk and fruit, milk and meat, milk and foods having sour tastes). Such disease-provoking dietary practices engender the metabolic toxin called *Ama*, which not only obstructs the proper flow of the *doshas* but also the distribution and assimilation of nutrients. *Ama* correlates with excess free radical production and inflammation, especially at the endothelial cell level.

*Vata*-aggravating lifestyle (for example, excess travel and physical activity, and excessive preoccupation with electronic media), microbial causes (*krimi*), trauma, genetic predisposition (*sahaja hetu*), and older age add to *Vata* vitiation and progression of disease. Improper breathing may limit the body's adequate intake and absorption not only of oxygen but also of *Prana* in the lungs and the colon, both subsequently affecting bone. Proper oxygenation is a typical benefit of Ayurvedically-prescribed deep breathing practices. This contributes to natural infection control. Although *Vata* is the principal *dosha* associated with bone pathology, *Pitta* may also become involved and manifest as inflammation; when *Kapha* becomes involved, edema, osteophytes, and tumors emerge.

The specific form taken by bone pathology is the result of genetic, constitutional, and lifestyle factors, as well as acquired pathology. After careful assessment of the aforementioned factors and delineation of the course of pathogenesis, a specific treatment plan is constructed. To give a general idea of treatment guidelines, the following protocol is outlined. It may not be universally applicable since each patient and each disease process presents

with unique features. Specific decompensations dictate the specifics of an individualized treatment regimen. Lower back pain with radiation to the leg (*gridhrasi*), for example, is well known in Ayurveda and its treatment follows protocols established thousands of years ago. A qualified practitioner, not self-help guidebooks, is needed to formulate diagnosis and treatment recommendations. Treatments may take place in a clinic and through outpatient recommendations for dietary protocols, herbo-mineral prescriptions, and other adjunctive techniques.

Ayurvedic treatments typically begin with procedures that target *Ama* detoxification and optimize the digestive process. In the context of a *Vata*-pacifying diet, various detoxifying herbs are used. These may include triphala (*Emblica officinalis*, *Terminalia chebula*, and *Terminalia belerica*), turmeric (*Curcuma longa*), guduchi (*Tinea cordifolia*),[9] castor oil (*Ricinus communis*), and ginger (*Zingiber officinale*). Substances that reduce inflammation include Boswellia (*Boswellia serrata*) and guggul (*Commiphora mukul*). In osteoarthritis (*Sandhigatavata*) where degeneration is prominent, ashwaganda (*Withania somnifera*) and other highly tonic/nutritive herbs are given after a period of stabilization to promote healing and rebuild tissue. Turmeric (*haridra* in Sanskrit; *jiang huang* in Chinese) is used in Ayurveda and Chinese medicine to stimulate blood flow and reduce inflammation. Single herbs and compounds with several herbs are typically given.

Ayurvedic physicians recommend *ghee*, very modest amounts of highly-clarified butter, to facilitate the assimilation and efficacy of herbs. Ghee or butter oil is regarded as a medicine, not similar to ordinary butter with its possible deleterious effects on lipid profiles and cardiovascular system. Ghee has specific therapeutically targeted effects and is an adjuvant and potentiator of other medicinal substances. Ghee contains up to 27% mono-unsaturated and about 66% short-chain fatty acids along with about 3 % conjugated linoleic acid (CLA). This composition is a beneficial profile. Taken in moderation, ghee demonstrates antioxidant, antimicrobial, anti-carcinogenic, and lipid nondysregulation properties.[10] Ghee contains a fat-soluble fraction of vitamin K, K-2, or meanquinone-7 or menaquinone-7 (MK-7). K-2 produces gamma-carboxylated osteocalcin and facilitates the incorporation of calcium into bone matrix. In Japan, MK-7 is highly concentrated in a soybean food, "natto," fermented by *Bacillus subtilis*. People with osteoporosis and those who might benefit from natto's significant blood-thinning properties eat this food.

Ayurvedic treatment includes dietary recommendations that follow classically-established *Vata*-pacifying guidelines. These consist of regular, moderately-sized meals; food choices that include warm, moist foods emphasizing sweet, salty, and sour tastes in moderation; sweet fruits; most cooked vegetables excluding mushrooms and excess legumes (beans, peas, and lentils); rice; all nuts and seeds; dairy products in moderation; and mild spices such as cinnamon (*Cinnamomum zeylanicum*), basil (*Ocinum spp.*), cardamom (*Eletarria cardamomum*) and fennel (*Foeniculum vulgare*). These dietary guidelines are not mere culinary suggestions. They come from Ayurveda's detailed and exacting analysis of the complex actions and therapeutic properties of food, herbal, and spice substances. Calcium-rich foods, a normal part of the Ayurvedic diet, include chickpeas, okra, almonds, sesame seeds, and milk drinks. Traditional cooking techniques for grains and legumes include presoaking and adequate cooking time to reduce excess phytic acid (inositol hexakisphosphate, IP6) that tends to chelate calcium and inactivate niacin. Although not a standard food in traditional Ayurveda, American practitioners recommend many marine macroalgae or seaweeds as dietary additions. For example, wakame (*Undaria pinnatifida*) frequently used in Japan (*ito-wakame*), China (*qundaicai*), and Korea (*miyeok*) as food and medicine contains about 980 to 1,300 mg assimilable calcium per 100 grams. Besides calcium, sea vegetables contain generous amounts of potassium, sodium, and magnesium; hence, judicious use of high-quality, guaranteed pure seaweed may be beneficial in patients whose sodium intake is not restricted.

In addition to diet and herbs, oils specially prepared for therapeutic massage (*abhyanga*) coupled with topical moist heat fomentation (*swedhana*) are a regular part of treatment protocols. Such intermittent mild temperature elevations aid in infection control. Commonly used therapeutic massage oils include sesame, castor, and a special compound called *Mahanarayan*. Efficacy lies in the mobilization of contracted tissues, alleviating pain, and reducing swelling and induration. Oil massage is a highly regarded treatment intervention, and one that patients perceive as helpful and valuable. In India, specially prepared herbalized oil enemas (*basti*) are also a regular part of specialized anti-*Vata* treatments.

## CONCLUSION

The psychology of aging is an important consideration in understanding the needs of the rapidly emerging generation of older citizens in society. Physical illnesses, particularly orthopedic problems, cause distortions in body image, and diminish self-esteem. Limitations in functioning and pain force patients to become less productive personally, socially, and occupationally. Recent scientific advances in Western medicine provide many rational choices for remediation and repair. Eastern medical traditions, such as Ayurveda with its favorable record of accomplishment, have emerged as complementary adjuncts. Although currently unexplored by modern scientific methods, they offer relief and restoration of functioning. For these reasons, the complete physician, not to mention his or her patients, can benefit from a familiarity with newly emerging medical systems and their applications. A greater yield of sustained positive outcomes resulting in mental and physical wellness may be attainable.

## References

1. F.J. Ninivaggi, Malingering, in: B.J. Sadock, V.A. Sadock (Eds.), Kaplan & Sadock's comprehensive textbook of psychiatry, ed 9, Lippincott Williams and Wilkins, Baltimore, 2010.
2. J.J. Clayton, Nutraceuticals in the management of osteoarthritis, Orthopedics 30 (8) (2007) 624–629.
3. D. Khanna, G. Sethi, K.S. Ahn, M.K. Pandey, A.B. Kunnumakkara, B. Sung, A. Aggarwal, B.B. Aggarawal, Natural products as a gold mine for arthritis treatment, Curr Opin Pharmacol 7 (3) (2007) 344–351.
4. F.J. Ninivaggi, Ayurveda: a comprehensive guide to traditional Indian medicine for the west, Praeger, Westport, Conn, 2008.
5. A.C. Kaviratna, Charaka Samhita, 4 vols, Girish Chandra Chakravarti Deva Press, Calcutta, 1902–1925.
6. J. Trikamji, N. Ram, Sushruta Samhita of Sushruta, Chaukhambha Orientalia, Varanasi, India, 1980.
7. K.R.S. Murthy, translator:Ashtanga Samgraha of Vagbhata, Chaukhambha Orientalia, Varanasi, India, 2005.
8. K.R.S. Murthy, translator: Madhava Nidanam, Chaukhamba Orientalia, Varanasi, India, 1987.
9. T.S. Panchabhai, U.P. Kulkarmi, N.N. Rege, Validation of therapeutic claims of Tinospora cordifolia: a review, Phytother Res 22 (4) (2008) 425–441.
10. H. Sharma, Butter oil (ghee) – myths and facts, Ind J Clin Pract 1 (2) (1990) 31–32.

# PART 2

# Basic Science of the Aging Spine

# Biomechanics of the Senescent Spine

*Boyle C. Cheng*

| K E Y   P O I N T S |
| --- |
| • Not all patients diagnosed with osteoporosis by current bone mineral density levels will experience vertebral fracture, nor will patients above the osteopenic level necessarily be free of fracture. |
| • The use of bone mineral density as an indicator for outcome success related to instrumented procedures is inconsistent, particularly in predicting complex failure loads. |
| • Additional parameters, including Modic changes, are important in the identification of additional vertebral fracture risk factors for patients. |

## INTRODUCTION

The microstructural effects of aging on the spine may have dramatic consequences on both the individual vertebrae and the vertebra as a constituent within an osteoligamentous structure, that is, a functional spinal unit (FSU). Additionally, the cervical, thoracic, and lumbar regions of the spinal column may be adversely affected by the deleterious effects of senescence. The consequences may cover a spectrum of physical quality-of-life factors ranging from the relatively benign to those that dramatically alter the health of a patient. When clinicians are faced with deteriorating conditions severe enough to warrant surgical intervention, additional considerations must be made for the properties of senescent spines. Therefore, the biomechanical capabilities of the spine should be examined with careful consideration for age along with this caveat: biomechanical changes do not necessarily become symptomatic.

Biomechanical measurements can be affected by numerous indicators, and it is important to distinguish which are related to global measures, for example, body mass index, and which may be relevant specifically to the local spinal elements, e.g., friability of a vertebral body. Two distinct but related indicators should be evaluated with spinal pathologies: the advancement of age and degenerative changes resulting in anatomical transmutation that potentially leads to abnormal loading of the spine. Anatomical changes may be attributed to the primary degenerative conditions associated with age. Miller et al reported an approximate 10% occurrence of severely degenerated intervertebral discs in 50-year-old males, with an increase to 60% in 70-year-olds.[1] The degenerative conditions result in several anatomical changes and, of particular importance to an aging population, is the potential for constriction of the spinal canal diameter. The cause of the constriction may be from a single specific etiology or from a combination of factors, including spinal canal stenosis, disc herniation, osteophyte growth into the canal, hypertrophy of the ligamentum flavum, and calcification of the posterior longitudinal ligament and the ligamentum flavum.

A combination of interrelated mechanobiological conditions and associated kinematic response of the spine due to degenerative diseases is also known to occur with age. Changes in proteoglycan concentration within the intervertebral disc along with matrix disorganization result in a cascade of events over time that affect the anatomical structures within an FSU. The range of motion (RoM) and the ability to absorb and transmit load in the spine are biomechanical capabilities that may be compromised by microstructural changes within the anterior and posterior columns. Under the worst conditions, the degenerative pathology within a FSU results in a significantly different kinematic response to physiologic motion, and abnormal loading may occur.

## AGING AND DEGENERATIVE CHANGES ON THE EFFECTS OF BIOMECHANICAL RANGE OF MOTION

The relationship between age, degeneration, and RoM has been studied both in human cadaveric FSU testing and in clinical studies. The instability of the lumbar spine was proposed by Kirkaldy-Willis and Farfan to be categorized into three diskrete stages of degenerative change. In order of progression, the clinical assessment of the lumbar spine categorized pathologic changes as temporary dysfunction, the unstable phase, and finally, stabilization.[2] Well-defined, controlled, biomechanical testing and clinical studies involving well-documented patient profiles have tested various aspects of this initial hypothesis on spinal instability.

Traditional methods of comparing the effects of age, degeneration, or subsequent treatments have been subjected to biomechanical characterization through the flexibility test method. The methodology of flexibility testing has been well described in the literature, originating with Panjabi's early description of load input utilizing pure moments.[3] Subsequent comparisons, particularly relevant in fixation instrumentation via flexibility testing, have described the performance of these devices relative to the intact spine. often with high mean age donor specimen. Additionally, comparisons between fixation treatments, as well as comparison of fixation treatments from laboratory to laboratory, have been possible. The standardization of the pure moment test protocol by Goel et al has contributed to the repeatability despite biologic variability inherent in cadaveric testing.[4]

It is important to understand the rationale of the test methodology when considering clinically relevant biomechanical studies. The basis of the traditional flexibility test, or pure moment testing, is to apply a uniform moment across all FSUs in a given specimen. Figure 8-1 is an example of a mounted lumbar specimen that will be subjected to flexion-extension bending. The ability to extrapolate the biomechanical effects to clinical outcomes is dependent on study design and successful interpretation of the resulting data. Clinically relevant biomechanical testing in the appropriate form is an important parameter for clinicians to consider in the triage of patients with spinal pathologies.

In a cadaveric human lumbar study by Mimura et al, the authors were able to demonstrate a statistically significant difference between RoM in lateral bending, but not in flexion-extension bending, for intervertebral discs with degenerative ratings in whole lumbar specimens under a flexibility protocol.[5] Biomechanical studies involving age as a variable in the analysis are often shown to be correlated to RoM. Board et al reported on the results of a human cadaveric cervical biomechanical study. Their results suggest that biomechanical flexion-extension in pure moment loading decreases the RoM as a function of the age of the specimen.[6] These findings agreed with published articles, when extrapolated and compared to equivalent test parameters. In a similar clinical evaluation on bending in the cervical spine involving only males, Sforza et al concluded that young adult males exhibited statistically significant larger flexion-extension RoM compared to their middle-aged counterparts who participated in the study.[7] Similarly, in a clinical cervical study involving multiple factors including both age and degeneration, Simpson et al determined age to be the most significant factor on RoM.[8]

Confounding these results are clinical considerations in which surgical treatment may be warranted, but subsequent conditions and outcomes related to the specific implant or procedure for the elderly patient may not

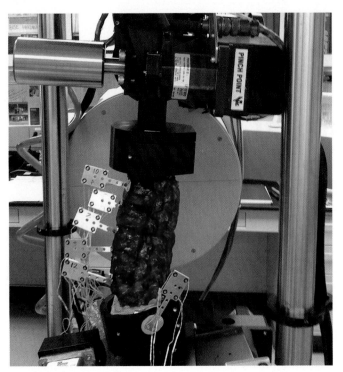

■ **FIGURE 8-1**   Biomechanical test setup subjected to flexibility protocol, with a lumbar specimen mounted in flexion-extension test.

be clear. For example, symptomatic spine pathology resulting in instability of a FSU and suitable for an instrumented fusion procedure must consider the interaction of the hardware and the patient's local host tissue. In addition to global metrics of bone quality, the local bone purchase dependent upon the microstructural integrity of bony trabeculation at the index FSU may have undergone severe anatomical changes. These differences affect the load response, exacerbate degenerative pathologies, and require additional considerations for the type of instrumentation suitable for the patient preoperatively. Intraoperatively, additional factors may further alter the structural integrity of the FSU, for example, endplate preparation or pilot hole drilling combined with tapping.

The biomechanical changes inherent to aging are complex in nature. Many steps have been taken toward the understanding the fundamental process of maintaining a healthy spine, including bone healing, the role of the intervertebral disc, and the significance of endplate changes. However, understanding the nature of biomechanical measurement and the clinical relevance of each metric may help further elucidate the suitability of the treatment for the senescent patient and, ultimately, improved treatment options may be developed.

## ASSESSING ANATOMICAL CHANGES

Accurate measurements of bone strength are essential to the clinical management of a diseased spine. Both the diagnosis of disease, such as osteoporosis, and also its triage, such as the surgical treatment of an unstable spinal motion segment with hardware, would benefit from explicit descriptions of vertebral bone quality. Dual-energy x-ray absorptiometry(DXA)–obtained measures of bone mineral density are widely regarded across many medical diskiplines as the gold standard for assessing fracture risk. The guidelines set by the World Health Organization based on the standard deviation units of bone mineral density (BMD), referred to as T-scores, have limitations that are documented in the literature. Also, BMD has not consistently supported correlations with patient fracture in all risk groups, and additional indicators to further enhance DXA scores would be particularly beneficial to lower-risk patients with higher T-scores.

Two primary reasons for the frequency of DXA measurements are the relatively noninvasive, nondestructive nature of the test and documented correlations associated with DXA measurements. Imaging modalities that

assist in the classification of degeneration have been useful in FSU pathophysiology and could be useful in understanding the relationships between aging, degeneration, and biomechanics of the FSU. Therefore, through the use of known techniques in detecting degeneration of the osteoligamentous structures, such as magnetic resonance imaging (MRI) and the Modic classification of vertebral endplate change, stronger correlations may be established between age and degeneration. Ideally, earlier fracture diagnostic capabilities for all risk groups may be added to a clinician's armamentarium.

## OSTEOPOROSIS, AGING, AND BIOMECHANICAL PROPERTIES

The use of clinical guidelines based primarily on BMD results has been widely accepted. The ability to identify patients with high risk of fracture via low BMD measurements, defined by T-scores of −2.5 or lower, and to subsequently provide effective pharmacological treatments, has been proved through large double-blinded placebo-controlled trials. Several challenges remain in identifying low-risk population and ultimately a means in cost effectively managing fracture risk. In an examination of 149,524 postmenopausal women 50 years of age and older with fractures, 82% had T-scores above the threshold criterion of −2.5.[9] Thus, it has been suggested that the value of BMD would be enhanced with additional risk factors for improved diagnostic capabilities.

Vertebral fracture is the most common result of osteoporosis in postmenopausal women older than 60 years of age. Surgical management through vertebral body augmentation involving the injection of polymethylmethacrylate (PMMA) has been diskussed as a method of fracture treatment in the literature. Understandably, the preferred course should be prevention, as opposed to surgical intervention. In addition, iatrogenic effects from vertebral body augmentation, including adjacent level implications, have not been assessed in well-controlled studies.

Analysis of available data regarding fracture in moderate-risk patient populations shows that the increase in fracture risk with decreasing age-adjusted BMD and other factors, including a prior history of fractures, are also important considerations. In short, not all patients diagnosed with current threshold values for osteoporosis will go on to fracture. Moreover, not all patients above the osteopenic level will be free of fracture related to bone structure and density.

## BMD AND IMPLICATIONS ON INSTRUMENTED PROCEDURES

Another use for BMD as measured by DXA is to determine the quality of bone for screw purchase. BMD has been shown to be correlated to pull-out strength, and for many fixation devices, screw purchase plays an important role in providing immediate stability and longer-term fixation. The screw-bone interface is integral to many constructs, such as anterior cervical plating and lumbar pedicle screw fixation, and adequate screw purchase is necessary for treatment of any spinal pathology depending on such instrumentation for stabilization and fixation. In patients showing an insufficient BMD, purchase becomes cause for concern. For the osteoporotic spine, the screw-bone interface may be augmented through various techniques in order to provide additional purchase strength. However, methods such as augmentation through PMMA should be exercised with caution, as complications may arise from the use of bone cement.

Biomechanical measures used to test screw-bone interfaces have been evaluated in a number of different ways. Axial pull-out strength has been frequently reported in the literature, including in human cadaveric spines that would be considered osteoporotic. Figure 8-2 illustrates a common test method for determining axial screw-bone interface strength. However, cyclical loading has been suggested to mimic more realistic modes of failure for implanted constructs. Studies have examined bending failure as an appropriate method of loading.[10]

The limitation of any test protocol is the ability to directly compare against native human conditions. Several of the published studies have considered various test materials including both cadaveric and synthetic test specimens. The utility of such tests should still be recognized but it must be tempered with an appropriate understanding of the clinical ramifications. Testing on cadaveric animal models is a consideration that should be taken

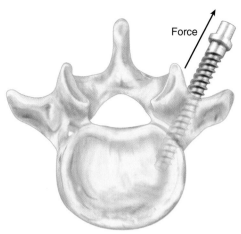

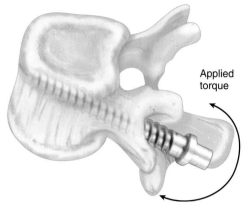

■ **FIGURE 8-2** Method of testing the screw-bone interface strength in axial pull-out.

■ **FIGURE 8-3** Application of cyclical bending moments necessary for creating "windshield-wiper" failures.

into account when evaluating screw-bone interface results. Bending modes of failures are considered more realistic complications, but test protocols are more difficult to execute. This is often due to the difficulty in defining the appropriate test methodology.

The bending moment and the associated load levels are one set of test parameters. A depiction of testing the effects of the screw-bone interface through bending moments in vertebrae is shown in Figure 8-3. The construct configuration is another study design consideration with implications for unilateral versus bilateral constructs with and without crosslinks. Fatigue is also another major factor difficult to mimic in a cadaveric test environment during biomechanical testing. Screw pull-out tests can be performed along the bone screw axis, but the flexion-extension type of bending should be executed under a cyclical protocol that eventually fails the screw-bone interface through off-bone screw axis loading. This results in a markedly different biomechanical response at the FSU and, in turn, may have different complications, for example, screw loosening. Gau et al reported modes of radiological failure in a clinical radiographic study that examined implanted constructs that exhibited "windshield-wipering," which may be an indication of bending fatigue at the screw-bone interface, and classified them accordingly.[11] Interestingly, these were not symptomatic complications.

The ability to derive a specific BMD measurement has been published in a study by Wittenberg et al[12] The authors hypothesized an equivalent mineral density of 90 mg/ml from quantitative computed tomography (qCT) as a threshold level to expect complications associated with screw loosening and 120 mg/ml as a threshold for fewer problems. This has not been validated in a clinical outcomes trial. Often, it is surgeon perception on the adequacy of bony purchase that governs the decision to instrument a patient with hardware. Additional data to provide a validated standardized DXA metric with positively correlated clinical outcomes for specific threshold levels would provide a higher confidence in BMD measurements as a preoperative indicator for instrumented procedures.

## DUAL ENERGY X-RAY ABSORPTIOMETRY AND MECHANICAL STRENGTH

The mechanical properties of both a FSU and its components may be analyzed by a number of different measurements and techniques. For ultimate strength and stiffness property studies, both localized indentation studies as well as compressive failure tests of vertebral bodies en bloc and complete FSUs have been reported in the literature. Due to differences used in the test protocols to determine strength, the correlation between bone mineral content (BMC) and BMD as reflected by DXA measurements have varied with failure loads.

Studies have shown the failure strength of vertebral bodies as measured by indentation testing differs between superior and inferior endplates; and also between locations on the same vertebral body endplate; for example, posterolateral regions tend to have the highest relative strength. With exceptions, the authors concluded from their study that a decrease in BMC correlated to a decrease in strength. In addition, the same research

group[13] later reported removal of the endplate resulted in a significant decrease in compressive failure strength. However, it was not clear if removal of the endplate affected DXA measurements.

DXA is a measurement reflective of the underlying bone mineralization. In order to determine the effects of surgical site preparation, for example., removal of the cartilaginous endplate for intervertebral spacer implants, the effects of surgical approaches on the structural integrity should be understood. DXA and vertebral strength have been shown to correlate closely in the native state. Vertebral body endplates have been shown to affect failure strength. When overly manipulated, the endplates can potentially result in the collapse of a vertebral body, but the relationship between iatrogenic complications due to surgical preparation and implant stiffness coupled with low BMD patients has not been studied.

The consistency of DXA measurements, particularly as it relates to strength, is dependent upon a number of factors, including artifacts from soft tissue. The correlations are especially problematic with higher BMD content. In a study utilizing DXA and cadaveric spine positioning, Myers et al suggested clinical studies to confirm supine lateral patient positioning would be more effective in determining BMD measurements.[14] The aging phenomenon that occurs within every human body may potentially cause global osteoarthritic changes, including BMC and BMD within the spine, that subsequently affect local DXA measurements. Utilizing animal models to control the homogeneity of specimens has not resulted in more significant correlations between BMD and strength. Contrarily, in a study involving porcine cervical spines,[15] the investigators reported no significant correlation between BMC or BMD with compressive failure strength. Furthermore, large animal models rarely exhibit vertebral body fractures even with reduced BMD levels, and thus would not be characterized into high risk for low-trauma fracture categories.

In conclusion, DXA has been a widely used indicator for osteoporotic patients and for assessing the risk of fracture. Potentially, it has validity as a gauge for the screw-bone interface in axial pull-out, but the more complex modes of loading often found in bone-anchoring devices require a better understanding of the failure modes. In addition, with the current DXA standard as an indicator for bone strength, the implications of implant failures and resistance to fracture are not well defined for T-scores above −2.5. However, other modalities exist that may augment the current metrics in quantifying the usefulness of current BMD measurements.

## MODIC CLASSIFICATION OF VERTEBRAL ENDPLATE CHANGE

Degenerative changes of the lumbar spine have been observed with MRI techniques. Specific signal changes from vertebral body endplates and marrow have been differentiated through imaging techniques that increased tissue contrast. A classification system of MRI scans using two different pulse sequences was published by Modic et al[16] Optimizing T1 and T2 relaxation times in pulse sequences during MRI studies helped define and characterize the imaged tissues. Three different types of change were recognized from T1-weighted and T2-weighted MRI scans of the same spine segment. The following is the accepted classification used for Modic changes:

Type 1: hypointense on T1-weighted and hyperintense on T2-weighted MRI signal

Type 2: hyperintense on T1-weighted and hyperintense on T2-weighted MRI signal

Type 3: hypointense on T1-weighted and hypointense on T2-weighted MRI signal

The interobserver and intraobserver error in a clinical study has been documented and the consistency of this imaging classification system was confirmed.[17] The study involved five independent observers of various clinical spine experience who graded 50 sagittal T1-weighted and T2-weighted MRI scans. The evaluation of the same scans was repeated by each participant following a 3-week interval with no reference to the first assessment. The intraobserver agreement, or consistency between the first and second evaluations by the same observer, was assessed based on Landis and Koch's use of the kappa statistic,[18] which was equal to 0.71. Additionally, interobserver agreement or consistency among all the observers was calculated to be 0.85 for the study. This study demonstrated the intraobserver agreement was substantial while interobserver agreement was excellent for the Modic classifications.

Although the original imaging studies were designed to investigate degenerative disc disease, the impact of these changes is not well understood nor is the clinical implication. One of the early findings of Modic type 1 change was fissures in the endplates, which were confirmed by histological findings. The intensity changes from MRI scans have been deduced to reflect osteocartilaginous fracture signs. Disc herniations that include components of the endplate, namely hyaline cartilage, are then suggestive of avulsion-type disc herniations. Reportedly, this form of intervertebral disc herniation is predominant in the elderly and may warrant investigations into failure strength.

## Magnetic Resonance Imaging and Modic Changes in 40-Year-Old Men and Women

A 5-year prospective study was conducted on a large sample of 40-year-old men and women drawn from the general population.[19] In this study, every ninth person born in the county of Funen, Denmark between May 27, 1959 and May 26, 1960 was selected by the Central Office of Civil Registration. Of the 625 selected study subjects, 412 agreed to participate (66%). The study included 199 males and 213 females.

Of the total number of participants, 92 patients (22%) had Modic changes. This was considered as a rare event when compared to other measured factors. For example, irregular nucleus shape was found in 306 patients (74%). Nonetheless, Modic changes were strongly associated with lower back pain (LBP) occurring within the year prior to the study. Of the 92 patients exhibiting Modic changes, 81 had LBP in this time interval while the remaining 11 did not.

## Significance of the Modic Classification to the Degenerative Process in the Spine

The changes within the Modic classification are generally accepted to signal a change within the FSU, which is composed of both vertebral bodies and the intervertebral disc. The structural components of the FSU include the superior vertebral body as well as the inferior body. In addition, a normal intervertebral disc can also be considered structural and is capable of transmitting load from one vertebral body to the other. However, over time, this capability within a patient's FSU may become diminished due to aging and its effects.

The complex loading vectors absorbed and transmitted by a FSU will change as the aging process affects specific components of the FSU. Vertebral bodies are subjected to changes that include fissuring, regenerating chondrocytes, and granulation tissue. Morever, the hydrostatic condition of the intervertebral disc may become altered and potentially result in reduction of hydration in the disc. From an imaging standpoint, an MRI study has shown a T2-weighted image was reduced in intensity when correlated to a loss of hydration and proteoglycan content. Such changes may eventually

lead to abnormal distribution of load at the endplates and thus potentially result in morphological change, e.g., amorphous fibrocartilage within the nucleus, as well as loss in functionality.

Changes to FSUs are sufficiently widespread that they are considered a part of the normal phenomenon of senescence. From a clinical perspective, the Modic type 1 changes are considered more acute changes, with fissures in the vertebral endplates. Type 2 changes are consistent with fatty degeneration of the bone marrow. Type 3 changes are observed in vertebral bodies exhibiting sclerotic changes. Additionally, Modic has shown that type 1 changes may convert to type 2 changes within 1 to 3 years. However, it remains to be proven whether type 2 and type 3 changes must first take on the characteristics of a type 1 change. Due to these known changes within the vertebrae, failure strength studies on the vertebral bodies exhibiting Modic changes would seem logical.

Studies should combine DXA measurement with imaging classifications, i.e., Modic changes of the vertebral body endplates, to enhance prediction based on relationships with compressive failure strength and subsequent intraoperative and postoperative implications. Current DXA-based osteoporosis measures are good models for high-risk patients, but all at-risk patient groups may benefit from more comprehensive indicators. Modic changes have not been tested for correlations to BMD or compressive vertebral strengths, but have been studied relative to degenerative changes within the spine. Understanding the relationship between Modic changes and vertebral strength could potentially augment DXA measurements for bone quality and subsequent risk of fracture with patients outside the current high-risk category. Finally, the ability to assist in determining appropriate treatments for low BMD patients at risk of traumatic fracture and predicting the clinical outcome is the end goal of clinically relevant biomechanics of the senescent spine.

## References

1. J.A. Miller, C. Schmatz, A.B. Schultz, Lumbar disc degeneration: correlation with age, sex, and spine level in 600 autopsy specimens, Spine 13 (1988) 173–178.
2. W.H. Kirkaldy-Willis, H.F. Farfan, Instability of the lumbar spine, Clin. Orthop. Relat. Res. 165 (1982) 110–123.
3. M.M. Panjabi, Biomechanical evaluation of spinal fixation devices: I. A conceptual framework, Spine 13 (1988) 1129–1134.
4. V.K. Goel, M.M. Panjabi, A.G. Patwardhan, et al., Test protocols for evaluation of spinal implants, J. Bone Joint Surg. Am. 2 (88 Suppl) (2006) 103–109.
5. M. Mimura, M.M. Panjabi, T.R. Oxland, et al., Disc degeneration affects the multidirectional flexibility of the lumbar spine, Spine 19 (1994) 1371–1380.
6. D. Board, B.D. Stemper, N. Yoganandan, et al., Biomechanics of the aging spine, Biomed. Sci. Instrum. 42 (2006) 1–6.
7. C. Sforza, G. Grassi, N. Fragnito, et al., Three-dimensional analysis of active head and cervical spine range of motion: effect of age in healthy male subjects, Clin. Biomech. (Bristol, Avon) 17 (2002) 611–614.
8. A.K. Simpson, D. Biswas, J.W. Emerson, et al., Quantifying the effects of age, gender, degeneration, and adjacent level degeneration on cervical spine range of motion using multivariate analyses, Spine 33 (2008) 183–186.
9. E.S. Siris, Y.T. Chen, T.A. Abbott, et al., Bone mineral density thresholds for pharmacological intervention to prevent fractures, Arch. Intern. Med. 164 (2004) 1108–1112.
10. R.F. McLain, T.O. McKinley, S.A. Yerby, et al., The effect of bone quality on pedicle screw loading in axial instability: a synthetic model, Spine 22 (1997) 1454–1460.
11. Y.L. Gau, J.E. Lonstein, R.B. Winter, et al., Luque-Galveston procedure for correction and stabilization of neuromuscular scoliosis and pelvic obliquity: a review of 68 patients, J. Spinal Disord. 4 (1991) 399–410.
12. R.H. Wittenberg, M. Shea, D.E. Swartz, et al., Importance of bone mineral density in instrumented spine fusions, Spine 16 (1991) 647–652.
13. T.R. Oxland, J.P. Grant, M.F. Dvorak, et al., Effects of endplate removal on the structural properties of the lower lumbar vertebral bodies, Spine 28 (2003) 771–777.
14. B.S. Myers, K.B. Arbogast, B. Lobaugh, et al., Improved assessment of lumbar vertebral body strength using supine lateral dual-energy x-ray absorptiometry, J. Bone Miner. Res. 9 (1994) 687–693.
15. R.J. Parkinson, J.L. Durkin, J.P. Callaghan, Estimating the compressive strength of the porcine cervical spine: an examination of the utility of DXA, Spine 30 (2005) E492–E498.
16. M.T. Modic, P.M. Steinberg, J.S. Ross, et al., Degenerative disc disease: assessment of changes in vertebral body marrow with MR imaging, Radiology 166 (1988) 193–199.
17. A. Jones, A. Clarke, B.J. Freeman, et al., The Modic classification: inter- and intraobserver error in clinical practice, Spine 30 (2005) 1867–1869.
18. J.R. Landis, G.G. Koch, An application of hierarchical kappa-type statistics in the assessment of majority agreement among multiple observers, Biometrics 33 (1977) 363–374.
19. P. Kjaer, C. Leboeuf-Yde, L. Korsholm, et al., Magnetic resonance imaging and low back pain in adults: a diagnostic imaging study of 40-year-old men and women, Spine 30 (2005) 1173–1180.

# 9

# Non-Invasive Strength Analysis of the Spine Using Clinical CT Scans

*Tony M. Keaveny*

**K E Y   P O I N T S**

- Most spine surgery candidates over age 50 are either osteopenic or osteoporotic.

- Biomechanical computed tomography (BCT) techniques can be used on clinical CT scans to provide measures of both vertebral density and strength.

- Clinical research studies have shown that the biomechanical outcomes from BCT are more highly associated with fracture risk for the spine than is bone mineral density.

- Vertebral strength as measured by BCT can provide earlier and additional insight compared to dual-energy absorptiometry (DXA) for monitoring therapeutic treatment effects at the spine.

- It may be possible in the future to use BCT to assess the strength and stability of various bone-implant systems for surgical planning and patient monitoring.

## INTRODUCTION

Osteoporosis is widely recognized as an underdiagnosed and undertreated disease. According to the National Osteoporosis Foundation and the National Institutes of Health, 10 million Americans are estimated to have osteoporosis, and another 34 million are at increased risk due to low bone mass, but only about 20% of those eligible to be screened are actually tested and only a fraction of those are positively diagnosed and treated. Above age 50, the density of vertebral trabecular bone decreases at a rate of about 2.2% to 3.0% per year for women, depending on age, and by about 1.7% to 2.5% per year for men,[1] with about 700,000 osteoporotic spine fractures occurring annually in the united States[2].

Management of osteoporosis in the over-50 age group is important both to avoid such fractures and to optimize spine surgery outcomes. A recent study from Taiwan[3] estimated that for all major spine surgical cases, not including vertebroplasty or kyphoplasty, 47% of women and 46% of men over age 50 had low bone mass or "osteopenia" — a BMD T-score of between −1.0 and −2.5 — and 44% of women and 12% of men had osteoporosis — a BMD T-score of less than −2.5. As the size of the aging population continues to increase, a huge and growing proportion of spine surgery patients may have compromised bone strength. This presents a challenge to the spine surgeon using any sort of instrumentation or implant for stabilization, since the underlying bone and the bone-implant interface need to be strong enough to sustain the stresses both from daily activities and spurious overloads.

From a patient-management perspective, it would be desirable clinically to be able to identify more patients at high risk of vertebral fracture. These patients can then be placed on an appropriate therapeutic treatment, which typically reduces fracture risk by about 50%. For spine surgery, surgical planning and postoperative patient management might be improved by identifying patients with compromised bone strength. Improved information on vertebral strength on a patient-specific basis might provide an objective basis for evaluation of actual surgical options, including type and size of implant. In addition to the condition being treated surgically, many spine surgery patients have compromised vertebral strength, which, if recognized, could be treated postoperatively with appropriate therapeutic agents.

A number of different types of imaging modalities are now available for noninvasive assessment of bone density, structure, and strength.[4] The dual-energy x-ray (DXA) scan is the current clinical standard for bone density assessment. However, DXA for the spine has a number of limitations. Being a 2D imaging modality, a DXA scan combines all bone morphology in the anterior-posterior direction. Thus, arthritic changes in the posterior elements, degenerative osteophytic growths around the endplates, and aortic calcification all produce bone mineral density increases in the DXA scan — increases that confound the measurement of bone mineral density in the load-bearing vertebral body. DXA scans also provide very limited information on the morphology, density, or strength of the pedicles. As a result of these limitations, DXA of the spine is less predictive of the risk of osteoporotic fractures than is DXA of the hip, DXA of the spine can be highly misleading in terms of measuring actual bone mineral density of the vertebrae or pedicles, and there remains a need for improved strength and fracture risk assessment of the spine.

Computed tomography (CT), being a 3D imaging modality, provides a powerful alternative to DXA and is preferable to magnetic resonance imaging (MRI) for bone strength assessment since it provides quantitative information on bone mineral density.[4] One limitation with CT analysis is the difficulty of interpreting the large amount of information in the scan in terms of a clinically relevant outcome such as bone strength. This is because a low value of bone mineral density at a particular location within the bone does not necessarily indicate a problem with overall bone strength. Conversely, such a local decrease in density may not show up in an averaged measure of bone mineral density, but may be problematic if that local decrease in density occurs in such a location as to appreciably compromise strength. To overcome this limitation, a sophisticated engineering structural computational analysis technique known as "finite element analysis" can be applied to CT scans to provide an estimate of vertebral strength,[5] in much the same way as engineers perform computational strength analysis of such complex 3D structures as bridges, aircraft components, and engine parts (Figure 9-1). The resulting "biomechanical computed tomography" (BCT) technology, which represents a post hoc analysis of a clinical CT exam, is now being used in a variety of clinical research studies that address vertebral strength, aging, osteoporosis and its various therapeutic treatments. Because BCT creates a mechanical model of the patient's bone, it can also be adapted to include a virtual implant and in that way provide estimates of strength and stability of various bone-implant constructs — all from analysis of a patient's preoperative CT scan.

## Clinical Case

The following analysis of proximal junction kyphosis is a *hypothetical case* to illustrate how strength estimates from BCT analysis could eventually be used clinically to provide spine surgeons with quantitative information as part of the decision-making process in preoperative surgical planning. This case also illustrates how BCT can currently be used for diagnosis of vertebral osteoporosis using clinical CT scans.

A 68-year-old woman presented with an overtly unstable spine involving circumferential disruption of the spinal column around the level of the thoracolumbar junction, including insults to both the vertebral body and posterior elements. Based on a physical exam and review of x-rays and CT and MRI scans of T10 through L2, the surgeon decided to decompress and fuse the T12-L1 disc and provide support by rigid pedicle screw fixation. Because of the patient's age, the surgeon was unsure about the possibility of osteoporosis. A review of this patient's medical record revealed that she had a DXA exam of both the hip and spine two years previously, which showed a T-score at the hip (femoral neck) of −2.2 and of the (total) spine of −1.8. Thus, this patient just missed being diagnosed as having osteoporosis as defined by WHO guidelines (any T-score of less than −2.5), but it was unclear as to the status of her osteoporosis classification at the time of surgery, particularly for her spine which had appeared to have a more normal T-score than the hip. To address these issues, the surgeon ordered a BCT analysis to be performed on the preoperative CT exam, focusing on the undamaged levels in order to assess risk of vertebral fracture for the postoperative situation.

The BCT analysis was used to estimate the vertebral strength for T10 and L2 in order to better assess the osteoporotic status of the vertebrae (Table 9-1). Analysis of the scans showed substantial posterior arthritic changes and that the bone strength was three standard deviations lower than the mean value for a young reference population. The volumetric density scores of the trabecular bone based on the CT data indicated low trabecular bone density — almost in the osteoporosis range — but they did not reflect that this patient had low cortical density and relatively small bones, both of which also contributed to her very low bone strength. The DXA spinal T-scores were therefore misleading because of the substantial posterior calcification, arthritic changes, low cortical density, and small bone size. Calculations of the strength-capacity — which take into consideration the expected magnitude of the in vivo forces acting on the patient's spine (see later in the chapter for more details) — were in the 60% range, indicating that the strength of this patient's vertebra was only about 60% of what it should be in order to safely lift a 10-kg object with back bent (a "worst case" strenuous loading condition). Based on these findings, the surgeon instrumented from T12-L1, advised the patient of her elevated risk of vertebral fracture, and referred her for an endocrine consultation.

## BASIC SCIENCE

### Aging of the Spine

Substantial changes occur to vertebrae with aging. Cadaver studies have shown that whole vertebral strength decreases by about 12% per decade from ages 25 to 85 (Figure 9-2). Although these changes are due primarily to a loss of bone density, which is offset in part by subtle increases in bone size, the loss of cortical bone is generally not as pronounced as the loss of the trabecular bone.[1] DXA generally is unable to distinguish between cortical and trabecular bone in the spine, due to its projectional nature. Aging of the spine is also accompanied by osteoarthritic changes (formation of osteophytes, etc.) around the disc and endplates. Again, due to projectional limitations, such degenerative changes are manifested as increases in BMD on DXA exams — effectively adding noise to the BMD signal from the more

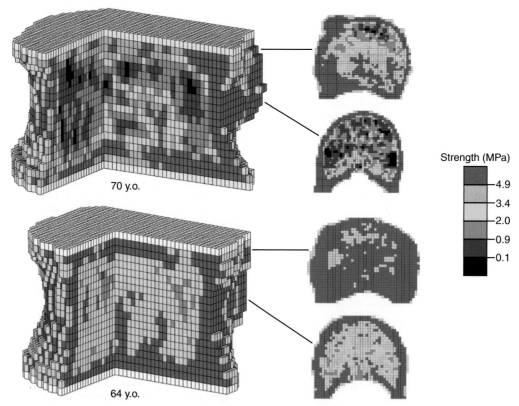

Strength (MPa)

— 4.9
— 3.4
— 2.0
— 0.9
— 0.1

70 y.o.

64 y.o.

■ **FIGURE 9-1** Details of BCT models for two women, showing sectioned view of the finite element model and two cross-sections for each. The colors indicate different values of material strength assigned to the individual finite elements within each model, which are obtained from quantitative analysis of the calibrated gray scale information in the patient's CT scan. *(Reproduced from Melton LJ, Riggs BL, Keaveny TM, Achenbach SJ, Hoffmann PF, Camp JJ, Rouleau PA, Bouxsein ML, Amin S, Atkinson EJ, Robb RA, Khosla S: Structural determinants of vertebral fracture risk, J Bone Miner Res 22:1885-1892, 2007, Fig 1.)*

biomechanically relevant vertebral body portion of the spine. There is also substantial heterogeneity in trabecular strength across the population at any age (Figure 9-2). Thus, although advanced age is associated with low bone strength, age, sex, and DXA information are inadequate for clinical assessment of vertebral strength for an individual patient.

## Finite Element Analysis of CT Scans — Biomechanical Computed Tomography

Because of the above-mentioned concerns over the fidelity of DXA scans for the spine and the substantial heterogeneity across patients in vertebral bone, quantitative CT is preferred for bone density assessment in the spine.[4] However, CT alone provides density measures in preselected regions of interest within the vertebra, e.g., trabecular centrum vs. trabecular bone near the endplates vs. all trabecular bone vs. all trabecular bone plus the cortex, etc., and such outcomes can be difficult to interpret with respect to actual strength of either the isolated vertebra or a vertebral bone-implant construct. In addition, use of CT-derived density data alone would be difficult for assessment of different surgical options because there would be no way to measure any biomechanical effect of the implant on stresses in the bone. To overcome these limitations, clinical CT scans can now be converted into biomechanical structural models of the patient's bones in a highly automated and repeatable fashion using a combination of sophisticated imaging processing and finite element modeling. This technology, termed biomechanical

computed tomography (BCT) because it represents a biomechanical analysis of a CT scan, has the main advantage of providing a strength outcome that is integrative in nature, not requiring specification of any particular region of interest with the bone. It can also account for typical in vivo loading conditions and can be used on isolated vertebrae, motion segments, or bones with virtually implanted prostheses. With appropriate comparison versus population reference values and biomechanical threshold values, such information can be used to assist the physician in various stages of the decision-making process during patient management.

The BCT technique, first introduced clinically in the early 1990s but substantially refined since then, starts by converting the gray scale Hounsfield Unit data in the standard DICOM-formatted CT image into calibrated values of bone mineral density. External calibration phantoms are typically placed underneath the patient during imaging in osteoporosis research studies, but phantomless calibration can be used clinically. After calibration of the gray scale values, the bone of interest is separated from the surrounding tissue via a variety of image processing techniques. The finite element mesh is then created from this processed bone image in which each finite element is assigned local material properties based on the calibrated gray scale information in the CT scan. Such material properties-density relations are derived from cadaver experiments. The final step is to apply loading conditions typical of habitual activities or more spurious overloads, depending on the clinical application. A finite element stress analysis is performed to compute the strength of the vertebra under the applied loading conditions — in essence, a virtual stress test. Models can be created of the vertebra alone, of the vertebra with surrounding soft tissue, of multiple vertebrae, or of a vertebra with a virtually implanted prosthesis, and analyses can be run for single or multiple loading conditions.

BCT has been used for over two decades in orthopedic laboratory research to study the mechanical behavior of such bones as the femur, humerus, radius, tibia, cranium, and vertebra, with and without implants, and more recently has found use in a number of clinical research studies. It has been well validated in cadaver studies, for both the hip and spine, and has consistently been found to be a better predictor of measured cadaveric strength than is BMD as measured by either DXA or quantitative CT alone. The technique is now undergoing extensive clinical validation for a variety of osteoporosis clinical applications. In the first published study of clinical BCT,[6] it was found that a measure of lumbar vertebral strength better discriminated between osteoporotic and non-osteoporotic subjects

**TABLE 9-1   Output Data from the BCT Analysis for Levels T10 to L2**

| Level | CT Density mg/cm³ | CT Density T* | BCT Strength Newtons | BCT Strength T* | Strength Capacity % |
|-------|-------|-----|-------|-----|-----|
| T10 | 105 | −2.3 | 1050 | −2.9 | 62 |
| L2 | 102 | −2.4 | 1140 | −3.0 | 60 |

*T-scores calculated as number of standard deviations below young reference mean.

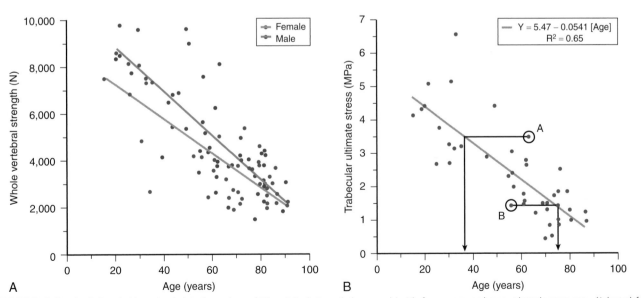

■ **FIGURE 9-2   A,** Cadaveric biomechanical testing values of L2 vertebral strength (expressed in N), for women and men, plotted versus age. *(Adapted from Mosekilde L, Mosekilde L: Sex differences in age-related changes in vertebral body size, density and biomechanical competence in normal individuals, Bone 11:67-73, 1990.)*

**B,** Ultimate compressive stress of human vertebral trabecular bone cores (expressed in MPa), versus age, obtained by biomechanical testing of cadaveric material. Despite the clear trend for decreasing strength with advancing age, age is not a very sensitive indicator of bone strength for any given individual. For example, subject A, although older than subject B, has trabecular strength more typical of a 37-year-old, whereas subject B's trabecular strength is closer to that of a typical 75-year-old. *(Adapted from Mosekilde L, Mosekilde L; Normal vertebral body size and compressive strength: relations to age and to vertebral and iliac trabecular bone compressive strength, Bone 7:207-212, 1986.)*

than did bone density (Figure 9-3). In a more recent study, BCT has been shown to differentiate those with prevalent vertebral fractures from those without, after accounting for age and despite areal BMD not being able to differentiate the fracture from no-fracture groups.[7] BCT has also been used to assess the effects of various drug treatments at the spine and can detect statistically significant between-treatment effects in the spine earlier than can DXA. [8]

In addition to providing measures of vertebral density and strength, BCT can also be used to implement controlled variations of the patient-specific models to produce additional strength outcomes of potential clinical significance. For example, by virtually peeling away the outer layer of bone and then running a second virtual stress test for strength analysis of the remaining bone, it is possible to quantify the strength effects associated with just the trabecular or cortical compartment.[8] Such studies have shown, for example, that strength associated with the outer two millimeters of bone in the vertebral body (which encompasses the cortical shell) is highly predictive of fracture at the spine groups[7] and can be differentially affected versus the trabecular compartment by various drug treatments.[8,9] The BCT technique so far has been used only in clinical research studies and is not yet FDA-approved.

## CLINICAL PRACTICE GUIDELINES

Given that there are no clinical practice guidelines available yet for BCT, a number of general issues related to interpretation are discussed instead. Results from the BCT analysis can be interpreted in a number of ways. As with the approach for bone density analysis with DXA or quantitative CT, values of bone strength can be compared against age-matched population values (so-called Z-scores) and against young normal reference values (so-called T-scores). A Z-score of −2.0, for example, indicates that the patient has a bone strength of two standard deviations below the mean of their sex-matched age group. A T-score of −2.0 indicates that the patient has a bone strength of two standard deviations below the mean of their sex-matched "young" (aged 20 to 30 years) reference group. A decision to treat can be based on where a patient stands with respect to such population reference values. Bone density values, which are measured as part of the BCT analysis,

can also be used in the patient evaluation. Another approach is to treat based on biomechanical threshold values, much as a DXA BMD T-score of −2.5 is commonly used to define osteoporosis.

Another outcome from the BCT analysis beyond strength is the "strength-capacity" (aka the "safety factor" in engineering analysis), defined as the ratio of the strength of the bone to the magnitude of the estimated applied in vivo force acting on the bone. This is the reciprocal of the "load-to-strength" ratio often used in biomechanics research studies.[10] The lower the value of the strength-capacity, the higher is the likelihood of fracture in the event of the simulated event, e.g., for the spine, bending over and lifting 10 kg. For example, if the vertebral strength for a patient's L2 was computed to be 2000 N, and the estimated in vivo force for lifting a 10 kg object with back bent was 3000 N, the strength-capacity of the patient's L2 vertebra for this activity would be 2000/3000 = 66%. This indicates that the patient's bone has only 66% of the strength necessary to safely engage in this lifting activity. While, in theory, strength-capacity values less than 100% would indicate that the bone is too weak to withstand the applied in vivo forces, because of the difficulty of estimating in vivo forces in an absolute accurate sense, strength-capacity values are, at present, best interpreted in relative terms. The in vivo force for a given activity can be calculated as part of the BCT analysis using such patient-specific information as weight and height, and various skeletal measurements obtained from the patient's CT exam including muscle size and location.

A third approach is to base treatment decisions on an absolute risk of fracture, which can be obtained based on analysis of fracture surveillance or other clinical outcome studies. Based on cost-effectiveness or other criteria, the physician can decide to treat if the absolute risk exceeds some critical value. As with all new technologies, as BCT is used more in the clinic, the accumulated evidence in support of how the outcomes can be best used for clinical decision making will accumulate, which in turn should lead to more objective and evidence-based guidelines for patient management and surgical planning.

## CLINICAL CASE EXAMPLES

A number of examples are presented to illustrate how BCT has been used so far in clinical research studies to assess vertebral strength responses to different types of drug therapies for osteoporotic and rheumatoid arthritis patients, and also to assess risk of osteoporotic vertebral fracture.

### Comparing Teriparatide and Alendronate for Treatment of Osteoporosis

Teriparatide and alendronate increase bone mineral density through opposite effects on bone remodeling, namely via anabolic and antiresorptive actions, respectively. In this study[8], two randomly assigned groups of postmenopausal osteoporotic women (N=28 teriparatide; N=25 alendronate) who had quantitative CT scans of the spine at baseline and postbaseline (6 months and 18 months) were analyzed with BCT for L3 vertebral compressive strength. At 18 months, patients in both treatment groups had increased vertebral strength, the median percentage increase being over five-fold greater for teriparatide (Figure 9-4). Larger increases in the ratio of strength to density were observed for teriparatide, and these were primarily attributed to preferential increases in trabecular strength that occurred only for this treatment. At 6 months, the between-treatment effect was statistically significant for vertebral strength but not for BMD, demonstrating the ability of BCT to differentiate treatment effects earlier than DXA. Further, median changes in the BCT-measured vertebral strength for the teriparatide and alendronate groups were 4.9% and 13.0%, respectively, and for DXA-measured spine BMD were 2.0% and 3.4%, respectively, indicating that changes were generally much larger for BCT than for DXA.

### Alendronate Treatment in Rheumatoid Arthritic Patients

In this study,[9] BCT analysis was applied to 29 rheumatoid arthritic patients, randomly assigned to be treated or not with either alendronate for their osteoporosis, but most of whom were on some sort of steroidal medication for their rheumatoid arthritis. Results indicated that, after 12 months

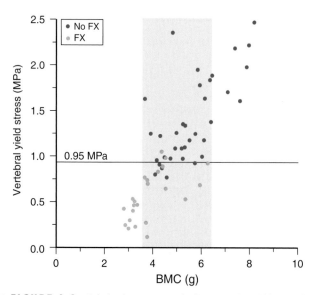

■ **FIGURE 9-3**    Relation between vertebral compressive yield stress (vertebral strength divided by its cross-sectional area) as measured by BCT and total bone mineral content of the vertebra as measured by quantitative CT, for individuals either having a radiographically confirmed osteoporotic vertebral fracture (FX) or having normal bone without any vertebral fracture (No FX). Note that between BMC values of about 4 to 6 g, most patients with osteoporosis had lower values of vertebral yield stress. A threshold point of 0.95 MPa for vertebral yield stress (shown above) was identified as having greater diagnostic accuracy than a traditional trabecular bone mineral density threshold. *(Adapted from Faulkner KG, Cann CE, Hasegawa BH: Effect of bone distribution on vertebral strength: assessment with patient-specific nonlinear finite element analysis, Radiology 179:669-674, 1991.)*

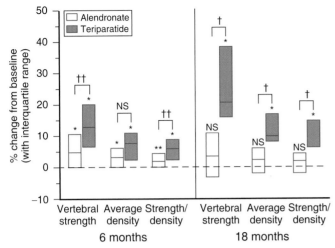

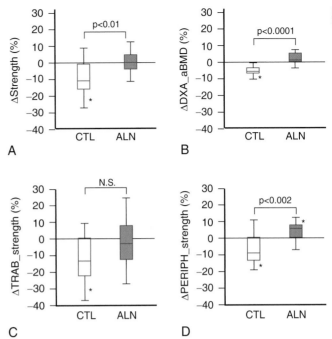

■ **FIGURE 9-4** Median percent change in BCT-predicted whole vertebral compressive strength, average vertebral density as measured by quantitative CT, and the ratio of whole vertebral compressive strength to average vertebral density in teriparatide-treated and alendronate-treated women, after 6 and 18 months of treatment. In each box, the line represents the median, the upper end of the box is the 75th interquartile range, and the lower end of box is the 25th interquartile range. *$p < 0.001$ and **$p < 0.05$ within group from baseline; †$p < 0.001$, ††$p < 0.01$ between group; NS, nonsignificant. At 6 months, between-treatment effects were statistically significant for strength but not for average density. Changes in the ratio of strength to density were also statistically different between treatments, indicating a between-treatment effect beyond an average density effect. *(Adapted from Keaveny TM, Donley DW, Hoffmann PF, Mitlak BH, Glass EV, San Martin JA: Effects of teriparatide and alendronate on vertebral strength as assessed by finite element modeling of QCT scans in women with osteoporosis, J Bone Miner Res 22:149-157, 2007.)*

of treatment, there was on average a loss in the nontreated group of 10.6%, which was completely arrested with alendronate treatment, primarily by its positive effect on the outer 2 mm of vertebral bone (Figure 9-5). These results demonstrate the substantial loss of vertebral strength that can occur in RA patients and the usefulness of alendronate treatment for arresting such loss.

## Assessing Risk of Vertebral Fracture in Postmenopausal Women

Data from a cross-section study on vertebral fracture prevalence were used to compare the abilities of BMD by DXA vs. vertebral strength and the strength-capacity by BCT for vertebral fracture risk assessment[7]. Forty postmenopausal women with a clinically-diagnosed vertebral fracture (confirmed semiquantitatively) due to moderate trauma (cases: mean age, 78.6 ± 9.0 years) were identified from an age-stratified sample of Rochester, MN women, and were compared to 40 controls with no osteoporotic fracture (70.9 ± 6.8 years). Results indicated that DXA-based BMD for the spine or total hip were not significantly different between fractures and controls, but age-adjusted BCT-measures of vertebral strength and load-to-strength ratio (the reciprocal of strength-capacity) were 23% lower and 36% higher, respectively. The age-adjusted odds ratio per standard deviation increase for the load-to-strength ratio measure was 3.2 ($p < 0.05$), versus a nonsignificant value of 0.70 for spine region BMD by DXA. Thus, if an individual presented to the clinic with a load-to-strength ratio that was 2.5 SD above the age-matched average value for his or her sex, she or he would be at an 18-fold (= $3.2^{2.5}$) elevated risk of fracture compared to the age-matched average. This study demonstrates the ability of the BCT-measured load-to-strength ratio (and thus its reciprocal, the strength-capacity) to provide additional fracture predictive ability compared to DXA-measured BMD.

## DISCUSSION

The combination of finite element modeling with clinical CT scans — biomechanical computed tomography — is a powerful research technique to noninvasively assess vertebral strength and is now finding its way into

■ **FIGURE 9-5** Percent change over 12 months from baseline in BCT-predicted vertebral strength (**A**), DXA-measured areal BMD (**B**), trabecular compartment (TRAB) strength (**C**) and peripheral compartment (PERIPH) strength (**D**), in alendronate-treated (ALN) and not-treated (CTL) groups of rheumatoid arthritic patients. The peripheral compartment comprises the outer 2 mm of bone, including the thin cortical shell and adjacent trabecular bone. Data are presented as box plots, where the boxes represent the 25th to 75th percentiles, the lines within the boxes represent the median, and the lines outside the boxes represent the 10th and 90th percentiles. *$P < 0.05$ versus baseline, NS — not significant; between-treatment effects shown with other p-values, when present. These data indicate that there is more variation seen in the patient response as captured by BCT-strength compared to DXA-BMD. Further, the protective effect of alendronate treatment is due primarily to its positive effect on the peripheral bone. Note also the substantial loss in vertebral strength for the untreated group: just over 10%, on average, and much higher for some individuals. *(Adapted from Mawatari T, Miura H, Hamai S, Shuto T, Nakashima Y, Okazaki K, Kinukawa N, Sakai S, Hoffmann PF, Iwamoto Y, Keaveny TM: Vertebral strength changes in rheumatoid arthritis patients treated with alendronate, as assessed by finite element analysis of clinical computed tomography scans: a prospective randomized clinical trial, Arthritis Rheum 58:3340-3349, 2008.)*

clinical studies. Well supported by cadaver studies, the technique is providing substantial new insight into drug treatment effects in the spine and can show treatment effects earlier than DXA. Early clinical results are providing evidence of the superiority of BCT over DXA for fracture risk assessment, although additional clinical studies are necessary to establish this more definitively. The technique is well suited for clinical use since it can be performed on preoperative and most preexisting CT exams. It also has the potential to be used in various surgical planning applications.

One clinical challenge with using BCT for fracture risk assessment is the actual need for a CT scan and the associated cost and radiation exposure. For an assessment of osteoporosis fracture risk, this leads to more radiation and a more expensive test than a traditional DXA exam. However, if the technique is used to analyze a *previously-acquired* CT exam, then the BCT fracture risk assessment analysis per se becomes less expensive than a DXA exam, more convenient than a DXA exam, and requires no extra radiation, because no new CT exam is required. Such previously-acquired CT exams would include a pelvic, spine, or abdomen CT, or such specialized CT exams as CT colonography, CT angiography, or CT for calcium scoring. Further development could lead to the application of BCT to such low-energy CT scanning techniques as intraoperative C-arm and O-arm scanning, which would be advantageous particularly for intraoperative osteoporosis screening and surgical planning.

For monitoring purposes, given the substantial advantage of using BCT to monitor treatment effects compared to DXA, performing a follow-up BCT analysis on just one vertebral level or just the proximal femur would be well-justified and could be performed earlier than a DXA exam to provide faster feedback on the patient's response to treatment. One important limitation of any CT-based exam, including BCT, is that the CT scan can be corrupted by the presence of metal hardware due to streaking artifacts, although it may be possible in the future to alleviate such artifacts within the 3D reconstruction algorithms. For the purposes of surgical planning, it is currently possible with BCT to virtually implant a prosthesis into the bone in a research setting, and in that way compute the stability or strength of the resulting bone-implant construct. Basic cadaver and clinical research studies are required to further develop such applications of BCT to the clinic and validate them with clinical outcomes. Related clinical applications for BCT include stability assessment of fracture healing and fusion constructs and strength assessment of metastasized or otherwise structurally compromised vertebrae. Given recent advances in CT technology, computer hardware power, and 3D image processing, it is expected that a variety of such advanced analysis techniques for CT scans will be available in the near future. Their integration into clinical practice where CT scans are being used should help improve management of patients with suspected osteoporosis or otherwise compromised vertebral strength.

## Acknowledgements

The author acknowledges support from the National Institutes of Health (grant AR49828). Dr. Keaveny has a financial interest in O.N. Diagnostics, and both he and the company may benefit from the results of this work.

## References

1. B.L. Riggs, L.J. Melton, R.A. Robb, J.J. Camp, E.J. Atkinson, L. McDaniel, et al., A population-based assessment of rates of bone loss at multiple skeletal sites: evidence for substantial trabecular bone loss in young adult women and men, J. Bone Miner. Res. 23 (2) (2008) 205–214.
2. L.J. Melton, Epidemiology of spinal osteoporosis, Spine 22 (Suppl. 24) (1997) 2S–11S.
3. D.K. Chin, J.Y. Park, Y.S. Yoon, S.U. Kuh, B.H. Jin, K.S. Kim, et al., Prevalence of osteoporosis in patients requiring spine surgery: incidence and significance of osteoporosis in spine disease, Osteoporosis Int. 18 (9) (2007) 1219–1224.
4. M.L. Bouxsein, Technology insight: noninvasive assessment of bone strength in osteoporosis, Nat. Clin. Pract. 4 (6) (2008) 310–318.
5. R.P. Crawford, C.E. Cann, T.M. Keaveny, Finite element models predict in vitro vertebral body compressive strength better than quantitative computed tomography, Bone 33 (4) (2003) 744–750.
6. K.G. Faulkner, C.E. Cann, B.H. Hasegawa, Effect of bone distribution on vertebral strength: assessment with patient-specific nonlinear finite element analysis, Radiology 179 (3) (1991) 669–674.
7. L.J. Melton, B.L. Riggs, T.M. Keaveny, S.J. Achenbach, P.F. Hoffmann, J.J. Camp, et al., Structural determinants of vertebral fracture risk, J. Bone Miner. Res. 22 (12) (2007) 1885–1892.
8. T.M. Keaveny, D.W. Donley, P.F. Hoffmann, B.H. Mitlak, E.V. Glass, J.A. San Martin, Effects of teriparatide and alendronate on vertebral strength as assessed by finite element modeling of QCT scans in women with osteoporosis, J. Bone Miner. Res. 22 (1) (2007) 149–157.
9. T. Mawatari, H. Miura, S. Hamai, T. Shuto, Y. Nakashima, K. Okazaki, et al., Vertebral strength changes in rheumatoid arthritis patients treated with alendronate, as assessed by finite element analysis of clinical computed tomography scans: a prospective randomized clinical trial, Arthritis Rheum. 58 (11) (2008) 3340–3349.
10. T.M. Keaveny, M.L. Bouxsein, Theoretical implications of the biomechanical fracture threshold, J. Bone Miner. Res. 23 (10) (2008) 1541–1547.

# 10

# Kinematics of the Aging Spine: A Review of Past Knowledge and Survey of Recent Developments, with a Focus on Patient-Management Implications for the Clinical Practitioner

*Adam K. Deitz, Alan C. Breen, Fiona E. Mellor, Deydre S. Teyhen, Kris W.N. Wong, Monohar M. Panjabi*

## KEY POINTS

- Functional testing of the spine (the flexion/extension and lateral bending x-rays that have been the standard of care for over 60 years) is used clinically in the detection of hypermobility and pseudarthrosis.

- Over the years, many investigators have published normative ranges of intervertebral range of motion (RoM) from asymptomatic subjects using the current standard of care; however, all of these studies have been conducted at a single clinical site and thus have not accounted for the RoM variability attributable to use of different imaging equipment and testing methods that can be found in today's clinical practice.

- By performing a meta-analysis of these studies to account for this variability among clinical sites, the authors put forward a new set of lumbar and cervical RoM thresholds for both ruling in and ruling out normal motion, hypermobility, and hypermobility.

- Many new technologies for assessing spine function have been proposed in the literature, and several of these have demonstrated the ability to deliver improved diagnostic efficacy. These newer technologies have also revealed important new insights into the function of the aging spine that have implications for the clinical practitioner.

- The authors put forward a set of suggested guidelines for the clinical use of functional testing, including suggested guidelines for the current standard of care for functional testing as well as for the newer technologies that have been proposed in the literature.

## AN INTRODUCTION TO FUNCTIONAL DIAGNOSTICS OF THE SPINE

Generally speaking, functional diagnostics are used to assess organ systems for the purpose of detecting dysfunction, identifying the underlying physiological defects, and indicating options for therapeutic intervention. For example, blood chemistry tests are used to assess liver function, while pulse rate monitoring and blood pressure testing are used to assess cardiovascular function. The spine is a series of multiarticulating joints whose primary functions are threefold: (1) to allow multidirectional motions between individual vertebrae, (2) to carry multidirectional external and internal loads, and (3) to protect the delicate spinal nerves and spinal cord. Therefore, functional diagnostics of the spine focus on the assessment and measurement of intervertebral motion under various environmental and movement conditions. The results are then used to help guide the management of patients suffering from various conditions of the spine.

In discussing spinal function as it relates to the aging spine, it is worthwhile to begin with a critical analysis of past knowledge and recent developments regarding spinal functional testing to establish a baseline understanding of the current state of orthopedic science. Such an analysis reveals that the functional testing method used in today's clinical practice — the standard flexion/extension and lateral side bending radiographs with which all practitioners are familiar — fails to deliver much useful diagnostic information, and is particularly poorly suited to the management of the aging spine. This analysis further reveals that there has never before been a comprehensive set of evidence-based guidelines put forward for the interpretation of functional testing results. This lack of a comprehensive set of evidence-based guidelines is especially problematic given that the clinical standard of care for functional testing has been part of the medical practice for seven decades, has been widely adopted by the vast majority of spine practitioners, and is routinely used on a large number of patients suffering from a wide array of spine diseases.

Therefore the objectives of this chapter are to present this critical analysis of past knowledge and recent developments regarding functional testing of the spine for the purpose of highlighting for the clinical practitioner: (1) recommendations on how best to interpret functional testing results, (2) how the interpretation of these testing results is best applied to gain insights into the kinematics of the aging spine, and (3) how newer functional testing technologies should be assessed and adopted to improve the management of the aging spine.

## THE CURRENT STATE OF THE ART: DIAGNOSTIC EFFICACY OF TODAY'S FUNCTIONAL TESTING METHOD

The current clinical standard of care for performing functional testing of the spine was introduced in the 1940s[1] and has since been the subject of scores of published investigations. Today's method is beset by multiple performance problems[2,3] and, although many practitioners are unaware of the fact, has been proven useless in differentiating normal from abnormal spinal function.[4–7] In holding true to the tenets of evidence-based medicine it is critical that, as a starting point, practitioners understand the limitations of this method so testing results are interpreted appropriately.

### Range of Motion (RoM) Measurements

Today's method for conducting functional testing of the spine (flexion/extension and lateral bending radiographs, which are referred to in this text as the clinical standard of care) involves capturing standard radiographs of the spine as subjects bend, and then hold their spines fixed in the extremes of motion in either the sagittal (in the case of flexion/extension) or coronal (in the case of lateral bending) planes. These studies are separate to, but often used as an adjunct with, other medical imaging studies such as plain radiographs or CT scans in the diagnostic assessment of a patient's spine. When performing these motions, each subject bends in each direction to his or her own maximum voluntary bending angle (MVBA).

These two images taken at the extremes of trunk bending within a single plane are then interpreted — either manually using a pen, ruler, and protractor or more recently, with the advent of digital imaging, an imaging workstation — to derive range of motion (RoM) measurements. RoM measurements represent the total displacement between any two vertebrae during MVBA bending, and are expressed as both angulations, as measured in degrees and referred to in this text as the intervertebral angle (IVA) in either the coronal or sagittal plane, and translations in the sagittal plane, measured in millimeters and referred to in this text as the intervertebral translation (IVT). See Figure 10-1 for a simplified diagram showing how IVA and IVT are derived from radiographic images.

RoM is defined by the rotation of the body (IVA) *and* the translation of a point on the body (IVT). While the rotation is unambiguous, the translation is not. The translation is different for different points of the vertebral body and, additionally, it is subject to magnification and distortion on radiographs. This ambiguity has led to: (1) the introduction of multiple techniques for selecting points on the vertebral body and measuring IVT;[2,4,8,21,22] (2) attempts to define standardized displacement thresholds for what constitutes translational instability;[9] and (3) the proposal of multiple systems for scoring and classifying translational instabilities (there have been the Myerding scale,[10] the Newman Scale,[11] and the modified Newman scale[12] for scoring translational instabilities, as well as the Wiltse[13] system for classifying them).

Despite the multiplicity of different methods that have been proposed over the years, the Myerding system has become the most widely used in clinical practice and has thus emerged as the standard system by which translational instability is graded. The Myerding system categorizes the severity of a translational instability based upon IVT measurements expressed as a percentage of the total superior vertebral body length (also measured in millimeters): grade 1 is 0% to 25%, grade 2 is 25% to 50%, and grade 3 is 50% to 75%;

Grade 4 is 75% to 100%; over 100% is spondyloptosis, when the vertebra completely falls off the supporting vertebra. One key advantage of the Myerding system is that it is a *relative* grading system, meaning that it helps to control for distortion and magnification errors that can be associated with *absolute* measurements of displacement (millimeters) derived from radiographic images.

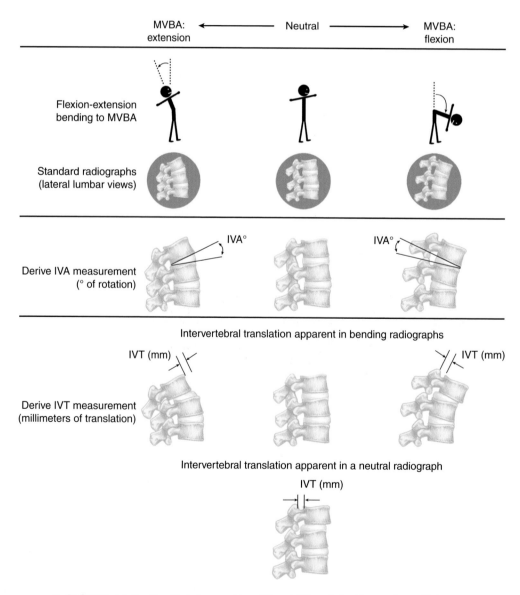

■ **FIGURE 10-1**  Simplified diagram of how IVA and IVT are derived from radiographic images.

Although IVT measurements have been the subject of intense investigation over the years, it is not a topic about which there is currently much debate. This topic was thoroughly explored in studies published in the 1970s through 1990s; however, in the past 15 to 20 years a de facto consensus has emerged with respect to the use of the Myerding system as the clinical gold standard for grading translational instability cases. The same is not true for IVA measurements, as no consensus has emerged with respect to the clinical application of IVA despite a very large volume of recent investigational activity. Therefore the remainder of this chapter will present a review of past and current knowledge with respect to IVA, with a particular focus on patient-management implications for treatment of the aging spine.

IVA is used clinically to assess intervertebral articulation in either the sagittal or coronal planes, and as such should *theoretically* be capable of detecting six specific types of intervertebral functional presentations (see Figure 10-2):

1. **Normal Motion:** IVA that is considered normal (i.e., between the second and ninety-eighth percentile of what is observed among normal healthy subjects)
2. **Hypomobility:** IVA that is abnormally low (i.e., below the second percentile). Note that stiffness and hypomobility are not the same thing; stiffness is a mechanical characteristic of the functional spinal unit (FSU), while hypomobility is a measurement representing the observed response of the FSU to gross spine bending. In that sense, hypomobility can be viewed as a proxy measurement of stiffness.*
3. **Rotational Hypermobility:** IVA that is abnormally large (i.e., above the ninety-eighth percentile). In today's medical practice, rotational hypermobility is considered a form of instability.
4. **Immobility:** The lack of any motion at all (IVA = 0°). In practice, the U.S. Food and Drug Administration (FDA) considers any IVA in the lumbar or cervical spine of up to 5° as effectively immobile for the purpose of evaluating arthrodesis status following a fusion, although the literature is equivocal and contradictory regarding the use of this 5° threshold,[14,15] and recently published treatment guidelines endorse this use of IVA in assessing arthrodesis status only as an adjunct.[16]
5. **Pseudarthrosis:** The presence of motion in a level for which a fusion has been previously attempted. Although theoretically this would include any IVA greater than 0°, according to the FDA standards described above, this only includes IVA of greater than 5°.
6. **Paradoxical Motion:** The presence of motion in the direction opposite to that of the spine bend (IVA < 0°). The term "paradoxical motion" was coined by Kirkaldy-Willis,[17] although it was first observed by Knutsson. It has been more recently discussed in other published studies.[18] In today's medical practice, paradoxical motion would be considered a form of instability.

However, there is a large gap between those six presentations that should *theoretically* be detectable, and those that are *actually* detectable with the current clinical standard of care. This gap is thoroughly explored in the following sections, and must be understood by the clinical practitioner in order to properly interpret functional testing results.

## Measurement Variability in Range of Motion (RoM) Measurements

As with any quantitative diagnostic measurement parameter, measurement variability is the key driver of diagnostic efficacy in the application of such measurements to differentiate between the various types of patient presentations. Simply stated, measurement variability is the enemy of effective diagnosis: the higher the measurement variability, the less effective the resulting diagnosis. In the case of RoM measurements, it has been shown that measurement variability is high[2,3] and diagnostic efficacy is low.[4–7] The causes and effects of this measurement variability are well understood; however, the implications for the clinical practitioner have rarely been discussed

---

*In engineering terms, stiffness is measured in Newton-meters per degree (N·m/°) while hypomobility is measured in degrees (°). However if one views the motion response of the FSU to a spine bend as an indicator of the mechanical stiffness of the FSU, then hypomobility can be viewed as a proxy measurement of stiffness.

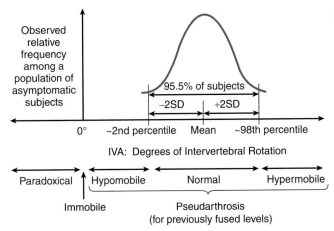

**■ FIGURE 10-2**  Theoretical framework for the detection of six functional presentations based on IVA measurements.

in the published literature. Therefore one of the main goals of this section is to present a data-driven analysis of RoM measurement variability and how this variability should be taken into account in the interpretation of functional testing results used in the diagnosis of spine disease and management of the aging spine.

RoM measurement variability is composed of variability between/within *observers*, and variability between/within *subjects*. Variability between observers is referred to as *interobserver variability*, while variability associated with a single observer taking multiple measurements at different points in time is called *intraobserver variability* (also called test/re-test variability). Similarly, variability between patients is referred to as *intersubject variability*, while the variability of any given patient between multiple tests taken at different points in time is referred to *intrasubject variability*. For example, *intersubject* variability can include the effects of physiologic differences from patient to patient, whereas *intrasubject* variability can include variability in the willingness of a patient to perform bending motions from test to test (which can often be due to the influence of pain and/or fear of pain among other things).

There is also a third component of RoM measurement variability that relates to the variability that exists between different testing sites. Different testing sites utilize different radiography platforms, and different imaging platforms can produce different types of image distortion, magnification, and other image variants. Further, different sites utilize different practices for patient positioning and image analysis. These variations among testing sites can directly contribute to RoM measurement variability and therefore must also be taken into account. For the purpose of this discussion, this variability among different testing sites will be referred to as *intersite variability*.

The different types of RoM measurement variability mentioned in the preceding paragraphs are interrelated in several ways that can be best understood through the concept of "accumulating" variability. As previously discussed, *intra*-subject variability is a measurement of the test/re-test variation within a given subject, while *inter*-subject variability is a measurement of the variability across a population of subjects. However, since the RoM measurement from any given subject is affected by *intra*-subject variation, then any measurement of *inter*-subject RoM variability across multiple subjects would necessarily "accumulate" the combined effects of *intra*-subject variation and *inter*-subject variation. The same concept holds true for measurements of *inter*-observer RoM variability, namely that these measurements accumulate the effects of both *intra*-observer and *inter*-observer variation.

This concept of "accumulation" of variability also applies to the overall relationship between observer-related variability (interobserver and intraobserver variability) and subject-related variability (intersubject and intrasubject variability). Subject-related variation in intervertebral motion exists as an inherent property of the physiology of the spine. In other words, there is a certain amount of variation that is inherent to the way the spines of different people move, or in the way a given person's spine moves at different points in time. For this discussion, we will refer to this inherent variation as the "pure" intrasubject and intersubject variability. However it is impossible to measure

**Diagram of "Accumulating" Measurement Variability**

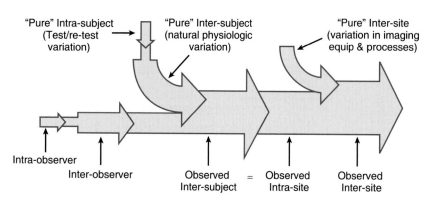

■ **FIGURE 10-3** Simplified conceptual diagram of the "accumulation" of RoM measurement variability, which applies to both IVA and IVT measurements. Note that this diagram is considered simplified because it does not represent every possible type of measurement variability. For example, observed intrasubject variability is not represented. This simplified diagram represents the interrelationships between those types of measurement variability that are most important for the clinical practitioner to understand in evaluating the performance of today's in vivo methods of spinal functional testing.

this "pure" intrasubject and intersubject variability without constructing an observational system to take measurements, and any observational system constructed to take measurements is also subject to both intraobserver and interobserver variability. Therefore any measurement of intersubject variability, for this discussion called "observed intersubject variability," necessarily "accumulates" the combined effects of both observer-related variability and subject-related variability.

See Figure 10-3 for a simplified conceptual diagram of how selected types of RoM measurement variability interrelate through the accumulation of measurement variability.

## Using Normative IVA Data to Detect Normal Motion, Hypomobility, and Hypermobility

As previously discussed, it is *theoretically* possible to use normative IVA data from a population of asymptomatic subjects to differentiate normal from hypomobile and hypermobile intervertebral motion (see Figure 10-2). However, with the current standard of care for conducting spinal functional testing, only hypermobility and pseudarthrosis can be detected with an acceptable level of statistical confidence. This fact, although not widely discussed, has very significant implications in terms of patient management, which are discussed later in this section. However as a starting point to this discussion, it is necessary to first re-examine the conventional wisdom regarding what is currently considered "normal healthy" intervertebral rotation.

As a general biostatistical principle, a quantitative diagnostic value is considered an outlier and therefore abnormal if it lies above or below two standard deviations of the mean value that is observed among a representative sample of normal healthy subjects (the mean plus and minus two standard deviations represents approximately 95.5% of all observed values). Therefore, the magnitude of such standard deviations will determine the specific ranges or IVA that should be considered normal versus hypomobile or hypermobile. Many investigators over the years have conducted studies of IVA values across asymptomatic populations for the purpose of producing such ranges, yet all of these investigators are plagued by the same Achilles' heel: they are all single-site studies and therefore fail to account for intersite variability. Thus every single-site study underestimates IVA measurement variability and therefore produces unreliable ranges of what constitutes normal versus hypomobile or hypermobile intervertebral rotation. However, by conducting a meta-analysis of these studies it is possible to account for this intersite variability and produce more representative ranges of what constitutes normal IVA.

In conducting this meta-analysis, a total of 22 published IVA datasets were identified (15 lumbar and 7 cervical). Each dataset was carefully examined and screened to ensure that: (1) the method for measuring IVA was consistent with the current clinical standard of care, and (2) the variability (standard deviation, or SD) among observed IVA values was published along with the mean. After applying this screen, three lumbar datasets and four cervical datasets qualified for this meta-analysis. See Table 10-1 for a list of all 22 datasets that were considered.

After including all qualifying datasets, the following values were tabulated for the mean and standard deviation of observed IVA values taken from multiple populations of asymptomatic subjects across multiple sites

(Table 10-2). The standard deviation values in the "Aggregated Across Sites" column at the far right of each table represent the standard deviation of the superset created by combining the observed values from all sites, and represents the observed intersite variability associated with the current standard of care for measuring IVA at each level, while the standard deviation values for each investigator represent that investigator's site's observed intersubject/intrasite variability.

Using these normative values that account for the effects of intersite variability, it is possible to produce threshold IVA values that represent hypomobility and hypermobility, as given in Table 10-3.

## Effects of IVA Measurement Variability on the Diagnostic Efficacy of Functional Testing of the Spine

To quantitatively assess the diagnostic efficacy of using IVA to detect different functional presentation (hypomobility, hypermobility, normal motion, etc.), it would be necessary to have a gold standard method for identifying true positives and true negatives for each type of functional presentation. If such a gold standard method existed, it would then be possible to quantitatively assess diagnostic efficacy with the traditional diagnostic efficacy parameters of sensitivity (Sn), Specificity (Sp), and the positive/negative likelihood ratios (+LR and –LR). however, the authors are unaware of that any such gold standard exists* and it is therefore impossible to measure these traditionally used diagnostic efficacy parameters. Therefore in this discussion of diagnostic efficacy associated with IVA measurements, these efficacy parameters will be described *qualitatively* in lieu of being able to *quantitatively* measure them.

As reflected in the hypomobility and hypermobility thresholds given in Table 10-3, the current standard of care for measuring IVA involves a high degree of measurement variability. This high degree of measurement variability, in turn, has disastrous consequences on the diagnostic efficacy of using IVA to detect intervertebral motion dysfunction. The first problem lies with the very low thresholds for detecting intervertebral hypomobility. Vertebral levels with IVA measurements of less than 2° to 5° are generally considered to be fused.[14,15] As previously discussed, the FDA considers any IVA of up to 5° as effectively immobile for the purpose of evaluating arthrodesis status following a fusion. Therefore, because the hypomobility thresholds are all *below* the FDA's 5° threshold for what is considered a fused FSU (except at C4/C5; Table 10-3), it is impossible to use IVA to differentiate hypomobile motion from a fusion, effectively rendering hypomobility an undetectable condition. A second consequence of this overlap between what is considered normal and hypomobile motion with what is considered a fused FSU is that one is guaranteed reduced specificity in detecting immobility *as well as* reduced sensitivity in detecting normal motion (because a "true normal" with an observed IVA of less than 5° is both a false

---

*This is true for immobility, hypomobility, normal motion, and hypermobility. However, there is a "gold standard" available for the detection of pseudarthrosis, which involves the intraoperative examination of a previously fused level during a revision surgery. Using this "gold standard," Sn, Sp, -LR and +LR for the use of IVA in detecting pseudarthrosis have been measured and reported.

## TABLE 10-1    IVA Datasets Consulted and Screened in This Analysis, and the Reason for Exclusion[*]

| Lumbar IVA Datasets | | | |
|---|---|---|---|
| **Investigator** | **Year** | **Included?** | **If not, why?** |
| Knutsson | 1944 | No | SD not published |
| Tanz | 1953 | No | Method not Standard of Care |
| Kapandji | 1974 | No | SD not published |
| White & Panjabi | 1978 | No | SD not published |
| Twomey | 1979 | No | SD not published |
| Pearcy | 1984 | Yes | |
| Tibrewal | 1984 | No | SD not published |
| Boden | 1989 | Yes | |
| Russell | 1993 | No | SD not published |
| Greene | 1994 | No | SD not published |
| Frobin | 1996 | Yes | |
| Van Herp | 2000 | No | SD not published |
| Troke | 2001 | No | SD not published |
| Wong | 2004 | No | Method not Standard of Care |
| Wong | 2006 | No | Method not Standard of Care |

| Cervical IVA Datasets | | | |
|---|---|---|---|
| **Investigator** | **Year** | **Included?** | **If not, why?** |
| Aho | 1955 | Yes | |
| Bhalla | 1969 | No | Outlier dataset[*] |
| Penning | 1986 | No | SD not published |
| Dvorak | 1988 | Yes | |
| Lind | 1989 | Yes | |
| Frobin | 2002 | Yes | |
| Reitman | 2004 | No | Method not Standard of Care |

[*]The Bhalla cervical dataset from 1969 had a published standard deviation that was four times lower than the average reported for other datasets, and was therefore considered an outlier and excluded from the meta-analysis. All other published standard deviations consistently fell within a narrow band of within about ± 25% of the average across all studies.

negative in the detection of normal motion as well as a false positive in the detection of immobility).

The second problem lies with the thresholds for detecting both intervertebral hypermobility and hypomobility. The thresholds for hypermobility are so high because IVA measurement variability is so large. Having such a high threshold for hypermobility (the average threshold for lumbar levels is 22° and for cervical levels is 26°, from Table 10-3) ensures that only the grossest of rotational hypermobilities will register as being definitively hypermobile; thus subtle hypermobilities remain undetected and register as "normal." Similarly, with hypomobility, high IVA variability makes the hypomobility thresholds so low that only the grossest of hypomobilities could register as being definitively hypomobile. As a consequence, the sensitivity of using IVA to detect hyper/hypomobility as well as the specificity of using IVA to detect normal motion are both reduced (those patients who register as normal but who have a subtle hyper/hypomobility are a false positive in the detection of normal motion as well as a false negative in the detection of hyper/hypomobility).

A third problem arises when one tries to use IVA to rule out hypomobility or hypermobility. It is theoretically possible to rule out hypomobility if observed IVA is sufficiently high. For example, if IVA is confirmed to be above the mean for any level, then it would be possible to rule out hypomobility (even the subtle hypomobilities described in the previous paragraph). It is similarly possible to rule out hypermobility if observed IVA is sufficiently low. However, one must consider the effects of interobserver variability in IVA measurements to be sure that a measurement is above or below the mean in producing threshold values to rule out hypomobility and hypermobility. In quantifying the interobserver variability at one investigational site, Lim et al.[3] reported that the 95% confidence interval for the interobserver variability in lumbar IVA measurements is ±5.2°. However, as this study took place at only one site, it almost certainly underestimates the actual interobserver variability that exists across different clinical sites. Nonetheless, if one uses the Lim estimate and assumes that an IVA measurement must be 5.2° above/below the mean to be 95% confident that the observed IVA is actually above/below the mean, and if one further assumes that any IVA measurement above/below the mean rules out hypo/hypermobility, then one can produce the "rule-out" thresholds for hypomobility and hypermobility given in Table 10-4. However, there are some limitations associated with the data used to create these threshold values (as described in the caption for Table 10-4), so therefore they should be considered nondefinitive until these limitations are addressed and new thresholds can be produced.

In conclusion, the diagnostic efficacy of using IVA to detect the following conditions can be summarized as:

- **Immobility:** Low specificity (high rate of false positives), so immobility should not be "ruled in" for IVA of 5° or less. May be definitively "ruled out" for IVA greater than 5°.
- **Pseudarthrosis:** May be definitively ruled in for IVA greater than 5°. Low sensitivity (high rate of false negatives) so pseudarthrosis should not be ruled out for IVA less than 5°.
- **Hypomobility:** Effectively undetectable (thresholds below what is considered fused). A nondefinitive rule-out diagnosis for hypomobility can be made if IVA is above the threshold values listed in Table 10-4.
- **Normal Motion:** Rule in diagnosis of normal motion should be considered non-definitive, because both sensitivity and specificity are low. May be ruled out with a high degree of confidence if IVA is above hypermobility thresholds (i.e., if hypermobility is ruled in).
- **Hypermobility:** May be definitively ruled in for IVA values above the hypermobility thresholds given in Table 10-3. Low sensitivity (i.e., high rate of false negatives), so hypermobility should not be ruled out if IVA is below the thresholds. May be nondefinitively ruled out if IVA is less than the threshold values given in Table 10-4.

The root cause of this poor diagnostic efficacy in the use of IVA in the detection of different functional presentations is the high degree of measurement variability associated with the current standard of care for measuring IVA. As a consequence, any reduction to IVA measurement variability would serve to increase the diagnostic efficacy of using IVA in the detection of the functional presentations given earlier.

## Conclusions: Implications for the Practitioner Regarding the Clinical Application of RoM Measurements

The current standard of care for functional testing of the spine provides IVA results that can be *overinterpreted* if measurement variability is not properly accounted for. Based on a comprehensive analysis of the effects of this variability, it is possible to put forward a set of clinical practice suggestions that are consistent with the published literature and that properly account for the effects of all sources of measurement variability:

1. Definitive diagnoses that can be made using the current standard of care for functional testing of the spine:

   - When an instability is suspected, any IVA measurement *above* the hypermobility thresholds given in Table 10-3 should be considered definitively hypermobile.
   - When pseudarthrosis is suspected in a previously fused segment, any measurement *above* 5° should be considered definitive pseudarthrosis.

**TABLE 10-2**    Normative IVA Data That Account for the Effects of Intersite Variability, Thereby Allowing for a More Representative Account of Mean IVA Values Than Has Ever Been Published in Any Single-Site Study[*]

| Lumbar Level | Pearcy '84 (n = 11) | | Boden '89 (n = 40) | | Frobin '96 (n = 61) | | Aggregated Across Sites | |
|---|---|---|---|---|---|---|---|---|
| | Mean | SD | Mean | SD | Mean | SD | Mean | SD |
| L1/L2 | 13.0° | 5.4° | 8.2° | 3.6° | 11.8° | 2.7° | 10.6° | 3.8° |
| L2/L3 | 13.0° | 2.8° | 7.7° | 3.9° | 13.9° | 3.0° | 11.6° | 4.4° |
| L3/L4 | 13.0° | 2.2° | 7.7° | 5.0° | 14.2° | 3.7° | 11.8° | 5.1° |
| L4/L5 | 15.0° | 4.1° | 9.4° | 6.5° | 16.4° | 4.1° | 13.8° | 6.0° |
| L5/S1 | 14.0° | 7.2° | 9.4° | 6.1° | 13.2° | 6.1° | 11.9° | 6.4° |
| Avg. | | 4.3° | | 5.0° | | 3.9° | Intersite variability (aggregated SD, averaged across levels) | 5.2° |

Average of the three sites' intersubject/intrasite variability (the average SD across all levels at each site, averaged across all three sites): 4.4°

| Cervical Level | Aho '55 (n = 15) | | Dvorak '88 (n = 28) | | Lind '89 (n = 70) | | Frobin '02 (n = 128) | | Aggregated Across Sites | |
|---|---|---|---|---|---|---|---|---|---|---|
| | Mean | SD | Mean | SD | Mean | SD | Mean | SD | Mean | SD |
| C2/C3 | 12.0° | 5.0° | 10.0° | 3.0° | 10.0° | 4.0° | 8.2° | 3.3° | 9.3° | 3.8° |
| C3/C4 | 15.0° | 7.0° | 15.0° | 3.0° | 14.0° | 6.0° | 14.2° | 4.7° | 14.3° | 5.1° |
| C4/C5 | 22.0° | 4.0° | 19.0° | 4.0° | 16.0° | 6.0° | 16.3° | 5.3° | 16.9° | 5.5° |
| C5/C6 | 28.0° | 4.0° | 20.0° | 4.0° | 15.0° | 8.0° | 16.6° | 6.7° | 17.3° | 7.4° |
| C6/C7 | 15.0° | 4.0° | 19.0° | 4.0° | 11.0° | 7.0° | 10.9° | 6.5° | 12.9° | 6.9° |
| Avg. | | 4.8° | | 3.6° | | 6.2° | | 5.3° | Intersite variability (aggregated SD, averaged across levels) | 5.8° |

Average of the four sites' intersubject/intrasite variability (the average SD across all levels at each site, averaged across all four sites): 5.0°

[*]All values are degrees of intervertebral rotation in the sagittal plane. Note the average intersubject/intrasite variability (i.e., the average of all four individual sites' variability averaged across all levels) is 4.4° for lumbar levels and 5.0° for cervical levels, while the average intersite variability (i.e., the aggregated variability from the superset of all sites averaged across all levels) is significantly higher at 5.2° (an 18% increase as compared to the average single-site variability) for lumbar levels and 5.8° (a 16% increase) for cervical levels. This represents the effects of variability between different clinical sites.

**TABLE 10-3**    IVA Thresholds for Hypomobility and Hypermobility[*]

| Lumbar Level | Hypomobile Threshold (Mean − 2*SD) | Hypermobile Threshold (Mean + 2*SD) | Cervical Level | Hypomobile Threshold (Mean − 2*SD) | Hypermobile Threshold (Mean + 2*SD) |
|---|---|---|---|---|---|
| L1/L2 | 3.0° | 18.3° | C2/C3 | 1.7° | 17.0° |
| L2/L3 | 2.8° | 20.4° | C3/C4 | 4.1° | 24.5° |
| L3/L4 | 1.6° | 22.0° | C4/C5 | 5.8° | 28.0° |
| L4/L5 | 1.7° | 25.8° | C5/C6 | 2.4° | 32.1° |
| L5/S1 | -1.0° | 24.8° | C6/C7 | -0.8° | 26.7° |

[*]All values are degrees of intervertebral rotation in the sagittal plane.

- Any measurement *below* −5° (i.e., 5° of motion in the direction opposite the bend) should be considered definitively paradoxical.

2. Nondefinitive diagnostic results possible with IVA measurements

- Due to the significant false negative rate when it comes to the detection of hypermobility, any IVA measurement above 5° but below the hypermobility thresholds given in Table 10-3 should be considered nondefinitive, but potentially normal. It is currently impossible to definitively rule in normal motion using today's clinical standard of care.
- Any IVA measurement ranging from −5° to 5° should be considered nondefinitive, but potentially hypomobile, immobile, paradoxical, or normal. If pseudarthrosis is suspected and an IVA of less than 5° is

observed, a corroborative spine CT view can be used to assist in the detection of pseudarthrosis.[16][*]

- Hypomobility and hypermobility may be nondefinitively ruled out based on the threshold values given in Table 10-4.

[*]Standard axial CT scanning cannot adequately reveal the hairline defect which frequently characterizes a pseudarthrosis after posterior fusion, especially in the frequent presence of metal fixation, or when the graft is irregular in shape and thickness. However, there is evidence that thin-section helical CT is currently the most successful method of proving fusion or pseudarthrosis in interbody fusions with carbon cages. (*See:* Hutter CG: Posterior intervertebral body fusion: a 25-year study, Clin Orthop 179:86-96, 1983. *Also see:* Lang P, Genant HK, Chafetz N, Steiger P, Morris JM: Three-dimensional computed tomography and multiplanar reformations in the assessment of pseudarthrosis in posterior lumbar fusion patients, Spine 13:69-75, 1988.)

**TABLE 10-4    IVA Thresholds for Ruling In/Out Hypomobility and Hypermobility***

| Lumbar Level | Hypomobile | | Hypermobile | | Cervical Level | Hypomobile | | Hypermobile | |
|---|---|---|---|---|---|---|---|---|---|
| | Rule In (IVA <) | Rule Out (IVA >) | Rule In (IVA >) | Rule Out (IVA <) | | Rule In (IVA <) | Rule Out (IVA >) | Rule In (IVA >) | Rule Out (IVA <) |
| L1/L2 | N/A | 15.8° | 18.3° | 5.4° | C2/C3 | N/A | 14.5° | 17.0° | 4.1° |
| L2/L3 | N/A | 16.8° | 20.4° | 6.4° | C3/C4 | N/A | 19.5° | 24.5° | 9.1° |
| L3/L4 | N/A | 17.0° | 22.0° | 6.6° | C4/C5 | N/A | 22.1° | 28.0° | 11.7° |
| L4/L5 | N/A | 19.0° | 25.8° | 8.6° | C5/C6 | N/A | 22.5° | 32.1° | 12.1° |
| L5/S1 | N/A | 17.1° | 24.8° | 6.7° | C6/C7 | N/A | 18.1° | 26.7° | 7.7° |

*All values are degrees of intervertebral rotation in the sagittal plane. It should be noted that the Lim et al.[3] estimate of interobserver variability that was used to create these thresholds was derived specifically for the lumbar spine (although it was also applied to the cervical spine in the Table 10-4 dataset) and does not include any effects of intersite variability. Therefore these threshold estimates should be considered nondefinitive until better data are available.

## TECHNOLOGICAL ADVANCES THAT IMPROVE THE DIAGNOSTIC EFFICACY OF SPINAL FUNCTIONAL TESTING

As stated throughout this text, the current standard of care for measuring IVA includes a high degree of both observer-related and subject-related variability. Technological developments in recent years have been effective at reducing both of these types of variability, and are discussed in this section. However, this section only includes those methods which could feasibly be adopted by the clinical practitioner and thus it does not discuss techniques which are purely investigational or are otherwise infeasible for immediate adoption (such as Roentgen Stereophotogrammatric Analysis,[19] external skin-marker–based motion measurement techniques,[20] as well as a variety of in vitro measurement methods).

### Reducing IVA Observer-Related Variability by Improving the Reliability of Image Analysis Techniques

With respect to observer-related variability, previous studies have confirmed widely variable IVA results from measurements of the same images taken by different observers. Lim et al. demonstrated that a difference of 9.6 degrees must exist between the IVA measurements from two observations in order to be 95% confident that there really is a difference in IVA.[3] This high degree of interobserver variability is a major contributor to overall observed measurement variability. However, recent advances have successfully reduced this interobserver variability through several novel techniques.

There have been improvements over the years with respect to the methods for landmarking the radiographic images and deriving IVA and IVT measurements from these images. Variability in IVA and IVT measurements can be introduced through distortion errors inherent to all radiographic images. Further, if patients move out of plane or have any significant axial rotation in their spines during imaging, the resulting IVA and IVT measurements can become more variable. A group led by W. Frobin found that interobserver variability in IVA and IVT measurements could be reduced simply by using a more sophisticated method of landmarking radiographic images.[21,22] This technique was found to significantly reduce the variability in IVA and IVT measurements associated with radiographic image distortion and with out-of-plane positioning of the subject during imaging.

There have been multiple groups who have successfully developed software-based image analysis tools that have been shown to reduce this interobserver variability. For example, one of the authors of this chapter, Kris Wong, recently developed a software algorithm for automatically deriving IVA measurements from bending images. Wong et al. published two datasets of normative values, one dataset that was derived manually,[23] and a second dataset that was derived using automated software image processing algorithms.[24] Both datasets were measured from active flexion-extension bending of the lumbar spine. The average standard deviation across the lumbar levels measured in this study (a measurement of the observed

intersubject/intrasite variability) decreased over 50%, from 2.8° to 1.3°, as a result of using automated software-driven image analysis versus manual image analysis. Other groups have been able to demonstrate similar results using commercially available image analysis software. Using an automated image analysis software program operated as a core lab service (QMA software operated by Medical Metrics, Inc., Houston, Texas) instead of a manual image analysis process, Reitman et al. published a cervical IVA dataset[25] of 155 asymptomatic subjects and Hipp & Wharton published a lumbar IVA dataset[26] of 67 asymptomatic subjects. The Reitman study reported an average standard deviation across cervical levels of 4.0°, while the Hipp & Wharton study published an average standard deviation across all lumbar levels of 3.6. While these are the lowest published standard deviation among different cervical or lumbar IVA datasets, these do represent a 20% (cervical) and 18% (lumbar) reduction relative to the average value for intersubject/intrasite variability (i.e., the average of all individual sites' average standard deviation) from the datasets listed in Table 10-2 (5.0° cervical and 4.4° lumbar). From the Wong , Hipp & Wharton, and Reitman datasets it can be shown that using automated software image analysis methods as opposed to manual methods for measuring IVA can reduce interobserver variability and thus also reduce observed intersite variability.

### Collecting Dynamic Images "During the Bend" through the Diagnostic Use of Fluoroscopy for Functional Testing of the Spine

With the current standard of care for conducting functional testing of the spine, only static images are collected while subjects hold static posture in their MVBAs; no dynamic images are collected, and no images are collected during the bend. There have been several research groups who have addressed this potential shortcoming by collecting dynamic images at points throughout spine bending by using fluoroscopy.[27–33] The principal advantage of using fluoroscopy instead of standard radiographs is that if a functional problem is only present dynamically, or if it is only visible at positions other than MVBA, it would never be detectable using the current standard of care. However, although arguably superior to the current standard of care, this method of functional imaging has never become widely used in the United States, because most major American payer organizations have refused to reimburse practitioners for such a use of diagnostic fluoroscopy.

### Reducing the Subject-Related IVA Variability Introduced through Uncontrolled Bending During Imaging

Subject-related variability is perhaps the largest contributor to overall IVA measurement variability. A large amount of subject-related variability is introduced as a result of the way patients bend during imaging. According to the current clinical standard of care, patients are instructed to bend their spines to their MVBA in both flexion and extension, and then hold those postures static while standard radiographs are captured. However, MVBA bending is highly variable, as subjects have different bending abilities and therefore bend to highly variable MVBAs. Further, the willingness of the subject to bend consistently to the same MVBA from test to test is also dependent upon the patient's perception of or fear of pain, which can be highly variable and unpredictable. One study examined the intrasubject variability in MVBA bending of the lumbar spine, and found that for the average patient, total gross lumbar spine bending varies about 26% from morning to evening.[34] Because gross spinal motion can be devolved into the sum of the individual motions at each intervertebral level, it stands to reason that any variability in overall gross spine bending will be reflected in intervertebral motion.

In addition to the diurnal variation that any given patient exhibits in spine bending MVBAs, there is also a high degree of variability in MVBA from subject to subject. This variability can be expected to be considerable, given the range of sensitivity or stoicism of subjects, their level of pain, and their fear or resilience in the face of it. In the cervical spine, there is a wide range of MVBA observed in normal asymptomatic subjects. The 95% confidence interval on observed sagittal plane cervical spine MVBA was measured to range from 34° to 82° of total gross motion — a very large range. The authors of that study, which measured both total gross cervical spine motion and cervical intervertebral motion (IVA), observed that "… this variation in gross motion between individuals had a highly significant effect on all measures of IVM [intervertebral motion]."[25] Variation in MVBA has also been measured in the lumbar spine among sufferers of chronic back pain.[34] The 95% confidence interval on observed sagittal plane lumbar MVBA was reported to range from 25° to 93° of total gross motion, an even larger range than was observed in the cervical spine among asymptomatics.

Clearly, this high degree of variability in MVBA plays a large role in driving the high levels of overall variability in IVA measurements. As discussed previously in this chapter, it is the high degree of variability in IVA that renders these measurements so clinically ineffective. Controlling the variability associated with MVBA bending therefore should be expected to reduce IVA measurement variability, and thus increase the diagnostic efficacy of functional testing of the spine.

One means of addressing the variability in MVBA bending is to normalize IVA measurements against the measurements of total range of motion between an entire spinal region. For example, in the lumbar spine the IVA from any given level can be divided by the total bending that occurs between L1 and S1 to express IVA as a percentage of total lumbar range of motion. By doing this, it is possible to reduce the effects of the variability introduced by MVBA bending. In the case of the lumbar spine, this method has been shown to be an effective means of addressing the variability inherent in MVBA bending.[29,30] This method has also been shown to be successful in studies involving the cervical spine.[25]

Another means of addressing IVA measurement variability caused by MVBA bending is through the use of *passive* rather than *active* spine bending. Dvorak and Panjabi (one of the authors of this chapter) published a study in 1991 in which they used a *passive* bending technique to decrease the variability in MVBA.[8] In this study, an assistant applied a pulling force to subjects as they bent into flexion. The assistants attempted to pull the patients into *passive* flexion with as constant a force as possible, and in so doing provided a level of standardization in the bending angles of the patients. In this study of 41 patients, the authors reported an average standard deviation of 2.8° in the IVA measurements across the lumbar levels from *passive* lumbar bending, which represents a 36% reduction to the observed intersubject/intrasite variability as compared to the mean value of 4.4° for the average standard deviation across lumbar levels from the MVBA datasets listed in Table 10-2.

Another means of addressing the IVA variability caused by MVBA bending is to take IVA measurements from standardized bending angles (SBA). For the remainder of this text, IVA measurements taken from SBA will be referred to as sIVA, while IVA measurements taken from MVBA will be referred to as IVA. Wong (an author of this chapter) et al. developed a novel method of measuring sIVA that involved the use of an electrogoniometer connected to a fluoroscope, such that the electrogoniometer could trigger the capturing of images of the lumbar spine at every 10° of lumbar bending.[23,24,31] Once images were collected, automated image analysis software was utilized to derive sIVA measurements from the fluoroscopic images. In that study, the authors reported an average standard deviation of 1.3° in the measurements of sIVA across the lumbar levels, which

represents a 72% reduction to the observed intersubject/intrasite variability as compared to the mean value of 4.4° for the average standard deviation across lumbar levels from the IVA datasets listed in Table 10-2.

## Motion Control Technology Used in Combination with Digital Videofluoroscopy and Automated Image Analysis Software

A group in Bournemouth, England led by Alan Breen, one of the authors of this chapter, has developed a patient handling system intended to reduce subject-related variability by controlling and standardizing the bending of the subject during imaging. This system involves a powered articulating device that is capable of rotating the subject's spine through a controlled and standardized sweep of spine bending during imaging. These devices are capable of providing controlled standardized spine bending in flexion/extension and lateral bending, cervical and lumbar spine motion, and standing active (weightbearing) as well as recumbent passive (nonweightbearing) spine bending. Using this device, sIVA can be measured in recumbent passive spine bending and both sIVA and IVA can be measured in standing active spine bending.

Breen et al. have integrated other recent technological developments — namely the use of digital videofluoroscopy plus the development of automated image analysis software to track vertebral bodies in sequential fluoroscopic images — together with these patient handling devices to produce a new system for conducting functional testing of the spine. Breen et al. have called this the OSMIA system, which stands for Objective Spinal Motion Imaging Assessment. Various components of this system have been discussed in a string of publications starting in 1988.[32,35–39] Performance and validation testing of the passive recumbent integrated system was published in 2006.[40] The results from this performance and validation testing suggest that the OSMIA system provides several important technical performance advantages relative to the current clinical standard of care.

The OSMIA system is intended to integrate all of the key technical performance benefits associated with other recent innovations in spinal functional testing into a single, integrated system. First, by measuring sIVA, the OSMIA system is intended to reduce subject-related variability similar to that observed by Wong et al. Second, by using digital videofluoroscopy imaging rather than standard radiographic imaging, the OSMIA system collects data "during the bend" in a way similar to previous investigators. Third, by using digital image-processing software to automatically track and measure movements of vertebral bodies, the OSMIA system is also intended to reduce observer-related variability.

See Figure 10-4 for an example of how the OSMIA system plots sIVA against the gross lumbar bending angle (the angle between the thorax and the pelvis). The OSMIA system has been tested on a normative cohort of 30 asymptomatic subjects, and among these subjects, motion patterns were generally similar to that depicted in Figure 10-4.

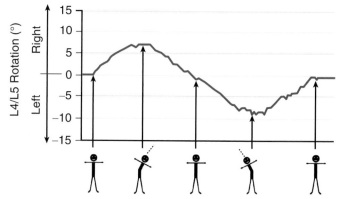

**L4/L5 Intervertebral Motion Plot (Asymptomatic Subject)**

■ **FIGURE 10-4** An example of a plot of sIVA vs. the gross lumbar bending angle from the OSMIA system. The graph depicts a typical sinusoidal curve moving in the same direction as the trunk bend taken from sIVA collected at L4/L5 from a patient tested with the OSMIA system in passive recumbent lateral side bending to 40° in each direction.

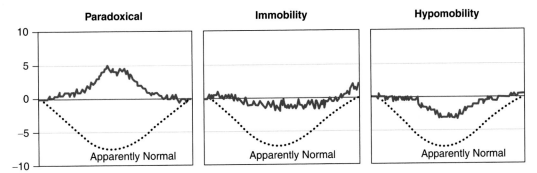

■ **FIGURE 10-5**   Case evidence of patients with lumbar degenerative disc disease presenting with apparent paradoxical motion, immobility, and apparent hypomobility. These plots depict motion at the index level as measured directly presurgical to a fusion or dynamic stabilization procedure. These motion plots represent sIVA measurements from passive recumbent side bending. In contrast to the motion plot depicted in Figure 10-4, which includes both the left and right phases of lateral lumbar spine bending, these motion plots represent intervertebral motion from only right lateral bending (to 40° of right lateral bending). The dashed "Normal" line on each graph is representative of the motion plots that were observed among the asymptomatic cohort.

In addition to the asymptomatic subjects tested with the OSMIA system, symptomatic patients have been tested prior to surgical fusion or dynamic stabilization procedures. Among this patient cohort, there is case evidence that many of the "theoretically detectable" functional presentations depicted in Figure 10-2 are detectable with the OSMIA system. See Figure 10-5 for case evidence of patients presenting with paradoxical motion, immobility, and intervertebral hypomobility.

## NEW INSIGHTS INTO THE BIOMECHANICS OF THE AGING SPINE

Making use of these recent advances in functional testing technology, it is now possible to begin to sharpen our understanding of the biomechanics of the aging spine. Having these new capabilities opens up a new world of insights into in vivo spine biomechanics that has been effectively off limits due to the prohibitively high variability in IVA measurements associated with the current clinical standard of care.

### Physiologic Variation in sIVA among Normal Subjects Is Very Low

By producing such a dramatic reduction to the observed measurement variability, the Wong et al. data yield two profound discoveries. First, it is clear that there is actually very little physiologic variation in the sIVA measurements among asymptomatic subjects. This fact has remained obscured by the high variability inherent in today's standard of care for functional testing of the spine. In fact, there is such little physiologic variation that it becomes possible to define very tight ranges for the 95% confidence interval of observed sIVA values. These ranges are narrow enough that it is possible to dramatically outperform the current clinical standard of care by: (1) being able to differentiate hypomobility from immobility, (2) differentiating hypomobility from normal motion, (3) detecting hypo/hypermobility with much tighter thresholds, which improves both the sensitivity of hypomobility/hypermobility detection as well as the specificity of the detection of normal motion. See Table 10-5 for the ranges for the detection of flexion-extension hypomobility and hypermobility for the measurement system devised by Wong et al.

### Rethinking the Conventional Wisdom Regarding Intervertebral Hypomobility and Age

A second profound finding of Wong et al. is that when sIVA is examined, vertebral levels in normal subjects became *less* hypomobile as normal subjects experience healthy aging, not *more* hypomobile, as has been the conventional wisdom. See Figure 10-6 for these results as reported by Wong et al. This has very significant implications for the management of the aging spine. While it has been shown that a patient's MVBA decreases with progressing age,[41-43] Wong et al. have proved that this is not due to a decreased motion response of lumbar FSUs to gross lumbar bending. Therefore, intervertebral hypomobility as observed with sIVA should be considered to be the result

**TABLE 10-5**   Mean sIVA, sIVA Standard Deviation (SD), and Hypomobility and Hypermobility sIVA Thresholds for the Measurement System Described by Wong et al.[*]

| Lumbar Level | Mean sIVA | SD | Hypomobile Threshold (Mean − 2*SD) | Hypermobile Threshold (Mean + 2*SD) |
|---|---|---|---|---|
| L1/L2 | 14.7 | 1.2 | 12.3 | 17.1 |
| L2/L3 | 12.1 | 1.3 | 9.5 | 14.7 |
| L3/L4 | 10.0 | 1.0 | 8.0 | 12.0 |
| L4/L5 | 7.2 | 1.1 | 5.0 | 9.4 |
| L5/S1 | 5.2 | 1.7 | 1.8[†] | 8.6 |

[*]All values represent degrees of intervertebral rotation in the sagittal plane associated with SBA bending from 10 degrees of extension to 40 degrees of flexion.
[†]Note: Because the generally accepted threshold for fusion is 5°, it might not be advisable to attempt to differentiate hypomobility from "functional fusion" at L5/S1. However, because Wong et al.[24] have demonstrated a much lower interobserver variability than is associated with the current clinical standard of care, it is debatable whether or not the threshold for "functional fusion" of 5° should apply.

of a pathological change, rather than a result of the normal aging process. Because intervertebral hypomobility is often associated with older patients with compromised disc height, it is important for practitioners to recognize intervertebral hypomobility observed with sIVA as being pathological, and not assume that intervertebral hypomobility in older patients is to be expected as part of the normal aging process.

### Age-Related Differences in the Functional Presentations of Degenerative Spondylolisthesis Patients

After conducting a study of sIVA in normal asymptomatic subjects, Wong et al. used this new measurement system to examine sIVA in 91 degenerative spondylolisthesis sufferers. Among these 91 patients, Wong et al. found the following spinal segmental mobility patterns:[44]

- 12/91: (13%): Immobility
- 27/91: (30%): Hypomobility
- 13/91: (14%): Normal
- 39/91: (43%): Hypermobility

A multiple regression analysis was then conducted to compare the predictive power of gender, age, grade of slippage, and disc height (as measured in the anatomical starting position) in predicting the mobility patterns that were observed among this population of degenerative spondylolisthesis sufferers. This analysis revealed that grade of slippage, followed by age, was a significant

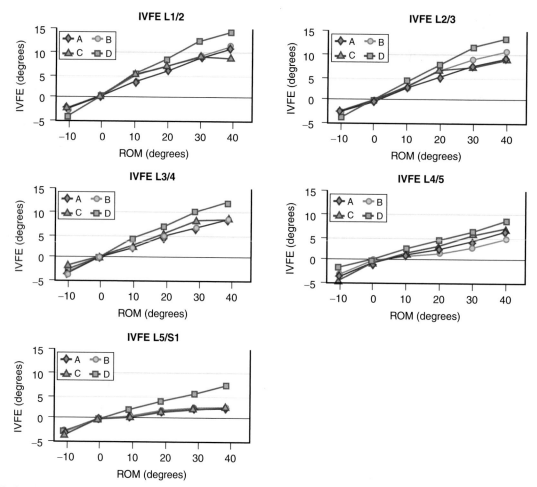

■ **FIGURE 10-6** Plot of sIVA versus gross lumbar bending angle for four age-defined cohorts. Wong et al. took sIVA measurements from 100 asymptomatic volunteers, subdividing this group into four 25-patient age-defined cohorts (Group A = 21 to 30; Group B = 31 to 40; Group C = 41 to 50; and Group D = 51 and above). Note that in each graph, the *oldest* cohort appeared to have the *greatest* sIVA values.

predictor of the observed mobility patterns. Specifically, younger patients with grade 1 L4/5 degenerative spondylolisthesis predicted hypermobility, whereas elder patients with grade 2 or above predicted a hypomobility pattern. These findings are consistent with the findings of Takayanagi et al,[33] who found that IVT and IVA in bending radiographs are both reduced in degenerative spondylolisthesis patients as compared to asymptomatic controls, and that both IVT and IVA decrease as the grade of slippage increases.

## SUGGESTIONS FOR THE CLINICAL USE OF FUNCTIONAL TESTING METHODS

A review of past knowledge shows that the current standard of care for assessing spinal function is poorly suited to the management of the aging spine. Hypomobility appears to be a condition that is more often associated with the diseased aging spine than with diseased younger patients; however, this is the one mobility pattern that is completely undetectable with the current standard of care. Further, while the current standard of care is arguably more effective in detecting hypermobility than any other mobility pattern, this condition is most commonly associated with younger patients as opposed to older patients. With respect to the use of functional diagnostics to assist in the management of the aging spine, there is a strong case to be made for the adoption of improved methods.

### Suggestions Regarding the Clinical Use of the Current Standard of Care

The current standard of care for conducting functional testing of the spine using standard radiographs and MVBA spine bending is the only method that is widely available to all practitioners, and will remain so until improved

methods become commercially available. Therefore the authors put forward the suggestions given in Table 10-6 regarding the use of the current clinical standard of care for conducting functional diagnostics of the spine.

### Suggestions Regarding the Clinical Use of Recently Developed Methods for Conducting Functional Testing of the Spine

There have been innovations in functional testing technology that offer the promise of definitively detecting those functional presentations most relevant to the aging spine (immobility, hypomobility, and normal motion). These innovations involve a set of three potential changes to the current clinical standard of care:

- The use of automated image analysis software to derive IVA measurements from radiographic images (as opposed to manual landmarking methods).
- The use of fluoroscopy to capture dynamic data regarding intervertebral motion during spine bending (as opposed to taking standard radiographs of patients holding static postures at the extremes of spine bending).
- The use of sIVA and IVA rather than IVA alone.

The authors have already put forward the improvements to diagnostic efficacy that are potentially attainable through the adoption of these improved methods. However, if any of these newer methods is to be adopted, it is critical that all issues affecting patient safety are fully explored. The authors have put the key considerations regarding patient safety associated with the adoption of these new methods for functional testing in Table 10-7.

**TABLE 10-6    Summary of Suggestions for the Clinical Use of the Current Standard of Care for Spinal Functional Testing**

| Suspected Condition | Functional Testing Results (using the current clinical standard of care) | | Diagnosed Result (Definitive diagnoses are in bold) | Comments |
|---|---|---|---|---|
| | IVA Greater Than | IVA Less Than | | |
| Rotational instability | IVA hypermobility thresholds in Table 10-3 | ∞ | **Rotational Hypermobility** (or more generally, an **"instability"**) | Very low false positive rate; can base treatment decision on this result alone. High rate of false negatives, so IVA below the hypermobility threshold should not be used to rule out a rotational hypermobility. |
| | 5° | IVA hypermobility thresholds in Table 10-3 | Inconclusive: "Potentially normal" | Suspect normal motion in these patients; however. do NOT base treatment decision solely on this result. |
| | Negative 5° (i.e., motion in the direction opposite the spine bend) | 5° | Inconclusive: "Potentially hypomobile, Immobile, Paradoxical, or Normal" | Suspect lower-than-normal motion in these patients; however, do NOT base treatment decision solely on this result. |
| | negative ∞ | Negative 5° (i.e. motion in the direction opposite the spine bend) | **Paradoxical Motion** (or more generally, an **"instability"**) | Can base treatment decision on this result alone. |
| Pseudarthrosis in previously fused patients | 5° | ∞ | **Pseudarthrosis** | Can base treatment decision on this result alone. |
| | Negative 5° (i.e., motion in the direction opposite the spine bend) | 5° | Inconclusive: "Potential pseudarthrosis" | Corroborative CT scan is suggested before considering a revision surgery although CT scans can have low sensitivity. |
| | negative ∞ | Negative 5° (i.e., motion in the direction opposite the spine bend) | **Pseudarthrosis** | Can base treatment decision on this result alone. |

**TABLE 10-7    The Authors' Suggestions Regarding the Key Patient-Safety–Related Issues Related to the Adoption of Any of the Newer Methods for Conducting Functional Testing of the Spine**

| Change to Functional Testing Method | Key Patient-Safety Issues and Authors' Suggestions |
|---|---|
| The use of automated image analysis software instead of manual landmarking techniques | • The software's observer-related variability in IVA measurements must be validated to be lower than what has been reported for manual landmarking techniques.<br>• The accuracy and precision of the software in measuring IVA must be known.<br>• If the observer-related variability is low enough, and if the accuracy and precision are good enough, it may be feasible to institute different thresholds for the detection of pseudarthrosis, immobility, and paradoxical motion than are currently used. |
| The use of fluoroscopy to capture dynamic images of intervertebral motion during spine bending instead of standard radiographs to capture images of statically held spine bending postures | • Fluoroscopy imaging may be substituted for standard radiographic imaging for the purpose of conducting functional testing.<br>• However, as image contrast for fluoroscopy can be poorer than that of standard radiographs, fluoroscopic images may fail to detect certain conditions that require the high contrast provided by standard radiographs (such as infection, skeletal neoplasia, etc.).<br>• Therefore, for any patient for whom fluoroscopy is substituted for standard radiographs for conducting functional testing of the spine, a recently taken standard radiograph of the spine should also be available.<br>• The total dose of radiation to the patient associated with any fluoroscopy-based protocol for conducting functional testing should be measured and compared to that which would be received by the patient with standard radiographic imaging. Any increase in effective dose to the patient needs to be carefully evaluated. |
| The use of sIVA and IVA rather than IVA alone | • Using SBA instead of MVBA from which to take IVA measurements has been shown to reduce the subject-related variability in these measurements (i.e., sIVA has less measurement variability than IVA).<br>• The total observed intersite variability associated with sIVA would need to be validated before new thresholds for detecting hypomobility, normal motion, and rotational hypermobility are adopted.<br>• Testing protocols would likely need to include assessments of sIVA as well as IVA, as there are potentially valuable diagnostic insights to be gained from observing IVA at the physiologic operating ranges of gross trunk motion. |

# References

1. F. Knutsson, The instability associated with disc degeneration in the lumbar spine, Acta. Radiol. 25 (1944) 593–608.
2. M. Panjabi, D. Chang, J. Dvorak, An analysis of errors in kinematic parameters associated with in vivo functional radiographs, Spine 17 (1992) 200–205.
3. M.R. Lim, R.T. Loder, R.C. Huang, S. Lyman, et al., Measurement error of lumbar total disc replacement range of motion, Spine 31 (10) (2006) E291–E297.
4. J. Dvorak, M.M. Panjabi, J.E. Noventoy, D.G. Chang, D. Grob, Clinical validation of functional flexion-extension roentgenograms of the lumbar spine, Spine 16 (8) (1991) 943–950.
5. S.D. Boden, S.W. Wiesel, Lumbosacral segmental motion in normal individuals. Have we been measuring instability properly? Spine 15 (6) (1990) 571–576.
6. L. Penning, J.T. Wilmink, H.H. van Woerden, Inability to prove instability: a critical appraisal of clinical-radiological flexion-extension studies in lumbar disc degeneration, Diagn. Imaging Clin. Med. 53 (4) (1984) 186–192.
7. W.O. Shaffer, K.F. Spratt, J. Weinstein, T.R. Lehmann, V. Goel, 1990 Volvo award in clinical sciences. The consistency and accuracy of roentgenograms for measuring sagittal translation in the lumbar vertebral motion segment: an experimental model, Spine 15 (8) (1990) 741–750.
8. J. Dvorak, M.M. Panjabi, D.G. Chang, R. Theiler, D. Grob, Functional radiographic diagnosis of the lumbar spine: flexion-extension and lateral bending, Spine 16 (1991) 562–571.
9. A.A. White III, R.M. Johnson, M.M. Panjabi, W.O. Southwick, Biomechanical analysis of clinical stability in the cervical spine, Clin. Orthop. 109 (1975) 85–96.
10. H.W. Myerding, Spondylolisthesis, Surg. Gynecol. Obstet. 54 (1932) 371–377.
11. P.H. Newman, The etiology of spondylolisthesis, J. Bone Joint Surg. [Br] 45 (1963) 39–59.
12. R.C. DeWald, Spondylolisthesis, in: K.H. Birdwell, R.C. DeWald (Eds.), The textbook of spinal surgery, second ed., Lippincott-Raven, Philadelphia, 1997.
13. L.L. Wiltse, The etiology of spondylolisthesis, J. Bone Joint Surg. Am. 44-A (1962) 539–560.
14. P.C. McAfee, S.D. Boden, J.W. Brantigan, R.D. Fraser, et al., Symposium: a critical discrepancy–a criteria of successful arthrodesis following interbody spinal fusions, Spine 26 (3) (2001) 320–334.
15. J.A. Hipp, C.A. Reitman, N. Wharton, Defining pseudoarthrosis in the cervical spine with differing motion thresholds, Spine 30 (2) (2005) 209–210.
16. D.K. Resnick, T.F. Choudhri, A.T. Dailey, M.W. Groff, et al., Guidelines for the performance of fusion procedures for degenerative disease of the lumbar spine. Part 4: radiographic assessment of fusion, J. Neurosurg. Spine 2 (2005) 653–657.
17. W.H. Kirkaldy-Willis, Instability of the lumbar spine, Clin. Orthop. Relat. Res. (165) (1982) 110–123.
18. S.A. Park, N. Ordway, A. Fayyazi, B. Fredrickson, H.A. Yuan, Measurement of paradoxical and coupled motions following lumbar total disc replacement, SAS Journal 2 (2008) 137–139.
19. G. Selvik, Roentgen stereophotogrammetry: a method for the study of the kinematics of the skeletal system, Acta Orthopaedica. Scandinavica. 232 (Suppl. 60) (1989) 1–51.
20. X. Zhang, J. Xiong, Model-guided derivation of lumbar vertebral kinematics in vivo reveals the difference between external marker-defined and internal segmental rotations, J. Biomech. 36 (2003) 9–17.
21. W. Frobin, P. Brinckmann, M. Leivseth, M. Biggemann, O. Reikerås, Precision measurement of segmental motion from flexion-extension radiographs of the lumbar spine, Clin. Biomech. (Bristol, Avon) 11 (8) (1996) 457–465.
22. W. Frobin, P. Brinckmann, M. Biggemann, M. Tillotson, K. Burton, "Precision measurement of disc height, vertebral height and sagittal plane displacement from lateral radiographic views of the lumbar spine." Clin. Biomech. (Bristol, Avon) 12 (Suppl. 1) (1997) S22–S30.
23. K.W.M. Wong, J.C. Leong, M.K. Chan, K.D. Luk, W.W. Lu, The flexion/extension profile of 100 healthy volunteers, Spine 29 (15) (2004) 1636–1641.
24. K.W.M. Wong, K.D. Luk, J.C. Leong, S.F. Wong, K.K. Wong, Continuous dynamic spinal motion analysis, Spine 31 (4) (2006) 414–419.
25. C.A. Reitman, K.M. Mauro, L. Nguyen, J.M. Ziegler, J.A. Hipp, Intervertebral motion between flexion and extension in asymptomatic individuals, Spine 29 (24) (2004) 2832–2843.
26. J.A. Hipp, N.D. Wharton, Quantitative motion analysis (QMA) of motion-preserving and fusion technologies for the spine, In Yue JJ et al (eds). Motion Preservation Surgery of the Spine: Advanced Techniques and Controversies. Saunders, Philadelphia, 2008.
27. H. Hino, K. Abumi, M. Kanayama, K. Kaneda, Dynamic motion analysis of normal and unstable cervical spines using cineradiography: an in vivo study, Spine. 15 24 (2) (1999) 163-8.
28. A. Okawa, K. Shinomiya, H. Komori, Y. Muneta, Y. Arai, O. Nakai, Dynamic motion study of the whole lumbar spine by videofluoroscopy, Spine 23 (16) (1999) 1743–1749.
29. D.S. Teyhen, T.W. Flynn, J.D. Childs, et al., Fluoroscopic video to identify aberrant lumbar motion, Spine 32 (7) (2007) E220–E229.
30. Harada, et al., Cineradiographic motion analysis of normal lumbar spine during forward and backward flexion, Spine 25 (15) (2000) 1932–1937.
31. S.-W. Lee, K.W.N. Wong, M.-K. Chan, H.-M. Yeung, J.L.F. Chiu, J.C.Y. Leong, Development and validation of a new technique for assessing lumbar spine motion, Spine 27 (2002) E215–E220.
32. A.C. Breen, R. Allen, A. Morris, Spine kinematics: a digital videofluoroscopic technique, J. Biomed. Eng. 11 (1989) 224.
33. K. Takayanagi, K. Takahashi, M. Yamagata, H. Moriya, H. Kitahara, T. Tamaki, Using cineradiography for continuous dynamic-motion analysis of the lumbar spine, Spine 26 (17) (2001) 1858–1865.
34. F.B. Ensink, et al., Lumbar range of motion: influence of time of day and individual factors on measurements, Spine 21 (11) (1996) 1339–1343.
35. A.C. Breen, et al., An image processing method for spine kinematics—preliminary studies, Clin. Biomech. 3 (1988) 5–10.
36. A.C. Breen, et al., A digital videofluoroscopic technique for spine kinematics, J. Med. Eng. Technol. 13 (1-2) (1989) 109–113.
37. K. Humphreys, A. Breen, D. Saxton, Incremental lumbar spine motion in the coronal plane: an observer variation study using digital videofluoroscopy, Eur. J. Chiropractic. 38, 56–62 1990.
38. A.C. Breen, Integrated spinal motion: a study of two cases, JCCA 35 (1) (1991) 25–30.
39. J.M. Muggleton, et al., Automatic location of vertebrae in digitized videofluoroscopic images of the lumbar spine, Med. Eng. Phys. 19 (1997) 77–89.
40. A.C. Breen, et al., An objective spinal motion image assessment (OSMIA): reliability, accuracy, and exposure data, BMC Musculoskel. 7 (2006) 1.
41. G.K. Fitzgerald, et al., Objective assessment with establishment of normal values for lumbar spinal range of motion, Phys. Ther. 63 (1983) 1776–1781.
42. J. Dvorak, et al., Normal motion of the lumbar spine as related to age and gender, Eur. Spine J. 4 (1995) 18–23.
43. M.S. Sullivan, C.E. Dickinson, J.D. Troup, The influence of age and gender on lumbar spine sagittal plane range of motion: a study of 1126 healthy subjects, Spine 19 (1994) 682–686.
44. K.W.N. Wong, et al: Different lumbar segmental motion patterns in patients with degenerative spondylolisthesis were detected with digital videofluoroscopic videos and distortion compensated roentgen analysis system. Presented at ISSLS 2007.

# Causes of Premature Aging of the Spine  11

*Florence P. S. Mok, Dino Samartzis, Kenneth M. C. Cheung, and Jaro Karppinen*

### KEY POINTS

- Various age-related factors are involved in the degenerative process of the spine.
- Premature aging of the spine can be affected by biochemical, biomechanical, cardiovascular, lifestyle, and genetic factors.
- Interactions between various etiological factors contributing to the premature aging of the spine may be present.
- Although premature aging of the spine may occur, such changes may not be synonymous with clinical symptoms.

## INTRODUCTION

The spine is the grand architect of the human body. Working in close symbiotic interplay between soft and bony tissues, the spine is responsible for structure and function, as well as protection of the spinal cord and associated neural elements. Aging is an inevitable process that affects almost every structure of the human body, including the spine. Age-related changes of the spine are an expected facet of life with the progression of age. However, it is not uncommon for physicians to encounter young patients presenting with characteristics of advanced aging of the spine, the so-called premature aging or degenerative changes.

Premature aging of the spine is a salient concern, in that if it achieves clinical relevance associated with symptoms and impaired function, it has the potential to incur severe socioeconomic consequences. To identify such degenerative changes, advanced imaging, such as magnetic resonance imaging (MRI), has been a popular mainstay in the armamentarium of the physician for diagnostic and therapeutic interventions. However, numerous studies have also documented that the severity of radiological changes is not always associated with clinical symptoms (Figure 11-1).[1] Nonetheless, it is essential to determine whether degenerative changes of the spine are a part of the natural evolution of the spine because of age, or if they result from a disease process (Figure 11-2) heralded by risk factors, possibly preventable, that prematurely change the spine. In this chapter, the authors will discuss the numerous factors that may contribute to premature aging of the spine.

## PREMATURE AGING FACTORS

### Biochemical

In humans, the notochordal cells in the nucleus pulposus (NP) dramatically decrease after birth, and they eventually disappear, probably through apoptosis, and are replaced by chondrocyte-like cells by the first decade. The reduction in notochordal cell population with maturity could decrease proteoglycan production and contribute to the degenerative process. Furthermore, the naturally occurring cellular senescence, via telomere shortening, plays a role in disc aging as well as degeneration. However, degenerated discs are prone to increased cell senescence as the exposure to various factors, such as interleukin-1 (IL-1), reactive oxygen species, and mechanical load, further accelerate disc degeneration. Therefore exposure to such factors could induce premature senescence of the disc.[2]

In addition, degenerated discs have been shown to have higher concentrations and activities of degradative enzymes than normal discs, which could be due to the phenotypic changes of disc cells in response to various stimuli such as chemical mediators and mechanical loading. The alteration in disc cell phenotype leads to a cascade of biochemical changes that include the following: (1) decrease in matrix synthesis (e.g., aggrecan, decorin, type II and type IX collagens); (2) downregulation in the expression of growth factors and their receptors, which impairs the regenerative processes; and (3) upregulation of the catabolic metabolism through the increase in concentration and activity of matrix metalloproteinases (MMPs), reduction in tissue inhibitors of metalloproteinases (TIMP) levels, as well as the increase in proinflammatory cytokines and their receptor levels. Among all the cytokines, interleukin-1β in particular seems to play a central role, because it suppresses matrix synthesis and also stimulates the production of other inflammatory mediators, which further enhances matrix catabolism.[2,3]

### Biomechanical

Clinically, disc degeneration is generally more prevalent and severe in the lower lumbar discs, suggesting that higher mechanical loading in this region may be a strong causative factor. Mechanical insults to the disc could induce fatigue failures in the endplates or annulus, which accelerate the catabolic cascade. However, mechanical loading is not a deleterious factor in itself as loading within physiological range stimulates disc matrix turnover and enhances anabolic factors, such as proteoglycan synthesis and TIMP production, whereas loading outside this range (less or more than optimal) is detrimental to disc metabolism. In vivo animal studies showed that high magnitudes or frequencies of dynamic and static compression induced cell apoptosis, structural failure and increased catabolism, whereas downregulation of anabolic gene expressions has been shown in the discs exposed to immobilization.[4-7]

A cadaveric investigation by Videman et al[8] reported that history of occupational physical loading was related to disc degeneration and pathological changes of the lumbar spine, but a clear linear dose-dependent relationship was not established. In former elite athletes, more spinal degenerative findings were presented in those who engaged in heavier loading exercises versus light exercises, yet it only accounted for less than 10% of variability of MRI findings, despite the extreme difference in loading conditions.[9] In fact, heavier lifetime physical loading, involving both occupational and leisure time activities, accounted only for small amounts of variance in disc degeneration in MRI, being 7% over T12-L4 and 2% over L4-S1.[10] Moreover, when accounting for individual anthropometric parameters, such as body weight, lifting strength, and axial disc area in relation to disc degeneration, although all with modest effect, the lifelong continuous loading associated with these parameters was more influential than extrinsic physical loading related to occupation and leisure activities.[11]

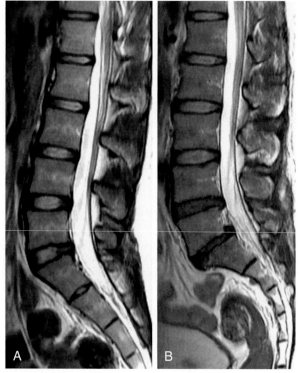

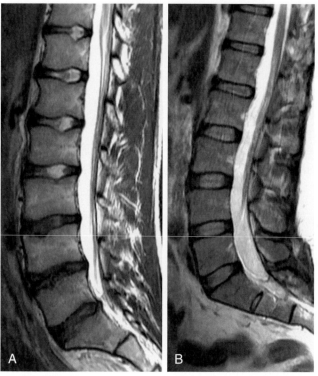

■ **FIGURE 11-1** **A,** An 18-year-old nonsmoking female presented with chronic low back pain for more than 2 years without history of lumbar injury. Sagittal T2-weighted MRI shows no evidence of disc degeneration or other radiological abnormalities. **B,** A 37-year-old female, who has never experienced low back pain. Sagittal T2-weighted MRI of the lumbar spine shows severe disc degeneration at L4-L5 and L5-S1, radial tear at L4-L5, and Grade I spondylolisthesis at L5-S1.

■ **FIGURE 11-2** **A,** A 16-year-old nonsmoking male presented with low back pain but had no history of lumbar injury. T2-weighted MRI of the lower thoracic and lumbar spine shows severe disc degeneration at L3-S1 and endplate irregularities over thoracic and lumbar spine. **B,** A 53-year-old asymptomatic female. Sagittal T2-weighted MRI shows no signs of disc degeneration or other radiological abnormalities.

## Atherosclerosis

The blood supply to the lumbar spine is derived from the abdominal aorta, which gives off branches to supply regional vertebral segments (Figure 11-3).[12] The nutritional supply to the intervertebral disc (IVD) depends on the diffusion potential through the endplates of the vertebral bodies. Therefore disc nutrition could be impeded by factors that diminish blood flow to the vertebrae, by defects or calcification of the endplates, or a combination of the three. An autopsy study by Kauppila et al.[13] determined that the severity of disc degeneration was significantly associated with the grade of stenosis of the segmental arteries supplying the disc, and this association was stronger in the upper three lumbar levels than the lower two levels. Moreover, the degree of disc degeneration also increased in line with the complexity of the atherosclerotic lesions in the abdominal aorta. In accordance to the cadaveric studies by Kauppila et al.[13] in vivo MRI studies have confirmed the association between impaired lumbar artery blood flow and diminished disc diffusion in both healthy subjects[14] and patients with low back symptoms.[15] It is generally thought that the reduced disc diffusion could in turn cause disc degeneration, but no definite answer to this hypothesis is available. Furthermore, clinical low back symptoms were also found to be associated with the presence of lumbar arterial stenosis.[16-18] An atherosclerotic contribution to back symptoms is further substantiated in a long-term prospective study by Leino-Arjas et al.[19] in which high baseline serum total cholesterol and triglyceride levels were associated with incident radiating low back pain among Finnish industrial employees. The increased risk of abnormal levels of cholesterol and triglycerides on radiating pain was independent of other potential risk factors, such as age, gender, occupational class, work history, exercise habits, smoking, and body mass index (BMI). The mechanism through which atherosclerosis and occlusion of arteries affect disc degeneration may be directly related to diminished blood flow, and hence decreased nutritional supply to the IVD, and also by the systemic inflammatory effect associated with atherosclerosis.

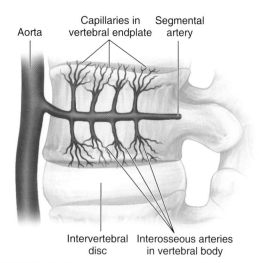

■ **FIGURE 11-3** The segmental artery provides blood supply to the vertebral body. *(Adapted from Raj PP. Intervertebral disc: anatomy-physiology-pathophysiology-treatment.* Pain Pract *2008;8:18-44.)*

In a long-term follow-up study of 98,407 female nurses, cardiovascular risk factors, such as smoking, diabetes, hypertension, high cholesterol, obesity, and family history of myocardial infarction before the age of 60 years, were significantly associated with an increased risk of lumbar disc herniation. Moreover, after adjustment for other cardiovascular risk factors, the increased risk of symptomatic disc herniation exhibited a dose-dependent relationship with smoking ($p = .003$) and overweight ($p = .01$).[20] However, in an observational study of 270 Japanese elderly with a mean age of 68.4 years, high-levels of LDL cholesterol was only associated with increased risk of disc degeneration at L4/5 (adjusted odds ratio = 2.65; 95% confidence interval = 1.33-5.52), but not at other levels. In the Japanese study, increased disc degeneration was not associated with their atherosclerosis index or with hyperglycemia.[21] However, the presence or severity of atherosclerosis at lumbar arteries was not properly assessed, and therefore the general interpretation of "atherosclerosis" in this study could be problematic. Nevertheless, the cited studies highlight the complexity of cardiovascular risk factors and their role upon disc degeneration.

## Lifestyle Factors

Disc degeneration had been previously regarded as an accelerated aging process caused by mechanical insults, such as encountered in physically demanding occupations or sports. However, lifestyle factors, such as smoking and obesity are regarded nowadays as risk factors of low back pain on the basis of meta-analyses.[22] In recent decades, a series of exposure-discordant twin studies using MRI to assess the association between disc degeneration and environmental risk factors exposure has been conducted. By comparing the differences of interest between twin siblings in these studies, the effects of genetics and early childhood exposures between subjects were better understood, providing a new perspective regarding disc degeneration.[23] On the basis of these twin studies, detrimental lifestyle factors may have negligible effect upon disc degeneration.

### Smoking

Battie and associates[24] assessed the effect of smoking on disc degeneration in 20 pairs of monozygotic (MZ) male twins and found that the disc degeneration score was 18% higher in smokers than in nonsmoking siblings. Additionally, smoking seemed to exert a systemic effect, because both upper and lower lumbar discs had higher disc degeneration scores, and the smokers had significantly more carotid atherosclerotic changes than nonsmoking co-twins. It was suggested that atherosclerotic changes associated with smoking could decrease the blood supply to vertebral vessels and structures, and hence could reduce disc nutrition and promote degeneration. However, despite the extraordinary discordance in smoking exposure with a mean difference of 31.6 smoking years between co-twins in this study, the effect of smoking was very trivial because it only explained 2% of the total amount of variance in disc degeneration scores.[24] In addition, in their later exposure-discordant study in 115 pairs of male MZ twins, smoking failed to demonstrate a significant association with disc degeneration.[10] The contradicting results were regarded to be due to the large differences in the mean smoking discordance between co-twins recruited in these two studies and the overall minor effect of smoking itself.[23] Nevertheless, more recent studies showed that smoking (nicotine) could, indeed, directly mediate the disc cells metabolism by inhibiting cell proliferation and their synthetic activity of extracellular matrix in vitro,[25] as well as increase the local production and release of inflammatory cytokines[26] and downregulate the expression of collagen genes in vivo.[27] These cellular responses of smoking provide evidence for the association of smoking with the degenerative process of the intervertebral discs. In clinical perspective, a recent prospective study among adolescence also demonstrated that regular smoking was associated with low back pain with an exposure–response relationship among young females.[28]

### Obesity

In a recent study, a BMI above 25 kg/m² was found to be significantly associated with lumbar disc degeneration at the lower four discs levels among elderly Japanese subjects.[21] The importance of obesity was also reported by Liuke et al,[29] who investigated the progression of disc degeneration in 129 middle-aged males. They found that persistent overweight (BMI above 25 kg/m² at both 25 and 40 to 45 years) significantly increased the risk of disc degeneration by 4.3-fold, whereas other lifestyle variables, such as smoking, occupation, driving, and the presence of historical back injuries, were not associated with disc degeneration. Moreover, obesity at young age was particularly detrimental, because subjects with BMI of 24 to 25 kg/m² and above 25 kg/m² at the age of 25 years had 3.5- and 4.5-fold increased risk of disc degeneration, respectively.[29] Furthermore, data of this chapter's authors (Samartzis et al, unpublished) identified that obesity was the

strongest risk factor associated with juvenile disc degeneration in a population-based cohort of Southern Chinese, because adolescents with BMI over 25 kg/m² had an 18-fold increased risk associated with disc degeneration. In addition, in a study assessing the association of BMI and lumbar disc degeneration in 2252 Southern Chinese adults, Samartzis and colleagues (unpublished observation) further noted that an increased BMI was associated with the presence and severity of disc degeneration, noting a significant linear dose–response association. In fact, the authors further noted that a positive linear relation with an increase in BMI to that of the number of degenerated disc levels.

The exact mechanism by which obesity or overweight causes lumbar disc degeneration is yet to be elucidated, but it could partly be due to the excess mechanical load acting directly on the intervertebral discs, and indirectly through systemic risk factors associated with obesity.[29] Obesity has been regarded as a low-grade systemic inflammatory condition, in which serum levels of C-reactive protein, interleukin-6 (IL-6), and tumor necrosis factor-α (TNF-α) were shown to be increased in obese individuals.[30] The increased levels of proinflammatory cytokines in obese subjects can be explained by the observation that both macrophages residing in adipose tissue and adipocytes are metabolically active, secreting proinflammatory cytokines, such as IL-6 and TNF-α, and adipocytokines (leptin, adiponectin, resistin).[31] Cytokines, in particular IL-1, not only enhance degradation of the disc matrix[3] but also are implicated in the pathophysiology of atherosclerosis.[32] Therefore, disc dsegeneration could be accelerated in obese subjects through inflammatory pathways. In fact, it has been shown that gene polymorphisms could have an interaction with obesity to increase the risk of disc degeneration.[33]

## Genetic Factors

The association between lifestyle factors and disc degeneration has been rather weak and even somewhat controversial as previously discussed, which suggest that other factors may potentially be more influential. Genetic determinants related to disc degeneration have received considerable attention in recent years. However, an accurate phenotype definition of disc degeneration is an absolute prerequisite for studies that evaluate the association between genetic factors and degenerative changes.[34] Nonetheless, it is not surprising that evidence from twin studies suggests a key role for familial aggregation, which includes the influences by both genetic factors and early environmental exposure. Overall, the reported heredity estimate ranges from 50% to 74%.[23] In an MRI study on monozygotic male twins, Battie et al[10] reported the disproportion of variance in disc degeneration explained by familial aggregation to be 61% and 34% in the upper versus lower lumbar spine, respectively. The combined effect of age and physical loading only accounted for less than 16% of the total variance. The disproportional variance across spinal levels was suggested to be due to the interactions between genetic influences and mechanical loading with spinal anthropometrics. Yet in a study of predominantly female British and Australian twins, heritability prevalence was almost identical in the lumbar (74%) and cervical spines (73%). However, heritability estimates varied for different degenerative phenotypes, such as lumbar osteophytes (54%), disc bulging (65%), and disc height narrowing (79%).[35]

Heredity may determine the development of the spinal structures, therefore, affecting their mechanical strength and properties. It could also affect the biochemical properties by influencing the homeostasis between matrix synthesis and degradation. In turn, the structural integrity of the tissue and the vulnerability of the spinal structures to withstand external loading could be compromised with genetic defects, and predispose the spinal structures to accelerated degeneration. To date, several genes associated with disc degeneration as well as endplate changes have been identified, which entail genes coding for collagens (e.g., COL1A1 gene for collagen I, and COL9A2 and COL9A3 genes for collagen IX),[36-42] aggrecan,[43-45] cartilage intermediate layer protein (CILP),[46-48] vitamin D receptor (VDR),[49-51] inflammatory mediators such as IL-1,[43,52-56] and degradative enzymes such as MMPs.[43,47,54,57-60] Although the association of disc degeneration with gene polymorphisms was evident, inconsistent results between studies were reported even when accounting for the same gene (e.g., COL9A2 and COL9A3 among Finns, Chinese, Japanese, and Greek). This could be due to the disparities in allelic frequencies according to ethnicity. Nevertheless, the identification of genetic predisposition was undoubtedly an important breakthrough in understanding the cause in affecting the premature aging of the spine.

## DISCUSSION

Aging is an inevitable process that affects all spinal structures; disc degeneration has been described as an age-dependent, cell-mediated matrix degradation process that results in progressive structural failure.[61] It is a complex condition that is determined by multiple biomechanical, environmental, lifestyle, and genetic factors and the interactions between these factors.

Numerous environmental factors have been suggested to be related to disc degeneration, as mentioned in previous sections, yet inconsistent results have been reported. On the contrary, the importance of genetic predisposition has been put forward by the twin and gene association studies in the recent decade.[23] In the aforementioned genetic studies, it is evident that disc degeneration is associated with multiple gene polymorphisms with substantial ethnicity variance, yet the difference in study methodologies, particularly the difference in phenotypic definition, between these studies make it difficult to appreciate which genes and the interactions between them would exert a dominant role in specific degenerative changes. Solovieva et al[62] provided evidence of gene–gene interaction, with an effect of a particular gene polymorphism on disc degeneration that would be modified by the presence of another gene polymorphism. It was found that an eightfold increased risk of higher disc degeneration score was associated with polymorphisms of COL9A3 in the absence of interleukin IL-1βT(3594), but no association was found with their joint occurrence. The gene programs the disc matrix turnover by coding for particular matrix synthesis and controlling its degradation. The effect of gene polymorphism should therefore, in theory, act systemically as long as the same gene polymorphism is coding for the same component, and producing the abnormal matrix identically in every disc across the whole spine. However, regional variations in disc degeneration are evident, with lower lumbar discs involved more commonly than the upper lumbar, suggestive of a gene–environment interaction affecting the vulnerability of a disc to degenerate. In fact, the notion of regional differences and gene–environment interactions have been confirmed by a recent twin study by Battie et al,[63] which noted that considerable differences were found in the genetic and environmental influences for upper versus lower lumbar levels. Moreover, three common unique environmental factors and two common genetic factors were found to influence the disc signal intensity across the lumbar levels. Interestingly, of the two identified genetic factors, it seemed that the first factor influenced all lumbar levels, but the second factor appeared to be specific for L4-S1 only. Besides that, approximately two thirds of the genetic influences were found to be shared among disc degeneration phenotypes studied (disc signal intensity, and disc height narrowing and bulging), suggesting that they have a common pathogenesis pathway in association with disc degeneration.

In a study among middle-aged occupationally active Finnish men by Solovieva et al,[33] the authors noted that 45% to 71% of the individuals with disc degeneration also presented with COL9A3 polymorphism and persistent obesity. The copresence of these two previously identified risk factors acted synergistically to increase the risk of having multilevel posterior disc bulge and multilevel decreased disc height, threefold and fourfold, respectively. In addition, they also found that the deleterious effect of occupational physical loading could be modified by the presence of IL-1 gene polymorphism.[55] Additionally, recent study by Virtanen et al[64] further substantiates the notion of gene–environment interactions, whereby a whole-body vibration was found to exert additive effect with all the polymorphisms analyzed (COL9A2, COL9A3, COL11A2, IL-1α, IL-1β, IL-6, MMP-3, and VDR) to increase the risk for symptomatic disc degeneration.

Histological evidence has illustrated that diminished blood supply to the disc is detrimental, appearing to initiate disc matrix degradation as early as in the first decade of life.[65] Moreover, the effect of various gene mutations on disc degeneration, such as the Trp2 allele of collagen IX,[37,38] D allele of the MMP-1 gene,[59] and the t allele of vitamin D receptor gene,[49] were also shown to exhibit an age-dependent effect.

## CLINICAL RELEVANCE

Degenerative changes of the spine can lead to low back pain and associated clinical symptoms, with the potential to severely impair function and quality of life. Premature aging of the spine further compounds this scenario by potentially debilitating an individual early on in the course of life. Moreover, such aging effects may usher further deleterious spine changes throughout one's lifespan due to the nature of the degenerative process. As such, factors contributing to premature aging of the spine leading to clinically relevant pathology are a global concern that can affect every population worldwide with potentially severe compounded socioeconomic effects.

Identification of various etiological risk factors contributing to premature aging of the spine is of paramount importance. Such knowledge may provide insight to address measures to prevent premature spine-related changes. In addition, therapeutic interventions may also be addressed to halt or reverse the effects brought upon by the aging process. With the increase of knowledge related to premature aging of the spine and emerging technologies to treat spine-related conditions, the quality of life and productivity of an individual will improve, and associated health care costs will diminish.

## References

1. J.P. Urban, C.P. Winlove, Pathophysiology of the intervertebral disc and the challenges for MRI, J. Magn. Reson. Imaging 25 (2007) 419–432.
2. C.Q. Zhao, L.M. Wang, L.S. Jiang, et al., The cell biology of intervertebral disc aging and degeneration, Ageing Res. Rev. 6 (2007) 247–261.
3. A.G. Hadjipavlou, M.N. Tzermiadianos, N. Bogduk, et al., The pathophysiology of disc degeneration: a critical review, J. Bone Joint Surg. Br. 90 (2008) 1261–1270.
4. I.A. Stokes, J.C. Iatridis, Mechanical conditions that accelerate intervertebral disc degeneration: overload versus immobilization, Spine 29 (2004) 2724–2732.
5. M.K. Elfervig, J.T. Minchew, E. Francke, et al., IL-1beta sensitizes intervertebral disc annulus cells to fluid-induced shear stress, J. Cell Biochem. 82 (2001) 290–298.
6. H. Miyamoto, M. Doita, K. Nishida, et al., Effects of cyclic mechanical stress on the production of inflammatory agents by nucleus pulposus and anulus fibrosus derived cells in vitro, Spine 31 (2006) 4–9.
7. J.A. Ulrich, E.C. Liebenberg, D.U. Thuillier, et al., ISSLS prize winner: repeated disc injury causes persistent inflammation, Spine 32 (2007) 2812–2819.
8. T. Videman, M. Nurminen, J.D. Troup, 1990 Volvo Award in clinical sciences. Lumbar spinal pathology in cadaveric material in relation to history of back pain, occupation, and physical loading, Spine 15 (1990) 728–740.
9. T. Videman, S. Sarna, M.C. Battie, et al., The long-term effects of physical loading and exercise lifestyles on back-related symptoms, disability, and spinal pathology among men, Spine 20 (1995) 699–709.
10. M.C. Battie, T. Videman, L.E. Gibbons, et al., 1995 Volvo Award in clinical sciences. Determinants of lumbar disc degeneration. A study relating lifetime exposures and magnetic resonance imaging findings in identical twins, Spine 20 (1995) 2601–2612.
11. T. Videman, E. Levalahti, M.C. Battie, The effects of anthropometrics, lifting strength, and physical activities in disc degeneration, Spine 32 (2007) 1406–1413.
12. P.P. Raj, Intervertebral disc: anatomy-physiology-pathophysiology-treatment, Pain Pract 8 (2008) 18–44.
13. L.I. Kauppila, A. Penttila, P.J. Karhunen, et al., Lumbar disc degeneration and atherosclerosis of the abdominal aorta, Spine 19 (1994) 923–929.
14. M. Kurunlahti, L. Kerttula, J. Jauhiainen, et al., Correlation of diffusion in lumbar intervertebral discs with occlusion of lumbar arteries: a study in adult volunteers, Radiology 221 (2001) 779–786.
15. O. Tokuda, M. Okada, T. Fujita, et al., Correlation between diffusion in lumbar intervertebral discs and lumbar artery status: evaluation with fresh blood imaging technique, J. Magn. Reson. Imaging 25 (2007) 185–191.
16. A. Korkiakoski, J. Niinimaki, J. Karppinen, et al., Association of lumbar arterial stenosis with low back symptoms: a cross-sectional study using two-dimensional time-of-flight magnetic resonance angiography, Acta. Radiol. 50 (2009) 48–54.
17. L.I. Kauppila, K. Tallroth, Postmortem angiographic findings for arteries supplying the lumbar spine: their relationship to low-back symptoms, J. Spinal Disord. 6 (1993) 124–129.
18. M. Kurunlahti, J. Karppinen, M. Haapea, et al., Three-year follow-up of lumbar artery occlusion with magnetic resonance angiography in patients with sciatica: associations between occlusion and patient-reported symptoms, Spine 29 (2004) 1804–1808.
19. P. Leino-Arjas, L. Kaila-Kangas, S. Solovieva, et al., Serum lipids and low back pain: an association? A follow-up of a working population sample, Spine 31 (2006) 1032–1037.
20. B.S. Jhawar, C.S. Fuchs, G.A. Colditz, et al., Cardiovascular risk factors for physician-diagnosed lumbar disc herniation, Spine J. 6 (2006) 684–691.
21. M. Hangai, K. Kaneoka, S. Kuno, et al., Factors associated with lumbar intervertebral disc degeneration in the elderly, Spine J. 8 (2008) 732–740.
22. R. Shiri, J. Karppinen, P. Leino-Arjas, et al., The association between smoking and low back pain: a meta-analysis. Am. J. Med. 123 (2010) 87.e7–e35.
23. M.C. Battie, T. Videman, J. Kaprio, et al., The Twin Spine Study: contributions to a changing view of disc degeneration, Spine J. 9 (2009) 47–59.
24. M.C. Battie, T. Videman, K. Gill, et al., 1991 Volvo Award in clinical sciences. Smoking and lumbar intervertebral disc degeneration: an MRI study of identical twins, Spine 16 (1991) 1015–1021.

25. M. Akmal, A. Kesani, B. Anand, et al., Effect of nicotine on spinal disc cells: a cellular mechanism for disc degeneration, Spine 29 (2004) 568–575.

26. H. Oda, H. Matsuzaki, Y. Tokuhashi, et al., Degeneration of intervertebral discs due to smoking: experimental assessment in a rat-smoking model, J. Orthop. Sci. 9 (2004) 135–141.

27. H. Uei, H. Matsuzaki, H. Oda, et al., Gene expression changes in an early stage of intervertebral disc degeneration induced by passive cigarette smoking, Spine 31 (2006) 510–514.

28. P. Mikkonen, P. Leino-Arjas, J. Remes, et al., Is smoking a risk factor for low back pain in adolescents? A prospective cohort study, Spine 33 (2008) 527–532.

29. M. Liuke, S. Solovieva, A. Lamminen, et al., Disc degeneration of the lumbar spine in relation to overweight, Int. J. Obes. (Lond) 29 (2005) 903–908.

30. U.N. Das, Is obesity an inflammatory condition? Nutrition 17 (2001) 953–966.

31. H. Tilg, A.R. Moschen, Adipocytokines: mediators linking adipose tissue, inflammation and immunity, Nat. Rev. Immunol. 6 (2006) 772–783.

32. H.R. Girn, N.M. Orsi, S. Homer-Vanniasinkam, An overview of cytokine interactions in atherosclerosis and implications for peripheral arterial disease, Vasc. Med. 12 (2007) 299–309.

33. S. Solovieva, J. Lohiniva, P. Leino-Arjas, et al., COL9A3 gene polymorphism and obesity in intervertebral disc degeneration of the lumbar spine: evidence of gene-environment interaction, Spine 27 (2002) 2691–2696.

34. D. Chan, Y. Song, P. Sham, et al., Genetics of disc degeneration, Eur. Spine J. 15 (Suppl. 3) (2006) S317–S325.

35. P.N. Sambrook, A.J. MacGregor, T.D. Spector, Genetic influences on cervical and lumbar disc degeneration: a magnetic resonance imaging study in twins, Arthritis Rheum. 42 (1999) 366–372.

36. S. Annunen, P. Paassilta, J. Lohiniva, et al., An allele of COL9A2 associated with intervertebral disc disease, Science 285 (1999) 409–412.

37. K. Higashino, Y. Matsui, S. Yagi, et al., The alpha2 type IX collagen tryptophan polymorphism is associated with the severity of disc degeneration in younger patients with herniated nucleus pulposus of the lumbar spine, Int. Orthop. 31 (2007) 107–111.

38. J.J. Jim, N. Noponen-Hietala, K.M. Cheung, et al., The TRP2 allele of COL9A2 is an age-dependent risk factor for the development and severity of intervertebral disc degeneration, Spine 30 (2005) 2735–2742.

39. S.N. Kales, A. Linos, C. Chatzis, et al., The role of collagen IX tryptophan polymorphisms in symptomatic intervertebral disc disease in Southern European patients, Spine 29 (2004) 1266–1270.

40. J. Karppinen, E. Paakko, S. Raina, et al., Magnetic resonance imaging findings in relation to the COL9A2 tryptophan allele among patients with sciatica, Spine 27 (2002) 78–83.

41. P. Paassilta, J. Lohiniva, H.H. Goring, et al., Identification of a novel common genetic risk factor for lumbar disc disease, JAMA 285 (2001) 1843–1849.

42. S. Seki, Y. Kawaguchi, M. Mori, et al., Association study of COL9A2 with lumbar disc disease in the Japanese population, J. Hum. Genet. 51 (2006) 1063–1067.

43. J. Karppinen, I. Daavittila, S. Solovieva, et al., Genetic factors are associated with modic changes in endplates of lumbar vertebral bodies, Spine 33 (2008) 1236–1241.

44. P. Roughley, D. Martens, J. Rantakokko, et al., The involvement of aggrecan polymorphism in degeneration of human intervertebral disc and articular cartilage, Eur. Cell Mater. 11 (2006) 1–7.

45. S. Solovieva, N. Noponen, M. Mannikko, et al., Association between the aggrecan gene variable number of tandem repeats polymorphism and intervertebral disc degeneration, Spine 32 (2007) 1700–1705.

46. S. Seki, Y. Kawaguchi, K. Chiba, et al., A functional SNP in CILP, encoding cartilage intermediate layer protein, is associated with susceptibility to lumbar disc disease, Nat. Genet. 37 (2005) 607–612.

47. A.M. Valdes, G. Hassett, D.J. Hart, et al., Radiographic progression of lumbar spine disc degeneration is influenced by variation at inflammatory genes: a candidate SNP association study in the Chingford cohort, Spine 30 (2005) 2445–2451.

48. I.M. Virtanen, Y.Q. Song, K.M. Cheung, et al., Phenotypic and population differences in the association between CILP and lumbar disc disease, J. Med. Genet. 44 (2007) 285–288.

49. K.M. Cheung, D. Chan, J. Karppinen, et al., Association of the Taq I allele in vitamin D receptor with degenerative disc disease and disc bulge in a Chinese population, Spine 31 (2006) 1143–1148.

50. Y. Kawaguchi, M. Kanamori, H. Ishihara, et al., The association of lumbar disc disease with vitamin-D receptor gene polymorphism, J. Bone Joint Surg. Am. 84-A (2002) 2022–2028.

51. T. Videman, J. Leppavuori, J. Kaprio, et al., Intragenic polymorphisms of the vitamin D receptor gene associated with intervertebral disc degeneration, Spine 23 (1998) 2477–2485.

52. C.L. Le Maitre, A.J. Freemont, J.A. Hoyland, The role of interleukin-1 in the pathogenesis of human intervertebral disc degeneration, Arthritis Res. Ther. 7 (2005) R732–R745.

53. C.L. Le Maitre, J.A. Hoyland, A.J. Freemont, Catabolic cytokine expression in degenerate and herniated human intervertebral discs: IL-1beta and TNFalpha expression profile, Arthritis Res. Ther. 9 (2007) R77.

54. V.K. Podichetty, The aging spine: the role of inflammatory mediators in intervertebral disc degeneration, Cell Mol. Biol. (Noisy-le-grand) 53 (2007) 4–18.

55. S. Solovieva, S. Kouhia, P. Leino-Arjas, et al., Interleukin 1 polymorphisms and intervertebral disc degeneration, Epidemiology 15 (2004) 626–633.

56. S. Solovieva, P. Leino-Arjas, J. Saarela, et al., Possible association of interleukin 1 gene locus polymorphisms with low back pain, Pain 109 (2004) 8–19.

57. D.M. Dong, M. Yao, B. Liu, et al., Association between the -1306C/T polymorphism of matrix metalloproteinase-2 gene and lumbar disc disease in Chinese young adults, Eur. Spine. J. 16 (2007) 1958–1961.

58. P. Goupille, M.I. Jayson, J.P. Valat, et al., Matrix metalloproteinases: the clue to intervertebral disc degeneration? Spine 23 (1998) 1612–1626.

59. Y.Q. Song, D.W. Ho, J. Karppinen, et al., Association between promoter -1607 polymorphism of MMP1 and lumbar disc disease in Southern Chinese, BMC Med. Genet. 9 (2008) 38.

60. M. Takahashi, H. Haro, Y. Wakabayashi, et al., The association of degeneration of the intervertebral disc with 5a/6a polymorphism in the promoter of the human matrix metalloproteinase-3 gene, J. Bone Joint Surg. Br. 83 (2001) 491–495.

61. M.A. Adams, P.J. Roughley, What is intervertebral disc degeneration, and what causes it? Spine 31 (2006) 2151–2161.

62. S. Solovieva, J. Lohiniva, P. Leino-Arjas, et al., Intervertebral disc degeneration in relation to the COL9A3 and the IL-1ss gene polymorphisms, Eur. Spine J. 15 (2006) 613–619.

63. M.C. Battie, T. Videman, E. Levalahti, et al., Genetic and environmental effects on disc degeneration by phenotype and spinal level: a multivariate twin study, Spine 33 (2008) 2801–2808.

64. I.M. Virtanen, J. Karppinen, S. Taimela, et al., Occupational and genetic risk factors associated with intervertebral disc disease, Spine 32 (2007) 1129–1134.

65. N. Boos, S. Weissbach, H. Rohrbach, et al., Classification of age-related changes in lumbar intervertebral discs: 2002 Volvo Award in basic science, Spine 27 (2002) 2631–2644.

# 12

# Osteoporosis and the Aging Spine: Diagnosis and Treatment

*Aasis Unnanuntana, Brian P. Gladnick, and Joseph M. Lane*

**K E Y   P O I N T S**

- Osteoporosis fractures markedly increase morbidity and mortality; therefore, strategies for diagnosis, prevention, and treatment of this condition are needed.

- Once a patient has been diagnosed with osteoporosis, a complete evaluation should be obtained. This includes a thorough medical history with particular attention paid to the risk of osteoporosis, a physical examination, and essential laboratory investigations. If secondary osteoporosis is suspected based on the clinical findings, further investigations are required directed at the secondary cause.

- All patients with osteoporosis should be tested for vitamin D deficiency. If inadequate, vitamin D supplementation is needed. The requirement for vitamin D intake in an adult is approximately 1000 to 2000 IU/day.

- Bisphosphonates are strong antiresorptive agents that have been shown to reduce both vertebral and nonvertebral fracture risks. Therefore they are the first-line drugs for the treatment of postmenopausal osteoporosis, unless contraindicated.

- Bisphosphonates might have an adverse effect on spinal fusion, whereas teriparatide facilitates fusion and increases the fusion mass. In addition, anabolic agents enhance fracture healing. We therefore recommend initiating an anabolic agent (PTH 1-34) when bone healing is required. If bisphosphonate therapy is considered, refrain 4 or more weeks before commencing therapy.

Osteoporosis is a systemic debilitating disease of the skeleton, characterized by significantly decreased bone mass in combination with the deterioration of bone microarchitecture. This process results in weakened bone with a great propensity for fracture with low-energy stress. As the average life expectancy and median age of the population rises, fractures secondary to underlying osteoporosis are becoming increasingly commonplace. More than 1.5 million osteoporotic fractures occur annually in the United States, the majority of which occur in the spine, hip, and wrist.[1] Women are predominantly affected; a recent study estimates that as many as one in two women who are older than 50 years of age will suffer an osteoporotic fracture.[2] These fractures can result in marked morbidity and mortality. For example, a single vertebral compression fracture in women is associated with a 1.2-fold increased age-adjusted mortality rate, and the presence of five fractures increases that risk to 2.3-fold.[3] In addition, a vertebral fracture increases the risk of a second vertebral fracture by 5-fold, and a hip fracture by 2-fold. Among patients with osteoporotic hip fractures, only 25% of patients ever make a full recovery, while 20% die within the year secondary to complications. Thus, spine surgeons must be increasingly suspicious of this disease in certain patient demographics, achieve a firm understanding of the pathogenesis of osteoporotic bone and the conditions that result in bone fragility, and become familiar with the current strategies for diagnosis, prevention, and treatment of osteoporosis.

## PHYSIOLOGY OF BONE REMODELING AND BONE TURNOVER

Bone is a dynamic, living tissue that continuously remodels itself throughout the lifetime of the patient. Bone homeostasis consists of three phases. The initial *resorption* phase is mediated primarily by osteoclasts, which are activated through the interaction of an osteoclast surface protein, receptor activator of nuclear factor-$\varkappa$B (RANK), with its ligand (RANKL). RANKL is primarily expressed by the osteoblast lineage and by stromal cells. During the *reversal* phase, osteoclasts become less numerous on the bony surfaces and are increasingly replaced by mononuclear cells. These mononuclear cells prepare the bony surface for the introduction of bone-forming osteoblasts and provide cytokine signaling, which stimulates the differentiation of osteoblasts and their subsequent migration to the surface of the bone. During the final *formation* phase, osteoblasts lay down newly formed woven bone to replace bone that had been previously resorbed.

Bone remodeling is a complex process that is regulated both locally and systemically. As previously mentioned, RANKL/RANK interactions at the local level promote induction of osteoclast activity and subsequent remodeling. Conversely, osteoprotegerin (OPG) is a soluble receptor for RANKL that acts as an antagonist to decrease osteoclastic activation and thereby reduce the rate of bone resorption. Interestingly, there are a number of systemic signaling mechanisms that act through the RANKL/RANK/OPG pathway to regulate bone homeostasis.[4] For example, parathyroid hormone (PTH) and the glucocorticoids both act to increase local expression of RANKL but decrease concomitant expression of OPG, resulting in a net increase in osteoclast activation and bone resorption. Alternatively, estrogens act to increase the local expression of OPG and decrease RANKL, which results in a net decrease in osteoclast activity and bone resorption (Figure 12-1). Derangement of these pathways can alter the delicate balance between bone resorption and bone formation, and may result in a net decrease of bone formation that contributes to the development of osteoporosis.

Based upon the varying influences of bone resorption and formation, osteoporosis is subdivided into two categories: low-turnover and high-turnover osteoporosis. The *low-turnover* state describes a situation in which normal bone homeostasis is altered by decreased osteoblast activity; however, the osteoclast activity remains normal. Low bone mineral density (BMD) in this setting, therefore, is a result of reduced bone formation. Conversely, the *high-turnover* state is characterized by increased activity of both osteoblasts and osteoclasts. However, osteoclasts are activated to a greater extent. The bone remodeling process is shifted toward bone resorption, resulting in an imbalance of bone turnover that causes osteoporosis. High turnover osteoporosis is the most common form and appears at menopause, while low turnover osteoporosis occurs following drug interventions including chemotherapy, steroids, and prolonged bisphosphonate use.

## DIAGNOSIS OF OSTEOPOROSIS

Although a good clinical understanding of osteoporosis takes into account the pathophysiology of bone remodeling, mineralization changes, and variable bone quality of the patient, the diagnosis of osteoporosis until recently

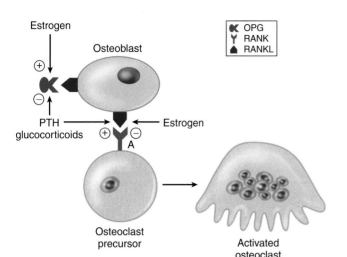

■ **FIGURE 12-1** Receptor activator of nuclear factor-κB (RANK) on the osteoclast precursor's surface interacts with its ligand (RANKL), expressed by the osteoblasts and stromal cells, thereby activating the differentiation of the osteoclast precursor to activated osteoclast and subsequent bone resorption. Osteoprotegerin (OPG) is a soluble receptor for RANKL that competitively inhibits the RANKL-RANK interaction. Various systemic modulators (estrogen, parathyroid hormone [PTH], or glucocorticoids) influence the activation of the osteoclasts via their effects on the RANK/RANKL/OPG pathway. (+), Activation; (–), Inhibition.

**TABLE 12-1    WHO-Based Criteria for Diagnosis of Osteoporosis**

| T-Score | Diagnosis |
| --- | --- |
| – 1.0 or above | Normal bone |
| Below –1.0 to above –2.5 | Osteopenia |
| – 2.5 or below | Osteoporosis |
| – 2.5 or below with fracture | Severe osteoporosis |

has relied upon a single criterion: the bone mineral density. The current gold standard of measuring BMD is dual-energy x-ray absorptiometry (DXA), which uses an x-ray beam to calculate the patient's BMD. The most preferred skeletal sites for evaluation of BMD are the spine and hip, because these two locations provide the best data for correlating low BMD with the risk of future fracture BMD is reported as the T-score, which is a measurement of how many standard deviations the patient's bone density is below the mean of young, healthy individuals at their peak bone mass. Based on this T-score, the World Health Organization (WHO) developed a classification system to define osteoporosis (Table 12-1).

Generally, osteoporosis is classified as either primary or secondary. Primary osteoporosis is further subdivided, based on its pathogenesis. Type I, or postmenopausal osteoporosis, is related to the abrupt decline of estrogen levels that occurs in menopausal women. Type II osteoporosis, known as senile or age-related osteoporosis, is due to the progressive decrease of BMD in both men and women that occurs with aging. Patients may suffer from both subtypes of primary osteoporosis.

Secondary osteoporosis is defined by the presence of some preexisting disease process or other causative factor, which causes a secondary decline in BMD (Table 12-2). Forty-five percent of osteoporotic women and 66% of osteoporotic men have their osteoporosis secondary to some underlying condition. Therefore patients with secondary osteoporosis must be identified because definitive treatment of the underlying cause is necessary to prevent further bone loss, and thus lower the risk of fracture. In this regard, it is important to consider the patient's BMD using the Z-score. The Z-score indicates how many standard deviations the patient's BMD is below the

**TABLE 12-2    Causes of Secondary Osteoporosis[5]**

**Hormone Excess**
- Parathyroid (primary or secondary)
- Thyroid
- Cortisol

**Hormone Deficiency**
- Estrogen (premenopausal or postmenopausal)
- Testosterone

**Diseases**
- Inflammation (rheumatoid arthritis, ulcerative colitis)
- Tumor or malignancy (multiple myeloma, lymphoma)
- Collagen vascular disease
- Renal osteodystrophy
- Others (liver diseases, immobilization)

**Drugs**
- Corticosteroids
- Thyroxine
- Alcohol
- Anticonvulsants (barbiturates, phenytoin)
- Anticoagulants (heparin, warfarin [Coumadin])
- Antimetabolites (methotrexate, cyclosporin)

expected value for his or her own age. The Z-score cannot be used to diagnose osteoporosis, but it is useful for screening the patient for secondary causes. A Z-score of –2.0 or lower should increase the index of suspicion that underlying medical problems, medications, or other factors may be responsible for the patient's low BMD.[6]

## EVALUATION FOR OSTEOPOROSIS

Once diagnosed with osteoporosis, a complete medical history should be obtained with particular attention to the risk factors for osteoporosis. These include age of 65 years or older, a history of vertebral fracture or any fracture during childhood, a family history of hip fracture, low body weight (BMI < 21 or weight < 127 lb), cigarette smoking, and use of corticosteroids for more than 3 months.[6] The physical examination should be performed particularly at the spine region. Height should be measured and compared with the greatest known height to determine height loss, which is an indicator of the presence of vertebral compression fractures. Balance and walking gait should be observed in each individual. The assessment of functional balance is performed by using the single limb stance test and the 6-minute walking test.

### Screening for Osteoporosis with Bone Mineral Density Measurement

A number of risk factors for osteoporosis have been identified by the International Society for Clinical Densitometry (ISCD),[7] and should be used to guide the screening process in a cost-effective manner. The current indications for BMD testing include any patient who is one or more of the following:

1. A female aged 65 or older
2. A postmenopausal female younger than 65 years who has clinical risk factors for fracture, such as low body mass index, prior fracture, or use of a high-risk medication
3. A woman during the menopausal transition with clinical risk factors for fracture
4. A male aged 70 years or older
5. A male younger than 70 years with clinical risk factors for fracture
6. An adult with a history of a fragility fracture
7. An adult with an illness known to cause bone loss or low BMD
8. An adult taking a medication known to cause bone loss or low BMD
9. Any patient being considered for pharmacologic treatment of bone loss
10. Any patient currently being treated for low BMD in order to monitor the treatment effect
11. Any patient not receiving therapy in whom evidence of bone loss would lead to pharmacologic treatment

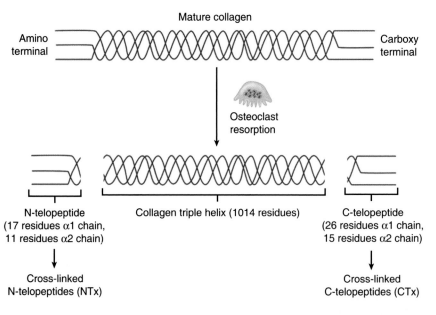

■ **FIGURE 12-2** The normal structure of a single human collagen molecule is shown. The collagen molecule is a triple helix consisting of two pro-α1 chains (red) and a single pro-α2 chain (blue). During osteoclast-mediated bone resorption, the bone collagen molecule is degraded, producing an amino-terminal (N)-telopeptide, a carboxy-terminal (C)-telopeptide, and a central region of intact triple helix. Cross-linked N-telopeptides (NTx) and cross-linked C-telopeptides (CTx) are specific for bone and achieve a measurable concentration in blood and urine. When osteoclast activity increases, bone is resorbed and more collagen is degraded, which coincides with an increased measured concentration of NTx and CTx.

In addition to these guidelines, it is important to take into account other factors that may increase a patient's propensity for low BMD or fracture. Patients with poor general health, alcoholism, dementia, frailty, recent discontinuation of estrogen replacement therapy, or long-term history of estrogen deficiency should be considered for DXA scanning even if they do not fit the ISCD criteria.

## Laboratory Investigations for Osteoporosis

Generally, laboratory investigations other than BMD measurement are not required for the diagnosis of osteoporosis. Some routine tests, however, should be performed to obtain baseline values as part of the initial workup. These include complete blood count with differential cell count, urinalysis, and blood chemistry profiles with serum calcium and phosphate. Some special laboratory tests are available to measure the balance between bone resorption and bone formation from serum and urine samples. These assays are called "bone markers."

Bone markers can be classified into two groups: bone formation and bone resorption markers. Bone specific alkaline phosphatase and serum osteocalcin are both produced when bone is formed and can be used as markers for bone formation. On the other hand, during bone resorption, human collagen is broken down and released into the bloodstream and subsequently secreted into the urine. By assaying the amount of collagen breakdown products, such as the cross-linked amino-terminal telopeptides of bone collagen (NTx) in urine or blood, the rate that bone is being resorbed can be determined (Figure 12-2). Measurement of bone markers is helpful for following a patient's response to treatment over time. Therefore it is advisable to get a baseline value as part of the initial workup. The goal of treatment of osteoporosis is to keep the NTx levels close to the normal range for premenopausal women.

Vitamin D deficiency is very common among elderly, with a prevalence of approximately 50%; however, many patients are asymptomatic. In addition, serum calcium and phosphate levels in this group of patients may not necessarily be abnormal. All older individuals, therefore, should be tested for vitamin D deficiency by measuring levels of 25-hydroxy vitamin D. If low, adequate vitamin D supplementation is encouraged. Values below 20 ng/mL are associated with poor muscle function as well as mineralization defects.

## Evaluation for Secondary Osteoporosis

When secondary osteoporosis is suspected on the basis of clinical findings or because the patient is relatively young and presented with fragility fracture, specific tests should be considered to evaluate contributing causes that may require additional medical attention. These include basic laboratory investigation of a complete blood count with differential, erythrocyte sedimentation rate, serum calcium and phosphate level, liver function tests, thyroid-stimulating hormone level, testosterone level in men, and a serum

**TABLE 12-3    Laboratory Investigations for Secondary Osteoporosis**

| Medical Diseases | Diagnostic Study |
|---|---|
| *Endocrine* | |
| • Hyperparathyroidism | serum calcium, serum phosphate, parathyroid hormone level |
| • Hyperthyroidism | TSH, T3, free T4 |
| • Hypogonadism | LH, FSH, estrogen, testosterone (men) |
| • Diabetes | blood glucose |
| *GI Disorders* | |
| • Crohn disease, Ulcerative colitis | CBC, ESR, CRP, serum albumin, colonoscopy |
| *Liver Disease* | |
| • Primary biliary cirrhosis, Chronic active hepatitis | Liver function test, antimitochondrial antibody, antibody for hepatitis A,B and C |
| *Bone Marrow Disorders* | |
| • Multiple Myeloma, Leukemia, Lymphoma | CBC with differential, serum calcium, serum protein electrophoresis |
| *Collagen Vascular Disease* | |
| • Osteogenesis imperfecta, Ehlers-Danlos syndrome, Marfan syndrome | Genetic testing for collagen defects |
| *Others* | |
| • Rheumatoid arthritis | CBC, ESR, CRP, rheumatoid factor |
| • Renal Failure | BUN, creatinine |

TSH = thyroid stimulating hormone; LH = luteinizing hormone; FSH = follicle stimulating hormone; CBC = complete blood count; ESR = erythrocyte sedimentation rate; CRP = c-reactive protein; BUN = blood urea nitrogen

protein electrophoresis if myeloma is considered (Table 12-3). When abnormalities are detected, the patient should be referred to a specialist for further evaluation and specific treatment.

## Assess for Risk of Falls and Fractures

Certain comorbidities associated with the aging population, such as unsteady gait, use of sedative or hypnotic medications, and impaired visual or neuromuscular function may predispose a patient to falls. By identifying patients at particularly high risk for falls early in the course of treatment, it is possible to prevent a subsequent fracture. It is well recognized that the fracture rate

**TABLE 12-4    Ten-Year Probability for Osteoporotic Fracture Based on FRAX Calculations[8]**

| Clinical Risk Factors* | 10-Year Fracture Probability (%)† |
|---|---|
| None | 8.6 |
| Current smoker | 9.2 |
| Alcohol (≥3 drinks/day) | 10.4 |
| Rheumatoid arthritis | 11.7 |
| Oral glucocorticoids | 13.7 |
| Parent with history of hip fracture | 16.0 |
| Previous fragility fracture | 16.4 |

*Assume in a female patient, aged 65 years, with BMI = 25 kg/m².
†Probabilities are given in absence of a known T-score.

**TABLE 12-5    Antifracture Efficacy of Agents for Treatment of Osteoporosis*[9]**

| Pharmacologic Agent | Fracture Type | | |
|---|---|---|---|
| | Vertebral | Hip | Nonvertebral† |
| **General** | | | |
| Calcium monotherapy | B | C | C |
| Vitamin D monotherapy and analogs (Calcitriol, alfacalcidol, etc) | C | C | C |
| Calcium plus vitamin D | C | A | A |
| **Antiresorptive** | | | |
| Estrogen replacement therapy | A | A | A |
| SERMs (Raloxifene) | A | C | C |
| Calcitonin, intranasal (Miacalcic) | A | C | C |
| Bisphosphonates | | | |
| Alendronate (Fosamax) | A# | A | A |
| Risedronate (Actonel) | A | A | A |
| Ibandronate (Boniva) | A | - | A |
| Zoledronic acid (Reclast) | A | A | A |
| **Anabolic** | | | |
| Teriparatide (Forteo) | A | - | A |

*Data from randomized, placebo-controlled clinical trials of women with prior vertebral fractures or with osteoporosis.
†Nonvertebral fractures; osteoporotic fractures exclusive of the spine.
#Also seen in men. A = convincing evidence of antifracture efficacy. B = inconsistent results. C = ineffective, or insufficiency evidence of efficacy. SERMs = selective estrogen receptor modulators

is highest among patients with osteoporotic bones (T-score −2.5 or below). However, a much larger proportion of patients reside in the range of osteopenia (below −1.0 to above −2.5). Consequently, more total fractures occur in this osteopenic group (55% of hip fractures). To adjust for the disparity, a new vehicle called the Fracture Risk Assessment Tool (FRAX) has been developed that adds additional risk factors to the calculation, and offers a better assessment of fracture risk than DXA scanning alone. This instrument calculates the patient's 10-year fracture risk based on age, sex, weight, height, previous fracture, parent with fractured hip, current smoking, use of glucocorticoids, presence of rheumatoid arthritis, secondary osteoporosis, alcohol use (>3 drinks/day), and BMD at the femoral neck area.

Each risk factor is weighted differently in the calculation depending on its importance. For example, in the absence of BMD measurements, a prior history of fracture is considerably more predictive of a patient's future fracture risk than is a history of smoking, and is weighted as such in the FRAX calculation (Table 12-4). As the patient accrues more risk factors, the FRAX score increases in a predictable manner.[8]

## TREATMENT IN OSTEOPOROSIS

### Nonpharmacologic Treatment

A multidisciplinary approach is critically important in the management of osteoporosis.[9] Nonpharmacologic treatment is used concurrently with pharmacologic therapy to optimize fracture risk reduction. Thus, every patient should be considered for nonpharmacologic management. Commonly used nonpharmacologic treatments include, but are not limited to, calcium and vitamin D supplementation, fall prevention, and balance and exercise programs.

### Calcium and Vitamin D Supplementation

Calcium and vitamin D supplementation is the cornerstone of all treatment modalities for osteoporosis. Literature clearly shows that adequate calcium and vitamin D intake reduces the risk of fractures. For optimal treatment, adequate calcium intake of 1000 to 1500 mg/day should be maintained in all patients on any type of treatment. To maximize the absorption of calcium across the small bowels, no more than 500 to 600 mg of elemental calcium should be taken at any given time. Among all calcium formulations, calcium citrate is the preferred form. Calcium citrate binds to oxalate, reducing its intestinal absorption, and citrate in urine inhibits crystal formation, thus reducing the incidence of kidney stones. In addition, calcium citrate does not require low pH for salt dissociation; therefore the absorption of this calcium formulation is reliable in patients taking $H_2$ blockers or proton pump inhibitors.

The current recommended dosages of vitamin $D_3$ from the Institute of Medicine are 200 to 600 IU/day. However, many experts consider these recommendations to be too low and suggest that the minimum adult intake should be 1000 to 2000 IU/day. The appropriate amount of vitamin D intake should be evaluated by monitoring 25-hydroxy vitamin D level

and serum PTH. Patients with vitamin D insufficiency will have low levels of 25-hydroxy vitamin D and elevated serum PTH from secondary hyperparathyroidism. At the Hospital for Special Surgery, 45% of patients undergoing elective surgery and 66% of patients presenting with fractures have vitamin D insufficiency. Higher doses of vitamin D are required in these patients to replenish depleted total body stores. Fifty thousand international units of vitamin $D_2$ can be taken orally once a week or every other week for 6 to 8 weeks, followed by a maintenance dose of vitamin $D_3$ of 1000 to 2000 IU/day. Toxicity is rare even if a dosage of 10,000 IU/day is given for up to 5 months.

## Pharmacologic Treatment

Osteoporosis has been divided into two categories, high-turnover and low-turnover osteoporosis. The pharmacologic agents currently available are commonly divided into antiresorptive and anabolic groups. Antiresorptive agents have been developed to address the high-turnover state. These include estrogen, selective estrogen receptor modulators (SERMs), calcitonin, and bisphosphonates. The anabolic agent, parathyroid hormone, provides active building of bone mass and has been suggested to treat the low-turnover state. Both antiresorptive and anabolic agents have demonstrated antifracture efficacy in many studies (Table 12-5).

### Antiresorptive Agents

**Estrogen** is an antiosteoporotic agent that has been shown to increase bone mass and thus decrease the risk of vertebral and hip fracture by approximately 30% to 40% as compared with patients taking placebo. Estrogen, however, has been found to increase rates of stroke and deep vein thrombosis, whereas combined estrogen and progesterone therapy is associated with increased risks of cardiovascular disease, breast cancer, dementia, and gallbladder disease. As a consequence, estrogen is mainly used in the early postmenopausal period to treat postmenopausal syndrome and then lowered to the least effective dose to control symptoms. Because of the risks of estrogen formulations, this precludes their use as primary agents in the treatment of osteoporosis.

**TABLE 12-6    Bisphosphonates Recommended to Treat Osteoporosis**

| Generic Name | Trade Name | Recommended Dose | Route of Administration | Instructions |
|---|---|---|---|---|
| Alendronate | Fosamax | 10 mg per day<br>70 mg per week | Oral | **Oral bisphosphonates:** |
| Risedronate | Actonel | 5 mg per day<br>35 mg per week<br>50 mg per month | Oral | Take with 8 ounces of water and waiting at least 30 min in an upright position before eating or drinking anything |
| Ibandronate | Boniva | 150 mg per month | Oral | **Intravenous bisphosphonates:** |
| Zoledronic acid | Reclast | 5 mg per year | Intravenous | Infusion over 15 to 45 min and co-administration with benadryl and tylenol |

All bisphosphonates: Precaution in patients with severe renal insufficiency and hypocalcemia

**SERMs** are a class of agents that bind to estrogen receptors. They have a significant effect on breast tissue and bone cells; however, they act as antagonists in the other receptor sites. Of the SERMs currently being used for clinical settings, only raloxifene has been approved for the prevention and treatment of osteoporosis. Early data suggest that raloxifene decreases the risk of breast cancer by 70%, which made raloxifene a preferred agent in this particular indication. Although raloxifene has been shown to reduce the risk of vertebral fracture, there was no significant reduction in the overall risk of nonvertebral fracture. In addition, by stimulating estrogen receptors, raloxifene increases the risk of pulmonary emboli and thrombophlebitis and may cause profound postmenopausal symptoms. Therefore clinicians must weigh the benefits of the reduced risks of vertebral fracture and invasive breast cancer against the increased risks of venous thromboembolism and fatal stroke when considering this agent for osteoporosis management.

**Calcitonin** is available as both a parenteral injection and nasal spray. The intranasal spray is the most commonly used formulation because of its superior compliance and ease of use. Calcitonin reduces the risk of vertebral fracture, but there is only a modest increase in BMD. Additionally, calcitonin treatment shows no benefit for reducing the risk of hip and other nonvertebral fractures. There are some data suggesting the analgesic effect of calcitonin. Although there is a hypothesis that calcitonin-induced analgesia may be mediated by increased beta-endorphins and may directly affect pain receptors in the central nervous system, the exact mechanism is still unknown. Therefore the current indication for calcitonin treatment is for alleviating painful vertebral compression fractures. It should be discontinued as soon as pain has been controlled, because other pharmacologic agents are much more effective at preventing future fractures.

**Bisphosphonates** are a class of antiresorptive agents that have been shown to be extremely efficacious in high-turnover osteoporosis. Currently, four bisphosphonates have been approved by the U.S. Food and Drug Administration for the treatment of posmenopausal osteoporosis: alendronate (Fosamax), risedronate (Actonel), ibandronate (Boniva) and zoledronic acid (Reclast).[10] These drugs differ in their potency, mode of administration, and dosing schedules. Alendronate and risedronate are administered orally, whereas zoledronic acid is administered by intravenous injection. Ibandronate is available in both oral and intravenous formulations (Table 12-6).

The mechanism of action of bisphosphonate involves interposition of a nondegradable drug barrier between osteoclasts and Howship's lacunae, thus interfering with resorption. The drug is then ingested by osteoclasts and disrupts the cellular membrane mevalonate synthesis pathway, leading to premature osteoclast death. Bisphosphonates slow the bone turnover rate, which has been reported to be decreased within 6 weeks with the oral formulations and within 3 days with the intravenous formulations. All oral bisphosphonates reduce the risk of both vertebral and nonvertebral fractures. The intravenous zoledronic acid appears to be effective in increasing bone mass and decreasing both the vertebral and nonvertebral fracture risk. In addition, when given within 3 months of an acute hip fracture, zoledronic acid lowers mortality by more than 20% and does not interfere with fracture healing.

The adverse effects of oral bisphosphonates are their inherent toxicity to epithelial cells lining the gastrointestinal tract. The results are irritation of the esophagus, acid eructation, nausea, and heartburn. Patients with a significant background of gastrointestinal intolerance, therefore, are not suitable

for prescribing oral formulations. However, clinicians may improve patients' tolerance by giving oral bisphosphonates in small doses and slowly increasing the dosage until full dose is achieved. This will lead to better compliance even with individuals who have a past history of dyspepsia. The other potential complication is osteonecrosis of the jaw. Osteonecrosis of the jaw is defined as exposed bone in the musculofacial region that fails to heal within 8 weeks after identification by a health care provider. The group of patients who carry the greatest risk for developing this complication are those with multiple myeloma or metastatic carcinoma of the skeleton who are being treated with relatively high doses of intravenous bisphosphonates. Therefore, before starting bisphosphonate treatment, especially with an intravenous formulation, patients should complete any dental work and should establish meticulous oral hygiene. In addition, intravenous bisphosphonates can cause a release of cytokines from osteoclasts and result in flulike symptoms. These include fever, muscle pain, headache, and bone pain. Most of the symptoms resolve within 3 days. Co-administration of diphenhydramine (Benadryl) and acetaminophen (Tylenol) can minimize these side effects.

The sequelae of long-term bisphosphonates on bone metabolism remain unclear. There is a hypothesis that prolonged treatment with bisphosphonates may lead to adynamic, fragile bone. In this state of oversuppression, microfractures generated through the wear and tear of normal daily life begin to accumulate and coalesce, leading to insufficiency fractures. Accumulation of microdamage is associated with a reduction in bone toughness. Many studies report low-energy subtrochanteric or mid shaft fractures after prolonged treatment with alendronate. This type of fracture is caused by minimal or no trauma and is characterized by (1) simple or transverse fracture, (2) breaking of the cortex on one side, and (3) hypertrophied diaphyseal cortices, Currently, the recommendation for bisphosphonate therapy is a 5-year period of treatment. Once the BMD is in its plateau and the urine level of NTx is in therapeutic range (20-40 nmol bone collagen equivalents/mmol of creatinine), changes in treatment, such as a rest period from bisphosphonates or the use of an anabolic agent, should be considered.

### Anabolic Agents

Teriparatide, parathyroid hormone (1-34), is the only anabolic agent available in the United States for the treatment of postmenopausal osteoporosis. It is administered subcutaneously once a day. When given intermittently, teriparatide can lead up to a 13% increase in bone mass over 2 years of therapy. This increase is greater than that achieved with bisphosphonate therapy. The risk of fracture was reduced by 65% and 53% for vertebral and nonvertebral fracture, respectively. Other benefits of teriparatide have been proposed. Many studies reported the possible benefits of teriparatide on fracture healing. Callus formation was accelerated by the early stimulation of proliferation and differentiation of osteoprogenitor cells and increases in production of bone matrix proteins. Teriparatide should be considered in the following conditions:

1. Patients with low-turnover osteoporosis
2. Patients who have been on bisphosphonates and still have fragility fracture
3. Patients with declining bone densities
4. Premenopausal women with osteoporosis

Contraindications include active Paget's disease of bone, metastatic cancer in the skeleton, history of skeletal irradiation, and children with open epiphyses. The adverse reactions associated with teriparatide are nausea, headache, dizziness, leg cramps, swelling, pain, weakness, erythema around the injection site, and elevation of serum calcium. There is a concern regarding osteosarcoma due to evidence showing that rodents, exposed to prolonged high doses of teriparatide, developed osteosarcoma. Therefore teriparatide should be discontinued after 2 years of treatment. After that, bisphosphonate therapy should be initiated to maintain its results.

## Pharmacologic Agents and Spinal Fusion

There are no clinical studies that evaluate pharmacologic agents for osteoporosis in the setting of vertebral fractures or spinal fusion. Bisphosphonates increase fracture callus size during endochondral repair but cause delay in maturation. Some animal studies have demonstrated that bisphosphonates delayed fusion. Therefore until clinical studies are available, we recommend that bisphosphonates should be started a few weeks after spinal fusion or vertebral fracture to reduce the possible adverse effects to the early biological processes of fracture healing. Teriparatide in all animal studies facilitated fracture healing. In both rat and rabbit models of spinal fusion, the administration of teriparatide speeded fusion, and increased the fusion mass. Based on these animal studies, teriparatide offers superior biology for spinal indications, when compared to bisphosphonates and a control group that only took calcium and vitamin D. However, the application of this agent in patients still awaits evidence-based studies.

## FUTURE DIRECTIONS

The available pharmacologic agents used to treat osteoporosis have their own limitations at some degrees. Understanding of cellular mechanism regulating bone formation and remodeling is critically important to developing new agents which will reduce the adverse effects or improve the outcome of treatment. Denosumab, a human monoclonal antibody against RANKL, has been shown in preclinical trials to increase bone mineral density and decrease bone resorption in postmenopausal women with osteoporosis. It is now awaiting approval for entry into the market. Cathepsin K inhibitors are another group of antiresorptive agents that were designed to reduce the activity of cathepsin K (a powerful osteoclast protease). Theoretically, this agent can limit the enzymatic degradation of bone matrix proteins.

Strontium ranelate is an agent that has both antiresorptive and anabolic action. Treatment of postmenopausal osteoporotic women with strontium ranelate has been shown to decrease fracture risk and increase bone mineral density. The long-term effects, however, remain unknown. The development of new formulations of teriparatide (noninjectable forms) or development of alternative parathyroid hormone analogs that possess longer half-life, leading to less frequent dosing, are also under investigation.

## SUMMARY

In general, the program for spinal care in elderly patients, particularly with osteoporosis/osteopenia, should include a thorough medical history and physical examination, appropriate diagnostic tests, maintenance of adequate nutrition including calcium, vitamin D, and the use of appropriate osteoporotic therapeutic agents. In the setting of spinal fusion and fracture healing, an anabolic agent such as parathyroid hormone may be advantageous in the early steps to enhance appropriate biological responses. Patients with osteoporosis require a multidisciplinary approach.

## References

1. R.W. Keen, Burden of osteoporosis and fractures, Curr. Osteoporos. Rep. 1 (2003) 66–70.
2. J.M. Lane, M.J. Gardner, J.T. Lin, M.C. van der Meulen, E. Myers, The aging spine: new technologies and therapeutics for the osteoporotic spine, Eur Spine. J. 12 (Suppl. 2) (2003) S147–S154.
3. J.T. Lin, J.M. Lane, Osteoporosis: a review, Clin. Orthop. Relat. Res. (425) (2004 Aug) 126–134.
4. D.J. Hadjidakis, Androulakis II, Bone remodeling, Ann. N. Y. Acad. Sci. 1092 (2006) 385–396.
5. E. Stein, E. Shane, Secondary osteoporosis, Endocrinol Metab. Clin. North Am. 32 (2003) 115–134.
6. J.D. Kaufman, S.R. Cummings, Osteoporosis and prevention of fractures: practical approaches for orthopaedic surgeons, Instr. Course Lect. 51 (2002) 559–565.
7. International Society for Clinical Densitometry. 2007 Official Positions & Pediatric Positions of the International Society for Clinical Densitometry. Available at http://www.iscd.org/Visitors/pdfs/ISCD2007OfficialPositions-Combined-AdultandPediatric.pdf. Accessed October 23, 2008.
8. J.A. Kanis, O. Johnell, A. Oden, H. Johansson, E. McCloskey, FRAX and the assessment of fracture probability in men and women from the UK, Osteoporos. Int. 19 (2008) 385–397.
9. M.L. Bouxsein, J. Kaufman, L. Tosi, S. Cummings, J. Lane, O. Johnell, Recommendations for optimal care of the fragility fracture patient to reduce the risk of future fracture, J. Am. Acad. Orthop. Surg. 12 (2004) 385–395.
10. L. Gehrig, J. Lane, M.I. O'Connor, Osteoporosis: management and treatment strategies for orthopaedic surgeons, J. Bone Joint Surg. Am. 90 (2008) 1362–1374.

# 13

# Osteoarthritis and Inflammatory Arthritides of the Aging Spine

*Kai-Ming G. Fu, Shu Man Fu, and Christopher I. Shaffrey*

**K E Y   P O I N T S**

- Osteoarthritis is the most common of the arthritides affecting the spine.
- Osteoarthritis has increased prevalence in the elderly.
- Conservative therapy can be effective in treating symptoms of spinal osteoarthritis.
- Operative intervention can benefit patients with intractable pain and/or neurological deficit.
- Other inflammatory arthritides should be excluded in the management of a patient with spinal osteoarthritis.

Because of space limitations, osteoarthritis of the aging spine will be primarily considered in this review. Certain inflammatory arthritides will be considered as a part of the differential diagnosis. Osteoarthritis is an almost ubiquitous disease and a significant source of morbidity. Although it can affect every age demographic, it has an increasing prevalence in the elderly population.[1] In the elderly, osteoarthritis is a significant source of disability and has a deleterious effect on a patient's quality of life. Although a majority of studies have examined the effect of osteoarthritis on hip, knee, and hand joints, osteoarthritis can affect any joint in the body, including those in the spine. Spinal osteoarthritis commonly manifests with back or neck pain. The degeneration caused by spinal osteoarthritis can also result in central canal or neural foraminal stenosis, or both, which may cause neurological deficit, including radiculopathy, neurogenic claudication, or myelopathy.

The treatment of spinal osteoarthritis is a significant burden on health care systems globally. Patients with spinal osteoarthritis are major consumers of pharmaceuticals and allied health resources. Although most patients are treated conservatively, as the population ages, spine surgeons will become increasingly involved in the treatment of spinal osteoarthritis in the elderly. A fuller understanding of the disease, including its risk factors and pathophysiology, is therefore imperative to properly counsel patients on their options for treatment. The following three case examples present patients with severe manifestations of osteoarthritis requiring consultation for possible surgical intervention.

## CLINICAL CASE EXAMPLES

### Clinical Case #1 (Degenerative Lumbar Spondylolisthesis)

Figure 13-1 presents lumbar magnetic resonance imaging (MRI) of a 67-year-old woman with a 30-year history of progressive lower back pain. This pain was exacerbated by activity and relieved by rest. She reported no associated radicular symptoms. Past medical history was significant for morbid obesity, diabetes, and osteoarthritis. Physical exam did not reveal

a neurological deficit. The patient had failed to improve despite intensive conservative therapy which included high dosage opiates, physiotherapy, epidural steroid injections, and facet blocks. MRI and plain radiography (see Fig. 13-4) revealed degenerative spondylolisthesis, central canal stenosis, and bilateral synovial cysts. Lateral flexion and extension films demonstrated a 10-mm anterolisthesis of L4 on L5 with 9 mm in extension and 11 mm in flexion. Due to increasing disability and lack of response to conservative measures, the patient was referred for evaluation for surgical intervention.

### Clinical Case #2 (Degenerative Cervical Spondylosis)

Figure 13-2 presents axial computed tomography (CT) myelogram images of a 79-year-old woman with moderate neck pain and progressive difficulty with ambulating during the past 4 years. At presentation, the patient was wheelchair bound with limited ability to transfer. Past medical history was significant for osteoarthritis, atrial fibrillation, and multiple peripheral neuropathies. Physical examination revealed gross lower extremity hyperreflexia and weakness and was consistent with myelopathy. Her sensation was diffusely diminished in her hands and arms, but she did have normal sensation in the C4-C5 distribution. She did not have a Hoffman sign, but had extensive hand intrinsic muscle atrophy. She did have crossed adductor reflexes. She was able to flex and extend her neck to 35 degrees and laterally rotate to 40 degrees. The patient's CT myelogram demonstrated severe spinal cord compression at the C4-C5, C5-C6, and C6-C7 levels. There was anterolisthesis and osteophytic bulging, which resulted in severe spinal canal narrowing.

### Clinical Case #3 (Atlantoaxial Instability)

Figure 13-3 presents images from a CT scan of an 85-year-old woman with severe neck pain and occipital neuralgia. The pain had been progressively worsening during the past 12-month period despite analgesia. Past medical history included hypertension, hypothyroidism, and osteoarthritis resulting in bilateral knee arthroplasties. On physical exam no weakness or evidence of myelopathy was detected. Dynamic imaging revealed a C1-C2 atlantodens interval of 4 mm in neutral, increasing to 5 mm in flexion and in extension. CT imaging (see Figure 13-3) demonstrated gross evidence of atlantoaxial instability including pannus. The patient received temporary relief with a greater occipital nerve block. Because of the overwhelming disability attributable to her neck pain and occipital neuralgia, the patient was considered for surgical intervention.

## BASIC SCIENCE

Osteoarthritis is a complex disease and may represent a series of diseases rather than one specific disease entity.[1] The consensus definition states that osteoarthritis is a result of both mechanical and biological events that destabilize the normal coupling of degradation and synthesis of articular

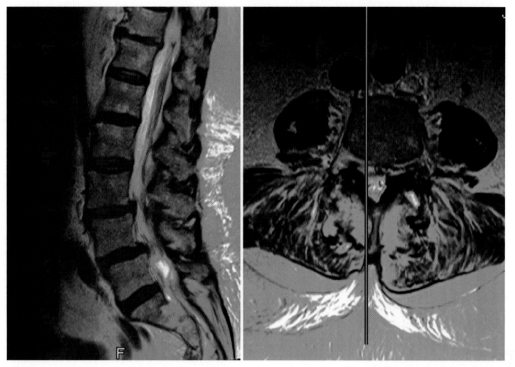

**■ FIGURE 13-1**    MRI of Case #1 demonstrating significant spondylosis and spondylolisthesis.

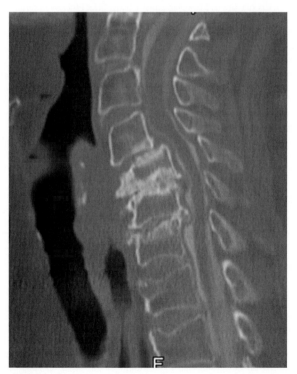

**■ FIGURE 13-2**    CT myelogram of Case #2 demonstrating advanced degenerative changes.

cartilage, extracellular matrix, and subchondral bone. When clinically evident, osteoarthritis is characterized by joint pain, tenderness, limitation of movement, crepitus, and variable degrees of inflammation without systemic effects.[1] Osteoarthritis affects articular joints including the knees and hips. The zygapophyseal or facet joints are the synovial joints in the spine and therefore susceptible to osteoarthritis. Spinal osteoarthritis is therefore a disease of the facet joints due to degeneration, resulting in facet joint incompetence.

## EPIDEMIOLOGY AND RISK FACTORS

Spinal osteoarthritis has been demonstrated through radiographic and cadaver studies to affect every adult age group.[2,3] The prevalence of clinical spinal osteoarthritis increases with age, with elderly patients having the highest radiographic and symptomatic prevalence.[1,3] There is also a significant gender difference in prevalence. Females are more likely than males to suffer from osteoarthritis in general. The gender difference is exacerbated after menopause and therefore greater in the elderly.[1]

Other risk factors besides age and gender have been reported to be associated with the development of osteoarthritis. Obesity has a strong correlation with developing osteoarthritis. This likely represents added mechanical stress to the facet joints. Previous trauma from sports activities and occupations requiring strenuous physical labor have also been associated with the development of spinal osteoarthritis.[1]

## PATHOPHYSIOLOGY

Osteoarthritis is a disease of the articular cartilage and underlying subchondral bone. Although the exact etiology of osteoarthritis is not known, one theory is that cartilage matrix turnover is negatively affected by degenerative forces. This disrupts the balance between cartilage synthesis and degradation. Evidence suggests that collagenase, gelatinase, and stromelysin, which are enzymes involved in cartilage degradation, are increased in osteoarthritic joints.[1] The cause for this imbalance is not clear. One proposed theory is that changes to the subchondral bone instigate changes to the cartilage matrix. Radiographic evidence of subchondral bone changes is often present in patients with osteoarthritis. It is theorized that stiffening of the subchondral bone due to microtrauma results in an abnormal environment for the overlying cartilage. This increases cartilage turnover and leads to further degradation of the joint. However, the debate as to whether subchondral bone changes are a result or cause of cartilage degeneration is not settled.[1]

Also unsettled is the role of the inflammatory response in the pathogenesis of osteoarthritis. Localized inflammation has been demonstrated in certain stages of osteoarthritis, including mononuclear cell infiltrate and synovial hyperplasia. The exact role of this inflammation, be it causative or reactionary, is not clear. Markers of inflammation such as C-reactive protein (CRP) may be elevated as well.[1] However, in general, systemic inflammation is not characteristic of osteoarthritis. Its presence would indicate that another pathology such as rheumatoid arthritis or gout should be considered.

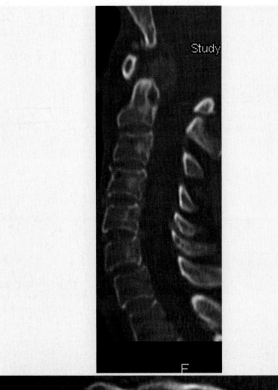

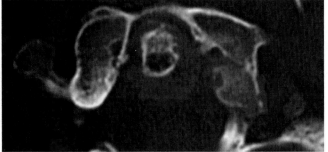

■ **FIGURE 13-3** CT images of Case #3 demonstrating pannus related to C1-C2 instability.

## DEGENERATIVE MECHANICS

Osteoarthritic changes at the facet joints can have a cascading effect on a patient's overall spinal health. The facet joints function as the posterolateral articulation between vertebral segments. As such, they bear weight, restrict anterior and posterior movement of the anterior column, and restrict axial rotation. Arthritic changes in these joints can promote abnormal spine mechanics, increasing degeneration. It is commonly held that facet joint arthrosis is a sequela of disc degeneration.[4] However, there is evidence to suggest that facet arthrosis is a long-standing phenomenon present before evidence of disc degeneration.[2] Either way, the coupling of facet joint arthritis with disc degeneration can lead to progressive degenerative changes. In the normal spine, facet joints bear between 18% and 25% of the segmental weight load.[4,5] Facet joints in degenerative spines can bear upwards of 47% or more in extension.[5] This leads to progressive stress on a weakened joint. Sequelae of continued stress on the weakened facet joint include osteophytosis and synovial cyst formation. These can cause radiculopathies if affecting the lumbar or cervical foramina. Specific symptoms vary by levels, with L4-L5 being the most commonly affected.[5] Large osteophytes or synovial cysts coupled with anterior osteophytic change can lead to central canal stenosis. This stenosis can result in symptoms of neurogenic claudication when located in the lumbar spine, or symptoms of myelopathy when located in the cervical spine.

Severe osteoarthritis in the facet joints can lead to changes in spinal alignment. Competent facet joints prevent forward sliding of one vertebra upon another. When damaged by osteoarthritis, facet joint incompetence contributes to degenerative spondylolisthesis. This spondylolisthesis is generally mild and

asymptomatic but can cause neurological symptoms when the degree is severe. Symptoms may include intractable neck or lower back pain or radiculopathy due to compression of the neural foramen. Osteoarthritic changes of the facet joints can also exacerbate other deformities of the spine, including degenerative scoliosis, as these joints serve as a stabilizing influence on spinal alignment.

The atlantoaxial junction is a common site for arthritic changes, most commonly seen in rheumatoid arthritis. Although classically not associated with osteoarthritis, atlantoaxial osteoarthritis has been reported to have a prevalence ranging between 5% and 18% of patients with spinal osteoarthritis.[6] True symptomatic prevalence is probably much smaller. Arthritic changes can affect the lateral mass articulations and the atlantodens articulation. Degeneration at the atlantodens articulation can produce a pannus, similar to that seen in rheumatoid arthritis, causing myelopathic symptoms due to cord compression. More commonly, osteoarthritis at the atlantoaxial junction results in neck pain. This pain generally originates in the suboccipital region. It can radiate both cranially and caudally and can present with severe occipital pain. In general, occipital pain or subaxial neck pain without a suboccipital component most likely does not represent pain from atlantoaxial osteoarthritis, and other sources of pain should be excluded. In cases where the pain generator is difficult to locate based upon symptomatology, C1-C2 facet blocks can be a diagnostic aid if they relieve the neck pain.

## NATURAL HISTORY

The natural history of spinal osteoarthritis is difficult to define. Most patients will present with back or neck pain, the etiology of which can be hard to determine. Some investigators feel that facet joints are a significant pain generator. Facet joints are innervated by branches of the dorsal rami of the same level and, the level above. After the capsule of the facet joint is innervated with nociceptive fibers. However, studies using facet blocks to examine facet joint contribution to spinal pain report varying prevalence from 7% to 75%.[5] In addition, a large study of the prevalence of spinal osteoarthritis in women demonstrated a peak in incidence of osteoarthritis in the mid thoracic spine region. However, this radiographic peak did not correlate with any clinical symptoms. The same study did demonstrate a peak at the L4-L5 segment, which correlated with increased symptom scores.[3] This study underlines the variability of clinical symptoms with significant radiographic findings.

In general, osteoarthritis is a progressive disease. Whereas disease modifying agents are currently employed in the treatment of gout, rheumatoid arthritis, and psoriatic arthritis, the treatment of osteoarthritis is primarily symptomatic. This treatment may be beneficial to most, but some patients still develop enough spinal degeneration to result in significant morbidity and disability. Decreased mobility coupled with deconditioning portends significant physical decline. Thus, while most patients will stabilize with current therapy, some patients will progress to developing significant pain, neurological deficit, and disability. These patients are the most likely to present to a spine surgeon for evaluation and treatment.

## CLINICAL PRACTICE GUIDELINES

### Evaluation

Elderly patients presenting with significant neck or back pain should be evaluated with plain radiographs to look for evidence of facet joint arthrosis. Those presenting with neurological deficit should be evaluated with MRI or CT myelogram to determine the extent and location of neural compromise. MRI offers a noninvasive assessment of soft tissue disease, whereas CT myelograms can provide additional information on bony compression and provide for surgical planning for instrumentation.

Rheumatological consultation may be necessary to exclude other inflammatory disorders. Diffuse idiopathic skeletal hyperostosis (DISH) has a high prevalence in the elderly. It commonly manifests with calcification and ossification of soft tissues including ligaments and affects the spine. Symptoms usually involve pain and stiffness. Although it may be present concomitantly with osteoarthritis, DISH is usually radiographically distinct and recognizable by osteophytic change, often affecting the anterior longitudinal ligament, with preservation of the disc space. Rheumatoid arthritis can also cause signs and symptoms similar to osteoarthritis. Cervical degeneration with pannus formation is seen with advanced rheumatoid arthritis.

Exclusion of other pain generators is imperative. Radiographic evidence of arthrosis does not necessarily correlate with symptoms. Patients with significant back and hip pain should be evaluated for such conditions as trochanteric bursitis. Treatment via steroid injection may alleviate both hip and back pain. Evaluation of hip osteoarthritis should also be undertaken. A hip–spine syndrome has been postulated for several years as a cause of spine pain in patients with severe hip osteoarthritis. Recent evidence has suggested significant improvement in back pain scores and improvement in Oswestry disability scores in patients undergoing hip replacements for hip osteoarthritis.[7] Because osteoarthritis commonly affects multiple joints, evaluation of the hip should be performed in patients with lower back and hip pain.

## Conservative Therapy

Conservative therapy for spinal osteoarthritis consists of reduction of risk factors and amelioration of symptoms. Obesity worsens symptoms of osteoarthritis, likely by increasing the load on the stressed facet joints. Weight loss should therefore be included in any treatment regimen. Lack of activity can lead to deconditioning and weight gain. Encouragement of physical activity is important in treating symptomatic cases of spinal osteoarthritis. Patients with severe obesity or deconditioning may find it difficult to begin an exercise regimen. Our group has had success with aquatic exercise therapy, which promotes increased activity while lessening the axial load on the spine. A trial of physiotherapy should be considered in patients before becoming operative candidates.

Analgesia for spinal osteoarthritis commonly includes nonsteroidal antiinflammatory drugs. Elderly patients may have multiple comorbidities and the risks of these medications should be evaluated before they are prescribed. Local application of heat may have some benefit in controlling symptomatic neck or back pain. Opiates may also play a role in management of the disease. These should be carefully prescribed in the elderly because they may have significant side effects. Pain treatment procedures also may benefit patients, especially those who are not candidates for surgery. Facet joint blocks can provide symptomatic relief of facet-mediated pain. They also may serve to elucidate those facets contributing to spinal pain. Epidural steroid injections can also be beneficial in treating spinal pain and radicular symptoms.

Conservative therapy of spinal osteoarthritis is generally symptomatic. Recent evidence has suggested that alendronate and other bisphosphonates may have a role in disease modification. Alendronate can reduce osteophyte progression and disc space narrowing in patients with spinal osteoarthritis. In a randomly selected subgroup of the Fracture Intervention Trial, which examined the effectiveness of alendronate, patients receiving alendronate demonstrated a significantly reduced increase in osteophyte progression and disc space narrowing from T4 to L5.[8] However, this was a secondary analysis and not a primary endpoint of the main study. After the results suggest that alendronate as a modifier of spinal osteoarthritis progression should be given further consideration.

## Operative Therapy

The surgical treatment of painful spinal osteoarthritis remains controversial. No large-scale randomized trials exist to support intervention for neck or back pain or even mild neurological deficit.[9,10] Evaluation for surgery should be tailored for each individual patient. Those patients with progressive neurological deficits or those who have failed extensive conservative therapies would seem to be better candidates for intervention. The type of intervention offered should be customized, because the goals of surgery will be different for each patient.

### Neurological Decompression

Decompressive surgery may be indicated when the goal of surgery is to halt the progression of neurological deficit in patients with spinal osteoarthritis. Decompression of the central canal can alleviate symptoms of neurogenic claudication. Foraminotomies can reduce radicular pain. However, studies to date on lumbar and cervical decompression have not proved any significant benefit versus conservative therapy.[9,10] Most studies are small, have poor outcome measures, and are retrospective. In the absence of significant supporting evidence, decompression may be indicated in cases of focal neurological element compromise, such as single level Foraminotomy. They may also be considered in patients who may not be good candidates for extensive procedures because of medical comorbidities. It should be stressed that decompressions have a poor track record in treating axial spinal pain.[9,10]

Decompressive surgery should not be considered in patients with evidence of gross instability. Spinal osteoarthritis affects the facet joints, decompensating the posterior element support structure. Further iatrogenic stress on incompetent facet joints via foraminotomy and facetectomy can lead to progressive spinal deformity, including spondylolisthesis, scoliosis, and abnormal kyphosis. This can exacerbate axial spinal pain and create new or worsen existing neurological deficits.

### Instrumented Spinal Fusion

In recent years, the number of instrumented spinal fusion procedures has increased, despite a lack of evidence of their effectiveness at treating axial spinal pain and radicular pain.[9,10] Conceptually, fusion procedures are attractive, because spinal osteoarthritis leads to facet joint instability. Those patients with axial spine pain demonstrably caused by facet arthrosis (i.e., improved with facet anesthetic blocks) may benefit from stabilization. However, there is no conclusive evidence to support this indication for fusion.[9,10] Patients with extensive neurological compression may be candidates for instrumented fusion procedures. More extensive decompression can be performed without concern for posterior element instability. Patients with significant deformity due to osteoarthritic changes may also benefit from corrective procedures.

Most degenerative spondylolisthesis may be successfully treated conservatively. However, those with significant axial pain or neural compression may benefit from surgical intervention if they have failed conservative therapy. Our group has had success in reduction of degenerative grade I or grade II spondylolisthesis using transforaminal interbody allograft and posterior segmental instrumented fusion. This technique allows for aggressive neural foraminal decompression and reduction of listhesis, and forgoes the associated morbidity of an anterior approach procedure.

Atlantoaxial instability may be another indication for surgical intervention. Patients with intractable neck. occipital pain, or both that is attributable to C1-C2 instability may be good candidates for surgical intervention. Recent case series data suggest that C1-C2 fusion can effectively reduce pain by 65%.[6] Atlantoaxial fusion would also be indicated in patients with significant pannus and myelopathy secondary to cord compression.

### Minimally Invasive Alternatives

In elderly patients with multiple medical comorbidities, minimally invasive procedures hold great promise. Decreased blood loss and trauma are positives, whereas increased operative times and limited procedure offerings are potential negatives. The body of evidence regarding minimally invasive alternatives while comparatively small continues to grow. Recent evidence suggests that minimally invasive decompression may be safe and beneficial to elderly patients. In a group of 50 patients aged 75 and over, minimally invasive lumbar decompression was performed without major perioperative complication and with improvement in disability and pain, at least in the short term.[11] This would suggest that minimally invasive decompressions may be an alternative for elderly patients not candidates for more traditional procedures.

## CLINICAL CASE EXAMPLES

### Discuss Treatment, Clinical Challenges, and Future Treatments

#### Case #1

This patient had failed conservative therapy, but had multiple medical comorbidities. Despite this, operative intervention was felt to be of benefit as the patient's current state of obesity and deconditioning prevented any further meaningful physiotherapy or exercise program. The patient was treated with decompressive laminectomies L3-L5 with complete L3-L4 and L4-L5 facetectomies. Bilateral placement of L3-L5 pedicle screws and right-sided L3-L4 and L4-L5 transforaminal interbody fusions were also performed. The fusion was supplemented with rhBMP-2 (recombinant human bone morphogenic

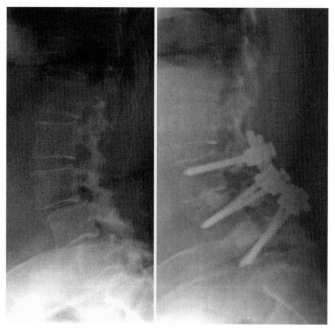

**■ FIGURE 13-4** Preoperative and postoperative lateral neutral radiographs of case 1 demonstrating degenerative spondylolisthesis and correction.

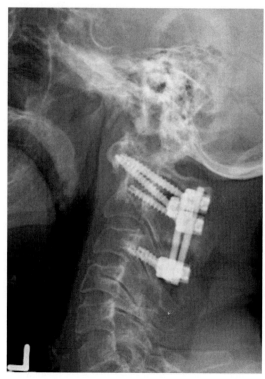

**■ FIGURE 13-5** Postoperative radiographs of Case #3 demonstrating C1-C3 fusion.

protein 2) anterior to the interbody spacer which represents off-label use. Challenges with this patient included obesity and multiple medical comorbidities. Preoperative medical consultation was undertaken to identify and to minimize potential risks. Great care was taken in positioning the patient to prevent pressure-related complications. Postoperatively the patient obtained significant pain relief. Radiographs confirmed improved alignment (Figure 13-4).

### Case #2

Because of the patient's progressive decline in ambulation and ability to perform activities of daily living, the patient was offered surgical intervention after being fully counseled on the attendant risks. The patient was treated with a two-stage reconstructive procedure performed in 1 day. Stage I included anterior exposure of the cervical spine with C5 and C6 corpectomies and realignment of the spine with C4 through C7 arthrodesis, using dual fibular allografts with C4 through C7 anterior instrumentation using a plate. Stage II was a C3 through T1 posterior segmental instrumented fusion using a combination of local bone graft (corpectomy bone from anterior decompression), rhBMP-2, and cancellous allograft. The patient recovered initially in the intensive care unit. No significant postoperative complications occurred. The patient had subsequent improvement in her symptoms of myelopathy.

### Case #3

This 85-year-old patient was treated with posterior exposure of the upper cervical spine, C1 through C3 arthrodesis, including C1 lateral mass screws, right-sided C2 pedicle screw, and C3 lateral mass screws. C1-C3 arthrodesis was performed with a combination of rhBMP-2 and cancellous allograft bone. The fusion was extended to C3 because of concern for placing a left-sided C2 pedicle screw (Figure 13-5). Decompression was not performed because the patient did not demonstrate evidence of myelopathy. The patient tolerated the procedure well and had near complete resolution of neck pain 1 year post surgery.

### CONCLUSIONS AND DISCUSSION

Spinal osteoarthritis is a progressive and potentially debilitating disease in the elderly. Therapies to date have focused on symptomatic relief. The sequelae of long-standing spinal osteoarthritis can lead to intractable pain

or neurological symptoms. These patients are often referred to the spine specialist. Great care must be taken in decision making in these patients. Many elderly patients are not good surgical candidates because of comorbidities. However, those failing conservative therapy may have few other options besides surgical intervention. Despite the risks, elderly patients regularly undergo spinal surgery and can improve symptomatically. Because the literature is inconclusive and long-term follow-up data are scarce, each patient must be assessed individually. Goals for surgery need to be clearly defined, and patient education and informed consent are paramount. In the future, minimally invasive alternatives may be beneficial in alleviating symptoms of advanced spinal osteoarthritis while reducing risks of intervention in patients not considered candidates for traditional procedures.

### References

1. P. Creamer, M.C. Hochberg, Osteoarthritis, Lancet 350 (9076) (1997) 503–508.
2. J.D. Eubanks, M.J. Lee, E. Cassinelli, et al., Does lumbar facet arthrosis precede disc degeneration? A postmortem study, Clin. Orthop. Relat. Res. 464 (2007) 184–189.
3. P.A. Kramer, Prevalence and distribution of spinal osteoarthritis in women, Spine 31 (24) (2006) 2843–2848.
4. C.A. Niosi, T.R. Oxland, Degenerative mechanics of the lumbar spine, Spine J. (Suppl. 6) (2004) 202S–208S.
5. L. Kalichman, D.J. Hunter, Lumbar facet joint osteoarthritis: a review, Semin. Arthritis Rheum. 37 (2) (2007) 69–80.
6. S. Schaeren, B. Jeanneret, Atlantoaxial osteoarthritis: case series and review of the literature, Eur. Spine J 14 (5) (2005) 501–506.
7. P. Ben-Galim, T. Ben-Galim, R. Nahshon, et al., Hip Spine Syndrome: The effect of total hip replacement surgery on low back pain in severe osteoarthritis of the hip, Spine 32 (19) (2007) 2099–2102.
8. T. Neogi, M.C. Nevitt, K.E. Ensrud, et al., The effect of alendronate on progression of spinal osteophytes and disc space narrowing, Ann. Rheum. Dis. 67 (2008) 1427–1430.
9. I.P. Fouyas, P.F. Statham, P.A. Sandercock, Cochrane review on the role of surgery in cervical spondylotic radiculomyelopathy, Spine 27 (7) (2002) 736–747.
10. J.N. Gibson, G. Waddell, Surgery for degenerative lumbar spondylosis: updated Cochrane Review, Spine 30 (20) (2005) 2312–2320.
11. D.S. Rosen, et al., Minimally invasive lumbar spinal decompression in the elderly: outcomes of 50 patients aged 75 years and older, Neurosurgery 60 (3) (2007) 503–509. discussion 509-510.

# 14

# Spinal Stenosis Without Spondylolisthesis

*Rob D. Dickerman*

Aging in the lumbar spine is most commonly manifested in the form of spinal stenosis, which is referred to as degenerative lumbar spinal stenosis. With the advances in medicine extending life spans, degenerative lumbar spinal stenosis is likely to be an ever-increasing problem. Spinal stenosis was first described over 50 years ago by Verbiest as a radicular syndrome from developmental narrowing of the lumbar vertebral canal.[1]

## CLINICAL CASE EXAMPLE

A 60-year-old man presents with progressive back and leg pain that is worse with standing and walking. On further discussion the patient admits to decreasing ability to walk for longer than 10 minutes, and he feels relief with sitting. The patient answers positively when asked if he can walk longer if he leans forward on a grocery cart. The patient admits to prior physical therapy and epidural steroid injections without relief. On examination the patient has a normal gait, with positive distal pulses at 70 beats per minute and no cyanosis or edema in the lower extremities. His reflexes are rated 2/4; strength is rated 5/5; he exhibits negative straight leg raise, no radiculopathy, and no myelopathy with no focal neurological deficits. Review of his T2-weighted magnetic resonance imaging (MRI) axial images of the lumbar spine demonstrates significant stenosis at the L4-L5 level secondary to hypertrophied ligamentum flavum and facet hypertrophy (Figure 14-1).

## BASIC SCIENCE

The pathogenesis of lumbar stenosis is an interesting degenerative cascade that eventually leads to the pathognomonic signs and symptoms. In brief, the degenerative cascade begins at the level of the intervertebral disc, which consists of an inner nuclear core called the nucleus pulposus and an outer supporting layer of the disc called the annulus fibrosus. Beginning early in life, the nucleus pulposus loses its vascular supply and depends on diffusion for its nutrient base, which slowly becomes insufficient. This change in vascular supply leads to dehydration and altered proteoglycan matrix, thus altering the mechanical properties of the disc and the pressure distribution within the disc and leading to a stressed and bulging annulus with loss of disc height.[2]

Vascular regression within the disc is thought to occur as the child moves from quadrupedal to bipedal motion, thus increasing the load on the disc space in the vertical position. The increasing intradisc pressure leads to involution of the blood supply. By 4 years of age the disc largely depends on cellular diffusion for survival.[2] With increasing age the metabolic strain to the intervertebral disc increases, yet the vascular supply is insufficient and diffusion cannot maintain the demands. The altered metabolism in the disc changes the overall electrolyte balance in the disc space, decreasing the net inward flow of fluid and decreasing water content from 90% to 70%; this change ultimately leads to loss of disc height and expandability.[2]

The aforementioned degeneration of the intervertebral disc leads to altered local and segmental mechanics, generating a cascade of compensatory changes within the facet complex, bones, and ligaments.[2] Along with degenerative changes occurring with the normal aging spine, the surrounding support structures are also aging and thus degenerating. The most important of the surrounding structures are the core muscles, which include the paraspinal musculature and the abdominal muscles.[3] As these supporting muscles lose tone, the spinal column stability depends more on the facet joints, ligaments, and intervertebral discs leading to compensatory hypertrophy of the ligaments, hypertrophied facet joints, and calcified annular-vertebral osteophytes (Table 14-1).[3]

Each patient develops unique symptoms based on his or her particular pathology, but in general, this degenerative process leads to central stenosis, foraminal stenosis, or both.[3] The most common levels affected are L4-L5 followed by L3-L4.

Recent histological and biochemical studies were performed to assess the pathomechanism of ligamentum flavum hypertrophy in degenerative spinal stenosis.[4] In 2005, Saiyro et al analyzed 308 specimens of ligamentum flavum from patients with spinal stenosis and concluded that fibrosis of the ligamentum flavum was the primary cause of the hypertrophy, and the fibrosis is a result of the mechanical stresses occurring with the degenerative cascade. The authors found high levels of transforming growth factor (TGF) and concluded that endothelial release of TGF in the early stages of degeneration may lead to the initial ligamentum flavum hypertrophy.[4] In 2007, Saiyro et al examined the amount of elastic fibers versus fibrosis or "scar tissue" in 21 ligamentum flavum specimens retrieved from patients with lumbar stenosis and compared them to normal controls. The authors found a significant amount of fibrosis in the ligamentum flavum from patients with stenosis and concluded that fibrosis or "scarring" causes hypertrophy of the ligamentum flavum.[5]

The spinal canal dimensions are not constant and are influenced by dynamic and postural factors.[3] Axial loading of the intervertebral disc causes bulging of the annulus, which in turn further compromises the central canal and the foramen. There can also be osteophyte formation from a degenerated facet joint, which can induce lateral recess or foraminal stenosis.[3]

Degeneration and aging is ubiquitous in the human, and the lumbar spine is not exempt. Degeneration is manifested as osteoarthritis in the lumbar spine and is largely responsible for the high prevalence of low back pain in the population; however, the resulting spinal stenosis is not totally responsible for "back pain" in the human population. In general, any patient in the seventh decade of life will exhibit radiographic evidence of spinal

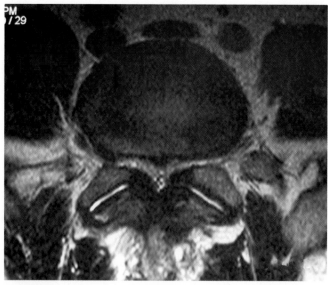

**■ FIGURE 14-1** Axial T2-weighted MRI of L4-L5 demonstrating significant lumbar stenosis secondary to hypertrophied ligamentum flavum, bulging annulus, and facet hypertrophy.

**TABLE 14-1** The Basic Degenerative Cascade for Lumbar Stenosis

Biochemical alterations in the intervertebral disc begins around 4 years of age.
Biochemical changes lead to biomechanical and structural alterations of the disc.
Disc structural and functional changes lead to compensatory alterations of the ligaments, facet joints and cartilaginous end-plates.
Hypertrophied ligamentum flavum and facet joints narrow the central canal and foramen.
Lumbar stenosis.

stenosis, but only a small percentage of these patients ever suffer from the symptoms of spinal stenosis.[6]

As previously discussed, degeneration is part of the life cycle and degeneration in the lumbar spine begins very early in life, with loss of the vascular supply to the intervertebral discs, and subsequent radiographic degenerative changes follow. Boden et al examined 67 individuals without back pain, neurogenic claudication, or radiculopathy.[7] Of the patients examined, 20% of the patients younger than 60 years had MRI evidence of herniated discs or stenosis. In the group of patients older than 60 years, 57% demonstrated degenerative changes including herniated discs and spinal stenosis. In fact there was radiographic evidence of degenerative disc disease in 35% of patients younger than 40 years, and in over 99% of the subjects older than 60 years. Thus, in our practice we follow the philosophy of "never treat films, treat the patient," which is particularly applicable when dealing with degenerative lumbar stenosis.

The classic pathognomonic symptom complex for lumbar spinal stenosis is termed "neurogenic claudication." In brief, patients with spinal stenosis will not suffer or exhibit symptoms while sitting or at rest. Once a patient stands or begins walking, they will begin to sense a heaviness or aching in their lower extremities, or both, which is relieved with sitting. Patients will inherently discover that if they maintain a slightly flexed posture in the lumbar spine, they can walk farther because the central canal and foraminal space is opened with flexion; for example, when leaning on the grocery cart while shopping. As the stenosis progressively worsens, the patients lose the ability to walk several feet or even stand upright. Symptoms may vary depending on whether the patient is suffering central canal stenosis or foraminal stenosis or both. Neurogenic claudication and radiculopathy secondary to spinal stenosis can basically be attributed to either direct mechanical compression from hypertrophied ligamentum flavum, bulging discs, and so on, or indirect vascular insufficiency from inadequate oxygen

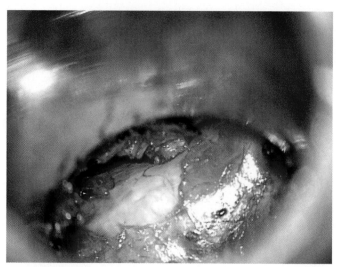

**■ FIGURE 14-2** Unilateral dilator approach under microscopic guidance demonstrating contralateral hypertrophied ligamentum flavum in the lateral recess.

delivery to the nerve roots.[8] Upon standing vertically, the lumbar lordotic angle increases, thus increasing the degree of stenosis by inducing an inward buckling of the hypertrophied ligamentum flavum into the central canal or lateral recess. This compression may act directly on neural elements or on the neurovascular supply.[3] The venous congestion is highly visible in some patients at the time of surgery. Whereas in the sitting position, the lordotic angle decreases, allowing the ligamentum flavum to relax, opening the canal and lateral recess and allowing adequate oxygen delivery.

## CLINICAL PRACTICE GUIDELINES

Current practice guidelines for patients with lumbar spinal stenosis without spondylolisthesis are multifactorial and are generally categorized into non-surgical and surgical options. Obviously, conservative care (nonsurgical) is recommended in all patients without intractable pain or a significant neurological deficit. This chapter is focused on surgical treatment options.

### Surgery

Surgical options are dependent on many factors including patient's clinical state, body habitus, type of pathology and surgeon's expertise. In this chapter we are only considering surgical options for lumbar spinal stenosis without spondylolisthesis and assumption of "classic neurogenic claudication" symptoms secondary to central and foraminal stenosis.

Decompressive lumbar laminectomy has been the classic approach for the treatment of spinal stenosis. Numerous surgical techniques have subsequently been developed since the advent of the classic open approach, including but not limited to minimally invasive surgeries. Rahman et al[9] compared multiple variables in patients who underwent "classic" open decompressive lumbar laminectomy versus minimally invasive surgery (MIS) for lumbar decompression. The MIS approach allowed for bilateral decompression through a unilateral dilator and use of the microscope (Figures 14-2 and 14-3). Results demonstrated that MIS patients had shorter operating room times, less blood loss, shorter length of hospital stay, and fewer complications. In addition, the MIS patients had better mobility in the immediate postoperative period.

One of the newer MIS techniques is the "interspinous process spreader," which is currently on the market and in development by several companies worldwide.[10] In simplistic terms, the devices are designed to be placed between the lumbar spinous processes and force the spinous process into a flexed posture, thus indirectly decompressing the spinal canal. Siddiqui et al analyzed the one-year outcomes after placing an interspinous process spreader in 40 patients with spinal stenosis and found that 54% of patients reported clinically significant improvement in their symptoms, 33% reported improvement in function, and 71% expressed satisfaction with the surgery.[10]

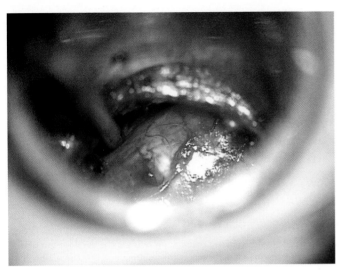

■ **FIGURE 14–3**  Unilateral dilator approach under microscopic guidance demonstrating contralateral decompression of lateral recess after removal of ligamentum flavum.

## CONCLUSIONS AND DISCUSSION

Lumbar spinal stenosis is a ubiquitous process that occurs with normal aging. The pathogenesis of lumbar spinal stenosis is part of the degenerative cascade, which is complex and mulifactorial. While spinal stenosis is not considered hereditary, many components that lead to spinal stenosis such as degenerative disc disease demonstrate a strong genetic component. With advances in medicine increasing the average lifespan, lumbar spinal stenosis will continue to become a more common problem and fortunately we have numerous minimally invasive surgical treatment options.

## Acknowledgments

Special thanks to Dr. Mark Eisenberg, Neurosurgery Section Chief, Long Island Jewish Hospital, New Hyde Park, New York.

## References

1. H. Verbiest, A radicular syndrome from developmental narrowing of the lumbae vertebral canal, Journal of Bone and Joint Surgery 36 (1954) 230–237.
2. R.D. Dickerman, J.E. Zigler, Discogenic Back Pain. In: Spivak JM, Connolly PJ, eds. Orthopaedic Knowledge Update Spine, American Academy of Orthopaedic Surgeons, Rosemont, IL, 3rd eds (2005) 319–329.
3. N.E. Epstein, Lumbar spinal stenosis. In: H.R. Winn eds, Youmans neurological surgery, Saunders, Philadelphia, PA, 5th eds, 2005, pp. 4521–4539.
4. K. Sairyo, A. Biyani, V. Goel, et al., Pathomechanism of ligamentum flavum hypertrophy: a multidisciplinary investigation based on clinical, biomechanical, histologic, and biologic assessments, Spine 30 (2005) 2649–2656.
5. K. Sairyo, A. Bivani, V.K. Goel, et al., Lumbar ligamentum flavum hypertrophy is due to accumulation of inflammation-related scar tissue, Spine 32 (2007) 340–347.
6. J.F. Healy, B.B. Healy, W.H. Wong, et al., Cervical and lumbar MRI in asymptomatic older male lifelong athletes frequency of degenerative findings, J. Comput. Assist. Tomogr. 20 (1996) 107–112.
7. S.D. Boden, D.O. Davis, T.S. Dina, et al., Abnormal magnetic-resonance scans of the lumbar spine in asymptomatic subjects. A prospective investigation, J. Bone Joint Surg. Am. 72 (1990) 403–208.
8. R. Watanabe, W.W. Parke, Vascular and neural pathology of lumbosacral spinal stenosis, J. Neurosurg. 64 (1986) 64–70.
9. M. Rahman, L.E. Summers, B. Richter, et al., Comparison of techniques for decompressive lumbar laminectomy: the minimally invasive versus the "classic" open approach, Minim. Invasive Neurosurg. 51 (2008) 100–105.
10. M. Siddiqui, F.W. Smith, D. Wardlaw, One-year results of XStop interspinous implant for the treatment of lumbar spinal stenosis, Spine 32 (2007) 1345–1348.

# Spinal Stenosis with Spondylolisthesis

**15**

*Vincent J. Miele, Sumeet Vadera, and Edward C. Benzel*

---

**K E Y   P O I N T S**

- In the majority of cases patients with spinal stenosis and degenerative spondylolisthesis may undergo a traditional laminectomy.

- Several factors, including the mobility of the listhesis, character of the slip (lateral listhesis), presence of an associated degenerative scoliosis, and the presence of axial pain are weighted in favor of adjunct fusion.

- If fusion is required, it can be performed with or without instrumentation. Generally, instrumentation increases the morbidity of the patient.

- Factors to consider when deciding on instrumentation include the amount of instability, age of the patient, bone quality, presence of comorbidities, amount of levels requiring decompression, and factors that predict worsening of listhesis (see previous point).

- New technologies, such as biologics used to promote fusion, minimally invasive techniques, and motion preservation technology are promising but have limited data proving efficacy.

---

Spinal stenosis accompanied by spondylolisthesis is a common diagnosis encountered by the spinal surgeon. Although nonoperative treatment consisting of antiinflammatory medications and epidural steroid injections is effective in some patients, many patients with severe symptoms are not helped by this strategy.[1,2] In the group that fails conservative therapy, decompression has been shown to be an effective treatment modality.[2-4] Although numerous studies have clearly demonstrated the beneficial effects of decompressive laminectomy, the fear of creating instability often limits this procedure's application. The concomitant presence of spondylolisthesis increases this likelihood. Controversy also persists regarding the virtues of concomitant spinal fusion in this patient population, which is often elderly. When fusion is chosen, the decision of whether or not to use instrumentation must be made. Fortunately, the management of this condition has evolved over the past several decades and numerous prospective randomized trials have been performed assessing the influence of fusion and instrumentation following decompression.

To treat a patient with spinal stenosis with degenerative spondylolisthesis, the clinician should have a basic knowledge of the epidemiology, diagnosis, and management of this condition. This chapter addresses specific situations in which individuals will have a high incidence of instability and progression of deformity without fusion. In addition, laminectomy without fusion may be considered. It will also discuss certain patient populations in which the better part of valor might be a limited decompression without fusion or a fusion without instrumentation. Finally, new techniques such as the use of biologics, motion preservation devices, and soft tissue stabilization will be discussed.

## PART ONE: UNDERSTANDING THE CONDITION

### Pathophysiology

As the spine ages, the accumulation of years of axial loading and rotational strains may lead to disc degeneration, facet arthrosis with hypertrophy, thickening or buckling of ligamentum flavum, and osteophyte formation.

This cascade of degenerative changes can result in the development of central canal or foraminal narrowing with resulting neural compression characterized by low back, buttock, and lower extremity pain.[1] They can also result in varying degrees of spinal instability and, depending on the anatomic predisposing factors, the vertebra develops either anterolisthesis or retrolisthesis. Spondylolisthesis, the slippage of one vertebra relative to the adjacent vertebrae, often results from asymmetric degeneration of the disc, the facet joints, or both.

Once degenerative spondylolisthesis begins, the imbalance in stress can lead to an asymmetric deformity, which further aggravates the asymmetric loading and results in a vicious circle that promotes progression of instability. As the listhesis progresses with the narrowing of the intervertebral disc, subsequent changes in the motion segment include spur formation, subchondral sclerosis, ligamentous hypertrophy and ossification, together with hypertrophic facet arthrosis. These secondary changes have a natural tendency to restabilize the motion segment.

The deformity may occur in any of three axes: axial rotation on the vertical axis, lateral translation, and anterior translation in the sagittal plane. The types of spondylolisthesis that can occur are therefore rotatory olisthesis (rotational subluxation of one vertebral body upon another), lateral subluxation, and translatory shift. A listhetic segment is defined as fixed if less than 2-mm translation occurs on flexion/extension radiographs. If a translation occurs that is greater than 2 mm, the listhetic segment is considered mobile.

Degenerative spondylolisthesis is commonly associated with symptomatic stenosis as well as degenerative scoliosis. The primary pathology in degenerative scoliosis is lateral listhesis, coupled with lateral wedging of the vertebral body and angulation secondary to asymmetric degeneration of the facet joints.

### Epidemiology

Degenerative spondylolisthesis is a relatively common pathology. A recent study involving a large series in an Asian population reported an overall incidence of 8.7%. It typically is found in individuals older than 50 years. It is also more common in women than men, which is thought to be secondary to the increased ligamentous laxity in the former.

The level L4-L5 is most commonly affected overall by degenerative spondylolisthesis. Anterolisthesis is more common in the lower lumbar segments in females, whereas retrolisthesis in the upper lumbar segments is equally common in both sexes. When disc degeneration occurs, the motion segment often settles into an anterolisthesis.

### Natural History

The majority of patients with a history of significant neurogenic claudication or vesicorectal symptoms have been shown to have poor outcomes without intervention. A prospective observational cohort study assessing the long-term outcomes (8- to 10-year follow-up) of patients with lumbar spinal stenosis treated either surgically or nonsurgically has demonstrated increased leg pain relief and greater back-related functional status in patients who initially received surgical treatment. Although degenerative spondylolisthesis has been shown to progress in 25% to 30% of patients, it fortunately rarely progresses to more than 30% of the subjacent vertebra. Some studies have demonstrated that as the pathology progresses and the disc space collapses, back pain can improve spontaneously.

## PART TWO: CLINICAL DECISION MAKING

### Evaluation

Patients with spinal stenosis and degenerative spondylolisthesis present with neurogenic claudication, radiculopathy, intermittent episodes of axial mechanical back pain, and vesicorectal disorder. L5 is the most commonly associated radiculopathy. This is because for a patient with spondylolisthesis at L4-L5 (the most commonly affected level), the L5 nerve root is usually compressed in the lateral recess. Less frequently, the vertebral body movement causes narrowing of the foramen and L4 nerve root compression. Specifically, this foraminal stenosis is the result of anterosuperior subluxation of the caudad superior articular facet from decreased disc height, hypertrophied ligament and disc material, and osteophyte formation in the posterolateral corner of the vertebral end plate. This can compress the exiting nerve root against the superior pedicle. The origin of the axial mechanical back pain component of the disorder can be primarily discogenic or related to facet degeneration, which is often difficult to distinguish. Generally, if the discomfort is primarily secondary to disc disease, it worsens with forward bending. Additionally, the patient often complains of a catching pain in the low back that tends to climb up the body that occurs when rising from a forward bent posture. The patient also often supports his or her weight by placing his or her hands on the knees and thighs. Pain that arises primarily from the facet joints is often worsened by extension and rotation of the spine and is often associated with paravertebral tenderness.

Obviously, a thorough vascular examination is imperative to identify a peripheral vascular component of the symptoms. A patient presenting with atypical symptoms (e.g., night pain, rest pain) should be evaluated for other etiologies, such as a tumor, acute compression type fracture, or infection.

### Imaging Studies

Imaging studies used to evaluate spinal stenosis with degenerative spondylolisthesis should focus on two goals. First, determining the extent of central and foraminal stenosis and secondary neural impingement. Magnetic resonance imaging (MRI) is most useful in this regard and can help differentiate between varying causes of stenosis, such as synovial cysts and ligamentum flavum hypertrophy. If MRI is contraindicated, a computed tomography (CT) myelogram can also be used. This information is needed to design an appropriate strategy to treat the patient's radicular complaints. Secondly, imaging should focus on quantifying the amount of instability present in the spondylolisthetic segment and specific characteristics that portend an increased risk of progression. This information is necessary when determining how aggressive a decompression should be attempted and if additional stabilization techniques will need to be employed. These studies should include upright weight-bearing anteroposterior and lateral radiographs of the lumbar spine and pelvis, as well as flexion and extension views. An alternative method is to compare standing lateral radiographs with radiographs taken with the patient in supine hyperextension using a pillow. Lack of motion suggests a component of secondary stabilization. Though it is unclear what magnitude of slip is considered unstable, most studies define instability as listhesis greater than 2 mm.

### Specific Patient Populations and Situations

#### Elderly

The aging baby boomer generation is leading a shift in demographics toward a "gray society," and over the next 25 years a significant proportion of the population in industrialized societies will be over 65 years old. Since both symptomatic spinal stenosis and spondylolisthesis typically appear between the fifth and seventh decades of life (40-60 years), these conditions frequently coexist in this populace, and many patients with these conditions will become surgical candidates. While decompression of disabling lumbar spinal stenosis may lead to a significant improvement in quality of life, concerns about potential medical complications in this sometimes fragile population

and uncertainty about the expected outcome of operative treatment make many surgeons apprehensive about big surgeries, such as decompression with arthrodesis.

Some controversy exists as to whether age should be considered an independent risk factor for surgery. Many authors report no difference in outcome or rate of complications between elderly and younger patients of comparable health.[7] Therefore advanced age alone should not be a contraindication for surgery. Some studies, on the other hand, have demonstrated that increasing age can be an independent risk factor for surgery, especially if the patient is older than 60 years.[5] One such study noted a 41% complication rate (14% major and 27% minor) for patients 41 to 60 years of age and a 64% complication rate (24% major and 40% minor) for those 61 to 85 years of age (27). Pulmonary complications were the most common major complications and genitourinary problems were the most common minor complications. Age more than 60 years was therefore found to be a significant risk factor for perioperative complication.

It has also been reported that decompressive surgery in the elderly population can be effective without the need for supplemental fusion, and many authors therefore do not recommend fusion in patients older than 70 years. This is partly because the risk of developing postoperative instability in this age group appears to be small because of some intrinsic stability afforded by the spondylosis and spondylarthrosis that occur as the spine ages as well as the decreased activity level of this population.[5]

If decompression without supplemental fusion is performed in this population, care should be taken to limit the number of levels decompressed. It has been shown that the probability of developing postoperative spondylolisthesis increases with the number of levels decompressed; (6% for 2 levels progressing to 15% for 3 or more levels). Other strategies (which will be discussed later in this chapter) that may be employed in the elderly include noninstrumented fusions and minimal bone removal.

#### Multiple Comorbidities

Patients who have multiple comorbidities, such as cardiac disease, vascular disease, or diabetes have an increased risk for postoperative complications.[6,7] The preoperative evaluation and optimization of patients with these conditions is critical. The addition of an arthrodesis increases the length of anesthesia as well as the amount of blood loss. Both of these factors can delay recovery time, and patients with multiple comorbidities are therefore more likely to require an extended rehabilitation period. These factors should all be considered when deciding upon the advisability of supplemental fusion with decompression. Finally, for patients with a limited life expectancy, treatment should be focused on obtaining an immediate improvement in quality of life without subjecting the patient to a prolonged and painful recovery period.

Several studies in the literature have examined the relationship between preoperative comorbidities and postoperative complications. Although there is a link between certain risk factors and postoperative mortality, increasing American Society of Anesthesiology (ASA) physical status class has been shown to be one of the best independent predictors of mortality. Previous studies have reported an increasing rate of postsurgical mortality with increase in the ASA class. In fact, increasing morbidity and mortality rates have been prospectively demonstrated with an increase in the ASA class in a large population where the mortality rate increased from zero to 7.2% from ASA class 1 to ASA class 4, respectively.[7]

#### Osteoporosis

Bone quality is a major determinant of success in all fusion procedures, especially those involving instrumentation. A mild spondylolisthesis can progress and become more symptomatic as osteoporosis worsens, as commonly occurs in postmenopausal females. As the vertebrae weaken, the asymmetric load can cause increasing deformity and de novo scoliosis, which can increase the patient's symptoms.

Osteoporotic bone is a relative contraindication to instrumented fusion because of the difficulty in obtaining and maintaining adequate fixation at the bone–screw interface. Although variations in technique such as the use of larger diameter screws, screw threads with more aggressive pitch to improve pull-out strength, and augmentation of the bone–screw interface with methylmethacrylate have been advocated, failures of fixation are still likely.[6]

A conundrum thus exists with respect to treatment of symptomatic stenosis in a patient with spondylolisthesis: the structural integrity of an already unstable motion segment can be further compromised by laminectomy, and it can be difficult to reliably achieve fixation with instrumentation. Therefore an already challenging situation can be made more difficult, and care should be taken to minimize disruption of posterior supporting structures during the procedure.

## Indications for Fusion

The indications for surgical management are persistent or recurrent back pain with leg pain or neurogenic claudication, leading to a significant reduction in quality of life, despite a reasonable trial of nonsurgical treatment (>3 months); progressive neurologic deficit; and bladder or bowel symptoms resulting from neurologic compression.[5] Surgical options vary from decompression alone to fusion with or without instrumentation. More recent additions to the surgical armamentarium include ligament stabilizers and biologic agents. There continues to be a tremendous amount of controversy regarding the efficacy of fusion in degenerative disease resulting in low back pain (LBP).[8,9]

### Lateral Listhesis

Though several forms of degenerative spondylolisthesis commonly occur in association with stenosis, of particular concern is the lateral subluxation of one vertebral body upon another. This requires both minimizing structural disruption during decompression and also close follow-up for progression of deformity if instrumented fusion is not performed.

### Concomitant de Novo Scoliosis—Significant Curve and Progressing Curve

Degenerative de novo scoliosis (DDS) refers to the development of spinal curvatures in adults without a previous history of scoliosis. This occurs secondary to degeneration of facet joints, joint capsules, discs, and ligaments, which may create monosegmental or multisegmental instability. The curvatures in DDS are generally slowly progressive and not severe, but are commonly associated with back and radicular leg pain, as well as neurogenic claudication. DDS and stenosis commonly occur in tandem for several reasons. They both have high individual frequency as patients age and therefore commonly occur together. In addition, the scoliotic spine responds to the stresses of being biomechanically compromised with facet arthrosis and ligamentum flavum buckling or thickening, both of which decrease foraminal and central canal diameter.

When nonoperative management of patients with this combination of pathologies fails, decompressive procedures are often required. Patients with DDS who undergo laminectomy commonly require concomitant fusion since removal of the posterior elements can compromise spinal stability. In addition, the traditional aim of surgery is to both decompress the compromised neural elements and to create a balanced and stable spine in both the coronal and sagittal planes. As with other conditions, the surgical morbidity of DDS is significantly greater when the decompressive surgery is combined with fusion.[5,6]

Consideration must be given to both the magnitude of the DDS curve and whether or not it is progressive. Although slow curve progression may occur without surgery, more significant and rapid progression is likely following decompression without instrumented fusion.

The location and amount of decompression within the DDS curve can influence its stability. For instance, if decompression is performed at the apex of the curve, particularly on its concavity, progression of the curve is more likely than if it occurs further from the apex. Similarly, instability can also be compromised when a decompression is performed at the bottom of a rigid curve, where it transitions to a mobile part of the lumbar spine— for example, at L4-L5 or L5-S1. In this case, the presence of a rigid curve above a decompressed segment may result in translation of the fused segment, causing the spine to fall out of balance.

### Axial Pain

Although the progression of spondylolisthesis is usually slow it commonly results in significant axial and radicular pain. One of the most frequent indications for its surgical treatment is intractable pain. As is generally true in

spinal surgery, success is more likely with radicular pain than with axial pain. The treatment of axial pain often involves correction or stabilization of the deformity. Thus, fusion with instrumentation is usually required.

Radicular pain accompanying axial back pain is commonly the result of nerve root compression in the concavity of the curve as a result of foraminal narrowing. It may also result from traction of the nerve root in the convexity of the curve. While this type of radicular pain may be treated with decompressive procedures, such as laminectomy or foraminotomy, it can be difficult to assure adequate foraminal decompression within the concavity without distraction via instrumentation.

## Nonfusion Decision Making

Laminectomy is the initial surgical treatment for degenerative spondylolisthesis. Several studies have shown the clinical effectiveness of performing a laminectomy, with up to 80% good or excellent outcomes. Degenerative spondylolisthesis may progress beyond 50% following laminectomy without concomitant fusion. Even when the listhesis has not progressed, a revision decompression at the same level often requires significant removal of the remaining facet joints, necessitating instrumented fusion.

Decompressive surgery without instrumented fusion has less perioperative morbidity than when combined with fusion and can be performed in some fragile populations. Two such groups that are an increasing segment of society are the elderly and those with multiple comorbidities. Decompression alone may also be considered in the patient with osteoporotic bones.

Evaluation of these patients should include determining whether the patient has any associated spondylolisthesis—especially lateral listhesis. In addition the magnitude of the curve and signs of progression must be considered. Finally, the patient's symptoms must be taken into account. Those without a significant axial pain component may be better candidates for decompressive surgery without fusion than patients with axial pain.

## PART THREE: MANAGEMENT

### Nonsurgical

As with the majority of spinal disorders, it is appropriate to attempt a nonsurgical solution first. Most patients with symptomatic spinal stenosis and degenerative spondylolisthesis respond to nonsurgical management and do not require surgery. Conservative treatments for spinal stenosis with degenerative spondylolisthesis include nonsteroidal antiinflammatory drugs, membrane stabilizer medications (e.g., gabapentin, pregabalin), activity modification, and physical therapy.[10]

The mainstay of physical therapy for this condition emphasizes flexion exercises, back strengthening, and aerobic conditioning. Aerobic conditioning can be somewhat problematic in this population, but exercises performed in flexion, such as stationary bicycle, enlarge the neural foramen and central canal, minimizing the symptoms of neurogenic claudication. Passive modalities such as ultrasound, massage, heat, and spinal manipulation are useful in that they may temporarily improve symptoms, but their efficacy has not been verified by prospective studies with long-term follow-up.[10]

### Surgical

#### Fusion Options with or without Instrumentation

Although surgical decompression alone often improves symptoms in the patient with spinal stenosis and degenerative spondylolisthesis, numerous studies have demonstrated the benefits of concomitant fusion, either noninstrumented or instrumented.[4,5,11] For stabilizing the spine, instrumented fusions are superior to uninstrumented fusions. However, they are not always feasible, especially in the elderly population with osteoporotic bones. When a fusion is desired but instrumentation is contraindicated, the benefit of noninstrumented fusions are that they generally require less dissection and blood loss and require less surgical time under anesthesia.

#### Decompression and Noninstrumented Posterolateral Fusion

Concomitant fusion improves long-term outcomes when a decompressive laminectomy is performed for spinal stenosis with degenerative spondylolisthesis. The placement of instrumentation increases morbidity, as well. It seems logical that un-instrumented posterolateral fusion could provide a good compromise between the two options.[9] Though much of the morbidity associated with preparation of the fusion bed would remain (increased dissection and pain, increased anesthesia time, and blood loss), the additional trauma and time of instrumentation placement would be avoided. Prospective studies of patients with degenerative spondylolisthesis who underwent decompression and uninstrumented dorsolateral fusion versus patients undergoing decompression alone have in fact demonstrated significantly better outcomes. Of note, although this procedure is associated with a high pseudoarthrosis rate (up to 36%), this did not affect patient outcomes. This is thought to be the result of stiffening of the spine and motion restriction due to a stable pseudoarthrosis.[11,12]

The procedure does have some disadvantages. As mentioned above, the patient must still undergo the extensive dissection of the lateral areas over the transverse processes. The fusion itself is negatively impacted by the relatively poor vascularity of the transverse processes as well as the constant intertransverse graft motion during activities of daily living secondary to the intervening juxtaposed paraspinous and quadratus lumborum muscles. Finally, dorsolateral fusion requires consolidation of bone over a fairly large distance (several centimeters) between transverse processes.

## Fusion with Biologics

Newer biologics have given the surgeon the advantage of relatively improved fusion rates using less invasive techniques. Numerous prospective randomized studies of recombinant bone morphogenetic proteins (recombinant human bone morphogenetic protein-2 [rhBMP-2] and recombinant human bone morphogenetic protein-7 [rhBMP-7]) have been performed. The safety, effectiveness, and radiographic outcomes of OP-1 (BMP-7) putty with autogenous iliac crest bone graft used for laminectomy and noninstrumented posterolateral fusion for symptomatic lumbar stenosis associated with degenerative spondylolisthesis have been reported and are encouraging.

A prospective randomized controlled multicenter clinical study with a 2-year follow-up has reported clinical success, defined as a 20% improvement in the preoperative Oswestry score. Success was achieved in 85% of patients treated with OP-1 putty versus 64% of patients treated with autograft. In addition, a successful posterolateral fusion was achieved in 55% of patients treated with OP-1 putty and in 40% of patients treated with autograft. Importantly, a 36-item Medical Outcomes Study Short-Form General Health Survey (SF-36). SF-36 scores showed similar clinical improvement in both groups.

A second prospective randomized clinical study has evaluated the use of rhBMP-2 to achieve posterolateral spine fusion in patients with a grade I spondylolisthesis and single level degenerative disc disease that were scheduled to undergo single level posterolateral lumbar arthrodesis. The study compared patients undergoing autogenous iliac crest bone graft with pedicle screw instrumentation, rhBMP-2 with pedicle screw instrumentation, and rhBMP-2 only with no instrumentation. The study demonstrated a radiographic fusion rate of 40% in the autogenous iliac crest bone graft with pedicle screw instrumentation, 100% in patients that received rhBMP-2 with pedicle screw instrumentation, and 100% in the rhBMP-2–only group.[13] More importantly, the clinical outcomes improved faster and to a greater degree in the rhBMP-2–only group. The surgical time was significantly less secondary to the elimination of the time required for bone graft harvest and placement of internal fixation.

## Decompression and Posterolateral Fusion with Instrumentation

The most effective method of achieving "stability" following decompression is the addition of instrumentation.[11] A prospective randomized study comparing the results of decompression and arthrodesis alone with those of decompression and arthrodesis combined with instrumentation has shown that the addition of spinal instrumentation improved the fusion rate (82%, instrumented versus 45%, noninstrumented).[4] Although achieving a solid fusion appeared to be less important, since no significant difference was found in clinical outcomes, more recent longer term (5- to 14-year) follow-up studies have reported that patients with pseudarthrosis did not do as well as those that achieved solid fusion.[4,11] The complication rates, revision rates, radiographic results, and patient satisfaction at 5-year follow-up were reviewed for patients following segmental posterior instrumented fusion with decompression in patients with lumbar degenerative spondylolisthesis and showed that no patient had a neurologic deficit, evidence of symptomatic pseudarthrosis (i.e., pain, lucency, loose instrumentation), or recurrent stenosis at the fused segment.[7]

Unfortunately, posterolateral fusion requires a large dissection for the preparation of the fusion bed, which is associated with increased pain, bleeding, time in surgery, and recovery. In addition to this, instrumentation further increases the morbidity of the surgery.[12]

## Facet Fusion

Facet joints normally function by bearing load and allowing motion, while restricting excessive motion. Fusion of the facet can be accomplished with or without instrumentation, and can substantially reduce the pain and morbidity associated with posterolateral fusion. Though studies have demonstrated that instrumented facet fusions can have a 96% fusion rate by CT scan, this is not as strong as a posterolateral fusion, and a functional outcome assessment was not reported.

Uninstrumented facet fusions are becoming more popular because of their simplicity and minimal additional dissection requirement. They can be performed using locally harvested autograft placed into the facet joint or with allograft bone dowels that are currently available from several companies. Unfortunately, no powerful studies are available on the effectiveness of uninstrumented facet fusion in stabilizing the spine.

Because a varying degree of disruption of the facet capsule (which in itself is stabilizing) must occur to perform a facet fusion, a negative to this procedure is that if a fusion does not occur, the spine will have in fact lost stability from the procedure. Additionally, if wide decompressions are performed, the added stress placed on the facet joint can lead to fracture of the thinned pars interarticularis and complete incompetency of the joint. Obviously, if any type of facet fusion is going to be attempted, care should be taken to preserve as much of the pars interarticularis as possible bilaterally.

## Fusion with Transforaminal Lumbar Interbody Graft

The addition of interbody support helps to restore the biomechanical advantages of a solid anterior column and provides an increased fusion surface area. These advantages could translate into an increased rate of fusion and improved patient outcomes. Unfortunately, no prospective randomized studies have been performed comparing decompression with transforaminal lumbar interbody fusion to decompression with instrumented posterolateral fusion. Until such a study is performed, it will be more difficult to justify the added dissection and anesthesia time required in an older patient population.

### Nonfusion Options

## Laminectomy

Many studies have demonstrated the efficacy of dorsal decompression for alleviating the symptoms of spinal stenosis.[1-3] Although laminectomy is a relatively well-tolerated procedure, the incidence of postoperative instability (increased translation and loss of alignment) has been reported to be as high as 50% in patients undergoing laminectomy for spinal stenosis and even higher in patients with degenerative spondylolisthesis.[5,10]

The standard surgical treatment for lumbar spinal stenosis consists of a decompressive laminectomy accompanied by partial medial facetectomy and foraminotomy, as needed. It is important to preserve as much of the facet joint as possible. Similarly, preservation of the pars interarticularis is essential to maintain stability and minimize the need for instrumentation. Therefore it is often helpful to expose and visualize the pars interarticularis in order to avoid its inadvertent disruption during the decompression.

When performed properly, the risk of postoperative instability following this procedure is less than 2% in patients without degenerative scoliosis. The risk of instability increases in patients with degenerative scoliosis, especially as the magnitude of the curve increases. Patients with curves greater than 20 degrees are at a higher risk of curve progression and often require prophylactic fusion. The risk of worsening postoperative spondylolisthesis also increases with the number of levels decompressed, ranging from 6% for 2 levels to 15% for 3 or more levels.

## Laminotomy or Interlaminar Fenestration

Interlaminar fenestration or laminotomy can provide significant neural decompression in select patients with minimal structural disruption, and can be especially useful in the treatment of lateral recess stenosis. These procedures emphasize the preservation of stabilizing structures such as the interspinous and supraspinous ligaments, spinous processes, and functionally important parts of facet joints. Interlaminar fenestration is accomplished by trimming bone around the interlaminar spaces of involved segments along with removal of the ligamentum flavum and medial portion of the facet joint. The fenestration extends laterally to decompress affected nerve roots with the preservation of the adjoining laminae, spinous processes, interspinous ligaments, and facet joints.

## Foraminotomy

Foraminotomy is often required when the neural foramen is narrowed as a result of disc space collapse or facet arthropathy. As with other decompressive procedures, aggressive foraminotomy can destabilize the spine, especially in the presence of degenerative scoliosis or spondylolisthesis, and can result in an increase in the magnitude of slip or rate of curve progression. Therefore care must be taken to minimize facet disruption by limiting the facetectomy to the medial one third of the facet joint and to preserve the pars interarticularis if possible. Decompression of the nerve root on the concavity of a curve, which often has significant foraminal narrowing, is often challenging and may not be feasible.

## Restorative Laminoplasty

Biomechanically, the vertebral arch, supraspinous and interspinous ligaments provide a tethering constraint during anterior flexion and support for the dorsolumbar fascia and muscles. In order for the posterior elements to provide support, the supraspinous and interspinous ligaments with their bony attachments must be intact. It has been demonstrated that extensive laminectomy can lead to instability if these points of attachment are removed.

Spinal canal enlargement by restorative laminoplasty, in which osteotomized vertebral arches are repositioned rather than removed, can provide an acceptable alternative to fusion. Theoretically, this method of decompression could be more effective in preventing postoperative instability than multilevel fenestration, because it involves less extensive dissection of the laminae and facet joints. As an alternative to decompression with fusion, it has been used in patients with both degenerative spondylolisthesis and degenerative scoliosis with 2-year follow-up studies showing no exacerbation of spondylolisthesis or scoliosis, nor the onset of other instability

Whereas favorable results have been demonstrated using laminoplasty, 2-year outcome studies have demonstrated that symptomatic improvement is less likely in patients with degenerative scoliosis, particularly with more severe scoliosis. Notably, the number of restored vertebral arches has not been found to have significant correlations on overall improvement rate. Similarly it has not been shown to be effective in patients with degenerative spondylolisthesis. Its benefit in lateral spondylolisthesis has not been evaluated.

## Minimally Invasive Techniques

Minimally invasive surgery (MIS) is becoming more popular in the treatment of many spinal disorders. With these techniques, a decompressive laminectomy, laminotomy, or foraminotomy is performed with minimal tissue dissection via the use of special retractor systems, unilateral approaches, and endoscopes. These techniques can be used to insert spinal instrumentation, or for decompression procedures alone. Although MIS decompression has many theoretical advantages with respect to minimizing tissue disruption and preserving stability, such benefits have not been conclusively proven. In addition, they can be associated with a steep learning curve and prolonged operative time, which may be an important issue in the elderly and medically fragile patient. As with any surgical procedure performed through a small portal, orientation can be difficult, and therefore an unintentionally aggressive facet resection or damage to the pars interarticularis could occur if landmarks are not properly recognized.

## Motion-Sparing Technologies

Recently, new technologies have become available that are primarily categorized as "motion preservation devices" but may have some use in minimizing destabilization while decompressing the stenotic patient. The literature is sparse and has mixed results on many of these device's efficacy. More follow-up is needed to determine their ultimate role and utility in patients with spondylolisthesis.

The goal of surgery with many of these devices is to provide semirigid stabilization, interspinous widening, or both, in an attempt to stabilize the spine, provide for neural decompression, and avoid the need for fusion. They mainly come in two varieties: interspinous process distraction devices and semirigid fixation between pedicle screws. A prospective study of patients with degenerative spondylolisthesis who underwent decompression of the spine, with and without stabilization, using the Graf system (Surgicraft, Worcestershire, UK) reported no statistically significant difference between decompression alone and decompression with stabilization using the Graf system. Additionally, stabilization using the Graf system was not effective in reducing the recurrence of leg symptoms. Another prospective clinical study evaluated whether elastic stabilization with the Dynesys system (Zimmer Spine, Minneapolis, Minn.) provided enough stability to prevent progression of spondylolisthesis after decompression for spinal stenosis with degenerative spondylolisthesis. Radiographically, no significant progression of spondylolisthesis was detected. The authors concluded that in an elderly population with spinal stenosis and associated degenerative spondylolisthesis, dynamic stabilization with this system in addition to decompression results in clinical outcomes similar to those seen with established protocols using decompression and fusion with pedicle screws. Of note, although the implant failure rate was fairly high (17%), none of these instances were clinically symptomatic.

Interspinous distraction devices prevent extension of the instrumented level and try to replicate the relief the patient obtains when they lean forward in flexion. A randomized controlled study of such a device, X STOP (St. Francis Medical Technologies, Alameda, Calif.), in patients with neurogenic claudication and degenerative spondylolisthesis, reported overall clinical success in 63% of the patients treated with the X STOP versus 13% success in the nonsurgical group. A common cause of failure of these devices is that their modulus of elasticity is usually far greater than the adjacent spinous processes, which leads to subsidence of the device into the spinous processes as well as fracture of the bone.

## CONCLUSION

Degenerative spondylolisthesis and spinal stenosis commonly occur in tandem and often cause back and radicular leg pain or neurogenic claudication. It is most common in elderly women at L4-L5. It is also most common in a patient population with multiple comorbidities and poor bone quality. Though many with this condition who undergo laminectomy also require fusion, decompressive surgery without instrumented fusion is an option in select patients and is better tolerated with less perioperative morbidity in this population of medically fragile patients.

The severity of a patient's symptoms and the presence of any neurological deficits must be taken into account. Evaluation of these patients should include determining the presence or absence of associated degenerative scoliosis and characteristics of the listhesis that portend less stability (lateral listhesis). In patients with an associated scoliosis, the magnitude and progression of the curve must be determined.

While traditional laminectomy can usually be performed without destabilizing the spine, care must be taken to spare the pars interarticularis and as much of the facet(s) as possible. Procedures such as laminotomy, interlaminar fenestration, foraminotomy, and restorative laminoplasty may be sufficient for neural decompression without significantly compromising structural integrity. Likewise, newer minimally invasive techniques have the potential to preserve more structurally important soft tissue. The ultimate role that these procedures play in the surgical treatment of patients with spinal stenosis and degenerative scoliosis remains to be proven.

When decompressive procedures are performed without fusion, a radical decompression should be avoided at the base or apex of a curve in order to minimize risk of curve progression. Curves that are greater than 20 degrees, demonstrate progressive deformity, or fit both criteria, are not good candidates for decompression without fusion. Finally, patients with significant axial pain are less likely to experience improvement in their back pain without concomitant fusion. Recent short-term studies have also shown the efficacy of adding biologics to aid in obtaining a solid fusion. Future technologies, such as dynamic stabilization and interspinous distraction devices, will require long-term prospective studies to prove their role in managing the patient with degenerative scoliosis and spondylolisthesis.

## References

1. D.K. Sengupta, H.N. Herkowitz, Lumbar spinal stenosis. Treatment strategies and indications for surgery, Orthop. Clin. North Am. 34 (2003) 281.
2. J.N. Katz, S.J. Lipson, M.G. Larson, et al., The outcome of decompressive laminectomy for degenerative lumbar stenosis, J. Bone Joint Surg. Am. 73 (1991) 809.
3. A.J. Caputy, A.J. Luessenhop, Long-term evaluation of decompressive surgery for degenerative lumbar stenosis, J. Neurosurg. 77 (1992) 669.
4. K.H. Bridwell, T.A. Sedgewick, M.F. O'Brien, et al., The role of fusion and instrumentation in the treatment of degenerative spondylolisthesis with spinal stenosis, J. Spinal Disord. 6 (1993) 461.
5. S. Matsunaga, K. Ijiri, K. Hayashi, Nonsurgically managed patients with degenerative spondylolisthesis: a 10- to 18-year follow-up study, J. Neurosurg. 93 (2000) 194.
6. R.J. Benz, Z.G. Ibrahim, P. Afshar, et al., Predicting complications in elderly patients undergoing lumbar decompression, Clin. Orthop. Relat. Res. (2001) 116.
7. M.Y. Wang, B.A. Green, S. Shah, et al., Complications associated with lumbar stenosis surgery in patients older than 75 years of age, Neurosurg. Focus 14 (2003) e7.
8. J.S. Fischgrund, The argument for instrumented decompressive posterolateral fusion for patients with degenerative spondylolisthesis and spinal stenosis, Spine 29 (2004) 173.
9. F.M. Phillips, The argument for noninstrumented posterolateral fusion for patients with spinal stenosis and degenerative spondylolisthesis, Spine 29 (2004) 170.
10. D.R. Murphy, E.L. Hurwitz, A.A. Gregory, R. Clary, A non-surgical approach to the management of lumbar spinal stenosis: a prospective observational cohort study, BMC Musculoskelet. Disord. 7 (2006) 16.
11. M.B. Kornblum, J.S. Fischgrund, H.N. Herkowitz, et al., Degenerative lumbar spondylolisthesis with spinal stenosis: a prospective long-term study comparing fusion and pseudarthrosis, Spine 29 (2004) 726.
12. Z. Ghogawala, E.C. Benzel, S. Amin-Hanjani, et al., Prospective outcomes evaluation after decompression with or without instrumented fusion for lumbar stenosis and degenerative Grade I spondylolisthesis, J Neurosurg Spine 1 (2004) 267.
13. S. Boden, J. Kang, H. Sandhu, et al., Use of recombinant human bone morphogenetic protein-2 to achieve posterolateral lumbar spine fusion in humans: A prospective, randomized clinical pilot trial 2002 Volvo Award in clinical studies, Spine 27 (2002) 2662.

# Imaging of the Aging Spine

16

*Colin S. Poon, Navid Zenooz, and Gordon Sze*

**KEY POINTS**

- Radiography is suited for evaluation of spine alignment. Lateral flexion and extension views are commonly used for assessment of segmental instability.

- MRI provides the most comprehensive imaging evaluation of the aging spine. Fat-suppressed imaging sequences are particularly valuable for imaging of spine trauma, inflammation, infection, and neoplasm. For inflammation, infection, and neoplasm, contrast enhanced T1-weighted imaging sequences can provide additional information.

- Nuclear bone scan is sensitive but not specific for evaluation of most active spine diseases.

- Radiography with lateral flexion and extension views is most commonly used for follow-up of postoperative spine. CT provides better assessment of hardware placement and postoperative complications. MRI and nuclear bone scan can be used for problem solving in patients with postoperative complications, and persistent or new symptoms.

Although the aging spine can be affected by a wide spectrum of diseases including neoplasm, infection, trauma, and degenerative disease, the latter by far is the most important in terms of disease burden and socioeconomic impact in the aging population. Back pain, with or without radiculopathy, is the most common indication for imaging of the spine. Patients with debilitating degenerative disease are often treated by surgery or other interventional procedures. Many of these patients will continue to have active complaints and require imaging follow-up. For these reasons, this chapter will focus on imaging of degenerative disease. Many other pathological conditions including trauma, infection and neoplasm can also affect the aging spine. An awareness of the imaging application in these diseases is important because a major role for early imaging of back pain is the exclusion of these "red flag" conditions. The imaging of these other diseases and postoperative spine, as well as a discussion of imaging techniques, are included in the Appendix (on the website) to serve as an introduction to these topics.

## IMAGING OF DEGENERATIVE SPINE DISEASE

Correlation between imaging morphology of degenerative disease and clinical symptoms can be poor, particularly for the most common complaint of pain. The reasons of the discrepancy are not clear, but several factors may come into play. Subjective complaints such as pain may be due to inflammatory response in the surrounding soft tissues, rather than mass effect that can be visualized directly on imaging. In addition, degenerative changes may indirectly compress the nerve roots by distorting their normal surrounding soft tissue structures, such as epidural fat, rather than compress the nerves directly. Imaging usually provides only a static snapshot of the anatomical structures. For example, most imaging studies are acquired with the patient supine, which is most likely different from the posture of the patients when they experience their symptoms. Although specialized units such as upright MRI scanners are now available to address these issues, their use is not yet widely adopted. Notwithstanding its limitations, imaging provides an important means for evaluation of the spine.

Degenerative disease of the spine most commonly involves the lumbar spine, followed by the cervical spine. Manifestations of degenerative spine disease include intervertebral disc degeneration, disruption of the annulus fibrosus, herniation of the nucleus pulposus, vertebral endplate changes, osteophyte formations, facet arthropathy, formation of juxta-articular cysts, degenerative spondylolisthesis, and spinal stenosis.

## Intervertebral Disc Degeneration

On radiography (Figure 16-1), intervertebral disc degeneration is indirectly inferred from loss of the normal disc space height. Gas may be seen in the disc space, due to a negative pressure within the degenerative disc causing extraction of nitrogen from extracellular space. This is commonly referred to as vacuum phenomenon. The vacuum phenomenon can be accentuated during extension of the spine and reduced during flexion. Vertebral endplate irregularity is often seen, with or without associated sclerotic changes at the endplates.

With the wide availability of MRI, CT is rarely requested for the primary evaluation of degenerative disc disease, except in patients with contraindications for MRI examination. Similar to radiography, CT can demonstrate

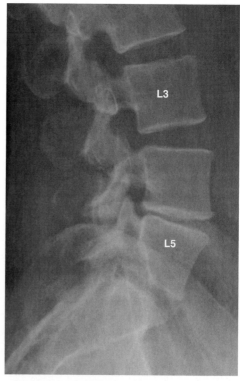

**FIGURE 16-1** Radiographic features of degenerative disc disease. Disc space narrowing and subtle cartilaginous endplate sclerosis are present at L4-L5.

disc space loss, endplate irregularity or sclerotic changes, and vacuum phenomenon. However, CT also allows direct visualization of disc bulging and disc herniation (Figure 16-2) , although with a lesser soft tissue contrast compared to MRI. When more accurate depiction of disc bulging and disc herniation is required, CT myelography can be performed (Figure 16-3) .

MRI provides the best soft tissue details of degenerative disc disease. In young healthy patients, the intervertebral discs demonstrate hyperintensity on T2-weighted images. With aging, there is loss of this hyperintensity due to a decrease of water content and changes in proteoglycan composition (Figure 16-4). There is decreased disc height and the endplates may become irregular. Gas from vacuum phenomenon may fill the space of a degenerative disc, which may demonstrate hypointensity on both T1- and T2-weighted images. Alternatively, the space may be filled with fluid, which is seen as hyperintensity on T2-weighted images. A degenerative disc may also calcify, which can give hypointensity or hyperintensity on T1-weighted images, depending on the type and concentration of calcification. A degenerative disc may also enhance secondary to the presence of granulation tissues.

Fissures of the annulus fibrosus may be seen in the intervertebral discs. On MRI, annular disruptions (also referred as fissures) may be seen as a small high intensity zone within the outer annulus (Figure 16-5) .

One of the primary advantages of MRI is the direct visualization of disc bulging or herniation, and its associated mass effect on the nervous structures. At a particular disc level, a disc can have bulging and one or more areas of herniation seen on the same occasion. In 2001, multiple societies reached a consensus to standardize the nomenclature and classification of disc pathology.[1] This work is currently being revised (A. Williams, S. Rothman, R. Murtagh, G. Sze, in progress). The consensus was initially developed for lumbar disc disease but is generalized to disc disease in the rest of the spine. Normal disc space is defined craniocaudally by the vertebral body endplates, and circumferentially by the ring apophysis of the vertebral bodies. In the newly revised consensus, a disc bulge refers to diffuse displacement of disc material beyond the normal disc space, and covers greater than 25% of the normal disc space circumference (i.e, greater than 90 degrees of the circumference) (Figure 16-6, A) . Disc displacement covering 25% or less of the circumference is called herniation. When the width of the base of the disc herniation is greater than any other measurements in the same plane of the herniation, it is called a protrusion (Figure 16-6, B). When any of the measurements of the herniation is greater than the width at its base, the herniation is described as an extrusion (Figure 16-6, C and D). In essence, a protrusion is a disc herniation with a wide base, whereas an extrusion is a narrow-based disc herniation with appearance sometimes resembling toothpaste that is squeezed out of its container. Migration refers to herniated disc material that is displaced above or below the level of the disc. When the disc extrusion is separated from the parent disc, it is referred to as a sequestration. Sequestered disc often demonstrates T2 hyperintensity

compared to its disc of origin. This may be secondary to the presence of granulation tissue, immune response, or inflammation.[2] Most disc sequestrations are seen in the epidural space, but rarely, they may migrate into the intradural space or posterior to the thecal sac. Herniated disc may be contained by the annulus fibrosus (subannular) or the posterior longitudinal ligament (subligamentous) (Figure 16-6, D), although the distinction sometimes can be difficult.

Disc material can also herniate through the vertebral cartilaginous endplates into the adjacent vertebral bone marrow. Intravertebral (intraosseous) herniation is often called Schmorl's node (Figure 16-7) and has been reported in 38% to 75% of the population. Most of these are seen as incidental findings.

## Vertebral Marrow Changes and Osteophyte Formation

Disc degeneration often leads to changes of the bone marrow adjacent to the cartilaginous endplates bordering the disc. MRI can demonstrate three patterns of bone marrow signal changes that have been classified by Modic et al[3] (Figure 16-8) . The vertebral marrow changes can convert from one type to another with time. In many patients, the vertebral marrow changes actually appear in a mixed pattern. The clinical and pathophysiological significance of vertebral marrow changes have been subject to debate. Some reports have suggested that type I change is likely to be inflammatory in origin and is more strongly associated with active low back symptoms and segmental instability.[4] It has also been suggested that patients with type I marrow changes respond better to fusion compared to those without or with other types of endplate changes, and that persistence of type I marrow changes after fusion is associated with a worse outcome.[5]

Osteophyte formation is commonly seen in the aging spine. Osteophytes refer to abnormal bony outgrowth that is believed to be induced by abnormal mechanical stress. They are often located at the edge of the annulus fibrosus and adjacent apophyses, and are best seen on radiographs or CT. Osteophytes at the outer rim of the vertebral endplates and associated with degenerative disease are commonly referred to as spondylosis deformans.

## Facet Arthropathy

Degenerative changes of the facet joints in the spine resemble that of other synovial joints in the rest of the body. Although radiography can demonstrate the bone changes associated with osteoarthritis, including joint space narrowing as a result of thinning of articular cartilage, subchondral sclerosis, marginal osteophyte formation, facet hypertrophy, and hyperostosis, these findings are best demonstrated on CT (see Figures 16-2 and 16-3). Very often, gas from vacuum phenomenon can also be seen on radiography or CT. MRI does not provide as much bony detail, but facet hypertrophy is

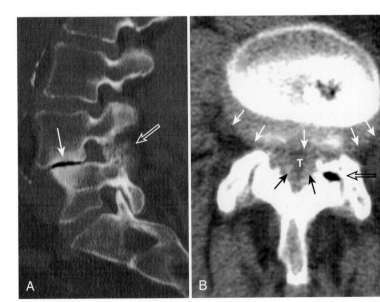

■ **FIGURE 16-2** CT of intervertebral disc degeneration. **A,** Reformatted sagittal CT image in bone window showing severe disc degeneration including severe disc space loss, lucency within the disc space consistent with gas (vacuum phenomenon), and sclerosis at the adjacent endplates (*white arrow*). The facet joint also demonstrates irregular hypertrophy, osteophytes and loss of joint space (*open arrow*). Degeneration of these structures lead to instability, resulting in anterolisthesis of L4 over L5. **B,** Axial image in soft tissue window demonstrates diffuse disc bulging (*white arrows*), thickening of the ligamentum flavum (*black arrows*), and facet arthropathic changes that include joint space narrowing, facet hypertrophy, and vacuum phenomenon in the facet joints (*open arrow*). These changes lead to severe spinal canal stenosis, with the thecal sac (*T*) severely compressed anteriorly and posterolaterally.

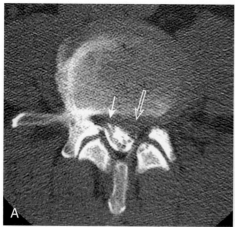 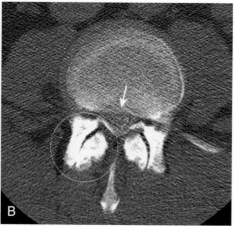

■ **FIGURE 16-3** CT myelogram. **A,** Axial image at the L3-L4 intervertebral level demonstrates a left central disc protrusion (*open arrow*), causing stenosis and impingement of the nerve roots at the left lateral recess. By comparison, the right L4 nerve root at right lateral recess (*white arrow*) is floating freely within the thecal sac. **B,** At the L2-L3 level, there is severe spinal stenosis as a result of disc bulging, ligamentum flavum hypertrophy, and facet arthropathic changes that include facet hypertrophy and sclerosis (*circle*), resulting in almost complete obliteration of the cerebrospinal fluid space (*arrow*).

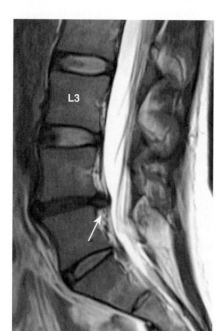

■ **FIGURE 16-4** Disc degeneration seen on MRI (T2-weighted image) (same patient as Figure 16-1). There is disc space narrowing and loss of the normal T2 hyperintensity of the L4-L5 disc. Bulging of the disc with a small protrusion into the spinal canal is also shown (*arrow*). Compare the L4-L5 disc with the normal appearance of the discs at L2-L3 and L3-L4 levels.

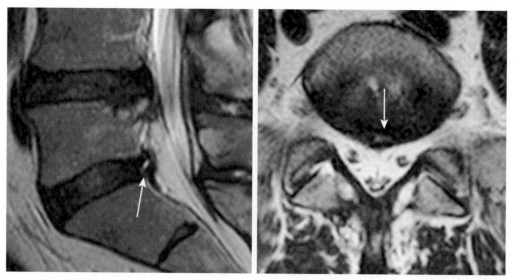

■ **FIGURE 16-5** Annular disruption seen as a high intensity zone (*arrow*) on T2 weighted images.

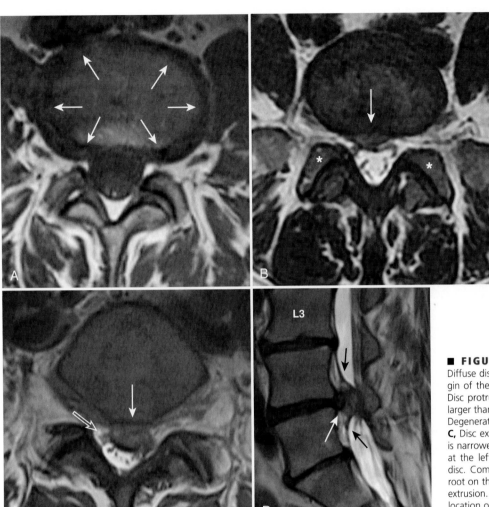

■ **FIGURE 16-6** Disc bulging and herniation. **A,** Diffuse disc bulging. The disc extends beyond the margin of the ring apophysis (*arrows*) circumferentially. **B,** Disc protrusion. Note the width of the base (*arrow*) is larger than any other dimensions of the disc herniation. Degenerative facet hypertrophy is also noted (*asterisks*). **C,** Disc extrusion. The width of the base (*white arrow*) is narrower than any other dimensions. The nerve root at the left lateral recess is impinged by the extruded disc. Compare this with the corresponding free nerve root on the right (*open arrow*). **D,** Subligamentous disc extrusion. Note the narrow width of the base and the location of the disc extrusion (*white arrow*) underneath the lifted posterior longitudinal ligament (*black arrows*).

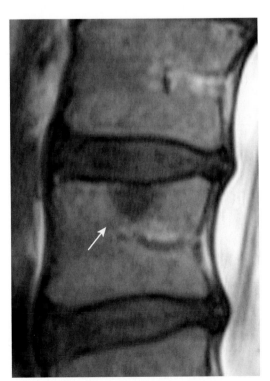

■ **FIGURE 16-7** Schmorl's node (*arrow*) at superior endplate of L4 vertebra. On this sagittal T2-weighted image, loss of the normal bright signal and bulging of the L3-L4 and L4-L5 discs are also noted.

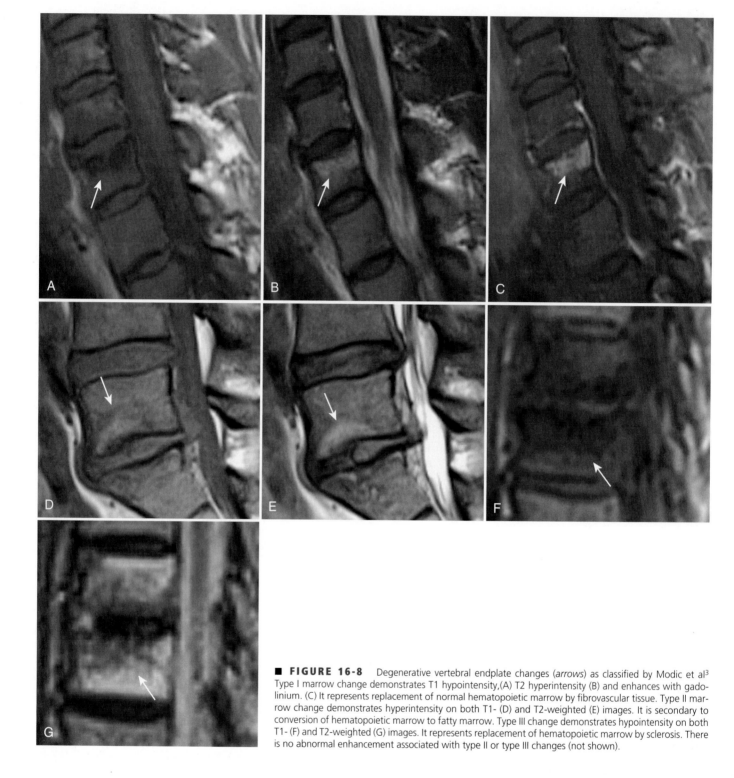

■ **FIGURE 16-8** Degenerative vertebral endplate changes (*arrows*) as classified by Modic et al[3] Type I marrow change demonstrates T1 hypointensity,(A) T2 hyperintensity (B) and enhances with gadolinium. (C) It represents replacement of normal hematopoietic marrow by fibrovascular tissue. Type II marrow change demonstrates hyperintensity on both T1- (D) and T2-weighted (E) images. It is secondary to conversion of hematopoietic marrow to fatty marrow. Type III change demonstrates hypointensity on both T1- (F) and T2-weighted (G) images. It represents replacement of hematopoietic marrow by sclerosis. There is no abnormal enhancement associated with type II or type III changes (not shown).

easily demonstrated (see Figure 16-6, *B*). In addition, MRI may demonstrate joint space effusion and inflammatory changes (synovitis) that can be associated with osteoarthritis (Figure 16-9). Synovitis is best demonstrated on fat-suppressed T2-weighted or postgadolinium MRI sequences.

The uncovertebral joints associated with the lower five cervical vertebral bodies are also commonly associated with arthropathic changes. The uncinate process may undergo hypertrophy and spur formation that can project into the neural foramina and spinal canal, leading to narrowing of the neuroforamina and spinal canal stenosis (Figure 16-10) .

Juxta-articular cysts are often seen associated with facet arthropathy. They include synovial and ganglion cysts. Compared to synovial cysts,

ganglion cysts do not have synovial lining and do not communicate with the joint space. However, on imaging, it is difficult to make the distinction and they are often simply referred to as juxta-articular cysts. The cysts are usually located in the posterolateral epidural space of the spinal canal. Occasionally, they may be completely outside of the spinal canal (Figure 16-11). They can calcify and sometimes can be confused with other pathological entities such as a disc herniation or a mass. However, the recognition of continuity of a lesion with adjacent degenerative facet joint should strongly suggest the diagnosis. On MRI, their signal intensity is variable and depends on whether they contain proteinaceous material or hemorrhage. Gas may be present in synovial cysts, as they communicate with facet joints that may contain gas from vacuum phenomenon. The cyst walls may contain hemorrhage or calcification. There may be contrast enhancement in the cyst wall or surrounding soft tissues if inflammatory response is present.

## Spondylolisthesis and Segmental Instability of the Spine

Spondylolisthesis, scoliosis, and segmental instability can result from degeneration of the stabilizing structures in the spine, including intervertebral discs, vertebral bodies, facet joints, joint capsules, and ligaments (see Figure 16-2). It is important to exclude other underlying pathologies, such as defect of the pars interarticularis or fracture. This consideration is particularly important when the anterolisthesis is greater than grade 1 (25% of the vertebral body diameter), or the degenerative changes are disproportionately mild to account for the high grade spondylolisthesis. Pars interarticularis defect can be detected using oblique radiography or CT. For occult pars defect or occult fracture, a nuclear bone scan may aid in their detection.

Segmental instability of the spine can be seen as spine deformity or spondylolisthesis that increases with spine motion and progresses over time. Standing radiography that includes anteroposterior and lateral projections

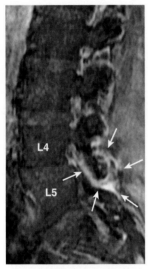

**FIGURE 16-9**  Enhancement may be present in degenerative disease of the facet joints (*arrows*). Other degenerative changes of the facet joints may also include facet hypertrophy, joint space narrowing, and joint effusion.

with flexion and extension of the spine provides the most easily available imaging tool for evaluation of spine instability.[6]

There are currently no standardized methods or criteria for diagnosis of spine instability.[7] However, values of 10 degrees for sagittal rotation and 4 mm for sagittal translation have been used to infer instability in some studies.[6] Sagittal rotation is measured as the variation of angle between two opposite vertebral endplates observed during flexion and extension on lateral projection, and sagittal translation is measured as the variation of distance between the lines that follow the posterior cortices of two adjacent vertebrae. To minimize the effect of radiographic magnification, the absolute distance can be given as a percentage of the anteroposterior width of the superior vertebra.

Reproducibility of measurement of segmental instability is difficult, and is subject to many factors, including patient positioning, angulation of x-ray beam, radiographic magnification effect that varies with the distance of the anatomical structures from the x-ray detector, and patient's level of cooperation.

Radiography can also demonstrate other indirect signs of instability, such as vacuum phenomenon and traction osteophytes. Traction osteophytes appear as horizontal osteophytes that arise typically on adjacent vertebral bodies below the rims of the endplate, approximately 2 to 3 mm from the edge of the intervertebral disc[8] (Figure 16-12) .

Instability is difficult to demonstrate directly on routine MRI and CT. Many imaging features can suggest instability indirectly, including spondylolisthesis, degenerative endplate changes, vacuum phenomenon, and degenerative disc disease. However, these imaging features are neither sensitive nor specific and can also be seen in degenerative spine disease without instability.

## Spinal Stenosis

Spinal canal stenosis and foraminal stenosis are common consequences of degenerative disease of the spine. Patients with congenital anomalies, such as short pedicles, are particularly at risk of developing spinal stenosis. Spinal stenosis is best evaluated with MRI because of its ability to assess both bony and soft tissue structures that can narrow the spinal canal or neural foramina (Figures 16-13 and 16-14). Direct impingement on the spinal cord or nerve roots can be easily seen on MRI. Disc bulging, disc herniation, degenerative changes of the facet and uncovertebral joints, thickening of the ligamentum flavum, epidural lipomatosis and spondylolisthesis can all lead to narrowing of the spinal canal and neural foramina. Although sagittal images can provide a general overview of spinal canal stenosis, axial images are essential for an accurate assessment of the degree of stenosis.

The central spinal canal can be narrowed anteriorly by disc bulge or herniation and vertebral osteophytes. Posterolaterally, it may be narrowed by facet disease and ligamentum flavum hypertrophy. Epidural lipomatosis tends to favor the posterior epidural space but may also be seen

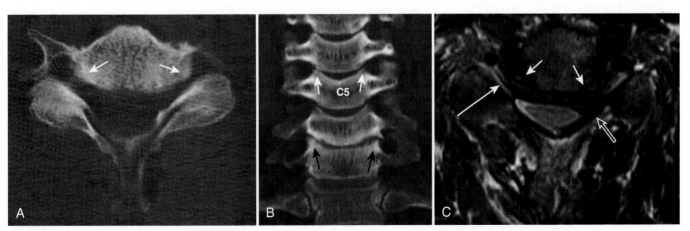

**FIGURE 16-10**  Uncovertebral joint degenerative disease causing neural foraminal narrowing. Axial CT image (**A**)and reformatted coronal CT image (**B**) at C6-C7 intervertebral level demonstrate spur formation at the uncovertebral joints (*black arrows*) projecting into the neural foramina, causing foraminal stenosis. Compare this with the normal uncovertebral joints at the other levels (*white arrows*). **C,** Axial T2-weighted MR image in a different patient demonstrates osteophytes at the posterior vertebral margin and uncovertebral joints (*short arrows*). A small disc protrusion is also noted at the left lateral recess (*open arrow*). There is narrowing of the bilateral neural foramina, worse on the left, causing impingement of the left exiting nerve root. *Long arrow,* right exiting nerve root.

circumferentially. These abnormalities lead to distortion of the normally round or oval shape of the spinal canal and thecal sac. With worsening stenosis, the spinal canal and thecal sac may become triangularly shaped or flattened. There may be effacement of cerebrospinal fluid space located between the degenerative processes, causing spinal stenosis and impingement of the spinal cord or nerve roots.

Grading of spinal canal stenosis can be performed according to the recommendation of the Combined Task Forces of the North American Spine Society, American Society of Spine Radiology, and American Society of Neuroradiology.[1] Spinal canal compromise of less than one third of the normal canal is graded as "mild," between one third and two thirds is "moderate," and over two thirds is "severe." Neural foraminal stenosis can be assessed on axial images and lateral sagittal images, using a grading scheme similar to that for central spinal canal.

Severe spinal canal stenosis can lead to compression of the spinal cord. This can result in ischemia and edema, which may eventually lead to irreversible damage and myelomalacia (Figure 16-15). Myelomalacia can be seen as T2 hyperintense signal of the spinal cord. Cystic changes and

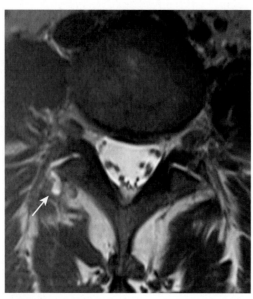

■ **FIGURE 16-11** **Synovial cyst.** Axial T2-weighted MR image demonstrates degenerative changes of the bilateral facet joints, which contain a small amount of effusion. On the right; a small synovial cyst (*arrow*) is seen in continuity with the right facet joint.

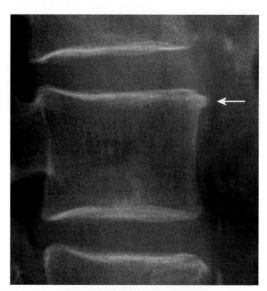

■ **FIGURE 16-12** Lateral radiography of lumbar spine demonstrates a traction spur (*arrow*), which is an indirect sign of segmental instability. (*From Leone A, Guglielmi G, Cassar-Pullicino VN, Bonomo L. Lumbar intervertebral instability. Radiology 2007; 245(1): 62-77, Figure 5.*)

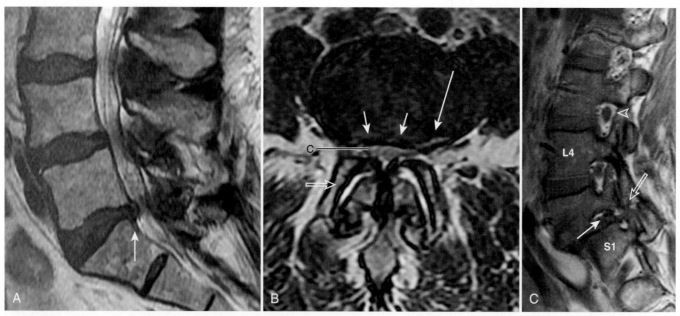

■ **FIGURE 16-13** **Spinal canal and neuroforaminal stenosis. A,** Sagittal T2-weighted image demonstrates disc bulging at the L5-S1 level and spinal stenosis (*arrow*). **B,** Axial T2-weighted image at L5-S1 level demonstrates severe spinal stenosis with nerve root impingement as a result of congenital shortening of the pedicles (note the short distance between the facets and the vertebral body) and superimposed degenerative changes including disc bulging and facet arthropathic changes. *Small arrows,* disc bulging; *long arrow,* annular disruption; (*open arrow*), facet hypertrophy and joint effusion. **C,** Sagittal T1-weighted image in another patient demonstrates anterolisthesis of L5 over S1 secondary to spondylolysis at L5 (*open arrow*). The L5 nerve root exiting the L5-S1 neuroforamen is compressed (*arrow*). Compare this with the free L3 nerve root exiting the L3-L4 neuroforamen (*open arrowhead*), which is completely surrounded by normal epidural fat.

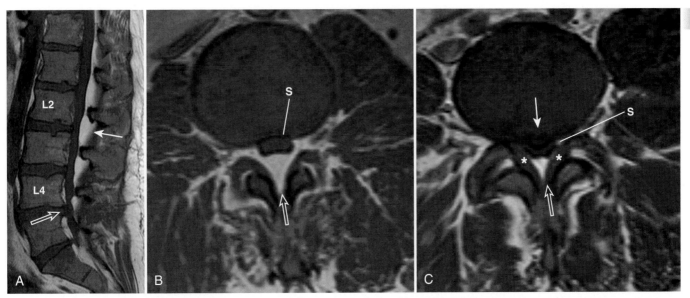

■ **FIGURE 16-14**    Severe spinal stenosis secondary to epidural lipomatosis and other degenerative changes. **A,** Sagittal T1-weighted image. **B,** Axial T1-weighted image at L3-L4 level. **C,** Axial T1-weighted image at L4-L5 level. Excessive epidural fat (*open arrows*) in conjunction with facet hypertrophy, ligamentum flavum hypertrophy (*asterisks*), and disc bulging and protrusion (*white arrows*) result in severe spinal stenosis. The thecal sac (*S*) is severely compressed.

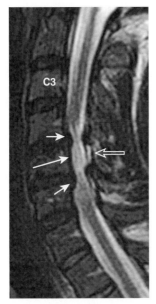

■ **FIGURE 16-15**    Myelomalacia at level of C4-C5 to C5-C6 is seen as increased T2 signal (*long arrow*) on this sagittal T2-weighted image. The cord is atrophic with small areas of cystic changes. This patient had traumatic injury and degenerative disease of the spine. Note the disc bulging and ligamentum flavum hypertrophy at C4-C5 and C5-C6 levels (*short arrows*) resulting in spinal canal stenosis. There is thinning of the ligamentum flavum at C5 level (*open arrow*), probably from previous hyperflexion injury.

tethering of the cord to the dural sac may also be present. Differentiation of myelomalacia from reversible edema or ischemia can be difficult when atrophy associated with the myelomalacia is not evident.

## SUMMARY

Imaging is an essential component of the evaluation of the aging spine. Proper patient management hinges on correct diagnosis. Imaging facilitates this by providing accurate depiction of the morphological changes associated with diseases. Plain film radiography, CT, and MRI constitute the mainstay of imaging evaluation of the spine. Ancillary techniques such as nuclear imaging, myelography, and discography are often used for problem solving in selective cases. Appropriate use and proper performance of the imaging techniques are prudent to maximize the benefits of imaging.

Degenerative disease is the most common reason for spine imaging. Standardized nomenclature for description of degenerative spine disease has been developed,[1] and further revision is now underway. A universal adoption of this nomenclature is encouraged to facilitate more effective communication among all who provide spine care to patients. Neoplasm, infection, and trauma are also important indications for imaging. Imaging is particularly important in patients presenting with the so-called red flags that suggest a higher risk of these diseases, such as increasing age, osteoporosis, and persistent or progressive symptoms. In patients who have received spine surgery, imaging is required to assess hardware placement, postsurgical complications, and disease progression after surgery.

Many issues in spine imaging warrant further research. The correlation between clinical presentation, imaging findings, and clinical outcomes is still not well understood. In addition, continuing advances in imaging technology will provide increasingly explicit anatomical details of the diseased spine, as well as new physiological and dynamic imaging data that have not been captured by the more traditional imaging technology. Some of these examples include high-resolution 3D MR imaging, special MR units that allow patients to be imaged in different positions, and ultrafast volumetric CT that can image the spine in flexion and extension. It is without doubt that imaging will play an ever-increasing role in the care of the aging spine.

## References

1. D.F. Fardon, P.C. Milette, Nomenclature and classification of lumbar disc pathology, Spine 26 (5) (2001) E93–E113.
2. T.J. Masaryk, J.S. Ross, M.T. Modic, et al., High resolution MR imaging of sequestered lumbar intervertebral discs, AJNR Am J. Neuroradiol. 9 (1988) 351–358.
3. M.T. Modic, P.M. Steinberg, J.S. Ross, et al., Degenerative disc disease: assessment of changes in vertebral body marrow with MR imaging, Radiology 166 (1988) 193–199.
4. R. Rahme, R. Moussa, The Modic vertebral endplate and marrow changes: pathologic significance and relation to low back pain and segmental instability of the lumbar spine, AJNR Am. J. Neuroradiol. 29 (2008) 838–842.
5. G.R. Buttermann, K.B. Heithoff, J.W. Ogilvie, et al., Vertebral body MRI related to lumbar fusion results, Eur. Spine. J. 6 (1997) 115–120.
6. A. Leone, G. Guglielmi, V.N. Cassar-Pullicino, L. Bonomo, Lumbar intervertebral instability, Radiology 245 (1) (2007) 62–77.
7. R.S. Nizard, M. Wybier, J.-D. Laredo, Radiologic assessment of lumbar intervertebral instability and degenerative spondylolisthesis, Radiol. Clin. North Am. 39 (1) (2001) 55–71.
8. I. Macnab, The traction spur: an indicator of segmental instability, J. Bone. Joint Surg. Am. 53 (1971) 663–670.

# Conservative Treatment Modalities

# 17

# Land Based Rehabilitation and the Aging Spine

*Jack Miletic and Avrom Gart*

| K E Y   P O I N T S |
| --- |
| • Review the pathophysiology of the "degenerative cascade" in the aging spine. |
| • Identify appropriate therapeutic movements for specific spinal pathology. |
| • Understand patient comorbidities and how they affect the rehabilitation of the aging spine. |
| • Understand the physiology behind the stability of the lumbar spine. |
| • Review the core stabilization exercises. |

Before focusing on the rehabilitation essentials, we will dedicate some time to reviewing the pathophysiologic basis of the degenerative spine, as has been elegantly described by Kirkaldy-Willis.[1] A thorough understanding of spinal anatomy and the process of degeneration will better equip us to grasp the focus of rehabilitation exercises tailored for specific pathologic findings in the degenerated spine. Comorbidities are a significant factor influencing the shape and depth of rehabilitation, therefore it is necessary to review common comorbidities encountered when determining a rehabilitation program, and how to adjust it based on these confounding factors. Finally, before reviewing the essential core stabilization exercises, we would like to touch on the normal physiology involved in stabilizing the spine. With this background, we can better understand the kinematics and kinesiology of the exercises reviewed.

## THE "DEGENERATIVE CASCADE"

The spine is dynamic and is constantly modeling and remodeling, a process greatly influenced by the physical stresses placed upon it. These changes can positively or negatively impact neurological status and spinal biomechanics. There are a certain set of conditions associated with degeneration of the aging spine. Most commonly seen disorders include degenerative disc disease, segmental dysfunction or instability, zygapophyseal arthropathy, spinal stenosis, cervical spondylotic myelopathy, and radiculopathy. To better understand these conditions and which therapeutic approach would be most appropriate, we need to understand the pathophysiology of the degenerating spine.

Currently, the most widely accepted theory of intervertebral disc degeneration pathophysiology is a three-stage approach described by Kirkaldy-Willis.[1] Stage I describes the acute pain of an initial insult occurring in the early 20 to 30 years of life. This is the beginning of what Kirkaldy-Willis described as the "degenerative cascade." Repetitive microtrauma to the vertebral endplates results in ischemic events that can compromise the nutritional and metabolic transport to the disc. This microtrauma may also be responsible for an alteration in proteoglycan content resulting in decreased disc hydration and subsequent load-bearing capacity. Clinically, the patient will present with intermittent and self-limiting pain. However, the pain experienced may be extremely debilitating because of the innervation of the outer third of the annulus by the sinuvertebral nerve.

Stage II, or the instability stage, represents continued disc dehydration and loss of disc height. Increased force transfer to the annulus occurs with the subsequent loss of disc height.[1] This stage occurs later in life, between 30 and 50 years of age, and the patient presents with periods of low back pain which is usually more intense and protracted in duration.

Stage III, known as the stabilization stage, usually occurs in the 60 and older population. There is continued end-stage tissue damage and attempts at repair. Disc resorption leads to disc collapse, endplate destruction, fibrosis, and osteophyte formation. The patient usually presents with symptoms of neurogenic claudication or radiculopathy from central, lateral recess, and/or foraminal stenosis.[1]

## THE FOCUS OF REHABILITATION

Aging is a normal process, and understanding the anatomic and physiological changes that occur with normal aging will allow for optimal rehabilitation. Some age-related bodily changes may be misunderstood and can unnecessarily limit daily activities; however, when designing an exercise program for older adults, the possibility of a latent or active disease process must be taken into consideration. The exercise prescription must be individualized based on the health status and the goals of the individual.

The focus of rehabilitation in the aging population should consist of the following: (1) increasing, restoring, or maintaining range of motion, physical strength, flexibility, coordination, balance, and endurance; (2) recommending adaptations to make the home accessible and safe; (3) teaching positioning, transfers, and walking skills to promote maximum function and independence within an individual's capability; (4) increasing overall fitness through exercise programs; (5) preventing further decline in functional abilities through education, energy conservation techniques, joint protection, and use of assistive devices to promote independence; and finally, (6) improving sensation, and joint proprioception, and reducing pain.

A conservative approach is usually warranted, considering the patient population's comorbidities. Any form of aerobic activity should be structured to provide adequate rest and minimal imposition of joint stress.[2] Initiating resistance training under close supervision with the least amount of resistance can provide significant benefit in the aging population.[3] As with younger individuals, functional range of motion is extremely important and all aspects of physical therapy should be preceded by appropriate stretching and warm-up to prevent further injury.

Much has been reported on the appropriate amount of rest a patient with acute back pain should adhere to. What has become clear is that excessive immobility will translate to decreased aerobic capacity, impaired flexibility, loss of muscle strength, and promotion of bone demineralization, all of which will exacerbate and promote further pain and disability.[4] Ultimately limiting bed rest to a short period proves to be less detrimental than extended periods of bed rest, even in the population of patients who exhibit radiculopathic symptoms.[5]

## PATHOPHYSIOLOGIC BASIS FOR REHABILITATION

The goal of exercise for the treatment of acute back pain is pain control. Therefore initiating exercises based on which direction of motion either increases or reduces pain will provide more positive outcomes.[6,7] Movement into flexion or extension will centralize low back pain and reduce the patient's symptoms.

Extension-based exercises, or McKenzie exercises, may be effective in reducing discogenic pain[8] by alleviating pressure on the posterior annular fibers and thereby altering intradisk pressure,[9] which will concurrently allow anterior migration of the nucleus pulposus[10] and subsequent decreased tension on the nerve root.[11] Contraindications to extension-based exercises include segmental instability, bilateral sensory or motor deficits, large or uncontained herniations, or an increase in radiculopathic symptoms. If the patient responds well to extension exercises and demonstrates centralization of his or her pain, repeated extension posturing while standing and use after sitting or forward bending is stressed. If the patient does indeed have segmental instability, manual blocking of extension at that level can be achieved by the therapist, and the patient can be educated on preventing segmental mobility.

Flexion-based exercises, or Williams exercises, may be effective in decreasing zygapophyseal joint compressive forces, thus alleviating the compressive load to the posterior disc, decompressing the intervertebral foramen, stretching hip flexors and paraspinal musculature, and strengthening core stabilizers, such as the abdominals.[12] Included in flexion-based exercises are pelvic tilts, which can be performed either with bent knees, straight legs, or standing, depending on the comfort level of the patient. These exercises will help decompress the zygapophyseal joint and help mobilize the pelvis for sacroiliac joint dysfunction.

When dealing with patients with idiopathic scoliosis it is widely understood that therapeutic exercises cannot prevent the progression of the curvature; however, there is a clear role for rehabilitation in this setting. The fundamental goal is to prevent the progression of secondary morbidities. Exercises to restore range of motion and strength should begin early. The patient will benefit from exercises that focus on improving trunk posture and alignment, which may prevent the development of a pathological curve. Abdominal and gluteal strengthening helps prevent deconditioning and atrophy, whereas lower extremity hip flexor stretching works well to prevent contractures.[13]

## COMORBIDITY INFLUENCE ON REHABILITATION

The key to a successful rehabilitation approach in any patient population is conservatism and understanding the patient's limitations. Interaction between exercise and the medical condition is essential to grasp so that deleterious exercise effects can be avoided, particularly when dealing with patients that may have cardiac disease, diabetes mellitus, obesity, osteoarthritis, peripheral vascular disease, or cancer.

In patients who have cardiac comorbidities, a typical rehabilitation approach would include isotonic, aerobic, and rhythmic exercises involving large muscle groups, as well as isometric and resistive exercises, particularly for patients with left ventricular dysfunction. Instituting heart rate and systolic and diastolic blood pressure parameters varies depending on the pathology.

Patients that have pulmonary comorbidities such as chronic obstructive pulmonary disease (COPD) respond to controlled breathing techniques to improve pulmonary function parameters with diaphragmatic breathing exercises. The need to monitor for hypercapnia is an essential indicator for the need for muscle rest periods to be added to the exercise program. As with cardiac precautions, pulmonary precautions are instituted with regard to respiratory rate and oxygenation.

Osteoporosis must be considered when therapeutic exercises are instituted. Physical therapy should be tailored to individual fitness level and anticipated propensity to fracture or current fractures. Precautions include avoiding spine flexion exercises, which may predispose to vertebral compression fracture.

## PHYSIOLOGIC FACTORS OF SPINAL STABILIZATION

Stability of the lumbar spine requires both passive stiffness, through the osseous and ligamentous structures, and active stiffness, through musculature. Any injury to the passive supporting network of the spine will result in instability.[14] That is why optimal muscle strength can protect the damaged spine from repetitive shear forces or nonphysiologic weight bearing. The thoracolumbar fascia acts as a physiologic corset, in essence providing a link between the lower limb and the upper limb, supporting the spinal segments and providing proprioceptive feedback to the individual. Therefore a comprehensive stabilization or facilitation of the abdominal, pelvic, and trunk

muscles, which attach to the thoracolumbar fascia and provide for flexion, extension, and rotation of the spine, is a key component to improving trunk strength and preventing future exacerbation of pain.

Stabilization of the spine progresses through a sequence of events that begins with strengthening of the smaller intersegmental local muscles of the lumbar spine, such as the multifidi and transversus abdominis. The multifidi usually span a few segments and thereby have a poor mechanical advantage as a significant mover of the spine, but they do play a role in rotational movement and balancing of the shear forces of the spine.[15,16] Initial exercises focus on obtaining isolated control of these muscles without substitution.

The next phase of stability training focuses on neutral spine stabilization exercises, regarded as the "safe," pain-free position.[17] A neutral spine position decreases tension on ligaments and joints, appropriate segmental forces with respect to the disc, and the zygapophyseal joint provides optimal stability with axial loading and gives the patient the greatest level of comfort. The neutral spine is located through various body positions, which is followed by lower extremity exercises initially without resistance, then with resistance while maintaining a neutral spine. This approach will help facilitate coordination, endurance, and strength.

Finally, the prime movers, including the rectus abdominis, erector spinae, and latissimus dorsi, are strengthened. Traditionally abdominal exercises have been emphasized as part of a low back exercise program, as well as lower extremity strengthening because of their integral association with the trunk. This is particularly important during lifting, where education in proper bending and lifting techniques is stressed to prevent new-onset low back pain. Lower extremity muscular flexibility is extremely important for optimal physiologic lumbar motion. Hip flexors and extensors attach to the pelvis and will essentially dictate lumbar positioning, which can result in excessive stress on lumbar segments and the sacroiliac joint. If a patient has tight hip flexors, this will result in extension of the lumbar spine and subsequent shear forces on the intervertebral disc. A slight alteration in the kinetic chain biomechanics will promote pain and disability. Self-stretching techniques should be initiated as early as possible in the neutral pelvic position.

## CORE STABILIZATION EXERCISES

The most common stabilization exercises incorporated in a routine rehabilitation program include (1) finding the neutral position, (2) sitting stabilization, (3) prone gluteal squeezing exercises, (4) pelvic bridging progression, (5) kneeling stabilization, (6) wall slide quadriceps strengthening, (7) position transition with postural control, (8) curl-ups, (9) diagonal curl-ups, (10) side bridging, and (11) straight leg lowering. Fitness programs that follow core-strengthening principles include Pilates, yoga, and taichi—all of which must first be determined appropriate in the aging population with certain limitations.

Figures 17-1 and 17-2 demonstrate abdominal strengthening exercises, showing proper activation of the muscles around the abdominal area to

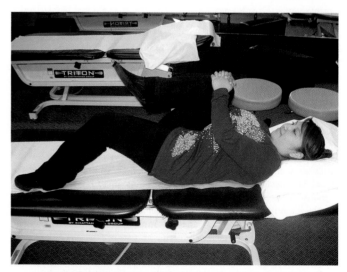

**■ FIGURE 17-1**   Abdominal exercises: single leg curl.

support the low back in static and dynamic positions. Daily dynamic load bearing causes the muscles to contract around the viscera to form a stable core region against which the forces are balanced, in coordination with posture.

Figures 17-3 to 17-5 demonstrate back and buttock exercises, which along with abdominal training help control movement, transfer energy, shift body weight, and move in any direction. Weak core muscles result in loss of lumbar lordosis and postural deficiency. Stronger, more balanced core musculature helps maintain appropriate posture and reduce strain on the spine.

Figures 17-6 to 17-8 demonstrate trunk and full body exercises, which are important for proper coordination patterns and abdominal and low back endurance.

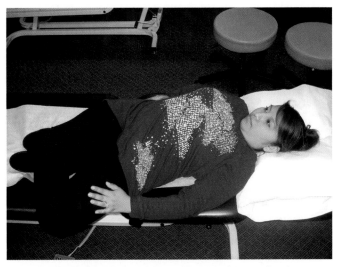

■ **FIGURE 17-2**   Abdominal exercises: lying trunk twist.

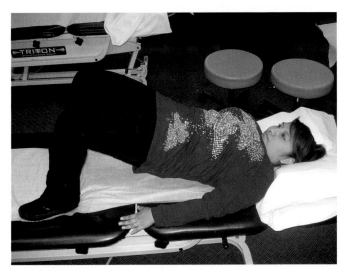

■ **FIGURE 17-3**   Buttock and back exercises: floor bridging.

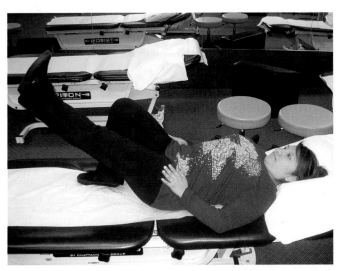

■ **FIGURE 17-4**   Buttock and back exercises: single-leg bridging.

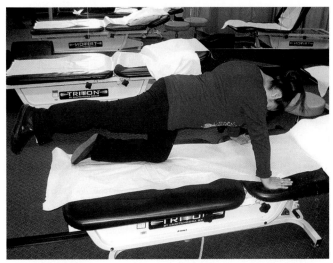

■ **FIGURE 17-5**   Buttock, back, and abdominal exercises: horse stance.

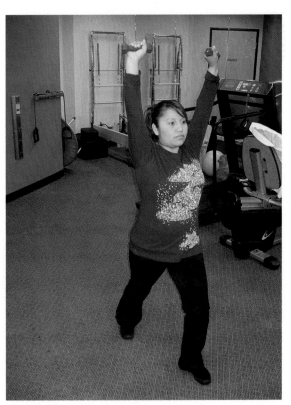

■ **FIGURE 17-6**   Trunk and full body exercises: modified weighted lunges.

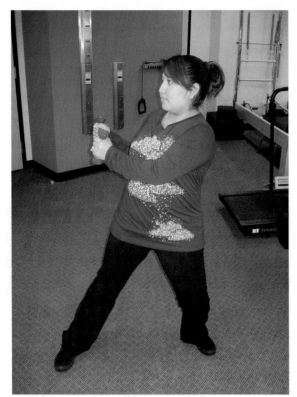

■ **FIGURE 17-7** Trunk and full body exercises: standing weighted obliques.

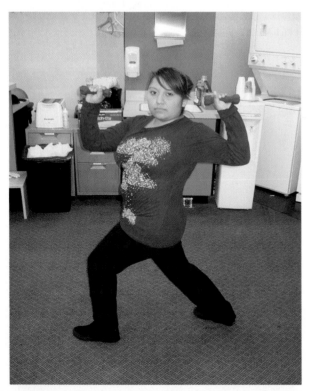

■ **FIGURE 17-8** Trunk and full body exercises: standing weighted obliques.

The ultimate goal of core stabilization is to achieve optimal task performance while maintaining appropriate trunk position and control, which will help ensure the prevention of recurrent injury. As always, consideration must be given to individual musculoskeletal response to the exercise and the overall metabolic demands.

### References

1. W.H. Kirkaldy-Willis, et al., Pathology and pathogenesis of lumbar spondylosis and stenosis, Spine 3 (1978) 319–328.
2. American College of Sports Medicine, ACSM's guidelines for exercise testing and prescription, sixth ed., Lippincott Williams & Wilkins, Philadelphia, 2000.
3. M.A. Fiatarone, et al., Exercise training and nutritional supplementation for physical frailty in elderly people, N. Engl. J. Med. 330 (1994) 1769–1775.
4. V.A. Coveretino, et al., Symposium: physiological effects of bed rest and restricted physical activity: and update, Med. Sci. Sports Exerc. 29 (1997) 187–206.
5. P.C.A.J. Vroomen, et al., Lack of effectiveness of bed rest for sciatica, N. Engl. J. Med. 340 (1999) 418–423.
6. R. Donelson, et al., Pain response to sagittal end-range spinal motion. A prospective, randomized, multicenter trial, Spine 16 (1991) S206–S212.
7. R. Stankovic, et al., Conservative treatment of acute low back pain. A prospective randomized trial: McKenzie method of treatment versus patient education in mini back school, Spine 15 (1990) 120–123.
8. R. Melzack, et al., Pain mechanism: a new theory, Science 150 (1965) 971–979.
9. A. Nachemson, et al., Intravital dynamic pressure measurements in lumbar discs: a study of common movements, maneuvers and exercises, Scand. J. Rehab. Med. (Suppl. 1) (1970) 1–40.
10. R.A. McKenzie, The lumbar spine: mechanical diagnosis and therapy, Spinal Publications, Waikance, New Zealand, 1981.
11. B.E. Schnebel, et al., The role of spinal flexion and extension in changing nerve root compression in disc herniation, Spine 14 (1989) 835–837.
12. P. Williams, Low back and neck pain: causes and conservative treatment, third ed., Charles C Thomas, Springfield, Ill, 1974.
13. K.J. Noonan, Adolescent idiopathic scoliosis: nonsurgical techniques: The pediatric spine: principles and practice, second ed., Lippincott Williams & Wilkins, New York, 2001, pp. 371–383.
14. G.R. Ebenbichler, et al., Sensory-motor control of the lower back: implications for rehabilitation, Med. Sci. Sports Exerc. 33 (2001) 1889–1898.
15. J.J. Crisco, et al., The intersegmental and multisegmental muscles of the lumbar spine. A biomechanical model comparing lateral stabilization potential, Spine 16 (1991) 793–799.
16. M.M. Panjabi, et al., Spinal stability and intersegmental spinal forces. A biomechanical model, Spine 14 (1989) 194–200.
17. J.A. Saal, Dynamic muscular stabilization in the non-operative treatment of lumbar pain syndromes, Orthop. Rev. 19 (1990) 691–700.

# 18

# Aquatic Physical Therapy

*Thomas Cesarz and David Speach*

**KEY POINTS**

- Swimming skill is not required for patients to safely engage in water-based therapies.
- Aquatic exercises are generally as safe as land-based exercises but health contraindications exist that may prohibit water-based therapy.
- Aquatic physical therapy is indicated when an individual cannot tolerate land-based therapies.
- Pain relief and improved function are the most common reasons for prescribing aquatic-based physical therapy.
- Scientific literature supporting purported benefits of aquatic therapy is limited. Extrapolated research in patients with knee arthritis and ankylosing spondylitis do demonstrate modest benefits in pain reduction and well-being following aqua therapy.

For millennia people have used water for healing and for rituals, traditions continuing through the present. Today, water is applied in a variety of therapies, with proponents of each often making broad and unsubstantiated claims of health benefits. Commonly used terms for water-based therapies include hydrotherapy, aquatic therapy, balneotherapy, and spa therapy.

Hydrotherapy and aquatic therapy are often used interchangeably to refer to physical therapy performed in water. Spa therapy refers to physical modalities applied in a relaxing atmosphere that may be purely commercial, devoid of oversight from a licensed practitioner at point of delivery. Spa therapies can include land-based modalities such as massage and electrotherapy, as well as water-based forms such as balneotherapy and whirlpool. Spa treatments, even when water-based, are typically passive.[1] Studies of spa interventions prove difficult. Balneotherapy refers to the immersion of patient or limb in a natural thermal mineral water, defined as at least 20° C, and containing a concentration of specific salts in excess of 1 g/L.[1]

This chapter focuses on aquatic therapy exercises that are analogous to land-based physical therapy. It will cover the theoretical underpinning of aquatic exercise with appropriate indications and contraindications.

## CLINICAL CASE EXAMPLES

A 78-year-old woman with advanced bilateral knee osteoarthritis and leg and back pain occurring only when walking and standing has been unable to tolerate land-based aerobic exercise due to pain.

A 68-year-old obese male smoker with chronic axial low back pain and poor endurance presents to a chronic pain center with markedly reduced daily function and pain with any movement or prolonged positioning.

## BASIC SCIENCE

For such a widely used and presumably safe activity, immersion in water has far-reaching physiological effects that help explain the patient's relief of symptoms but also raise the flag of specific contraindications. Water differs from air in density, buoyancy, and viscosity, rendering it of different therapeutic value.

Water is nearly 800 times as dense as air.[2] The bottom of a mass of material exerts a pressure based on the density of the material. For example, at sea level, effectively at the "bottom" of the earth's atmosphere, patients are exposed to the pressure of air. When a patient enters a body of water, be it a hot tub, swimming pool, or ocean, the water exerts pressure that increases with increasing depth. Water affects the cardiovascular and renal systems. Water's hydrostatic pressure compresses veins, increasing venous return and pushing blood centrally, leading to a rise in central blood volume, cardiac blood volume, and cardiac output.[3] Compression of veins can reduce edema. Healthy individuals seated for 2 hours in water from the renowned spa at Bath, England, showed a doubling of diuresis and 50% increase in cardiac index. The increase in diuresis is not due to an increase in creatinine clearance, though alteration of renally active hormones may play a role.[4] It is unclear if hydrostatic pressure is the primary mechanism underlying all of these systemic effects.

Water is a viscous substance that resists movement. The resistance offered by the water increases as speed of movement increases, so when the patient first starts exercising in water, a slower velocity is naturally used. As strength and endurance improve, faster movement is possible with greater challenge. Because of the mechanics of fluid, resistance is maximized if the patient performs exercises in a continuous movement in which the limb is kept below the water surface. Resistance can be strategically lessened to accommodate the patient's strength level with partial submersion and pausing during the movement. For the stronger patient, water mitts and hand paddles can be added to increase drag of the limb.[5] Training in water has several advantages compared to land. Movements against water are inherently more difficult than identical movements against air because of water's viscosity, making virtually any movement against water a resistance training exercise. Performing resistance training movements in water puts less stress on joints because they are unloaded of gravitational forces compared to land.

Pain decreases in water through several mechanisms. The natural buoyancy of water unloads joints and supports the body so less muscle activation and coordination is required to maintain balance. Standing upright with water up to the neck, the upward buoyant force counteracts gravity so that about 10% of the normal gravitational force is exerted on the body. Discs, facets, and peripheral joint structures are unloaded allowing for functional movements such as walking with less stress.[6] Reduction of muscle activity to maintain balance allows for easier control of proper pelvic tilt and lumbar curvature. Body support from buoyancy in positions of spinal flexion and extension means the patient can actively range through normally painful spinal load movements with less compression on the spine. Normal range of motion may be achieved in a pain-free manner in the aquatic environment before trying similar exercises on land.[5] A negative effect of buoyancy is a decrease in body stability with water levels above the T8 spinal level. Shallower water may be indicated if the patient has difficulty keeping his or her feet planted on the pool floor.[5] An additional factor in aquatic therapy pain relief is that water acts as a diffuse sensory stimulus that can alter or suppress the typical pain experience.[5]

## Case Studies

### TREATMENT, CLINICAL CHALLENGES, AND FUTURE TREATMENTS

A 78-year-old woman with bilateral knee osteoarthritis and leg and back pain occurring only when walking and standing has been unable to tolerate land-based aerobic exercise. For this individual, her knee arthritis interferes with her ability to bear weight and train her spine on land. Evidence exists showing that aquatic exercises decrease pain from peripheral joint arthritis. The unloading effect that occurs in water allows for strength training and aerobic conditioning while in a supportive environment that protects from falls. Her history is suggestive of neurogenic claudication from lumbar spinal stenosis, a condition where the patient often obtains relief while in positions of flexion. In water a flexion posture is achieved with less compressive force on the vertebral bodies, limiting the risk of an exercise-induced osteoporotic compression fracture or aggravation of mechanical low back pain. Eventually, this patient can try transitioning to a land-based program with the goal of improving her walking tolerance.

A 47-year-old obese male smoker with chronic axial low back pain and poor endurance presents to a chronic pain center with markedly reduced daily function and pain with any movement or prolonged stationary position. Chronic low back pain is very challenging to treat. Once an individual becomes deconditioned, land-based exercises can be too challenging, particularly in patients with limited pulmonary capabilities as in obstructive pulmonary disease. Water is an ideal environment to begin recovery of strength, endurance, and flexibility. The prescribing physician must pay attention to any contraindications for aquatic therapy that are present in this patient, such as comorbid severe heart disease or open wounds. The primary goal for this patient will be to decrease the pain associated with movement. The buoyant aquatic environment reduces axial load on his spine. Limb exercises performed quickly under water will be more difficult than on land. An aquatic-based conditioning program must be titrated to his endurance, which will increase over the course of therapy.

## CLINICAL PRACTICE GUIDELINES

### Physician Evaluation and Prescription

While obtaining the history and physical the practitioner will pay special attention to factors that will make aquatic therapy uniquely beneficial, as well as to contraindications. Evaluation includes a focused neurologic and musculoskeletal examination with a focus on spinal range of motion, strength, sensation, and gait. A common example of an aquatic therapy regimen is that outlined by Dr. Andrew Cole.[7] Static and dynamic exercises of progressive difficulty are used for development of spinal stabilization. Examples include sitting against the pool wall with neutral spine posture, walking forward and backward, abdominal crunches, a host of exercises designed for the facilitation of neutral spine posture, flexibility, conditioning and core strength.

### Indications

Indications for water therapy are similar to those for land-based therapies with the most important criterion being unsuitability for a fully land-based program. The patient may need extra support due to weakness or proprioceptive loss and concurrent land-based spinal rehabilitation is possible if the patient can tolerate some land-based exercises.[7] Ultimately the patient needs to function on land in an air atmosphere without the support and comfort of water. Aquatic therapy can be used to decrease pain, and improve gait, strength, endurance, or coordination. In water, skills can be simulated in a less challenging setting than land with the ultimate goal being improved function and pain level while on land. The water milieu can serve as a bridge to improved land function.[5]

### Contraindications

There are general contraindications for use of any form of water immersion including home bathing. These include open wounds, fever, severe heart disease, bowel or bladder incontinence, open ports such as tracheostomy, feeding tube, or colostomy, and extreme cognitive or functional impairment rendering a water environment unsafe.[5]

### Evidence Base

High quality evidence supporting the efficacy of water therapy for pain relief and functional restoration in patients with spinal disorders has been limited, with the practice supported primarily by anecdotal reports and extrapolation from studies of peripheral joint arthritis. The purported special ability of aquatic therapy to reduce pain has been challenged in a recent meta-analysis. Hall et al.[8] conducted an exhaustive search of 18 databases for studies of water therapy in the treatment of pain for neurologic or musculoskeletal conditions. The authors distilled the 793 identified studies down to 19 that were of adequate quality with sufficient data to analyze. Three of the included studies were of chronic low back pain, while the remaining were of rheumatoid arthritis, osteoarthritis, fibromyalgia, and multiple sclerosis. The authors found that in aggregate there was no additional pain-relieving effect of aquatic therapy compared to land-based therapies. When compared with no treatment at all, aquatic therapies provide a small amount of pain relief.[8] These results do not eliminate the possibility of water-specific pain-relieving properties. The pain-relieving effect may be the same for land- and water-based therapies yet their mechanisms may differ. For the individual unable to tolerate land-based therapies aquatic therapies are a means to seek a pain-relieving effect.

A useful resource for clinicians interested in exploring the evidence base for water therapies is http://aquaticnet.com/index.htm, an online repository of references for scholarly and non-scholarly writings on water therapies.

## CONCLUSIONS AND DISCUSSION

Aquatic therapy is an alternative form of physical therapy that is indicated when land-based exercises are prohibitively challenging. Exercise in water can be performed with lower requirements of strength, balance, and coordination. Buoyancy reduces forces across joints, making movement less painful. Despite these theoretical advantages there has been limited literature evidence especially in the form of randomized controlled trials to show that exercising in water translates to decreased pain and improved function on land. For special populations, however, such as those with peripheral joint comorbidities, severe edema, and deconditioning, water-based therapy is useful when land-based exercise is intolerable.

## References

1. T. Bender, Z. Karagulle, G.P. Balint, C. Gutenbrunner, P.V. Balint, S. Sukenik, Hydrotherapy, balneotherapy, and spa treatment in pain management, Rheumatol. Int. 25 (3) (2005) 220–224.
2. P.A. Tipler, Physics for scientists and engineers, third ed, Worth Publishers, New York, 1991.
3. B.E. Becker, Cole, J. Andrew, Aquatic rehabilitation, in: J.A. DeLisa (Ed.), 4 ed., Physical medicine and rehabilitation, Vol. 1. Lippincott Williams & Wilkins, Philadelphia, 2005, pp. 479–492.
4. J.P. O'Hare, A. Heywood, C. Summerhayes, G. Lunn, J.M. Evans, G. Walters, et al., Observations on the effect of immersion in Bath spa water, BMJ (Clin. Res. Ed.) 291 (6511) (1985) 1747–1751.
5. R.L. McNeal, Aquatic therapy for patients with rheumatic disease, Rheum. Dis. Clin. North Am. 16 (4) (1990) 915–929.
6. C. Konlian, Aquatic therapy: making a wave in the treatment of low back injuries, Orthop. Nurs. 18 (1) (1999) 11–18; quiz 19–20.
7. J. Andrew, R.E.E. Cole, Marilou Moschetti, Edward Sinnett, Aquatic rehabilitation of the spine, Rehab. Management (April/May) (1996) 55–62.
8. J. Hall, A. Swinkels, J. Briddon, C.S. McCabe, Does aquatic exercise relieve pain in adults with neurologic or musculoskeletal disease? A systematic review and meta-analysis of randomized controlled trials, Arch. Phys. Med. Rehabil. 89 (5) (2008) 873–883.

# 19

# The Role of Spinal Injections in Treating the Aging Spine

*Jason Marchetti*

**K E Y   P O I N T S**

- Understand the indications, contraindications, and current evidence support for commonly performed spinal procedures.
- Understand the utility and limitations of spinal procedures in the overall management of patients with degenerative conditions.
- Improve patient selection for spinal procedures in the management of degenerative conditions of the spine.

The use of invasive procedures for spinal conditions has proliferated over the years, particularly with the advent of fluoroscopic guidance. The most common spinal targets for injection are the epidural space, nerve root sheath, facet joints, and the sacroiliac joints. There is much controversy regarding the utility of these injections, however, both as diagnostic and as therapeutic tools. For the surgeon, diagnostic considerations are important for determining a true "pain generator" before offering specific surgical recommendations. This is vitally important because history, physical exam, and imaging studies are often limited in specificity for individual pain conditions.[1,2] The therapeutic value of interventions is important as an adjunct to other nonsurgical treatments, particularly to help patients avoid surgery or to alleviate pain in patients who are otherwise poor surgical candidates.

Modern guidelines and recommendations from various societies suggest that the use of fluoroscopic (or CT) guidance is mandatory (when not contraindicated) to improve the accuracy and safety of these procedures.[1,2] Although ultrasound guidance has been explored, this modality is limited in its ability to detect intravascular uptake.[3] Despite "blind" techniques being described for all types of injections, the only ones that may be done without image guidance with any acceptable chance of safe, proper needle placement include lumbar interlaminar and caudal epidural steroid injections (ESIs).

Contraindications to steroid injections (and other invasive spinal procedures) include bleeding diathesis, anticoagulation, local or systemic infection, uncontrolled diabetes or glaucoma, hypovolemia, and medical instability; and high doses of local anesthetics should be avoided in patients with multiple sclerosis.[1] Acute fracture and malignancy should also be avoided. Contraindications to fluoroscopy include pregnancy.

The purpose of this chapter is to review the current pertinent literature regarding these interventions, particularly as they relate to degenerative spinal conditions.

## EPIDURAL STEROID INJECTIONS

Epidural steroid injections are one of the most commonly performed interventions for the management of painful spinal conditions. Approaches to the epidural space include interlaminar, transforaminal (or selective nerve root), catheter directed, and the caudal approach for the lower lumbar segments.

A recent systematic review of relevant ESI literature by Salahadin et al.[4] highlights the variability in quality and relevance of studies looking at ESI

efficacy. A common pitfall when studying invasive procedures is considering the efficacy of the comparator procedure. For instance, many studies evaluating ESI compare the procedure to epidural saline,[5] epidural anesthetic without steroid,[6] injections into nearby tissues,[7] alternative injected medications (e.g., hyaluronic acid and Sarapin) or a combination of these strategies.[8,9] Many of these comparator procedures have demonstrated therapeutic efficacy and are therefore not truly placebo. Matthews et al.[7] compared caudal ESIs to local anesthesia over the sacral hiatus (some were at "tender spots," however). This may be most consistent with a true placebo comparator.

Considering the proposed mechanism of action of steroid injections (reducing inflammatory chemicals at the site of injury/pathology and possibly contributing to neuronal stability), the expectation that any type of steroid injection, done one time, will result in more than 6 months of relief or benefit is unrealistic.[1] Therefore the number and frequency of injections are other variables that must be considered when assessing the long-term efficacy of injections.[1,10] Consistency of outcome measures must also be considered: improvement in both reported pain and functional ability should be considered when judging the efficacy of any procedure, including ESI.

In their review, Salahadin and colleagues[4] considered anything less than 6 weeks as "short term" and any time beyond 6 weeks as "long term." Their analysis, using commonly accepted "evidence-based medicine" definitions for literature review, yielded ratings for each approach as outlined in Table 19-1. Interlaminar and transforaminal ESIs in the low back and neck had "indeterminate" evidence for use in axial spine pain, postlaminectomy syndrome, lumbar disc extrusions, and lumbar stenosis. Interestingly, caudal ESIs have "moderate" evidence for short- and long-term improvement for chronic, axial low back pain, and their "strong" and "moderate" short- and long-term ratings for radicular pain also include patients with postlaminectomy syndrome.[4]

From the surgeon's standpoint, avoidance of surgery is an important outcome consideration. In this regard, at least transforaminal injections (lumbar and cervical) have shown efficacy.[11] This approach, in the lumbar spine, has also been shown to be more effective for radicular pain than interlaminar ESIs.

There is no significant evidence to suggest a specific, fixed timing regimen of injections. Current guideline recommendations (including Official Disability Guidelines and International Spine Intervention Society[ISIS]) suggest that repeated injections should be considered as symptoms recur, and the repeated injections should not be considered in patients who do not demonstrate significant (usually defined as >50% short-term relief) transient improvement following an initial injection. Similarly, the maximum number of injections that an individual may undergo during a specific amount of time (such as during 1 year) has not been adequately studied, but consensuses from various guidelines and societies suggest that no more than four injections should be considered over the course of a year and that repeated injections should be separated by at least one to two weeks. Riew et al.[6] found that up to four lumbar transforaminal ESIs were required to optimize therapeutic benefit (in this case, avoidance of surgery) beyond 15 months, and the interval between injections ranged from 6 days to 10.5 months. This is also the only lumbar injection study[12] to require

**TABLE 19–1    Summary of Literature Support for Various ESI Approaches for the Treatment of Lumbar and Cervical "Radicular Pain" as Outlined by Salahadin et al.[4]**

|  | Short-term Benefit | Long-term Benefit |
| --- | --- | --- |
| Lumbar interlaminar ESI | Strong | Indeterminate |
| Lumbar transforaminal/SNRB | Strong | Moderate |
| Caudal ESI | Strong | Moderate |
| Cervical interlaminar ESI | Moderate | Moderate |
| Cervical transforaminal/SNRB | Moderate | Moderate |

a failure of 6 weeks of other nonoperative interventions including physical therapy, nonsteroidal anti-inflammatory drugs (NSAIDs), bracing, or a combination of the three. The integration of these other treatments with injection therapies is therefore also poorly understood.

Complications of epidural injections include generic considerations for any invasive procedure (local tissue trauma, bruising, pain, infection) as well as those specific for trauma to the local spinal tissues, medication or steroid related side effects, and those associated with x-ray exposure during fluoroscopy. Minor complications including dural puncture with subsequent "spinal headache," increased pain, elevated blood sugar level or blood pressure, sympathetic mediated symptoms such as flushing or vasovagal response and acute insomnia have been described and occur infrequently. Botwin et al reported an overall complication rate during fluoroscopically guided ESIs as occurring in less than 10% for lumbar injections[13] and approaching 17% for cervical ESIs.[14] Caudal injections had a rate of minor complications of 15.6%,[15] and for the thoracic spine, a 20.5% rate was reported.[16] Intravascular needle placement has been noted in about 10% to 20% of lumbar injections.[17] Subarachnoid needle placement is also a concern, because it may cause spinal anesthesia or arachnoiditis.[1]

Major or severe complications are fortunately very rare when injections are performed with fluoroscopy and by experienced interventionalists.[1] Potentially catastrophic injury can occur, however, including infarction of central nervous system tissues (causing paraplegia, tetraplegia, or stroke syndromes), compression of neural elements or spinal cord by hematoma, CNS infections, pneumocephalus, and chemical meningitis, to list a few. Transforaminal approaches, particularly in the cervical spine, likely carry the greatest risk of these rare yet serious complications.[4]

Predictors for negative outcome following ESI include poor education, unemployed status, smoking, chronic or constant pain, high medication usage, high number of previously attempted treatments, pain that is not increased with activity or coughing, psychological disturbances, and nonradicular diagnoses.[18]

## FACET JOINT PROCEDURES

Approximately 20% of low back pain complaints can be attributed to the zygapophyseal joints in the lumbar spine[1,19-22] and likely account for even higher rates of pain in the cervical and thoracic spines.[19,20,22] Also known as facet or z-joints, these joints become arthritic and potentially painful as with any joint in the body, and consequently, older individuals may be expected to be more likely to respond to facet blocks than younger patients.[20,21,23] In fact, in a study of older Australians with non–injury-related chronic low back pain, 30% of individuals reported at least 90% relief following placebo-controlled facet blocks.[21]

Over the past 40 years, our understanding of the innervation of facet joints and their potential as pain generators has greatly expanded.[2] We now know that even referred leg pain and hamstring tightness can be associated with facet joint pain and thus mimic features of sciatica. Cervical facet joints may refer pain to the head, neck, and shoulder areas and have well-described referral pattern "maps," whereas thoracic facet joints may produce mid back pain with accompanying neuropathic symptoms as well.[22] Along

with the evolution of this knowledge, so too have interventional approaches in dealing with facet-mediated pain.

The specific diagnosis of facet-mediated pain is difficult and controversial, however, because there are no reliable factors of patients' history, physical exam, or imaging studies to otherwise effectively determine pain of facet origin. Several studies have evaluated the use of single photon emission CT (SPECT) to determine if abnormalities can predict facet joint disease and therefore predict favorable response to joint injections. One study example by Pneumaticos et al[24] determined that patients who had "hot" facet joints treated with steroid injection responded more favorably than patients who also had non–hot joints injected (joints were selected clinically by the attending physician as is done in typical practice). Despite this and other positive results, SPECT is not routinely used, perhaps because of limited availability and expense.

For diagnostic injections, there is a high false-positive rate for single sets of lumbar injections.[19] Therefore two positive diagnostic injections are felt to be required before considering pain to be truly of facet origin, at least for the purposes of clinical research. These injections should be low volume and demonstrate a specific response based upon the expected duration of the anesthetic used.[23,25] In clinical practice, this "double block" approach may not be required, or practical, given the relatively similar morbidity of rhizotomy (the procedure that should be considered if diagnostic blocks are positive) compared to injections. Others also argue that the improved specificity of double blocks reduces the sensitivity and therefore denies a potentially therapeutic procedure (rhizotomy) to some patients who would otherwise benefit. Again, this approach assumes that the risks and comorbidity of performing rhizotomy in patients with false-positive results is not significantly greater than performing the second diagnostic block.

Potential complications of facet joint procedures include those described in the section on ESI that may be related to needle placement; side effects of sedation, injected medication, or both; and radiation associated with image guidance.[22] Septic joints have been reported after intra-articular injections,[26] whereas radiofrequency (RF) neurotomy procedures have been associated with painful dysesthesia, anesthesia dolorosa, hyperesthesia, and nerve root injury[22]; however, the overall rate of even minor complications is very low.[27]

Over the years, conflicting results have emerged regarding efficacy of facet joint procedures.[22] One of the most recent systematic reviews by Bogduk et al[2] only considered prospective, double blind, randomized, placebo-controlled trials in their evaluation, and determined that controlled, diagnostic medial branch blocks are the only validated method of diagnosing facet mediated pain and that properly performed neurotomy is the only validated treatment for facet joint pain. A more encompassing review was done by Boswell et al.,[22] and their results are included in Table 19–2. Their process was similar to the Salahadin et al. review discussed in the section on ESI,[4] and short-term and long-term relief were defined as 6 weeks or less versus longer than 6 weeks duration for injections, respectively, and less than or more than 3 months duration, respectively, for neurotomy procedures. Of note, achievement of long-term relief with injection therapy often requires multiple injections. For instance, in their study of cervical facet pain, Manchikanti et al.[28] noted an average of 3.5 injections over the course of a year with an average duration of effect of approximately 3.5 months per injection. Interestingly, this benefit of medial branch blocks was noted with or without steroid. Findings, including number of injections and duration of effect, were similar in their studies of lumbar and thoracic medial branch blocks as well.[29]

Medial branch blocks (MBB) in the lumbar spine have been repeatedly validated for diagnostic utility.[2] ISIS guidelines[23] suggest that patients should be evaluated for at least 2 hours postinjection, or until relief ceases (whichever occurs first). To be truly diagnostic, relief should also be noted while the patient is attempting activities that are typically aggravating. There is debate regarding the amount of relief required to consider blocks successful,[2,20] but 80% pain relief has typically been accepted as the standard for a "positive" response. A recent retrospective study by Cohen et al.[20] however, indicates that the patients who reported 50% to 79% improvement following a single diagnostic block did as well with subsequent rhizotomy as those who reported 80% or more relief following diagnostic block. It is also unclear how much secondary factors, including the use of sedation, anesthesia, or both, during diagnostic blocks, affect the results.[20]

The use of steroids and Sarapin have also been studied for medial branch blockade both in the neck and low back. These substances have not

**TABLE 19-2    Summary of Literature Support for Various Facet Joint Procedures for the Treatment of Chronic Facetogenic Pain as Outlined by Boswell et al[22]**

| Procedure | Short-term Relief | Long-term Relief |
|---|---|---|
| Cervical intra-articular | Limited | Limited |
| Thoracic intra-articular | Indeterminate | Indeterminate |
| Lumbar intra-articular | Moderate | Moderate |
| Cervical MBB | Moderate | Moderate |
| Thoracic MBB | Moderate | Moderate |
| Lumbar MBB | Moderate | Moderate |
| Cervical MBN | Strong | Moderate (Strong*) |
| Thoracic MBN | Indeterminate | Indeterminate |
| Lumbar MBN | Strong | Moderate |

*Long-term relief for cervical facet pain has strong evidence when a multiple lesion per level strategy is used, as reported by Lord et al and advocated by others.[23,35] This procedure is not commonly done in the United States and significantly increases operative time.

demonstrated improved or longer lasting efficacy as compared to bupivacaine alone in subjects identified as having facet-mediated pain with double blocks.[28,29]

Intraarticular steroid injections have been shown to be no more effective than saline injections into the facet joints.[26,30] Unfortunately the only prospective, double-blind, randomized, placebo-controlled trial for intraarticular cervical facet injections was limited to MVC-related whiplash sufferers.[30] The authors screened patients for facet-mediated pain with double blocks and found no benefit from intraarticular steroid versus anesthetic. Results of this study, however, should not be applied to degenerative cervical facetogenic pain, which should be studied separately. A study by Kim et al.[31] evaluated intraarticular cervical facet injections in a variety of diagnoses and found that those with "disc herniation" responded better than those with myofascial or whiplash pain syndromes. Intraarticular hyaluronic acid injections were compared to lumbar facet joint steroid injections by Fuchs et al,[32] and no difference in efficacy was noted.

Radiofrequency neurotomy of the medial branch nerves (MBN) (and dorsal ramus of L5) has been used extensively to denervate suspected painful facet joints and remains the only available intervention that has demonstrated substantial, long-term relief.[2] Early techniques, where an RF probe is placed perpendicular to the path of the target nerve, have been criticized and often demonstrate limited efficacy.[2] The more modern approach of placing the probe along the length of the suspected nerve path is recommended by the International Spine Intervention Society[23] and has been shown to coagulate a greater length of the target nerves. Because repairing a greater length of nerve will take longer than a shorter lesion, it can be expected that the "parallel probe" technique can result in long-lasting improvement, as has been suggested in reviews of these techniques and studies.[2] With parallel probe placement, significant benefit (60%-80% improvement) may last 6 to 12 months or even longer.[33] Benefit has also been demonstrated with up to three repeated treatments, and no limit has yet been established as to how many treatments may result in diminished returns.[33] Usual RF ablation involves lesioning at 80° C for 90 seconds at each site, but benefit has also been demonstrated with "pulsed" RF current at 2 Hz for 4 minutes at 42° C.[34]

In the cervical spine, one prospective, double-blind, randomized, placebo-controlled trial has been conducted for assessing medial branch neurotomy.[35] The authors determined that this treatment is effective in patients who have MVC-related whiplash with demonstrated facet pain (at C3-C4 and C6-C7) using a triple block technique. This technique is similar to the aforementioned double block, with the addition of a single placebo block as well.

When done according to recommended ISIS guidelines,[23] no significant complications of lumbar medial branch neurotomy have been described.[2]

Debate exists as to whether it is acceptable to perform the procedure under general anesthesia. This may increase the risk of nerve root injury with improper probe placement, because the patient cannot sense and thus warn of impending injury.[2] Testing the probe with varied frequency stimulation is important to perform regardless of use of general anesthesia. This allows the interventionalist to assess for motor activation of the nerve root, an important warning sign of probe misplacement.

Other studies have evaluated alternative means for neurotomy, including cryoneurolysis[36] and percutaneous laser denervation.[37] All three studies have shown promising initial results for short- and long-term relief when performed in the lumbar spine and may become more widespread options in the future.

## SACROILIAC JOINT PROCEDURES

Similar to facet joints, up to 20% of low back pain complaints can be attributed to the sacroiliac (SI) joint.[1,38] The sensitivity and specificity of diagnostic blocks, however, remain controversial because of insufficient study and high false positive rates.[38] Similarly, the only prospective, double-blind, randomized, placebo-controlled trial involving SI joint injections involved 10 patients with low back pain and spondylarthropathy, and they did not use diagnostic blocks to screen patients. This study[39] compared intraarticular injections of steroid versus saline and revealed statistically significant benefit of steroid at 1 month.

Various radiofrequency denervation techniques have been described for the SI joint, but little high-quality evidence exists to support their use. A recent study by Cohen et al.[40] describes a novel "cooled-probe" RF denervation technique of the lateral branches as they exit the upper sacral foramen (instead of along the SI joint line, as is done in traditional techniques). The benefit of the cooled RF lesion is that a larger "sphere" of tissue may be lesioned, theoretically improving the chances that the desired nerve branch may be included in the lesioned area. The results of the study demonstrate greater than 50% pain relief, and significant functional improvement, in the majority of patients at 6 months compared to only 14% of patients receiving a sham treatment. Results were similar, however, at 1 month between the two groups. Further study is obviously needed before more widespread acceptance (and coverage) of this technology is seen.

## SPECIFIC DEGENERATIVE CONDITIONS

### Degenerative Disc Disease

Approximately 40% of low back pain can be attributed to internal disc disruption[1]; however, there is controversy in this diagnosis because there is no universally accepted gold standard diagnostic test for discogenic pain. When strict interpretive criteria[41] are used (Table 19–3), however, discography has proven itself useful in identifying patients who benefit from treatment.[42] Not all degenerative discs are painful, however, and it is typical for sufferers of degenerative discogenic pain to have worse complaints during the early or middle stages of degeneration (typically 4th-6th decades) followed by relative pain relief in later years when degenerative pathology is most severe. Painful degenerative lumbar discs are noted to have higher concentrations (relative to nonpainful discs) of sensory fibers at the endplates and nucleus and have higher concentrations of proinflammatory chemicals.[1] For this reason, it makes sense to consider local injection of steroid for therapeutic effect, either within or just posterior to the annulus. Transforaminal lumbar ESIs have demonstrated excellent delivery to the anterior epidural space, whereas lumbar interlaminar ESIs achieve ventral flow in just over one third of attempts, and caudal ESIs have significantly variable delivery locations.[43]

Intradiscal procedures such as intradiscal electrothermal therapy (IDET) and percutaneous radiofrequency neurotomy of the ramus communicans have shown modest benefit at 6 and 4 months (respectively) in carefully selected patients. Intradiscal steroid injections have very limited data and have not been shown to be more effective than intradiscal saline or bupivacaine injections.[44]

As discussed in the ESI section, only caudal ESIs have been studied sufficiently and demonstrated some benefit for axial LBP; however, a study by

**TABLE 19-3** International Spine Intervention Society Guidelines for Discography Interpretation, 2004[23]

| Discogenic Pain | Concordant Pain | Psi Pain Induction | Control Discs |
|---|---|---|---|
| Unequivocal | ≥7/10 | <15 above opening pressure | 2 pain-free discs |
| Definite | ≥7/10 | <15 above opening pressure | 1 pain-free disc |
| Definite | ≥7/10 | <50 above opening pressure | 2 pain-free discs |
| Probable | ≥7/10 | <50 above opening pressure | 1 pain-free disc & 1 with noncon- cordant pain at >50 psi |

Manchikanti et al.[45] revealed no difference in the improvement between discogram positive or negative patients. Although not well studied for axial low back pain, because of their superior placement of medication in the ventral epidural space, a trial of one to three transforaminal ESIs may be considered for discogenic spine pain before consideration of surgery.[1]

## Degenerative Lumbar Spondylolisthesis

As lumbar degenerative spondylolisthesis is an anatomic condition with variable symptomatology, it could be argued that diagnostic spinal injections, and possibly discography, could be helpful in determining specific, structural pain generators (i.e., facetogenic vs. discogenic pain) in patients with this entity. Similarly, ESIs or SNRBs could be helpful for those patients who suffer with radicular or neurogenic claudication symptoms. The efficacy of these injections, however, particularly within the specific context of spondylolisthesis, is uncertain.

A recent (2008) literature review that yielded clinical guidelines regarding lumbar degenerative spondylolisthesis from the North American Spine Society (NASS),[46] found a paucity of evidence to make any recommendations regarding such procedures in this setting. Unfortunately, the same was true for all usual nonsurgical treatments including physical therapy, manipulation, bracing, TENS, or medications. Many of the studies to date have compared "conservative" care to surgical interventions, but there have not been any studies comparing injections to placebo. This includes the recent SPORT study, which has provided significant evidence regarding surgery for the condition.[47] Furthermore, data are lacking to accurately describe the natural course of spondylolisthesis.

The NASS guideline developers suggest that spondylolisthesis should be further studied according to symptom subsets (e.g., axial vs. radicular pain, neurogenic claudication/stenosis).

## Degenerative Lumbar Spinal Stenosis

With spinal stenosis, we again have an anatomic description of a problem with variable symptomatology and an unclear natural history. It is well accepted that those who present with significant neural compromise should be considered quickly for surgery. For ethical reasons, this category of patients, therefore, will not likely be studied in placebo-controlled trials and may not even be studied outside of surgical interventions (such as with bona fide cauda equina). Spinal injections, however, may be considered for diagnostic and therapeutic purposes for those who present without significant neurological compromise. Symptom subsets may again be considered for further research to determine treatment response for axial pain, radicular pain, or neurogenic claudication.

As with spondylolisthesis, many studies have concentrated on comparing conservative care with surgical intervention, including the recent SPORT study.[48] In 2007, clinical guidelines regarding degenerative spinal stenosis were also developed by NASS.[49] This group's review of the available

literature led to a Grade B recommendation in favor of a single transforaminal ESI for short-term relief of radicular symptoms associated with stenosis. A Grade C recommendation was made for multiple transforaminal or caudal ESIs to prolong pain relief from radiculopathy or neurogenic claudication associated with spinal stenosis. It should be noted that "multiple" in this setting refers to repeated injections at times when the patient's symptoms return or worsen following initial injection(s). This is in contrast to previously described "series of 3" injections in which the intervention is repeated at specified time intervals regardless of initial response. This approach had been used extensively in the past when most injections were done without image guidance in order to improve the rate of success. As discussed earlier in the chapter, a fixed schedule for a series of 3 is no longer considered standard of care and is not supported by the literature.

## CONCLUSION

Regardless of the underlying degenerative pathology, in patients who lack emergent or urgent surgical indications, diagnostic or therapeutic spinal injection therapy should be considered before surgical interventions. These may help in identifying specific pain generators, may provide substantial long-term pain relief in some patients (and therefore help avoid surgery), and may identify patients who might respond to alternative interventions, such as RF neurotomy.

## References

1. DePalma, et al., Evidence-informed management of chronic low back pain with epidural steroid injections, Spine J. 8 (2008) 45–55.
2. N. Bogduk, Evidence-informed management of chronic low back pain with facet injections and radiofrequency neurotomy, Spine J. 8 (2008) 56–64.
3. Galiano, et al., Real-time sonographic imaging for periradicular injections in the lumbar spine: a sonographic anatomic study of a new technique, J. Ultrasound Med. 24 (2005) 33–38.
4. Salahadin, et al., Epidural steroids in the management of chronic spinal pain: a systematic review, Pain Physician 10 (2007) 185–212.
5. Karppinen, et al., Periradicular infiltration for sciatica, Spine 26 (2001) 1059–1067.
6. Riew, et al., The effect of nerve-root injections on the need for operative treatment of lumbar radicular pain, J Bone Joint Surg. Am. 82 (2000) 1589–1593.
7. Matthews, et al., Back pain and sciatica: controlled trials of manipulation, traction, sclerosant and epidural injections, Br. J. Rheumatol. 26 (1987) 416–423.
8. Devulder, et al., Nerve root injections in patients with failed back surgery syndrome: a comparison of three solutions, Clin. J. Pain. 15 (1999) 132–135.
9. Manchikanti, et al., Caudal epidural injections with sarapin steroids in chonic low back pain, Pain Physician 4 (2001) 322–335.
10. Kolstad, et al., Transforaminal steroid injections in the treatment of cervical radiculopathy: a prospective outcome study, Acta Neurochir. (Wien) 147 (2005) 1065–1070.
11. G.R. Butterman, Treatment of lumbar disc herniation: epidural steroid injection compared with discectomy: a prospective, randomized study, J. Bone Joint Surg. Am. 86-A (2004) 670–679.
12. DePalma, et al., A critical appraisal for the evidence for selective nerve root injection in the treatment of lumbosacral radiculopathy, Arch. Phys. Med. Rehabil. 86 (2005) 1477–1482.
13. Botwin, et al., Complications of fluoroscopically guided transforaminal lumbar epidural injections, Arch. Phys. Med. Rehabil. 81 (2000) 1045–1050.
14. Botwin, et al., Complications of fluoroscopically guided interlaminar cervical epidural injections, Arch. Phys. Med. Rehabil. 84 (2003) 627–633.
15. Botwin, et al., Complications of fluoroscopically guided caudal epidural injections, Arch. Phys. Med. Rehabil. 80 (2001) 416–424.
16. Botwin, et al., Adverse effects of fluoroscopically guided interlaminar thoracic epidural injections, Arch. Phys. Med. Rehabil. 85 (2006) 14–23.
17. Furman, et al., Incidence of intravascular penetration in transforaminal lumbosacral epidural steroid injections, Spine 25 (2000) 2628–2632.
18. Hopwood, et al., Factors associated with failure of lumbar epidural steroids, Reg. Anesth. 18 (1993) 238–243.
19. Manchukonda, et al., Facet joint pain in chronic spinal pain: an evaluation of prevalence and false-positive rate of diagnostic blocks, J. Spinal Disord. Tech. 20 (2007) 539–545.
20. Cohen, et al., Lumbar zygapophyseal (facet) joint radiofrequency denervation success as a function of pain relief during diagnostic medial branch blocks: a multicenter analysis, Spine 8 (2008) 498–504.
21. Schwarzer, et al., Prevalence and clinical features of lumbar zygapophyseal joint pain: a study in an Australian population with chronic low back pain, Ann. Rheum. Dis. 54 (1995) 100–106.
22. Boswell, et al., A systematic review of therapeutic facet joint interventions in chronic spinal pain, Pain Physician 10 (2007) 229–253.
23. Bogduk, et al., International Spine Intervention Society Practice Guidelines for spinal diagnostic and treatment procedures, 1st ed., San Francisco, 2004.
24. Pneumaticos, et al., Low back pain: prediction of short-term outcome of facet joint injection with bone scintigraphy, Radiology 238 (2) (2006) 693–698.
25. N. Bogduk, Diagnostic nerve blocks in chronic pain, Best Pract. Res. Clin. Anaesthesiol 16 (2002) 565–578.

26. Lilius, et al., Lumbar facet joint syndrome: a randomized clinical trial, J. Bone Joint Surg. 71B (1989) 681–684.

27. Kornick, et al., Complications of lumbar facet radiofrequency denervation, Spine 29 (2004) 1352–1354.

28. Manchikanti, et al., Therapeutic cervical medial branch blocks in managing chronic neck pain: a preliminary report of a randomized, double-blind, controlled trial: clinical trial NCT0033272, Pain Physician 9 (2006) 333–346.

29. Manchikanti, et al., Evaluation of lumbar facet joint nerve blocks in the management of chronic low back pain: preliminary report of a randomized, double-blind controlled trial: clinical trial NCT00355914, Pain Physician 10 (2007) 425–440.

30. Barnsley, et al., Lack of effect of intraarticular corticosteroids for chronic pain in the cervical zygapophyseal joints, N. Engl. J. Med. 330 (1994) 1047–1050.

31. Kim, et al., Cervical facet joint injections in the neck and shoulder pain, J. Korean Med. Sci 20 (2005) 659–662.

32. Fuchs, et al., Intraarticular hyaluronic acid versus glucocorticoid injections for nonradicular pain in the lumbar spine, J. Vasc. Interv. Radiol. 16 (2005) 1493–1498.

33. J. Schofferman, G. Kine, Effectiveness of repeated radiofrequency neurotomy for lumbar facet pain, Spine 29 (2004) 2471–2473.

34. Tekin, et al., A comparison of conventional and pulsed radiofrequency denervation in the treatment of chronic facet joint pain Clin. J. Pain 23 (2007) 524–529.

35. Lord, et al., Percutaneous radiofrequency neurotomy for chronic cervical zygapophyseal-joint pain, N. Engl. J. Med. 335 (1996) 1721–1726.

36. Birkenmaier, et al., Percutaneous cryodenervation of lumbar facet joints: a prospective clinical trial, Int. Orthop. 2006.

37. Mogalles, et al., Percutaneous laser denervation of the zygapophyseal joints in the pain facet syndrome, Zh. Vopr. Neirokhir. Im. N N. Burdenko 1 (2004) 20–25.

38. S.P. Cohen, Sacroiliac joint pain: A comprehensive review of anatomy, diagnosis, and treatment, Anesth. Analg. 101 (2005) 1440–1453.

39. Maguars, et al., Assessment of the efficacy of sacroiliac corticosteroid injections in spondylarthropathies: a double-blind study, Br. J. Rheumatol. 35 (1996) 767–770.

40. Cohen, et al., Randomized placebo-controlled study evaluating lateral branch radiofrequency denervation for sacroiliac joint pain, Anesthesiology 109 (2008) 279–288.

41. Derby, et al., The ability of pressure-controlled discography to predict surgical and non-surgical outcomes, Spine 24 (1999) 364–371.

42. W.S. Oh, J.C. Shim, A randomized controlled trial of radiofrequency denervation of the ramus communicans nerve for chronic discogenic low back pain, Clin. J. Pain 20 (2004) 55–60.

43. Bryan, et al., Fluoroscopic assessment of epidural contrast spread after caudal injection, ISIS, 7th Annual Scientific Meeting, Las Vegas, NV, August 1999.

44. Khot, et al., The use of intradiscal steroid therapy for lumbar spinal discogenic pain: a randomized controlled trial, Spine 29 (2004) 833–836.

45. Manchikanti, et al., Effectiveness of caudal epidural injections in discogram positive and negative chronic low back pain, Pain Physician 5 (2002) 18–29.

46. North American Spine Society Evidence-Based Clinical Guidelines for Multidisciplinary Spine Care: Diagnosis and Treatment of Degenerative Lumbar Spondylolisthesis. 2008.

47. J.N. Weinstein, J.D. Lurie, T.D. Tosteson, et al., Surgical versus nonsurgical treatment for lumbar degenerative spondylolisthesis, N. Engl. J. Med. 356 (22) (2007) 2257–2270.

48. Weinstein, et al., Surgical vs nonsurgical therapy for lumbar spinal stenosis, N. Engl. J. Med. 358 (8) (2008) 794–810.

49. North American Spine Society, Evidence-Based Clinical Guidelines for Multidisciplinary Spine Care: Diagnosis and Treatment of Degenerative Lumbar Spinal Stenosis. 2007.

# 20

# Acupuncture in Treatment of Aging Spine–Related Pain Conditions

*Chunbo Cai, Weibin Yang, Linqiu Zhou, Wei Huang, and James J. Yue*

**K E Y   P O I N T S**

- History of acupuncture and its development in Europe and North America.
- Basic knowledge of operation and techniques of acupuncture treatment.
- Application of acupuncture in treatment of spine-related pain conditions.
- The concept of meridians and their application in acupuncture treatment of spine-related pain conditions.
- The limitation of this chapter in its scale to include the available information on evidence-based medicine to demonstrating the efficacy of acupuncture in management of spine-related pain conditions.

Acupuncture is an important component of Traditional Chinese Medicine (TCM), which has been used in China and other regions for over 5000 years. A Chinese classic, Huang Di Nei Jing (黄帝内经), *Yellow Emperor's Inner Canon* in English translation, has been regarded as the earliest source on acupuncture in writing. Compiled in circa 100 bc, this treasured classic contains eighty-one treatises organized into two parts: Su Wen (素问) and Lin Shu (灵枢). The latter is considered the bible for the application of acupuncture. The principles stated in the treatises still guide the practitioners in modern times.

Acupuncture was introduced to Europe in the eighteenth century by returning missionaries and was mentioned in a history of surgery published in 1774 in France. In North America, widespread public and professional awareness of acupuncture commenced in 1971 when James Reston reported his observations in Beijing, as a sports journalist on a ping-pong tournament trip, in *The New York Times*.[1] There has been a substantial increase in the use of complementary and alternative medicine in the United States since then.[2] Acupuncture is the most frequently used modality in complementary and alternative medicine for the treatment of symptoms of osteoarthritis,[3] and especially in the treatment of back and neck pain, or other related pain conditions, including radiculopathy resulting from disc herniations or spinal stenosis. Despite the vast application of acupuncture, evidence-based clinical research in English publications, in which most authors used the approaches of "Western style of acupuncture," has show an inconsistent conclusion on the effectiveness of acupuncture. The Western approach of acupuncture was defined as conventional diagnosis followed by individualized acupuncture treatment using a combination of prescriptive tender, local, and distal points. This is in contrast to the approach in TCM, which would formulate an individualized diagnosis based on TCM theories of meridians and energy (or qi).[4]

Acupuncture is the procedure of inserting and manipulating filiform needles into various points (called acupuncture points) to relieve pain or for other therapeutic purposes. According to TCM, acupuncture points are the sites through which the vital energy, or "qi" and "blood," are transported throughout the body surface. In the basic framework of TCM, there is a channel system with meridians connecting most of the acupuncture points regulating the functions of the internal organs and musculoskeletal system in a human body. The meridian system is believed to transport energy to every part of the body to keep the physiological function in balance. Health is regarded as a state of balanced homeostasis of the yin and the yang. Any creature, including human beings, is presumed to suffer from diseases when the energy is not flowing smoothly because it is blocked or stagnant along the meridians, which in turn would result in disharmony in the body as a whole. The etiology of disharmony is usually categorized as internal pathological excess, such as sadness, anger, or fear; and external assaults, such as cold, heat, or dampness. Acupuncture is reports to restore the flow of vital energy and to bring the human body to a new balanced state (homeostasis). Despite the long history in the application of acupuncture in many clinical conditions, the mechanism behind it has not been fully understood and explained within the framework of the Western medical system.

## DESCRIPTION OF THE NEEDLE

An acupuncture needle is divided into five parts (Figure 20-1): tip, body, root, handle, and tail. The tip and body of a needle are the parts being inserted into the body of a subject on the acupuncture points. The handle and tail of a needle are the parts used by a practitioner to manipulate the needle. The root connects the body and handle of a needle. Commonly used acupuncture needles are made of stainless steel, with sizes from 26 to 40 gauge and lengths from 0.5 inch to 2.5 inches. Because of the small size, quite often people describe an acupuncture needle as a "painless needle." The tip of an acupuncture needle is blunt, even though it is very tiny. Compared with the tip of a regular needle in the same gauge number, the tip of an acupuncture needle has less chance of cutting the tissue.

## OPERATIVE TECHNIQUES

Depending on the location of acupuncture points, a patient can be placed in supine, prone, recumbent, or sitting positions. Lying position is usually preferred due to the possibility of fainting in some patients from needling (Figure 20-2 ).

### Needle Insertion Techniques

There are four common ways to insert a needle: finger pressing insertion, pinching needle insertion, pinching skin insertion, and tight skin insertion. The skin at the insertion site is cleaned with an alcohol pad. The needle insertion angle can be perpendicular, oblique, or horizontal to the skin surface with various depths, depending on the location of the acupuncture points, the medical conditions being treated, and the patient's general health.

**Finger pressing insertion.** This technique is used when a short needle is used. Before inserting, the practitioner uses one fingertip (guiding finger) of the assisting hand to gently press the acupuncture point. The needle is then inserted into the skin of the acupuncture point along the edge of the guiding finger.

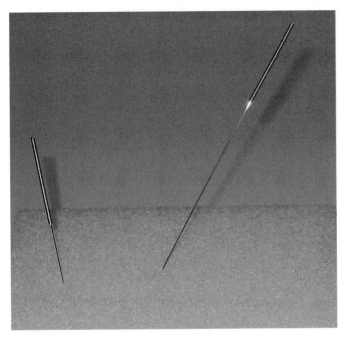

■ **FIGURE 20-1** Acupuncture needle.

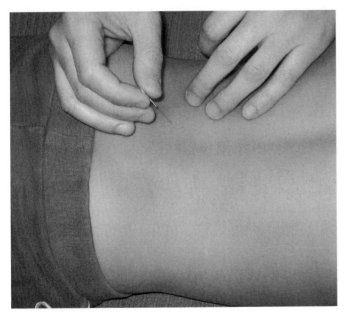

■ **FIGURE 20-2** A needle is inserted in a patient in the lying position.

**Pinching needle insertion.** This technique is used when an acupuncture point is deep and a long needle is used. Once the acupuncture point is identified, the thumb and index finger of the assisting hand hold the distal part of the needle with sterile gauze or sterile cotton ball, and the dominant hand holds the handle of the needle. The needle is then inserted with both hands.

**Pinching skin insertion.** This technique is used when the skin and muscles of the insertion site are thin or if the insertion point is close to important organs, such as lungs or eyeballs. Once the acupuncture point is identified, the skin and muscles are pinched or picked up with the thumb and index fingers of the assisting hand. The needle is then inserted through pinched skin with the dominant hand.

**Tight skin insertion.** This technique is used when the skin over the acupuncture point is loose. Once the acupuncture point is identified, the skin over the acupuncture point is stretched and tightened with the thumb and index fingers. The needle is inserted with the dominant hand.[5]

## Needle Manipulation

In TCM, the outcomes of acupuncture treatment are believed to rely heavily on the means of stimulations to the needles after insertion. There are two basic methods of stimulating the needles: manual manipulation and electrical stimulation.

There are various techniques in manipulating the needles manually to achieve the desired effects, which have been developed by generations of acupuncturists over thousands of years. The techniques are grouped by the needle effects, which are categorized as tonification (to treat deficiency), sedation (to treat excess), or neutral. For example, in *tonification*, the needle is inserted so that the angle of the needle is in the direction of energy flow on a specific meridian, and then advance the needle slowly, turning it with slow yet firm clockwise rotations as the needle is being advanced, and not penetrating too deeply. The needle can be continuously manipulated or left alone. When withdrawn, the needle should be removed quickly and the skin at the insertion point should be covered by a finger and massaged in a clockwise fashion. *Sedation* is the opposite of tonification. The needle is angled against the direction of energy flow on the meridian and is inserted quickly and deeply with rapid counterclockwise rotations. The needle should be withdrawn slowly and the surface should not be touched after removal of the needle. The duration of the treatment is usually 20 to 40 minutes.[1]

Electric stimulation became available in modern times. The electrodes are connected to the needles. The negative lead is attached to the needle(s) where the electron flow is started, whereas the positive lead is attached to the needle(s) where the flow is directed to. The low-frequency impulse, between 2 and 8 Hz, is considered to have the tonification effect. Higher frequency impulse, between 70 and 150 Hz, is used on the points surrounding the painful area, especially in musculoskeletal pain conditions.[1]

## Other Modalities and Techniques Related to Acupuncture and the Meridian System

In addition to the commonly used body acupuncture needles and needling techniques, there are other subsystems, such as ear acupuncture (auricular acupuncture), scalp acupuncture, hand acupuncture, three-sided needle bleeding method, and seven star needle (brush of needles) tapping. Moxibustion, guasha, and cupping are also the techniques used in the comprehensive acupuncture regimen. One of the most commonly used techniques is called Tui Na. According to one of the most popular teaching textbooks used by many TCM medical schools in China, Tui Na is regarded as an equally important method as acupuncture in the treatment of musculoskeletal disorders, especially in spine-related pain conditions.[8] Tui Na involves deep tissue manipulation on the acupuncture points along meridians, also manipulation of the joints, muscles, and tendons. The goal of Tui Na is to restore the flow and balance of energy along the meridians and the biomechanical alignment. The application of Tui Na is essential in the treatment of spine-related pain and other organ diseases, especially in the pediatric population.[8] Presently, because of various reasons, Tui Na has been introduced to Western societies only as "acupressure" and categorized as a massage therapy with limited medical content.

## Application of Meridian Theory in Spine-Related Pain Conditions

In TCM, the framework of diagnosis and point selection for treatment is based on the theoretical network of the meridian system and the internal organ subsystem related to the meridian system, where the names of the internal organs are regarded as the names for the subsystem with particular functionalities rather than the actual anatomic entities. For instance, Spleen in TCM represents a functional subunit in the body to facilitate digestion and transportation of the nutrients to the rest of the body via the meridians in general, not the actual organ called the spleen in Western medicine. The names of the internal organ subsystems that are used to name the meridians include Lung, Pericardium, Heart, Large Intestine, San Jiao (Triple Heater), Small Intestine, Bladder, Gallbladder, Stomach, Spleen, Kidney, and Liver. These twelve principal meridians are the primary subcircuits of the structure and functions throughout the body, which consists of three pairs of yin and yang meridians in a limb:

Hand Tai Yin—Lung, Hand Yue Yin—Pericardium, Hand Shao Yin—Heart;

Hand Yang Ming—Large Intestine, Hand Shao Yang—San Jiao, Hand Yai Yang—Small Intestine;

Foot Tai Yin—Spleen; Foot Yue Yin—Liver, Foot Shao Yin—Kidney;

Foot Yang Ming—Stomach, Foot Shao Yang—Gallbladder, Foot Tai Yang—Bladder.

The three yin meridians of the hand begin on the chest and travel along the medial and volar aspect of the arm to the hand. The three yang meridians of the hand begin on the hand and travel along the lateral and dorsal aspect of the arm to the head. The three yin meridians of the foot begin on the foot and travel along the frontal and medial aspect of the leg to the torso. The three yang meridians of the foot begin on the face, and travel down the body and along the lateral and posterior aspect of the leg to the foot. There are two meridians along the midline of the body corresponding to the anterior and posterior sagittal plane of the torso: the one on the posterior surface of the body is called Du meridian (Governing Vessel) and the one on the anterior surface is called Ren meridian (Conception Vessel), both of which are very important meridians in the treatment of almost all medical conditions, especially spine-related medical conditions.

Based on the framework described previously, clinical information is analyzed by clinicians to make TCM diagnoses of specific medical conditions and to identify appropriate points to treat. For example, the symptoms and signs of lumbar intervertebral disc herniation at a given spinal segment can be considered as pathological changes on Du meridian (on the midline in the back), Gallbladder meridian of Foot Shao Yang (on the lateral aspect of the leg), Bladder meridian of Foot Tai Yang (on the posterior aspect of the back down the leg), or Kidney meridian of Foot Shao Yin (on the medial aspect of the leg). The TCM diagnosis can be classified into blood stagnation syndrome of Du meridian, damp-heat excess syndrome of Gallbladder meridian, wind-cold-damp syndrome of Bladder meridian, and Kidney-Yang deficiency syndrome.[6] Then the acupuncture treatment is delivered to the points on the related meridian(s).

Moreover, the core principle of TCM is to view a specific medical condition as a particular manifestation of imbalance in the whole body at a certain level rather than only the disorder of a particular anatomic site or organ. Take an example of the radiculitis resulting from a lumbar disc herniation consistent with the Kidney-Yang deficiency, the points used are usually not limited to the ones on the Kidney meridian of Foot Shao Yin. The points on other synergistic meridians having the function of enhancing the Kidney-Yang energy would also be considered. For instance, the points on the Spleen meridian of Foot Tai Yin are used to enhance the digestion system to supply sufficient nutrients to correct the Kidney-Yang deficiency. Furthermore, acupuncture treatment, as in other components in TCM, is highly individualized. The treatment approaches are dynamically modified throughout the course of follow-up visits according to the prognosis of the patient.

The therapeutic effect could also be enhanced by methods of Tui Na, moxibustion, and Chinese medicinal herbs, under the guidance of the meridian and internal organ subsystem.

## Hua Tuo Jia Ji Points

Another set of points that is also commonly used for treatment of spine-related medical conditions are the points at each vertebra along the spine, slightly lateral to the midline bilaterally, called Hua Tuo Jia Ji (华佗夹脊; HTJJ) points. Hua Tuo Jai Ji points are believed to be named after Hua Tuo, one of the most famous ancient Chinese physicians (110 ad to 207 ad) and is regarded as the father of surgery in ancient Chinese medicine. Those points are not only important in the treatment of spine-related pain condition, but also commonly used in treating other internal organ disorders. However, HTJJs were only documented in a few books historically, despite their vast clinical application. Hua Tuo Jai Ji points are described as the points located from the first thoracic vertebra to the fifth lumbar vertebra. It was recently proposed that the landmarks of HTJJ points are the facet joints along the spine, including the cervical region (Figure 20-3 ).[7] The application of the HTJJ system is relatively straightforward, because of its segmental distribution along the spine. The targeting points usually correspond to the level of the vertebrae and nerve

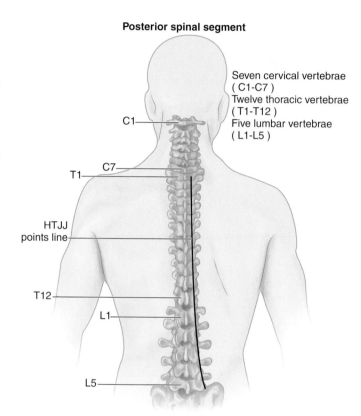

■ **FIGURE 20-3** The landmarks of HTJJ points are the facet joints along the spine, including the cervical region.

roots involved in the pathological processes. The hypothesized mechanism is that stimulation of the HTJJ points affects not only the nerve roots but also the paraspinal muscles and the chain of sympathetic ganglia along the spine.[7]

## RESEARCH BACKGROUND OF BASIC SCIENCES AND CLINICAL OUTCOMES

From the late 1950s, there has been a considerable amount of government-funded research in basic sciences and clinical outcomes of TCM in China, especially of acupuncture. Since the early 1970s, more and more studies on acupuncture have been published in the English literature from many disciplines of basic and clinical sciences. Acupuncture is probably the most thoroughly researched physical modality in medicine for its analgesic effects. The analgesic events observed from electrical acupuncture stimulation were found to be related to the activities of the endogenous opioid peptide system. Animal studies also suggest that acupuncture-induced analgesia may be mediated by substances released in the cerebrospinal fluid. Both low-frequency and high-frequency electric stimulation in rats could induce analgesia, but different frequencies produce different effects in terms of the types of endorphins released. The animal studies indicate that the analgesic effect of acupuncture can be considered a general phenomenon in the mammalian world.[1]

The development of neuroimaging tools, such as positron emission tomography (PET) and functional magnetic resonance imaging (fMRI), has taken the study of acupuncture's effects on the activity of human brain to another level. Studies using PET have shown that thalamic asymmetry present among patients with chronic pain was reduced after acupuncture treatments. There are studies that reported the relationships between particular acupuncture points and visual cortex activation on the fMRI. These powerful new tools open the possibility to new scientific studies on this ancient therapy.[9]

There has been a large volume of reports and cohort studies reporting the effectiveness of acupuncture treating spine-related pain conditions, especially neck and back pain.[1] It is difficult to design a double-blind study because of the lack of a true sham acupuncture technique. Only a few randomized, controlled studies have reported that acupuncture is more effective in the treatment of back pain than controls or placebo, in which medications or usual care including physical therapy are used as the control[10]; whereas some other studies reported no better effectiveness of acupuncture compared to controls or placebo.[4] The large-scale studies are mostly conducted using the Western style of acupuncture. Some case reports and cohort studies included the diagnoses of disc herniation, spinal stenosis, and spondylolisthesis. However, most of the randomized and controlled studies in large cohorts focused on nonspecific neck and back pain, and yet the objectives of the studies were the treatment of pain rather than the possible pain generators or pathologies of the spine.[4,10] A recent study demonstrated long-term pain relief by needle acupuncture compared with placebo in patients with chronic low back pain. The authors concluded that acupuncture did not seem to be a suitable treatment modality for neuropathic pain and it was sometimes indicated for the treatment of chronic nociceptive pain.[11]

## COMPLICATIONS

Like other procedures using needles, such as trigger injections, there are possible adverse events during acupuncture treatment: fainting, hematoma, pneumothorax, and injuries to the nerve tissue, including spinal cord. Other reported events include needlestick, bent needle, or broken needle left in the body.

## CLINICAL PRESENTATION AND DISCUSSION

### Case One

A 45-year-old otherwise healthy white man who was an electrician presented with a 6-week history of low back pain radiating to the lateral aspect of the left leg and down to the dorsum of the left foot and the great toe. His visual analog pain score (VAS) was 6-8/10. He had temporary relief from taking methylprednisolone (Medrol) for 7 days. On examination, he was neurologically intact. The active range of motion in the lumbar spine was limited in flexion, extension, and side flexion. His gait was antalgic. A lumbar spine MRI was ordered, which showed a large central and paracentral disc herniation at L4-L5, encroaching on the left L5 root. He declined to consider an epidural steroid injection or surgery because he preferred holistic health care. He also declined to consider pain medications and preferred to seek acupuncture treatment. He then underwent acupuncture twice a week for 2 weeks, with 50% reduction of pain, and then continued the treatments once a week for 4 weeks. At the follow-up visit in 6 weeks, he had only residual pain with a VAS of 1-2/10 and planned to return to work. He was advised to continue regular home exercises for spine conditioning.

### Case Two

A 53-year-old white woman who was an anesthesiologist presented with a 4-month history of neck pain radiating into the medial aspect of the right arm, with numbness, tingling, and hot sensation in the right hand. Her VAS was 5-7/10. She had one cervical epidural steroid injection and a course of physical therapy, which provided about 40% reduction of the pain temporarily. She had tried taking cyclobenzaprine (Flexeril) without much relief. On physical examination, she was neurologically intact. The active range of motion in her cervical spine was limited in flexion and side flexions, with pain and a feeling of tightness on the right side of her neck. There was significant tightness in the paraspinal muscles and trapeziums on the right side of her neck. A cervical spine MRI showed mild to moderate degenerative changes, with moderate foraminal stenosis at multiple levels from C4-C5 to C7-T1. She decided to try acupuncture treatment. Her symptoms subsided after acupuncture treatments once a week for six sessions.

### Case Three

A 75-year-old Asian man who was a retired accountant presented with an 8-month history of persistent recurrent low back pain radiating in the frontal aspect of his right thigh. He felt somewhat weak in the right knee.

He had tried pain medications and a prolonged course of physical therapy without much relief. He had three lumbar epidural steroid injections, the first two of which provided 70% pain reduction for 1 month each time. The third injection did not provide any relief.

A lumbar spine MRI showed moderate to severe central stenosis with grade I anterolisthesis at L3-L4 resulting in moderate foraminal stenosis. Lumbar spine x-rays showed 5-mm slippage at L3-L4 without evidence of instability on the flexion and extension views.

On physical examination, the active range of motion of the lumbar spine was limited in extension because of the pain. The right knee reflex was diminished. The muscle strength was tested at 4/5 in the right knee flexors compared to the left ones. He was referred to see a spine surgeon, who recommended a spinal decompression and intervertebral fusion surgery. The patient decided not to have the surgery and wanted to try any other regimen that could possibly be helpful. He started acupuncture treatment once a week for 6 sessions, which provided 60% pain reduction. He was advised to increase the intensity of the strengthening exercises learned from physical therapy. He then decided to have Tui Na treatments with acupuncture once a week. His pain improved almost 90% at the follow-up visit 4 weeks later. The strength was 5/5 in the right knee flexors. He was happy with his progress.

### Case Discussions

The three cases presented are to illustrate the typical scenarios in clinical practice, in which acupuncture and other related techniques, such as Tui Na, could play a role in the treatment of spine-related pain conditions. The process in TCM diagnosis and the details in the treatment of acupuncture and Tui Na are not within the scope of this chapter.

In Case One, it is apparent that the symptoms were related to a herniated disc. Besides the analgesic effect, the acupuncture treatment might have played a role in the antiinflammatory and healing process through its effect on blood circulation as reported in other articles that are not discussed in this chapter. However, one can argue that the improvement could well be the part of the natural course of the symptomatology of lumbar disc herniation. In Case Two, it is possible that the pain was not directly related to the assaults on the nerve roots from the spinal pathology. The tightness and spasm of the muscles and other soft tissues in the neck and shoulder region could affect the nerves, or blood or lymphatic circulations in the vicinity. All these factors discussed, alone or jointly, would result in the symptoms in the arm and hand. Hence, in this case, the effect of acupuncture treatment might have been from the relaxation of the local muscles and other soft tissues. In Case Three, the effects of acupuncture treatment might have been achieved from the combination of the possible mechanisms discussed previously with the addition of the mechanical enforcement from Tui Na treatment, which might have also corrected the micro biomechanical dislocation or malalignment of the tendons, ligaments, or even facet joints despite the lack of evidence of a gross instability on the x-rays.

Given the limitation of the scale of this chapter, it is impossible to include all the information on the evidence-based medicine in demonstrating the application of acupuncture in the management of spine-related pain conditions. Readers are referred to other sources in the references.

## CONCLUSIONS

Although the effectiveness of acupuncture in the treatment of spine-related pain conditions remains controversial in English publications, the clinical practice guideline from the American College of Physicians and the American Pain Society favors the use of acupuncture. For patients who do not improve with self-care options, clinicians should consider the addition of nonpharmacologic therapy with proven benefits: for acute low back pain, spinal manipulation; for chronic or subacute low back pain, intensive interdisciplinary rehabilitation, exercise therapy, acupuncture, massage therapy, spinal manipulation, yoga, cognitive-behavioral therapy, or progressive relaxation (weak recommendation, moderate-quality evidence).[12]

# References

1. Joseph M. Helmes, Acupuncture energetic—a clinical approach for physicians, second ed., Medical Acupuncture Publishers, Berkeley, California, 1997.
2. D.M. Eisenberg, R.B. Davis, et al., Trends in alternative medicine use in the United States, 1990-1997: results of a follow up national survey, JAMA 289 (1998) 1569–1575.
3. E. Ernst, Acupuncture as a symptomatic treatment of osteoarthritis—A systematic review, Scand. J. Rheumatol. 26 (1997) 444–447.
4. P. White, G. Lewith, P. Prescott, J. Conway, Acupuncture versus placebo for the treatment of chronic mechanical neck pain, Ann. Intern. Med. 141 (12) (2004) 911–919.
5. Zhang Enqin, Chinese acupuncture and moxibustion, Publishing House of Shanghai College of Traditional Chinese Medicine, , 1990, pp. 340–364.
6. L.P. Wang, Meridian differentiation of lumbar intervertebral disc herniation (Article in Chinese), Zhongguo Gu Shang 22 (10) (2009 Oct) 777–778.
7. Chunbo Cai, Revisit of the anatomy of Hua Tuo Jai Ji points, Med. Acupunct. 19 (3) (2007) 125–128.
8. Dafang Yu, Tui Na Xue (in Chinese), Publishing House of Shanghai Sciences and Technology (1984) 7–22.
9. J. Shen, Research on the neurophysiologic mechanisms of acupuncture: review of selected studies and methodological issues, J. Altern. Complement. Med. 7 (Suppl. 1) (2001) S121–S127.
10. D.C. Cherkin, K.J. Sherman, A.L. Avins, J.H. Erro, L. Ichikawa, W.E. Barlow, K. Delaney, R. Hawkes, L. Hamilton, A. Pressman, P.S. Khalsa, R.A. Deyo, A randomized trial comparing acupuncture, simulated acupuncture, and usual care for chronic low back pain, Arch. Intern. Med. 169 (9) (2009 May 11) 858–866.
11. C. Carlsson, et al., Acupuncture for chronic low back pain: a randomized placebo-controlled study with long-term follow-up, Clin. J. Pain 17 (4) (2001) 296–305.
12. R. Chou, A. Qaseem, V. Snow, D. Casey, J.T. Cross Jr., P. Shekelle, D.K. Owens, Clinical Efficacy Assessment Subcommittee of the American College of Physicians; American Pain Society Low Back Pain Guidelines Panel, Diagnosis and treatment of low back pain: a joint clinical practice guideline from the American College of Physicians and the American Pain Society, Ann. Intern. Med. 148 (3) (2008 Feb 5) 247–248.

# 21

# Tai Chi, Qi Gong, and Other Complementary Alternative Therapies for Treatment of the Aging Spine and Chronic Pain

*Wei Huang, Alice Fann, Linqiu Zhou, Weibin Yang, Chunbo Cai, and James J. Yue*

---

## KEY POINTS

- Various complementary alternative therapies based on movements, energy, and mind-body interactions are used in the treatment of older patients with spine conditions and chronic pain to decrease pain, improve function, and maintain general health. Many times, they are used in combination with more traditional treatment modalities.

- Movement-based therapies such as Tai Chi ("Tai Ji Quan") incorporate balance training, mind concentration, breathing techniques, and core muscle strengthening to improve spine function and to promote general health.

- Energy-based therapies and mind-body interactions may take advantage of the use of attention in their effective management of chronic nonmalignant pain in older patients.

- Clinical application of these complementary alternative therapies is promising, but requires diligent guidance and monitoring from providers to ensure safety and benefits, as there are no definitive practice guidelines that are supported or not supported by currently available clinical trials.

- Mechanistic research on these modalities is challenging, due to the complex interplay of central, autonomic, and peripheral nervous systems when these therapies are applied.

## INTRODUCTION

Among patients with spine conditions and chronic pain, there is an increasing use of complementary alternative therapies that are considered to be "holistic," noninvasive, and nonpharmaceutical. Such therapies are either used as alternative options or as complementary modalities to medical techniques and/or pharmaceutical agents that are known and accepted by the majority of "conventional" medical practitioners. This chapter will introduce some of these referred complementary alternative therapies, including therapies based on movements, energy, and mind-body interactions. Although complete understanding of the physiologic basis for these therapies is still limited, this chapter provides basic concepts and clinical guidelines about Tai Chi, Qi Gong, and other energy-based therapies, as well as some mind-body interaction practice such as mindfulness meditation, guided imagery, and spirituality practice. It will also delineate some basic science studies that may explain some of their clinical effects. Using a clinical case example, we will demonstrate the selective use of such therapies in a comprehensive pain management plan to improve clinical success. Certain clinical practice-related issues will be reflected in case discussion. Readers are advised to view this chapter only as an introduction to these complementary alternative therapies; by no means do we try to cover all inspirations, debates, and scientific investigations of the topic.

## TAI CHI

It is easy to associate Tai Chi with those slow, deliberate movements performed in synchronization by groups of elderly people in parks. Strictly speaking, so-called Tai Chi in the Western world should be Tai Ji Quan in the Chinese Pinyin system or Tai Chi Chuan in Wade-Giles transliteration. "Tai Chi" itself is, rather, a concept in Chinese Taoist philosophy where Yin and Yang, although being the two opposite "supreme ultimate" forces, infiltrate and reconcile each other to unite as a single universe. Tai Chi Chuan originated in China about 600 years ago as a form of martial arts and was once one of the most powerful forms of combat. It was named after Tai Chi as "the Supreme Ultimate Boxing" because its movements are based on Yin-Yang Tai Chi philosophy to feature a defense system that applies the force from an assailant to fend off the attack without deliberate killing. By convention, the term Tai Chi will be used to refer to Tai Chi Chuan in this chapter.

There are five main styles of Tai Chi: Chen, Yang, Wu (or Hao), Wu, and Sun. Although each style has different speeds and forms of movements, practicing any style of Tai Chi requires similar fundamentals, including (1) concentration with internal stillness and quick reaction time, (2) deep breathing skills to enhance its aerobic component, (3) strong leg support and good balance for constant body weight shifting during movements, (4) correct posture and spine alignment with relaxed muscles to maintain stability without unnecessary muscle tension, and (5) an agile torso (lumbar spine) with coordination among all body parts to perform the movements gracefully. Masters of Tai Chi build up internal energy that gives them not only the power needed during combat, but also health and longevity. The latter is the main reason why Tai Chi is widespread in the world, with many participants being attracted to it not for its combative content but for its health benefits. When it is performed for health reasons, the movements can be slow and deliberate with low exercise impact and, therefore, can be tolerated well by the elderly (Figure 21-1).

Compared to other types of exercises, Tai Chi involves more weight bearing and strength training than yoga and a wider range of coordinated movements than other aerobic exercises. Even in low-impact Tai Chi, emphasis is placed on correct posture and spine alignment with appropriate muscle relaxation. Such features make Tai Chi a good therapy for patients with chronic back pain. Although no randomized controlled clinical trial was found in the literature using Tai Chi for spine conditions, clinical benefits have been observed including strengthened core muscles, increased functional range of motion, decreased pain level, and improved quality of life.

Even with simplified Tai Chi exercises, studies have demonstrated improvement in balance, reduced fear of falling, and decreased risk of falls in older adults.[1] Tai Chi, like other forms of exercise, can also reduce blood pressure, improve heart failure, normalize blood lipids and glucose levels,[2] and positively affect bone mineral density in postmenopausal women.[3] In the older population, when compared to age and body size-matched

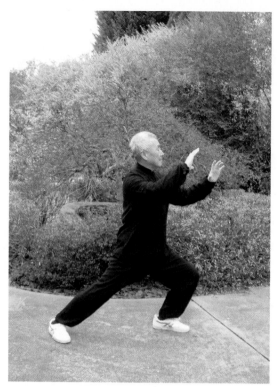

■ **FIGURE 21-1**   When performed for health reasons, the movements of Tai Chi can be slow and deliberate, with low exercise impact.

sedentary controls, Tai Chi practitioners have higher oxygen uptake, greater flexibility, and a lower percentage of body fat.[4]

## Clinical Practice Guidelines

Because there are different levels of Tai Chi forms, from those commonly practiced by the elderly to those practiced by combat martial artists, recommendations for patients with spine conditions have to be individualized. Basic Tai Chi forms can be tolerated well by the elderly who are not active or do not have good balance or coordination; these forms focus on lower body strength and good posture that will improve balance and coordination. Intermediate levels of Tai Chi forms can improve core muscle strength, cardiovascular tolerance, and pulmonary function. Combat levels of Tai Chi forms are not recommended until patients have developed excellent balance and coordination as well as strong core muscle strength; this form should only be practiced under the guidance of Tai Chi masters and with close monitoring of physicians because some of these forms can cause sports-related injuries.

Tai Chi instructors are certified after undertaking a certain amount of training and participating in teaching for a certain number of hours; however, the amount of each needed varies with the different certifying institutions. The certification process is not regulated by legislation. A good reference is important before sending your patients to a particular instructor, preferably one with experience in teaching patients with spine conditions.

## FROM QI GONG TO ENERGY-BASED THERAPIES

Qi Gong ("Training of Qi") is a form of energy therapy, energy therapies being those that use and/or manipulate bioenergy or "Qi" fields for medical treatment purposes. The concept of energy therapy is based on the theory that there are patterns of Qi flow in human bodies; the disruption of such patterns of flow can lead to dysfunction and disorders. No one can observe Qi itself, but it has been claimed to be able to "move" around the body and to defend certain body areas. For example in Qi Gong performance, a practitioner resists a sharp weapon, such as the tip of a piercing spear, at his throat by moving his Qi towards that area. Qi has also been perceived when there is "blockage." A clinical example of such is when a patient presents

with a complaint of "having poor circulation." The symptoms typically are cold, numb fingers and toes; conventional medical tests for nerve function, blood flow, vitamin levels, and endocrine pathology all turn out to be normal. In Traditional Chinese Medicine, such a patient has a problem of Qi "blockage"; therefore energy cannot "flow" toward the distal extremities. The principle of energy therapy is to restore the normal "flow" of Qi or the human bioenergy field for disease prevention or treatment.

Qi Gong originated in China, under the influence of meditation and martial arts practices. Qi Gong masters claim to be able to move energy along meridians for their own health and possibly to heal others' illnesses. However, driven by financial profit, some inauthentic Qi Gong "masters" also claim to be able to heal and may fool the public. In those cases, certain clinical improvements of the treated patients are likely contributed by acupressure massage, mind-body interactions, psychological placebo effects, and/or the benefits of touch. Some personal conversation between one author (WH) and a well-known Qi Gong master revealed that using energy to heal others hurts the practitioners themselves and thus is rarely practiced except in emergency situations. Therefore, Qi Gong masters usually would rather teach people how to control their own Qi to run smoothly along meridians to maintain health and achieve self-healing.

Besides Qi Gong, other main types of energy-based therapies include Reiki (Japanese), Breema (American), and therapeutic touch (American). Some of these are critically questioned by the research community. For instance, in therapeutic touch, practitioners with their hands placed several inches to feet away from a patient claim that they can feel the energy field emanated by a human body and detect certain patterns of disruption; however, in one clinical investigation, they could correctly detect only 44% of the time (less than chance) the position of a child's hand.[5] Although this illustrates certain doubts on energy-based therapies for their bioenergy base, we are not rejecting their clinical effects as the possible effects may be achieved in other ways.

## Clinical Practice Guidelines

Energy-based therapies have been used in chronic back pain in the elderly for myofascial release, pain relief and coping, and improvement of depression. Whether such therapies are truly bioenergy based is currently not clear. Clinical application should be practiced cautiously according to each individual's condition.

Some forms of energy therapy such as Qi Gong are not recommended for self-practice without guidance. Cases of "energy maltracking during practice" with psychological reactions have been reported around the world. These cases present with symptoms interpreted by mainstream psychiatrists as psychosis or schizophrenia. In bioenergy-based theory, such incidences are thought to be induced by energy invasion into certain meridians without proper guidance. In the clinical psychiatry point of view, such incidences occur with meditation psychosis.

## MIND-BODY THERAPIES

Mind-body therapies use the power of the mind to make positive changes in the body and improve health. The practice of such power might be traced back to ancient Buddhist philosophy and practice; the use of it for healing has been recent, with various approaches. We will introduce here a few of the available therapies that are better known to the public.

## Mindfulness Meditation

The mindfulness-based stress reduction (MBSR) program was developed at the University of Massachusetts Medical Center. Mindfulness meditation has three purposes: knowing the mind, training the mind, and freeing the mind. It calls for awareness of conscious and unconscious thoughts, feelings, and behaviors that underlie emotional, physical, and spiritual health, and cultivates greater awareness of one's own bodily functions for the unity of mind and body. The mind is known to be a factor in stress and stress-related disorders. In mindfulness meditation, patients learn to distinguish between mind and awareness, learn to see how the mind dwells on anxiety and fear that burns up energy, learn to stay in the present moment while experiencing high levels of pain, and learn to distinguish between pain sensations and the mind's creation of the experience of suffering. The practice thus brings nonjudgmental moment-to-moment awareness to thoughts, sensations, or emotions as they arise.

In one qualitative study, 27 older adults with chronic low back pain participated in a MSBR program.[6] The authors found a report of improved attention, improved quality of sleep, and improved quality of life along with reduction in pain. In another randomized controlled study of 37 older adults with chronic pain, subjects were randomized into MSBR or wait-list control groups. MSBR participants were found to have improvement in pain acceptance, activity engagement, and physical functioning after 6 months.[7] Both studies showed that MSBR was feasible and effective in the older adult population with spine conditions and chronic pain.

Mindfulness meditation is usually taught in weekly group classes that require daily practice outside the group setting for an intensive 8 weeks. It can include sitting, walking, loving-kindness, or body-scan type of meditation. The students are usually given guided meditation tapes for assisting with meditation techniques and are required to practice daily afterwards.

## Guided Imagery

Guided imagery is based on the belief in the power of imagination and visualization, a healing tool used by ancient Greeks, by Tibetans, and later by Freud. It is the conscious use of imagination that occurs naturally to create positive images and bring about healthy changes in both body and mind. It uses imagery in a more purposeful and directed way and can control negative thoughts such as fears and concerns. The practice usually begins with a relaxation exercise, either with an individual trained in guided imagery or through the use of audiotapes/CDs, to focus the attention and relieve tension before the actual guided imagery. It involves a breathing exercise and, to start with, visualization of a safe place, followed by the creation of more specific guided images in the mind's eye. Imageries can be used over and over again or change each time. Five types of guided imagery are usually practiced: (1) pleasant imagery such as imagery of a peaceful location; (2) physiologically-focused imagery such as imagery of white cells fighting disease or cancer cells; (3) mental rehearsal such as successfully performing a public task; (4) mental reframing such as imagery that reinterprets a past experience and its associated emotions; and (5) receptive imagery that involves scanning the body for diagnostic or reflective purposes.

There have been few studies on guided imagery in older subjects with pain. Morone and Greco[8] reviewed two studies that were done over a short period of time with small numbers of subjects. Both found that guided imagery was feasible in older adults using the techniques at home, without difficulty and with good compliance, and the practice reduced pain and increased mobility in these subjects.

## Spirituality and Religiousness

Spirituality and religiousness is the belief in a higher power than humans. Whereas spirituality may be practiced within an organized religion but, for some, may lack social context; religious beliefs tend to be practiced in a community of like-minded believers. These beliefs may increase social support, improve health behaviors, and improve psychological states. Stronger religious beliefs have been shown to decrease depression and to decrease stress, increase relaxation, and/or provide distraction from pain. Religious and spiritual beliefs improve outlook and function in people with chronic pain.

The role of spirituality and religiousness in health, viewed from a scientific perspective, has been yielding interesting, perhaps intriguing, results. In general, studies have reported fairly consistent positive relationships with physical health, mental health, and substance abuse outcomes, mostly using cross-sectional or prospective designs.[9] There were few studies found in the literature regarding spirituality/religiousness in older patients with nonmalignant chronic pain. Baetz and Bowen[10] polled 37,000 Canadians and found that those who reported stronger religious beliefs had fewer reports of pain and increased reports of psychological well being. Of those with chronic pain, those who reported more religious and/or spiritual beliefs were more likely to use positive coping mechanisms including attitudinal and activity strategies, and reported increased control and self-efficacy, which led to an increase in pain tolerance. They were also more likely to exercise.

## BASIC SCIENCE

The search for the underlying mechanisms of these complementary alternative therapies is challenging using conventional biological and pharmacological research models. However, breakthroughs in brain imagery and neural network have provided some insights in our understanding of the power of our mind. The well-studied autonomic nervous system in Western medicine is also getting renewed interests due to its involvement in many of these holistic therapies.

## Attention and Pain

Chronic pain is associated with impairment of attentional processes. Attention can be thought of as the preferential processing of various types of cognitive information. The function of attention is the appropriate selection of stimuli, maintenance of concentration, and interactions with space and time.[11] The anterior cingulate cortex (ACC) is needed for sustained attention, because it modulates one's ability to concentrate over time by coordinating and integrating task-specific processes. The ACC has a pivotal role in executive processes, motivation, allocation of attentional resources, premotor functions, and error detection. It is activated by moderate-to-intense painful stimulation, and positron emission tomography studies have revealed a large concentration of opiate receptors in this region.[12] The more intense and the longer the duration of painful stimuli, the more active the ACC becomes.

Pain may interrupt complex cognition and capture attention that might otherwise be allocated elsewhere; chronic pain may result in a person sustaining focus on the pain rather than other stimuli. Various studies have shown that persons reporting greater attention to pain also report higher pain intensity; persons engaging in attention-demanding tasks report lower pain intensity. Directing attention away from the pain decreases the perception of pain; this distraction away from pain decreases activity in the ACC, insular cortex, thalamus, and somatosensory regions.[12-14]

Another area of interest is the periaqueductal gray (PAG), which receives major inputs from the frontal cortex, hypothalamus, frontal granular, insular cortex, and amygdala. The PAG projects to the rostral ventromedial medulla, which in turn sends projections to pain-transmitting neurons in the dorsal horn of the spinal cord and the trigeminal nucleus caudalis.[15] Within this complex neuronetwork, PAG plays an important role in the descending modulation of pain and in defensive behavior. A study using functional MRI assessed changes in the PAG region in normal subjects.[15] Noxious and warm thermal stimuli were applied to the subjects, who were told whether or not to attend to pain. Increased activity within the PAG correlated with perceptual decreases in pain intensity; a greater change in PAG activity was found with a larger decrease in reported pain intensity. Activation difference in the PAG significantly correlated with the total pain score change, using visual analogue scale (VAS), between conditions; a greater change in PAG activity was found with a larger decrease in reported pain intensity. Increased activity within the PAG correlated with perceptual decreases in pain intensity.

Mind-body therapies are likely to exert their clinical effects through modulation of such attentional and emotional modulation. Mindfulness meditation calls for awareness of various conscious and unconscious thoughts, feelings, and behaviors; guided imagery focuses on peaceful and pleasant images; and spirituality engages people in giving up control over one's life and giving in to a higher power. All these distract from painful, unpleasant physical experiences and potentially produce more positive feelings and less pain. Even Tai Chi and some energy-based therapies emphasize the experience of moving/regulating Qi, a strong distraction from a focus on focal illness or pain. We mentioned earlier some doubts on healing touch by the scientific community; however, from attention and distraction aspects, healing touch could still be effective in producing some pain relief by distracting patients' attention and inducing positive feedback.

## Regulation of the Autonomic Nervous System

Tai Chi, Qi Gong, and other energy-based therapies, as well as mind-body interaction, all claim to be able to lower blood pressure, provide a sense of relaxation and serenity, improve sleep, strengthen the immune system, and improve pain, physical activities, and quality of life. These can be viewed as

## Clinical Case Example

A 67-year-old man was referred by his primary care physician for a consultation on chronic back pain that started during his military service and was present intermittently during his younger years. For the 10 years prior to being seen, the pain increased and became more constant; the pain intermittently radiated to his right gluteal region. It was exacerbated by bending either forward or backward, lifting, prolonged standing or walking, and was ameliorated with rest, topical heat application, or massage. At his initial visit, he reported more stiffness in the morning, difficulty with his usual back stretching, and intolerance to standing or walking for greater than 15 minutes. His average daily pain was rated at 9/10. Physical therapy that focused on a back program made the pain worse and he stopped going after one session. He took over-the-counter ibuprofen and acetaminophen until they were no longer effective. His primary care physician prescribed gabapentin 300 mg three times a day and tramadol 50 mg three times a day with reported minimal pain relief; he reported an increase in daytime drowsiness and two falls in the week prior to his presentation.

Past medical history was also significant for diabetes, hypertension, post-traumatic stress disorder (PTSD), and chronic insomnia due to a combination of pain, and nocturia. He had been successfully employed as a manager of a hardware store until 3 months prior to his presentation, when he was laid off due to the economy. At work, he had divided his time between a more sedentary desk job and a more active component in which he had to walk around the store, occasionally lifting some objects of no more than 60 pounds. He used to smoke cigarettes 2 packs a day for 25 years and quit about 20 years ago; he drank beers socially and denied a history of illicit drug use except for experimental marijuana use in high school.

Review of systems revealed chronic constipation that was treated with senna and fiber supplements. He had night sweats but without cough or fever. Chest x-ray was negative for pathology. There had been worsening depression since he lost his job; lately he rarely left the house, per him, due to pain.

On physical examination, he appeared his stated age. He had abdominal obesity and walked with a slow, wide-based gait that was not antalgic. He was able to stand on tiptoes and heels, although standing on heels aggravated his pain. He turned very slowly and lost his balance once during the turn. Lumbar spine had loss of normal curvature and range of motion was limited due to pain with flexion to about 60 degrees (complaining of "deep pain" in the L4-5 area, midline as well as paraspinals), extension to only about 10 degrees (complaining of "sharp pain" all over the low back), lateral rotations to about 45 degrees (complaining of "aching pain" all over the low back). Facet loading on the right reproduced radiating pain down the right lower extremity, traveling from the back to gluteal region and then stopped at the back of the knee.. Paraspinal muscles were tender to palpation in a diffuse area across the back. Straight leg raise produced pain in the posterior knees only. Neurological examination demonstrated manual muscle testing limited by pain; symmetrical deep tendon reflexes in both lower extremities; and intact pinprick sensation. Psychologically, he engaged in conversation with poor eye contact.

Magnetic resonance imaging (MRI) of the lumbar sacral spine showed multilevel lumbar spinal stenosis with L4-5 and L5-S1 degenerative discs. There was also bilateral L3-4, L4-5, and L5-S1 facet hypertrophy with mild neuroforaminal narrowing at L4-5 on the left. Cord signals were normal.

The assessment was a combination of myofascial and facetogenic pain. Although he also had degenerative disc disease, the clinical presentation did not suggest an acute lumbar radiculopathy. He was taught basic back/leg stretching exercises in the supine position and was referred for chiropractor manipulation of his lumbar spine.

At follow-up, he reported that the stretching exercises reduced his pain to a level of 7/10 and that he continued those daily. He also received two sessions of chiropractor manipulation, with significant symptom relief after the first session; however, the pain returned to baseline after only 2 days. He went back the second time and did not get much relief.

He was given trigger point injection and reported immediate 90% pain relief. However, a week later, he called and reported pain back to baseline after 3 days and sounded very distressed. He was referred for right L5-S1 facet injection.

Two weeks later, he reported only 1 week of 60% pain relief from the facet injection; therefore, he was not interested in injections any more. And, he reported, he was not happy with his psychiatrist who diagnosed him with severe depression. He stated, "Who wouldn't be depressed with this kind of pain and nothing has helped." He was more interested in holistic medicine but did not wish to get acupuncture since needles would be involved.

He was then referred to a basic Tai Chi class that involved mainly slow, coordinated hand and back movements while standing, and to a pain group headed by a psychologist who used coping strategies for pain and depression, including meditation and relaxation techniques.

He went to the Tai Chi class once a week (1 hour each) and practiced the movements 5 times per week (20 minutes each) at home, and attended the pain group therapy twice a month. Sleep hygiene was reviewed in the clinic and education about sleep schedule and environment was provided. He was also instructed to apply the learned relaxation skills prior to bedtime. After a month, he felt that he could transfer better in the morning time, sit longer, and had better tolerance of prolonged standing and walking. After 3 months, his pain was down to 1-2/10 with occasional exacerbation to 5-6/10 pain; therefore, he cut out all pain medications, except for occasional ibuprofen or acetaminophen. He felt stronger in his legs and back, and reported no more falls.

A year later, he reported a 30-lb weight loss; his pain was gone most days except during changes in weather. At night, it took less time for him to fall asleep, although his sleep was still fragmented. He also felt more energetic, with less need for diabetic medication, and experienced fewer nighttime sweats.

He started a higher level of Tai Chi with movements such as single-leg standing, turning, and stooping, walked 30 minutes a day, and continued meditation three times per week. He also found a part-time job and was extremely satisfied with the results.

positive effects on a range of autonomic physiological processes, confirmed by research studies that examined Tai Chi and mind-body interactions.[16, 17] The aforementioned neuronetwork, i.e., ACC and PAG, has also been found to modulate autonomic function.[18, 19] Therefore, future mechanistic research may help further understand the interplay among the central, peripheral, and autonomic nervous systems with the resultant clinical effects from these holistic therapies.

## Case Discussion

This case illustrates a common approach that has been adopted by many pain specialists: the application of a comprehensive pain management program that is layered, staged, and integrated. The treatment modalities were selected at different stages according to the progression of the symptoms, the responses the patient achieved, the invasiveness of the therapies, and the patient's preferences.

It appears that the patient finally improved with the introduction of Tai Chi and pain group therapy. However, the patient already had some short-lasting pain relief from various modalities, such as stretching and topical heat. The return of his pain after various injections, regular physical therapy, and chiropractic manipulation, and the loss of his job fortified his misconception that his pain was very significant and permanent. Tai Chi became an appropriate choice of therapy as its movements and exercises were well tolerated by the patient and gradually built up his flexibility and strength; with noticeable functional changes, Tai Chi provided positive feedback to the patient and "started" the success.

Tai Chi is an exercise that is considered to be holistic because it integrates mind concentration with a high level of internal engagement and external movements. However, it is not the only exercise that should be considered holistic. In fact, any exercise, sport, or activity that requires such integration of mind and body would produce similar effects. The selection of the type lies in the provider's experience and the patient's preference. For instance, if the patient preferred to learn dancing, which also requires concentration, graceful posture, and poised movements, the clinical effects might be as significant as seen with Tai Chi.

Even with the improvements achieved by Tai Chi exercises, treatment of depression also played an important role in clinical progress. The contribution of depression to pain is often not recognized by patients. Depression can worsen pain symptoms, and effective treatment of depression can improve chronic pain.[20] Active treatments and socialization are extremely important for treatment of depression as well as pain, to break the cycle of pain and depression. The socialization at the Tai Chi classes, along with pain group therapy that introduced chronic pain coping strategies that diverted the patient's attention from pain to more positive images of his own health and condition, all contributed to his improvements in this clinical case.

The impact of sleep in chronic pain management has been often underestimated even by pain specialists. However, there are strong correlations between chronic pain and sleep difficulties.[21] Education on sleep hygiene and the use of relaxation techniques helped improve this patient's sleep, which contributed to decreased pain at morning time. Improved pain and function further provided improved sleep at night.

Most of these complementary alternative therapies require the active participation of patients and are, therefore, different from other medical modalities such as procedures, passive therapies, and medications. Because of this characteristic, they can pose certain clinical challenges in their delivery. Active engagement of patients in their own healthcare becomes an important task for providers to enhance the clinical efficacy of treatments.

## CONCLUSION

The holistic concept has been the focus and attraction of most complementary alternative therapies that have demonstrated their clinical effects in the aging spine and chronic pain. Their promising clinical effects have earned their place in a comprehensive clinical management program as an integral part of reducing pain and improving function. Complementary and alternative medical practices can be blended with traditional evidence-based medicine to optimally promote a healing environment and overall patient well-being.[22] Their underlying mechanisms prompt further investigation; however, use of the simple pharmacological model must be avoided due to their complicated involvement of multiple aspects of healing, such as active exercises, concentration, mind-body interaction, attention modification, and autonomic regulation.

## References

1. H.M. Taggart, Effects of Tai Chi exercise on balance, functional mobility, and fear of falling among older women, Appl. Nurs. Res. 15 (4) (2002) 235–242.
2. G.Y. Yeh, C. Wang, P.M. Wayne, et al., Tai chi exercise for patients with cardiovascular conditions and risk factors: a systematic review, J. Mol. Signal. 29 (3) (2009) 152–160.
3. P.M. Wayne, D.P. Kiel, D.E. Krebs, et al., The effects of Tai Chi on bone mineral density in postmenopausal women: a systematic review, Arch. Phys. Med. Rehabil. 88 (5) (2007) 673–680.
4. C. Lan, J.S. Lai, M.K. Wong, et al., Cardiorespiratory function, flexibility, and body composition among geriatric Tai Chi Chuan practitioners, Arch. Phys. Med. Rehabil. 77 (6) (1996) 612–616.
5. L. Rosa, E. Rosa, L. Sarner, et al., A close look at therapeutic touch, JAMA 279 (13) (1998) 1005–1010.
6. N.E. Morone, C.S. Lynch, C.M. Greco, et al., "I felt like a new person." The effects of mindfulness meditation on older adults with chronic pain: qualitative narrative analysis of diary entries, J. Pain 9 (2008) 841–848.
7. N.E. Morone, C.M. Greco, D.K. Weiner, Mindfulness meditation for the treatment of chronic low back pain in older adults: a randomized controlled pilot study, Pain 134 (2008) 310–319.
8. N.E. Morone, C.M. Greco, Mind-body interventions for chronic pain in older adults: a structured review, Pain Med. 8 (2007) 359–375.
9. C.E. Thoresen, Spirituality and health, J. Health Psych. 4 (1999) 291–300.
10. M. Baetz, R. Bowen, Chronic pain and fatigue: associations with religion and spirituality, Pain Res. Manage. 13 (2008) 383–388.
11. D.R. Gitelman, Attention and its disorders, BriMed. Bulletin 65 (2003) 21–34.
12. S.J. Bantick, R.G. Wise, A. Ploghaus, et al., Imaging how attention modulates pain in humans using functional MRI, Brain 125 (2002) 310–319.
13. P. Petrovic, K.M. Petersson, P.H. Ghatan, et al., Pain-related cerebral activation is altered by a distracting cognitive task, Pain 85 (2000) 19–30.
14. S.E. Longe, R. Wise, S. Bantick, et al., Counter-stimulatory effects on pain perception and processing are significantly altered by attention: An fMRI study, Neuroreport 12 (2001) 2021–2025.
15. I. Tracey, A. Ploghaus, J.S. Gati, et al., Imaging attentional modulation of pain in the periaqueudctal gray in humans, J. Neurosci. 22 (2002) 2748–2752.
16. W.A. Lu, C.D. Kuo, The effect of Tai Chi Chuan on the autonomic nervous modulation in older persons, Med. Sci. Sports Exercise 35 (12) (2003) 1972–1976.
17. H.D. Critchley, Psychophysiology of neural, cognitive and affective integration: fMRI and autonomic indicants, Int J. Psychophysiol. 73 (2) (2009) 88–94.
18. Y.Y. Tang, Y. Ma, Y. Fan, et al., Central and autonomic nervous system interaction is altered by short-term meditation, Proc. Natl. Acad. Sci. U.S.A. 106 (22) (2009) 8865–8870.
19. R. Bandler, K.A. Keay, N. Floyd, et al., Central circuits mediating patterned autonomic activity during active vs. passive emotional coping, Brain Res. Bull. 53 (1) (2000) 95–104.
20. L.H. Lunde, I.H. Nordhus, S. Pallesen, et al., The effectiveness of cognitive and behavioural treatment of chronic pain in the elderly: a quantitative review, J. Clin. Psychol. Med. Settings 16 (3) (2009) 254–262.
21. F. Stiefel, D. Stagno, Management of insomnia in patients with chronic pain conditions, CNS Drugs 18 (5) (2004) 285–296.
22. J. Geimer-Flanders, Creating a healing environment: rationale and research overview, Cleve, Clin. J. Med. 76 (Suppl. 2) (2009) S66–S69.

# 22

# Oral Analgesics for Chronic Low Back Pain in Adults

*Kathleen Abbott and Amy Folta*

---

**KEY POINTS**

- Back pain can impair function and quality of life.
- Oral analgesic medication can be used, if needed, in addition to physical modalities and topical treatments.
- The main classes of medications used include NSAIDs (nonsteroidal antiinflammatory drugs), muscle relaxants, opioid analgesics, and adjuvant medications, such as antidepressant and anticonvulsant drugs.
- The elderly and people with medical illnesses are more susceptible to adverse drug reactions.
- The risks versus benefits must be weighed for any medication used.

---

## INTRODUCTION

The most common type of pain for which patients seek medical attention is back pain. Chronic back pain is associated with a reduced quality of life, depression, loss of sleep, and reduced psychosocial and physical function. Analgesic medications are used to treat chronic pain, in conjunction with traditional physical modalities and therapy. Treatment with analgesic medications can help to restore physical and social function, while improving sleep, mood and concentration. Side effects should be minimized as best as possible.[1] Acetaminophen and nonsteroidal antiinflammatory drugs (NSAIDs), along with pain modulators, are on the first step of the analgesic ladder to treat mild to moderate pain, as recommended by the World Health Organization (WHO). Opioid analgesics are added as a second-line treatment for moderate to severe pain.[2] Adjuvant medications are used to treat conditions contributing to pain such as altered neuronal function or muscle spasm. An example would be an antidepressant or anticonvulsant medication to treat neuropathic pain from a lumbar radiculopathy. Muscle relaxants can be used to treat muscle spasm.[2,3]

When treating the elderly, it is important to use a medication with the shortest possible half-life as well as the lowest effective dose, as the elderly population is more prone to side effects. Sedative effects of medications can cause significant confusion and thereby impair function and increase the risk of falling. In the elderly, metabolism of medications is reduced with reduced renal clearance. Therefore, buildup of medication is more likely, placing patients at a higher risk of side effects, especially when combined with other drugs. However, when pain is continuous, a long-acting analgesic medication should be considered[5]. Elderly and medically ill patients are more prone to toxic renal and hepatic side effects. Also, drugs have variable effects on the liver's cytochrome P450 system, which vary between individuals; therefore it is important for medications to be obtained from one pharmacy, which can then monitor for medication interactions.

Pharmacologic changes with age include:

- Changes in the ratio of fat to lean body mass can increase the volume of distribution and may result in a longer effective half-life for fat-soluble drugs, such as methadone.

- Slower gastrointestinal transit time can prolong the effects of continual release medications.
- Liver oxidation function may be reduced, contributing to a longer medication half-life.
- Renal excretion may be reduced, which can prolong the effects of renal metabolites.
- The risk for anticholinergic side effects such as confusion, constipation, movement disorders, and incontinence, is increased.[5]

## NONOPIOID ANALGESIC AGENTS: ACETAMINOPHEN, NSAIDs, ASPIRIN

### Acetaminophen

Acetaminophen (Tylenol) is one of the most commonly used medications both by prescription and over the counter, either by itself or in combination with other products. Acetaminophen is used for the treatment of mild to moderate pain. It is also an antipyretic, but does not have significant antiinflammatory properties. Although considered a safe drug, acetaminophen has a very narrow therapeutic index, thus making a safe dose and a dose able to contribute to liver toxicity very close to each other. The once recommended 1000 mg per dose or 4000 mg a day are being reconsidered. The FDA now recommends a lower dose of a max of 3250 mg per day, which can be divided into 5 doses of 650 mg a day. Studies have shown that a 650 mg dose is almost as effective as the 1000 mg for pain and may be a lot safer for patients.[17] Due to acetaminophens effects on the liver, chronic use of acetaminophen should be avoided in patients with hepatic impairment, and patients should limit usage of alcohol products (1-2 drinks per day). Long-term overdosing of acetaminophen may result in hepatic necrosis and can be fatal. Patients should be made aware of the possible ease of overdose if they are on many pain medications, such as Percocet®, Vicodin®, and Darvocet®, all of which contain varying doses of acetaminophen.[3,5,6]

### Nonsteroidal Antiinflammatory Drugs (NSAIDs)

All NSAIDs have antiinflammatory, analgesic, and antipyretic properties.[3,4,6,7] They are commonly used to treat inflammatory conditions, and are used for analgesia in low back pain as well as for the pain and inflammation of many types of arthritis. NSAIDs are characterized as either selective or nonselective COX-2 inhibitors.

The inflammatory cascade can be triggered by a number of causes such as a physical injury or response to infection. In response, at the cellular level, prostaglandins are synthesized by cyclooxygenase. NSAIDs inhibit the cyclooxygenase (COX) enzyme and therefore reduce production of prostaglandin, usually nonselectively via COX-1 and COX-2 pathways.[12] Prostaglandins are thought to sensitize the pain receptors and are involved in peripheral and central pain transmission. The enzyme COX-1 (cyclooxygenase-1) is prevalent, located in most normal cells, and involved in many aspects of physiologic function. COX-2 is more involved in the inflammatory process. COX-2 is expressed in parts of the kidney, brain, and endothelial cells. COX-1 is found in the gastric epithelium and is involved in the formation of cytoprotective prostaglandin. The COX-2–specific inhibitory NSAIDs were formulated to be gastric-protective; however, they do not reduce the risk of other effects of traditional NSAIDs.[3,4,6,7,12] The NSAIDS and aspirin do not affect the lipoxygenase pathway, therefore they do not reduce the formation of an important inflammatory mediator, the leukotrienes.[3,4,6,7,12,18]

The NSAIDs have a black box warning that includes cardiovascular disease, myocardial infarction, stroke, and hypertension. The nonselective NSAIDs, such as ibuprofen at low doses, also can interfere with the cardioprotective effect of aspirin. NSAIDs, such as ibuprofen at doses as low as 400 mg, should be taken either 8 hours before or 30 minutes after aspirin, if the aspirin is taken on a daily basis for its cardioprotective effect. If they are taken together then the cardioprotective effect of aspirin may be negated.[12] Also, NSAIDs are contraindicated for the perioperative pain of coronary artery bypass grafts, because platelet adhesion and aggregation can be disrupted.[4,5,6]

NSAIDs may increase the risk of renal and hepatic impairment, as well as of gastrointestinal irritation including bleeding and ulceration. GI bleeding risk is increased in the elderly; in smokers; when NSAIDs are used with aspirin; with corticosteroid use, ethanol use, anticoagulation, debilitation, and history of peptic ulcer. The risk of gastric ulceration can be reduced with the use of a proton pump inhibitor, or a prostaglandin analog such as misoprostol. However, despite that there is still an important risk of developing a severe life threatening gastrointestinal bleed. NSAIDs should be taken with food or a large volume of milk or water to reduce GI side effects.[4–6]

Congestive heart failure can be aggravated by the increased action of antidiuretic hormone due to NSAID use. Renal circulation is reduced due to reduced prostaglandin synthesis. This can affect the electrolytes at the renal level and lead to fluid retention and edema, a common side effect. Central nervous system side effects include headache and dizziness. NSAIDs should be discontinued if a rash develops from their use, due to the risk of Stevens-Johnson syndrome.[4,6]

Contraindications to NSAID use include hypersensitivity or allergic reaction to the drug used or any component of its formulation, aspirin, NSAIDs, as well as perioperative use for coronary artery bypass grafting. There is a cross-sensitivity to NSAIDs in those patients who have bronchial asthma, aspirin intolerance, and rhinitis. Avoid NSAIDs in severe hepatic and renal failure. Use caution for uncontrolled hypertension. See Table 22-1 for individual drug descriptions.[4,6]

## Cyclooxygenase Inhibitors (COX-2)

Cyclooxygenase-2 inhibitors are NSAIDs that specifically inhibit cyclooxygenase-2 and not the cyclooxygenase-1 enzyme at therapeutic concentrations. This effect does give some gastric protection. There still needs to be caution when used in the presence of renal and hepatic disease. The liver enzyme cytochrome P2D6 is inhibited, causing a significant interaction with fluconazole and lithium. COX-2 inhibitors share the same black box warning that the other traditional NSAIDs have.[4,6] (See Table 22-1.)

## Aspirin

Aspirin prevents the formation of thromboxane A2, which then prevents platelet aggregation by irreversible COX-1 inhibition. Prostaglandin formation is inhibited, as with other NSAIDs.[6] (See Table 22-1.)

## Flavocoxid (Limbrel®)

A newer product that is used for its antiinflammatory properties is flavocoxid, which, although given by prescription, is considered a medical food product. Limbrel® acts partially on the COX-1, COX-2, and 5-LOX pathways. There is a balanced inhibition of metabolism of the COX pathways, with inhibition of leukotrienes in the 5-LOX (lipid oxygenase) pathways. There is an antiinflammatory effect, with minimal effect on organ function. Arachidonic acid is still produced to maintain organ function.

Limbrel® also has antioxidant properties. Its efficacy has been similar to that of naproxen in a comparison study for treatment of osteoarthritis of the knee. Limbrel® has been used with patients who are anticoagulated with warfarin. It is recommended to check the prothrombin time 1 to 2 weeks after its initiation. Limbrel® is contraindicated if there is hypersensitivity to it or to flavonoids.[8]

## Opioid Analgesics

Sometimes the use of nonopioids may not be enough to control moderate to severe pain. At this point, according to the WHO, a narcotic analgesic may be a good choice for the patient. These medications have a higher potential for abuse and addiction; therefore they are controlled substances in the United States, and require a prescription. The goals of treatment with an opioid include reduction of pain and improved functional status, with no alteration of cognition and compliance with its use.[2,9] The three primary opioid receptors are mu, kappa, and delta receptors. Most analgesic medications are selective for the mu receptor, consistent with their similarity to morphine. The mu receptors are located in the central nervous system and in peripheral tissues.[9]

These receptors have analgesic properties and can also cause drowsiness, clouded cognition, and altered mood. Opioids have rewarding properties associated with their addiction potential as well.[6] It is important to be familiar with signs of addiction, physical dependence, and tolerance when prescribing opioid medications.[9] Patients also need to be monitored for opioid-induced hyperalgesia, in which opioids can potentially contribute to abnormal pain sensitization.[9] The elderly with no history of or current substance abuse are at low risk of addiction.[5] The opioids may cause fewer life-threatening events than chronic NSAID use in the elderly.[2]

When prescribing opioid medications it is important to be aware of the following commonly used terms. Tolerance is physiologic responce when there is a reduction in effectiveness of a drug with repeated administration.[9,18] A patient with tolerance would need a higher dose of medication to get the same effect.

Physical dependence is present when there is physical withdrawal from a medication, such as when discontinuing the medication or from rapid dose reduction or when given an antagonist to that medication.[9] Addiction has been defined as the compulsive use of a drug despite physical harm.[9] Other findings with addiction may also include poor control of drug usage, and cravings.[9] Compliance with the use of these medications is done to monitor for abuse, misuse, and drug diversion. A controlled substance agreement is suggested for use. The agreement should state that opioid medication be obtained from one physician, only one pharmacy used, and urine or serum toxicology be done when asked. The agreement should include patient responsibilities and list the risks of treatment. No early refills are recommended, and a police report should be required for lost or stolen prescriptions.[9]

There are opioid-antagonistic, partial agonist/antagonist medications that have variable binding to the opioid receptors. These medications are reserved for use by the clinician experienced in their use in the patient with opioid addiction.[10]

Opioid prescriptions are titrated to try to maximize analgesia while minimizing side effects.[4] Common side effects to opioid prescriptions (to which a tolerance usually develops) include nausea, mental clouding, and sedation. An antiemetic is commonly needed transiently. Pruritus (itching) and sweating are also common. Caution should be used for the potential risk of respiratory depression, especially when used in patients with respiratory compromise and when added to other CNS depressants. Elderly patients require careful monitoring and should be on the lowest possible dose. Constipation is a common side effect that generally requires long-term treatment. Alcohol use should be avoided when taking this class of medications. It is essential that alcohol be avoided when on some long-acting formulations, as the time release component can be disrupted and lead to fatality. For chronic pain, long acting opioids should be used as maintenance therapy with limited use of short acting opioids to control breakthrough pain. When discontinuing opioids, they should be tapered to avoid withdrawal symptoms from physical dependence. Pain, blood pressure, mental status, and respiratory status should be monitored while on these medications.[4,6]

Opioids carry a black box warning to be alert for problems of abuse, misuse, and diversion.[3] See Table 22-2 for descriptions of individual drugs.

**TABLE 22-1  NSAID classes: Proprionic acids, Acetic acid derivatives, Oxicams, Salicylates, Cox 2 inhibitors**

| Drug | Common Starting Dose | Max Dose | T1/2 (hours) | Comments |
|---|---|---|---|---|
| Acetaminophen (APAP) Tylenol® | 325-650mg q 4-6 h | 4gm/day | 2 | Caution other APAP containing products, caution in hepatic disease, and alcohol use[3,6] |
| **Propionic Acid Derivatives** | | | | |
| Ibuprofen Advil®, Motrin® | 200-800mg 3-4 times/day | 3200mg/day | 2-4 | Avoid use directly with aspirin; may negate antiplatelet effect of aspirin [3,4,5] |
| Naproxen Naprosyn®, Aleve®, Anaprox® | 250-500 mg q12h. If >65 yr old 200mg q12h | 1,500mg/day | 12-15 | GI bleeding can occur with no warning when on NSAIDS[3,4] |
| Ketoprofen Oruvail® | IR- 25-75mg q6-8h analgesic ER- 100-200 mg/day | 200mg/day | 2 | 100mg/day in severe renal disease, 150mg/day in mild renal disease Lower dose analgesic; higher dose anti-inflammatory.[3,6] |
| Flurbiprofen Ansaid® | 100mg q12h | 300mg/day | 6 | [6] |
| Oxaprozin Daypro® | 600-1200mg/d | 1800mg/day or 26mg/kg/day | 40-56 | Slow onset of action,600mg/day for renal impairment Adjust dose for hepatic impairment False positive urine toxicology for benzodiazepines has been reported.[3,6] |
| **Acetic acid derivatives** | | | | |
| Diclofenac Voltaren® | IR- 50mg q8-12h DR- 50-75 mg q 8-12h ER- 100mg/d | IR:200mg/day DR: 200mg/day ER: 100mg/day | 1-2 | Arthrotec® Diclofenac with misoprostal (200mcg) to prevent gastric and duodenal ulceration from NSAIDS dose- start 50mg 2-3x/day 200mg/day or 75 mg twice daily[3,4] Topical gel and patch available |
| Etodolac: Lodine® | IR: 200-400 mg q6-8h XL: 400-600mg/day | 1000mg/day | 7 | Has some cox-2 selectivity[3,6] |
| Ketorolac Toradol® | 10mg q4-6h | 40mg/day | 2-8 | 5 day use ONLY. Commonly used in IM form. Used for moderate to severe pain. High risk of GI and renal side effects [3,5] |
| Nabumetone Relafen ® | 500-1,000mg 1-2 times/day | 2,000mg/day | 24 | Has some cox 2 selectivity. Can take several days for onset of action to occur. Relatively low risk of GI toxicity, less antiplatelet effect[3,5,6] |
| **Enolic Acids [Oxicams]** | | | | |
| Meloxicam Mobic® | 7.5mg/day | 15mg/day | 15-20 | Has some cox 2 selectivity at low doses, less gastric side effects at 7.5mg[3,6] |
| Piroxicam Feldene® | 10-20mg/day | 20mg/day | 45-50 | Significant reduction of lithium excretion[6] |
| **COX 2 Inhibitors** | | | | |
| Celecoxib Celebrex® | 100mg qd-bid | 400mg/day | 6-12 | Selective cox 2 inhibitor[6] |
| **Salicylates** | | | | |
| Aspirin | 325-650mg q4-6h | 4g/day | 2-3 (High dose 15-30) | Increased risk of bleeding. Avoid use in children with viral illness due to risk of Reyes syndrome. Discontinue for tinnitus and hearing loss <100mg/day cardioprotective.[3,6] |
| Salsalate Amigesic, Disalcid | 500-750mg q12h | 4000mg/d 2-3 divided doses | Low dose 7-8h, high dose 15-30h | Less antiplatelet effect, may need to check salicylate levels in frail patients[3,5] |
| Diflunisal Dolobid® | 250-500mg q8-12 h | 1500mg/day | 8-12 | Less antiplatelet and GI side effect compared with aspirin[3] |
| Choline Magnesium trisalicylate: Trilisate® | 500-1000 mg q 8 h | 4500mg/day | Low dose: 2-3 High dose: 30 | QD or BID dosing when steady state is reached. No significant effect on platelet aggregation.[3,5] |

**TABLE 22-2**   Narcotic Analgesics

| Opioids | | | | |
|---|---|---|---|---|
| **Drug** | **Starting Dose** | **Max Dose** | **T1/2** | **Comments** |
| Propoxyphene Darvon® With acetaminophen= Darvocet® | Hydrochloride form 65mg q 4-6h Napsylate form 50-100mg q4-6h Darvocet-N® | Hydrochloride form 390mg/day Napsylate form 600mg/day | 6-12 parent drug Norpro- poxyphene 30-36metabolite | Avoid in severely depressed, suicidal, or addiction prone patients. Metabolized to an active metabolite norpropoxy-phene. May give false positive for methadone on a urine toxic screen. |
| Tramadol Ultram® | 50-100mgq 4-6h Can start at 12.5 -25mg dose ER 100mg qd | max-400mg/day 300mg/day for ultram ER | 6 | Slightly inhibits reuptake of serotonin, caution in combina-tion with selective serotonin reuptake inhibitors (SSRIs) Avoid use within 14 days following MAO inhibitor use. Avoid ER formulation in severe renal and hepatic impair-ment. Increased risk of seizure if on SSRI, TCA, anorectics, cyclobenzaprine, promethazine, neuroleptics, and drugs or conditions that lower the seizure threshold, and history of seizure.[4,5] |
| Tapentadol Nucynta® | 50mg q4-6 hour (equivalent to 10mg of Oxycodone) | | | Less gastric side effects |
| Morphine | Start dose: Immediate Release- 5-15mg q3-4h prn Control release- 15mg bid or qd | titrate to effect | 2-4 | Contraindication: hypersensitivity to morphine sulfate or any part of its formulation, increased intracranial pressure, severe respiratory depression, paralytic ileus, and acute or severe asthma. In renal insufficiency use cautions due to toxic build up of the metabolite.[3,4] |
| Kadian® Avinza® | sustained release morphine-10-20mg qd or bid extended release morphine-30mg qd | Max dose 1600mg/ day | | Can sprinkle kadian and avinza on applesauce Avoid alcoholic beverages as it can disrupt the control release mechanism which can be fatal. |
| Morphine Sulfate and Naltrexone Hydro-chloride Embeda® | extended release-20 mg/day has morphine 20mg and sequestered naltrex-one 0.8mg | Has 100mg/4mg capsule for opioid tolerant patients | | Avoid alcohol. When crushed, chewed, or dissolved the naltrexone is released and can precipitate withdrawal if opioid tolerant. Naltrexone is a pure opioid antagonist that competes for mu receptor with morphine if released/drug tapered with, negates effect of morphine[16] |
| Codeine Codeine with acet-aminophen Tylenol with codeine | 15-30mg q4-6h prn Control release 50mg q12h | 120mgq12h Control release: 300mgq12h | 2-4 | Contraindicated in hypersensitivity to codeine or to other phenanthrene derivative opioids Note: 10% of caucasions are unable to convert codeine to morphine due to polymorphisms in CYP2D6. This causes codeine to be ineffective for analgesia[3,4] Monitor liver enzymes and reduce dose in renal impairment. |
| Hydromorphone Dilaudid® | 2-4mg q3-4h prn | 8mg q3-4h | 1-3 | Used for breakthrough pain[3] |
| Hydrocodone Vicodin®, Norco®, Lortab®, Lorcet® | 5-10mg q4-6h prn Start 2.5-5mg q4-6h in elderly | max hydrocodone-60mg/day | 3-4 | Comes with acetaminophen, aspirin, or ibuprofen prepara-tion. CYP2D6 activity may be important for analgesic effect.[3,4] |
| Methadone Dolophine® | start 2.5-10mg q8-12h Cau-tion to increase dose In elderly start 1mg q 12h and titrate weekly | High dose up to 200mg increases risk of QT prolongation and fatal arrhythmia, prescription experi-ence helpful with its multiple drug interactions | Mean 20-35 Range 5-130 | For analgesia dose is q8-12h, with analgesic effect Shorter than half life. Accumulation can occur with repeated doses. Has renal and fecal excretion, can use in renal failure. Titration must be done slowly. Daily dose given to suppress withdrawal symptoms in physically dependant people.[14] |
| Oxycodone Percocet® (with acet-aminophen) | IR: 2.5-5mg q6h Increase to 10-30mg q6h as needed | | 2-4 | Black box warning-risk includes abuse, misuse, and diversion Available with Tylenol, aspirin, or alone[3,4] |
| Oxycodone ER Oxycontin® | ER: 10mg q 12h | Highest dose tablet 160mg | ~5 | Black box warning- problem of abuse, misuse, and diver-sion. CYP2D6 liver enzyme deficiency may Limit effectiveness Avoid with fatty meals [3, 4] |

*Continued*

**TABLE 22-2    Narcotic Analgesics—cont'd**

| | Opioids | | | |
|---|---|---|---|---|
| Drug | Starting Dose | Max Dose | T1/2 | Comments |
| Oxymorphone Opana® | IR- 5-20mg q4-6h increase 5-10mg every 3-7days ER- 5mg q12h titrate q3-7days by 5-10mg q12h | | IR: 7-9 ER: 9-11 | Contraindicated for morphine analog hypersensitivity. Same contraindication as in morphine. Avoid use in moderate to severe hepatic failure. Take 1h before or 2h after a meal swallow whole [3,4] |
| Fentanyl Transdermal Patch Duragesic® | start 12-25 micrograms q72h, adjust first dose after 3-6days | | 17 | May require q 48h dosing. Do not use in opiod naive patients Black box warning- use with CYP3A4 inhibitors such as diclofenac, may increase effects and potential respiratory depression. Serious or life threatening hypoventilation can occur. Remove for fever as amount released will be increased. May contain metal and should be removed prior to MRI. The fentanyl patch may be preferred in asthma patient. Common side effects include drowsiness and nausea and vomiting.[4] |

**TABLE 22-3    Muscle relaxants**

| Drug | Starting Dose | Max Dose | T1/2 | Comments |
|---|---|---|---|---|
| Tizanidine Zanaflex® | 2-4mg TID or hs, increased by 2mg q1-3 days | 36mg in divided doses q6-8h | 2.5 | Alpha adrenergic agonist. Increases presynaptic inhibition of motor neurons Avoid use with CYP1A2 inhibitor, such as ciprofloxacin, fluvoxamine Caution: sedation, hypotension and weakness. Monitor liver enzymes at baseline, 1,3, and 6 months and periodically, monitor renal function and blood pressure.[3,4,5] |
| Baclofen Lioresal® | 5mg TID, increase dose 5mg q 3d | 200g/day | 3.5 | Avoid abrupt withdrawal due to risk of seizure and rebound spasticity. Caution when used with TCA and MAOI. Caution with seizure history. Monitor for dizziness, headache, and confusion [3,4,5] |
| Metaxalone Skelaxin® | 400-800mg TID prn | 800mg QID | 9 | Common side effects: Headache, dizziness, nervousness/irritability, nausea and vomiting. Taking with food increases the CNS depressant effects. Adverse reaction includes hemolytic anemia and leukopenia Contraindicated with impaired hepatic or renal function or history of drug induced hemolytic anemia or other anemias. [4,11,12] |
| Methocarbamol Robaxin® | 500mg QID prn | 1.5g QID | 1-2 | Caution with renal or hepatic impairment Side effects: dizziness, metallic taste, bradycardia, headache, hypotension, nausea, nystagmus, confusion, renal impairment [3,4] |
| Orphenadrine Norflex® | 100mg bid prn | | | Antihistamine derivative Side effects: anticholinergic, nystagmus, weakness of muscle Caution: patients with arrhythmia or cardiovascular disease or in elderly Contraindicated in glaucoma or myasthenia gravis [3,4] |
| Cyclobenzaprine Flexeril® [immediate release] Amrix® [extended release] | IR: 5mg TID prn ER: 15mg QD prn | IR: 10mgTID ER: 30mg QD | IR: 18 ER: 32 | Pharmacologically related to tricyclic antidepressants Contraindication: Avoid usage with or within 14 days of an MAO inhibitor. Avoid with moderate to severe hepatic impairment, hyperthyroidism, CHF, arrhythmia, recent MI Caution: elderly, cardiovascular disease, angle closure glaucoma, urinary hesitancy/retention, increased ocular pressure, Tramadol may increase risk of neuroexcitablility and seizure Common side effect- somnolence and dry mouth, headache, and fatigue [3,4,11,12] |
| Carisprodol Soma® | 250mg-350mg TID and HS prn | | 2.4 Metabolite= 10h | Metabolite meprobamate is anxiolytic and sedating Side effects: CNS depression Caution: If poor metabolizer of CYP2C19 can get high dose High potential for abuse and dependence. Meprobamate has been classified as a controlled substance by USA federal law, schedule IV. Contraindicated: acute intermittent porphyria[4] |

## MUSCLE RELAXANTS AND ANTISPASTICITY MEDICATIONS

Medications used to treat muscle pain include muscle relaxants and antispasticity medications. The exact mechanism of action of skeletal muscle relaxants is not fully understood. They are thought to disrupt the spasm-pain-spasm cycle, and are recommended to be used for up to 2 weeks at a time. The antispasticity medications tizanidine and baclofen can be used for longer periods of time, and act centrally to reduce hypertonicity in upper motor neuron syndromes. These medications can cause sedation with CNS depression, which may disrupt physical and mental function. Caution must be taken when a patient is also on other medications that can suppress the CNS, and with the use of alcohol.[11,12] See Table 22-3 for individual drugs.

**TABLE 22-4   Antidepressants**

| Drug | Starting Dose | Max Dose | T1/2 hrs | Comments |
|---|---|---|---|---|
| **TCA** | | | | |
| Amitriptyline-elavil®, Nortriptyline-pamelor®, and Desipramine-norpramine | 10-50mg qhs Increase to 50-150mg qhs, as tolerated | 300mg 150mg 300mg | 30 30 7-60 | Avoid use with an MAOI within past 14 days, acute recovery phase after MI, or narrow angle glaucoma. Avoid concurrent use of cisapride on amitriptyline. Nortriptyline is less cardiotoxic than other TCA. Caution with hyperthyroidism, urinary hesitancy, or seizure disorder.[3,4] |
| *Norepinephrine-serotonin reuptake inhibitors* | | | | |
| Duloxetine Cymbalta® | 30mg QD Lowest dose 20mg QD | 120 mg QD or divided doses | 12 | Weak inhibitor of dopamine Indicated to treat general anxiety disorder, major depressive disorder, fibromyalgia, diabetic neuropathic pain. Monitor blood pressure and cognition and dizziness. Risk serotonin syndrome with other antidepressants, ritonavir, tramadol, buspirone sibutramine[3,4,5] |
| Venlafaxine Effexor® | XR: 25mg QD IR: | 225mg QD | 3-7 | Has been found to be more effective to treat diabetic peripheral neuropathic pain at higher doses, which puts patients at risk for elevated BP and pulse rate. Risk for serotonin syndrome as above. Indicated for major depressive disorder, generalized anxiety disorder, panic disorder, social anxiety disorder Use caution with concomitant hypertension or seizure disorder. [3,4] |
| *Norepinephreine-dopamine reuptake inhibitor* | | | | |
| BupropionSR Wellbutrin SR® | 75-150mg QD | 400mg QD or divided doses | 21 Metabolite-20-37 | Contraindicated for seizure disorder, anorexia/bulimia. Avoid use of MAOI within 14 days. Can assist in smoking cessation. CNS depressants and amantadine may increase toxic effects of drug. Adverse reactions include tachycardia, headache, insomnia, hypertension, agitation, tremor, nausea, somnolence, weight loss, and dry mouth.[3,4] |

## ANTIDEPRESSANTS

Antidepressants have been found to have analgesic properties in the treatment of fibromyalgia and neuropathic pain. Tricyclic antidepressants (TCAs) have also been found to be effective for headaches. The TCAs act by inhibiting the reuptake of norepinephrine and serotonin at the presynaptic neuronal membrane in the CNS. TCAs have anticholinergic side effects that can cause dry mouth, constipation, dizziness, tachycardia, blurred vision, and urinary retention. The risk of cerebral and cardiac intoxication increases with high doses and when combined with selective serotonin reuptake inhibitors (SSRIs). There is a risk of death from overdosage as well. Avoid use of TCAs after myocardial infarction, in the presence of bundle branch block, with cardiac depressant medications, or in narrow-angle glaucoma. The use of a secondary amine such as nortriptyline is preferred to the use of a tertiary amine such as amitriptyline, due to weaker anticholinergic effects.[2,3,12] See Table 22-4.

Selective serotonin reuptake inhibitors have fewer side effects and are a better choice for patients with cardiovascular disease. Side effects include nausea, headache, nervousness, and sexual dysfunction. The SSRIs also can cause SIADH with hyponatremia. Alcohol should be avoided with their use. Their use should be avoided in the treatment of bipolar disorder or with an MAO inhibitor. Caution should be used if there is a potential of seizure disorder. The risk of serotonin syndrome is increased when combined with tramadol, MAOIs, TCAs, other SSRIs, bupropion, buspirone, venlafaxine, ritonivir, and sibutramine.[3] (See Table 22-4.)

The norepinephrine-serotonin reuptake inhibitors (NRIs) have side effects including sedation, confusion, hypertension, nausea, sexual dysfunction, constipation, tremor, dry mouth, nervousness, and diaphoresis. Caution must be used due to the risk of serotonijn syndrome when taken with MAOIs, SSRIs, buproprion, buspirone, tramadol, sibutramine, and ritonivir. Their use should be avoided within 14 days of use of an MAOI.[3] (See Table 22-4.)

All antidepressants have a black box warning for increased risk of suicidal thinking and behavior in children, adolescents, and young adults with major depressive disorder and other psychiatric disorders. The response to treatment should be monitored. Antidepressants should be tapered when discontinued.[2-4]

## ANTICONVULSANTS

Adjuvant therapy for pain with anticonvulsants is often seen. Drugs in this class most commonly used for the treatment of pain include gabapentin, topiramate and pregabalin (Table 22-5). Gabapentin (neurontin®) is indicated for the treatment of partial seizures, epilepsy, and postherpetic neuralgia, and has off-label uses for chronic pain and and social phobias. Gabapentin's mechanism of action is not fully understood, but its effects are thought to be due to its ability to increase the inhibitory neurotransmitter effect associated with an increase in GABA. When used for pain, the dose of gabapentin is often higher than its FDA-indicated doses. A normal starting dose is 100 to 300 mg three times a day, increased by 100 mg three times a day every 3 days, to achieve a maintenance dose of 300 to 600 mg/day in divided doses. However, doses of 1200 mg/day up to 3600 mg/day in divided doses have been shown to be the most effective in the treatment of pain.[13]

Gabapentin is renally eliminated and therefore has fewer side effects than those medications metabolized by the cytochrome P enzyme system in the liver. Common side effects include somnolence, dizziness, fatigue (should subside within 2 weeks of treatment), ataxia, edema, and weight gain. Patients should not expect relief right away; 6 to 8 weeks of titration to maximize dose and then 1 to 2 weeks of stable levels typically provide some relief. Gabapentin is a preferred treatment for adjuvant therapy because of its low incidence of side effects and drug interactions, and its proof of efficacy in many clinical trials.

Topiramate (Topamax®), another anticonvulsant, also increases the inhibitory effect of GABA. Topiramate is most often used to treat several seizure disorders, but is also commonly prescribed for prophylactic treatment for migraine headaches as well as for neuropathic pain. The initial dose is 50 mg/day, titrating over 8 weeks to reach a peak of

**TABLE 22-5    Anticonvulsants**

| Drug | Starting Dose | Max Dose | T1/2 hrs | Comments |
|---|---|---|---|---|
| Gabapentin Neurontin® | 100mg TID | 3,600mg/day | 5-7 | Renal adjustment dose is necessary for those with renal disorders Abrupt discontinuation could potentiate seizures |
| Topiramate Topamax® | 50mg/day 25mg lowest dose tablet | 800mg/day | 21 | Use with acetazolamide may increase risk of kidney stones, drink plenty of water Doses as low as 50mg/d has been associated with metabolic acidosis |
| Pregablin Lyrica® | 150mg/day 25mg lowest dose | 600mg/day | 6 | Edema/weight gain |

400 mg in divided doses. Doses of 300 mg/day have been shown to be effective in treating back pain.[14] Like gabapentin, topiramate is eliminated renally; therefore, dose adjustment is needed for those who are renally impaired. Common side effects include dizziness, somnolence, ataxia, impaired concentration, confusion, fatigue, weight loss, memory difficulties, and speech difficulties. First doses of topiramate can be taken at bedtime to help with the dizziness and somnolence. Topiramate inhibits carbonic anhydrase; therefore there is a higher risk of nephrolithiasis. Patients on this medication should drink plenty of water.[18] Topiramate may increase concentrations of phenytoin and decrease levels of valproic acid.

Pregabalin (Lyrica®), one of the newer anticonvulsants/analgesics, is FDA approved for the treatment of diabetic neuropathy, fibromyalgia, and postherpetic neuropathy. Pregabalin interferes with sodium channels in the CNS, inhibiting excitatory neurotransmitter release. Like gabapentin, pregabalin has few drug interactions and a limited side-effect profile, making this drug a popular choice for the adjuvant treatment of pain. The most common side effects associated with pregabalin include dizziness, somnolence, ataxia, dry mouth, edema, and blurred vision. Doses start at 150 mg/day in divided doses and go to a maximum of 600 mg/day. As with the two other anticonvulsants, doses of pregabalin must be adjusted for those with renal impairment, and, if stopped abruptly, there may be a chance for seizures; therefore patients should always be tapered off all of these adjunct medications. Pregabalin differs from the other two anticonvulsants in that pain reduction has been shown as early as one week after starting treatment with pregabalin, unlike gabapentin, which can take several weeks to have an effect. Pregabalin also differs from topiramate in that it has been associated with weight gain and edema, whereas topiramate has been shown to decrease weight.

## CONCLUSION

It can be challenging to treat patients with chronic pain. There are multiple facets to every individual person's pain syndrome, ranging from psychosocial issues to physical deformity. It is important to treat these patients with a team approach involving the patient, his or her family, and the treating providers. The nonopioid medications are commonly used to treat mild to moderate pain. Opioid medications are sometimes used when pain is moderate to severe, usually in combination with adjuvant medications. With all medications, it is important to weigh the risk of side effects versus the benefit of use. This chapter is meant to be an overview of some of the medications more commonly used to treat pain, as well as discussing some of the potential risks to their use. Beyond this review,

the following references can be used to get more detailed information. Additional resources include:

1. American Academy of Pain Medicine: http://www.painmed.org/clinical_info/guidelines.html
2. American Pain Society: http://www.ampainsoc.org & http://www.ampainsoc.org/links/clinician1
3. Federation of State Medical Boards: http://www.fsmb.org/PAIN/resource.html[5]

## References

1. C.A. Miaskowski, R. Payne, W.K. Jones, Breakthroughs and challenges in the pharmacologic management of common chronic pain conditions, Clinician 23 (3) (2005) 1–17.
2. D. Lussier, Management of chronic pain in older persons: focus on safety, efficacy, and tolerability of pharmacologic therapy, Clinical Courier 23 (27) (2005) 1–8.
3. P. Beaulier, A. Huskey, R.K. Portenoy, D. Fishbain, 2009 Overview of analgesic agents, Pain Medicine News Special Edition (2008) 27–50.
4. C.F. Lacy, L.L. Armstrong, M.P. Goldman, L.L. Lance, Drug information handbook: a comprehensive resource for all clinicians and healthcare professionals, seventeenth ed., Lexi-Comp, Hudson, OH 2008.
5. Pharmacologic, management of persistent pain in older persons, J. Am. Geriatr. Soc. 57 (2009) 1331–1346.
6. L. Brunton, K. Parker, et al., Goodman & Gilman's manual of pharmacology and therapeutics, McGraw Hill NY, NY, 2008.
7. M. Abramowicz, G. Zuccotti, Drugs for Pain, Treatment guidelines from the medical letter, Med. Lett. Drug. Ther. 5 (56) (2007) 23–32.
8. Physicians' desk reference, sixth ed., Montvale, NJ, 2009.
9. A.M. Trescot, M.V. Boswell, et al., Opioid guidelines in the management of chronic noncancer pain, Dugs for Pain 9 (2006) 1–40.
10. S. Helm II, A.M. Trescot, J. Colson, N. Sehgal, S. Silverman, Opioid antagonists, partial agonists, and agonists/antagonists: the role of office-based detoxification, Pain Physician 11 (2008) 225–235.
11. P.P. Toth, J. Urtis, Commonly used muscle relaxant therapies for acute low back pain: a review of carisprodol, cyclobenzaprine hydrochloride, and metaxalone, Clin. Ther. 26 (2004) 1355–1367.
12. M.K. Freedman, M.F. Saulino, E.A. Overton, M.Y. Holding, I.D. Kornbluth, Interventions in chronic pain management. 5. Approaches to medication and lifestyle in chronic pain syndromes, Arch. Phys. Med. Rehabil. 89 (Suppl. 1) (2008) S56–S60.
13. K. Yildirim, M. Sisecioglu, S. Karatay, et al., The effectiveness of gabapentin in patients with chronic radiculopathy, Pain Clin. 15 (2003) 213–218.
14. M. Muehlbacher, M.K. Nickel, C. Kettler, K. Tritt, C. Lahmann, P.K. Leiberich, et al., Topiramate in treatment of patients with chronic low back pain: a randomized, double blind, placebo-controlled study, Clin. J. Pain. 22 (2006) 526.
15. R. Gallagher, Methadone: an effective, safe drug of first choice for pain management in frail older adults, Pain Med. 10 (2) (2009) 319–326.
16. Embeda CII (morphine sulfate and naltrexone hydrochloride) extended release capsules prescribing information. King Pharmaceuticals, Inc, Bristol, Tenn, 2009.
17. Anon. Acetaminophen overdose and liver injury-background and options for reducing injury. Food and Drug Administration: http://www.fda.gov/ohrms/dockets/ac/09/briefing/2009-4429b1-01-FDA.pdf
18. Laurence L. Brunton, Goodman & Gilman's The Pharmacologic Basis of Therapeutics, eleventh ed. (2006) New York.

# Yoga and the Aging Spine

# 23

*Jason A. Berkley and Anand A. Gandhi*

---

| K E Y   P O I N T S |
| --- |
| • Define yoga. |
| • Know different types of yoga. |
| • Learning yoga postures for the aging spine. |
| • Benefits of yoga for the aging spine. |
| • Muscles involved in postures. |

## INTRODUCTION

Yoga is a physical and mental discipline that originated many centuries ago in ancient India. It is derived from a Sanskrit word meaning to "take control" or "to unite." Yoga incorporates the body, mind, and spirit to achieve harmony and balance with a universal consciousness. It is now associated with a form of exercise in which techniques are learned to control the body and mind through a series of asanas (postures).

There are five principles of yoga that form the basis of teachings and disciplined methods for attaining these goals: proper exercise (asanas), proper breathing (pranayama), proper relaxation (savasana), proper diet, and meditation (dhyana). Proper exercise is achieved through asanas or postures that stretch and tone the muscles and ligaments, increase spine and joint flexibility, and ease physical tensions though movement. Proper relaxation relieves muscle tension, conserves energy, and regulates body and mind function. Proper breathing provides for good health, by using all parts of the lung to increase vital oxygen uptake. Yoga breathing exercises control of prana, the life force, which in turn increases energy levels and focuses the mind. Proper diet, consumed in moderation, nourishes the body and mind. Positive thinking and meditation facilitate a peaceful mind, while relaxing the body[1].

## CLINICAL AND BASIC SCIENCE

Yoga is classified by the National Institutes of Health as a form of Complementary and Alternative Medicine. There are many well-documented benefits to yoga, including improved flexibility and range of motion, improved posture, increased strength, decreased pain, improved balance, and improved coordination.[2] Individuals with an aging spine benefit from yoga because it "promotes a full range of motion, helps to restore flexibility, and improve circulation in muscles and around joints."[2] Yoga therapy also creates a sense of well-being through the release of beta-endorphins, breaks up chronic muscle tension and stress, and prevents osteoporosis through weight-bearing exercises.

Yoga places "an emphasis on standing poses to develop strength, stability, stamina, concentration, and body alignment."[3] Abnormalities of the deep spinal intrinsic muscles lead to postural and functional imbalances. Yoga therapy goals for the treatment of the aging spine include educating patients on proper body mechanics, correcting underlying internal malfunctions, and preventing recurrence of pain through healthy postural movement patterns. According to yoga philosophy, a person's age is determined by the flexibility of the spine and not by the number of years lived.[4] Yoga benefits the aging spine by imparting flexibility to the spine, firming up the skin, eliminating tension from the body, and strengthening abdominal muscles.

There are many different types of yoga that are practiced throughout the world. Hatha Yoga is what most people in the West associate with the word "yoga," and is practiced for mental and physical health throughout the West. In the aging spine, individuals should focus their attention on the following types of Hatha Yoga: Iyengar, Ashtanga, Bikram, and Vini. Iyengar Yoga places great attention to detail and precise focus on body alignment with the use of props, such as cushions, benches, blocks or straps. It focuses on the structural alignment of the physical body through the development of postures with use of props to assist individuals that lack flexibility or compensate for injuries. Ashtanga Yoga allows for individual specialization of yoga moves that link breath and movement in flowing exercises. This form of yoga focuses on powerful flowing movements that increase flexibility, balance, and concentration to rehabilitated spines. Bikram Yoga is conducted in a very warm environment, which maintains body heat, making the spine more flexible by allowing the tissues to stretch. Room temperatures average 105°F (40°C), which is not always suitable for individuals with significant heart disease. Vini Yoga involves synchronizing the breath with progressive series of postures, which in turn produce intense internal heat and a profuse, purifying sweat that detoxifies muscles and organs. The flowing movements create heat in the body, which removes toxins and improves tendon, tissue, and muscle flexibility.[5]

Limited scientific research exists examining the benefits of yoga therapy for individuals with low back pain and aging spines. One study by Vidyasagar et al. looked at the effect of Hatha Yoga therapy in individuals with nonspecific low back pain. Their findings reveal that after completing 9 weeks of yoga therapy, the majority of the selected participants noted pain relief, although the study lacked long-term follow-up and a description on assessment of pain status.[6] Another study by Williams et al. looked at chronic low back pain patients who participated in a 16-week Iyengar Yoga therapy. Their results show less pain, less functional disability, and a decrease in pain medication usage after 3 months.[7] A more recent study by Tekur et al. examined the effect of short-term intensive yoga therapy versus physical exercise therapy in individuals with chronic low back pain. Their findings show that 7 days of intensive yoga therapy improved spinal flexibility in terms of flexion, extension, and lateral rotation better than physical therapy in individuals with chronic back pain.[8] Another study by Sherman et al. compared 12 weeks of home yoga therapy with 12 weeks of a home exercise program and educational material. Their findings show that over 3 to 6 months, yoga is more effective than traditional exercises or an educational reference for improving function and pain in individuals with chronic low back pain.[9] One study by Greendale et al. showed that elderly women with an excessive curvature of the upper part of the spine may benefit from practicing yoga. They report that specific yoga postures that target the upper back appear to help straighten the spine and restore physical function in patients with hyperkyphosis.[10]

Yoga-based spinal exercises attempt to correct dysfunctions of head, spine, thoracic cage, and pelvis. Altering leg positions changes the movement at different levels of the spine; flexed legs target the thoracic region, while extended legs target the lumbar segments. Correct posture and proper breathing enhance spinal stability. Yoga therapy exercises require relaxation of the rib cage through complete activation of the diaphragm in inhalation. This will activate the deep spinal stabilizers, including the abdominal wall (core training), diaphragm, multifidi, and pelvic muscles, which will increase abdominal pressure while reducing axial pressure on the vertebral discs and spine. The goal of yoga-based spinal exercises is to restore normal motor function.[11] There are certain exercises that can be used for both strengthening and stretching of the spine. It is important to learn these postures correctly, as poor technique may cause injury (Tables 23-1 and 23-2).

As we now know, there are many factors that influence and are associated with degeneration of the spine. In addition to normal aging, high BMI, high LDLc, occupational lifting, and sports activities are associated with degenerative disease.[12] These factors can be either controlled or greatly reduced with the multi-pronged benefits of yoga, thereby curbing the progression of the aging spine. Aside from disc degeneration, other factors lend themselves to the overall process of the aging spine. Spinal stenosis, lumbar facet arthritis, and osteopenia/osteoporosis play a role in the spine as it ages. Although no modality can prevent these changes from occurring, the quality of life of the

patient is what is primarily at stake. Pain is the obvious result, yet the emotional toll is usually not taken into account. The benefit of yoga has been shown to not only positively influence the physical effects of the aging spine, but also the emotional aspect. The mind and body are connected in many ways. The pain cycle is a double-feedback loop: when a person experiences pain, his or her mood/depression worsens. As a result, he may experience more pain symptoms. This loop continues until the cycle can be broken. Yoga is one modality which can be used to accomplish this goal. Although further studies are needed, it seems "the initial indications are of potentially beneficial effects of yoga interventions on depressive disorders."[13]

Therapeutic benefits of Yoga in individuals with an aging spine uses a three headed approach to alleviate back pain, including yoga therapy, breathing, and relaxation. The tenets of yoga therapy include deep stretching postures that stretch and relax the spinal musculature, along with core strengthening that builds up muscles that support the spine (Figures 23-1 through 23-7). Yoga therapy postures also correct structural irregularities in the spine and increase flexibility of the spinal vertebrae. Specific yoga

### TABLE 23-1 Lumbar Exercises

| Muscles Involved | Yoga Stretching Exercises | Yoga Strengthening Exercises |
|---|---|---|
| Multifidi/ | Cobra | Extended Triangle |
| Lumbar paraspinals | Extended Triangle | Side Angle Pose |
| Abdominals | Upward Stretch Legs | Cobra |
| | Boat | Bow |
| Oblique/Intercostals | Extended Triangle | Extended Triangle |
| | Spinal Twist | Spinal Twist |
| | Abdominal Twist | Abdominal Twist |

### TABLE 23-2 Cervical Exercises

| Muscles Involved | Yoga Stretching Exercises | Yoga Strengthening Exercises |
|---|---|---|
| Sternocleidomastoid/ | Spinal Twist | Twisting Poses |
| Cervical paraspinals | Extended Triangle | |
| | Camel | |
| Trapezius | Camel | Bridge |
| | Cobra | Shoulder Stand |

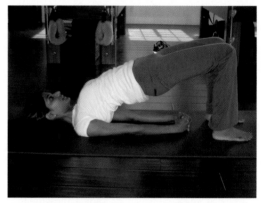

■ **FIGURE 23-2** The Bridge pose.

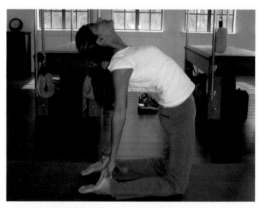

■ **FIGURE 23-3** The Camel pose.

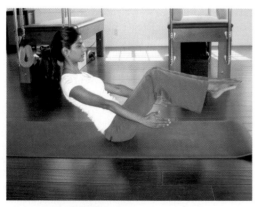

■ **FIGURE 23-1** The Boat pose.

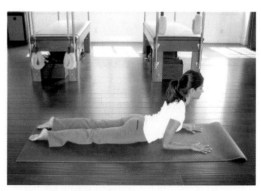

■ **FIGURE 23-4** The Cobra pose.

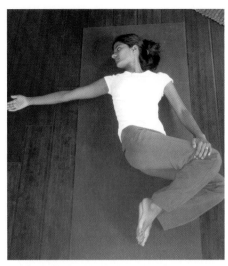

■ **FIGURE 23-5**   The Spinal Twist pose.

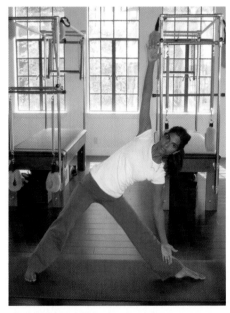

■ **FIGURE 23-6**   The Extended Triangle pose.

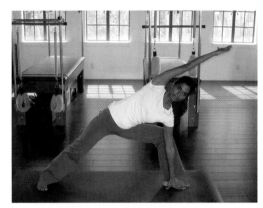

■ **FIGURE 23-7**   The Side Angle pose.

understanding of the fundamentals. There is concern that beginners will be unable to obtain correct alignment of the spinal vertebrae and musculature in certain poses without the guidance of an experienced teacher.[14] Patients who have been diagnosed with advanced spinal stenosis should avoid extreme extension of the spine, such as back bends in yoga. Patients with advanced cervical spine disease should avoid doing headstands and shoulder stands in yoga. It is extremely important to consult your physician before participating in a yoga regimen. You should also consult a yoga expert (yogi) to teach proper technique and limitations with the aging spine. Yoga therapy movements are fluid in nature. Great care must be taken if an individual experiences pain, which is not part of the normal yoga cycle.

## ACKNOWLEDGMENT

The authors thank Neha Shah, DPT, for demonstrating the postures in the illustrations.

## References

1. ABC of Yoga. http://www.abc-of-yoga.com Accessed February 1, 2010.
2. LC, Yoga basics for older adults, Functional 3 (6), 2005.
3. KW, LS, JP, Therapeutic application of iyengar yoga for healing chronic low back pain, Int J. Yoga Therapy 13 (2003) 55–67.
4. Yoga for Life. http://www.yoga-for-life.org Accessed February 1, 2010.
5. KB. http://www.spine-health.com/wellness/yoga-pilates-tai-chi/types-yoga Accessed February 1, 2010.
6. J. Vidyasagar, Bp, VR, Pr, MJ, KS, Effects of yoga practices in non-specific low back pain, Clin. Proc. NIMS. 4 (1989) 160–164.
7. K.A. Williams, J. Petronis, D. Smith, D. Goodrich, et al., Effect of Iyengar yoga therapy for chronic low back pain, Pain 115 (2005) 107–117.
8. P. Tekur, C. Singphow, H.R. Nagendra, N. Raghuram, Effect of short-term intensive yoga program on pain, functional disability and spinal flexibility in chronic low back pain: a randomized control study, J. Altern. Complem. Med. 14 (6) (2008) 637–644.
9. K.J. Sherman, D.C. Cherkin, J. Erro, D.L. Miglioretti, R.A. Deyo, Comparing yoga, exercise, and a self-care book for chronic low back pain: a randomized, controlled trial, Ann. Intern. Med. 143 (12) (2005) 849–856.
10. G.A. Greendale, A. McDivit, A. Carpenter, L. Seeger, M.H. Huang, Yoga for women with hyperkyphosis: results of a pilot study, Am. J. Public Health 92 (10) (2002) 1611–1614.
11. C. Liebenson, Rehabilitation of the spine, Lippincott Williams & Wilkins, Baltimore, 2007.
12. M. Hangai, K. Kaneoka, S. Kuno, S. Hinotsu, et al., Factors associated with lumbar intervertebral disc degeneration in the elderly, Spine J. 8 (5) (2008) 732–740.
13. K. Pilkington, G. Kirkwood, H. Rampes, J. Richardson, Yoga for depression: the research evidence, J. Affect. Disorders 89 (1-3) (2005) 13–24.
14. Get rid of your lower back pain with the help of yoga. www.yogawiz.com Accessed February 1, 2010.

therapy postures that are of benefit to the aging spine include: Trikona Asana (The Triangle), Tada Asana (Mountain Pose), Ek Pada Asana (One-Legged Posture), Bala Asana (Child Pose), Bhujanga Asana (Cobra Pose), and the Parivritta Parshvakona Asana (Half-Revolved-Belly Pose).[14] Breathing control techniques can eliminate additional stress that is placed on the spine and back due to irregular respiratory patterns. Meditation and relaxation alleviate back pain not only by removing tension and stress from the muscles, but also by battling pain on a psychological level.

## CONCLUSION

Yoga can benefit individuals with an aging spine in many different ways, if practiced under proper guidance. However, patients can actually do more harm than good by engaging in various yoga poses without a proper

# PART 4

# Surgical Treatment Modalities: Cervical Spine

# 24

# Cervical Stenosis: Radiculopathy – Review of Concepts, Surgical Techniques, and Outcomes

*Zachary A. Smith, Sean Armin, and Larry T. Khoo*

---

### KEY POINTS

- The clinical presentation of spondylosis can range from no symptoms to radiculopathy or severe myelopathy.

- Diagnostic imaging modalities include plain radiography and magnetic resonance imaging (MRI). Computed tomography with intrathecal contrast may play a role in evaluating certain disease processes poorly imaged by MRI.

- The role of neurophysiologic testing with motor and somatosensory evoked potentials is not clearly defined, but may prove beneficial in measuring subclinical disease and predicting outcome following surgery.

- Conservative medical management is indicated for patients with minimal symptoms, with surgical intervention reserved for patients with significant disability and/or a progressive clinical course.

- Surgical techniques include anterior and posterior decompression, which have demonstrated greater than 85% efficacy in the treatment of neurological symptoms. The addition of arthrodesis and instrumentation may yield better neck pain scores and radiographic lordosis at while increasing cost, morbidity, and adjacent segment degeneration (ASD).

- Preliminary data on cervical artificial disc replacement demonstrate equal efficacy to classic anterior cervical discectomy and fusion in relieving symptoms with trends toward improved recovery and decreased soft-tissue complications. As yet, the long-term ability of these prosthetic devices to decrease the incidence of ASD remains undefined.

## INTRODUCTION

Cervical spondylosis is a progressive degenerative process resulting in pathologic changes in the intervertebral discs and surrounding structures[1]. Such changes include intervertebral disc protrusion, osteophyte formation, and hypertrophy of the lamina, ligaments, and hypophyseal joints.[2,3] Clinical onset can begin as early as the third decade, with progression continuing into the eighth decade.[1] Radiographic signs of spondylosis are evident in 50% of the population by the fifth decade, while prevalence is estimated at 98% for people over 70.[4] Secondary myelopathy is considered to be the most common cause of spinal cord dysfunction in patients over 55.[5]

The effects of spondylosis can range from subclinical symptoms to primary root impingement (radiculopathy) and myelopathy. Proper diagnosis depends on meticulous history-taking, thorough physical examination, and the use of appropriate imaging, neurophysiologic, and laboratory tests. The natural history of cervical spondylosis is not well understood[6], and treatment of spondylosis includes both conservative medical management and surgical intervention. A variety of surgical procedures have been well described including anterior and posterior approaches with or without fusion. This chapter reviews the relevant anatomy, pathophysiology, symptomatology, diagnosis, natural history, and management of cervical spondylosis.

## REGIONAL ANATOMY OF THE CERVICAL SPINE

Normal anatomy of the cervical spine consists of vertebrae, intervertebral discs, ligaments and joints, neural elements, and surrounding soft tissue and vascular structures.

### Osseous Components

The bony cervical spine is composed of seven vertebrae (Figure 24-1A-C). The lower five segments (C3-C7) are similar in morphology, while the first two segments (C1 and C2) are anatomically distinct. The first cervical segment, the atlas (C1), is ring-shaped and articulates primarily with the occipital condyles above and the superior facets of the second cervical segment below. The second cervical segment, the axis (C2), has a cone-shaped projection (the odontoid process) that articulates with the anterior arch of C1. The remaining cervical vertebrae (C3-C7) share similar architecture; the vertebral bodies are roughly cylindrical in shape and increase in size from rostral to caudal. From each body projects an uncinate process superiorly, which indents the posterolateral margins of its respective intervertebral disc. The transverse processes project anterolaterally and house the foramen through which the vertebral arteries pass. The spinal cord runs through the spinal canal, which is formed by the posterior elements including the pedicles, the facet joints, the lamina, and the spinous process. At each level, nerve roots exit the canal between vertically adjacent pedicles (Figure 24-1C,D)

The unique morphology of C1 and C2, as well as the increasing vertebral body size of the lower segments, may contribute to the pathogenesis of spondylosis. The anteroposterior diameter of the canal is generally larger at C1 and C2 when compared to the lower vertebrae; thus the spinal cord is estimated to occupy only one third of the atlantal ring at C1, while it occupies up to three fourths of the canal in the lower segments. This variability may account for the predisposition for spinal stenosis with symptomatology at the C4-C7 levels.[7]

### Intervertebral Discs

The vertebrae are linked together by intervertebral discs, which provide a stable yet flexible architecture. The discs normally account for 22% of the height of the spinal column and function to spread axial loading forces. Each disc is composed of four elements: the nucleus pulposus, the anulus fibrosus, and the two cartilaginous endplates. The nucleus pulposus accounts for 40% of the cross-sectional area of the intervertebral disc and is located toward the posterior aspect of the disc. It consists of primarily of Type II collagen fibers and mucopolysaccharide ground substance. The anulus fibrosus is made of fibrocartilage that surrounds the nucleus pulposus in a concentric lamellar fashion. It is attached directly to the vertebral bodies via Sharpey fibers, which project from the outer lamella to the epiphyses. The anulus also attaches to the anterior and posterior longitudinal ligaments, but the posterior attachment weakens with age, which may lead to a predisposition

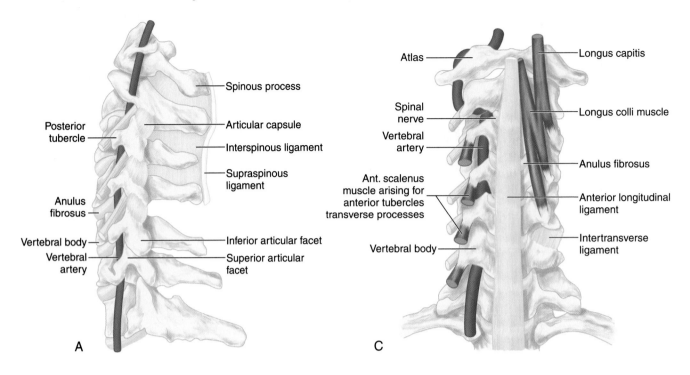

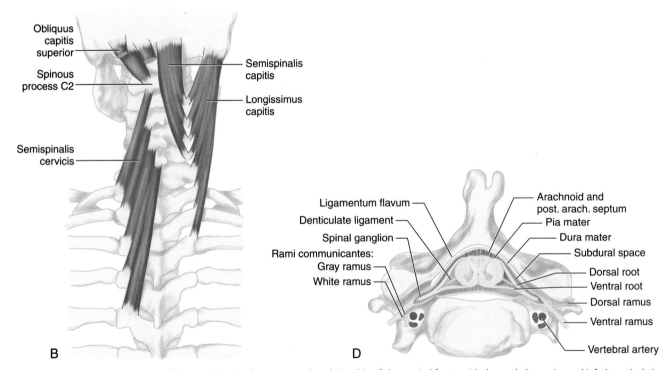

■ **FIGURE 24-1**   **A,** A lateral view of the cervical spine demonstrates the relationship of the cervical facets with the angled superior and inferior articulating facets and their encasing articular capsules. The anterior intervertebral discs and bodies are also seen. The spinous processes and dorsal arches are significantly stabilized by the dorsal interspinous and supraspinous ligaments. **B,** A posterior view of the cervical spine demonstrates the complex arrangement of the dorsal stabilizing musculoligamentous complex and its attendant musculature. **C,** An anterior view of the cervical spine demonstrates the anterior longitudinal ligament connecting the vertebral bodies at the level of the discs as well as the intertransverse ligaments between the transverse processes. The relationship of the vertebral arteries coursing rostrocaudally through the foramina transversaria is also shown. **D,** An axial view of a cervical segment shows the spinal canal containing the neural elements which are stabilized and held in place within the subdural space by the dentate ligaments. The nerve roots with their dorsal root, ventral roots, and spinal ganglia are shown as well. The dorsal arch of the ligamentum flavum lies directly below the neural elements. Again shown are the vertebral arteries within the foramina transversaria with their relationship to the nerve root and the uncinate joint.

toward central posterior disc protrusions. The endplates are cartilaginous structures situated between the nucleus pulposus and the trabecular bone of the vertebral bodies. Perforating fibers anchor the endplates to the nucleus and serve as a conduit for nutrients to enter the disc.

## Ligaments and Joints

The cervical spine allows for greater mobility than the thoracic or lumbar regions. Various ligaments reinforce the cervical spine during flexion, extension, and rotational movement. The anterior and posterior longitudinal ligaments extend the entire length of the spine and provide stability to the intervertebral joints. The anterior longitudinal ligament attaches to the ventral aspect of the vertebral column and is apposed to the intervertebral discs, while the posterior longitudinal ligament courses along the dorsal aspect of the vertebral column and merges fibers with the annulus as well as the adjacent endplates (see Figure 24-1C). The ligamentum flavum attaches to the anterior surface of each vertebral arch and to the superior edge of each lamina, and covers each facet joint. Its function is to stabilize the neck during flexion (see Figure 24-1D). Due to its considerable elastic capacity, the ligamentum flavum can normally stretch during flexion without compromising the integrity of the spinal canal. Additional ligaments such as the supraspinous and interspinous ligaments serve see further stabilize the spinal column (see Figure 24-1B).

The superior and inferior facets comprise the articular pillars (see Figure 24-1A). In the cervix, these joints are angled obliquely and inferiorly and are oriented perpendicular to the vertebral bodies. Each superior facet articulates anteriorly to its inferior process, forming synovial joints, each with a fibrous capsule.

## Vascular Supply

The cervical cord's vascularity is provided primarily by the paired vertebral arteries, which arise from the subclavian arteries in the thorax and course superiorly to form the basilar artery at the base of the pons. Branches from the vertebral arteries form the anterior spinal artery, which courses along the ventral median fissure of the spinal cord, and is responsible for supplying the anterior two thirds of the cord. The vertebral arteries also give rise to the paired, posterior spinal arteries, which travel along the dorsal aspect of the cord (see Figure 24-1D).[8] Cervical medullary arteries branching from the vertebral arteries create variable anastomoses within the canal and contribute additional vascular supplies.

## PATHOPHYSIOLOGY OF CERVICAL SPONDYLOSIS

Cervical spondylosis is a multifaceted degenerative process that can affect all components of the spine including the intervertebral discs, facet joints, ligaments, spinal soft tissues, and bony elements. The initial pathological changes in spondylosis originate in the disc space. The proposed mechanism of disc degeneration occurs secondary to an alteration in the protein composition of the disc matrix. With aging, the molecular weight of the glycoproteins in the disc decreases along with the chondroitin sulfate content. The net effect is a change in the osmotic properties of the disc, with decreased inflow of fluid. Dehydration of the disc leads to loss of height, as well as loss of expansion capability under axial loading. As the disc progressively loses the ability to distribute normal loads of pressure, the nucleus pulposus becomes predisposed to fragmentation. Fragmentation of the nucleus combined with increasing weakness in the annulus with aging can result in herniation of disc material into the spinal canal (Figure 24-2A).

Loss of disc height not only contributes to disc herniation, but also results in osteophyte formation. As the annulus bulges under the impaired function of the damaged disc, the periosteum of the adjacent vertebral bodies undergoes reactive processes. Hyperostosis of the subperiosteal bone generates a spondylotic ridge or osteophyte, which can impinge on the ventral canal to cause cord compression. Spondylosis also leads to hyperostosis of the posterior elements. In the dorsolateral spinal column, decreased disc height causes pathological changes in the facets with destruction of the joints and resultant hypertrophy. Abnormal mobility of the spine contributes to osteophyte formation in the neural foramina, leading to peripheral nerve compression and radiculopathy. As spondylosis progresses, the ligamentum

flavum becomes hypertrophic and loses elasticity. During hyperextension especially, the ligament tends to buckle inward, contributing additionally to canal compromise.[10]

The mechanism by which spondylosis leads to cord injury is not entirely understood; the pathophysiology is complicated by the common absence of symptoms in patients with radiographic evidence of significant disease.[11] Spondylosis with disc herniation, osteophyte formation, and ligament hypertrophy clearly reduces the anterior-posterior diameter of the spinal canal. As expected, patients with congenitally narrow canals are therefore more prone to be symptomatic. Studies have suggested that the normal canal diameter is 17 to 18 mm (C3 -C7) and that a reduction in axial diameter to 11 to 13 mm is more likely to lead to myelopathy.[10] Abnormal cervical motion and instability following degenerative changes may exacerbate cord injury. With neck flexion, the cord may move against the ventral spondylotic ridges causing cord damage. Extension may lead to cord strangulation between the folded ligamentum flavum posteriorly and osteophytes or herniated disc material anteriorly (Figure 24-2B).

There is considerable debate as to whether cord injury is due to direct compression of neural structures or secondary to extrinsic compromise of vascular supply. The vascular ischemia theory was first proposed in 1954 by Brain.[2] Breig noted later that in cervical flexion, mechanical flattening of the spinal cord occurred, with consequent decreased patency of the anterior sulcal and transverse arteries.[12] Other authors have noted that anterior-posterior compression of the spinal cord in both pathologic and experimental studies resulted in stretching of the transverse vessels and terminations of the anterior spinal artery with ischemia of the anterior two thirds of the cord.[8,13,14,15] Clinically, Allen noted that the cervical spinal cord blanched during flexion in patients with spondylosis.[16]

Human pathologic studies of cervical spondylosis demonstrate that canal compromise with cord compression results in characteristic histological changes. Ono et al. found that compression of the cord is associated with extensive destruction of both gray and white matter, with consequent demyelinization.[17] Interestingly, the areas of the cord most encroached upon tend to display histopathologic evidence of severe infarction. Ogino et al. demonstrated an association between localized infarction of the gray matter and a decrease in the anterior-posterior canal ratio to below 20%.[18] As cord injury secondary to spondylosis progresses, tissue destruction leads to gliosis, scarring, cystic degeneration, and neuronal cell loss.

In conclusion, the pathophysiology of spondylosis appears to be the result of several degenerative processes that occur in conjunction. The decrease in disc height leads to herniation, reactive hyperostosis with osteophyte formation, and hypertrophy of the ligaments. These events, along with abnormal cervical motion, compromise the cord within the canal. The mechanism of cord injury is still not well understood but appears to be related to impaired vascular supply leading to neuronal ischemia. As spondylosis becomes more severe, pathological changes of the cord become evident: demyelination, gliosis, cystic degeneration, and neuronal cell loss.

## CLINICAL PRESENTATION OF CERVICAL SPONDYLOSIS

Cervical spondylosis can present with a variety of clinical syndromes. Pain may be localized to the neck or display a radicular pattern. Weakness can occur as a mixture of upper and lower motor neuron findings. Lower motor signs generally predominate at the level of the lesion, while upper motor findings are present at segments below. Atrophy and diminished reflexes are common in the involved upper extremity. Lower segmental involvement presents as hyperactive reflexes, increased tone, clonus, or (most commonly) abnormal gait. Sensory impairment is highly variable, with patchy sensory loss in both the upper and lower extremities occurring along three neural pathways. Pain and temperature sense are often affected contralateral to the lesion, due to spinothalamic tract fibers crossing at levels near their entrance into the canal. The posterior columns, which convey position and vibration sense, decussate in the brain stem and therefore are often affected ipsilateral to the lesion. Spondylosis can also affect the dorsal root as it enters the canal, resulting in impaired dermatomal sensation.

Myelopathy is a common and severe manifestation of cervical spondylosis.[5] Symptoms may be slowly progressive and associated with intermittent periods of remission and exacerbation.[20] Clinical presentation generally

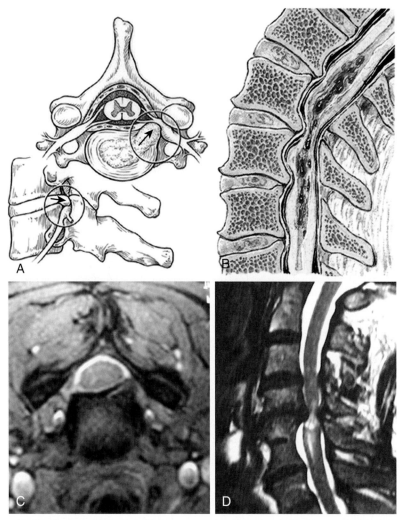

■ **FIGURE 24-2** **A,** A posterolateral disc herniation is shown in this spondylytic cervical spine segment, causing compression of the nerve root at the level of the foramen without compromise of the cord itself. When symptomatic, such lesions are typically associated primarily with radicular complaints. **B,** Multilevel spondylytic osteophytes combined with chronic disc herniations contribute to a severely narrowed central canal that can be associated with central hemorrhage and myelomalacia. Clinical syndromes include central cord syndrome and cervical myelopathy. **C,** A T2-weighted axial MR image of a cervical posterolateral disc herniation provides an example of root compression in cervical spondylosis. The cord, although displaced, is not significantly compressed. **D,** A T2-weighted sagittal MR image demonstrates multilevel spondylytic changes with disc herniations, ultimately causing significant canal stenosis and spinal cord compression. T2-signal changes within the parenchyma of the spinal cord demonstrate injury to the substance of the neural elements.

consists of lower motor neuron involvement at the level of the lesion, with upper motor neuron signs at segments below. Upper extremity involvement is often unilateral, while that of the lower extremity is bilateral. Lower motor neuron findings include weakness and atrophy with progressive loss of dexterity, particularly at the level of the lesion. The lower extremities may demonstrate spasticity, clonus, hyperreflexia, or abnormal gait, with a positive Babinski sign. Sensory disturbances are poorly localized, generally affecting the lower extremities and trunk, while rarely involving cervical levels.[20] Bowel and bladder impairment are rare, but indicate poor prognosis.

Due to the complex symptomatology of cervical degenerative disease, Crandall et al. described five clinical syndromes to aid in clustering various findings.[21]

1. Transverse myelopathy: involvement of the corticospinal, spinothalamic, and dorsal column tracts, as described earlier.
2. Principally motor symptoms: corticospinal tract involvement with minimal sensory deficit.
3. B rown-Séquard syndrome: hemi-cord disease affecting ipsilateral motor strength, ipsilateral proprioception and vibration sense, and contralateral pain and temperature sense. Generally reflects an asymmetric narrowing of the canal.

4. Central cord syndrome: motor and sensory deficit predominant in the upper extremity.
5. Radiculopathy: direct root compression secondary to a herniated disc or spondylotic change.[22] Patients typically present with sensory disturbances in a radicular pattern, specific motor group weakness, and decreased specific reflex. With chronic disease, profound weakness and atrophy may be present.

Among other possible findings is the "numb, clumsy hand."[23] This condition involves a glove-like distribution of primary sensory loss combined with motor loss. Tandem spinal stenosis simultaneously affects the cervical and lumbar regions, presenting with a trio of symptoms: neurogenic claudication, gait abnormality, and mixed upper and lower motor neuron signs.[24] Vertebral artery insufficiency can present with dizziness and unsteadiness when the head is rotated.[25] Rarely, large osteophytes can cause dysphagia due to direct compression of the esophagus.[5]

It is important to consider other neurological conditions that may exhibit symptoms mimicking cervical spondylosis. Any mass lesion within the spinal canal that compresses the cord or nerve roots can manifest with such findings. Extradural, intradural, and osseous tumors of the spine, as well as infectious processes such as epidural abscesses, can compromise canal integrity. Fortunately, these conditions can generally be distinguished from cervical spondylosis via effective MRI. Multiple sclerosis is another condition commonly confused with cervical spondylosis, and a mixed picture of upper and lower motor neuron signs is a hallmark finding in amyotrophic lateral sclerosis. Correctly diagnosing cervical spondylosis depends on detailed history-taking, complete neurological examination, and diagnostic measures including imaging, neurophysiology, and laboratory tests.

## DIAGNOSTIC MODALITIES

### Neuroradiology

Plain film radiographs of the cervical spine are traditionally performed with a series of anteroposterior, lateral, and oblique films. Relevant findings on lateral films include the height of disc spaces and evidence of osteophytes protruding into the spinal canal. Also of import is the anteroposterior diameter of the canal, as it is highly indicative of disease severity in patients with symptomatic spondylosis.[22] The diameter is determined to be the shortest distance from the dorsal aspect of the vertebral body (including any posteriorly projecting discs or spurs) to the spino laminar line, with 12 mm in the lower cervical region being the lowest normal value.[26] This calculation, however, is manipulated by the magnification of the film — an obstacle circumvented by an alternative method described as Pavlov's ratio.[27] This number represents the ratio of the anteroposterior diameter of the spinal canal divided by the anteroposterior diameter of the corresponding vertebral body. A normal value is approximately 1, with values of 0.8 or less suggesting compression. This method allows quick appraisal of the integrity of the canal without being influenced by magnification.

Computed tomography allows for better assessment of the spinal canal than plain radiography.[26] CT axial plane images have been shown to provide an accurate estimate of the canal diameter while also differentiating laterally projecting osteophytes and midline calcifications (i.e., as seen in OPLL).[28] CT scans alone, however, poorly visualize the soft tissue structures within the spinal canal. With the addition of intrathecal contrast, CT myelography can allow for quantification of cord compression at every level. CT myelography has been effective in correlating symptomatic disease with cross-sectional area of the canal.[29]

Magnetic resonance imaging is the most recent advancement in the radiographic evaluation of cervical spondylosis, offering the advantages of imaging in multiple planes and improved definition of neural and ligamentous elements. Disc herniations are readily demonstrated and often have associated signal changes (see Figure 24-2C). MRI also distinguishes cervical spondylosis from disease processes that mimic it clinically, such as tumors, epidural masses, demyelination, and syrinx. The complete neuraxis can also be easily imaged if necessary. In comparison to CT myelography, MRI is a safer, less invasive procedure, making MRI the procedure of choice for initial evaluation of radiculopathy or myelopathy.[28,30,31]

Unlike conventional x-ray technology, MRI allows for the demonstration of pathological processes within the spinal cord parenchyma. Intramedullary signal intensity changes have been noted at segments adjacent to areas of spondylotic compression[32] (see Figure 24-2D). In experimental models, histological confirmation of cord injury is found at levels demonstrating MRI signal change with maximum mechanical compression.[33] The cause of signal change is attributed to myelomalacia, gliosis, and edema.[32,34,35] Clinical data correlating the degree of signal change with outcome are confusing at best, but high-intensity lesions are thought to suggest poor prognosis.[34,36,37,38]

MRI still poses problems in diagnosing certain degenerative changes. Small, lateral osteophytes can be difficult to distinguish from lateral disc herniations.[28] Also, midline calcifications seen in ossification of the posterior longitudinal ligament (OPLL) may be poorly visualized. In addition to these limitations, the high incidence of degenerative abnormalities imaged in asymptomatic individuals also proves problematic. Teresi et al. found disc protrusions in 57% and spinal cord impingement in 26% of patients over 65 years of age when clinical evidence of cervical spondylosis was absent.[39] So although imaging techniques allow direct visualization of disease progression, determination of patient prognosis and indication for surgical intervention is not made by such modalities alone.

### Neurophysiology

Neurophysiological evaluation of cervical spondylosis may prove a valuable supplement to other findings. Recent interest in these functional diagnostic modalities stems from the difficulty in interpreting common radiographic abnormalities in asymptomatic patients. Neurophysiological testing may also assist in predicting prognosis and measuring response to treatment. In evaluating cervical spondylosis, electromyography (EMG) allows differentiation of radiculopathy from neuropathy, and peripheral from central nerve entrapment.[40] EMG also helps localize affected nerve roots by demonstrating conduction abnormalities in muscles innervated by adjacent cervical segments. This technique may assist in preoperative determination of levels requiring decompression. Somatosensory evoked potentials (SSEPs) involve electrical stimulation of peripheral sensory nerves while recording evoked activity from either the spinal cord or sensory cortex. Clinical studies showing spondylotic involvement of the posterior columns suggest that SSEPs may help appraise the functional status of the sensory system. Leblhuber et al. found that dermatomal SSEPs were altered at levels corresponding to cervical segments with degenerative changes.[44] Yet these neurophysiologic and radiographic abnormalities were also found in asymptomatic patients. Although experimental models have found a temporal relationship between changes in SSEPs and the onset of neurological deficit,[33] the diagnostic value of SSEPs has been challenged through studies that found median and ulnar nerve abnormalities in only a small percentage of patients with symptomatic cervical spondylotic myelopathy.[42,43]

Cortical motor evoked potential (MEP) recording has been suggested as a more sensitive test of spinal cord dysfunction than SSEPs,[44] due to the predominance of motor findings in patients with cervical spondylosis.[44] MEP abnormalities may also be detected in patients before the onset of clinical symptoms.[43-45] In comparison, MEP can detect abnormalities in 84% of patients with radiographic cord compression, while SSEPs show dysfunction in only 25%.[46]

The role of electrophysiological studies in diagnosing cervical spondylosis or predicting outcome is not entirely clear at this time. Cusick suggests that combining MEP and SSEP recordings allows for evaluation of long tract function of both ascending and descending white matter. These two tests provide insight into the integrity of two spinal cord areas often affected by spondylosis. By integrating electrophysiological studies and radiographs, patient vulnerability to neurological deficit may be estimated, as well as optimal timing of surgical intervention for patients with subclinical disease.[44]

## NATURAL HISTORY OF CERVICAL RADICULOPATHY

The natural history of cervical spondylosis is not well described. Since early descriptions of the condition, surgery was widely accepted as the treatment of choice, and no studies were made to determine long-term progression. Only a few investigators have attempted to formulate a likely picture using patients treated with a collar.

Lees and Aldren-Turner classified cervical spondylosis as a relatively benign condition.[19] The common course experienced by their patients was characterized by long periods of stable symptomatology interspersed with short bouts of deterioration; chronic, gradual deterioration was rare. They also found that myelopathy did not develop in a group of patients presenting solely with radiculopathy. In following studies, Nurick agreed with the findings of Lees and Aldren-Turner, and also found that patients who had undergone surgical laminectomy had no significant improvement over those with no treatment.[3] Thirdly, he realized that age of onset served to significantly determine the prognosis for later deterioration.

When comparing 48 patients who underwent surgery with those in Lees and Aldren-Turner's study, the other authors found that 70% of patients enjoyed improved conditions from cervical laminectomy. Their conclusion was that patients with moderate or severe symptoms due to cervical spondylosis benefit greatly from surgery, whereas those with mild disability are not likely to be significantly helped. Doubt was later cast upon Lees and Aldren-Turner's theories in that they were thought to have bias toward milder cases.

Scoville found that the best outcome of surgery was in patients treated within one year of onset of symptoms.[48] He further elaborated on Lees and Aldren-Turner's model in claiming that patients should be treated surgically, shortly after mild disability was noticed, and before further progression. He did admit that mild cases were adequately treated conservatively.

Smith and Robinson more recently described the course of cervical spondylosis that is most accepted today.[47] They found that motor complaints tended to be more permanent than neck, bladder, and sensory symptoms. Motor findings were also predominant in the lower extremities, and sensory in the upper. Although most of their patients followed an episodic but unpredictable pathway, one third of cases were found to be nonprogressive between acute episodes, while two thirds experienced a gradual increase in symptoms between intermittent, acute episodes of worsening. A minority of patients had a constant worsening in condition, and very few people enjoyed spontaneous improvement. Their conclusion was that although progression of the disease is usually slow, prognosis is poor, and improvement rare. They hypothesized that patients reporting improvement may simply be coping better, or may simply be reporting a slowing of progression.

Although many agree that there is a need to compare the outcome of different surgical treatments for cervical spondylosis with the natural history, such a study would be unethical. As surgery is widely accepted as incontrovertibly beneficial, it would prove difficult to randomize patients with severe or progressive disability to nontreatment.

## TREATMENT AND DECISION-MAKING

Two options exist for treating cervical spondylosis: conservative and surgical. Conservative treatment is aimed toward patients with milder symptoms and can range from simply monitoring the patient to isolating the neck with a hard or soft collar. The collar should hold the neck either neutral or slightly flexed, with duration of use varying between patients. Drug therapy is another option in nonsurgical treatment, consisting of analgesics, muscle relaxants, and nonsteroidal antiinflammatory drugs. Analgesics are used to relieve acute pain episodes, and muscle relaxants to reduce muscle spasm

(which can lead to pain and ischemia) and increase range of motion. The goal of antiinflammatory therapy is to reduce impingement upon nerve roots due to inflammation. It should be noted that drug therapy is recommended as a supplement to immobilization; rest is the best conservative way to reduce symptoms.

Surgical intervention is used when patients suffer moderate, severe, or progressive disability. A definite diagnosis must be made before surgery is used to reduce narrowing of the canal and stabilize the vertebral column.

## POSTERIOR CERVICAL SURGICAL TECHNIQUES

Cervical laminoforaminotomy and laminectomy is the classic posterior approach used in treating cervical spondylosis, and is still used in patients suffering posterior canal compression from a hypertrophic ligamentum flavum. In this procedure, the lamina is removed from the affected level and those adjacent to it; foraminotomies may also be performed to relieve radiculopathy. This surgery is contraindicated in patients lacking normal cervical curvature or suffering from cervical instability. In the latter case, laminectomy may be performed if preceded by anterior cervical fusion.

Laminoforaminotomy and laminectomy should be performed under general anesthesia, with the neck in a neutral position to prevent stretching of the spinal cord over any anterior protrusions within the canal. The patient can either sit or lie prone; the former allows a dry field, but increases the risk of an air embolism. After proper fixation of the head in pins and/or traction as noted above, radiographic assessment of the spinal alignment and confirmation of the neurological exam should be obtained prior to incision (Figure 24-3A). A midline incision is then made over the pathology in question. For occipitocervical fusions, this incision should typically extend from the inion on the skull to slightly above the C7 prominence. A more limited

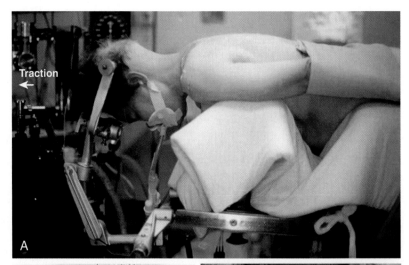

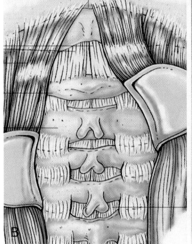

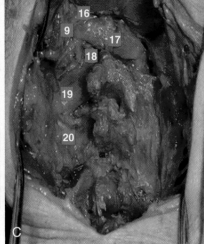

■ **FIGURE 24-3 A,** For posterior approaches, the patient is typically positioned prone, either on a horseshoe or in surgical Mayfield pins as shown here. The arms are typically tucked downward to maximize surgical exposure. **B-C,** Dorsal midline exposure of the posterior cervical musculature with section of the interspinous ligaments reveals the underlying dorsal bony arches with the lamina and spinous processes. Wider dissection exposes the pillars of the articular facets with their bodies and the articular capsules encasing the joint spaces themselves.

incision can be made for subaxial cases. Due to the narrowed interspaces and inferior inclination of the spinous processes, overdissection and stripping of the facets may lead to unwarranted fusion of uninvolved levels, leading to an excessive decrease in mobility.

The dissection is carried down sharply in the midline to the level of the posterior cervical musculature fascia. A midline raphe is formed from the union of the deep cervical fascia, prevertebral fascia, ligamentum nuchae, and the supraspinous ligaments (Figure 24-3B). By maintaining the exposure in this relatively avascular midline plane, blood loss can be minimized. Frequent palpation of the bony processes demarcating the midline is essential. Self-retaining retractors are placed to maintain the exposure, but excessive retraction can obscure the midline and lead to scything to either side.

After the ligamentum nuchae is encountered over the cervical spinous processes, a subperiosteal dissection is performed to mobilize the muscles off the processes. As the processes are often bifid, care should be taken to avoid accidental spinal canal entry. The exposure is then carried down to the lamina which are palpated and identified. Using gentle lateral retraction with a small Cobb elevator, electrocautery is used to dissect the muscles off the lamina (Figure 24-3C). Excessive downward pressure with the elevator must be avoided, as the cervical spine is highly mobile even in its normal state under anesthesia. The laminae of the cervical spine are angulated 45 degrees from medial to lateral and also in a cephalic direction. The interlaminar areas are also wide and should be exposed cautiously. It is here that the venous plexus overlying the vertebral artery is often encountered as the facet capsule is exposed. Bipolar cautery and gentle tamponade with Gelfoam are usually effective in obtaining hemostasis. For uninvolved levels, care should be taken to preserve the facet capsule (zygapophyseal joint). Self-retaining retractors to maintain exposure should be placed at or above the anteroposterior plane of the facets to avoid injury to the nerve roots and vertebral artery.

Alternatively, a minimally invasive paramedian tubular approach can be used as well. A stab incision is initially made approximately 1 cm off midline ipsilateral to and at the level of the pathology. Under fluoroscopic guidance, a small tubular dilator or pin is inserted through the posterior cervical musculature and fascia down to the facet or lateral mass of the target level. Although we have not routinely done so, anteroposterior radiographic images could be obtained to guarantee proper pin positioning (Figure 24-4A). Once the dilator has been docked on the facet in question, the skin incision is extended above and below the Steinmann pin for a total length of approximately 2.0 cm. The skin edges are retracted and the cervical fascia is incised using Metzenbaum scissors. Care should be taken not to cut muscle fibers during this procedure, as this can cause unnecessary blood loss. This sharp opening of the fascia allows for easier passage of the sequential dilating cannulas with a minimum of force (Figure 24-4B). A series of dilators is then sequentially inserted through the neck soft tissues, over which an 18mm tubular retractor is then inserted (Figure 24-4C). Real-time lateral radiographic images are obtained as often as needed to insure a proper working trajectory throughout this process (Figure 24-4A-C). The working channel (tubular retractor) is then attached to a flexible retractor affixed to the operating table side rail, and locked in position at the junction of the lamina and lateral mass (Figure 24-4D).

Once the standard or minimally invasive retractor is set in the desired position over the correct level as confirmed by fluoroscopic imaging, a Bovie cautery with a long tip is then used to remove the remaining muscle and soft tissue overlying the lateral mass and facet. Typically loupe magnification or an operating microscope is used for maximal visualization. With the bone well delineated, a small straight cervical curette is used to scrape the inferior edge of the superior lamina and the medial edge of the lateral mass/facet. This exposure is then carried underneath the lamina and facet with the use of a small angled curette. Proper placement of the curettes can be confirmed under fluoroscopy. Good dissection of the underlying flavum and dura from the bone defines the relevant anatomy and helps to prevent incidental dural tears. Bleeding from epidural veins and the edge of the flavum is controlled via long-tipped bipolar cautery. A small angled Kerrison rongeur is then utilized to begin the foraminotomy. Periosteal and bone bleeding is addressed with bone wax and cautery. In cases of marked facet arthropathy and enlargement, a drill with a matchstick-type bit is used to further thin the medial facet and lateral mass (Figure 24-5A,B). Dissection with an

angled curette facilitates safe use of the Kerrison rongeur. In this fashion, the decompression is continued.

The laminoforaminotomy is completed when the nerve root has been well exposed along its proximal foraminal course. The adequacy of the decompression should be confirmed by palpating the root along its course with a small nerve hook (Figure 24-5C). In cases in which a herniated disc was present, either a nerve hook or small #4 Penfield elevator is used to mobilize the nerve root superiorly to expose the disc space and fragment. For this maneuver, additional exposure is obtained by drilling a small portion of the superomedial portion of the pedicle directly below the exiting nerve root. With the root retracted, the disc fragment is then removed in a standard fashion with curettes and long endoscopic pituitary rongeurs (Figure 24-5D). Additional osteophytes encountered in this region can also be drilled or curetted as needed. Upon completion of the discectomy and decompression, the nerve hook is again passed along the exiting root to confirm its free passage and a lateral fluoroscopic image is obtained.

After inspection of the nerve root, hemostasis is obtained by bipolar cautery and gentle tamponade with thrombin-soaked Gelfoam pledgets. The area is then copiously irrigated with lactated Ringer's solution impregnated with bacitracin. A small piece of Gelfoam soaked with Solu-Medrol is gently placed over the laminoforaminotomy defect. A soft collar can be fitted for patient comfort, but is not necessary, as early mobilization is recommended. Major complications consist of wound healing and infection.

## ANTERIOR CERVICAL SURGICAL TECHNIQUES

Another surgical option is the anterior approach, which allows for fusion of the vertebral column concurrent with removal of osteophytes and prolapsed discs protruding into the anterior space of the canal. This approach

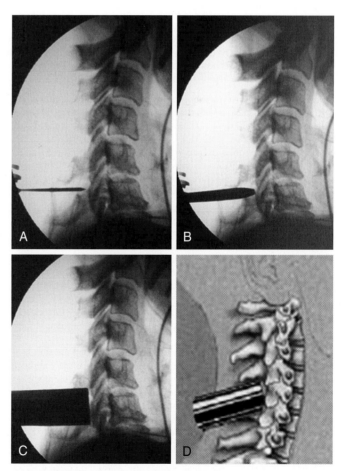

■ **FIGURE 24-4**  **A-D,** Lateral intraoperative fluoroscopic images demonstrate sequential tubular dilation of the dorsal musculoligamentous complex with ultimate docking of a working portal at the level of the C5/6 posterior laminofacet junction and disc level.

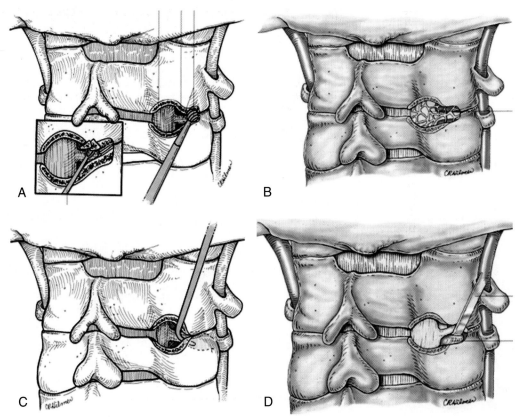

■ **FIGURE 24-5** **A-D,** After exposure and confirmation under fluoroscopy, a high-speed drill burr is used to decompress the laminofacet junction. The lateral aspect of the cord and the exiting nerve root are exposed **(A).** Immediately investing these structures is the epidural venous complex, which often requires hemostasis via tamponade and bipolar cautery **(B).** The decompression is confirmed with the use of a nerve hook or probe to palpate the course of the exiting nerve root **(C).** For cases where fragmentectomy is required, a small retractor is used to elevate the nerve root to gain access to the disc space **(D).**

is preferred in cases involving compression at one or two levels (although it is rarely performed in cases with three or four), and is particularly useful for patients with cervical instability. Several variations upon this method have arisen since its inception, with none having a distinct advantage.

As with laminectomy, this procedure is performed under general anesthesia, with the neck in a neutral position. The patient is placed in supine position with a roll placed transversely between the scapulae in order to extend the neck (Figure 24-6A). Following palpation of landmarks, a 2 to 3 cm skin incision is made along a skin crease at the level of interest between the sternocleidomastoid (SCM) and slightly off the midline (M) (Figure 24-6B). Finally, ensuring the correct level of the skin incision also prevents difficulty in dissection. Palpable landmarks in the neck aid in identifying the approximate level. The inferior angle of the mandible corresponds to C2-3; the hyoid bone to C3; thyroid cartilage to C4-5; the cricoid cartilage to C6, and the carotid tubercle to C7. Alternatively, a longer oblique or longitudinal incision can be made if an extensive decompression is planned (i.e., greater than 3-level corpectomy). Injection of lidocaine with epinephrine into the skin prior to incising may help diminish superficial bleeding.

Incise the superficial fascia overlying the platysma along the skin incision. The subsequent surgical course is through a potential space through the trajectory demonstrated in Figure 24-6C. The fibers of the platysma muscle are then either incised longitudinally along the direction of its fibers or split transversely. The deep cervical fascia underneath is then identified. Next, palpate the medial border of the sternocleidomastoid muscle and carefully split the fascia longitudinally. This allows one to retract the SCM laterally. The laryngeal strap muscles (sternohyoid, sternothyroid) as well as the midline structures immediately deep to them (trachea [T] and esophagus [E]) are then retracted medially. Deep to the SCM muscle, identify the carotid sheath (C) as well as the pretracheal fascia overlying it. Carefully incise the fascia medial to the sheath while protecting the midline structures. The carotid sheath can now also be retracted laterally.

Using blunt dissection, develop a plane toward the midline until the prevertebral fascia directly anterior to the vertebral bodies can be visualized. Identify the midline of the vertebral bodies (corresponding to the white stripe of the anterior longitudinal ligament) as well as the longus colli on each side. Using electrocautery, incise the prevertebral fascia longitudinally to the desired length. Use a periosteal elevator to then subperiosteally uncover the vertebral bodies and intervening disc spaces (A). Place retractors under each longus colli muscle to protect surrounding structures. The view of the field is provided by an operative microscope, which minimizes risk of injury during cord decompression. Place a spinal needle in a disc space and obtain a cross-table lateral film of the cervical spine to confirm the level. An assistant pulling axially on wrist straps depresses the shoulders and allows for a better radiograph. After confirming the level, a discectomy and/or corpectomy can be performed as indicated. Distraction pins can be placed in the appropriate vertebral bodies, and general distraction applied to facilitate discectomy and decompression, particularly in heavily collapsed spaces (Figure 24-7A).

The prolapsed disc and osteophytes are removed, and a bone graft is inserted within the interspace to provide stability and promote fusion. Typically, straight and angled curettes are used to free the disc and cartilaginous portions of the endplate from the bony vertebral body surfaces. Fragments of disc are then removed with pituitary rongeurs (Figure 24-7B). This process is gradually advanced down toward the level of the posterior longitudinal ligament (PLL). At times, drilling with a matchstick-type high-speed drill bit is useful to flatten irregular endplate osteophytes as well as to remove anterior closing lip osteophytes. Particular attention, however, should be taken to avoid excessive damage to the bony endplates, especially if grafting will be done, to prevent excessive subsidence of the graft. The PLL is then opened sharply with a small 1- or 2- mm Kerrison rongeur. Initial opening can be facilitated with the use of a small nerve hook probe. The PLL is then sectioned to reveal the underlying dura as needed, depending on the exact extent and location of the neurological

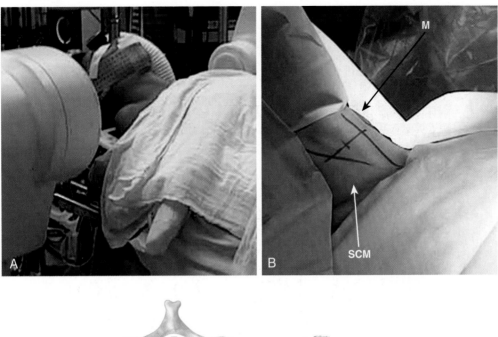

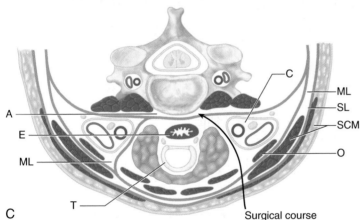

■ **FIGURE 24-6** **A-C,** For anterior cervical approaches, the patient is positioned supine, often with either a chin strap or traction tongs to optimize the exposure and the cervical lordosis. The C-arm can be draped in as well **(A).** The incision is marked at the level of the pathology, based on either anatomic landmarks or fluoroscopic guidance between the sterno-cleidomastoid [SCM] and the midline [M] **(B).** The surgical course is a lateral-to-medial type of trajectory passing through the skin, platysma, and the external cervical fascia **(C).** Once opened, this potential viscerocarotid space is split between the carotid sheath [C] laterally and the trachea [T] and esophagus [E] medially. The retractors are ultimately secured at the level of the prevertebral space at the anterior border of the spine (A).

compression as determined by the preoperative imaging and the patient's clinical symptoms. It is particularly important to extend the decompression rostrocaudally by undercutting the marginal endplate osteophytes in an hourglass shape to ensure that there is no residual canal or foraminal compression (Figure 24-8A). The majority of surgeons, therefore, choose to remove larger osteophytes from posterior and posterolateral canal surfaces. Some surgeons also choose to open and excise the posterior longitudinal ligament. Doing so allows prolapsed discs to be more easily identified for removal (which is useful in up to 35% of cases). Further, excision of the ligament provides prophylaxis against buckling, a possible source of post-operative pain.

Autologous bone grafts are usually taken from the iliac crest (over 70% of the time), with other options including the patient's tibia or fibula, bone banks, and calf bone (Figure 24-8B). Artificial grafts are also possible using methylmethacrylate, hydroxyapatite, or biopolymer. Although such materials do not necessarily provide a better outcome, donor site pain can be eliminated. Benefits of fusion include reduced risk of repeated spinal cord injury and pain by minimizing abnormal movement, as well as prevention and treatment of residual or recurrent nerve root compression via loss of disc space height. Another advantage of fusion is increased resorption of osteophytes, although complete resorption may take several years. A variety of specific interbody grafting techniques including

the Smith-Robinson impacted type, the Cloward dowel, and the Bailey-Badgely slot type grafts have been commonly employed over the years (Figure 24-8C).

The necessity of grafts is questioned, however, in that fusion occurs in over 75% of patients who do not receive a graft. The first reported anterior cervical decompression surgery without fusion was in 1960. In this procedure, the disc is resected to achieve decompression, and the space is left empty. The nonfusion anterior approach is used in patients suffering acute soft disc prolapse with minimal osteophyte formation, and neurological outcome is outstanding. Patients tend to have shorter recovery time with fewer complications. When osteophytes must be removed, the outcome is generally not as good as with fusion; many patients suffer new or recurrent pain symptoms. As such, the majority of modern surgeries now employ grafting with or without plating.

Vertebrectomy with strut grafting is a more recent surgical tool used in treating patients suffering from severe disease at many levels. Significant improvement is reported in 70% to 80% of cases, and many authors feel that this procedure is superior to other surgical options. When performing vertebrectomy, a trench is drilled out along the axes of the affected vertebra and disc spaces to achieve decompression, and the column is reconstructed using a graft from the iliac crest, rib, or fibula. In cases requiring immediate stabilization, titanium or PEEK implants can be used to reinforce the

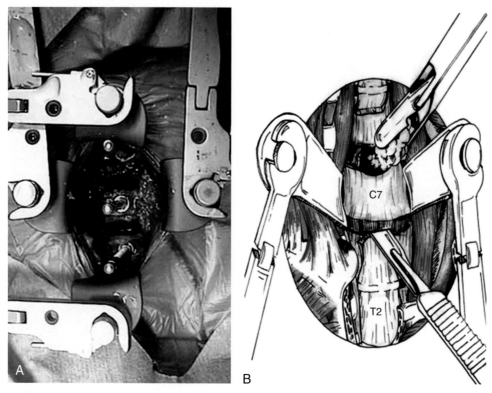

■ **FIGURE 24-7**   **A-B,** After developing flaps under the longus colli laterally, the retractor blades are then secured underneath them to provide exposure to the spine. If desired, Caspar-type distraction pins can be secured into the surrounding vertebral bodies **(A).** Annulotomies are then made with a scalpel blade and discectomy completed with a combination of angled curettes, drill, and Kerrison and pituitary rongeurs **(B).**

vertebral column, while also providing magnetic resonance imaging compatibility for postoperative imaging.

Anterior cervical microforaminotomy is a well-established minimally-invasive anterior cervical procedure and has the advantage of good decompression of the nerve root and maintenance of spinal stability without the need for fusion. Technically more demanding, decompression of the nerve root is achieved by removing the osteophytes from a lateral to medial trajectory with a focus on preserving the structural stability of the remaining joint and intervertebral disc (Figure 24-9A,B). Small slim retractors are docked at the junction of the lateral uncinate joint and the transverse process, immediately medial to the vertebral artery at the level of the disc and exiting nerve root (Figure 24-9C). With the vertebral artery retracted laterally, curettes and drill bits are used to expand the foramen and decompress the lateral aspect of the uncinate joint through the dorsolateral osteophyte (Figure 24-9D). Once exposed, the disc herniation is resected with micropituitary forceps (Figure 24-9E) to thereby ultimately decompress the neural foramen and exiting root (Figure 24-9F).

## SURGICAL OUTCOMES

Assessing the results of surgery for cervical spondylosis has proved difficult for many reasons. As the disease is heterogeneous in presentation, studies include a variety of cases disparate in age, extent of vertebral involvement, and severity of symptoms. To date, no prospective, randomized experiments have been published. Currently available publications consist mostly of retrospective reviews of different procedures performed at the same institution. Furthermore, there is no standardized method of assessment. The Japanese Orthopedic Association proposed a scale involving four-limb function and bladder symptoms. The Odum scale grades from excellent to poor, and the Nurick system assesses ability to walk. Magnetic resonance has been used to determine the underlying cause of poor postoperative results. In examining 56 patients, Clifton found that only 12 patients had adequate decompression at the correct levels, whereas 32 cases had either residual compression at operated levels or untreated compression at additional levels.[55] Batzdorf

and Flannigan similarly found patients with residual cord compression.[56] Harada found that when significant decompression was not achieved, recovery was significantly worse.[57] In light of these findings, the necessity of preoperative imaging for accurate determination of involved levels and best method of approach becomes apparent.

The effectiveness of posterior cervical laminoforaminotomy for decompression of the lateral recess and neural foramen has been well documented in numerous publications over the last four decades.[48, 49] When compared to standard anterior cervical techniques, the posterior approach via a "keyhole" type of osteotomy may provide better exposure for decompression of the exiting root and for removal of lateral osteophytes and discs. Previous work examining laminoforaminotomy has shown that adequate foraminal exposure can be accomplished without necessarily destroying the facet joint or causing iatrogenic instability.[50] As long as less than 50% of the facets are removed, there is little compromise of the sheer biomechanical strength of the cervical spine.[51] The posterior approach also avoids the additional risks of injury to the anterior structures of the neck including the trachea, esophagus, thyroid, thymus, carotid arteries, jugular veins, vagus nerve, recurrent laryngeal nerve, superior laryngeal nerve, ansa cervicalis, and thoracic duct. Lastly, cervical laminoforaminotomy is an operation that treats the offending pathology without necessitating a fusion. As longitudinal studies now demonstrate an increased incidence of adjacent level problems following cervical fusion, avoiding arthrodesis when possible seems particularly prudent.[52] Overall, no statistically-significant difference in results between anterior and posterior approaches for the management of isolated cervical radiculopathy has been demonstrated.[53] The overall clinical popularity of laminoforaminotomy was tempered by technical limitations including a limited surgical view, difficulty in resecting osteophytes, limited visualization of the distal foramen, and often generous epidural venous plexi and associated bleeding.[54] Furthermore, the muscle dissection often needed to obtain an adequate surgical exposure has been associated with increased postoperative muscle spasm, neck pain, and recovery time. When considering laminectomy, reported results tend to disagree. With respect to age, some investigators find a significantly better outcome in patients under 50, while others do

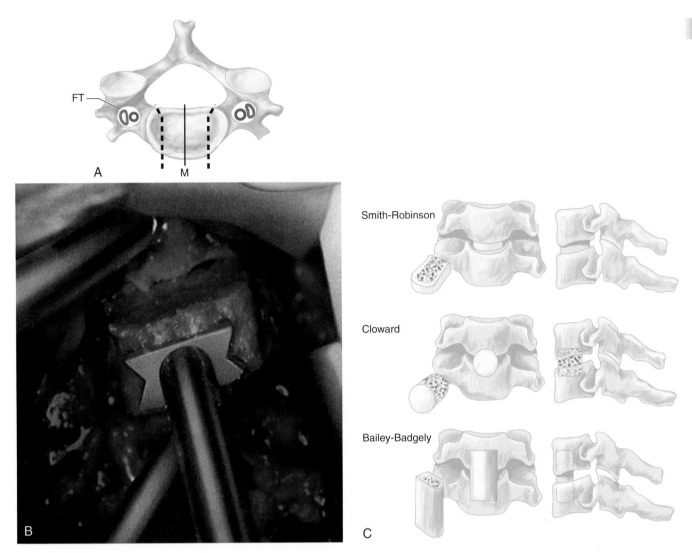

■ **FIGURE 24-8    A-C,** Typically a funnel or hourglass-shaped decompression is carried through the disc space to avoid inadvertent injury to the vertebral arteries, which are lateral at the level of the midbody **(A).** Widening of the exposure at the level of the canal and foramen is essential to ensure adequate decompression of the neural elements. Once the discectomy is completed, most surgeons opt to place an interbody graft comprised of either autograft bone, allograft bone, or synthetic material **(B).** A variety of specific interbody grafting techniques including the Smith-Robinson impacted type, the Cloward dowel, and the Bailey-Badgely slot type grafts have been commonly employed over the years **(C).**

not. Regarding general overall improvement, some studies reported benefit in over 80% of cases, whereas others found no significant advantage over conservative therapy. Finally, most authors agree that shorter duration of preoperative symptoms is a good prognostic factor, while some deny any significance. Possible confounding factors include the consideration of cases where osteophyte removal, opening of the dura, or sectioning of the dentate ligaments was performed concurrently with laminectomy (which tends to cause more complications due to neural injury). Despite the glaring differences, it is generally believed that younger patients who have less neurological involvement and a shorter duration of disease enjoy greater improvement.

Overall, clinical outcomes associated with the surgical treatment of degenerative disc disease by anterior cervical discectomy (ACD) or anterior cervical discectomy and fusion (ACDF) have been excellent. According to a literature review from 1991,[58] good clinical outcomes have been reported for 61% to 94% of ACDF cases and for 65% to 96% of ACD cases. These data showed that an interspace fusion is not mandatory for good clinical outcomes. The development of a fibrous union or pseudarthrosis has not been consistently associated with poor clinical outcomes. However, once pseudarthrosis is present, 67% of patients have associated symptoms.[59] Since then, the question of whether an interbody fusion is required has been unresolved.[60] Proponents of ACD favor its simplicity, low cost, and the absence of complications related to autograft harvest and interbody graft failure (e.g., graft

extrusion, collapse, subsidence, and pseudarthrosis). Advocates of ACDF stress that foraminal decompression by interbody distraction, prevention of disc space collapse, and stabilization of cervical alignment are key advantages compared with ACD alone. The resorption of dorsal osteophytes has been attributed to fusion and immobilization of the segment. The postoperative incidence of neck pain has been reported to be smaller with fusion than without. Furthermore, the incidence of kyphotic deformity is thought to be higher if fusion is omitted. Comparative, prospective clinical studies between ACD and ACDF, however, failed to find a clinical benefit to ACDF.[61-68]

Despite these findings, the overall trend in the United States and Canada has been toward increased application of anterior interbody fusion for the treatment of cervical degenerative disc disease.[69-71] Autograft from the iliac crest has usually been used for interbody fusion. However, its harvesting is associated with complications such as prolonged pain, cosmetic deformity, wound infection, hematomas, and peripheral nerve irritation or injury.

Unplated anterior cervical interbody fusion for degenerative disc disease has a higher tendency to fuse with autograft than allograft, sometimes with better clinical outcomes.[72-74] In contrast, other studies failed to demonstrate significant differences in radiological or clinical outcomes between allograft and autograft.[75-77] A meta-analysis of the literature comparing fusion outcomes of allograft and autograft for one- and two-level cervical interbody fusion without plating found a higher fusion rate for autograft and a lower

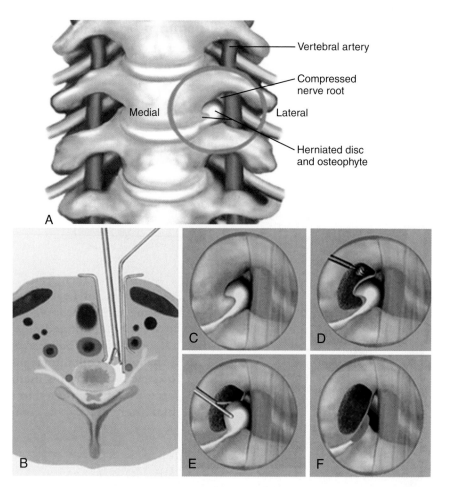

Vertebral artery

Compressed nerve root

Medial

Lateral

Herniated disc and osteophyte

■ **FIGURE 24-9** **A-F,** Anterior cervical microforaminotomy is a slightly more lateral approach than used in standard anterior midline cervical disectomy, and instead focuses on the lateral aspect of the disc space at the level of the neural foramen immediately medial to the vertebral artery **(A, B).** Once exposure is obtained with slimblade type retractors between the uncinate joint and the vertebral artery laterally **(C),** curettes and drills are used to complete the bony decompression and foraminotomy **(D).** The herniated fragment is exposed and resected with micropituitary forceps **(E)** to ultimately complete a good decompression of the neural elements **(F).**

incidence of graft collapse than for allograft. However, clinical outcomes were statistically similar.[78] A review of the literature failed to find allograft to be an adequate equivalent to autograft for anterior cervical interbody fusion.[79] However, the morbidity associated with autograft harvest was eliminated by the application of allograft. The possibility of transmitting infectious diseases like human immunodeficiency virus from tissues, including allograft, donated by a screened donor is exceptionally rare.[75,76]

A prospective study of ACDF comparing autograft and biocompatible osteoconductive polymers found significantly less graft protrusion and intersegmental kyphosis in the biocompatible osteoconductive polymer group. However, this study failed to demonstrate incorporation or biodegradation of biocompatible osteoconductive polymers.[80] In a prospective, nonrandomized study, Senter et al.[81] compared the outcomes of autograft ACDF with ACDF with hydroxyapatite. Fusion with the latter was equal or superior to that with autograft alone. In prospective comparisons of autograft and xenograft, clinical and radiological data favored the use of autograft.[82,83]

Recent prospective clinical trials of fusion with interbody titanium cages have found promising clinical results and radiological outcomes, with low rates of implant failure (e.g., backout and subsidence) or pseudarthrosis when compared with allograft or autograft. Even the fusion rates for cages are superior to those associated with autograft or allograft fusion.[84-86] Despite these recent data, some conclude that autograft remains superior to alternative interbody fusion materials.[87]

In the early 1960s, Bohler[88] applied an anterior cervical plate and screw construct to treat traumatic instability of the spine. After his report, anterior cervical plate constructs were applied using bicortical, nonlocked, variable-angle screws for fixation.[89,90] However, hardware failure was common,[91] and a unilateral locked, fixed-angle plate-screw anterior system was introduced by Morscher et al.[92] in 1986 (Figure 24-10A).

A variety of unicortical locked, dynamic, fixed, or hybrid plate-screw systems are now available for anterior cervical interbody fusion and plating[93] to increase stability of the cervical fusion segment (Figure 24-10B,C). As a result, fusion rates have increased, and the rates of graft failure and pseudarthrosis

have thereby decreased.[94,95] Furthermore, anterior cervical plate fixation for degenerative disc disease maintains sagittal balance more effectively,[96-98] thereby potentially limiting adjacent level biomechanical stress.[99] Postoperative loss of lordosis and cervical kyphosis have been associated with ACD and ACDF without plating. Yet, again, prospective randomized studies comparing single-level ACD, ACDF, and ACDF with plating have failed to show a clinical benefit associated with either procedure,[66,100] although a clinical benefit was found for two-level procedures.[101] Moreover, concern has been expressed about the cost and complication of cervical plating for the treatment of degenerative disc disease. Hardware failure has been a source of early and delayed morbidity. In a prospective clinical trial, patients undergoing ACDF with plating tended to have a more frequent incidence of dysphagia than patients without plating. Yet, in the same study, more multilevel procedures were performed in the plating group, which could also account for these findings.[102]

In more recent surgical series, refinements in the design of anterior cervical plating and more surgical experience have lowered the incidence of plate-related complications.[103-109] When all aspects, including possible reoperation and time to return to work, are considered, overall costs decrease when anterior cervical plating is added to fusion.[110] Plating also may increase fusion rates with allograft and thereby obviate the need for autograft.[111] The complications associated with autograft harvest would be decreased without compromising fusion rates. Again, experts are divided on the need for plating, in particular, for single-level disease.

## COMPLICATIONS OF SURGERY

The complications of these procedures are similar to those of any other type of surgery, with a mortality rate of less than 1.5%. Cardiac disorders, thrombophlebitis (with possible pulmonary embolism), and infection top the list. Vessels exposed to injury are the vertebral arteries, the carotid arteries, and the jugular vein; extradural or superficial hematomas may also occur. Nerves at risk include the paravertebral sympathetic chains, the superficial and recurrent laryngeal nerves, along with the spinal cord and nerve

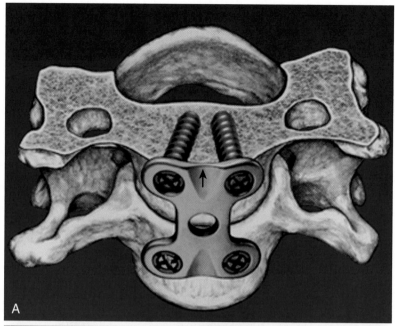

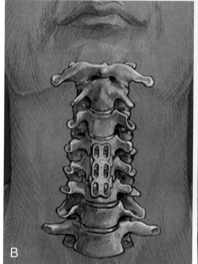

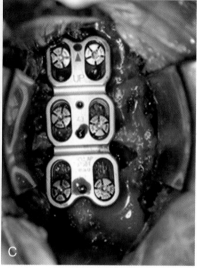

■ **FIGURE 24-10**    **A-C,** A classic Morscher type constrained construct is seen with converging screws that are constrained to the plate to prevent inadvertent backout **(A).** More modern anterior cervical plates are also constrained but allow more variability of the screws in the form of rotation and translation to facilitate screw placement, as well as to optimize long-term load sharing **(B, C).**

roots. Soft tissue complications may involve surgical injury to the trachea, esophagus, thoracic duct, and cervical pleura (Figure 24-11A). Often, the recurrent laryngeal nerve is injured from a combination of the anterior cervical retractor blades compressing the nerve against the endotracheal tube itself, thereby resulting in injury to the mucosal portion (Figure 24-11B). Infection runs the gamut from easily treated to discitis (leading to severe, lingering pain) or meningitis (also a complication of dural injury).

When comparing anterior and posterior approaches, neurological complications occur more commonly after laminectomy (2% to 8% of patients compared to the combined 1.04% average for both approaches). During the posterior procedure, displacement of the thecal sac and spinal cord after decompression can lead to cord or root damage. During the anterior procedure, bone grafts can result in displacement or nonunion. For iliac grafts, complications include donor site pain, hematoma, and infection, as well as possible injury to the lateral cutaneous nerve in the thigh.

## EMERGING TECHNOLOGIES: ARTIFICIAL Disc REPLACEMENT

After cervical spinal fusion, increased motion has been documented at adjacent levels,[112] and radiological data have shown degenerative disc disease to occur at adjacent cervical segments on long-term follow-up[113] (Figure 24-12A). Whether the increased incidence of adjacent level degeneration

(ALD) found in the cervical spine after fusion is caused by increased mechanical stresses on adjacent cervical segments or whether the observed degenerative cervical changes merely represent the natural history of degenerative disc disease of the cervical spine is unknown. Clinical studies estimate that the incidence of symptomatic degeneration above a fusion ranges from 2% to 3% per year above the expected natural history[114] (Figure 24-12B). The rationale underlying the use of artifical discs is to maintain physiologic segmental cervical motion after ACD and decompression of the neural structures. By maintaining cervical segmental motion, adjacent level motion is decreased.[115] Theoretically, this decrease should eliminate or reduce the incidence of ALD. Several artificial discs have been designed and applied clinically. Short-term follow-up data have shown equivalent clinical outcomes when cervical degenerative disc disease is treated with conventional fusion or an artificial cervical disc.[116-118] Earlier designers of artificial cervical joints showed a more frequent incidence of hardware failure when compared with more recent clinical evaluations of cervical artificial joints. [116-118] Placement of these discs is technically very similar to that of standard anterior cervical interbody grafting techniques. Authors describe the need for wider interbody exposure, discectomy, and more meticulous endplate preparation. Specific implantation techniques vary according to the specific design of the artificial disc. Whether these devices will be associated with superior clinical outcomes compared with standard surgical treatment options for cervical degenerative disc disease will only be

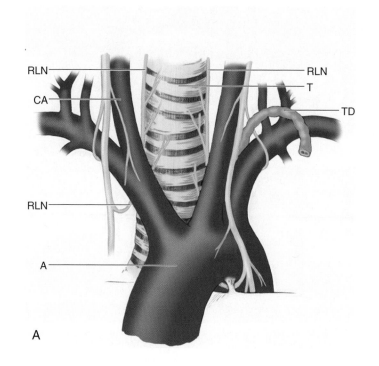

A

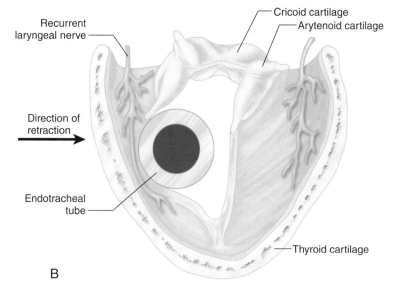

B

■ **FIGURE 24-11** **A-B,** The proximity of the recurrent laryngeal nerve [RLN] in relation to the trachea [T] and carotid sheath [CA] demonstrates the tenuous nature of this structure that can often be injured during anterior cervical approaches **(A).** The mucosal portion of the RLN can also be damaged by retraction of the midline structures causing the nerve to be sandwiched between the endotracheal tube and the retractor **(B).**

determined when sufficient long-term follow-up data have been gathered from ongoing clinical trials in the United States and Europe.

The BRYAN cervical disc (Medtronics; Minneapolis, MN) trial was published in 2009[119] (Figure 24-13A). This was a multicenter study in which patients with single-level cervical DDD were randomized to receive either the BRYAN cervical disc (n=242) or anterior cervical discectomy and fusion (n=221).[14] The main study hypothesis was that the outcomes from disc replacement would be at least equivalent to fusion. 465 patients were followed for two years. Initially, investigators and patients were blinded to the procedure. However, postoperatively, the investigational group was treated with a two-week course of nonsteroidal antiinflammatory drugs and was allowed to resume nonstrenuous activities as they pleased. Because of these postoperative differences, "further blinding was not practical or ethical." At 24-month follow-up there was a 91.6% retention rate. At 24 months, both groups had improvements in the clinical outcomes. Overall success in the intervention group was 82.6% compared with 72.7% in the fusion group (p=0.005). Neck Disability Index (NDI) scores were 16.2 in the intervention group and 19.2 in the control group (p=0.025). NDI success (defined as greater than 15 point improvement in the NDI) was 86% in the intervention group versus 78.9% in the fusion group (p=0.001). Improvements in SF-36 scores were comparable, as were measures of neck and arm pain. Patients who received the BRYAN artificial disc returned to work about two weeks earlier than those who had fusion. Given that this was a non-inferiority trial, an as-treated analysis was the primary analysis (versus an intention-to-treat analysis). There were 12 patients in the study who were randomly assigned to receive the artificial disc but who received the control treatment because of anatomic or technique difficulties during the surgery. Another important limitation is that 117 patients were randomly assigned but declined participation once receiving the assigned treatment, many because of dissatisfaction with the assigned treatment.

The Prestige trial (Medtronics; Minneapolis, MN) was published in 2007[120] (Figure 24-13B). This was a multicenter trial in which 541 patients with single-level cervical DDD were randomized to cervical disc arthroplasty with the Prestige disc (n=276) or cervical fusion (n=265). Participants were not blinded. Overall success at 24 months was actually higher in the intervention group than in the control group. The NDI scores and NDI success were not statistically significantly different. The rate of neurologic success was greater in the intervention group. SF-36 scores and neck pain

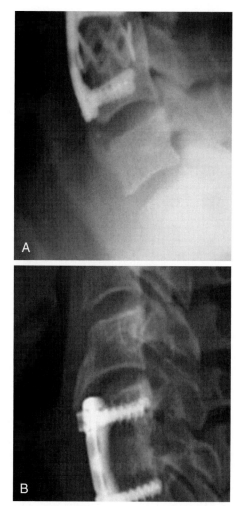

■ **FIGURE 24-12**  **A-B,** Adjacent segment degeneration can occur after successful anterior cervical discectomy and fusion. This can occur either from stress and/or motion transfer to the adjacent levels **(A)** or directly from hardware impingement **(B)**. This phenomenon can affect either the rostral or caudal level.

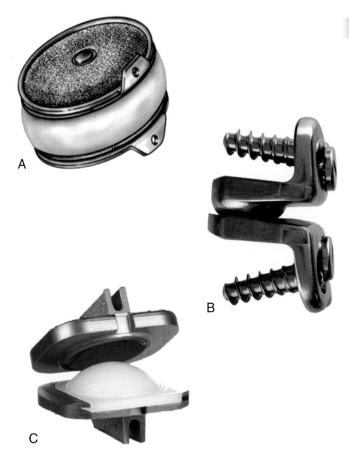

■ **FIGURE 24-13**  **A-C,** Examples of the three approved artificial cervical disc prostheses demonstrate significant differences in design, materials, biomechanical range of motion, constraint, fixation type, and dampening ability to axial load. The BRYAN disc is impacted within the disc space and has rounded endplates to conform to the native disc endplates which have been premilled to match the metal contours. Small optional fixation pinholes are provided **(A).** The Prestige disc prosthesis relies on standard constrained body screws for fixation **(B).** The ProDisc-C utilizes two keels to maintain stability within the disc space **(C).**

were improved more in the intervention group. There were fewer secondary surgeries in the intervention group.

The ProDisc-C (Synthes Inc; Paoli, PA) trial was published in 2009 and is the study upon which FDA approval was based[121] (Figure 24-13C). This was a multicenter study at 13 clinical sites. A total of 209 patients were randomized to receive either the ProDisc artificial disc replacement (n=103) or ACDF (n=106). All participants had single-level cervical disc disease that was unresponsive to conservative treatment. All participants were blinded until after the surgery. The main study hypothesis was that the outcomes from disc replacement would be at least equivalent to fusion. A secondary hypothesis was that disc replacement was superior to fusion. All of the patients were followed for 2 years. The primary outcomes of overall success and NDI success were comparable in the two groups. Overall success was 72.3% in the intervention group versus 68.3% in the control group. The results of the secondary outcomes were comparable. Fewer secondary surgeries were required in the intervention group. Few patients in the disc replacement group required narcotics at follow-up (10.1% vs. 18.5%; p = 0.073). At 24-month follow-up, safety and efficacy were comparable in those who had disc replacement compared with those who got fusion.

In all three studies, the rate of adverse events was not inferior to those seen in the fusion group and was often less than those seen in the fusion group. Adverse events included device-related complications, esophageal dysfunction, surgical complications, and the need for secondary surgeries. Study follow-up was not long enough to determine the effect of disc replacement versus surgery on the rate of development of DDD in adjacent discs. The results of the three trials showed that cervical disc replacement was

not inferior to cervical fusion based on 2-year clinical outcomes. The clinical outcomes evaluated are largely relevental. Although the 2-year follow-up data are promising, they do not provide information about the long-term impact of these procedures. The theoretic advantage of a decrease in the development of adjacent disc DDD has not been shown over the long term. Thus, given the lack of information about the long-term clinical impact of artificial cervical disc replacement, whether or not the technology ultimately improves net operative and disease outcomes is not known.

## CONCLUSION

Cervical spondylosis is a common degenerative disease resulting in pathological changes of the vertebrae, ligaments, joints, and soft tissues of the spinal column. Radiographic evidence of spondylosis has been demonstrated in at least 50% of patients over the age of 50. Pathophysiology includes a congenitally narrow canal, disc herniation, osteophyte formation, joint and ligament hypertrophy, and abnormal spine mobility. Cord injury is presumed to be either due to direct compression of neural elements, or compromise of vascular supply.

The clinical presentation of spondylosis can range from no symptoms to radiculopathy or severe myelopathy. Diagnostic imaging modalities include plain radiography and magnetic resonance imaging. Computed tomography with intrathecal contrast may play a role in evaluating certain disease processes poorly imaged by MRI. The role of neurophysiological testing with motor and somatosensory evoked potentials is not clearly defined, but may prove beneficial in measuring subclinical disease and predicting outcome following surgery. Conservative medical management is indicated for patients with minimal symptoms, with surgical intervention reserved for patients with significant disability and/or a progressive clinical course. Both anterior and posterior approaches with or without grafting and fusion have been described. Surgical outcome is variable and significant prognostic factors are not yet identified. The association between cervical degenerative disease and age suggests an increasing prevalence of cervical spondylosis as the elderly population expands. Understanding of cervical spondylosis is still limited and further research is necessary to better define criteria for patient selection for surgery, appropriate surgical procedures, prognostic factors, and outcome measures.

## References

1. W.F. Lestini, S.W. Wiesel, The pathogenesis of cervical spondylosis, Clin. Orthop. 239 (1989) 69–93.
2. R. Brain, Cervical spondylosis, Ann. Int. Med. 41 (1954) 439.
3. S. Nurick, The pathogenesis of the spinal cord disorder associated with cervical spondylosis, Brain 95 (1972) 87–100.
4. W.E. Hunt, Cervical spondylosis: natural history and rare indications for surgical decompression, Congress of Neurological Surgeons: Clinical neurosurgery, Williams and Wilkins, Baltimore, 1980.
5. F.A. Simeone, R.H. Rothman, Cervical disc disease, in: R.H. Rothman, F.A. Simeone (Eds.), The spine, W.B. Saunders, Philadelphia, 1982.
6. H. LaRocca, Cervical spondylotic myelopathy: natural history, Spine 13 (1988) 854–855.
7. W.W. Parke, Correlative anatomy of cervical spondylotic myelopathy, Spine 13 (1988) 831–837.
8. I.M. Turnbull, Micro vasculature of the human spinal cord, J. Neurosurg. 35 (2) (1971) 141–147.
9. A. Breig, Adverse mechanical tension in the central nervous system, second ed., John Wylie & Sons, New York, 1978.
10. H.H. Bohlman, S.E. Emery, The pathophysiology of cervical spondylosis and myelopathy,, Spine 13 (1988) 843–846.
11. J.F. Cusick, Monitoring of cervical spondylotic myelopathy, Spine 13 (1988) 877–880.
12. A. Breig, Adverse mechanical tension in the central nervous system, second ed., John Wylie & Sons, New York, 1978.
13. A. Breig, I.M. Turnbull, O. Hassler, Effects of mechanical stresses on the spinal cord in cervical spondylosis: a study of fresh cadaver material, J. Neurosurg. 25 (1) (1966) 45–56.
14. M.R. Gooding, Pathogenesis of myelopathy in cervical spondylosis, Lancet 2 (7980) (1974) 1180–1181.
15. M.R. Gooding, C.B. Wilson, J.T. Hoff, Experimental cervical myelopathy: effect of ischemia and compression of the canine cervical spinal cord, J. Neurosurg. 43 (1) (1975) 9–17.
16. K.L. Allen, Neuropathies caused by bony spurs in the cervical spine with special reference to surgical treatment, J. Neurol. Neurosurg. Psychiatr. 15 (1952) 20.
17. K. Ono, H. Ota, K. Tada, T. Yamamoto, Cervical myelopathy secondary to multiple spondylotic protrusions: a clinico-pathologic study, Spine 2 (1977) 109–125.
18. H. Ogino, K. Tada, K. Okada, K. Yonenobu, Y. Yamamoto, K. Ono, H. Namiki, Canal diameter, anteroposterior compression ratio, and spondylotic myelopathy of the cervical spine, Spine 8 (1983) 1–15.
19. F. Lees, J.W. Aldren-Turner, Natural history and prognosis of cervical spondylosis, BMJ 92 (1963) 1607–1610.
20. J.A. Epstein, N.E. Epstein, The surgical management of cervical spinal stenosis, spondylosis, and myeloradiculopathy by means of the posterior approach, in: The Cervical Spine Research Society, (Eds.), The cervical spine, second ed., J.B. Lippincott Company, Philadelphia, 1989.
21. P.H. Crandall, U. Batzdorf, Cervical spondylotic myelopathy, J. Neurosurg. 25 (1966) 57–66.
22. Z.B. Friedenberg, H.A. Broder, J.E. Edeiken, H.N. Spencer, Degenerative disc disease of cervical spine, JAMA 174 (1960) 375–380.
23. D.C. Good, J.R. Couch, L. Wacaser, "Numb, clumsy hand" and high cervical spondylosis, Surg. Neurol. 22 (1984) 285–291.
24. T.F. Dagi, M.A. Tarkington, J.J. Leech, Tandem lumbar and cervical spinal stenosis, J. Neurosurg. 66 (1987) 842–849.
25. J. Giroux, Vertebral artery compression by cervical osteophytes, Adv. Otorhinolaryngol. 28 (1982) 111–117.
26. G. Alker, Neuroradiology of cervical spondylotic myelopathy, Spine 13 (1988) 850–853.
27. Torg JS, Pavlov H, Robie B, Jahre C: Pavlov's ratio: A simplified, accurate and specific method for determining stenosis of the cervical spinal canal, Presented at the 15th annual meeting of the Cervical Spine Research Society, Washington D.C., December 5, 1987.
28. T.B. Freeman, C.R. Martinez, Radiological evaluation of cervical spondylotic disease: Limitations of magnetic resonance imaging for diagnosis and preoperative assessment, Perspect. Neurol. Surg. 3 (1992) 34–54.
29. L. Penning, J.T. Wilmink, H.H. van Woerden, E. Knol, CT myelographic findings in degenerative disorders of the cervical spine: clinical significance, AJNR Am. J. Roentgenol. 146 (4) (1986) 793–801.
30. P.F. Statham, D.M. Hadley, P. MacPherson, R.A. Johnston, I. Bone, G.M. Teasdale, MRI in the management of suspected cervical myelopathy, J. Neurol. Neurosurg. Psychiatry. 54 (1991) 484–489.
31. E.M. Larsson, S. Holtas, S. Cronqvist, L. Brandt, Comparison of myelography, CT myelography and magnetic resonance imaging in cervical spondylosis and disc herniation, Acta. Radiol. 30 (1989) 233–239.
32. M. Takahashi, Y. Sakamoto, M. Miyawaki, H. Bussaka, Increased signal intensity secondary to chronic cervical cord compression, Neuroradiology 29 (1987) 550–556.
33. O. Al-Mefty, H.L. Harkey, I. Marawi, D.E. Haines, D. Peeler, H.I. Wilner, R.R. Smith, H.R. Holaday, J.L. Haining, W.F. Russell, et al., Experimental chronic compressive cervical myelopathy, J. Neurosurg. 79 (1993) 550–561.
34. M. Takahashi, Y. Yamashita, Y. Sakamoto, R. Kojima, Chronic cervical cord compression: Clinical significance of increased signal intensity on MR images, Radiology 173 (1989) 219–224.
35. Y. Matsuda, K. Miyazaki, K. Tada, A. Yasuda, T. Nakayama, H. Murakami, M. Matsuo, Increased MR signal intensity due to cervical myelopathy, J Neurosurg 74 (1991) 887–892.
36. T.F. Mehalie, R.T. Pezzuti, B.L. Applebaum, Magnetic resonance imaging and cervical spondylotic myelopathy, Neurosurgery 26 (2) (1990) 217–226. Discussion 226-227.
37. K. Yone, T. Sakou, M. Yanase, K. Ljiri, Preoperative and postoperative magnetic resonance image evaluations of the spinal cord in cervical myelopathy, Spine 17 (1992) S387–S392.
38. O. Al-Mefty, L.H. Harkey, T.H. Middleton, R.R. Smith, J.L. Fox, Myelopathic cervical spondylotic lesions demonstrated by magnetic resonance imaging, J Neurosurg 68 (1988) 217–222.
39. L.M. Teresi, R.B. Lufkin, M.A. Reicher, B.J. Moffit, F.V. Vinuela, G.M. Wilson, J.R. Bentson, W.N. Hanafee, Asymptomatic degenerative disc disease and spondylosis of the cervical spine: MR imaging, Radiology 164 (1987) 83–88.
40. D.H. Clements, P.F. O'Leary, Anterior cervical discectomy and fusion for the treatment of cervical radiculopathy, in: M.B. Camins, P.F. O'Leary (Eds.), Disorders of the cervical spine, Williams & Wilkins, 1992.
41. F. Leblhuber, F. Reissecker, H. Boehm-Jurkovic, A. Witzmann, E. Deisenhammer, Diagnostic value of different electrophysiologic tests in cervical disc prolapse, Neurology 38 (1988) 1879–1881.
42. Y.L. Yu, S.J. Jones, Somatosensory evoked potentials in cervical spondylosis, Brain 108 (1985) 273–300.
43. M. De Noordhoot, J.M. Remade, J.L. Pepin, Magnetic stimulation of the motor cortex in cervical spondylosis, Neurology 41 (1991) 75–80.
44. V. Di Lazzaro, D. Restucia, C. Colosimo, P. Tonali, The contribution of magnetic stimulation of the motor cortex to the diagnosis of cervical spondylotic myelopathy: correlation of central motor conduction to distal and proximal upper limb muscles with clinical and MRI findings, Electroencephalogr. Clin. Neurophysiol. 85 (1992) 311–320.
45. A. Travlos, B. Pant, A. Eisen, Transcranial magnetic stimulation for detection of preclinical cervical spondylotic myelopathy, Arch. Physiol. Med. Rehab. 73 (1992) 442–446.
46. J. Dvorak, J. Herdmann, Janssen, Theiler R, Grob D: Motor-evoked potentials in patients with cervical spine disorders, Spine 15 (1990) 1013–1016.
47. G.W. Smith, R.A. Robinson, The treatment of certain cervical-spine disorders by anterior removal of the intervertebral disc and interbody fusion, J. Bone. Joint Surg. 40 (1958) 607–624.
48. W.B. Scoville, G.J. Dohrman, G. Corkill, Late results of cervical disc surgery, J. Neurosurg. 45 (1976) 203–210.
49. F. Murphey, J.C.H. Simmons, B. Brunson, Cervical treatment of laterally ruptured cervical discs: review of 648 cases, 1939-1972, J. Neurosurg. 38 (1973) 679–683.
50. A.J. Raimondi, in: Pediatric neurosurgery: theoretical principles, art of surgical techniques, Springer, New York, 1987.
51. R.B. Raynor, J. Pugh, I. Shapiro, Cervical facetectomy and the effect on spine strength, J. Neurosurg. 63 (1985) 278.
52. L.Y. Hunter, E.M. Braunstein, R.W. Bailey, Radiographic changes following anterior cervical spine fusions, Spine 5 (1980) 399–401.
53. Dillin W, Booth R, Cuckler J, et al: Cervical radiculopathy: a review, Spine 11 (1986) 988-991.
54. M.J. Ebersolf, R.B. Raynor, G.K. Bovis, et al., Cervical laminotomy, laminectomy, laminoplasty, and foraminotomy, in: E.C. Benzel (Ed.), Spine surgery: techniques, complication avoidance and management, Churchill Livingstone, Philadelphia, 1999.
55. A.G. Clifton, J.M. Stevens, P. Whitear, BE Kendall: Identifiable causes for poor outcome in surgery for cervical spondylosis: post-operative computed myelography and MR imaging, Neuroradiology 32 (6) (1990) 450–455.
56. U. Batzdorf, B.D. Flannigan, Surgical decompressive procedures for cervical spondylotic myelopathy: a study using magnetic resonance imaging, Spine 16 (1991) 123–127.
57. A. Harada, K. Mimatsu, Postoperative changes in the spinal cord in cervical spondylotic myelopathy demonstrated by magnetic resonance imaging, Spine 17 (1992) 1275–1280.
58. W. Grote, R. Kalff, K. Roosen, Surgical treatment of cervical intervertebral disc displacement, Zentralbl Neurochir 52 (1991) 101–108.
59. F.M. Phillips, G. Carlson, S.E. Emery, et al., Anterior cervical pseudarthrosis: Natural history and treatment, Spine 22 (1997) 1585–1589.
60. V.K. Sonntag, P. Klara, Controversy in spine care: Is fusion necessary after anterior cervical discectomy? Spine 21 (1996) 1111–1113.
61. N. Abd-Alrahman, A.S. Dokmak, A. Abou-Madawi, Anterior cervical discectomy (ACD) versus anterior cervical fusion (ACF), clinical and radiological outcome study, Acta. Neurochir. (Wien) 141 (1999) 1089–1092.
62. C.B. Bärlocher, A. Barth, J.K. Krauss, et al., Comparative evaluation of microdiscectomy only, autograft fusion, polymethylmethacrylate interposition, and threaded titanium cage fusion for treatment of single-level cervical disc disease: A prospective study in 125 patients, Neurosurg Focus 12 (Article 4) 2002.
63. G.C. Dowd, F.P. Wirth, Anterior cervical discectomy: Is fusion necessary? J. Neurosurg. Spine 90 (1999) 8–12.
64. A.N. Martins, Anterior cervical discectomy with and without interbody bone graft, J. Neurosurg. 44 (1976) 290–295.
65. J. Rosenorn, E.B. Hansen, M.A. Rosenorn, Anterior cervical discectomy with and without fusion: A prospective study, J. Neurosurg. 59 (1983) 252–255.
66. S. Savolainen, J. Rinne, J. Hernesniemi, A prospective randomized study of anterior single-level cervical disc operations with long-term follow-up: surgical fusion is unnecessary, Neurosurgery 43 (1998) 51–55.
67. M.J. van den Bent, J. Oosting, E.J. Wouda, et al., Anterior cervical discectomy with or without fusion with acrylate: a randomized trial, Spine 21 (1996) 834–839.
68. F.P. Wirth, G.C. Dowd, H.F. Sanders, et al., Cervical discectomy: a prospective analysis of three operative techniques, Surg. Neurol. 53 (2000) 340–346.

69. P.D. Angevine, R.R. Arons, P.C. McCormick, National and regional rates and variation of cervical discectomy with and without anterior fusion, 1990–1999, Spine 28 (2003) 931–939.

70. B. Drew, M. Bhandari, D. Orr, et al., Surgical preference in anterior cervical discectomy: a national survey of Canadian spine surgeons, J. Spinal Disord Tech. 15 (2002) 454–457.

71. S.M. Zeidman, T.B. Ducker, J. Raycroft, Trends and complications in cervical spine surgery: 1989–1993, J. Spinal Disord. 10 (1997) 523–526.

72. H.S. An, J.M. Simpson, J.M. Glover, et al., Comparison between allograft plus demineralized bone matrix versus autograft in anterior cervical fusion: a prospective multicenter study, Spine 20 (1995) 2211–2216.

73. R.C. Bishop, K.A. Moore, M.N. Hadley, Anterior cervical interbody fusion using autogeneic and allogeneic bone graft substrate: a prospective comparative analysis, J. Neurosurg. 85 (1996) 206–210.

74. J.C. Fernyhough, J.I. White, H. LaRocca, Fusion rates in multilevel cervical spondylosis comparing allograft fibula with autograft fibula in 126 patients, Spine 16 (1991) S561–S564.

75. B.L. Rish, J.T. McFadden, J.O. Penix, Anterior cervical fusion using homologous bone grafts: a comparative study, Surg. Neurol. 5 (1976) 119–121.

76. S. Savolainen, J.P. Usenius, J. Hernesniemi, Iliac crest versus artificial bone grafts in 250 cervical fusions, Acta. Neurochir. (Wien) 129 (1994) 54–57.

77. W.F. Young, R.H. Rosenwasser, An early comparative analysis of the use of fibular allograft versus autologous iliac crest graft for interbody fusion after anterior cervical discectomy, Spine 18 (1993) 1123–1124.

78. T. Floyd, D. Ohnmeiss, A meta-analysis of autograft versus allograft in anterior cervical fusion, Eur. Spine J. 9 (2000) 398–403.

79. C.C. Wigfield, R.J. Nelson, Nonautologous interbody fusion materials in cervical spine surgery: how strong is the evidence to justify their use? Spine 26 (2001) 687–694.

80. A.A. Madawi, M. Powell, H.A. Crockard, Biocompatible osteoconductive polymer versus iliac graft: a prospective comparative study for the evaluation of fusion pattern after anterior cervical discectomy, Spine 21 (1996) 2123–2129.

81. H.J. Senter, R. Kortyna, W.R. Kemp, Anterior cervical discectomy with hydroxylapatite fusion, Neurosurgery 25 (1989) 39–42.

82. G.L. Lowery, R.F. McDonough, The significance of hardware failure in anterior cervical plate fixation: patients with 2- to 7-year follow-up, Spine 23 (1998) 181–186.

83. J.N. Rawlinson, Morbidity after anterior cervical decompression and fusion: the influence of the donor site on recovery, and the results of a trial of surgibone compared to autologous bone, Acta. Neurochir. (Wien) 131 (1994) 106–118.

84. R.J. Hacker, J.C. Cauthen, T.J. Gilbert, et al., A prospective randomized multicenter clinical evaluation of an anterior cervical fusion cage, Spine 25 (2000) 2646–2654.

85. D.B. Moreland, H.L. Asch, D.E. Clabeaux, et al., Anterior cervical discectomy and fusion with implantable titanium cage: initial impressions, patient outcomes and comparison to fusion with allograft, Spine J. 4 (2004) 184–191.

86. C. Thomé, J.K. Krauss, D. Zevgaridis, A prospective clinical comparison of rectangular titanium cages and iliac crest autografts in anterior cervical discectomy and fusion, Neurosurg. Rev. 27 (2004) 34–41.

87. C.C. Wigfield, R.J. Nelson, Nonautologous interbody fusion materials in cervical spine surgery: how strong is the evidence to justify their use? Spine 26 (2001) 687–694.

88. J. Bohler, Immediate and early treatment of traumatic paraplegias [German], Z. Orthop. Ihre. Grenzgeb. 103 (1967) 512–529.

89. W. Caspar, D.D. Barbier, P.M. Klara, Anterior cervical fusion and Caspar plate stabilization for cervical trauma, Neurosurgery 25 (1989) 491–502.

90. R. Orozco Delclos, J. Llovet Tapies, Osteosintesis en las fracturas de raquis cervical: nota de tecnica, Rev. Ortop. Traumatol. Ed. Lat. Am. 14 (1970) 285–288.

91. C.G. Paramore, C.A. Dickman, V.K. Sonntag, Radiographic and clinical follow-up review of Caspar plates in 49 patients, J. Neurosurg. 84 (1996) 957–961.

92. E. Morscher, F. Sutter, H. Jenny, et al., Anterior plating of the cervical spine with the hollow screw-plate system of titanium, Chirurg 57 (1986) 702–707.

93. R.W. Haid, K.T. Foley, G.E. Rodts, et al., The Cervical Spine Study Group anterior cervical plate nomenclature, Neurosurg. Focus 12 (Article 15) (2002).

94. W. Caspar, F.H. Geisler, T. Pitzen, et al., Anterior cervical plate stabilization in one- and two-level degenerative disease: overtreatment or benefit? J. Spinal Disord. 11 (1998) 1–11.

95. J.C. Wang, P.W. McDonough, K.K. Endow, et al., Increased fusion rates with cervical plating for two-level anterior cervical discectomy and fusion, Spine 25 (2000) 41–45.

96. C.P. Geer, N.R.W. Selden, S.M. Papadopoulos, Anterior cervical plate fixation in the treatment of single-level cervical disc disease (abstract, paper #722), J. Neurosurg. 90 (1999) 410A.

97. A. Katsuura, S. Hukuda, T. Imanaka, et al., Anterior cervical plate used in degenerative disease can maintain cervical lordosis, J. Spinal Disord. 9 (1996) 470–476.

98. S.J. Troyanovich, A.R. Stroink, K.A. Kattner, et al., Does anterior plating maintain cervical lordosis versus conventional fusion techniques? A retrospective analysis of patients receiving single-level fusions, J. Spinal. Disord. Tech. 15 (2002) 69–74.

99. A. Katsuura, S. Hukuda, Y. Saruhashi, et al., Kyphotic malalignment after anterior cervical fusion is one of the factors promoting the degenerative process in adjacent intervertebral levels, Eur. Spine J. 10 (2001) 320–324.

100. B. Zoega, J. Karrholm, B. Lind, One-level cervical spine fusion: a randomized study, with or without plate fixation, using radiostereometry in 27 patients, Acta Orthop. Scand. 69 (1998) 363–368.

101. B. Zoega, J. Karrholm, B. Lind, Plate fixation adds stability to two-level anterior fusion in the cervical spine: A randomized study using radiostereometry, Eur. Spine J. 7 (1998) 302–307.

102. R. Bazaz, M.J. Lee, J.U. Yoo, Incidence of dysphagia after anterior cervical spine surgery: a prospective study, Spine 27 (2002) 2453–2458.

103. D.S. Baskin, P. Ryan, V. Sonntag, et al., A prospective, randomized, controlled cervical fusion study using recombinant human bone morphogenetic protein-2 with the CORNERSTONE-SR allograft ring and the ATLANTIS anterior cervical plate, Spine 28 (2003) 1219–1225.

104. B. Bose, Anterior cervical arthrodesis using DOC dynamic stabilization implant for improvement in sagittal angulation and controlled settling, J. Neurosurg. Spine 98 (2003) 8–13.

105. P.J. Connolly, S.I. Esses, J.P. Kostuik, Anterior cervical fusion: outcome analysis of patients fused with and without anterior cervical plates, J. Spinal Disord. 9 (1996) 202–206.

106. D. Grob, J.V. Peyer, J. Dvorak, The use of plate fixation in anterior surgery of the degenerative cervical spine: a comparative prospective clinical study, Eur. Spine J. 10 (2001) 408–413.

107. M.G. Kaiser, R.W. Haid Jr., B.R. Subach, et al., Anterior cervical plating enhances arthrodesis after discectomy and fusion with cortical allograft, Neurosurgery 50 (2002) 229–236.

108. A.A. Madawi, M. Powell, H.A. Crockard, Biocompatible osteoconductive polymer versus iliac graft: a prospective comparative study for the evaluation of fusion pattern after anterior cervical discectomy, Spine 21 (1996) 2123–2129.

109. S. Shapiro, P. Connolly, J. Donnaldson, et al., Cadaveric fibula, locking plate, and allogeneic bone matrix for anterior cervical fusions after cervical discectomy for radiculopathy or myelopathy, J. Neurosurg. Spine 95 (2001) 43–50.

110. M.R. McLaughlin, V. Purighalla, F.J. Pizzi, Cost advantages of two-level anterior cervical fusion with rigid internal fixation for radiculopathy and degenerative disease, Surg. Neurol. 48 (1997) 560–565.

111. G.L. Lowery, M.W. Reuter, C.E. Sutterlin, Anterior cervical interbody arthrodesis with plate stabilization for degenerative disc disease (abstract), Orthop. Trans. 18 (1994) 345.

112. C. Wigfield, S. Gill, R. Nelson, et al., Influence of an artificial cervical joint compared with fusion on adjacent-level motion in the treatment of degenerative cervical disc disease, J. Neurosurg. Spine 96 (2002) 17–21.

113. D.R. Gore, S.B. Sepic, Anterior discectomy and fusion for painful cervical disc disease: a report of 50 patients with an average follow-up of 21 years, Spine 23 (1998) 2047–2051.

114. A. Hilibrand, G. Carlson, Palumbo, et al., Radioculopathy and myelopathy at segments adjacent to the site of a previous anterior cervical arthrodesis, J. Bone Joint. Surg. 81A (1999) 519–528.

115. C. Wigfield, S. Gill, R. Nelson, et al., Influence of an artificial cervical joint compared with fusion on adjacent-level motion in the treatment of degenerative cervical disc disease, J. Neurosurg. Spine 96 (2002) 17–21.

116. B.H. Cummins, J.T. Robertson, S.S. Gill, Surgical experience with an implanted artificial cervical joint, J. Neurosurg. 88 (1998) 943–948.

117. J. Goffin, A. Casey, P. Kehr, et al., Preliminary clinical experience with the Bryan cervical disc prosthesis, Neurosurgery 51 (2002) 840–845.

118. B. Jollenbeck, R. Hahne, A. Schubert, et al., Early experiences with cervical disc prostheses, Zentralbl Neurochir 65 (2004) 123–127.

119. J.G. Heller, R.C. Sasso, S.M. Papadopoulos, et al., Comparison of BRYAN cervical disc arthroplasty with anterior cervical decompression and fusion: clinical and radiographic results of a randomized, controlled, clinical trial, Spine (Phila Pa 1976) 34 (2) (2009) 101–107.

120. P.V. Mummaneni, J.C. Robinson, R.W. Haid Jr., Cervical arthroplasty with the PRESTIGE LP cervical disc, Neurosurgery 60 (4 Suppl. 2) (2007) 310–314. discussion 314-315.

121. D. Murrey, M. Janssen, R. Delamarter, et al., Results of the prospective, randomized, controlled multicenter Food and Drug Administration investigational device exemption study of the ProDisc-C total disc replacement versus anterior discectomy and fusion for the treatment of 1-level symptomatic cervical disc disease, Spine J. 9 (4) (2009) 275–286.

# 25

# Cervical Stenosis

## Myelopathy

*Sathish Subbaiah, William Thoman, and Richard Fessler*

---

### KEY POINTS

- Cervical spondylosis is the primary cause of myelopathy in the elderly population

- Muscle-sparing posterior decompression of the cervical spine is a safe and effective treatment option in the elderly population, who often have significant comorbidities.

- The indications for cervical microendoscopic decompression of stenosis (CMEDS) are the same as for an open decompression procedure: radiographic evidence of stenosis and spinal cord compression with correlative clinical evidence of myelopathy.

- The advantages of the muscle-sparing approach include decreases in blood loss, length of stay, OR time, perioperative neck pain, and infectious risk as compared to open procedures.

- Utilizing a single incision and a unilateral approach, bilateral decompressions of up to three cervical levels can be achieved while preserving the posterior musculature and ligaments in order to help prevent progressive iatrogenic kyphotic deformity.

## INTRODUCTION

Cervical spondylotic stenosis is the number one cause of myelopathy in patients over the age of 55.[1] For this reason, the spine surgeon focusing on the care of the aging population must be adept in understanding the clinical presentation of cervical myelopathy and correlating these changes to the radiographic studies available. After this careful review, the appropriate management can be discussed with the patient as it relates to his or her overall medical health.

Axial neck pain and symptoms related to cervical stenosis are among the most common complaints of the elderly patient to the spinal surgeon. The cervical spine holds the formidable task of transferring the structural load of the fixed occiput to the relatively fixed thoracic spine. It does so while concurrently allowing a significant degree of motion in all three planes. This delicate balance between structural integrity and flexibility accounts for the significant degree of degenerative changes that occur as the spine ages.

Degenerative changes that begin in the cervical disk lead to a cascade of changes in the bony and soft tissue anatomy of the cervical spine. The disk height is diminished, and intrinsic changes in the disk prevent the natural distribution of axial and rotational forces.[2] These unnatural increased forces at the vertebral endplates, uncovertebral joints, and facet complexes lead to the formation of peripheral osteophytes that can diminish the diameter of the canal. Through repeated cycles of flexion and extension, the spinal cord can be stressed against these osteophytes. Posterior to the spinal cord, degenerative changes can lead to reactive hypertrophy of the ligamentum flavum as well as facet arthropathy.[2] Extension of the cervical spine can lead to buckling of the posterior ligaments and further compression on the spinal

cord.[3] The situation is further exacerbated in individuals with a congenitally narrowed spinal canal.[3] The average cervical spinal canal diameter on plain x-ray is 17 mm.[4] The diameter of the spinal cord itself, on average, is measured at 9 mm, while the CSF space and ligaments that surround the spinal cord are averaged at 4 mm. Patients are often thought to become symptomatic from cervical stenosis with diameters less than 13 mm.[5]

The pathophysiology of cervical myelopathy is still under investigation. Pathologic analysis of the injured cervical spinal cord reveals a flattening and indentation of the cord. These changes are most directly seen in the dorsal and lateral columns.[1] There is evidence to suggest that ischemic changes are the direct cause of the injury seen in the cervical spinal cord.[3] In severe cases of myelopathy, necrosis and cavitations are seen in the central spinal gray matter as well. Demyelination changes are also evident in the lateral columns at the level of compression, with further demyelination changes in the caudal corticospinal tract.[1] Furthermore, the cervical spinal cord between C5 and C7 is a watershed region and is acutely sensitive to any changes in vascular flow. Compressive forces that affect the delicate radicular arteries, anterior spinal artery, and dorsal spinal artery at these levels can lead to the central necrosis of the gray matter that is seen with myelopathy.[1]

The symptoms of cervical spondylotic myelopathy can be varied and subtle. A thorough history and a sensitive physical examination are as essential as the radiographic data. Initial signs of spinal cord injury often manifest in the lower extremities.[4] These symptoms include fatigue and subjective weakness in the legs as well as a worsening sense of imbalance and gait difficulties. Symptoms often progress to the upper extremities and manifest as difficulty manipulating objects with the fingers and loss of manual dexterity. Bowel and bladder dysfunction is a variable symptom, and its prognostic indication remains unclear. Pathologic reflexes and other symptoms of upper motor neuron injury are common, including increased tone in the extremities with associated hyperreflexia, clonus, and positive Hoffman and Babinski signs. In severe cases, abnormal sensory changes can also be appreciated.

Cervical spondylosis is considered the most common progressive degenerative disease of the cervical spine. It is seen in 10% of patients by the age of 25 years and 95% of patients by the age of 65.[1] Cervical spondylosis remains the most common cause of myelopathy in the aging individual, but there are numerous other causes that must be considered. Other causes of myelopathy include: ossification of the posterior longitudinal ligament, ossification of the ligamentum flavum, trauma, intrinsic/extrinsic tumors, compressive abscesses, or inflammatory disease processes including rheumatoid arthritis.[3]

Anterior and posterior decompressive procedures have been shown to be effective treatments in halting the progressive course of cervical myelopathy.[2] A prospective multicenter nonrandomized comparison of operative and nonoperative treatment for cervical myelopathy with a mean follow up of 11 months revealed that patients treated with operative management had significant improvement in functional status and neurologic symptoms.[6] Even with this information, patient selection for operative treatment of myelopathy remains key, as the natural history of the disease remains unpredictable.

Anterior approaches are often successful in treating focal anterior pathology such as a discrete cervical disk herniation. Although the anterior approach is safe and effective, there exist many potential risks that must be carefully understood. These risks include possible injury to the vascular structures (carotid and vertebral artery, jugular vein), neurologic structures (recurrent laryngeal nerve), and soft tissue structures (esophagus, trachea, lymphatic duct).[4] Furthermore, the fusion that is performed after an anterior cervical discectomy/corpectomy will limit cervical mobility and can lead to accelerated degenerative changes at the end of the fusion construct.

Posterior cervical decompression for cervical stenosis is a safe and effective treatment option, but can also have increased risks in the elderly population. The procedure requires a significant degree of muscle division and reflection off the cervical spine. These muscles can have the propensity to become denervated or devascularized when retracted for the long procedure. This can lead to postoperative pain and spasm that can be persistently disabling in 18% to 60% of patients.[7] The complete removal of the laminae, spinous process, interspinous ligaments, and a portion of the facets can have long-term negative effects on cervical sagittal balance.[2] Iatrogenic destabilization of the cervical spine and postoperative kyphosis can be limited by lateral mass fusion of the cervical segments, but this procedure leads to extended operative time, increased blood loss, and restrictive motion.[2] Furthermore, as discussed earlier, fusion can lead to adjacent segment degenerative changes.

By utilizing techniques developed for the posterior decompression of the lumbar spine, minimal access surgery can be performed in the cervical spine. The cervical microendoscopic decompression of stenosis (CMEDS) is a procedure that allows for bilateral posterior decompression of one to three cervical levels through a single 1.8 cm incision.[8] By utilizing a unilateral approach, the contralateral musculature and ligaments are preserved, leading to less perioperative pain and increased stability of the posterior "tension band." The limited studies in the use of this procedure have shown the potential for decreased blood loss, decreased length of stay, decreased use of pain medications, and preservation of normal cervical lordosis.[7]

## INDICATIONS/CONTRAINDICATIONS

The muscle-sparing techniques to decompress symptomatic cervical myelopathy hold key advantages in the elderly population. As with any surgery, the appropriate indications and patient selection are vital to favorable surgical outcomes. Most patients who are candidates for an open cervical decompression are candidates for a cervical microendoscopic decompression of stenosis (CMEDS). The primary indication for the CMEDS is clear radiographic evidence of cervical spondylosis with clinical evidence of myelopathy. Patients with a primary posterior pathology, hypertrophied ligamentum flavum, severe facet arthropathy, and hypertrophied cervical laminae are especially favorable candidates for surgery. Symptomatic anterior pathology at multiple levels due to moderate disk protrusion and disk osteophtye complexes are appropriate indications for surgery as well.

As described earlier, the natural course of cervical myelopathy remains unclear, but there appears to be a clear consensus that new onset of myelopathic symptoms or gradual worsening of myelopathic symptoms are indications for operative management. In regards to myelopathy of unknown duration, it is important to have a clear discussion with the patient regarding the uncertain nature of the natural history of the disease. Furthermore, it is important to discuss the effects of further worsening of myelopathic symptoms as well as the risks for any possible operative intervention. It is our opinion that surgical intervention should be strongly considered in these patients due to the devastating consequences of exacerbation of symptoms of cervical spondylotic myelopathy (CSM) and the low morbidity of the muscle-sparing posterior decompression.

Contraindications to the CMED would be similar to the contraindications for a posterior open cervical decompression of CSM. These contraindications would include primary anterior pathology with little evidence of posterior spondylotic changes. This would include patients with evidence of central disk herniation that may or not be calcified. Other disease processes that fit in this category include multilevel OPLL. Furthermore, clear preoperative evidence of cervical subluxation on flexion/extension plain films, or a significant degree of cervical kyphosis would be other contraindications

for a muscle-sparing posterior cervical decompression. In both these disease processes, the need for surgical fusion of the cervical spine should be considered.

## CLINICAL PRESENTATION AND EVALUATION

The patient is a 60-year-old man who has complained of worsening neck pain for the past 2 years. He states that the pain is worsened with any flexion or extension of his neck. He also states that at times with these movements he will experience a "shocklike" pain down his spine. He notes a new numbness in his feet and has had frequent falls in the last two years. He is hyperreflexic in his lower extremities bilaterally and has six beats of clonus on testing of his feet. His MRIs in Figures 25-1A and B eg reveal a mild loss of cervical lordosis with spondylotic changes throughout his cervical spine. There is loss of disk height, disk bulging, and anterior compression of the spinal cord, which is worse at the C3-4 disk space. There is severe ligamentum flavum hypertrophy and resulting cervical stenosis at this level as well. Preoperative flexion and extension x-rays were obtained, which revealed no abnormal subluxation. As this patient had clear symptoms of cervical myelopathy, surgical treatment was recommended.

For an elderly patient with significant comorbidity, it is imperative to have a full medical workup include cardiac risk stratification. The risks, benefits, and alternatives to surgery are discussed with each patient prior to any treatment.

## DESCRIPTION OF THE DEVICES

1. Tubular retraction system – e.g., METRx (Medtronic Somafor Danek, Memphis, TN) tubular system or any tubular retraction system
2. Endoscope that is compatible with the retracting system
3. Endoscope camera and monitor
4. Endoscopic spinal instrumentation

## OPERATIVE TECHNIQUES

The patient is seen in the preoperative area and his symptoms and physical exam are reviewed to evaluate for any clinical changes. His incision is marked and he is brought to the operating room. At the discretion of the anesthesiologist, a fiberoptic intubation is often employed to minimize any risk to the stenotic cervical spinal canal. Prophylactic antibiotics are administered prior to beginning the procedure. The use of preoperative corticosteroids is an option. The patient is then prepared for neurophysiologic monitoring throughout the procedure with somatosensory evoked potentials, motor evoked potentials, and electromyography of the appropriate cervical roots. Neuromuscular relaxants are used sparingly to prevent any iatrogenic changes in the neuromonitoring through the procedure. A urinary catheter is usually not placed. The patient is maintained at normotensive systolic pressures throughout the procedure. If the patient has a history of hypertension or other significant cardiac risk factors, an arterial line is placed for continuous monitoring. The patient will ultimately be placed in a sitting position. Measures to detect and treat air embolism are options, including a central venous access line or a precordial Doppler.

After the airway and lines are secured, the patient is rotated 180 degrees away from the anesthesiologist. The patient is placed in a Mayfield fixation device and is positioned in the seated position. The head is slightly flexed to straighten the cervical spine, with the ultimate goal of having the spine directly perpendicular to the floor. We have found this positioning to be very effective in decreasing epidural bleeding and minimizing pooling of blood in the operative field. In patients with large shoulders or thin necks, the ability to visualize the entire cervical spine with fluoroscopy is improved in this position as well. All pressure points are padded, and the arms are draped over the patient's lap. The neck is checked to prevent any hyperflexion, which can lead to obstruction of the airway or compromised venous drainage. In general, there should be at least two fingerbreadths distance from the chin to the chest. The C-arm is then positioned to achieve a true lateral image, with the arc swung either under the table or directly in front of the patient. The base of the C-arm is often placed ipsilateral to the side

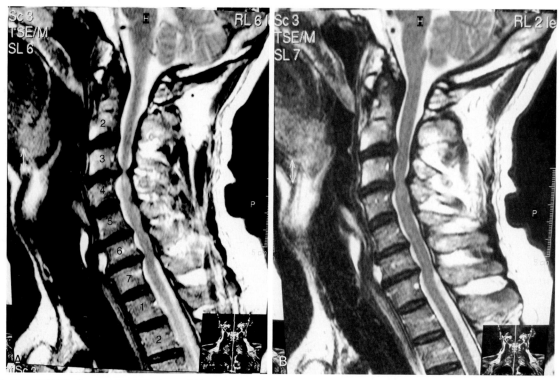

■ **FIGURE 25-1** **A and B,** MRIs show mild loss of cervical lordosis with spondylotic changes throughout the patient's cervical spine.

of the incision. The operative levels are identified and the skin incision is marked. The endoscope and monitor are checked to be in working condition. The monitor is placed above the patient or next to the patient's head contralateral to the incision site. The monitor is placed directly in the line of sight for the surgeon so that he or she can comfortably manipulate the instruments while observing the monitor.

The patient's posterior neck is shaved, scrubbed, and draped in the usual manner. Adhesive-lined drapes and an antibacterial adhesive layer (Ioban – 3M Health Care, St. Paul, MN) are used, as staples or metal stays will interfere with the fluoroscopy. The suction tubing, electrocautery, camera cables, and light source are passed and secured over the patient away from the field.

The operative level is rechecked by lateral fluoroscopic imaging with a sterile K-wire placed against the neck of the patient to approximate the level. The incision is 1.8 cm long running rostral to caudal and is 1.5 cm lateral to the midline. Local anesthetic is injected and the incision is made. The incision is opened to the cervicodorsal fascia under direct visualization, and the fascia is incised as well under direct visualization, to the size of the skin incision. The smallest tubular dilator is then introduced past the fascia and slowly docked against the rostral cervical lamina under fluoroscopic guidance. As the interlaminar space can be variable from individual to individual in the cervical spine, and as the ligamentum flavum is thinned out laterally, it is imperative to have precise control of the dilator as it spreads the dorsal cervical musculature. The dilator is carefully docked at the inferomedial edge of the lateral mass at the border of the lamina, and the positioning is reconfirmed with lateral fluoroscopy.

The tubular muscle dilators are serially inserted and the final 16-mm tubular METRx retractor is inserted and fixed in place to the table-mounted flexible retractor arm. The serial dilators are removed and the position of the retractor is confirmed by fluoroscopy. The 25-degree angled endoscope is then attached to the camera, white-balanced, and attached to the retraction tube via a cylindrical plastic friction-couple.

Upon initial view with the endoscope, there will be a layer of soft tissue and musculature over the lamina and lateral mass. A curette is used to carefully assess the bony anatomy under the soft tissue. The soft tissue is cleared away via monopolar cautery, bipolar cautery, and pituitary rongeurs over solid bone of the lamina. A small up-angled curette is placed under the inferior lip of the lamina, and the ligamentum flavum is carefully detached.

A 1 or 2-mm bayoneted Kerrison punch with a small footplate is then placed under the lamina to begin the laminotomy.

The laminotomy is continued with the use of the Kerrison punch, or a drill with a fine cutting bit can be utilized medially where the ligamentum flavum is thickest. It is important not to dissect or detach the ligamentum flavum and to allow it to cover and protect the dura during the bony decompression. There should never be any ventral manipulation or pressure placed against the ligamentum flavum or the dura underneath. After the ipsilateral laminotomy is completed, the tubular retractor is "wanded" and angled 45 degrees off the midline to visualize the contralateral side. The up-angled curettes are once again used to carefully dissect the ligamentum flavum off the spinous process and contralateral lamina. At this point, we use a drill with a fine cutting tip with a guarded sleeve extended to protect the vulnerable soft tissue on the opposite side of bony drilling. The undersurface of the spinous process and the contralateral lamina are carefully and methodically drilled away to decompress the spinal canal. The drilling is continued up to the contralateral facet to provide for adequate bilateral decompression.

After the bony decompression is completed, attention is then turned to carefully dissecting a plane between the hypertrophied ligamentum flavum and the dura. Angled curettes are used to carefully dissect away the ligament from the dura, and 2-mm Kerrison punches are used to dissect off the ligament. The decompression continues until a pulsatile decompressed dura is visualized (Figure 25-2 ). Any further bony compression from facet hypertrophy or osteophytes off the adjacent lamina are carefully drilled or resected with the Kerrison rongeurs. A fine probe is used to assess the contralateral foramen to reassure that there is no compression of the exiting nerve root. The tube is then returned to its original position. Once again, through the use of angled curettes and Kerrison rongeurs, the hypertrophied ligament is carefully dissected away from the ipsilateral field. Any further bony compression from osteophytes or facets that are visible after removal of the ligamentum flavum is drilled away. The ipsilateral foramen is also tested to assure that no foraminal stenosis remains. The cleared dura should be pulsatile and fully decompressed. The field is then irrigated with antibiotic saline and hemostasis is achieved. The tubular retractor is detached from the retractor arm and is slowly removed. The removal is carefully observed on the monitor to confirm no arterial bleeding in the musculature that must be addressed while removing the retractor system. If a second rostral or caudal level is to be decompressed, the smallest tubular dilator is reinserted through

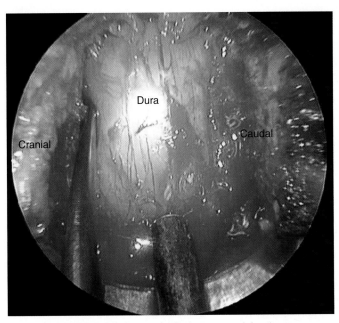

**■ FIGURE 25-2** A pulsatile decompressed dura is seen.

- Advantages
  1. In the elderly population with more significant comorbidities, the muscle-sparing CMEDS can be a safe, effective treatment option with significantly less blood loss, OR time, and length of hospital stay.
  2. As compared to an open decompressive procedure, the CMEDS provides patient with a significantly lesser degree of postoperative neck pain, thus limiting the quantity and duration of narcotics in the elderly population.
  3. By utilizing a unilateral incision and approach to achieve a bilateral decompression, the contralateral posterior musculature and ligaments are preserved. The preservation of this posterior tension band can help in preventing postlaminectomy kyphosis.
  4. The sitting position aids in decreasing epidural bleeding and pooling in the surgical field.
- Disadvantages
  1. The learning curve for any muscle-sparing technique can be steep, but is easily overcome with training in cadaveric specimens.
  2. In the elderly patient with symptomatic CSM and preoperative radiographic signs of kyphosis or subluxation, a muscle-sparing decompression will not allow adequate reduction or stabilization of deformities.

the same cervicodorsal fascial incision and similarly docked to the level of interest, and the decompression is repeated.

For wound closure, the fascia is closed with absorbable sutures. Inverted absorbable sutures are used for the subcutaneous layer. A running subcuticular stitch is placed, and then Dermabond is applied. There is no dressing placed over the wound. The patient is returned to the supine position and is awoken and extubated. The patient is observed for 2 to 3 hours in the recovery area prior to being discharged home. If the patient has significant medical comorbidities, we elect to admit the patient and observe overnight prior to discharge. The patients are discharged with a prescription for an opioid/acetaminophen pain reliever as well as a prescription for a muscle relaxant as needed.

## COMPLICATIONS AND AVOIDANCE

The major risk to any anterior or posterior surgery of the cervical spinal cord is injury to the spinal cord itself. There are two steps in the procedure where the risk of injury is highest. Careful attention must be paid during the initial serial dilation of the tubular retractors. Migration of the dilators between the interlaminar space would have disastrous consequences. For this reason, we do not recommend the use of the K-wire in this procedure. The fascia itself is incised under direct visualization and the smallest dilator is then used to localize the surface of the lamina/facet joint interface. The dilator must be advanced very carefully without any medial angulation to dock directly upon the border of the lamina and lateral mass.

The second high-risk step occurs during the decompression. Unlike in muscle-sparing lumbar decompression of stenosis, there can be no ventral compression of the ligamentum flavum or dura. It is important to use a curette to create a dissection plane between the ligaments and the ventral cervical laminae. After this is completed, the cervical lamina is drilled away to create more working room for the complete decompression.

Dural tears and CSF leak are a rare complication in cervical decompressive surgery. The ability to place a stitch into a small tear in the space provided through the tubular retractor can be very challenging. Treatment of a dural tear can be completed with a small piece of Duragen (Integra Lifesciences Corporation, Plainsboro, NJ) and a small drop of Duraseal (Confluent Surgical). With the removal of the Metrix retractor system at the end of the case, the muscles quickly return to their original position, leaving virtually no dead space for a pseudomeningocele to form.

## CONCLUSION/DISCUSSION

Cervical spondylosis is a common radiographic finding in the elderly population that in severe cases can lead to symptoms of progressive myelopathy. The treatment is decompression of the cervical spine through an anterior or posterior approach. Open anterior and posterior approaches can be very effective, but each poses risks that must be carefully addressed in the elderly population.

Cervical microendoscopic decompression (CMEDS) was developed by the modification of minimal-access techniques that were pioneered in the lumbar spine. Through the use of tubular retractors, the cervical musculature and ligaments are spared the dissection that is required in open posterior cervical approaches. The long-term effects of this muscle-sparing technique may provide multiple benefits over open decompressions while providing excellent clinical outcomes. These benefits include: decreased blood loss, decreased length of stay, decreased postoperative pain and muscle spasm, decreased disruption of the posterior tension band and risk of sagittal deformity, and decreased risk for infection.[7,9]

## References

1. D.B.E. Shedid, E.C. Benzel, Cervical spondylosis anatomy: pathophysiology and biomechanics, Neurosurgery 60 (S1) (2007) 7–13.
2. C.C. Edwards, K.D. Riew, P.A. Anderson, A.S. Hilbrand, A.F. Vaccaro, Cervical myelopathy: current diagnostic and treatment strategies, Spine J. 3 (1) (2003) 68–81.
3. D.C. Baptiste, M.G. Fehlings, Pathophysiology of cervical myelopathy, Spine J. 6 (2006) 190S–197S.
4. M. Geck, F.J. Eismont, Surgical options for the treatment of cervical spondylotic myelopathy, Orthop. Clin. N. Am. 33 (2002) 329–348.
5. B.S. Wolf, B. Khilnani, L. Malis, The sagittal diameter of the bony cervical spinal canal and its significance in cervical spondylosis, J. Mt. Sinai Hosp. NY. 23 (3) (1956) 283–292.
6. P. Sampath, M. Bendebba, J.D. Davis, T.B. Ducker, Outcome of patients treated for cervical myelopathy: a prospective, multicenter study with independent clinical review, Spine 25 (2000) 670–676.
7. J.E. O'Toole, K.M. Eichholz, R.G. Fessler, Posterior cervical foraminotomy and laminectomy, In A practical guide to the anatomy and techniques for minimally-invasive spine surgery, Springer, 2007.
8. M.J. Perez-Cruet, D. Samartzis, R.G. Fessler, Microendoscopic cervical laminectomy and laminoplasty, In An anatomic approach to minimally invasive spine surgery, Quality Medical Publishing, Inc, St. Louis, 2006.
9. R.G. Fessler, L.T. Khoo, Minimally invasive cervical microendoscopic foraminotomy: an initial clinical experience, Neurosurgery 51 (5 Suppl.) (2002) S37–45.

# 26

# Cervical Kyphosis

*Perry Dhaliwal and R. John Hurlbert*

- Cervical kyphosis can be caused by cervical disk disease, osteoporosis, or inflammatory arthritides.
- Patients with cervical kyphosis should be considered for surgery in the setting of intractable pain, neurological deficits, or progressive cervical deformity.
- Surgical decision-making depends on identifying the presence or absence of a fixed cervical deformity.
- In the majority of patients, cervical kyphosis may be corrected using an anterior approach.
- Posterior approaches to the cervical spine for correction of a kyphotic deformity are reserved for patients with a chin-on-chest deformity or an ankylosed spine.

## INTRODUCTION

Degenerative changes in the spinal column may lead to significant deformity and neurological compromise. Superimposed on these degenerative changes are age-related changes in soft tissue structures of the cervical spine. The cumulative effects lead to alterations in the way biomechanical forces are accommodated by the spine. Cervical kyphosis is one manifestation of deformity secondary to degenerative changes such as cervical disk degeneration, osteoporosis, and inflammatory arthritides. The complex biomechanics of the cervical spine, as well as the nature of degenerative disease, makes surgical management of cervical kyphosis a challenging endeavor.

Though cervical kyphosis is a well-recognized deformity in the setting of degenerative disease, it is generally poorly defined. This is in part due to the complex biomechanics of the cervical spine as well as the paucity of standardized methodology for evaluating cervical spine alignment. Therefore, identification of cervical kyphosis is dependent on clinical judgment applied to the presentation of a given patient. However, despite the absence of standardized definitions, cervical kyphosis has been observed and managed with success in a variety of clinical situations. Here, we diskuss basic biomechanical and surgical principles relevant to the management of cervical kyphosis in the setting of degenerative spine disease.

## BIOMECHANICS OF THE CERVICAL SPINE

Much literature is available that describes the normal anatomy and biomechanical processes of the cervical spine. The problem of cervical kyphosis deserves special interest, as it demonstrates the direct impact of degenerative spine disease on the anatomy, alignment, and kinematics of the cervical spine. Underlying any diskussion about cervical kyphosis are concerns regarding spinal cord damage as well as spinal instability.

## Cervical Motion and the Spinal Cord

Many studies have focused on the effect of neck motion on the spinal cord. These concepts become particularly important in the setting of cervical kyphosis as the spinal cord is stretched over the area of deformity. Cadaveric studies have demonstrated that neck motion may result in injury to the spinal cord when the tensile load on the spinal cord exceeds the strength of spinal cord fibers to bear this load. The mechanism of injury has been identified as loss of axonal integrity secondary to stretch-induced injury. This form of injury has significant consequences on the conduction of electrical signals through white matter. These conduction deficits are as follows[1]: transient ionic imbalances from altered axonal membrane permeability, conduction loss from myelin damage, and irreversible conduction loss in the setting of profound damage to axons. Furthermore, ischemic damage may result from impingement of transverse arterioles caused by anterior compression of the spinal cord.[2] Cervical kyphosis can aggravate this compression, placing the patient at risk of significant spinal cord damage with the potential for serious functional consequences. Prevention of further neurological injury is of primary consideration in the management of patients with cervical kyphosis.

## Degenerative Processes in the Cervical Spine

The evolutionary function of the cervical spine is to allow for support and orientation of the head. This places the head in an ideal position for use of all sensory modalities including vision, hearing, taste, and smell. The cervical spine also plays a crucial role in the protection of the spinal cord and nerve roots. In their review, Yoganandan and colleagues summarize how the various bones, muscles, tendons, ligaments, and connective tissue structures serve to maintain proper alignment throughout the various movements.[3] However, each of the different tissues contributes differently because of its unique structure and composition. Though an in-depth review of the soft tissue biomechanics is beyond the scope of this discussion, there are certain factors which are pertinent in the diskussion of cervical kyphosis.

Ligamentous structures are composed of collagen fibers and serve to resist tensile or distractive forces at extremes of motion. Each of the ligaments of the cervical spine resists different external forces due to its particular orientation and the components to which it is attached. Resistance to distraction is most effective when the force is applied along the direction of the fibers. As an example, interspinous ligaments are crucial for resisting excessive movement during flexion. Likewise, the anterior longitudinal ligament is most important for resisting motion during extension of the neck. With age, the composition of ligaments changes to contain proportionately more elastin than collagen.[4] As a result, the ligaments are not as resistant to distractive forces causing the spine to become less stable both at rest and during motion. With a kyphotic deformity, age and ligamentous laxity may contribute to progression of the deformity and cause abnormal stress on the posterior elements and disk spaces, leading to facet joint hypertrophy and osteophyte formation.

While ligaments serve to resist distractive forces, the structure of the intervertebral disk allows it to resist forces in several directions. The structure of the cervical disk is unique compared to the thoracic or lumbar spine, in that the annulus is not a circumferential structure.[5] In the cervical spine, the annulus is thickest at the anterior portion of the disk and tapers laterally toward the uncovertebral joints. Posteriorly, there is a small remnant of the annulus in the midline position (Figure 26-2). The primary function of the intervertebral disk in the cervical spine is to resist compressive forces. Through the aging process, the normal physiology of the intervertebral disk

## Clinical Case Example

A 45-year-old right-handed man with Klippel-Feil syndrome presented with complaints of neck pain since the age of 12. He had also developed concomitant pain and numbness in the left upper extremity over the course of several years, which was exacerbated by extension of his neck. On clinical examination, the patient was noted to have significantly reduced range of motion in his neck on flexion and extension. Head rotation was limited to 45 degrees on either side of midline. Extension of his neck provoked a feeling of numbness which radiated into the fourth and fifth digits of his left hand. On motor examination, the patient had normal strength in all major muscle groups of the upper and lower extremities bilaterally. Tone was increased in all four limbs. A Hoffman reflex was present in the right hand and plantar responses were down-going bilaterally. He was also noted to have increased reflexes in the upper and lower extremities. Finger-to-nose and heel-to-shin testing were both normal. MR imaging demonstrated segmental kyphosis from C2 to C6 with spinal cord compression secondary to degenerative changes in the cervical spine (Figure 26-1).

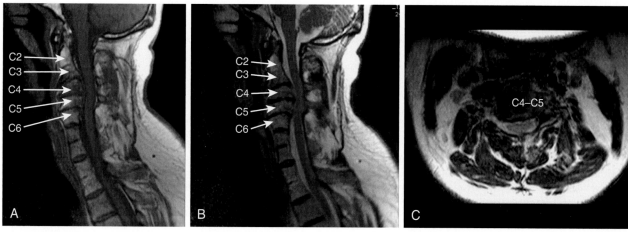

■ **FIGURE 26-1**  MR imaging of the cervical spine. **A,** T1W sagittal. **B,** T2W sagittal. **C,** T2W axial MR imaging demonstrating segmental kyphosis from C3-C6 with foraminal and canal stenosis.

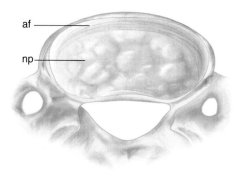

■ **FIGURE 26-2**  Cervical disk. Note the presence of the annulus fibrosus at the anterior rim and the median position posteriorly. The remainder of the cervical disk does not have an annulus fibrosus. *(Adapted from Bogduk N, Mercer S: Biomechanics of the cervical spine. Part 1: normal kinematics, Clin Biomech 15:633-648, 2000.)*

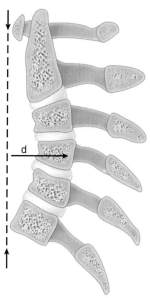

■ **FIGURE 26-3**  Progression of cervical kyphosis occurs through axial loading and bending along a moment arm in the setting of degenerative disease. *(Adapted from Steinmetz MP, et al: Cervical deformity correction, Neurosurgery Suppl 60(1):S1-90-97, 2007.)*

changes such that the equilibrium of matrix synthesis and degradation is altered. Moreover, the structure of the matrix becomes increasingly disorganized, water is lost, and there is narrowing of the intervertebral disk.[6] Progression of these degenerative changes is influenced by age-related changes to the vertebral body end plates which prohibit the passage of nutrients to the intervertebral disk. With the collapse of the disk comes concomitant loss of lordosis (Figure 26-3). Over time, these changes lead to wedging of the vertebral body and cervical kyphosis.

Although muscles, ligaments, and intervertebral disks all play vital roles in maintaining proper alignment of the cervical spine, the importance of the bony structures cannot be ignored. The vertebral bodies are composed of cortical and cancellous bone, the latter being most responsible for resisting compressive forces.[7] The vascularity of cancellous bone allows for alterations in bone composition consistent with systemic metabolic changes. Osteoporosis is one such degenerative disease which affects cancellous bone in the context of hormonal changes, lack of calcium and vitamin D, and reduced mobility. These factors may induce cellular changes to cancellous bone, causing osteoporosis and predisposing the patient to fractures of the vertebral bodies. Susceptibility to fractures is directly related to the structural changes that occur with osteoporosis.[8] In normal bone, the trabeculae are organized in horizontal and vertical planes, which reinforce the strength of the bone. In osteoporotic bone, there is loss of horizontal trabeculae,[8] which compromises the strength of bone and predisposes the patient to fractures in the setting of minor force loads. As degenerative changes in the ligaments and intervertebral disks progress, many of the forces are transferred to the vertebral bodies. With osteoporotic changes, the vertebral bodies are unable to provide the same strength against axial loading and wedging or fractures may result. Pathological fractures and wedging of the vertebral bodies are significant contributors to the development and progression of cervical kyphosis.

In summary, despite being subjected to the same physiological axial loads, the aged spine cannot withstand the same compressive or tensile forces as the juvenile spine. Numerous degenerative processes are at play that may contribute to the development of cervical deformity. Ligamentous laxity limits resistance to distractive forces and leads to abnormal forces on the vertebral bodies, intervertebral disks, and posterior elements. Collapse of the disk space causes axial loads to become concentrated on the anterior vertebral bodies, and concomitant changes to bone density result in vertebral wedging. The end result is cervical kyphosis accelerating further degenerative change through abnormal shear forces. Ultimately, alterations in the functional anatomy of the cervical spine lead to symptoms of axial neck pain, radiculopathy, and eventually myelopathy.

## Cervical Kyphosis and Inflammatory Arthritides

While biomechanical models demonstrate the complexity of organized motion within the normal cervical spine, degenerative diseases add an additional layer of complexity. Processes native to the anatomical structures of the cervical spine such as osteoporosis and cervical disk degeneration have been discussed in the aforementioned paragraphs. However, other less common but more pathological conditions have age-related effects on the cervical spine, such as rheumatoid arthritis and ankylosing spondylitis. These progressive inflammatory conditions have been known to alter the alignment and soft tissue structures of the cervical spine and are relevant when considering the surgical management of cervical kyphosis.

Inflammatory rheumatic disorders are considered uncommon causes of cervical kyphosis. Ankylosing spondylitis affects the entire axial skeleton from sacrum to the cervical spine and is classified as a seronegative arthropathy. Although the exact pathogenesis of ankylosing spondylitis is not well understood, an inflammatory mechanism is postulated, and a large majority of patients will test positive for human leukocyte antigen-B27. Though fewer women than men tend to be affected by ankylosing spondylitis, they will more commonly have disease involving the cervical spine. Clinically, the disease affects synovial and cartilaginous joints. Though the vertebral column is routinely involved, large appendicular joints may also be damaged by synovitis and enthesitis.[9] Due to the diffuse inflammatory changes seen with this condition, there is overall stiffening of the vertebral column and structural weakness. These changes affect the spine's ability to compensate for external loads, and a predisposition for spinal fractures results. Though fractures may occur in any location along the vertebral column, the most common location for a spinal fracture in the setting of ankylosing spondylitis is the lower cervical spine.[10] The fractures themselves may lead to kyphosis and neurological sequelae but the more common scenario is that of a chin-on-chest deformity due to severe kyphosis at the cervicothoracic junction.

Rheumatoid arthritis is another inflammatory condition, and generally affects the small joints of the feet, hands, elbows, wrists, hips, knees, ankles, and cervical spine in a variable fashion. There are numerous theories to explain the pathogenesis of rheumatoid arthritis, which are beyond the scope of this review. However, the clinical findings of painful, swollen, erythematous joints are the end result of destruction of synovial joints via the numerous pathways that have been described in the literature. These same inflammatory processes are responsible for facet joint erosion, disk space narrowing, and erosion of the vertebral bodies. As a result of these inflammatory processes, patients with rheumatoid arthritis are predisposed to three types of instability: atlantoaxial subluxation, cranial settling, and subaxial subluxation.[11] The combination of cervical instability and predisposition to fractures may make the rheumatoid patient prone to significant kyphotic deformity in the cervical spine.

Through the understanding of the biomechanics of the cervical spine, it is clear that normal cervical spinal alignment is maintained by a complex interaction between muscles, ligaments, bones, and intervertebral disks. When the effects of cervical disk disease, osteoporosis, or inflammatory arthritides manifest, they may alter the biomechanics of the cervical spine. The cumulative consequence of altered biomechanics and degenerative spine disease results in spinal deformity such as cervical kyphosis.

## MANAGEMENT OF THE PATIENT WITH CERVICAL KYPHOSIS

The management of patients with cervical kyphosis begins with careful patient assessment and adequate imaging. Currently there is no level I or II evidence to guide surgical decision-making. Basic biomechanical principles, clinical experience, and knowledge of the natural history of degenerative spine disease guide surgical management. In the following paragraphs, key points in the decision-making paradigm are brought forward to provide a basic framework for patient management.

### Patient Assessment

In the assessment of a patient with cervical degenerative disease, a thorough history and physical examination are crucial. It is important to characterize the type of pain experienced by the patient. Regardless of the nature of the degenerative disease, certain characteristics of pain originating from the cervical spine are associated with favorable surgical outcomes. A patient may complain of midline neck pain and/or radicular pain involving one or both upper limbs. A mechanical nature may be suggested by exacerbation with certain neck movements, coughing, or straining. Stiffness and discomfort may arise from muscles of the neck, adding a component of musculoskeletal pain difficult to treat through surgery alone. Nonspecific bodily pain is a major contributor to reported functional disability in patients with inflammatory arthritides.[12,13] In addition to pain, upper extremity dermatomal numbness may provide clues to symptomatic motion segments. With progressive cervical kyphosis, patients may also complain of forward gaze, dysphagia, or respiratory difficulties.

Cervical myelopathy is another manifestation of degenerative spine disease. In the setting of cervical kyphosis, myelopathy is usually a result of chronic stretch injury and compression to the spinal cord. Patients may describe numbness, clumsiness of the hands, gait unsteadiness, and bowel or bladder difficulties. Physical examination may reveal spasticity, ataxic gait, and the presence of pathologic reflexes such as the Hoffman or Babinski signs. These symptoms are usually insidious in onset and progressive in nature. It is important to note that rheumatoid patients have a high incidence of morbidity and mortality following the onset of myelopathic symptoms.[14]

In addition to myelopathy, patients with rheumatoid arthritis have several other unique issues which deserve attention. Many of these patients will typically have mechanical suboccipital pain that is worse when upright and relieved when lying in a recumbent position. Due to the predisposition for subluxation, these patients may be aware of excessive movement in their cervical spine and they may describe a sensation where the head feels as though it will fall forward with flexion. Because of the possibility of cranial settling, patients with rheumatoid arthritis may also present with symptoms of lower cranial nerve deficits such as shoulder weakness or dysphagia.

Important to consider is the differentiation of peripheral neuropathies from nerve root involvement. This is imperative as incorrect localization in the setting of cervical myelopathy or nerve root involvement will result in inappropriate management decisions. This can be particularly challenging for patients with rheumatoid arthritis, where muscle atrophy, tenosynovitis, tendon rupture, nerve entrapments, and peripheral neuropathies may be seen. A careful physical examination should allow the clinician to distinguish between these two forms of neurological dysfunction.

Physical examination in the setting of degenerative spine disease and cervical kyphosis is never complete without an assessment of the patient's overall spinal alignment. Normal alignment of the spine aims to center the head and neck over the shoulder girdle and pelvis. One should also examine the range of motion of the neck. Patients with ankylosing spondylitis may present with severe cervicothoracic kyphosis and marked limitation in range of motion of the neck. These patients will not have correction of the kyphosis while lying in a recumbent position. Patients with rheumatoid arthritis may also demonstrate significant limitation in neck movement due to pain and muscle stiffness. Any anticipated surgical correction must consider preoperative alignment and range of motion not only to establish surgical objectives but to help define realistic outcomes.

## Imaging

Radiographic studies complement the history and physical examination in helping to identify fractures, instability, and malalignment, as well as the potential for further neurological injury. Standard x-rays of the cervical spine include lateral, AP, and odontoid views. As well as providing initial screening for alignment and fractures, they are also helpful to assess bone quality. Flexion-extension views should be routinely performed in the setting of kyphosis to evaluate a fixed versus flexible deformity as well as to detect occult instability. CT scanning may also be undertaken to assess bone quality and further define spinal alignment, particularly in the relationship of the posterior elements.

Studies have addressed normal alignment of the cervical spine,[15] but none has provided a standardized definition of what constitutes normal cervical lordosis. Similarly, degree of kyphosis has not yet been systematically correlated with severity of presentation or natural history. As a result, decision making regarding correction of cervical kyphosis is dependent on the underlying degenerative disease and subjective clinical judgment about acceptable or unacceptable decompression and realignment. For example, kyphosis in the setting of rheumatoid arthritis often involves cranio-cervico-thoracic reconstruction whereas in the setting of ankylosing spondylitis, it typically involves segmental subtraction and reconstruction.

Magnetic resonance imaging has significantly improved the ability to examine soft tissue and neurological structures of the cervical spine. MR imaging provides structural information about the brainstem, vertebral bodies, ligaments, spinal cord, and nerve roots. In the setting of degenerative diseases of the cervical spine, an MRI should be obtained to confirm the pathology behind neurological signs or symptoms, or if any significant attempt is to be made at restoration of sagittal alignment.

## Surgical Decision-Making

Traditionally, the surgical management of cervical deformity has been considered primarily where there is evidence of radiographic instability. In their review, White and Panjabi[16] describe clinical stability as the ability of the cervical spine to prevent neurological impairment, pain, or gross deformity under physiologic loads. In keeping with this definition, surgical management for cervical kyphosis should be considered where there is evidence of clinical instability as determined by the presence of intractable pain, progressive neurological impairment, or progressive deformity.

Although the criteria for surgical intervention are generally accepted, the timing of surgical intervention is debatable. Where intractable pain and progressive neurological deficits are the predominant symptoms, common-sense principles advocate early surgical intervention. However, in those patients with progressive but otherwise asymptomatic deformity, the picture is less clear. In a small retrospective study[17] of thirteen patients, Iwasaki et al. examined predictive factors for the development of cervical kyphosis or myelopathy. The authors concluded that anterior osteophyte formation was representative of posterior ligamentous instability and predictive of progression of cervical kyphosis. In the same study, a ratio below 0.3 of the A-P diameter at the pontomedullary junction relative to the spinal cord diameter at the apex of kyphosis was felt to be predictive of progression of myelopathy. Despite this single study, there are no clear guidelines that serve to facilitate decision making.[18] Nonetheless, it is immediately obvious to any spinal surgeon that progressive cervical deformity can ultimately result in severe pain and irreversible neurological compromise. Therefore, common-sense principles dictate that early surgical intervention is warranted in patients with progressive cervical deformity.

## The Surgical Approach

Once a patient presents with intractable pain, neurological deficit, or progressive kyphotic deformity, a strategic surgical approach must be chosen. The approach must be such that the symptoms are relieved, cervical

alignment is improved, and overall stability is conferred to the cervical spine. An important consideration in surgical decision-making is the presence or absence of a fixed kyphotic deformity. A fixed kyphotic deformity is one in which the deformity does not reduce spontaneously as the patient attempts to extend the neck. This is usually the result of a combination of underlying degenerative changes including vertebral wedging, osteophyte formation, or facet hypertrophy. In contrast, a reducible kyphotic deformity is one in which motion is preserved through the kyphotic segment during flexion and extension. When a fixed kyphotic deformity is present, the surgical approach must accommodate intraoperative reduction of the cervical deformity.[19] In this circumstance, anterior osteophytes must be resected and disk spaces released in an attempt to reestablish sagittal alignment.

With reducible kyphotic deformities, partial motion may not allow for normal alignment of the cervical spine. In this case, a trial of traction may be warranted in an attempt to reestablish alignment of the cervical spine. If alignment is established, the patient should be maintained in this alignment with a halo device until the time of surgery.

Once the decision has been made to proceed with surgery, one must decide which surgical approach will be most suitable—anterior, posterior, or both. Several issues deserve consideration as the surgical approach is selected. First and foremost, the goal of surgery is to decompress or otherwise preserve integrity of the underlying nerve roots and spinal cord. Only then does the goal become to reestablish sagittal alignment. However, as mentioned earlier, there is no standardized definition for normal cervical lordosis. An additional principle is that because of the sensitive nature of the spinal cord, anterior pathology should be treated with an anterior approach whereas posterior pathology should be treated via a posterior approach. Steinmetz et al.[18] have proposed an algorithm for management of cervical kyphosis that considers each of these factors (Figure 26-4).

With this in mind, it is our experience that the majority of patients with cervical kyphosis can be managed through an anterior approach alone. This allows for superior correction of the deformity under distraction, is better tolerated by the patient, and does not violate the posterior tension band of the cervical spine. Also, if radicular pain is a major component of the patient's symptomatology, an anterior approach allows for superior decompression of the cervical nerve roots. Finally and inarguably, it allows reconstruction of a failed anterior column through provision of additional anterior column support. Given the success of multilevel fusion with anterior approaches,

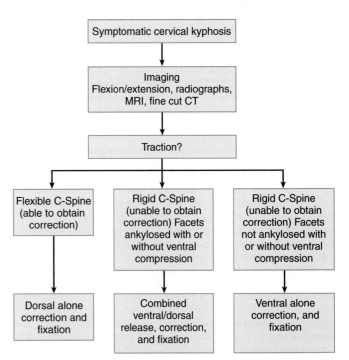

■ **FIGURE 26-4**   Treatment algorithm for correction of cervical deformity. *(Adapted from Steinmetz MP et al: Cervical deformity correction, Neurosurgery Suppl 60(1):S1-90-97, 2007.)*

the surgeon should not hesitate to perform multilevel diskectomies or, if necessary, corpectomies in order to ensure adequate decompression and alignment. If, due to the presence of severe kyphosis, a posterior approach is deemed necessary, this can often be combined with an anterior approach to ensure maximal decompression and fixation at the involved levels. Isolated posterior fixation is reserved for exceptional circumstances where a patient's physical stature limits access to the anterior cervical spine.

## Surgical Complications

Regardless of the surgical approach, there is a potential for adverse consequences as a result of surgery. Risks of anterior approaches to the cervical spine include dysphagia, vocal cord paralysis, injury to the carotid or vertebral arteries, upper airway obstruction, esophageal trauma, cranial nerve damage, and postoperative infection or hematoma. Similarly, the risks of posterior approaches to the cervical spine include injury to spinal cord or nerve roots, injury to the vertebral artery, epidural hematoma, and wound infections. With both anterior and posterior approaches, failure of hardware and fusion is a significant concern. Hardware and graft failure may be avoided by anterior approaches, use of autologous bone graft, and, where necessary, osteoinduction through the use of bone morphogenic proteins. Although fusion failure can be linked to construct length, it is important to plan reconstruction to incorporate all kyphotic segments.

Although biomechanical and surgical principles currently allow for appropriate decision making in patients with cervical kyphosis, further study is needed. Normal lordosis should be defined so that surgeons have a uniform definition from which to base their management. Natural history and randomized studies are necessary to assess predictive factors for progression of cervical kyphosis and may assist in determining the timing of surgery for these patients. Going forward, new technologies such as disk arthroplasty bear promise of a role in the management of cervical kyphosis.

## CONCLUSIONS/DiskUSSION

The organization of the cervical spine is complex, involving bone, ligaments, muscle and other soft tissues. Each of these structures contributes to normal alignment and serves to protect important neurological structures including the spinal cord and cervical nerve roots. Compromise of these tissues in the setting of degenerative disease compromises the structural integrity of the cervical spine and allows for deformity. Cervical kyphosis is one manifestation of weakened structural support and degenerative disease in the cervical spine.

In the management of cervical kyphosis, the clinical symptomatology of the patient and the nature of the kyphotic deformity must be considered. Surgical management is appropriate in the setting of intractable pain, neurological compromise, and progressive kyphotic deformity. Unfortunately, robust physiological studies do not exist, and therefore normal sagittal alignment

## *Clinical Case Example*

### TREATMENT AND CLINICAL CHALLENGES

In our case, the patient has presented with progressive symptoms of neck pain, numbness involving the left upper extremity and early signs of myelopathy. On MR imaging, abnormalities in sagittal alignment are immediately evident (see Figure 26-1). Reversal of cervical lordosis can be seen in the subaxial cervical spine with a kyphotic deformity from C3 to C5. Compression of the cervical spinal cord is associated with this, accounting for the patient's myelopathy. Fused segments can be appreciated at C2-C3, C7-T1, and T2-T3, consistent with a preexisting diagnosis of Klippel-Feil syndrome. Degenerative disk disease involving C2-C3, C3-C4, and C4-C5 is also noted. On axial imaging, left-sided foraminal stenosis is seen at the C3-C4 and C4-C5 levels. Given this patient's neurological deficits and radiological evidence of kyphosis, the patient was advised to undergo surgical intervention.

The treatment algorithm provided in this chapter recommends to first consider the presence or absence of a fixed kyphotic deformity. Close examination of the MR study demonstrates that the kyphotic deformity is segmental in nature and that osteophytes are absent. Extension radiographs confirmed reduction in deformity through the kyphotic segments. Hence traction was not considered a useful adjunct in this circumstance.

The first objective of surgery was to ensure adequate decompression of the spinal cord. MR sequences show the bulk of the stenosis to be located through the kyphosis at C3 to C5. Thus the overall surgical strategy had to permit correction of sagittal alignment as well as relief of nerve root and spinal cord compression. With these goals in mind, the patient was taken to the operating room and an anterior approach was undertaken. Extensive tissue dissection allowed for adequate exposure of C2 to C7, and distraction was applied through pins in the bodies of C3 and C6 respectively. Diskectomies were performed at the C3-C4, C4-C5, and C5-C6 levels and distraction tightened. Decompression of the nerve roots was obtained by ensuring exposure to the uncovertebral processes and removal of excess disk material laterally. Once decompression was complete, corpectomies were performed at the C4 and C5 levels by drilling away bone between the diskectomy sites. Thereafter, a single iliac crest graft was taken (measured under distraction) to reestablish anterior column support. Instrumentation was performed from C3 through C6 (Figure 26-5).

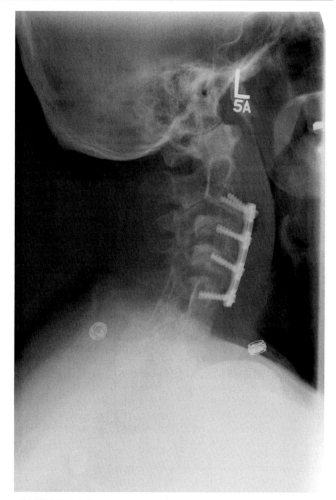

■ **FIGURE 26-5** Postoperative film demonstrating anterior cervical diskectomies and instrumented fusion. Note reestablishment of cervical lordosis from C3-C6.

of the cervical spine is not well defined. However, for the surgeon to provide adequate decompression of neural tissues, the underlying kyphotic deformity must be addressed through decompression followed by reconstruction. The exact surgical approach is dependent on the nature of the pathology and one's ability to use nonsurgical adjuncts such as traction to help realign the cervical spine, but almost invariably involves a primary anterior approach.

Cervical kyphosis is a complex surgical problem that requires an in-depth understanding of the natural history of degenerative diseases of the spine. However, careful patient selection and the use of appropriate surgical technique will ensure satisfactory surgical outcomes and symptomatic relief for the patient. Although current understanding allows for a rational approach to this particular problem, further research into the biomechanics of the cervical spine in the context of degenerative disease would certainly assist surgeons in developing new strategies to manage the problem of cervical kyphosis.

## References

1. R. Shi, J.D. Pryor, Pathological changes of isolated spinal cord axons in response to mechanical stretch, Neuroscience 110 (2002) 765–777.
2. D.C. Baptiste, M.G. Fehlings, Pathophysiology of cervical myelopathy, Spine J. 6 (2006) 190S–197S.
3. N. Yoganandan, S. Kumaresan, F. Pintar, Biomechanics of the cervical spine part 2: cervical spine soft tissue responses and biomechanical modeling, Clin. Biomech. 16 (2001) 1–27.
4. M. Panjabi, V.K. Goel, Takata K: Physiologic strains in the lumbar spine ligaments: in vitro biomechanical study, Spine 7 (1982) 192–203.
5. N. Bogduk, S. Mercer, Biomechanics of the cervical spine part 1: normal kinematics, Clin Biomech. 15 (2000) 633–648.
6. M. Aebi (Ed.), Aging spine, Springer-Verlag, Heidelberg, 2005.
7. M.J. Silva, T.M. Keaveny, W.C. Hayes, Load sharing between the shell and the centrum in the lumbar vertebral body, Spine 22 (1997) 140–150.
8. T.A. Einhorn, Bone strength: the bottom line, Calcif. Tissue Int. 51 (1992) 333–339.
9. D. Borenstein, Inflammatory arthritides of the spine, Clin. Orthop. Relat. R 443 (2006) 208–221.
10. M.J. Broom, J.F. Raycroft, Complications of fractures of the cervical spine in ankylosing spondylitis, Spine 13 (1988) 763–766.
11. F.H. Shen, et al., Rheumatoid arthritis: evaluation and surgical management of the cervical spine, Spine J. 4 (2004) 689–700.
12. M. Ward, Quality of life in patients with ankylosing spondylitis, Rheum Dis. Clin. North Am. Nov 24 (4) (1998) 815–827.
13. J.Y. Reinster, The prevalence and burden of arthritis, Rheumatology 41 (suppl.1) (2002) 3–6.
14. M. Reiter, S. Boden: Inflammatory disorders of the cervical spine, Spine 23 (24) (1998) 2755–2766.
15. J.W. Hardacker, et al., Radiographic standing cervical segmental alignment in adult volunteers without neck symptoms, Spine 22 (13) (1997) 1472–1479.
16. A. White, M. Panjabi, The role of stabilization in the treatment of cervical spine injuries, Spine 9 (1984) 512–522.
17. M. Iwasaki, et al., Cervical kyphosis: predictive factors for progression of kyphosis and myelopathy, Spine 27 (13) (2002) 1419–1425.
18. M.P. Steinmetz, et al., Cervical deformity correction, Neurosurgery 60 (1) (2007) S1-90-97.
19. O'Shaughnessy, et al., Surgical treatment of fixed cervical kyphosis with myelopathy, Spine 33 (7) (2008) 771–778.

# 27

# Surgical Treatment Modalities for Cervical Stenosis: Central Cord Syndrome and Other Spinal Cord Injuries in the Elderly

*Michael Fehlings and Randolph Gray*

**KEY POINTS**

- Central cord syndrome occurs more often in the elderly population.

- The pathophysiology of spinal cord injury involves a primary mechanical insult, followed by secondary injury that is multifactorial, though triggered by ischemia.

- Cord deformation and signal change are commonly seen in patients with central cord syndrome.

- There is currently no standard regarding the timing of surgery in patients with central cord syndrome.

- If surgery is elected, evidence suggests that surgery can be performed safely within the first 24 hours, which may positively influence neurological outcomes.

## INTRODUCTION

It is estimated that around 20% of the population of the United States will be over the age of 65 by the year 2040. This worldwide phenomenon of the aging baby boomer population is already having an impact on spine surgeons and spinal cord rehabilitation centers as older patients account for a larger proportion of the cases of spinal cord injury (SCI).

Patients presenting following cervical spinal cord injuries with disproportionate weakness of the hands and arms and relative preservation of lower extremity strength are often categorized as having either a cruciate paralysis or, more commonly, acute central cervical spinal cord injury (Box 27-1).

Acute central cord syndrome was first described in 1954 by Schneider, in a case series of 8 patients with neurological deficits following hyperextension injury to the cervical spine and a review of another 6 cases reported in the literature with a similar injury mechanism and neurological presentation.[1]

The leading causes of SCI are motor vehicle accidents, sports and recreational activities, accidents at work, falls in the home, and violence.

It is estimated that the annual incidence of SCI varies between 11.5 to 53.4 per million population.[2] In the United States, the annual incidence is around 40 per million. Central cord syndrome is the most common spinal cord injury pattern.[3] The relative distribution of other types of SCI is shown in Figure 27-1.

## MECHANISM

Based on radiographic, operative, and postmortem findings, Schneider postulated that during forceful hyperextension the anterior osteophytes and the bulging of the ligamentum flavum caused significant anteroposterior narrowing of the spinal canal and contusion of the spinal cord (Figure 27-2).

He noted in the postmortem findings that the maximum injury was in the central part of the spinal cord. The mechanism of central cord syndrome is a hyperextension injury, often on a background of long-standing cervical spondylosis, with no bony or ligamentous injury. Hyperextension of the cervical spine causes overlapping of the laminae and buckling of the ligamentum flavum, reducing the canal diameter by a further 2 to 3 mm. This compromise may cause significant acute cord compression in an aging spondylotic cervical spine with preexisting discoligamentous and osseous compression. It is estimated that this mechanism of hyperextension accounts for around 50% of cases of acute traumatic central cord syndrome (ATCCS).

**BOX 27-1  TYPES OF SPINAL CORD SYNDROMES**

Central cord syndrome
Brown-Séquard syndrome
Anterior cord syndrome
Posterior cord syndrome
Conus medullaris syndrome
Cauda equina syndrome

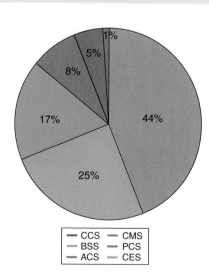

- CCS   - CMS
- BSS   - PCS
- ACS   - CES

■ **FIGURE 27-1** The relative distribution of syndromes in spinal cord injury. BSS, Brown-Séquard syndrome; CMS, Conus medullaris syndrome; ACS, Anterior cord syndrome; PCS, Posterior cord syndrome; CCS, Central cord syndrome; CES, Cauda equina syndrome.

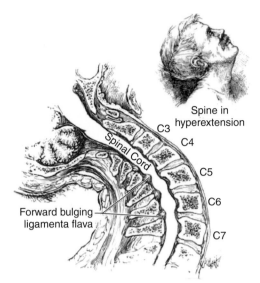

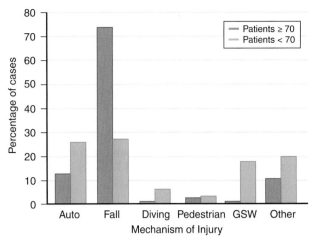

■ **FIGURE 27-3** Causes of cervical spinal cord injuries. GSW, gunshot wound.

■ **FIGURE 27-2** Original drawing of the hyperextension mechanism from Schneider's paper in 1954. *(From Schneider RC, Cherry G, Pantek H: The syndrome of acute central cervical spinal cord injury; with special reference to the mechanisms involved in hyperextension injuries of cervical spine [part 1], J Neurosurg 11:546-577, 1954.)*

---

**BOX 27-2    SALIENT FEATURES OF CENTRAL CORD SYNDROME**

- Acute cervical spinal cord injury caused by traumatic forceful hyperextension of the neck
- Disproportionate motor impairment of upper more than lower extremities
- Bladder dysfunction and urinary retention
- Varying degrees of sensory loss below the level of the lesion
- Recovery pattern is characterized by the return of lower extremity function first, followed by upper limb function, with finger movement being the last of the upper limb functions to return.

---

The other mechanisms are fractures and/or subluxations and herniated nucleus pulposus.[4] The most common mechanism of injury in the elderly population is a low-energy ground-level fall with impact on the head or chin causing forceful hyperextension of the neck. Typically this low-energy impact does not cause any bony injury.

## DEFINITION OF CENTRAL CORD SYNDROME

Central cord syndrome was described by Schneider in 1954: "It is characterized by disproportionately more motor impairment of the upper than the lower extremities, bladder dysfunction, usually urinary retention, and varying degrees of sensory loss below the level of the lesion." (Box 27-2).[1]

## INCIDENCE AND AGE

The average age of spinal cord injury (SCI) has increased from 28.7 to 38 years, and the percentage of spinal cord injury in people over 60 years of age has increased from 4.7% to 11.5%. After the age of 45 years, falls are the most common cause of cervical spinal cord injury, increasing in incidence with advancing age. In one series, 74% of injuries in patients 70 years of age or older were caused by falls (Figure 27-3).[5] SCI in the elderly typically results from a low-energy injury sustained from a fall at ground level. There is a bimodal pattern of the age distribution in ATCCS patients. The increase in age has had an impact on the pathogenesis, functional deficit, recovery, and rehabilitation of patients with spinal cord injuries.[6] In general, older patients demonstrate less recovery from spinal cord injury compared to younger patients (Box 27-3).[7] Experimental animal studies have shown that increased age increases the area of pathology and amount of demyelination, while demonstrating a significantly lower amount of endogenous remyelination following induced SCI.[6] These studies have

demonstrated that abnormalities in myelination and functional deficits secondary to SCI are age-related.

Advances in medicine seen over the past five decades have resulted in a dramatic increase in life expectancy following spinal cord injury. At present, the available data would suggest the mortality among spinal cord injury patients is around 3.8% in the first year post-injury, 1.6% in the second year post-injury, and approximately 1.2% a year over the next 10 years.[8] The chronological age, degree of injury severity, injury completeness, and neurological level are the most important predictors of mortality. The annual mortality rate varies between 0.4% and 0.5%.

---

**BOX 27-3    FACTORS PREDICTING MOTOR RECOVERY AND FUNCTIONAL OUTCOME**

Neurological deficit at presentation
Comorbidities
Formal education
Age at injury
Development of spasticity

---

## BASIC SCIENCE

### Pathophysiology of Acute Traumatic Central Cord Syndrome (ATCCS)

The peripheral compressive forces exerted on the spinal cord cause concussion, and contusion of the spinal cord results in a primary and secondary neuronal injury following the acute trauma. MRI and histopathological studies have shown that ATCCS is predominantly a white matter injury. Intramedullary hemorrhage, as was previously thought in the original descriptions, is not a necessary feature of the syndrome. However, rarely and in more severe trauma, bleeding into the central part of the cord may cause ATCCS, portending a less favorable prognosis. These histological changes reflect stasis of axoplasmic flow and both intracellular and extracellular edematous injury. The secondary injury is facilitated by a cascade of events mediated by systemic and local vascular insults, electrolyte shifts, edema, and excitotoxicity. The pathophysiological changes can progress in the first few days after the injury, both proximally and distally.[9]

Two theories have been postulated to explain the pathoanatomical basis of disproportionate involvement of the upper more than the lower extremities.

### Theory of Somatotopic Organization of Corticospinal Tracts (Neuroanatomical Theory)

Although the theory had been that central cord injury results in deficits that reflect the somatotopic organization of the corticospinal tracts (CST), recent axonal tracing data from primates and imaging-pathological data from humans have essentially discredited this theory.[10] This theory was based on early work done by Foerster (1937) and Schneider (1954), where it was postulated that the somatotopic organization of the human corticospinal tract (CST) resulted in the central injury of the spinal cord affecting the more medially organized CST fibers of the hand within the lateral columns in preference to the more laterally placed lower limb fibers. Foerster presented no evidence for his theory of somatotopic organization of the CST tracts. There has been no neuroanatomic evidence presented even subsequently to support these assertions.

## Theory of Increased Upper Limb and Hand Functional Representation of CST (Functional Theory)

The more recent theory postulated is that the CST in the human is more important for hand and arm function than it is for the lower extremity. It is believed that the CST has assumed a relatively greater importance for movement, particularly hand function, as humans ascend the phylogenetic scale, with more CST fibers synapsing with anterior horn cells innervating upper limb and hand function. Therefore any injury of the cervical cord involving the CST will preferentially affect more upper limb and hand function, as this pathway may be predominantly devoted to the motor function of the arms and hands in humans. The afferent fibers carried in the lateral and ventral descending pathways can mediate lower limb voluntary motor activity, and both must be substantially damaged to cause lower limb paralysis. More recent studies looking at the MRI scan findings in ATCCS have also concluded that the injury to the corticospinal tracts is global in nature and not confined to its medial part as has been described in the past. [10,11] All these more recent studies have suggested that the functional differentiation of the descending pathways of the upper and lower is the reason for the disproportionate involvement of upper limbs and hands in central cord syndrome.

## Neurological and Functional Recovery of Central Cord Syndrome in the Elderly

There is a significantly higher mortality and morbidity among elderly patients with SCI compared to younger patients. In one of the largest published series on acute admissions of SCI in geriatric patients, the mortality rate in the first year was eightfold more than in younger patients. The reasons for this increase in mortality and morbidity are multifactorial, including increased age, reduced physiological reserves, increased respiratory complications with prolonged periods of bed rest and inactivity, and a higher incidence of multiorgan failure.

Elderly patients with incomplete spinal cord injury do pose a significant challenge with regard to rehabilitation. Recent evidence suggests that most patients older than 60 years of age recover good function with rehabilitation. The group of patients with ATCCS has been shown to improve more significantly than in the other described spinal cord syndromes.

The influence of age alone on the neurological recovery is difficult to ascertain from the literature due to the heterogeneity of the outcome measures and the use of historical controls. In a more recent study, age alone has not been shown to be an independent predictor of poor neurological recovery following ATCCS. However, increased age has been shown to have an adverse effect as measured by the Functional Independence Measure (FIM).[12] Improved FIM has also been shown to improve with formal education, absence of spasticity, and with surgical treatment.

## IMAGING IN ACUTE TRAUMATIC SPINAL CORD INJURY[13]

## Imaging Modalities Used to Assess Cervical Spine Injury (Box 27-4)

- Lateral radiograph of cervical spine
- Computed tomography (CT)
- Magnetic resonance imaging (MRI)

A lateral radiograph of the cervical spine is useful for initial imaging in the setting of cervical trauma, especially in a neurologically intact patient.

---

> **BOX 27-4   THREE COMMON CLINICAL PRESENTATIONS OF ATCCS**
>
> 1. ATCCS with a background of segmental spinal canal stenosis secondary to disc/osteophyte complex and no discoligamentous or skeletal injury
> 2. ATCCS secondary to skeletal or ligamentous injury on a background of cervical spondylosis and spinal canal stenosis.
> 3. ATCCS secondary to acute disc herniation with no preexisting spinal canal stenosis

However, its limitations in detecting upper and lower cervical spine skeletal injuries are well recognized.

CT scan remains the most useful and informative imaging tool for skeletal trauma in the cervical spine. The advent of rapid-sequence spiral CT scans with multiplanar reconstruction has made the detailed evaluation of bony injury much easier.

Magnetic resonance imaging is the imaging modality of choice in investigating spinal cord injury. The parenchymal hemorrhage/contusion, edema, and spinal cord disruption seen on MRI in acute and subacute SCI correlate well with the predicted outcome. It has been shown to be useful in quantifying the extent of axonal loss in spinal cord injury.

### MRI Findings in Traumatic SCI

1. Prevertebral soft tissue injury
2. Skeletal injury
3. Extradural compression
4. Cord deformation and signal change within the cord

### Skeletal Injury

A change in the vertebral body morphology is the most reliable sign of fracture on MRI scan. Disruption of the cortical margins is best seen on T2-weighted and gradient echo images. There is also altered signal intensity of the medullary bone relative to the adjacent segments, which is a reliable sign of compression fractures of the vertebral body. Characteristically, the region of skeletal injuries shows a lower signal intensity on T1-weighted images and a higher intensity on T2-weighted images. Over 90% of patients over the age of 60 years will have changes of spondylosis, and hence the appreciation of subtle skeletal injuries on MRI can be extremely difficult.

CT scan is a much more sensitive method of detecting vertebral fractures, especially minor fractures involving the posterior elements. It is, however, not reliable for detecting the presence of cord swelling, disc herniation, and prevertebral edema.

### Extradural Compression

Extradural compression by herniated discs, elevation of the posterior longitudinal ligament, and infolded ligamentum flavum is best appreciated on T2-weighted images. The injured disc often has a higher signal intensity compared to the adjacent discs.

### Cord Deformation and Signal Change within the Cord

Edema of the cord is seen as areas of high signal intensity on proton-density and T2-weighted images. The area of increased signal is directly proportional to the severity of the injury. In the first week following injury, intramedullary hemorrhage is seen as low signal intensity on T2-weighted images and is centered in the region of cord edema. After the first week, the area of intramedullary hemorrhage consists mainly of methemoglobin, which is seen as an area of high signal intensity on T1-weighted images.[14] The presence of intramedullary hemorrhage not only reflects on the severity of the injury but also on the poor prognosis for neurological recovery.[15]

## TREATMENT

The debate on the optimal treatment of central cord syndrome continues around the controversies of the benefit of surgery, timing of surgery, and the use of high-dose intravenous steroids.

Spontaneous, though usually incomplete, recovery of neurological function in the setting of central cord syndrome is well recognized. There

## BOX 27-5  SUGGESTED CLINICAL PRACTICE GUIDELINES BASED ON CURRENT EVIDENCE

*ATCCS secondary to forced hyperextension with preexisting stenosis and no discoligamentous or skeletal injuries:*
- Observe for neurological improvement
- Decompressive surgery acutely if expected neurological recovery does not occur, or in a delayed fashion once neurological recovery plateaus out.

*ATCCS secondary to discoligamentous or skeletal injury:*
- Acute decompression and stabilization once patient is hemodynamically and medically stable
- Aim to perform surgery within 24 hours of injury

is no convincing evidence that acute decompressive surgery improves the neurological outcome of this group at this stage, although this remains an area of controversy. The University of Maryland, led by Aarabi, is currently undertaking a clinical trial to examine this question. However, in the absence of more definitive data, delayed surgical treatment of the stenosis once the neurological improvement has plateaued, or earlier if no significant neurological improvement occurs, is a reasonable algorithm for treating this subgroup. In patients with normal cervical sagittal balance, decompression through laminectomy, with or without posterior instrumented fusion, is an option. In cervical spines without instability, an open-door expansile cervical laminoplasty is another surgical intervention that can be safely applied with promising results. In kyphotic cervical spines, it is recommended that the decompression be performed from an anterior approach, with multilevel discectomies or corpectomies with internal fixation.

There is Class II and class III evidence to support early surgical decompression and stabilization in ATCCS caused by ligamentodiscal injuries and unstable skeletal injuries, the objective being relief of acute compression, stabilization, and correction of spinal alignment, thus preventing further secondary injury to the spinal cord. Early decompressive surgery in this group is more effective and has been shown to reduce length of ICU stay and improve overall motor recovery. The exact timing of surgery in this setting is, however, debatable. Currently there is no standard regarding the timing of decompressive surgery after SCI. The proposed guidelines, based on the recent literature, state that decompressive surgery can be safely performed in the first 24 hours of injury in a hemodynamically stable patient (Box 27-5). There is preliminary evidence that early decompression within 24 hours of injury may improve the neurological recovery.[16-18]

## Clinical Challenges

Clinical challenges include the following:

- Reduced physiological reserve and management of age-related comorbidity
- Delayed retrieval/referral to spinal trauma center
- Management of complications secondary to SCI, including respiratory failure
- Rehabilitation challenges that are unique to the elderly
- Increased costs/burden to society of geriatric SCI

## Future Treatments

Future treatments include:

- Role of neuroprotective treatments (e.g., the sodium-glutamate antagonist riluzole) to minimize secondary spinal cord injury
- Spinal cord regeneration/stem cell research
- Development of algorithm and standard of care for surgical decompression

## SUMMARY

Central cord injury describes a syndrome where patients present with disproportionate weakness of the hands and arms and relative preservation of lower extremity strength. The injury, which is the commonest form of cervical SCI accounting for 45% of such injuries, usually occurs as a result of a low velocity injury (eg a fall) in the setting of congenital or acquired cervical stenosis. The disproportionate involvement of the upper extremities reflects the fact that the corticospinal tract predominantly innervates motoneurons subserving volitional control of the hands and arms.

The management algorithm involves a precise diagnosis with appropriate CT and MR imaging, medical stabilization (including hypertensive therapy and consideration of the use of corticosteroids) and surgical decompression/stabilization. The latter is undertaken by the senior author in an acute manner (within 24 hours of the injury) only with severe injuries which do not show significant neurological recovery. Otherwise, surgical intervention is preferred once neurological recovery starts to plateau (around 6 weeks after injury). Future research will more precisely determine the appropriate role and timing of surgical intervention and will examine the role of novel neuroprotective approaches such as the sodium-glutamate antagonist riluzole.

## References

1. R.C. Schneider, G. Cherry, H. Pantek, The syndrome of acute central cervical spinal cord injury; with special reference to the mechanisms involved in hyperextension injuries of cervical spine (part1), J. Neurosurg. 11 (1954) 546–577.
2. L.H. Sekhon, M.G. Fehlings, Epidemiology, demographics, and pathophysiology of acute spinal cord injury, Spine 26 (2001) S2–12.
3. W. McKinley, K. Santos, M. Meade, K. Brooke, Incidence and outcomes of spinal cord injury clinical syndromes, J. Spinal Cord. Med. 30 (2007) 215–224.
4. B. Aarabi, M. Koltz, D. Ibrahimi, Hyperextension cervical spine injuries and traumatic central cord syndrome, Neurosurg. Focus 25 (2008) E9.
5. D. Fassett, J. Harrop, M. Maltenfort, S. Jeyamohan, J. Ratliff, D. Anderson, A. Hilibrand, T. Albert, A. Vaccaro, A. Sharan, Mortality rates in geriatric patients with spinal cord injuries, J. Neurosurg. Spine 7 (2007) 277–281.
6. M.M. Siegenthaler, D.L. Ammon, H.S. Keirstead, Myelin pathogenesis and functional deficits following SCI are age-associated, Exp. Neurol. 213 (2008) 363–371.
7. J. Furlan, M. Bracken, M. Fehlings, Is age a key determinant of mortality and neurological outcome after acute traumatic spinal cord injury? Neurobiol. Aging, 2008.
8. J.S. Krause, R.E. Carter, E.E. Pickelsimer, D. Wilson, A prospective study of health and risk of mortality after spinal cord injury, Arch. Phys. Med. Rehab. 89 (2008) 1482–1491.
9. C.H. Tator, Update on the pathophysiology and pathology of acute spinal cord injury, Brain Pathol, 1995.
10. C.T. Pappas, A.R. Gibson, V.K. Sonntag, Decussation of hind-limb and fore-limb fibers in the monkey corticospinal tract: relevance to cruciate paralysis, J. Neurosurg. 75 (1991) 935–940.
11. F. Collignon, D. Martin, J. Lénelle, A. Stevenaert, Acute traumatic central cord syndrome: magnetic resonance imaging and clinical observations, J. Neurosurg. Spine. supplement(2002) 29–33.
12. M.F. Dvorak, C.G. Fisher, J. Hoekema, M.C. Boyd, V. Noonan, Factors predicting motor recovery and functional outcome after traumatic central cord syndrome: a long-term follow-up, Spine. 31 (11) (2005) 2303–2011.
13. D. Lammertse, D. Dungan, J. Dreisbach, S. Falci, A. Flanders, R. Marino, E. Schwartz, Rehabilitation NIoDa: Neuroimaging in traumatic spinal cord injury: an evidence-based review for clinical practice and research, J. Spinal Cord Med. 30 (20) (2007) 205–214.
14. A.E. Flanders, D.M. Schaefer, H.T. Doan, M.M. Mishkin, Acute cervical spine trauma: correlation of MR imaging findings with degree of neurologic deficit, Radiology 177 (1) (1990) 25–33.
15. A.E. Flanders, C.M. Spettell, L.M. Tartaglino, D.P. Friedman, G.J. Herbison, Forecasting motor recovery after cervical spinal cord injury: value of MR imaging, Radiology 201 (1996) 649–655.
16. M.G. Fehlings, L.H. Sekhon, C.H. Tator, The role and timing of decompression in acute spinal cord injury: what do we know? What should we do? Spine 26 (2001) S101–10.
17. M.G. Fehlings, Perrin: The timing of surgical intervention in the treatment of spinal cord injury: a systematic review of recent clinical evidence, Spine 31 (11 supplement) (2006) 28–35.
18. J.S. Harrop, A.D. Sharan, J. Ratliff, Central cord injury: pathophysiology, management, and outcomes, Spine J. 6 (2006) S198–S206.

# 28

# Occipital-Cervical and Upper Cervical Spine Fractures

*Nduka Amankulor, Grahame Gould, and Khalid M. Abbed*

### K E Y   P O I N T S

- Understand occipital-cervical anatomy
- Identify injury types, bony and ligamentous, in the occipital-cervical region.
- Understand nonoperative and operative treatment options of specific occipital-cervical injuries.
- Learn surgical techniques used to treat occipital-cervical injuries.
- Be aware of potential complications of occipital-cervical injuries.

## OVERVIEW

The craniocervical junction and atlantoaxial spine is composed of a complex set of unique vertebrae, ligaments, and joints that function to maintain the mechanical stability and dynamic range of motion of the head and neck and protect the vital underlying neurovascular structures including the brainstem, cervical spinal cord, lower cranial nerves, and the vertebral arteries. Appropriate identification and treatment of injuries to this region requires a firm understanding of the normal anatomy and how it is affected by inflammatory, degenerative, traumatic, and neoplastic processes that can lead to neural compression and instability.

## ANATOMY

### Occipital Bone

The occipital bone is an anteriorly concave bone that forms the base of the cranium. The occipital condyles are paired kidney-shaped structures that form the base of the occipital bone and are the structural bases for the articulation of the skull with the cervical spine. This articulation is mainly formed by the atlanto-occipital joint, a paired synovial joint composed of the bilateral occipital condyles projecting inferiorly to articulate with the concave lateral masses of the atlas. The atlas, in turn, articulates with the axis anteriorly via the odontoid process, and laterally via the lateral masses, with associated synovial capsules at each articulation.[1]

### The Atlas

The atlas, or C1, is the first cervical vertebra and is shaped to allow articulation with the odontoid process of C2 and the skull. It is unique in that it has no vertebral body. In place of a vertebral body, the anterior portion of C1 is composed of an anterior tubercle, which forms the site of attachment for the longus colli and the anterior longitudinal ligament, and an anterior arch, which is roughly cylindrical and anteriorly convex. The anterior arches of C1 extend slightly laterally and posteriorly to join the lateral masses. The C1 lateral masses makeup the majority of the C1 surface area and articulate with the large occipital condyles. The posterior arches of C1 extend posteriorly and medially from the lateral masses to terminate

in the short posterior tubercle. The posterior tubercle is analogous to the spinous processes of the other cervical vertebrae; however, its small size allows for greater range of motion between the skull and C1 during neck extension.

### The Axis

The axis, or C2, is the unique second vertebra. It is widely described as a pivot joint because the skull and atlas rotate around C2 with significant freedom. The axis is a transitional vertebra and shares properties with the unique C1 vertebra and the relatively uniform vertebrae of the subaxial spine. The body of the axis gives rise to its most unique feature, the odontoid process, which is a peglike extension of bone that tapers superiorly and terminates in the midline just behind the anterior arch of C1. The tip of the odontoid process is perfectly situated for ligamentous connections with the atlas and the occipital condyles. The superior articular surface of C2 is rounded and flat, like its counterpart on C1; however, the inferior articular surface of C2 is similar to the rest of the subaxial spine. Unlike C1, the axis has a pedicle, or isthmus, and a true lamina.

### Ligaments of the Craniocervical Junction

The bony anatomy of the skull base, occipital condyles, atlas, axis, and odontoid process is of obvious importance in understanding biomechanical stability, fracture patterns, and surgical planning. The anatomy of the ligamentous structures of the craniocervical junction and upper cervical spine is also of crucial importance in maintaining biomechanical stability of the region, where injury to ligamentous structures can dramatically alter management of bony fractures. The nuchal ligament runs dorsally over the occiput and upper cervical spine, from the inion to the spinous processes of the cervical vertebrae. The ligamentum flavum runs underneath the laminae and projects superiorly to the base of the occiput. The anterior longitudinal ligament (ALL) has a dense arrangement of fibers and projects from the anterior tubercle of the axis inferiorly along the ventral surface of each cervical vertebral body. The anterior atlanto-occipital membrane, the superior extension of the ALL, is superficial, more loosely arranged, and connects the basilar part of the occiput to the atlas. The posterior longitudinal ligament runs along the dorsal surface of the cervical vertebral bodies and projects superiorly as the tectorial membrane, attaching to the skull base. The alar ligaments (attaching to the odontoid process, occipital condyles, and atlas), apical ligament (attaching the odontoid process to the clivus), and transverse atlantal ligament (restricting the odontoid to the anterior arch of the atlas) play a key role in maintaining the anatomic relationship of the odontoid process, the atlas, and the foramen magnum. Given the significant range of flexion-extension at O-C1 and rotation at C1-2, and the critical importance of the underlying neurovascular structures, biomechanical instability of this region can present with severe disability and must be treated aggressively.

## The Vertebral Artery

Knowledge of the vertebral artery (VA) anatomy at the craniocervical junction is extremely important for understanding the mechanisms and consequences of injury to this region. Injury to the vertebral artery in this region can occur as a result of blunt or penetrating trauma, C1 or C2 fractures (especially those traversing the foramen transversarium), and iatrogenic injuries caused by aggressive manipulation of the cervical spine, for example.

The paired VAs usually arise from each subclavian artery. They ascend posteriorly and superiorly between the longus colli and scalenus anterior and enter the foramen transversarium of the upper six cervical vertebrae. The foramen transversarium pierces the transverse processes of each of these cervical vertebrae. The VA travels superiorly through the lower five cervical vertebrae and then curves laterally and superiorly to enter the foramen transversarium of the atlas. The artery then curves anteriorly and superiorly to enter the foramen magnum, traveling along the lateral aspect of the medulla.

## INJURIES OF THE CRANIOCERVICAL JUNCTION

### Overview

As with any trauma patient, priority in management begins with the primary and secondary survey including craniospinal immobilization, hemodynamic stabilization, and radiographic evaluation. High-resolution computed tomography (CT) scans are indicated for any patients with clinical suspicion for cervical spine injury, including patients with altered sensorium or clinical evidence of head injury. Once identified, traumatic injuries of the craniocervical junction are triaged based on the clinical evidence of neural injury, vascular injury, and/or mechanical instability, and supplemental imaging such as angiography and magnetic resonance should be utilized liberally when indicated.

### Occipitocervical Instability

OC instability is one of the most dangerous conditions affecting the cervical spine. True OC instability is a clinical emergency. The pathophysiology of OC instability ranges from trauma to inflammatory/neoplastic conditions, but trauma is the most common reason for operative intervention.

### Occipitoatlantal Dislocation

Among traumatic injuries to the cervical spine and causes for OC instability, occipitoatlantal dislocation (OAD) is one of the most severe types of injuries. It is a hyperflexion-distraction injury which results in the ligamentous disconnection of the skull from the cervical spine. OAD is often immediately fatal because of associated neurological and vascular injuries. The first clue in the diagnosis of OAD is the mechanism of injury. High-impact injuries should always arouse the suspicion of OAD. Plain radiographs of the cervical spine reveal prevertebral soft tissue swelling and an increase in the basion-dens interval, which should measure 12 mm or less. More definitive diagnosis is made with reconstructed CT images of the craniocervical junction. MRI and CT of the craniocervical junction are comparable in terms of identifying OAD, but MRI can often identify the specific ligaments injured.

OAD injuries can be identified into three broad categories. Type I injuries are characterized by anterior displacement of the occipital condyles on the C1 lateral masses; type II injuries are characterized by displacement of the occiput and C1 in the vertical plane; and finally, type III injuries are marked by posterior displacement of occipital condyles compared to C1.

### Occipital Condyle Fractures

Occipital condyle fractures can be classified into three main types according to the Anderson and Montesano scheme.[2] These fractures are seen in 1% to 3% of cases of blunt trauma to the craniocervical region. Type 1 fractures usually result from axial loading injuries and are comminuted. Type II fractures are linear fractures that originate in the squama of the occipital bone and extend into the condyle. Type III fractures are avulsion fractures of the condyles; these fractures are most prone to instability and atlanto-occipital dislocation.

## C1 Fractures and Transverse Ligament Injuries

Fractures of the atlas are usually defined in relation to the lateral mass and extent of arch involvement.[3] They can involve any parts of the ring in isolation or in combination, ranging from single unilateral fractures to burst-type fractures involving all four aspects, which is known as a Jefferson fracture. Since isolated atlas fractures without ligamentous injury are stable and heal with simple immobilization, the clinical importance of fractures of the atlas is to understand the possible involvement of the transverse ligament, the vertebral artery, and other associated spinal fractures. The most commonly cited radiographic criteria indicating unstable disruption of the transverse ligament include the Rule of Spence[4] (lateral displacement of C1 lateral masses over C2 greater than 6.9 mm) and the atlantodental interval being greater than 3 mm. However, when feasible, this author prefers MRI evaluation of all atlas fractures to assess for concomitant ligamentous injury. Transverse ligament disruption, as with other cases of atlantoaxial instability, is an indication for surgical fixation.

Nontraumatic disruption of the atlantoaxial ligaments can also lead to gross atlantoaxial instability. C1-2 rotatory subluxation is a rare condition usually seen after inflammatory and/or infectious conditions of the pharynx and tonsils in the pediatric population. In the elderly, rheumatoid arthritis (discussed later) can lead to atlantoaxial instability requiring surgical stabilization.

## C2 Fractures

Odontoid process fractures affect the elderly far more often than younger people and are, unfortunately, relatively common. The most common classification scheme for fractures of C2, the Anderson and D'Alonzo scheme,[5] relies on the location of the fracture line within the odontoid process or body of C2. In this scheme, type I fractures involve the tip of the dens, type II fractures run through the junction of the dens and the body of C2, and type III fractures course through the vertebral body of C2.

Type I fractures are an avulsion of the alar ligament and are usually stable. Cervical collar immobilization for symptomatic management is usually sufficient.

Type II fractures (Figure 28-1) are the most common type of dens fracture and are more often subject to nonunion, especially in patients older than 50 years of age when displacement is greater than 5 mm. When choosing treatment strategies for type II odontoid fractures, the surgeon must consider the integrity of the transverse ligament, age and orientation of the fracture, displacement and/or angulation of the fractured process, and

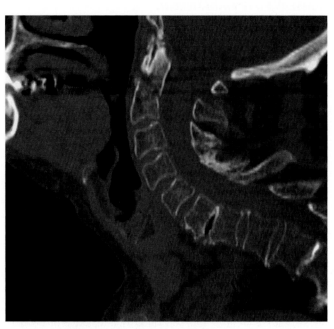

■ **FIGURE 28-1**  Type II dens fracture.

patient-specific factors such as medical comorbidities, and body habitus. For example, certain body habitus features, such as a barrel chest, can make anterior odontoid screw placement impossible.

Type III fractures extend into the C2 vertebral body. This fracture type can be mechanically unstable but usually heals well with immobilization. As such, treatment usually entails cervical immobilization in either a rigid cervical orthosis or a halovest for 12 weeks, and the majority of patients heal by bony union.

Fractures of the C2 pedicles (also known as traumatic spondylolisthesis or hangman's fractures) are often classified based on the mechanism of injury,[6,7] where flexion (type III) and flexion-distraction (type IIa) are often unstable and require surgical fixation, especially type IIa injuries with greater than 4 mm distraction and/or greater than 11 degrees of angulation. Other fractures of the axis can include isolated fractures of the C2 vertebral body or fractures of the C2 spinous process or lamina, which are usually stable and can achieve good union with nonoperative immobilization.

## Craniocervical Manifestations of Rheumatoid Arthritis

Between 10% and 85% of patients with rheumatoid arthritis (RA) have neck pain and 10% to 60% have neurological deficits.[8] Spinal column manifestations of RA are most often seen at the craniocervical junction. This is usually a late finding in the disease course; therefore, a significant proportion of RA patients with craniocervical abnormalities are elderly.

RA of the upper cervical spine, similar to RA in peripheral joints, is an inflammatory condition that results in degenerative synovitis, ligament laxity, pannus formation, and bony erosion. These pathological changes can lead to atlantoaxial subluxation and are present in up to 86% of patients with RA.[8] RA can also lead to degeneration of the occipital condyle-C1 joints, leading to cranial settling. Degeneration of the C1-2 and O-C1 joints can also lead to vertical migration of the odontoid process into the foramen magnum (basilar invagination), resulting in myelopathy from odontoid compression of the lower brainstem. Myelopathy can also be caused by pannus formation around the dens and consequent narrowing of the spinal canal.

Management of craniocervical abnormalities in patients with rheumatoid arthritis depends on the severity of clinical symptoms and the extent of craniocervical instability. Similar to craniocervical and atlantoaxial instability induced by traumatic events, measurement of the Powers ratio and the atlantodental interval can be used to assess occipitoatlantal and atlantoaxial instability, respectively. C2 vertical subluxation can be assessed by a number of radiographic lines (Chamberlain's, McRae's and McGregor's lines). Frank craniocervical instability requires surgical stabilization.

## CONSERVATIVE MANAGEMENT OF OCCIPITOCERVICAL INJURIES IN THE AGING SPINE

Once evidence of occipitocervical injuries is discovered in the aging spine, the treating clinician has to decide whether to pursue surgical or nonsurgical management of these conditions. The initial step in the management of all craniocervical region injuries is to determine whether the injury is stable or unstable. Some instances of craniocervical abnormalities, like occipitoatlantal dislocation, result in evidence of clear instability and are therefore surgical emergencies. However, stable injuries such as type I odontoid fractures can be managed with cervical orthoses while bony union is achieved.

Conservative management of upper cervical injuries is usually achieved with rigid immobilization of the cervical spine either with rigid cervical collars, such as the Philadelphia collar or Miami J collar, or with halo vests. Cervical collars provide good sagittal motion restriction in the upper cervical and subaxial spine. However, they are easy to remove and thus have variable rates of user adherence.

Halo vests provide good upper cervical and subaxial sagittal motion restriction. They also provide superior axial plane motion restriction compared to cervical collars. In addition, halo vests are secured to the skull and cannot be easily removed by users. Halo vests are associated with a higher morbidity and mortality rate, especially for elderly patients. For these reasons, halo vest use in the aging population, while sometimes unavoidable, should be approached with caution.

## SURGICAL APPROACHES AND TECHNIQUES

### Ventral vs. Dorsal Approaches

Isolated odontoid fractures, any large C2 pannus with ventral compression of the spinal cord, and bony tumors of C1 or C2 (especially those located in the midline and anterior to the spinal cord) can be approached ventrally. Ventral approaches to the high cervical spine can be accomplished through the neck, the posterior pharyngeal wall, the maxilla, or the mandible. The ventral retropharyngeal approach gains access to the ventral aspects of C1 and C2. With this approach, care must be taken to preserve the cervical branches of the facial nerve and the hypoglossal nerve as these structures traverse the neck. The transoral approach utilizes an incision in the dorsal pharyngeal wall and provides excellent access to the ventral midline cervical spine. It can be used for odontoid resection and for resection of clival lesions. Transoral approaches may be associated with relatively higher complication rates, including CSF leak, wound dehiscence, retropharyngeal abscess, and lingual edema. Extended maxillary approaches (described by Crockard and colleagues) and mandibular approaches can be utilized in cases where wider surgical corridors are required.

Dorsal approaches to the occipitocervical region are used far more frequently than ventral approaches. The patient is positioned in the standard prone position and common surgical principles such as dissection along the avascular midline plane and subperiosteal dissection are employed.

### Occipitocervical Fusion

The instrumented technique for achieving rigid fixation across the occipitocervical junction was popularized by Ransford and colleagues in 1986. They described the use of a contoured steel loop and sublaminar wiring to establish a fairly rigid fixation across the OC junction. Although the use of sublaminar wires increases the risk of injury to neural structures when compared to uninstrumented, onlay fusion procedures, the vast improvement in fusion rates after sublaminar wiring popularized its use. However, in spite of the improved level of fixation after sublaminar wiring, patients still required the use of halo vests before complete solid fusion could be established. The desire for fixation techniques that obviate the need for halo vests led to the techniques being used today. The most common surgical treatment for OC instability today involves the use of a contoured occipital plate that is connected by a rod to cervical screws (Figure 28-2).

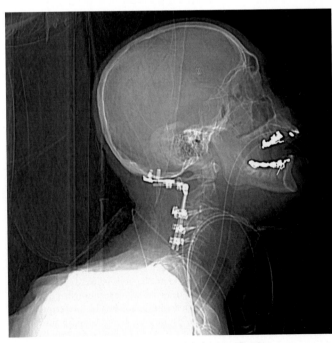

**■ FIGURE 28-2**  Occipital-cervical fixation.

Patients undergoing occipitocervical fusion are usually placed in a Mayfield clamp and secured in a prone position, taking care to avoid excessive motion at the craniocervical junction during positioning. Since fixation of the occiput to the cervical spine eliminates the natural range of motion at the OC-C1 joint, care must be taken to maintain the spine in a neutral position in order to prevent patients from assuming a permanent flexed or extended position after surgery. An incision is usually made from the external occipital protuberance down to C3 or C4 and a subperiosteal muscular dissection is performed at all levels where screws are to be placed. The occipital bone is thickest in the midline and thins out laterally, so the length of the occipital screws must be chosen carefully and in accordance with the shape of the bone. Depending on the integrity of the bony structures in the atlas and axis, lateral mass screws can be placed at C1 and translaminar or pedicle/pars screws may be used at C2. Transarticular C1-C2 screws are also an option. The cervical spine screws are then secured via a rod to the occipital plate.

## Odontoid Screw

When feasible, an excellent option for treatment of type 2 odontoid fractures is direct fixation of the fracture with an anterior odontoid screw (Figure 28-3). Preoperative considerations include intact transverse ligament, fracture line orientation, and acuity of injury (given concern for nonunion with sclerotic fracture edges). Depending on displacement of the fractured odontoid process, reduction can be first achieved with external immobilization prior to, or at the time of, surgery.

Practical preoperative considerations include patient anatomy and operative positioning to allow proper screw trajectory. Limiting factors can include barrel chest, short craniocaudal neck dimension, or rigid cervical spine preventing extension to achieve necessary trajectory. When discussing the operative plans and obtaining patient consent, possible plans for aborting screw placement and proceeding with C1-2 posterior fusion can be helpful.

Operative planning, positioning, and set-up are critical for appropriate odontoid screw placement. Patients are positioned and C-arm biplanar fluoroscopy is utilized to achieve adequate working views in the AP and lateral planes and optimal fracture reduction prior to incision.

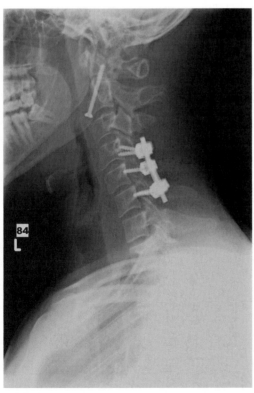

■ **FIGURE 28-3**  Anterior odontoid screw with C4-6 lateral mass fixation.

Skin incision is planned based on necessary screw trajectory and cosmesis, often centered around C5, and neck dissection should proceed with standard attention to developing a safe corridor between the carotid sheath and trachea/esophagus to access the anterior cervical spine. Placement of the screw is performed over a K-wire under fluoroscopic guidance and an appropriate entry point is chosen at the anterior-inferior body of C2, depending upon the planned screw trajectory. Optimal placement can be facilitated by drilling a recess into the body of C3 and removing a piece of the C2-3 disc to allow for the screw trajectory and entry point at C2. A single lag screw is utilized for fracture fixation and reduction, and an attempt should be made to achieve bicortical purchase through the odontoid fragment to maximize biomechanical stability of the construct. Great care is taken at the time of K-wire and screw placement to avoid injury to the vertebral-basilar complex and cervical cord/brainstem dorsal to the fracture fragment. Advantages of odontoid fracture fixation with an odontoid screw include direct fracture reduction/stabilization, preservation of some C1-2 motion, decreased time of immobilization, and decreased morbidity associated with halo placement or posterior surgical approach.

## C1-2 Harms

Multiple options exist for posterior C1-2 fixation. In cases of fractures involving both the atlas and odontoid, consideration must be given to the stability of the atlantal arch in immobilizing the C1-2 complex, and, when necessary, fixation can be extended to the occiput. Otherwise, posterior C1-2 fixation techniques are useful in cases of atlantoaxial instability including type II odontoid fractures, degenerative disease of the C1-2 complex, osteoinvasive malignancy of the C1-2 complex, and nonunion of odontoid fracture.

C1 lateral mass-C2 pars/pedicle screw fixation, known as the Harms construct[9], is an effective posterior fusion construct for appropriately selected patients, and, unlike an odontoid screw, it can be utilized in patients with a disrupted transverse ligament. Advantages include direct visualization of fusion surfaces, flexibility in timing of surgery (can be utilized in acute and chronic treatment of instability), and, as a polyaxial screw and rod construct, it can easily be extended to the occiput or subaxial spine, if necessary.

Operative planning is critical to safe and effective treatment and should include a preoperative cervical spine CT scan to delineate the bony anatomy; when necessary, this can be supplemented with vascular imaging to define vertebral artery anatomy. Patients are positioned prone with the head immobilized in a halo or Mayfield pins that are secured to the table. The neck is maintained in a neutral position, and C-arm fluoroscopy or other navigation tools are utilized.

If use of iliac crest autograft is planned, positioning, prepping, and draping the patient should be modified accordingly. Incision and dissection is carried through the midline ligamentum nuchae to expose the caudal edge of the occipital bone and the cephalad edge of the C3 lamina, and subperiosteal lateral dissection is extended to the C1-2 joint and the lateral aspect of C2 (while preserving the C2-3 facet capsule). Great care must be taken to avoid injuring the vertebral artery, including limiting lateral dissection to the medial one third of the cephalad atlantal arch and, when present, recognizing the ponticulus posticus identified on preoperative CT scan.

Screw placement requires adequate exposure of the lateral mass of C1, which requires identification, and often retraction, of the C2 (greater occipital) nerve, along with meticulous hemostasis, as there is often significant bleeding from a venous plexus. The middle of the C1 lateral mass at the junction with posterior atlantal arch is a reliable entry point for the C1 lateral mass screw. The screw is inserted with a slight medial trajectory as the medial wall of C1 is palpated to ensure maintenance of its integrity. Lateral fluoroscopy (or other navigation tool) should be utilized and the tip of the screw should be aimed at the anteriormost part of the anterior arch.

The superolateral quadrant of the C2 lateral mass is the approximate entry point for a C2 pedicle screw. The screw is placed with a medial and cephalad trajectory (about 30 degrees in each plane). A C2 pars screw is an alternative to the pedicle screw; it is very similar but has a more inferior and medial entry point and thus has a steeper cephalad trajectory and less medial trajectory. It is essential that preoperative CT scans be studied carefully, as there is a high variability in the position and course of the vertebral arteries in this area.

Placement of rods is performed in a standard fashion. Use of autograft and/or allograft is done at the preference of the surgeon, and careful attention is directed to decortication and preparation of the fusion surfaces including the C1-2 articulating surfaces.

## C1-2 Transarticular Screws

An alternative method for posterior atlantoaxial fixation is a C1-2 transarticular screw construct (Figure 28-4), where an appropriatelysized lag screw traverses the pars interarticularis of C2, the atlantoaxial joint, and the lateral mass of C1. The indications for its use and its biomechanical stability are similar to C1-2 posterior fixation screw-rod constructs.

Preoperative planning is similar to that for C1-2 posterior screw-rod fixation techniques, with an emphasis on the importance of vertebral artery anatomy. The patient should be positioned in Mayfield or halo pins rigidly fixed to the operating room table. C-arm fluoroscope should be positioned for AP and lateral imaging, and sterile prep and drape should include the caudal extension of the sterile field to the upper thoracic spine for possible percutaneous placement of the transarticular screws. Careful analysis of fluoroscopic visualization of atlantoaxial spine and ability to achieve appropriate alignment of C1-2 for screw placement should be performed prior to incision. Sublaminar wiring can augment the transarticular screw fixation construct, and may be employed at the surgeon's discretion.

The appropriate trajectory of the transarticular screw requires a steep cephalad angle that, depending upon individual patient anatomy, may not be technically feasible in the wound utilized for dissection of the atlantoaxial spine. Therefore, use of a percutaneous tunneling device through a separate stab incision over the lower cervical or upper thoracic spine may be necessary to achieve the optimal angle, under fluoroscopic guidance.

Beginning with a K-wire under fluoroscopic guidance, the entry point for the transarticular screw is approximately 3 mm lateral to the medial edge, and 3 mm superior to the inferior edge of the C2 inferior articular process. The trajectory proceeds in a steep cephalic and slightly medial angle across the pars of C2. After traversing the pars, the screw can be visualized in the surgical field prior to entering the lateral mass of C1, where attention should be directed toward retracting/protecting the C2 nerve and ganglion. For optimal placement, the tip of the screw should engage the cortex of the

anterior-superior lateral mass of C1. Use of a 4- to 5- cm lag screw (size can be planned based on preoperative CT) can achieve firm bony purchase and tight compression of the C1-2 joint for optimal fusion. Attention should be directed toward decortication of fusion surfaces, often including placement of a tricortical strut graft between lamina of C1 and process of C2 to augment fusion.

## C2 Laminar Screws

In 2004, Wright and Leonard reported a case series of C2 fixation using crossing laminar screws at C2 (Figures 28-5 and 28-6). Since then, the C2 laminar screw has emerged as a viable alternative to C2 pedicle/pars screws and C1/2 transarticular screw techniques. The growth of this technique can be attributed to ease of placement, lower incidence of vertebral artery injury, and a similar biomechanical profile when compared to C2 pedicle/pars or C1-2 transarticular screw placement.

The initial approach to C2 for translaminar screw placement is similar to the techniques described before. A midline incision is carried down to the posterior elements of C2 in the avascular midline plane. Subperiosteal dissection is used to free the muscular attachments to the lamina and spinous process of C2. The entry point for the laminar screws are on the opposite side of the spinous process (i.e., the left laminar screw starts on the right side of the spinous process). One entry site should start slightly more cephalad and the other should start slightly more caudad to allow crossing in the middle of the spinous process. A hand drill or small pedicle probe is used to cannulate the lamina, usually to a length of 26 to 30 mm. The undersurface of the lamina, within the cervical canal, should be palpated to ensure maintenance of the cortical wall. A 3.5 × 26-30 mm screw is placed in the predrilled lamina. These screws can then be attached via rods to C1 lateral mass screws, occipital plates, or subaxial screws, depending on the particular construct. If needed, lateral extenders are available to make rod placement easier.

## COMPLICATIONS

Injuries to the occipital-cervical region are associated with significant morbidity and mortality. Most often, death is due to neurologic injury or cerebrovascular insufficiency. The risk of death or serious morbidity is higher if instability

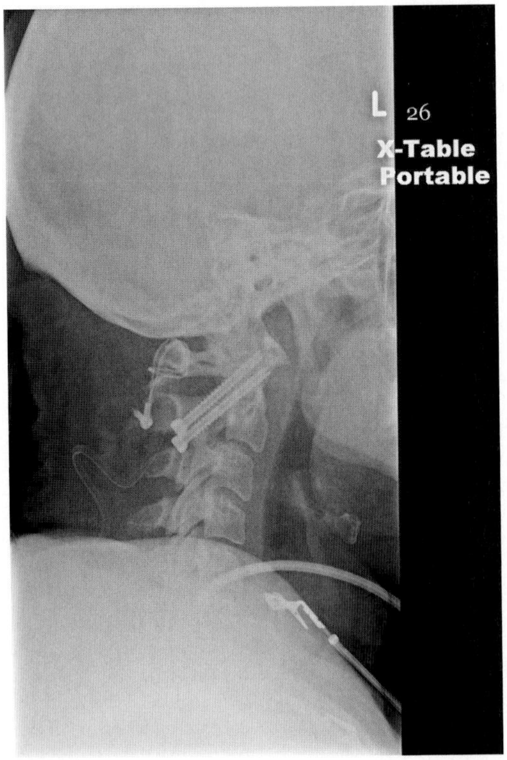

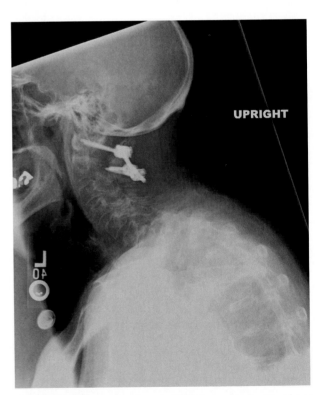

■ **FIGURE 28-4**   C1-2 transarticular screws with supplemental translaminar wiring.

■ **FIGURE 28-5**   C1 lateral mass–C2 laminar screw fixation of type II dens fracture seen in Figure 28–1.

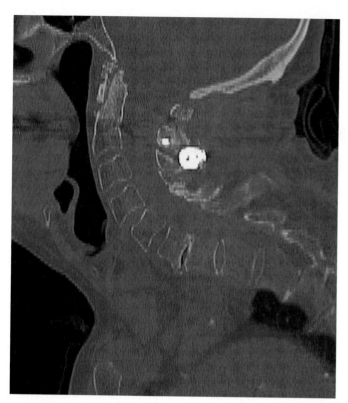

■ **FIGURE 28-6**  Type II dens fracture seen in Figure 28-1 healed after C1-C2 laminar screw fixation.

is missed or the diagnosis is delayed. With appropriate management, nonunion of bony injuries is uncommon, except for type II odontoid fractures.

## CONCLUSIONS

The craniocervical junction is a complex region with complex biomechanics and unique skeletal, ligamentous, and neurovascular anatomy. It is a commonly injured region with potential for significant morbidity and mortality. Initial treatment of these spine injuries requires attention to maintenance of airway and ventilation, cervical stabilization, diagnostic imaging, and reduction of vertebral displacement if malalignment is present. Definitive treatment is based on injury type, patient demographics such as age, and clinical presentation such as the presence or absence of neurologic deficit.

## References

1. R.S. Jackson, D.M. Banit, A.L. Rhyne, B.V. Darden, Upper cervical spine injuries, J. Am. Acad. Orthop. Surg. 10 (4) (2002) 271–280.
2. P.A. Anderson, P.X. Montesano, Morphology and treatment of occipital condyle fractures, Spine 13 (1988) 731–736.
3. C.D. Landells, P.K. Van Peteghem, Fractures of the atlas: classification, treatment and morbidity, Spine 13 (1988) 450–452.
4. K.F. Spence, S. Decker, K.W. Sell, Bursting atlantal fracture associated with rupture of the transverse ligament, J. Bone Joint Surg. Am. 52 (1970) 543–549.
5. L.D. Anderson, R.T. D'Alonzo, Fractures of the odontoid process of the axis, J. Bone Joint Surg. Am. 56 (1974) 1663–1674.
6. B. Effendi, D. Roy, B. Cornish, R.G. Dussault, C.A. Laurin, Fractures of the ring of the axis: a classification based on the analysis of 131 cases, J. Bone Joint Surg. Br. 63 (1981) 319–327.
7. A.M. Levine, C.C. Edwards, The management of traumatic spondylolisthesis of the axis, J. Bone Joint Surg. Am. 67 (1985) 217–226.
8. P.M. Pellicci, C.S. Ranawat, P. Tsairis, W.J. Bryan, A prospective study of the progression of rheumatoid arthritis of the cervical spine, J. Bone Joint Surg. Am. 63 (A) (1981) 342–350.
9. J. Harms, R.P. Melcher, Posterior C1-C2 fusion with polyaxial screw and rod fixation, Spine 26 (22) (2001) 2467–2471.

# 29

# Subaxial Cervical and Upper Thoracic Spine Fractures in the Elderly

*Jared T. Lee, Christopher C. Harrod, and Andrew P. White*

**KEY POINTS**

- Elderly patients are at increased risk of neurological injuries, including central cord syndrome, due to degenerative stenosis, spondylotic stiffness, and changes in spinal cord morphology and vasculature.

- Spinal ankylosis increases the risk of unstable fractures, which may not be diagnosed on initial imaging studies such as plain radiographs.

- For historical reasons, central cord syndrome has traditionally been treated nonoperatively or operatively after a period of observation, but early surgical treatment has been demonstrated to be advantageous for patients with traumatic instability, ongoing cord compression, or severe neurological deficits.

- Elderly patients with subaxial cervical and upper thoracic spine fractures have increased treatment risks as compared to young patients, related to medical comorbidities, ankylosed segments, osteoporotic bone, and preexisting stenosis.

- Spinal reconstruction in the setting of osteoporotic fractures may require specific operative techniques to prevent hardware failure.

## INTRODUCTION

The geriatric cervical spine is prone to injury. The susceptibility to bony, ligamentous, and neurological injury may be associated with age-related changes including osteoporotic bone, stiffened spinal articulations, preexisting stenosis, and altered spinal cord vasculature and morphology. Because of these factors, which influence injury susceptibility in the elderly patient, the majority of subaxial cervical and upper thoracic spine injuries occur secondary to low-energy mechanisms. Even within the geriatric population, age is an important predictor of injury location based on mechanism.

Although atlantoaxial fractures are more common than subaxial fractures in the elderly, there is considerable morbidity associated with subaxial cervical and upper thoracic spine fractures. These more caudal spine injuries are more likely to be associated with neurological deficits, in comparison to atlantoaxial injuries, and more likely to be associated with higher-energy mechanisms.[1]

Apart from the nearly ubiquitous osteoarthritic spondylosis seen in geriatric patients, other etiologies of severe cervical and thoracic spine ankylosis can alter the biomechanics of the cervical spine, causing increased susceptibility to fracture from minor traumatic events. These include ankylosing spondylitis (AS) and diffuse idiopathic skeletal hyperostosis (DISH). Both conditions result in a stiff and often osteoporotic spine. With injury, both the anterior and posterior columns may be completely disrupted, causing frank instability. Fractures of the ankylosed spine are associated with 50% morbidity and 30% mortality.[2] For this reason, a high level of suspicion is required not to overlook potentially unstable fracture patterns.

The lateral cervical spine radiograph is widely used as a screening tool in the nongeriatric trauma patient. Because of the susceptibility of injury, the significant consequences of injury, and the potential for occult injury in the geriatric population, however, more extensive imaging may be warranted. This is particularly relevant in the spondylotic or ankylotic spine, to avoid missing injuries.

The treatment of subaxial cervical and upper thoracic spine fractures continues to be evaluated. The subaxial cervical spine injury classification system (SLIC) has been established to provide clinicians with standardization for making nonoperative versus operative decisions and, ultimately, how to surgically approach the injuries.[3] The traditional thinking regarding the most optimal timing of surgical treatment of injuries is also changing. Specifically, there is now good evidence that early surgical treatment of central cord injuries is superior to late treatment for certain categories of patients. Geriatric surgical techniques are also evolving; the complex and overlapping pathologies of osteoporosis and ankylosis present challenges for which meticulous preoperative planning may prevent certain postoperative complications.

## BASIC SCIENCE

Cervical spine fractures occur in approximately 2% to 3% of blunt trauma patients. Subaxial fractures account for 40% to 60% of the cervical spine fractures. Of these, it has been found that nearly 20% involve the C7-T1 junction. Many subaxial cervical and upper thoracic spine fractures can be overlooked in the multiply-injured trauma patient. Geriatric patients, in particular, have characteristics that may make injury recognition difficult. These include preexisting spondylosis with or without degenerative deformities, as well as patient factors that make the physical examination difficult, including dementia, baseline weakness, and neuropathies. In the ankylosed spine, even minimally displaced segments can be unstable. The failure to recognize these sometimes subtle injuries can lead to devastating neurological consequences.

The radiographic and clinical evaluation of the cervical spine in the patient following trauma continues to be evaluated. There are ongoing modifications of recommendations regarding the role of radiographs, multiplanar CT, and MRI to rule out cervical spine injuries in the trauma patient. Multiplanar CT and MRI have been shown to have very high sensitivity for detecting cervical spine injury. Despite a high sensitivity, there are reports of cervical spine injury in obtunded patients with an unremarkable multiplanar CT.[4] Brandenstein and colleagues recently reported on four patients with negative cervical CT scans and MRIs who later had evidence of cervical instability.[5] They estimated that 0.2% to 0.4% of their patients would have cervical spine instability despite normal CT and MRI findings. Not surprisingly, three of the four patients with instability were geriatric. It is prudent to have a high degree of suspicion for cervical spine injuries in the geriatric patient despite seemingly normal imaging.

## ANKYLOSING SPONDYLITIS

Ankylosing spondylitis (AS) is a seronegative (RF-negative) spondyloarthropathy that predominantly affects the sacroiliac joints and spine. It typically, but not exclusively, affects HLA-B27–seropositive patients. The

*Text continues on p. 174*

## Clinical Case Examples

### CASE 1

A 58-year-old male fell from standing and struck the back of his head. This resulted in temporary loss of consciousness and neck pain. He was transferred from an outside hospital when abnormal neurological findings were appreciated. On presentation at our institution, he was immobilized in a rigid cervical collar and was hemodynamically stable. His exam revealed

weakness (4/5) of bilateral upper extremities muscle groups. He also had 4/5 strength in his quadriceps but other lower extremity strength was 5/5. His past medical history was significant only for hypertension.

Imaging evaluation revealed extensive degenerative changes. Posterior osteophytes from C3 to C7 and calcification of the posterior longitudinal ligament were demonstrated on CT scanning. There was no fracture, malalignment, or prevertebral edema appreciated (Figure 29-1). An MRI revealed C3-4 disc osteophyte complex associated with spinal cord compression and T2 hyperintensity of the cord. Additional disc protrusions were seen at more caudal cervical levels (Figure 29-2).

He was initially treated with cervical collar immobilization. His neurological examination was monitored. The patient showed no improvement in his neurological examination. The recommendation to decompress and stabilize the cervical spine was accepted by the patient. A posterior direct decompression with instrumented fusion was performed from C3 to T1 (Figure 29-3).

Postoperatively, his upper extremity weakness resolved. Two weeks later, however, he presented to the emergency department with recurrent weakness in elbow flexion bilaterally. His examination revealed 4/5 strength in bilateral deltoids and 3/5 strength in biceps and forearm supination. Otherwise his upper and lower extremity motor strength had improved to 5/5. He did not have any sensory deficits. Examination was consistent with C5 nerve palsy. He was treated with observation and analgesic medications. At latest follow-up, he is ambulatory with a fluid narrow-based gait and with resolved weakness in elbow flexion and supination.

### CASE 2

A 51-year-old male with known diffuse idiopathic skeletal hyperostosis (DISH) had a syncopal event and fell from the stands at Fenway Park, impacting his face and forehead. He had transient paralysis of bilateral upper extremities and severe neck pain. He was stabilized in a cervical collar at Fenway and transferred to our emergency department for evaluation.

On initial examination, he was found to have recovered motor function, and to have intact sensation to pain and light touch in bilateral upper extremities. He had persistent severe neck pain and severe burning pain and sensitivity to light touch in both hands, refractory to intravenous pain medications.

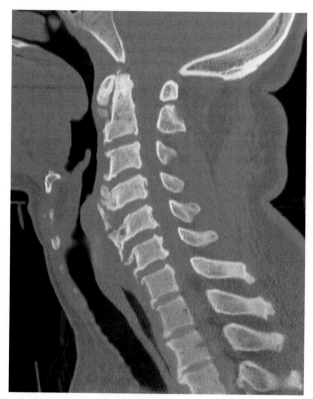

■ **FIGURE 29-1** Case 1: Midsagittal CT of cervical spine shows multilevel degenerative changes without evidence of fracture.

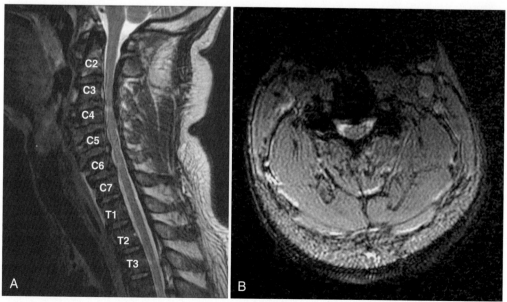

■ **FIGURE 29-2** Case 1: MRI performed after physical examination consistent with central cord syndrome. **A,** Midsagittal T2-weighted cervical spine MRI shows anterior cord compression from the C3-4 disc. **B,** Axial T2-weighted cervical spine MRI at the C3-4 disc level shows cord edema and central canal stenosis.

Imaging evaluation demonstrated several disc osteophyte complexes. The largest was observed at C3/C4, where there was 50% narrowing of the central canal. Extensive flowing nonmarginal osteophytes were also well characterized by CT scan (Figure 29-4). While no obvious unstable injuries were appreciated on CT, a subsequent MRI revealed extension distraction fractures with three column disruption at both C3-4 and C6-7. Each level of injury was associated with dissociation of the anterior longitudinal ligament and osteophytes (Figure 29-5). The spinal cord was compressed at C3-4 and C6-7.

A C3 to C7 laminectomy and C3 to T1 instrumented fusion were performed. He tolerated the procedure well and was extubated in the operating room (Figure 29-6). Since the patient's body habitus limited the adequacy of intraoperative radiographs, a CT scan was performed immediately postoperatively to evaluate the spinal alignment and instrumentation (Figure 29-7).

Postoperatively, the patient reported an immediate decrease in his burning hand pain. He was able to ambulate with PT and was discharged home on postoperative day 3. At his 6-week follow-up, he complained only of hyperesthesias of the right small and index fingers. He had no weakness and normal sensation, with resolution of his severe sensitivity to light touch.

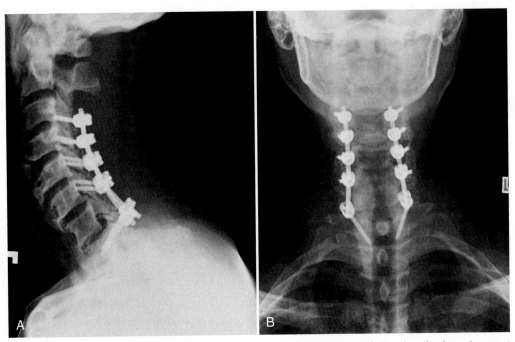

■ **FIGURE 29-3**  Case 1: C3-C7 laminectomy and C3-T1 instrumentation and fusion show hardware in correct position and adequate laminectomy. **A,** Lateral postoperative x-ray. **B,** AP postoperative x-ray.

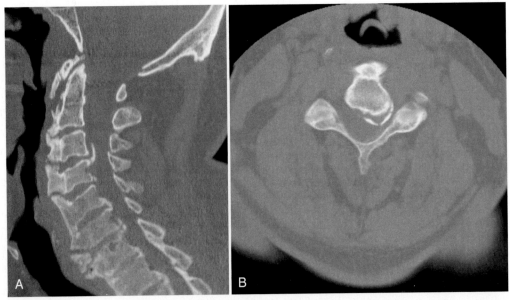

■ **FIGURE 29-4**  Case 2: Initial midsagittal and axial CT reveals many aspects of DISH. There are four continuous ankylosed vertebrae, the osteophytes are nonmarginal, and it spares the posterior elements, Due to the degree of DISH, it was difficult to say if there was a fracture or instability base on CT scan alone. **A,** Midsagittal CT scan. **B,** Axial CT scan at C3 level shows central cord compression from osteophyte.

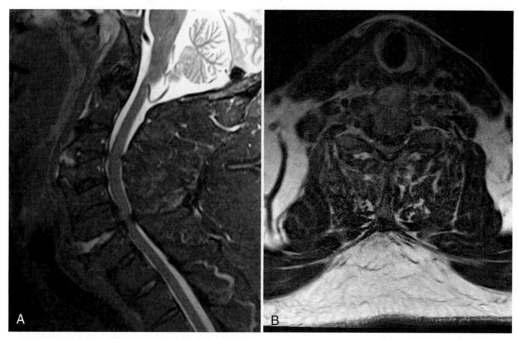

■ **FIGURE 29-5**    Case 2: **A,** Sagittal STIR MRI with increased signal at C3-4 and C6-7 consistent with acute injury. **B,** Axial T2-weighted image at C7 shows cord compression.

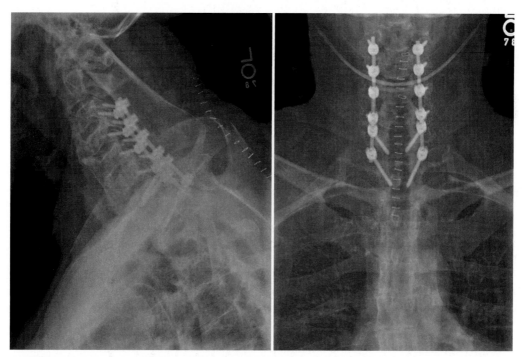

■ **FIGURE 29-6**    Case 2: Postoperative AP and lateral cervical spine x-rays with good sagittal and coronal alignment. Hardware in appropriate position without evidence of complications.

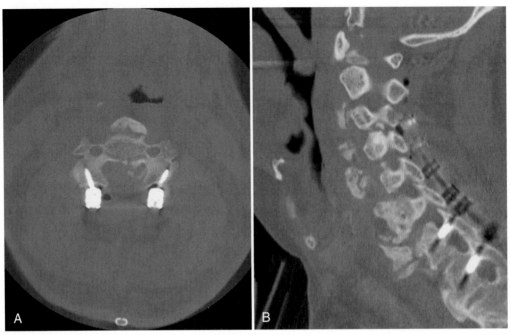

■ **FIGURE 29-7** Case 2: Postoperative CT scan. **A,** Axial CT at C3 level with lateral mass screws. **B,** Sagittal CT scan demonstrates pedicle screws within the C7 and T1 pedicles.

prevalence ranges from 0.1% in African and Eskimo populations to as high as 6% in Haida Native Americans in northern Canada. The white populations of the USA and UK have a prevalence of 0.5% to 1.0%. AS typically has its onset in the third decade of life, with a mean age of onset of 26. It rarely begins after the age of 40, although the diagnosis may be made at a later age because earlier symptoms are ignored or benign. A juvenile form of AS is described, but it does not affect the spine.

Sacroiliitis is the most common presenting symptom, with bilateral or unilateral buttock pain being the chief complaint. Spinal stiffness and discomfort typically progress gradually and affect all joints in the spine. Extraaxial involvement includes plantar fasciitis, insertional Achilles tendinitis, eye lesions, enteritis, colitis, prostatitis, aortitis, and, rarely, fibrosis of the upper lung.

The hallmark spinal pathology seen in AS is due to enthesitis. The enthesis is the site of tendon and ligament attachment to bone. Local inflammation at the enthesis may lead to radiographic lysis of bone. AS affects the insertions and attachments of the discovertebral, costovertebral, and costotransverse joints, as well as the other interspinal ligaments. The reactive bone formation at the sites of inflammation and the remaining lysis result in a stiff and osteoporotic spine. This combination results in an increased susceptibility to spine fractures.[6]

### DIFFUSE IDIOPATHIC SKELETAL HYPEROSTOSIS

Diffuse idiopathic skeletal hyperostosis (DISH) was first described by Forestier and Rotes-Querol in 1950, and it is often still referred to as Forestier disease. It has specific diagnostic criteria as outlined by Forestier. These include at least four contiguous vertebrae involved in ossification, without evidence of loss of disc height, and with relatively well-preserved facet joints and SI joints. The ossification is nonmarginal and flowing along the anterolateral vertebrae. Additionally, there are extraspinal manifestations such as increased heterotopic ossification after surgery.

DISH is not related to HLA-B27, and there has been no relationship found with other seronegative spondyloarthropathies such as AS. DISH has some relationship with HLA-8 and is relatively common, with prevalence as high as 28% in autopsy series. It is felt that 15% of women and 25% of men over the age of 50 have DISH, and the prevalence increases with age. There is no difference in prevalence between blacks and whites.

The thoracic spine is most commonly affected. The large syndesmophytes more often involve the right half of the vertebral body in the thoracic spine, contralateral to the aorta, whereas involvement is symmetric in the cervical or lumbar spine. DISH of the cervical spine usually involves the lower segments and can become large enough to exert a mass effect on the esophagus and cause dysphagia.

The bone morphology in DISH is different than in AS. Whereas vertebrae with inflammation-induced osteolysis adjacent to affected entheses are commonly seen in AS, in DISH, bone quality is relatively well preserved. Both conditions, however, are associated with increased risk of fracture through or adjacent to ankylosed vertebral segments. These patients can present a challenge in correctly identifying a cervical fracture.[7]

### BIOMECHANICS AND CLASSIFICATION OF SUBAXIAL SPINE FRACTURES

Ferguson and Allen reviewed 165 cases to develop a classification system for subaxial spine fractures based on the mechanism of injury. They developed six mechanisms with reproducible fracture patterns. The mechanisms described can be divided into three compression injuries (compression-flexion, compression, and compression-extension), two distraction injuries (distraction-flexion, distraction-extension), and lateral flexion. Each mechanism has varying degrees of severity based on radiographic findings. Although commonly used as a framework for fracture discussion, these results have never been validated in the current literature. Additionally, witnessed compression injuries have resulted in variable fracture morphology. This classification does not specifically grade the amount of ligamentous injury nor does it quantify the amount of neurological injury.

In addition to classification is the question of subaxial spine instability after injury. White and Panjabi published a biomechanic study evaluating clinical and radiographic markers of cervical spine instability. Their work focused on the ligamentous structures surrounding the vertebral bodies. They developed a checklist with point values, with a score of five or more indicating instability. The radiographic markers on plain film are sagittal plane translation of >3.5 mm, sagittal plane rotation >11 degrees, positive stretch test, and abnormal disc narrowing. Clinical criteria are cord damage, root damage, and if dangerous loading is anticipated. There are two additional criteria: anterior elements unable to function and posterior elements unable to function. While this checklist, published in 1976, is a tool

**TABLE 29-1 The Subaxial Cervical Spine Injury Classification System (SLIC)**

| | Points* |
|---|---|
| **Morphology** | |
| No abnormality | 0 |
| Compression + burst | 1+1=2 |
| Distraction (e.g., facet perch, hyperextension) | 3 |
| Rotation or translation (e.g., facet dislocation, unstable teardrop or advanced-stage flexion-compression injury) | 4 |
| **Discoligamentous complex** | |
| Intact | 0 |
| Indeterminate (e.g., isolated interspinous widening, MRI signal change only) | 1 |
| Disrupted (e.g., widening of anterior disc space, facet perch or dislocation) | 2 |
| **Neurological status** | |
| Intact | 0 |
| Root injury | 1 |
| Complete cord injury | 2 |
| Incomplete cord injury | 3 |
| Continuous cord compression (neuro modifier in the setting of a neurological deficit) | +1 |

*A score of 3 or less indicates nonoperative management. A score of 5 or greater indicates need for surgical intervention.

for evaluating spine instability, the commonplace use of CT and MRI has provided a level of detail and sensitivity that has made the point system infrequently used.

More recently, a classification system has been developed using the injury morphology, discoligamentous complex, and neurological status to classify injuries and to determine the need for surgical intervention. This subaxial cervical spine injury classification system (SLIC) by the Spine Trauma Study Group (STSG) was developed not only to classify subaxial spine fractures but also to predict the need for surgical stabilization and/or reduction. The system is based on assigning points according to the severity of injury in three categories: proposed mechanism of injury, discoligamentous complex injury, and neurological injury. If a patient's SLIC score is 1 to 3, then nonsurgical treatment is recommended. If the score is 5 or more, then surgical treatment is recommended (Table 29-1). To assess the reliability and validity of this classification system, 20 surgeons in two different settings used the system to classify 11 different spine fractures and clinical scenarios. They found the reliability to be slightly lower than that of the Ferguson and Allen classification. The validity was good in comparison to the Ferguson and Allen classification system. Of note is that 93% of the time, the surgical versus nonsurgical treatment recommended by SLIC was the treatment recommendation of the practicing clinician.

## INSTRUMENTATION OF OSTEOPOROTIC LOWER CERVICAL AND UPPER THORACIC SPINE

The mechanisms and fracture patterns of the cervical spine differ in the geriatric population as compared to the young trauma population. This is due in part to decreased bone mineral density, most typically related to osteoporosis. Osteoporosis is common and affects 55% of people older than 50 years old, with an increased prevalence in women. Osteoporosis is associated with preferential loss of trabecular (or cancellous) bone as compared to cortical bone. This pattern of bone loss has important bearing on spinal instrumentation and can preclude adequate screw purchase with traditional

fixation methods. When considering surgical intervention in the geriatric population it is necessary to consider the diminished bone quality and utilize techniques that limit complications. Potential complications related to instrumentation of the geriatric cervical spine include loss of fixation, nonunion with subsequent hardware failure, loss of deformity correction, and adjacent segment fracture.

While not yet FDA approved, lateral mass screws are commonly used for reconstruction of the subaxial cervical spine. These short small-diameter screws are typically placed using unicortical technique and, as such, rely on sufficient trabecular bone to prevent loss of fixation. While it may be associated with other risks, bicortical placement of lateral mass screws may be considered when trabecular quantity is compromised. Additionally, an alternative technique has been described to place screws across three or four cortices by traversing the cervical facet articular cortex, as well as the posterior (and possibly the anterior) cortex of the lateral mass. Placement of transfacet screws can be technically demanding, and requires an approximately 40-degree caudal insertion angle in the sagittal plane and 20 degrees lateral in the coronal plane. For this reason, the occiput can interfere with placement in cephalad cervical segments. Additionally, transfacet placement cannot be used in the most caudal instrumented segment as it will violate the normal unfused facet joint. This is a technique that can certainly be helpful in salvage scenarios, such as when lateral mass fixation has been found to be inadequate intraoperatively.

One may also consider augmenting a construct that uses lateral mass instrumentation to ensure adequate fixation. For example, cranial or caudal extension of the construct is frequently useful in the geriatric spine. By extending the fusion, additional points of fixation may be included to reduce the stresses on any particular screw-bone interface. Furthermore, cranial extension may allow placement of a C2 pars screw, while caudal extension may allow placement of a pedicle screw in C7 or in the upper thoracic pedicles. These screws have the benefit of improved cortical contact throughout the length of the screw, which typically is longer than a lateral mass screw and, as such, offers improved fixation. A CT scan is useful to plan the placement of either a C2 pars screw or a cervical or thoracic pedicle screw. The CT scan will provide preoperative assessment of pedicle diameter, orientation, and bone quality. In the spondylotic spine, the pedicles can be entirely sclerosed and may be unable to accept a blunt pedicle probe; they may require alternative techniques for cannulation, such as drilling. When considering C2 pedicle fixation, the course of the vertebral artery must be known in detail. Intraoperative fluoroscopy can be employed to avoid injury, and to allow for the placement of a long and well-fixed screw along the medial cortex of the canal. It is also useful to access the canal in these cases, to establish the exact location and morphology of the medial wall cortex.

Other techniques that can be used to improve fixation in osteoporotic bone include the use of instrumentation that relies on the (relatively well-preserved) cortical bone. These include hooks, sublaminar wires, and translaminar screws. Placement of these does require at least part of the lamina to remain intact, which can limit their use in cases that require multilevel posterior decompression of the injured neural elements. Placement of hooks and wires can often be accomplished at the same vertebral level as a concomitant screw, enhancing fixation of that vertebra. This may be particularly useful at the construct's terminal vertebra.

Until solid fusion has been achieved, stabilization can be augmented by use of rigid cervical orthosis. The duration of treatment should be based on the intraoperative assessment of the quality of fixation and the patient's ability to tolerate a rigid orthosis. The most common intolerance is due to skin breakdown under the mandible, mastoid, occiput, or shoulders. Additionally, patients may complain of dysphagia or diminished respiratory capacity. These risks must be weighed against the need for supplemental cervical stabilization.

There are several techniques that may be used when planning instrumentation of the osteoporotic spine. To prevent intraoperative frustration, delays, and complications, a meticulous preoperative plan must be made and communicated to the OR staff.

## CLINICAL PRACTICE GUIDELINES

The importance of identifying cervical spine fracture, instability, or injury in the geriatric trauma patient cannot be overstated. Many characteristics of the geriatric population make identifying these injuries difficult.

An accurate history of events surrounding the injury may be difficult, due to altered consciousness at the time of injury, associated head injuries, or baseline dementia. Additionally, a complete physical examination may be limited by altered mental status or by underlying medical conditions that alter the exam. Radiographic interpretation can, at times, be very difficult due to degenerative changes. Even when a diagnosis is made, there can be significant medical comorbidities that increase the morbidity and mortality related to these fractures.

Initial evaluation should consist of resuscitation as outlined by Advanced Trauma Life Support guidelines. Cervical spine precautions should be maintained even for perceived low-energy mechanisms. Patients with no complaints of neck pain but a history compatible with possible neck injury should have cervical collar stabilization until cleared. A thorough history and physical should be performed. An accurate history may require contacting family members or health care providers who can provide information regarding baseline function, impairments, and past medical history. Inspection of the face and cranium can give important clues to the mechanism of injury and energy transferred to the cervical spine. While maintaining cervical stability, the cervical orthosis should be removed and the posterior cervical midline palpated. With log roll, the entire spine should be palpated to assess for noncontiguous spine injuries that may be present in 10% to 15% of patients. Complete neurological examination must be performed.

Radiographic evaluation should be performed in all patients with suspected cervical spine injury. High-quality and complete images are required, and inadequate images cannot be accepted.. Standard radiographs that visualize from C1 to T1 can provide excellent information in regard to alignment, prevertebral swelling, disc height, and fractures. Standard radiographs, however, are often not adequate in the geriatric population because listhesis, spondylosis, ankylosis, and other degenerative changes make ruling out acute trauma difficult. As such, CT scan is often required to adequately evaluate the injured geriatric spine when radiographs are difficult to interpret. CT scans have much better sensitivity for detecting injuries and are also useful to aid in preoperative planning. MRI should be used in any patient with suspected ligamentous or neurological injury. MRI will provide the best information regarding neurological compression and is useful in determining if decompression is best performed from an anterior or posterior approach, or both.

Nonoperative treatment versus operative treatment of subaxial cervical and upper thoracic spine injuries is frequently based on instability and neurological injury. The SLIC score, although not a perfect tool, provides an excellent framework from which to build treatment strategies. An injured spine without neurological injury may be appropriate for nonoperative treatment in a rigid cervical orthosis, whereas the same injury with neurological injury may require decompression and stabilization to facilitate recovery or prevent further injury.

The timing of surgery, especially in regards to central cord syndrome, remains controversial. All patients with central cord syndrome should be treated aggressively with medical therapies. These therapies include rigid cervical orthosis, intensive care unit admission for monitoring, mean arterial pressure >85 mm Hg, intravenous pressors if needed to maintain blood pressure, and early involvement of physical and occupational therapy. Surgical intervention in central cord injury is indicated if there is progressive neurological deficit or overt spinal instability requiring reduction and fixation. If surgery is to be performed, there is new evidence that early surgical decompression (<24 hours after injury) improves neurological recovery more than late surgical decompression (>24 hours after injury). However, there is no current consensus on the timing of surgical intervention for central cord syndrome.[8]

To decrease overall morbidity and mortality of the injured geriatric patient, it is imperative to optimize his or her medical management. This starts with an accurate past medical history and medication list as well as obtaining prior ancillary studies such as cardiac studies and pulmonary function tests. This information is critical for perioperative risk stratification. Early communication with anesthesia, internal medicine, geriatric medicine, and other consult services can prevent delays in surgical treatment and allow sufficient time for necessary interventions. Postoperatively, special attention should be paid to mobilizing the patient to prevent decubitus ulcers, deep vein thrombosis, and pulmonary complications. Additionally, the cervical orthosis should be checked to ensure adequate fit and appropriate

distribution of contact pressure to prevent skin breakdown. Medical optimization and limited use of delirium-producing agents will allow the patient to rehabilitate from his or her injury. It must be communicated to patients and families that long-term care may be needed for patients with partial recovery from neurological injuries.

## CLINICAL CASE EXAMPLES: TREATMENT, CLINICAL CHALLENGES, AND FUTURE TREATMENTS

### Case 1

This patient had a low-energy mechanism resulting in central cord syndrome with no evidence of fracture or ligamentous injury on initial CT imaging. Historically, central cord syndrome has been treated medically with a limited role for operative decompression. Hadley reviewed the historical trends of central cord syndrome and showed that historical treatments are being revisited.[9] The age-old nonoperative treatment strategy was based on the case series reported by Schneider in the early 1950s. His initial series reported 50% mortality rate in two central cord patients surgically decompressed. The other patient had recovery similar to the nonoperatively treated patients. Four years later, in 1958, he published a second series in which 20 patients were reviewed. Three of the patients were treated surgically; one patient was treated early, and two patients weeks after their injury. The patient treated early had dramatic neurological improvement. Of the patients surgically decompressed later, one of the two late patients had neurological recovery similar to those managed medically. The other suffered neurological injury and was quadriplegic. Despite the fact that these patients underwent aggressive retraction of the injured spinal cord, with transdural approaches to resect anterior osteophytes, and with sectioning of the dentate ligaments, the conclusion from this series was to treat central cord syndrome medically. This guided much of the thinking toward treatment of central cord syndrome from that time forward. It was not until Brodkey, in 1980, published his results of seven operatively treated patients with traumatic central cord syndrome that surgical management was again revisited. These patients were selected for surgery because their neurological recovery had plateaued and myelography showed anterior compression of the spinal cord. Of the seven patients, all patients' trajectories of neurological recovery improved, and three patients had full neurological recovery. After reviewing the most recent data with regard to treatment of central cord syndrome, Hadley et al. concluded that early reduction of fracture-dislocation is recommended, and surgical decompression of the compressed spinal cord is warranted, especially if the compression is focal and anterior.

The operative technique highlights a well-reported complication of posterior cervical decompression. The incidence of C5 nerve palsy after posterior decompression is approximately 5%. Half of the patients have sensory deficits or pain, and the other 50% have motor weakness only. It is generally unilateral, but is seen bilaterally in about 10% of cases. A recent study showed the cervical spinal cord drifted posteriorly approximately 2.8 mm at 24 hours after surgery and then decreased to 1.9 mm, 2 weeks after surgery. Interestingly, the absolute posterior drift was at the C5-6 level. In their study of 19 patients, two patients developed C5 nerve palsy. These two patients had the largest degree of posterior drift seen at 24 hours and 2 weeks.[10] This C5 nerve palsy associated with posterior decompression generally has a good prognosis. Nearly all patients with a C5 palsy with 3/5 or 4/5 strength regain their strength by 6 months, with half having full recovery by 3 months.

### Case 2

The patient's fall from a standing height resulted in a significant cervical spine injury. The ankylosed cervical spine was extended on impact and resulted in a fracture of the anterior column at two noncontiguous cervical levels. This case exemplifies the necessity of maintaining a high suspicion for unstable injuries in the anklyosed spine.

The degree of osteophyte formation made interpretation of the CT scan difficult. It was unclear to both the consulting spine surgeon and the interpreting radiologist whether there had been a bony injury to the cervical spine. An MRI demonstrated the fracture through the C3-4 and C6-7 disc spaces. The degree of injury is significant, and even after further review, difficult to see on CT scan. In patients with degenerative spines that preclude accurate assessment by x-ray or CT, it may be warranted to perform dynamic cervical spine x-rays or an MRI. Clinical clearance of the ankylosed cervical spine should be done with caution, as evaluation of neck pain in the DISH patient is not a reliable clinical tool; many DISH patients have neck pain at baseline.

This case also highlights the complexity of operative planning, as it is a two-level fracture involving the anterior spine. The severe overgrowth of osteophytes distorts the normal anatomy, makes anterior dissection more difficult, and potentially destabilizes the spine when removed. Although anterior stabilization of a spine with an anterior column fracture provides the most stable fixation, in this case it would be technically very difficult. Stabilization would require a 3-level corpectomy and extensive debridement of anterior osteophytes for plate positioning. The risks of bleeding, esophageal injury, and nonunion would be significant with the described procedure. Furthermore, such a multilevel corpectomy would require a posterior fusion to reduce the nonunion risk. Therefore a posterior approach was employed, as imaging demonstrated adequate cervical lordosis for posterior decompression. The goal was to allow posterior drift of the spinal cord and stabilize the spine with instrumentation and lateral mass fusion. Whereas AS is associated with osteoporotic bone, DISH patients generally have well-maintained bone mineral density. Excellent purchase was obtained in lateral masses and in the pedicles of T1. The construct was felt to have adequate stability without crossbars or supplemental techniques. There was no evidence of loss of fixation at follow-up.

## CONCLUSION

The absolute number of geriatric cervical spine fractures and injuries will likely continue to increase as the population ages. The geriatric spine is prone to injury and to subaxial spine fractures, and more often has neurological injury with these in comparison to upper cervical spine fractures. The clinician should maintain a high degree of suspicion for lower cervical and upper thoracic spine injury, even with reportedly minor mechanisms of injury.

Two important disease processes that increase the susceptibility of the cervical spine to injury are AS and DISH. The stiffened and often osteoporotic vertebral segments can lead to devastating neurological injury. Central cord syndrome is often associated with trauma in the degenerative spine, and the indications and timing of surgery continue to be defined. Under specific circumstances, early decompression is associated with improved neurological recovery. The ankylotic and spondylotic changes in these cervical spines make diagnosis difficult with plain radiographs, and a very low threshold for ordering multiplanar imaging is indicated. It must be remembered that the most common severe complication of subaxial trauma is a missed injury.

Subaxial cervical spine fractures have had many classification systems developed over the past three decades. We have found the SLIC score to be very useful, in that it considers the neurological status, morphology of injury, and posterior ligamentous complex. It is our feeling that the reliability and validity of this scoring system will improve as more clinicians become familiar with its use. Surgical treatment of the injured geriatric spine requires meticulous planning and the use of techniques such as supplemental hooks and wires or screw techniques that rely more heavily on the screw and cortical bone interface. These techniques include C2 pedicle screws, laminar screws, and transfacet screws. A thorough understanding of the pathophysiology of subaxial and upper thoracic fractures in the geriatric patient, combined with conscientious treatment plans, will help prevent the morbidity and mortality so often associated with these injuries.

## References

1. M.J. Sokolowski, et al., Acute outcomes of cervical spine injuries in the elderly: atlantaxial vs subaxial injuries, J. Spinal Cord Med. 30 (3) (2007) 238–242.
2. P. Whang, et al., The management of spinal injuries in patients with ankylosing spondylitis or diffuse idiopathic skeletal hyperostosis: a comparison of treatment methods and clinical outcomes, J Spinal Disord. Tech. 22 (2) (2009) 77–85.
3. A.R. Vaccaro, et al., The subaxial cervical spine injury classification system, Spine 32 (2007) 2365–2374.
4. J.J. Como, et al., Practice management guidelines for identification of cervical spine injuries following trauma: update from the eastern association for the surgery of trauma practice management guidelines committee, J. Trauma 67 (3) (2009) 651–659.
5. D. Brandenstein, et al., Unstable subaxial cervical spine injury with normal computed tomography and magnetic resonance initial imaging studies: a report of four cases and review of the literature, Spine 34 (20) (2009) E743–E750.
6. E.N. Kubiak, et al., Orthopedic management of ankylosing spondylitis, Journal of the American Academy of Orthopaedic Surgeons 13 (2005) 267–278.
7. T.A. Belanger, et al., Diffuse idiopathic skeletal hyperostosis: musculoskeletal manifestations, JAAOS 9 (2001) 258–267.
8. D. Nowak, et al., Central cord syndrome, Journal of the American Academy of Orthopaedic Surgeons 17 (12) (2009) 756–765.
9. M.N. Hadley, et al., Management of acute central cervical spinal cord injuries, Neurosurgery 50 (3) (2002) S166–S172.
10. T. Shiozaki, et al., Spinal cord shift on magnetic resonance imaging at 24 hours after cervical laminoplasty, Spine 34 (3) (2009) 274–279.

# 30

# Infections of the Cervical Spine

*Kamal R.M. Woods, Samer Ghostine, Terrance Kim, and J. Patrick Johnson*

---

**K E Y   P O I N T S**

- Early diagnosis and treatment is pivotal to the management of cervical spine infections, given their propensity to cause rapid and severe neurological decline.

- Most patients with cervical spine infections complain only of vague neck pain, although fevers, radiculopathy, neck rigidity, and dysphagia may also be present.

- The diagnosis of cervical spine infection is typically made based on elevated erythrocyte sedimentation rate (ESR) and confirmatory imaging.

- In the absence of acute neurological deficit or spinal instability, pyogenic cervical osteomyelitis, and cervical discitis are usually treated with 4 to 8 weeks of intravenous antibiotics.

- Surgical treatment is recommended for cervical epidural abscesses, subdural empyemas, and intramedullary abscesses.

## INTRODUCTION

Evidence from Egyptian mummies suggests that infections of the spine predate the era of written history. In his textbook *On the Articulations*, Hippocrates (400 BC) included reports of vertebral deformity that likely resulted from what was later described by Pott as tuberculous spondylitis. Today, infections of the spine are relatively rare clinicopathologic entities. When they do occur, however, these infections still pose both diagnostic and therapeutic challenges to clinicians.

Spine infections predominate in the lumbar region, followed by the thoracic and then the cervical regions. Nonetheless, cervical infections are particularly problematic because of their propensity to cause more rapid and severe neurological deficits. The discussion that follows will examine the most surgically relevant cervical spine infections: pyogenic vertebral osteomyelitis, spinal epidural abscess, discitis, subdural empyema, and intramedullary abscess.

## BASIC SCIENCE

Cervical infections may be viewed from the perspective of the infectious organism: bacterial, viral, fungal, or parasitic. Alternatively, they may be approached based on the response of the host to the inciting organism: pyogenic ("pus-forming"), or granulomatous. The classic example of a granulomatous infection is tuberculous spondylitis (Pott disease), in which the histology shows caseating central necrosis surrounded by Langhans giant cells. Granulomatous infections may also be caused by fungi, such as aspergillosis, coccidiomycosis, blastomycosis, and cryptococcosis. Parasitic infections of the cervical spine, including cysticercosis, schistosomiasis, and echinococcosis, are extremely rare, and data on their management are limited to case reports.

Overall, the most common causative agent for spinal infections in the United States is *Staphylococcus aureus*, which is present in more than 50% of cases. When the spine infection is associated with a genitourinary or gastrointestinal infection, *Escherichia coli*, *Proteus*, and other gram-negative bacteria are frequently responsible. Patients who have a recent history of intravenous drug abuse are more likely to be infected with *Pseudomonas aeruginosa*. *Streptococcus* is a significant cause of intramedullary cervical abscesses, as it can spread through the lymphatic system from the retropharyngeal space.

There are several potential routes for the dissemination of infections to the cervical spine, including direct extension from contiguous structures, open spinal trauma or surgery, hematogenous, or lymphatic. Both venous and arterial mechanisms have been implicated in hematogenous spread. The Batson venous plexus was proposed as a valveless conduit through which infections of the pelvis, such as urinary tract infections, may spread to the spine. This venous mechanism has been largely refuted, and an alternative arterial route postulated.[1] In the case of vertebral pyogenic osteomyelitis, infection is thought to seed the metaphyseal (subchondral) bone near to the anterior longitudinal ligament via a rich arterial network. The posterior spinal arteries that branch off the dorsal artery entering the intervertebral foramen are probably responsible for cervical epidural abscesses. Infections of the retropharyngeal space can enter the lymphatics and spread along the spinal nerves to communicate with the spinal subarachnoid space and Virchow-Robin space, thus leading to cervical subdural empyemas or cervical intramedullary abscesses.

Interestingly, discitis is seen in two distinct patient populations: pediatric and adult. While discitis in the pediatric population is usually caused by a hematogenous source, adult discitis occurs in patients who have undergone prior surgery involving the disc space. The reason for this clear distinction is that, as the spine ages, there are changes that take place in its vascularity. Histologic studies have shown that an end-arteriolar supply of the disc is present during infancy and childhood, and these end arteries are obliterated by the third decade of life.[2]

## CLINICAL PRACTICE GUIDELINES

The guidelines that govern the diagnosis and treatment of cervical spine infections may vary on a case-by-case basis. However, there are certain common themes which ought to be emphasized.

### Risk Factors

Numerous risk factors for the development of cervical spine infections have been identified, including diabetes, intravenous drug usage (especially via the jugular vein), alcohol abuse, urinary tract manipulation or infection, immunocompromised state, steroid therapy, prior spine surgery, advanced age, and male gender. In the setting of diabetes, steroids, or other immunocompromised state, the diagnosis is usually delayed because of an impaired inflammatory response.

### Clinical Presentation

The most common chief complaint for all cervical spine infections is vague, nonspecific neck pain of a progressive nature. With pyogenic osteomyelitis and discitis, this pain is exacerbated by neck motion, and eventually becomes extremely debilitating. Radicular pain is frequently present in epidural abscesses, and results from either direct nerve root compression or inflammation.[3] If a cervical epidural abscess spreads to the retropharyngeal space, then dysphagia or even airway compromise may result.

The time course to presentation for cervical spine infections varies from acute (less than 1 week), to subacute (1 to 6 weeks), to chronic (more than 6 weeks). In the case of pediatric discitis, this pain is usually so severe at an early stage that a diagnosis is made before the infection spreads to the adjacent vertebral bodies.[4] For pyogenic vertebral osteomyelitis, the presentation tends to be subacute to chronic in 90% of cases, partly because of its more insidious onset. A definitive diagnosis of pyogenic vertebral osteomyelitis is made, on average, 8 weeks to 3 months after disease onset.[5] Patients who present acutely (less than 1 week) are more likely to be febrile, and to have other constitutional signs and symptoms.

Infections that result in the formation of a mass-occupying abscess have a greater chance of presenting with neurological deficit. This may be seen in vertebral osteomyelitis that extends into the epidural space, or with a primary spinal epidural abscess. Likewise, subdural empyemas and intramedullary abscesses cause neurological deficit at an early stage. In some instances of vertebral osteomyelitis, the bony quality is compromised to the extent that bony collapse may occur, leading to spinal instability and secondary neurological deficit. Sometimes, spinal epidural abscesses and subdural empyemas may cause neurological compromise that is out of proportion with the degree of compression. This is thought to be secondary to vascular compromise from venous compression, thrombosis, or thrombophlebitis.[6]

On physical exam, some patients with cervical infections may have local tenderness at the level of the infection, or diffusely in the cervical region. Given the paucity of other physical exam findings, such spine tenderness may seem somewhat dramatic. When the adjacent soft tissue is affected, the skin may show the typical signs of infection: erythema, swelling, warmth, induration, or even fluctuance. Meningitis may be associated with epidural abscesses and subdural empyemas, resulting in rigidity of the neck with passive flexion.

## Laboratory and Imaging Studies

Much like the physical exam findings, laboratory data for cervical spinal infections can be rather obscure. The peripheral white blood cell count is usually normal or just slightly elevated. For this reason, it is imperative to check the erythrocyte sedimentation rate (ESR) when cervical infection is under consideration. In the case of pyogenic osteomyelitis, the ESR may be elevated to 43 to 87 mm/hr (Westergren method).[7] Apart from its diagnostic value, the ESR is an important marker to assess the degree of response to treatment.

The next important diagnostic step is appropriate imaging of the spine. This investigation should begin with plain x-rays. In the case of discitis or vertebral osteomyelitis, narrowing of the disc space may be seen as early as 2 to 3 weeks after infection onset. By 10 to 12 weeks, there is sclerosis of the adjacent vertebral body endplates, due to the bony deposition caused by inflammation. This is likely related to the fact that the subchondral bone is highly vascular and, therefore, is the initial nidus of infection in the vertebral body.[8] With time, the sclerotic process gives way to lysis of the bone, and thus blurring of the endplates on x-ray. The infection eventually spreads to involve the remainder of the vertebral body. In approximately 5% of pyogenic spinal infections, the infection involves the dorsal elements. As the bone is progressively compromised, bony collapse can take place and lead to fracture and deformity of the spine. Plain x-rays are usually normal with spinal epidural abscesses, subdural empyemas, and intramedullary abscesses.

Computed tomography (CT) scans allow for examination of the bony details with greater clarity. For this reason, bone erosion and rarefaction may be detected earlier than on plain x-rays. CT is particularly useful in surveying the posterior elements for involvement by infection, and in assessing associated fractures. Additionally, CT may provide useful information when planning surgical instrumentation of an unstable cervical spine.

Magnetic resonance imaging (MRI) remains key to the diagnosis of cervical infections. For pyogenic osteomyelitis, the sensitivity and specificity rates of MRI are 96% and 93%, respectively.[9] MRI allows the spinal cord, nerve roots, and paraspinal soft tissue to be visualized to determine the extent of their involvement by the infection. Pyogenic osteomyelitis, discitis, epidural abscesses, subdural empyemas, and intramedullary abscesses

all usually appear hypointense on T1-weighted MRI, and hyperintense on T2-weighted MRI. T1-weighted MRI with contrast enhancement is also useful to delineate the margins of an abscess. Another important feature of infections that is clearly demonstrated by MRI is their tendency to span from one vertebral body to the other, through the intervening disc space. Tumors, on the other hand, usually involve the anterior vertebral bodies and skip the disc spaces.

In certain circumstances, myelography via lateral C1-2 punctures may be valuable in making a diagnosis of cervical spine infection. An advantage of myelography is that cerebrospinal fluid can be obtained in the same procedure for laboratory studies. At the same time, myelography carries a risk of introducing an extradural infection into the intradural spaces. Nuclear scans may be beneficial in detecting an infection in the early stages; however, with advances in MRI technology, the role of nuclear studies is diminished.

## Treatment

Patients with pyogenic cervical osteomyelitis and/or cervical discitis who lack acute (less than 72 hrs) neurological deficit or spinal instability are usually treated conservatively with 4 to 8 weeks of IV antibiotics. The commencement of antibiotics for these patients should be delayed until the causative agent has been identified, as prior treatment with antibiotics decreases the yield of subsequent cultures. In many cases, the infectious organism can be implied based on positive blood, urine, or sputum cultures. Blood cultures are most sensitive during the acute febrile stage of the infection. As the disease becomes more chronic, fever is less common and the sensitivity of blood cultures decreases.

When the extraspinal cultures are all negative, tissue culture is recommended before starting antibiotics. In the cervical spine, CT-guided needle biopsy is discouraged because of the close proximity of vital structures that are at risk of injury during percutaneous biopsy. Therefore, an open biopsy is usually required to obtain a tissue specimen in the cervical spine. Once tissue is obtained, broad-spectrum antibiotics may be started until final tissue cultures and sensitivities are available to fine-tune the antibiotic regimen. If the tissue culture is also negative, then the infection is treated with empirical broad-spectrum antibiotics.

Serial ESR and MRI are used to analyze the response to treatment. The ESR is expected to decrease by 50% by the end of antibiotic therapy. Failure to achieve this expected decrease in ESR is considered failure of medical management, and is an indication for surgical intervention. Other indications for surgical intervention in pyogenic cervical osteomyelitis and cervical discitis are acute (less than 72 hrs) neurological deficit at the initial presentation or at any point during medical therapy, and bony collapse leading to deformity or spinal instability.

Surgery for pyogenic cervical osteomyelitis and cervical discitis is usually done through the anterior triangle of the neck. Most cases of pyogenic osteomyelitis involve at least two adjacent vertebral bodies and the intervening disc space. Some authors recommend treating such an infection with a two-level corpectomy, three-level discectomy, and a strut graft between the remaining healthy endplates. However, it is important to evaluate surgical candidates on a case-by-case basis. If there is concern for the integrity of the posterior elements based on the CT, then posterior instrumentation may be indicated. For isolated cervical discitis without involvement of the adjacent endplates, anterior cervical discectomy and fusion is sufficient.

Surgical intervention should be regarded as the first-line treatment for cervical epidural abscesses, subdural empyemas, and intramedullary abscesses. Cervical epidural abscesses tend to be ventral, unlike in the thoracic and lumbar spines where they are more often dorsal. This allows such epidural abscesses to be drained after an anterior cervical discectomy, with or without corpectomy, depending on the extent of the abscess. When an epidural abscess extends into the retropharyngeal posterior triangle, such as commonly occurs with tuberculous infections, a posterior triangle exposure is needed. Rarely, an abscess at C1-C2 may require drainage using the retropharyngeal or transoral approach.

Posterior cervical laminectomy is used to treat cervical subdural empyemas and intramedullary abscesses. After durotomy, debridement or drainage of suppurative material is performed for subdural empyemas. For intramedullary abscesses, intraoperative ultrasound may be useful to localize the abscess. A midline myelotomy is then performed to access the abscess

## *Clinical Case Example*

### DISCITIS/SPINAL EPIDURAL ABSCESS

A 49-year-old male heroin abuser presented to the emergency department with progressive neck pain for 2 to 3 months, and inability to ambulate for the past 12 hours. His ESR was elevated, prompting imaging of the neck with plain x-rays (Figure 30-1A) followed by MRI (Figure 30-1B). A diagnosis of cervical discitis with an associated ventral epidural abscess was made, for which he underwent emergent anterior cervical decompression and drainage of the spinal epidural abscess. His kyphotic deformity corrected with extension of the neck on the operating table, and anterior reconstruction was achieved with allograft and anterior cervical plating (Figure 30-1C). Over the next several weeks, the patient gradually regained strength in his lower extremities and walked into his follow-up clinic visit at 6 weeks.

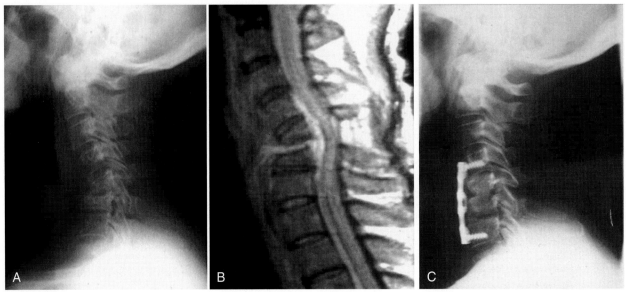

■ **FIGURE 30-1  A,** Lateral cervical x-ray demonstrating reduction in the height of the C5-6 disc space, erosion of the adjacent superior and inferior endplates, and kyphotic deformity with splaying of the spinous processes. **B,** T2-weighted MRI revealing increased signal in the C5-6 disc space, and extension of the infection into the epidural space causing cord compression and edema. **C,** Postoperative x-ray showing correction of the kyphotic deformity and the anterior C4-7 plate.

cavity. One must bear in mind that posterior cervical laminectomy has the potential to cause subsequent kyphotic deformity, especially in cases where the infection has also eroded the vertebral bodies anteriorly.

External immobilization has long been regarded as an important component of the treatment for pyogenic cervical osteomyelitis and/or discitis. However, the method and duration of immobilization has not been studied prospectively, and the exact role of immobilization has not been determined. Nonetheless, immobilization potentially accomplishes two goals: improved pain control, and stabilization of the spine. The orthosis that is selected depends on the affected cervical level and the degree of instability. Possible methods of immobilization include halo fixation, sternal-occipital-mandibular immobilizer (SOMI) brace, and hard cervical collar.

When spinal instability is present, it is necessary to consider internal fixation, with or without arthrodesis. Gross purulence was once considered an absolute contraindication to bone graft and instrumentation because of concern about recurrent infection. However, there are few practical solutions for an unstable cervical spine. Fortunately, there is now an increasing body of evidence that instrumentation and fusion may be safely performed after all grossly infected material is removed.[10]

### CONCLUSIONS/DISCUSSION

Infections of the cervical spine have a propensity to cause catastrophic neurological deterioration, underlining the importance of prompt diagnosis and treatment. Often, the clinical presentation is vague and insidious, leading to untoward delays in diagnosis. Therefore, a high index of suspicion is necessary, and appropriate laboratory and imaging investigations should be performed when clinically indicated.

It is widely accepted that most cases of pyogenic cervical osteomyelitis and cervical discitis may be treated conservatively with antibiotics, although the route and duration of antibiotics are yet to be studied in a prospective, randomized fashion. Some authors advocate early surgical intervention for all cervical spine infections in an attempt to avoid later complications, such as neurological decline or bony collapse. Well-designed clinical trials are needed to clearly define the role and timing of surgical intervention for infections of the cervical spine.

### References

1. A.M. Wiley, J. Trueta, The vascular anatomy of the spine and its relationship to pyogenic vertebral osteomyelitis, J. Bone Joint Surg. Br. 41 (1959) 796–809.
2. M.B. Conventry, R.K. Ghormley, J.W. Kernohan, The intervertebral disc, its microscopic anatomy and pathology: part I: anatomy, development and physiology, J. Bone Joint Surg. Am. 27 (1945) 105–112.
3. R.J. Martin, H.A. Yuan, Neurosurgical care of spinal epidural, subdural, and intramedullary abscesses and arachnoiditis, Orthop. Clin. North Am. 27 (1996) 125–136.
4. H.B. Kemp, J.W. Jackson, J.D. Jeremiah, A.J. Hall, Pyogenic infections occurring primarily in intervertebral discs, J. Bone Joint Surg. Br. 55 (1973) 698–714.
5. K.A. Vincent, D.R. Benson, T.L. Voegeli, Factors in the diagnosis of adult pyogenic vertebral osteomyelitis, Orthop. Trans. 12 (1988) 523–524.
6. N.A. Russell, R. Vaughan, T.P. Morley, Spinal epidural infection, Can. J. Neurol. Sci. 6 (1979) 325–328.
7. P.M. Ross, J.L. Fleming, Vertebral body osteomyelitis, Clin. Orthop. 118 (1976) 190–198.
8. E.H. Allen, D. Cosgrove, F.J. Millard, The radiological changes in infection of the spine and their diagnostic value, Clin. Radiol. 29 (1978) 31–40.
9. M.T. Modic, D.H. Feiglin, D.W. Piraino, F. Boumphrey, et al., Vertebral osteomyelitis: assessment using MRI, Radiology 157 (1985) 157–166.
10. D. Fang, K.M. Cheung, I.D. Dos Remedios, et al., Pyogenic vertebral osteomyelitis: treatment by anterior spinal debridement and fusion, J. Spinal Disorder 7 (1994) 173–180.

# 31

# Rheumatoid Arthritis of the Cervical Spine

*Amar D. Rajadhyaksha and Jeffrey A. Goldstein*

---

**K E Y   P O I N T S**

- Newer pharmacological therapies may decrease the inflammatory response in rheumatoid arthritis and may reduce the incidence and severity of musculoskeletal involvement.

- Plain radiographs are still the screening method of choice for cervical spine involvement. An AADI of greater than 9 mm is indicative of atlantoaxial instability and is a relative indication for surgical intervention.

- The PADI is a more reliable radiographic tool than the AADI. A PADI less than 14 mm has a high predictive value for predicting paralysis and is a more reliable criterion for cervical fusion. Patients with a PADI greater than 14 mm have a higher chance of neurological recovery after surgical intervention, whereas those with a PADI less than 10 mm tend to have poor neurological recovery.

- A combination of the Ranawat, Clark, and Redlund-Johnell measurements is the most sensitive and specific method for analyzing cranial settling.

- Patients with rheumatoid arthritis must be followed carefully, as progression of disease is common. Failure of fixation and adjacent level disease are common.

## INTRODUCTION

Rheumatoid arthritis (RA) is a chronic inflammatory disease that commonly presents with polyarthropathy, systemic symptoms, and cervical spine involvement. Some reports state that RA was first described by A.J. Landre-Beauvais, whereas others credit Robert Adams. Robert Adams described it as a separate entity from gout in the nineteenth century in Dublin. The term rheumatoid arthritis was coined by A.B. Garrod, and its predilection for the cervical spine was first highlighted by his son, A.E. Garrod.[1]

RA presents as a chronic disabling disease with intermittent flares and remissions. It reduces life expectancy, and half of all afflicted patients become disabled within 10 years of diagnosis. The cervical spine is the second most commonly affected site after the hands and feet. Cervical spine involvement is particularly concerning because of the neurological manifestations. Once the patient develops myelopathic symptoms, prognosis is poor.

The natural history can be modified by early and aggressive medical management. With the introduction of corticosteroids and DMARDs (disease-modifying antirheumatic drugs), people can be managed nonoperatively. However, once a patient starts developing myelopathic signs, surgical intervention becomes a consideration. Depending on each surgeon's philosophy and the individual case, the timing of surgery may be controversial. However, studies show that patients with progressive myelopathy benefit from an early decompression and stabilization.

Patients with RA have a complicated presentation and require a multidisciplinary approach. Patients can often present with inability to grasp fine objects. This could be caused by cervical myelopathy, peripheral joint involvement in the hand and fingers, or both. Therefore, a treating physician must have a comprehensive understanding of the natural history, physical exam, radiologic findings, and treatment strategies associated with RA.

## EPIDEMIOLOGY AND NATURAL HISTORY

The prevalence of RA is up to 1% to 3% of the United States population. It is commonly seen in those 40 to 70 years of age, and the male to female ratio is approximately 1:3. Symptomatic cervical spine disease is present in 40% to 80% of patients with RA. Up to 86% of patients have radiographic evidence of cervical spine involvement. In a study that evaluated patients with RA undergoing hip and knee arthroplasty, over 60% had cervical spine involvement.[2]

Cervical subluxation can be identified in 15% of these patients within 3 years of being diagnosed with RA. Atlantoaxial subluxation develops in 5% to 73% of patients within 10 years of diagnosis. Subaxial subluxation develops in 20% of patients and can be at multiple levels. Neurological symptoms are found in 17% of patients. Of those who develop myelopathy, 50% die within 1 year if left untreated. In those left untreated, patients with atlantoaxial subluxation may progress to more complex instability patterns like cranial settling. The natural history of cranial settling is more aggressive with a poorer prognosis than that of isolated atlantoaxial instability. Ten percent of myelopathic patients with RA die a sudden death. It is thought that this is due to brain stem compression or vertebrobasilar insufficiency.

Predictors of disease progression and severity of cervical involvement include disease duration, rapid joint erosion, arthritis mutilans, history of high-dose corticosteroid use, high seropositivity, subcutaneous nodules, vasculitis, and male sex. Other postulated factors include elevated C-reactive protein and certain HLA positivities.

## PATHOPHYSIOLOGY

Rheumatoid arthritis is a chronic immune-mediated response. Unknown antigens, perhaps viral, trigger a cell-mediated response resulting in the release of various inflammatory mediators. The inflammatory response is put into motion by the CD4+ lymphocytes, which activate the B lymphocytes to produce immunoglobulins that are found in the rheumatoid synovium. The rheumatoid synovium contains two distinct cell types: type A cells are morphologically similar to macrophages and type B cells are similar to fibroblasts. Type A cells are mainly for phagocytosis, whereas type B cells are highly metabolic and are equipped with organelles for protein synthesis. These cells produce multiple inflammatory mediators, such as TNF-α, metalloproteinases, collagenases, progelatinases, and IL-1.[3] These mediators are targets for DMARDs.

This inflammatory reaction has an affinity for synovial joints. In the cervical spine, these joints include the atlantooccipital, atlantoaxial, facets, and uncovertebral joints. The atlantooccipital and atlantoaxial articulations are the only two segments in the spine without intervertebral discs, which may account for the great tendency for instability at these regions. Once this inflammation, pannus formation, and ligamentous and bony erosions occur, progressive cervical instability ensues. It is seen in the cervical spine, in order of frequency, as atlantoaxial subluxation, subaxial subluxation, and cranial settling.

Atlantoaxial instability is the most commonly seen (40% to 70%) affliction in the rheumatoid spine. The formation of periodontoid pannus leads to erosion of the transverse, alar, and apical ligaments. The weight of the head combined with flexion and extension at this level leads to stretching and eventual rupture of these ligaments. The odontoid itself and the lateral atlantoaxial articulations are commonly eroded as well, leading to further instability. Depending on the pattern and location of bony and ligamentous erosion, the subluxation may present as anterior, posterior, lateral, or rotational. Anterior is the most common (70%). Anterior subluxation of 0 to 3 mm is normal in adults, 3 to 6 mm is suggestive of instability and rupture of the transverse ligaments, and greater than 9 mm suggests gross instability and incompetence of all periodontoid stabilizing structures. Posterior subluxation is rare and may be associated with a defect in the anterior C1 arch or fracture or erosion of the odontoid. Lateral subluxation is defined as 2 mm of lateral displacement at the atlantoaxial articulation.

Subaxial subluxation is the second most common (20% to 25%) manifestation in the cervical spine. Erosions of the facet joints, uncovertebral joints, and interspinous ligaments result in anterior subluxation of the subaxial vertebrae. It is most commonly seen at the C2-3 and C3-4 levels and typically affects multiple levels resulting in a "staircase" deformity. Subaxial subluxation also occurs at adjacent levels after an atlantoaxial fusion.

Cranial settling, or basilar invagination, is a late finding that is due not only to ligamentous and capsular erosion, but mainly to bone and cartilage destruction of the atlantoaxial and atlantooccipital articulations (Figure 31-1). Cranial settling carries an ominous prognosis. Anterior compression of the medulla oblongata can lead to injury to cranial nerve nuclei, syringomyelia, or obstructive hydrocephalus. Sudden death may also occur due to brainstem compression or vertebrobasilar dysfunction.

## CLINICAL PRESENTATION

Patients with RA present with general symptoms specific to RA as well as symptoms due to spinal involvement. General symptoms include fatigue, weight loss, malaise, morning stiffness, and anorexia. Rheumatoid arthritis of the cervical spine may often be asymptomatic. Neck pain, however, is the most common symptom (40% to 80%). Patients often have facial, temporal, and occipital pain due to irritation of the C1-2 nerve roots, trigeminal nerve, greater auricular nerve, and greater occipital nerve. Occasionally, patients may complain of a "clunking" sensation

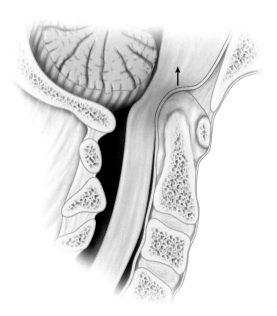

■ **FIGURE 31-1** Lateral view of the upper cervical spine, demonstrating basilar invagination *(arrow)* of the odontoid process into the foramen magnum. Note the compression of the spinal cord. *(Reproduced with permission from Boden SD, Dodge LD, Bohlman HH, Rechtine GR: Rheumatoid arthritis of the cervical spine: a long-term analysis with predictors of paralysis and recovery, J Bone Joint Surg Am 75:1282-1297, 1993.)*

on flexion and extension corresponding to subluxation and reduction at the C1-2 level (positive Sharp-Purser test).

Objective neurological signs occur in 7% to 34% of patients. Patients may present with simple radiculopathy or more complex myelopathy. Radiculopathy may manifest as paresthesias, numbness, or weakness in specific nerve root distributions. Myelopathic signs are seen, and significant spinal cord compression occurs. Clinical signs and symptoms include a wide-based spastic gait, clumsy hands (difficulty grasping coins or buttoning one's shirt), and change in handwriting. Loss of bowel and bladder function occurs late. Compression of the pyramidal tract may occur, leading to a "cruciate paralysis" with varying degrees of upper extremity weakness.

Physical examination reveals general signs of RA and those specific to cervical spine involvement. The general exam reveals peripheral joint involvement characterized by stiffness, redness, warmth, and bogginess. Some patients may have nodules over the extensor surfaces of joints (typically elbows); this occurs in 20% of patients. On exam of the cervical spine, the patient may present with torticollis, lateral head tilt, tenderness to palpation, and painful, restricted range of motion. Neurological abnormalities are seen in 7% to 10%. Patients may present with weakness or paresthesias. Myelopathic findings include hyperreflexia, hypertonia, clonus, positive Babinski test, and positive Hoffman sign.

Careful examination is necessary, as neurological deficit can be masked by weakness from peripheral joint involvement. Myelopathy is progressive and often goes unnoticed because of peripheral involvement. Fine motor skill deterioration may be mistaken for hand involvement, or decreasing ambulatory status may be mistaken for large joint involvement. As patients become more myelopathic, prognosis worsens. The Ranawat grading system for neural assessment may be used to appropriately classify the severity of myelopathy and can be used as a prognostic tool (Table 31-1).

## LABORATORY DATA

Abnormal laboratory findings include anemia, elevated erythrocyte sedimentation rate, and an increase in serum globulin level. Thrombocytosis may also be seen in patients with active disease. Rheumatoid factors (antibodies directed at other host antibodies) are present in 80% of patients. Antinuclear antibodies may be present in 30% of patients. Potential risk factors for cervical involvement include elevated C-reactive protein and HLA-Dw2 or HLA-B27 positivity.

## RADIOGRAPHIC ANALYSIS

### Plain Radiographs

Some authors recommend routine radiographic screening of all patients with rheumatoid arthritis. Others have set criteria for ordering radiographs. Standard radiographs include AP, lateral neutral, lateral flexion/extension, and open mouth. Indications for ordering radiographs include cervical symptoms greater than 6 months, neurological signs or symptoms, preoperatively, rapidly progressive peripheral joint deterioration, and rapid functional deterioration.

Radiographic criteria for RA, as defined by Bland, include atlantoaxial subluxation of 2.5 mm or more, multiple subaxial subluxations, disc space narrowing without osteophytes, vertebral erosions, eroded (pointed) odontoid, basilar impression, apophyseal joint and facet erosions, osteopenia, and secondary osteosclerosis from occiput to C2, which may indicate degenerative change.

| TABLE 31-1 | Ranawat Grading Scale for Myelopathy |
| --- | --- |
| **Grade** | **Severity** |
| I | Normal |
| II | Weakness, hyperreflexia, altered sensation |
| IIIA | Paresis and long-tract signs, ambulatory |
| IIIB | Quadriparesis, nonambulatory |

The lateral neutral, flexion, and extension films are an effective screening tool for detecting cervical involvement in RA. They allow for identification of static and dynamic instability in the upper and lower cervical spine. Anterior atlantodental interval (AADI) and posterior atlantodental interval (PADI) can be determined from these views. These two values are used to determine atlantoaxial instability. The AADI is measured from the posterior aspect of the anterior arch of the atlas to the anterior surface of the dens. Anatomically, the transverse ligament holds the odontoid process against the anterior arch of the atlas and acts as the primary stabilizer of the atlantoaxial articulation. As the transverse ligament attenuates, there is more motion between the odontoid and atlas, which manifests on flexion/extension films as dynamic instability. An AADI greater than 6 mm has been used as a sign of instability, whereas an AADI greater than 9 mm has been considered an indication for surgery. However, the use of the AADI in management has been questioned, as erosive changes and anatomic abnormalities may be present. Boden et al [4] showed that the PADI may be more reliable and a better predictor of neurological recovery after surgical stabilization. Patients with a PADI greater than 14 mm experienced a higher rate of neurological recovery, while those with a PADI less than 10 mm had no recovery (Figure 31-2). Posterior subluxation may also be seen on lateral radiographs and should raise the suspicion of an absent or fractured odontoid. The open-mouth view is useful to identify lateral subluxation, which is defined as greater than 2 mm of lateral displacement at the C1-2 lateral articulation.

Several radiographic measures have been described to define cranial settling or basilar invagination [5] (Figure 31-3). McRae's line is defined on the lateral radiograph as a line that connects the margins of the foramen magnum. If the odontoid tip migrates above this line, it is considered cranial settling. Chamberlain's line runs from the hard palate to the posterior edge of the foramen magnum. If the odontoid tip migrates 6 mm above this line, it is considered cranial settling. McGregor's line runs from the hard palate to the opisthion or posterior base of the occiput. Cranial settling is defined as odontoid tip migration greater than 4.5 mm above this line. Erosive changes in the odontoid have made these relationships difficult to reliably measure. Therefore, the Ranawat method was designed to assess the extent of collapse at the atlantoaxial articulation. In this technique, the distance along the odontoid was measured from the C2 pedicle to the transverse axis of the ring of C1. A distance of less than 15 mm in males and 13 mm in females is considered to be cranial setting. Redlund-Johnell also described a technique that measured the vertical line from the midpoint of the caudad margin of C2 to McGregor's line; cranial settling is diagnosed when the distance is less than 34 mm in males and 29 mm in females (Figure 31-4). Clark et al defined the "station of the atlas," which describes the relationship of the anterior ring of C1 to the body of the odontoid, which is divided into thirds. The atlas usually lies at station I which corresponds to the proximal third (Figure 31-5). Riew et al stated that no single measurement alone was reliable; however, the combination of the Ranawat, Clark, and Redlund-Johnell methods yielded sensitivity and negative predictive value of 94% and 91%, respectively.

Subaxial subluxation is the second most common instability pattern; it is characterized by sagittal plane listhesis in sequential vertebrae ("staircase") and posterior element changes (facet joint erosions and widening, whittling, and spindling of the spinous processes). Subaxial subluxation has been defined by Yonezawa as subluxation greater than 4 mm or 20% listhesis of vertebral body diameter. The space available for the cord should also be a consideration. Boden et al described 14 mm as critically stenotic canal in the rheumatoid subaxial spine compared to 13 mm in the spondylotic spine. This is due to the abundance of hypertrophic pannus in the canal.

## Magnetic Resonance Imaging

Magnetic resonance imaging (MRI) has become a mainstay in the workup of any cervical spine disease, including RA. It provides information about the bony structures, ligamentous structures, periodontoid pannus, brain stem and spinal cord integrity, space available for the cord (SAC), and the craniocervical junction. In some cases, the periodontoid soft tissue can be abundant and produce a mass effect. In such cases, the radiographic parameters listed earlier may underestimate the amount of brain stem and spinal cord involvement. Cord gliosis, edema, and myelomalacia may also be seen on MRI. These changes are associated with poorer neurological recovery after surgery. The cervicomedullary angle can also be measured on MRI. This angle is found between vertical lines drawn along the anterior surface of the brain stem and cord on the sagittal MRI. The angle is normally between 135 and 175 degrees. Myelopathic signs correlate with MRI findings of a cervicomedullary angle of less than 135 degrees.

## Computed Tomography

Computed tomography may also be used, especially in patients in whom MRI is contraindicated. CT adds valuable information about bony anatomy and osseous erosions. The use of contrast media helps provide information about inflammatory soft tissue changes and helps differentiate between effusions and hypervascular pannus.

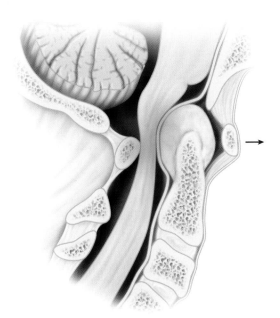

■ **FIGURE 31-2** Diagrammatic representation of atlantoaxial subluxation typically seen in patients with rheumatoid arthritis. The posterior atlantodental interval (PADI) is measured from the posterior margin of the odontoid process to the anterior margin of the posterior arch of C1. It demonstrates forward subluxation of the atlas on the axis, pannus formation around the odontoid process, and osseous erosions. There is severe compression of the spinal cord between the pannus anteriorly and the arch of the atlas posteriorly. *(Reproduced with permission from Boden SD, Dodge LD, Bohlman HH, Rechtine GR: Rheumatoid arthritis of the cervical spine: a long-term analysis with predictors of paralysis and recovery, J Bone Joint Surg Am 75:1282-1297, 1993.)*

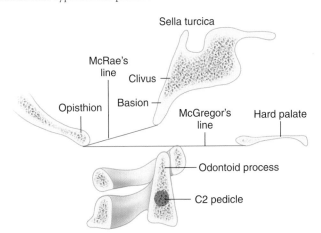

■ **FIGURE 31-3** Radiographic landmarks for assessing atlantoaxial impaction in patients with rheumatoid arthritis. On a lateral radiograph, atlantoaxial impaction is diagnosed by protrusion of the odontoid tip proximal to McRae's line or 4.5 mm above McGregor's line. *(Reproduced with permission from Kim DH, Hilibrand AS: Rheumatoid arthritis in the cervical spine, J Am Acad Orthop Surg 13(7):463-474, 2005.*

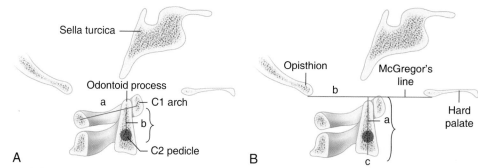

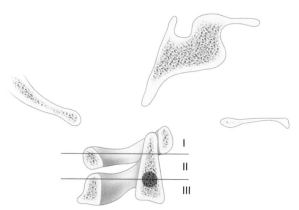

■ **FIGURE 31-4** Methods to assess atlantoaxial impaction on plain radiographs. **A**, Ranawat method. A line (a) is drawn across the transverse axis of the atlas, and a connecting line (b) is drawn through the vertical axis of the odontoid from the center of the C2 pedicle radiographic shadow. Values (x) <15 mm in men and <13 mm in women are diagnostic for atlantoaxial impaction. **B**, Redlund-Johnell method. A line (a) is drawn between McGregor's line (b) and the midpoint of the inferior endplate of C2 (c). A value (x) <34 mm in men and <29 mm in women is diagnostic for atlantoaxial impaction. *(Reproduced with permission from Kim DH, Hilibrand AS: Rheumatoid arthritis in the cervical spine, J Am Acad Orthop Surg 13(7):463-474, 2005.*

■ **FIGURE 31-5** Clark station. The station of the first cervical vertebra is determined by dividing the odontoid process into three equal parts in the sagittal plane. If the anterior ring of the atlas is level with the middle third (station II) or caudal third (station III) of the odontoid process, basilar invagination is diagnosed. *(Reproduced with permission from Riew KD, Hilibrand AS, Palumbo MA, Sethi N, Bohlman HH: Diagnosing basilar invagination in the rheumatoid patient: the reliability of radiographic criteria, J Bone Joint Surg Am 83-A(2):194-200, 2001.)*

## MANAGEMENT

### Nonoperative Management

The treatment of RA has been revolutionized by the introduction of newer pharmacological therapies that target the inflammatory mediators responsible for disease. The treatment of RA previously consisted of patient education, physical therapy, NSAIDs, remittive agents (gold, penicillamine, hydroxychloroquine, etc.), corticosteroids, and immunosuppressive agents (i.e., methotrexate). The newer drugs that are used in conjunction with the aforementioned regimen include antagonists to tumor necrosis factor-alpha (TNF-α) and interleukin-1 (IL-1).[6]

Infliximab is a chimeric IgG1 monoclonal antibody that binds soluble and membrane-bound TNF-α, thereby interfering with the binding of TNF-α to its receptor. Etanercept is a recombinant, fully human form of the p75 TNF receptor fusion protein. Adalimumab is a fully human monoclonal TNF-α antibody that binds to TNF-α. This interferes with TNF receptor binding, causing cell lysis to TNF-α expressing cells. These agents can be used in conjunction with methotrexate and corticosteroids to have a synergistic effect.

The concern with this class of drugs is the toxicity. TNF-α helps to maintain containment of organisms in granulomas. Therefore, blocking TNF-α can increase the risk of infections. New cases of tuberculosis as well as reactivation of old disease in patients undergoing anti-TNF-α therapy have been reported. The use of these agents in patients with active infections should be carefully considered. Although the mechanism is not clear, primary lymphomas have been reported in patients on TNF-α antagonists. There have also been reports of new-onset demyelinating disorders and exacerbations of previously known multiple sclerosis in patients using these drugs. Hypersensitivity reactions can occur. They may be local at the site of injection (redness or itching) or systemic (cardiopulmonary, itching, hypotension, etc.).

Interleukin-1 is mostly produced by monocytes and macrophages. Anakinra is a recombinant form of human IL-1 receptor antagonist that targets the type 1 IL-1 receptor. It may be used alone or in conjunction with methotrexate. The main adverse event is the increased risk of bacterial infection. The combined use of a TNF-α antagonist and anakinra is discouraged, due to the increased risk of infection.

Nonsurgical management also includes physical therapy and bracing. Cervical collars provide some pain relief, warmth, and a feeling of stability. Soft collars offer comfort but do not protect against progressive subluxations. Rigid collars can limit anterior subluxations but do not allow reduction of the subluxations in extension. Rigid collars, however, are poorly tolerated, especially in patients with temporomandibular disease and skin problems.

### Surgical Indications

Goals of surgical treatment are to relieve pain, and to achieve spinal stability through a solid fusion, and to decompress the involved neural structures. Surgery should be considered in any of the previously mentioned instability patterns (atlantoaxial instability, subaxial subluxation, and cranial settling) with or without pain, myelopathy, or neurological deficits.[7] Indications include progressive neurological deficit, mechanical neck pain in the setting of instability, radiographic risk factors of impending neurological injury (PADI less than 14 mm in the setting of atlantoaxial instability), cranial settling (as demonstrated by the combination of Clark station, Redlund-Johnell and Ranawat criteria), and a cervicomedullary angle less than 135 degrees.

The decision to undergo surgery should be individualized. The chronic systemic disease process and side effects of treatment often result in patients who are poor surgical candidates because of malnutrition, anemia, and osteopenia. However, surgery should be strongly considered in patients with intractable pain and neurological deficits who are good surgical candidates.

Shen et al[8] described an algorithm for the patient who is neurologically normal. In these patients, observation is acceptable if the plain radiograph lateral view shows a PADI of greater than 14 mm and there is minimal evidence of cranial settling. For patients with a PADI less than 14 mm, an MRI should be obtained to look for the true SAC (scrutinizing odontoid erosion and periodontoid pannus). If the SAC is less than 13 mm or the cervicomedullary angle is less than 135 degrees, prophylactic arthrodesis should be considered. In patients with atlantoaxial instability and associated cranial settling, they recommend a more aggressive approach because of a higher morbidity and mortality associated with this subgroup of patients. In the subaxial spine, a posterior canal diameter greater than 14 mm in the neurologically normal patient can be observed, whereas those with a posterior canal diameter less than 14 mm on x-ray should obtain an MRI. If the SAC is less than 13 mm or there is significant subluxation, stabilization should be considered.

## Preoperative Assessment

Preoperative assessment is imperative for all rheumatoid patients. Considerations include preoperative planning (bone stock, deformity, etc.), medical optimization (nutrition, anemia, etc.), and anesthesia evaluation (awake fiberoptic nasal or endotracheal intubation). Patients with severe basilar invagination may require preoperative cervical traction using a halo ring. This can improve alignment and improve neurological symptoms. Baseline somatosensory evoked potentials prior to positioning a myelopathic patient may help prevent further cord injury owing to malpositioning of the neck or operative maneuvers. Perioperative positioning is important, as many of the subluxations can be reduced under anesthesia and held in place with a positioning device (i.e., Mayfield skull clamp). Anterior and posterior approaches are available for addressing the craniocervical and subaxial pathologies. The surgical approach should be determined by the pathology and morphology of the spine. It is important to understand the radiographs, neurology, and patient symptomatology while planning surgical intervention.

## Operative Management

### Atlantoaxial Subluxation

Several methods have been described for atlantoaxial stabilization. The Gallie wiring technique was first described in 1939 for fracture fixation. Various approaches have been taken to instrument the upper cervical spine. The Gallie technique consists of passing sublaminar wires rostrally beneath the lamina of C1 or atlas and then around the spinous process of C2, with the addition of a clothespin-shaped bone graft. The Brooks-Jenkins modification of the Gallie technique consists of sublaminar wires beneath the lamina of atlas and axis, with two cortical bone graft struts as opposed to one. The atlas can be instrumented using hooks and claws as well. Harms described a rigid posterior construct for stabilization of the upper cervical spine.[9] This construct consists of C1 lateral mass screws and C2 pars interarticularis screws or C2 pedicle screws. Recently, pedicle screw fixation of C2 has become more common. The pedicle lies posterior and medial to the transverse foramen. The pedicle projection lies 5 mm caudal to the superior laminar edge of the axis and 7 mm lateral to the lateral border of the spinal canal. The pedicle axis is directed 30 degrees medial to the sagittal plane and 20 degrees rostral to the axial plane. The inferior pedicle width is approximately 3 mm less than the width of the superior pedicle. Therefore, to avoid vertebral artery injury and to maintain adequate purchase in the C2 pedicle, the screw should be directed to the superior medial portion of the pedicle.

The lateral C1-C2 articulation can also be fixed via the transarticular screw technique of Magerl. The transarticular screw traverses the isthmus of the axis and enters the posterior aspect of the atlantoaxial joint on its way to the lateral mass of the atlas (Figure 31-6). There are various contraindications to the transarticular screws, mostly focusing on the cord of the vertebral artery. When the transverse foramina are high-riding, this prevents placement of transarticular screws. The vertebral artery passes in a groove through the axis before entering the transverse foramina of the atlas. If the depth of the groove exceeds 5 mm, the remaining height of the lateral mass and pedicle width of C2 are both less than 2 mm. This would make it impossible to safely pass a 3.5 mm screw. Also, if the isthmus of the axis is less than 5 mm in height or width, the chance of penetration into the vertebral artery by a 3.5 millimeter transarticular screw increases. To be aware of these anatomical variations, it is necessary that preoperative CT scans (and CT angiograms) with 3D reconstructions be done prior to transarticular screw placement. An additional complication of transarticular screws is hypoglossal nerve injury. The twelfth cranial nerve courses anterior to the lateral tip of the C1 lateral mass. If the screws are too long or the lateral mass is overdrilled, injury to this nerve may occur, resulting in motor paresis of the tongue.[10]

### Cranial Settling

In cases of cranial settling, occipitocervical fusion may be necessary. This is the treatment of choice in patients with cranial settling and fixed atlantoaxial subluxation leading to posterior cord impingement from the ring of C1. Each case must be individualized. In the former case, if the subaxial spine is involved, fusion may have to be extended to T2 in order to support the rigid construct and the weight of the head. In the latter case, occiput to C2 fusion with a C1 laminectomy may be the procedure of choice. Sublaminar wires, hooks, screws, and bolts have been used for occipital fixation. Screws provide easy fixation with adequate purchase. Some authors have suggested that unicortical screw fixation is almost as good as bicortical fixation. Use of unicortical screws may also prevent damage to the intradural sinuses and brain matter. If the bone quality is good, suboccipital wires and hooks may be used and provide excellent fixation. However, in osteoporotic bone these two methods may not provide rigid occipital fixation. One proposed advantage to screw fixation is that in the case of dural leakage the osseous hole is completely filled by the screw, thus stopping the leakage of spinal fluid. Ideal placement of occipital screws is along the superior nuchal line or the external occipital crest below the inion. Ebraheim et al suggest that 8 mm screws can safely be placed 2 cm lateral to the midline at the level of the inion, 1 cm from the midline 1 cm below the inion, and 0.05 cm from the midline 2 cm below the inion. This will ensure optimum purchase in the occipital bone. This explains the rationale for a "T" plate for fixation of the occiput. Depending on the pathology, caudal fixation may include C2 pedicle screws, subaxial lateral mass screws, and C7-T2 pedicle screws to provide a stable, rigid construct.

### Subaxial Subluxation

In the case of subaxial subluxation, reducible subluxations can be fused anteriorly or posteriorly, but optimal treatment for irreducible subluxations is anterior decompression and fusion. This allows for release of tight anterior structures. Some authors recommend anterior and posterior fusions in this population because of the osteoporotic bone. Posterior fusion should be strongly considered following any laminectomy, to maintain sagittal balance. The extent of fusion is often not obvious, as RA is progressive. Instability patterns vary and postfusion adjacent level disease is common. Therefore, the need to extend the fusion to the occiput or T2 must be considered. Posteriorly, the lamina provide excellent fixation for sublaminar wires or hooks. Sublaminar wires, due to their low volumetric displacement, result mostly in segmental fixation. Hook constructs achieve segmental fixation as well, but also result in canal intrusion and large volumetric displacement.

Lateral mass screw techniques as described by Roy-Camille, Magerl, Anderson, and Ahn have been used and result in adequate fixation, either

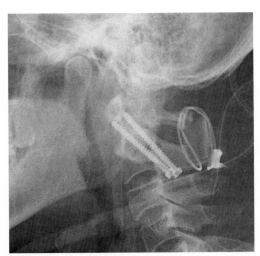

■ **FIGURE 31-6**   The postoperative cervical radiograph after the transarticular screw fixation revealed that the atlantoaxial complex was rigidly fixed with adequate purchase of the C1 lateral mass by the screw. *(Reproduced with permission from Lee JH, Jahng TA, Chung CK: C1-2 transarticular screw fixation in high-riding vertebral artery: suggestion of new trajectory, J Spinal Disord Tech 20[7]: 499-504, 2007.)*

unicortical or bicortical. The distance from the posterior midpoint of the lateral mass to the transverse foramen ranges from 9 to 12 mm. The lateral border of the artery lies 6 degrees lateral to the posterior midpoint of the lateral mass. Therefore, lateral mass screws are started at the posterior midpoint of the lateral mass and directed at least 10 degrees lateral to the sagittal plane. Trajectory parallels the facet joint, aiming toward the anterosuperior lateral corner of the lateral mass. Practically, this can be accomplished by laying the drill bit against the adjacent caudal spinous process. This will help ensure the required lateral angulation and anterosuperior trajectory. This will carry the tip of this screw superior to the exiting nerve root and lateral to the vertebral artery.

The lateral masses of C6 and C7 are often too small to place screws. At C7, the average pedicle height and width are 6.5 and 5 mm respectively. Therefore, these pedicles are typically large enough to accommodate 3.5 to 4.0 mm screws. At C7, the projection of the axis of the pedicle is 1 mm inferior to the middle of the transverse process and 2 mm medial to the lateral border of the lateral mass. Because of the projection of the pedicles onto the lateral masses, it is necessary to start laterally, close to the lateral "roll-over" of the lateral mass. Pedicles are angulated posterior superior to anterior inferior and directed approximately 45 degrees medially. The margin for error in cervical pedicle screws is very small. There is no space between the pedicle and the nerve root superiorly or between the pedicle and the dura medially.

Anterior fixation in the cervical spine is similar to that of the spondylotic spine. However, due to the osteoporotic rheumatoid bone, anterior fixation is often augmented by posterior fixation. Vertebral bodies can provide good screw fixation anteriorly. Because of the kidney-shaped vertebral body, screws placed in a converging orientation tend to be shorter than those placed in a diverging orientation. However, diverging screws could result in screw penetration into the neuroforamen or the transverse foramen, resulting in either nerve root or vertebral artery injury. The problem with converging screws is that they converge in the softer central cancellous bone

and may be prone to failure of fixation. Therefore, diverging screws may be preferred in certain situations, such as in patients with severe osteoporosis.

### Odontoid Resection

When severe cranial settling occurs, resection of the odontoid may be necessary. An anterior decompression may be indicated in cases where there is an irreducible anterior extradural compression of the cervicomedullary junction by pannus or a severely migrated odontoid. Odontoid resection may be performed with or without resection of the anterior ring of C1. Occasionally, a portion of the clivus may need to be resected to gain access to the odontoid. The transoral approach is associated with an increased risk of infection with mouth flora; therefore some surgeons prefer an extrapharyngeal approach. Odontoid resection may be combined with posterior occipitocervical fusion or anterior strut grafting and stabilization. Preoperative assessment is necessary and includes swallowing and respiratory analysis. The presence of a mobile and stable temporomandibular joint is crucial to allow 2.5 to 3 cm opening.

### CONCLUSION

Management for rheumatoid arthritis of the cervical spine has improved. This is mainly due to earlier diagnosis and screening, early surgical referral, and aggressive medical management. Surgical outcomes have improved, primarily due to newer techniques, improved preoperative and postoperative management, appropriate patient selection, and improved surgical timing. Most authors recommend surgery in patients with neurological deficits. Those without neurological compromise should be investigated and followed carefully. Once a patient becomes myelopathic, the long-term mortality increases and the potential for neurological recovery decreases. Cervical spine involvement is common in patients with rheumatoid arthritis. Management is complicated and a multidisciplinary approach must be used.

## Case Report

### HISTORY

This is a 65-year-old female who complains of neck pain and occipital headaches for the past 3 years. She denies any history of trauma, fever, chills, or weight loss. She denies any difficulty walking or buttoning her shirt. She has no bowel or bladder complaints. She has no pain radiating down the arms.

### PAST MEDICAL HISTORY

Rheumatoid arthritis diagnosed at age 17, hypertension, asthma, osteoporosis

### PHYSICAL EXAMINATION

She has obvious metacarpophalangeal joint deformities. She has no motor or sensory deficits in bilateral upper extremities and is normoreflexic. She has negative Hoffman and Babinski signs. She does have painful range of motion of the neck.

### RADIOGRAPHIC FINDINGS

See Figure 31-7A-C.

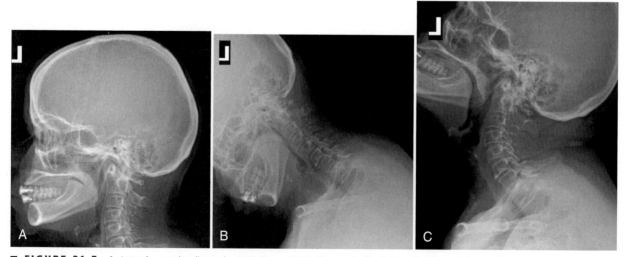

■ **FIGURE 31-7** **A,** Lateral neutral radiograph: AADI 8 mm, PADI 13 mm. Redlund Johnell: 28 mm (abnormal for women <29). Ranawat Index: 12 mm (abnormal for women <13), **B,** Lateral flexion radiograph: AADI 9 mm, PADI 12 mm, and **C,** Lateral extension radiograph: AADI 4 mm, PADI 17 mm.

## MRI

See Figure 31-8.

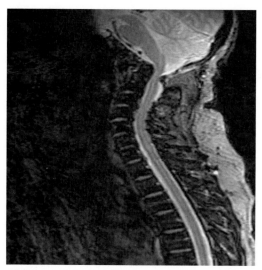

■ **FIGURE 31-8** Magnetic resonance imaging showing odontoid erosion, retrodental pannus, basilar invagination, and a compromised PADI.

## POSTOPERATIVE RADIOGRAPHS

See Figure 31-9.

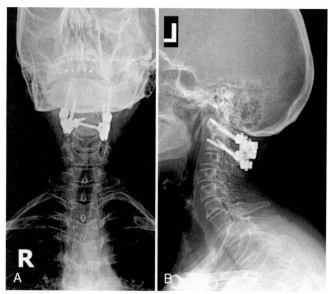

■ **FIGURE 31-9** Postoperative radiographs (AP and lateral) showing rigid Harm type posterior fixation consisting of C1 lateral mass screws and C2 pedicle screws.

## References

1. K. Chin, Surgical management of rheumatoid arthritis, in: Herkowitz, Garfin, Eismont, Bell, Balderston (Eds.), The spine, Elsevier, Philadelphia, 2006.
2. D. Borenstein, Arthritic disorders, in: Herkowitz, Garfin, Eismont, Bell, Balderston (Eds.), The spine, Elsevier, Philadelphia, 2006.
3. A.T. Casey, H.A. Crockard, J. Pringle, M.F. O'Brien, J.M. Stevens, Rheumatoid arthritis of the cervical spine: current techniques for management, Orthop. Clin. North Am. 33 (2) (2002) 291–309.
4. S.D. Boden, L.D. Dodge, H.H. Bohlman, G.R. Rechtine, Rheumatoid arthritis of the cervical spine: a long-term analysis with predictors of paralysis and recovery, J. Bone Joint Surg. Am 75 (9) (1993) 1282–1297.
5. H.V. Nguyen, S.C. Ludwig, J. Silber, D.E. Gelb, P.A. Anderson, L. Frank, A.R. Vaccaro, Rheumatoid arthritis of the cervical spine, Spine J. 4 (3) (2004) 329–334.
6. T. Doan, E. Massarotti, Rheumatoid arthritis: an overview of new and emerging therapies, J. Clin. Pharmacol. 45 (7) (2005) 751–762.
7. D.H. Kim, A.S. Hilibrand, Rheumatoid arthritis in the cervical spine, J. Am. Acad. Orthop. Surg. 13 (7) (2005) 463–474.
8. F.H. Shen, D. Samartzis, L.G. Jenis, H.S. An, Rheumatoid arthritis: evaluation and surgical management of the cervical spine, Spine J. 4 (6) (2004) 689–700.
9. J. Harms, R.P. Melcher, Posterior C1-C2 fusion with polyaxial screw and rod fixation, Spine 26 (22) (2001) 2467–2471.
10. T.J. Puschak, et al., Relevant surgical anatomy of the cervical, thoracic, and lumbar spine, in: Vaccaro, Betz, Zeidman (Eds.), Principles and practice of spine surgery, Mosby, Philadelphia, 2003.

# 32

# Tumors of the Cervical Spine

*Oren N. Gottfried, Scott L. Parker, and Ziya L. Gokaslan*

## KEY POINTS

- Spine tumors are divided into those occupying the intramedullary, intradural-extramedullary, and extradural regions.

- In adults, ependymomas are the most common cervical intramedullary tumor; the optimal treatment is a complete resection.

- Cervical schwannomas are usually located intradurally. They are approached by laminectomy, with a high rate of total resection; however, large tumors or those with a large extradural component often require additional surgical exposure.

- The most common epidural spine disease is metastasis, for which the best treatment is circumferential decompression of the spinal cord, reconstruction, and immediate stabilization, plus postoperative radiotherapy.

- Malignant primary spinal tumors are more common in adults. Chordoma is the most common solid primary tumor; it is locally aggressive, often involves the cervical region when it occurs in the mobile spine, and is best managed by a total resection.

## INTRODUCTION

Tumors of the vertebral axis are usually described and grouped based upon their location: intramedullary (IM), intradural-extramedullary (IDEM), and extradural (ED). IM lesions are found within the spinal cord parenchyma, comprise only 5% of all spinal lesions, and 50% of these tumors are located in the cervical spine. Ependymomas account for 60% to 70% of all IM tumors found in adults, followed by astrocytomas and hemangioblastomas. Extramedullary-intradural lesions comprise 40% of all spine tumors and may commonly extend to the spinal roots. IDEM tumors include meningiomas and nerve sheath tumors (neurofibromas and schwannomas); each occurs with similar frequency. Only 15% of meningiomas are located in the cervical spine, while nerve sheath tumors have an equal distribution throughout the cervical, thoracic, and lumbar spine. Extradural lesions arise in vertebral bodies or epidural space and comprise 55% of all spine lesions. Primary ED tumors are relatively uncommon, with the vast majority of tumors in this region being metastases. Primary ED tumors include osteoid osteomas, osteblastomas, osteochondromas, hemangiomas, osteosarcomas, chordomas, and chondrosarcomas. Metastatic ED tumors to the spine include breast, lung, prostate, gastrointestinal, and renal cell carcinomas; myeloma; and lymphoma; and they often invade the vertebral column. The cervical spine is the region least often involved by spinal metastases (10%).

In this chapter, we discuss tumors of the three compartments of the spine: IM, IDEM, and ED. We provide the basic presentation, imaging findings, details of surgery, and management of tumors with adjuvant therapies. Additional attention is placed on describing the more common cervical tumors found in adults as well as the most challenging tumors of the cervical spine. Specifically, there are more detailed discussions and case examples of the surgical management of intramedullary ependymomas, cervical schwannomas, and cervical chordomas.

## INTRAMEDULLARY SPINAL TUMORS

### General Information, Clinical Presentation, and Imaging

Patients with intramedullary glial spinal cord tumors may present with pain, sensory dysfunction, and weakness referable to the level of the lesion. A characteristic presentation of an intramedullary tumor is a central, dull aching of a gradual onset that is not referable to a specific neurological location. The symptoms can be of a longer duration for lesions that grow slowly. As the lesion increases in size, the symptoms may progress from the vague ones described above to more neurologically localizing sensory, and even later, motor changes. In contrast, in patients with malignant astrocytomas, symptoms occur rapidly with a mean duration of less than 6 months before diagnosis.

The diagnostic imaging modality of choice, to differentiate the three most common IM lesions (ependymomas, astrocytomas, and hemangioblastomas), to evaluate the possibility of malignancy, and for preoperative evaluation and planning, is gadolinium-enhanced magnetic resonance imaging (MRI). An MRI of the entire spine axis is indicated to evaluate for other lesions or metastasis. IM lesions commonly result in widening of the spinal cord. Also, MRI provides evaluation of associated findings commonly seen with IM lesions, such as edema, hemorrhage, cyst, syringomyelia, and cord atrophy. Intramedullary tumors may be difficult to see on T1-weighted images as they appear isointense to the adjacent spinal cord. T2-weighted images are the most diagnostic, as these tumors often appear hyperintense to the surrounding spinal cord. Although ependymomas often display homogeneous enhancement on MRI, astrocytomas are often much less uniform. This is caused by inconsistent contrast uptake as a result of their irregular margins and associated necrosis. Whereas ependymomas result in symmetric expansion of the spinal cord, astrocytomas are more infiltrative, have margins that are less sharp, and are eccentrically located. Hemangioblastomas can be differentiated from the other tumors by their origin and location on the posterior surface of the spinal cord with the tumor nodule on the pial surface and more intense enhancement than that of ependymomas.

### Ependymomas

Ependymomas account for the majority of all intramedullary spinal cord tumors found in adults. They comprise about 60% of all IM spinal cord tumors and are the most common glial tumors of the spinal cord. IM ependymomas arise from the ependymal cells lining the central canal. Ependymomas are benign and slow-growing, centrally located, well-circumscribed and sometimes encapsulated, and they cause symmetric expansion of the cord without infiltration into the surrounding neural tissue. Their arterial supply is most often derived from the anterior spinal artery. Ependymomas appear as reddish or purple-gray masses with many small blood vessels. Associated hemorrhage at the outer margins of the tumor and reactive cysts occur with many IM ependymomas.

Intramedullary ependymomas most commonly occur in the cervical and cervicothoracic regions of the spinal cord. The mean age at presentation is 42 years, and there is a slight female predominance. The most common presenting symptom is neck pain localized to the region of the spine, but patients may also present with dysesthetic pain or numbness and, with larger tumors, with symptoms from neural compression. Given the slow growth and well-circumscribed quality of these tumors, symptoms generally progress slowly, and patients often have a long history prior to diagnosis.

On T1-weighted images, ependymomas appear isointense relative to the neural parenchyma although, infrequently, they may appear hypointense. Heterogeneity and hyperintensity on T1-weighted images may reflect a hemorrhagic component. On T2-weighted images, ependymomas are commonly hyperintense relative to the normal spinal cord. Ependymomas are homogeneously and intensely enhancing with a well-defined border of enhancement. Hemorrhage at the cranial or caudal margin of ependymomas is common and T2-weighted images may demonstrate a low-signal-intensity rim. About half of ependymomas have nonenhancing reactive cysts with similar signal intensity to cerebrospinal fluid. Also, half of cervical ependymomas are associated with a syrinx. Cervical lesions average 4.2 vertebral segments in length.

## Astrocytomas

Astrocytomas of the spinal cord are rare in adults and arise from glial cells in the spinal cord. They are less common than ependymomas in the adult population. The majority of IM astrocytomas are low-grade tumors, but approximately 25% of adult spinal cord astrocytomas have anaplastic features. IM astrocytomas are commonly found in the cervical region of the spinal cord.

There is slight male predominance of IM astrocytomas. In adults, the incidence of spinal cord astrocytomas peaks between the third and fifth decades of life, but these tumors may occur in individuals of any age. As with ependymomas, patients often present with symptoms near the level of the tumor. The most common signs and symptoms of spinal cord tumors include localized pain, numbness and paresthesias, unilateral or bilateral weakness, bowel or bladder dysfunction, spasticity, and gait difficulties. Patients with malignant astrocytomas are more likely to present with neurological deficit, given the rapid growth of the tumor and subsequent neural compression.

On imaging, intramedullary astrocytomas of the spinal cord vary in size and length, with 6 vertebral-body segments being the average length. Spinal astrocytomas have variable and heterogeneous enhancement patterns. The tumor margin is often not well defined. Tumor cysts are a common finding, and reactive cysts may be observed at the cranial and caudal ends. IM astrocytomas may be associated with a syrinx. Spinal astrocytomas are more infiltrative, have less defined margins than the other IM lesions, and are more eccentric in location. Spinal astrocytomas are less prone to have extratumoral hemorrhage. MRI may demonstrate significant cord edema, drop metastasis, and leptomeningeal spread with malignant astrocytomas.

## Hemangioblastomas

Hemangioblastomas are benign tumors of vascular origin that arise from the erythrocyte precursor. They account for less than 5% of IM tumors. They may occur sporadically or in association with von Hippel-Lindau disease (20% to 30% of cases); these patients typically present with multiple lesions. Patients typically present by age 40 years. Often patients present with pain, weakness, or paresthesias. Hemangioblastomas are localized to the dorsal aspect of the spinal cord. Hemangioblastomas are characterized by prominent vascularity, large reactive cysts, the coexistence of a syrinx, and a widened, edematous cord. MRI signal intensity of hemangioblastomas is similar to those of ependymomas, but the tumor nodule, on the pial surface, commonly has more intense enhancement. Flow voids may be present and there may be local edema of the cord around hemangioblastomas.

## OPERATIVE TECHNIQUES (See Figures 32-1 and 32-2)

## Intramedullary Tumors

The patient is positioned prone on gel rolls in a Mayfield head holder with the arms tucked to the side, with care taken to pad all pressure points. We use intraoperative neurophysiologic monitoring with somatosensory evoked potentials, transcranial motor evoked potentials, and continuous electromyography for all IM cervical spine tumors. The use of total intravenous anesthesia allows for effective monitoring during tumor resection. We maintain the mean arterial pressure at a normal range to ensure adequate

spinal cord perfusion. A lateral x-ray with skin markers in place allows for identification of the relevant level of the spine and a precise skin exposure. A standard dorsal midline approach is used. A subperiosteal dissection of the paraspinal musculature exposes the lamina and spinous processes. Prior to laminectomy, the level is confirmed again with radiograph. Generally, we perform a joint-sparing laminectomy at the vertebral level above and below the area of the lesion. If there is a suspicion of a high-grade astrocytoma and we obtain biopsy confirmation of this lesion, we target the location of the greatest size of the mass, and may not require a laminectomy overlying the entire lesion. Prior to dural opening, the tumor is precisely visualized with ultrasound to confirm adequate exposure. A durotomy is made in the midline, and the dural edges are sutured to the soft tissues laterally, exposing the arachnoid overlying the spinal cord. Using an operating microscope, the arachnoid is opened and tacked laterally to the dural edges with vascular clips. Care is taken to avoid any blood rundown into the operative field by placing sponges along the outer dural margin. For ependymomas, or lesions not extending to the dorsal surface, we prefer approaching the tumor, if possible, with a midline myelotomy between the dorsal columns. For more lateral lesions, a myelotomy dorsal to the dorsal root entry zone approach is performed. We use neurophysiological monitoring to define the dorsal columns and midline sulcus, as the midline may be difficult to identify due to the tumor growth. A bipolar cautery is used on the pial surface, and it is sharply incised. The myelotomy is extended beyond both poles of the tumor to facilitate a gross total resection. We make the best attempt to preserve all veins and arteries. The dorsal columns are dissected apart. Commonly, we enhance exposure with retraction of the cord with a pial suture.

Demarcating and establishing a plane between the parenchyma and tumor is key to achieving a gross total or more aggressive resection. Regardless of the suspected tumor pathology, we always send tumor specimens early in the dissection for evaluation with frozen pathology. The bulkiest component of the lesion is often in the center, and thus a good place to begin the dissection, as there is decreased potential for harm to surrounding neural structures. As mentioned earlier, it is also important to have complete exposure to the poles of the tumor. For ependymomas, we generally can identify and develop a clear plane between cord and tumor, and the tumor capsule is dissected circumferentially from the spinal cord parenchyma. We recommend en bloc resection of the tumor whenever possible, as it reduces the potential for tumor spillage, avoids encountering excessive bleeding from the tumor during dissection, and thus allows maintenance of better surgical planes. Dissection along the anterior median raphe is usually the most difficult portion of the surgery, as the tumor tends to adhere to this thin segment of the cord. Because small branches of the anterior spinal artery penetrate the neoplasm along the anterior aspect of the cord, great care must be taken to avoid disrupting the anterior spinal artery. The final step in removing the ependymoma after dissection from the ventral surface is the separation from the anterior spinal artery.

For large tumors or ones with indistinct planes, it may be necessary to debulk the mass with an ultrasonic aspirator. When en bloc resection is not feasible due to an inability to clearly visualize the dissection planes, internal debulking may be performed to decrease the amount of traction on the cord. The major disadvantage of extensive debulking is fragmentation of the tumor, thereby destroying the correct dissection planes. For large tumors, after debulking, it may be possible to remove further tumor capsule and delineate the tumor margins from the cord.

Generally, for an ependymoma or low-grade astrocytoma, we will always attempt a total resection if there are no persistent changes on neurophysiological monitoring. If there are neurological changes on monitoring, we typically elect to perform a second staged resection at a later date. For biopsy-confirmed anaplastic astrocytomas we resect as much abnormal appearing tissue as possible and only attempt a total resection if there is no evidence of significant changes on monitoring, and the tumor is easily resectable with a visible cord-to-tumor interface and is not disseminated. The extent of resection may be confirmed via intraoperative ultrasonography. We do not perform more than a biopsy on a glioblastoma multiforme or a disseminated anaplastic astrocytoma. Gross total resection is the acceptable surgical option for a hemangioblastoma.

After tumor resection, we achieve hemostasis, avoiding the temptation to coagulate any of the surface vessels. The tacked sutures on the pia and

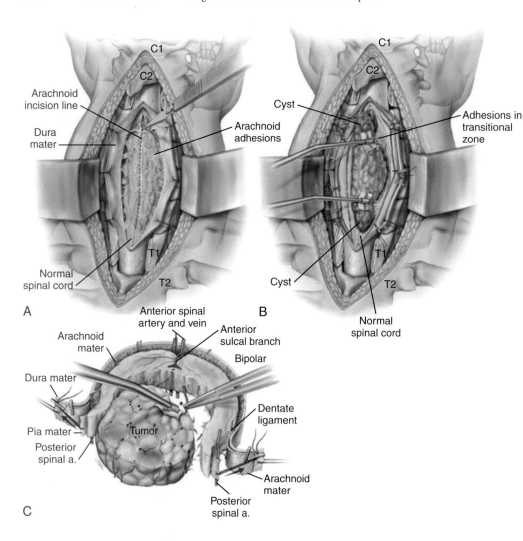

■ **FIGURE 32-1 A,** Intraoperative illustration of a patient with a C4–C7 ependymoma. The durotomy is completed, and the arachnoid is incised *(dashed line).* **B,** Tumor dissection is initiated in the middle portion of the tumor, which is the bulkiest. **C,** Great caution must be exerted while coagulating branches of the anterior spinal artery supplying the neoplasm along the anterior aspect of the cord to avoid occluding the anterior spinal artery. (a = *artery*) *(From Neurosurgery 51:1162-1174, 2002.)*

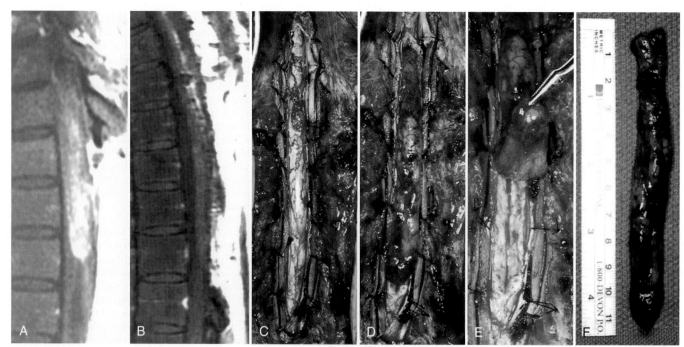

■ **FIGURE 32-2** Spinal cord ependymoma. **A,** Preoperative T1-intensity, gadolinium-enhanced MRI scan of a patient with a thoracic cord intramedullary ependymoma. **B,** Postoperative T1-intensity, gadolinium-enhanced MRI scan of the same patient showing complete resection of the neoplasm. **C,** Intraoperative photograph of the same patient showing the spinal cord before the myelotomy. **D,** Ependymoma mushrooming out of the myelotomy. **E,** Tumor elevated caudally, with a forceps used to dissect the anterior plane. **F,** En bloc resected ependymoma. *(From Neurosurgery 51:1162-1174, 2002.)*

dura are removed. The dura is closed primarily, in a watertight fashion. The subarachnoid space is irrigated to remove any blood prior to final closure, and a Valsalva maneuver confirms lack of CSF egress. Fibrin glue is placed over the dural closure. The wound is closed in the standard fashion and we leave a subfascial drain until there is limited output. We allow the patient to ambulate and sit up immediately after surgery.

In the authors' experience with intramedullary cervical tumor resection, patients presenting with myelopathic motor symptoms or those undergoing three or more levels of cervical laminectomy were found to have an increased likelihood of developing subsequent symptomatic instability requiring fusion, and we elect to fuse these patients with standard lateral mass and pedicle screws at the time of tumor resection. In the absence of myelopathy and/or the need for three-or-more-level laminectomies, we prefer laminoplasty or laminectomy if the majority of the facet is maintained.

## Postsurgical Management

The best current treatment of ependymomas consists of gross total resection without need for adjuvant therapy. The implementation of radiotherapy for ependymomas is warranted in cases of malignancy or disseminated tumor. In the case of a subtotal resection, we generally consider a secondary stage resection. The senior author (ZG) resected 26 spinal cord ependymomas, 11 of which had previous treatment with surgery and/or radiation therapy. A gross total resection was achieved in 88% of patients. Only one patient developed a recurrence over a mean follow-up period of 31 months. This study demonstrated that radical surgical resection of spinal cord ependymomas can be safely achieved in the majority of patients. A trend toward neurological improvement from a postoperative deficit can be expected between 1 and 3 months after surgery and continues for up to 1 year. The best predictor of outcome is the preoperative neurological status.

In the setting of residual ependymoma or low-grade astrocytoma that is not surgically resectable, radiotherapy is advocated. The dose is generally lower for these IM lesions compared to the adjuvant treatment of anaplastic astrocytomas (AAs) or glioblastoma multiforme. Higher grade lesions receive higher doses, and disseminated disease requires complete craniospinal radiation. There are no well-defined chemotherapeutic or radiosurgery regimens for IM tumors, but they remain possible treatment options for the future. In general, most authors only recommend biopsy for high-grade astrocytomas, followed by radiotherapy, but others have advocated for more aggressive surgical treatment of nondisseminated anaplastic astrocytomas. For example, in one large series of 35 high-grade spinal astrocytomas, radical resection of AAs was associated with a trend of increased overall survival in nondisseminated AA cases. The overall survival rate with these high-grade lesions remains poor.

## INTRADURAL-EXTRAMEDULLARY SPINAL CORD TUMORS

### General Information, Clinical Presentation, and Imaging

The two most common IDEM tumors, occurring with approximately equal incidence, are meningiomas and nerve sheath tumors, including neurofibromas and schwannomas. Meningiomas are more common in females and occur with the highest frequency in the thoracic spine, but approximately 20% present in the cervical spinal cord, with most localizing to the upper cervical spine near the foramen magnum. In comparison, schwannomas show no preference with respect to sex or region of the spinal cord. Whereas meningiomas and schwannomas commonly result in local pain or signs from mass effect on the spinal cord including myelopathy, nerve sheath tumors cause radicular pain from their involvement of the spinal roots.

Gadolinium-enhancing MRI is the imaging modality of choice for IDEM spinal tumors to differentiate between these two types of lesions and to identify the origin, location, and extent of the lesion. An MRI of the entire spine should be obtained to ensure there are not other lesions elsewhere. Preoperative imaging also is important to evaluate the tumor's relation to major vessels, including the vertebral artery (VA). Furthermore, a vascular study including CT angiography or MR angiography is indicated to evaluate whether a tumor extends into the transverse foramen or is adjacent to major vessels, including the VA.

### Nerve Sheath Tumors

The vast majority (85%) of nerve sheath tumors are comprised of schwannomas, with only 15% consisting of neurofibromas. Schwannomas may occur sporadically or as part of neurofibromatosis (NF) 2, while neurofibromas occur in NF1. Typically, schwannomas arise from Schwann cells of the dorsal sensory spinal roots (77%), and therefore often present localized to the posterolateral region of the spinal canal. The schwannoma often arises from a single nerve fascicle, with the remaining fascicles either displaced to one side or located around the tumor. Schwannomas appear grossly as a smooth globoid mass attached to a nerve, do not produce nerve enlargement, and are suspended eccentrically from the nerve. They are firm, encapsulated neoplasms and can be cystic, hemorrhagic, or fat-containing. Schwannomas can be localized completely intradurally, may extend intraforaminally with or without an extradural component, or may be entirely extradural. Dumbbell tumors are schwannomas with contiguous intraspinal, foraminal, and extraforaminal components. In general, 49% to 84% of schwannomas are intradural, 8% to 32% are completely extradural, 1% to 19% are both intradural and extradural, 6% to 23% are dumbbell, and 1% are intramedullary. While purely intradural schwannomas are more common in the thoracic and lumbar regions, dumbbell tumors occur predominantly in the cervical spine. The frequency of schwannomas occurring in the cervical spine is similar to the occurrence in the lumbar or thoracic regions.

Sporadic spinal schwannomas usually present between the fifth and sixth decades of life. Men and women are affected equally. Typically, patients present with local pain and signs of compression of adjacent neural structures, with neurological deficits developing late in the course of the illness. The symptoms are vague in the beginning and worsen gradually, primarily because of the slow growth of the lesions. Most patients present initially with segmental pain followed by local pain; gait ataxia, motor weakness, bladder paresis, and dysesthesia are less common. Patients usually report an average duration of symptoms from 2 to 3 years, but some may have had symptoms for more than 15 years.

On MRI, schwannomas can be differentiated from meningiomas by their heterogeneous and less avid enhancement. Also, schwannomas often appear isointense on T1-weighted images, but they can be distinguished from meningiomas by their increase in signal intensity seen in T2-weighted images. Schwannomas may be associated with an expansion of the intervertebral foramen of the involved nerve root, and thus CT images are valuable to evaluate the bony anatomy. Smooth bony expansion at the foramen with lack of significant erosion suggests this benign, slow-growing lesion. Overall, it is important to evaluate the degree of extraspinal extension of a tumor to help with surgical approach and preoperative planning.

### Meningiomas

Typically, spinal meningiomas are located in the intradural extramedullary space, grow slowly, and spread laterally in the subarachnoid space until they result in symptoms. Spinal meningiomas are typically IDEM (83% to 94%), but rarely (5 to 14%), tumors have an extradural component or are entirely extradural (3% to 9%). Most meningiomas are located laterally and a posterolateral location is more common than anterolateral location. Only a small proportion of meningiomas (<20%) are located in the cervical spine, but in younger populations the cervical location is more common. When located in the cervical spine, spinal meningiomas are commonly located in the upper cervical spine, are located more anterolateral and often result in motor dysfunction, especially in the hand and distal arm.

Meningiomas typically occur between the ages of 49 and 62 years. With their slow growth, there is commonly a significant delay between the onset of symptoms and diagnosis. The mean duration of symptoms prior to presentation is usually 1 to 2 years, but patients may have noted pain symptoms beginning 15 to 20 years prior to diagnosis. Patients often present with pain, sensorimotor deficits, and sphincter disturbances. Typically, back or radicular pain precedes the weakness and sensory changes; the sphincter dysfunction is always a late finding. Additionally, signs of myelopathy are present in most patients. Weakness is present in 64%, and 32% of patients are nonambulatory at the time of presentation.

MRI is the best imaging technique for diagnosing spinal meningiomas. It clearly delineates the level of the tumor and its relation to the cord, which is useful in planning surgery. Typically, spinal meningiomas are isointense to the normal spinal cord parenchyma on T1- and T2-weighted images, and they display intense enhancement after gadolinium injection. The characteristic sign of a meningioma is a "dural tail" of enhancement.

## OPERATIVE TECHNIQUES

### Intradural-Extramedullary Tumors

Many spinal meningiomas and schwannomas present eccentrically, dorsolateral to the spinal cord; therefore, they are accessible via a posterior or posterolateral approach and are easily seen after the dura is opened. Unilateral laminectomy, with or without facetectomy, may be used for eccentrically located ventral tumors. Ventrolaterally located tumors often require dentate ligament sectioning to obtain further ventral exposure and visualization, but some ventral tumors may provide the necessary spinal cord retraction to provide access via the standard posterior exposure. A divided dentate ligament or noncritical nerve root may be retracted to provide further ventral exposure. Intraoperative ultrasonography is used to establish the location of the tumor before dural opening. Tumor resection is performed with intraoperative electrophysiological monitoring, and additionally, for schwannomas, with intraoperative stimulation with motor-evoked potentials of nerve fascicles (at levels responsible for limb function) prior to sectioning.

IDEM tumors in the cervical area may present surgical challenges because of the need for extensive bony exposure, which results in the potential for spinal instability. In addition, large tumors of the cervical spine may compress adjacent neurovascular structures and cause tight adhesion between the tumor capsule and spinal cord, adjacent nerve roots, vertebral artery, cervical plexus, or carotid sheath, all of which may be injured with tumor resection. The majority of IDEM tumors are approached posteriorly; some midline ventral tumors may be approached anteriorly with a corpectomy and fusion. Some of the arguments against the use of the anterior approaches to ventrally located spinal tumors include inadequate access to the tumor because of a deep and constrained operative field, excessive bleeding from the epidural venous plexus, the need for spinal reconstruction, and the risk of postoperative cerebrospinal fluid leak. Access to ventrally located tumors by a posterior approach may not always be possible, however, because of the need to place undue retraction on the spinal cord. Thus a purely ventral approach or a combined anterior and posterior approach is indicated.

### Spinal Schwannomas

Many schwannomas that are located completely intradurally, with or without a small foraminal component, may be approached through a laminectomy, but very large tumors, tumors that are located extradurally, or those with an ED component often require an additional or different surgical approach to achieve gross total resection. For the standard midline exposure of an ID schwannoma, the schwannoma is exposed and the plane of dissection on the tumor surface must be identified. An arachnoid membrane often adheres to the tumor and must be incised and reflected off the tumor surface. Next, the tumor and its capsule are cauterized to decrease the size of the tumor and its vascularity. The normal proximal and distal aspects of the involved nerve are exposed, and the attachment to the involved nerve root is identified. Internal debulking may be performed with an ultrasonic aspirator. The schwannoma is then separated from the nerve. Although it is often necessary to section the fascicle involved with the tumor, in the majority of cases, it is possible to preserve all other fascicles of the nerve root. Functioning nerve fascicles often can be dissected free and swept circumferentially off the surface of an underlying schwannoma, thus preserving their function. Interestingly, sectioning of nerve fascicles at levels relevant for arm function often does not result in a deficit, as many fascicles are already nonfunctional.. Some proximally located schwannomas may be embedded in the pia, and resection of these tumors may require resection of a segment of the pia.

For dumbbell cervical schwannomas, one may perform a single-stage, modified posterior midline exposure. First, the ID component is resected as earlier, but a complete unilateral facetectomy is performed. Then the dural incision is extended laterally over the nerve root sleeve to gain access to the foraminal and extraforaminal tumor extension. The exposure extends up to 4 cm from the lateral dural margin; tumor extension beyond these limits often requires an additional anterolateral approach. If it is possible to preserve the nerve root, an intrafascicular tumor dissection is performed. If it

is necessary to sacrifice the nerve root, the lateral dural incision is extended around the dural root sleeve to disarticulate it from the dural tube. Next, the dural tube is reconstructed to be watertight. Removal of the foraminal and extraforaminal tumor components depends on their size and relation to the nerve root and nerve root sleeve. Generally, the tumor is followed distally along the nerve root to the lateral margin. Detaching the levator scapulae and posterior and middle scalene muscle attachments from the posterior tubercles of the transverse processes allows the exposure to extend 3.5 to 4 cm from the lateral dural margin. The rostral and caudal tumor margins are then defined. The VA is displaced ventromedially and separated from the dumbbell tumors by the tumor capsule or nerve sheath, the periosteum, and a perivertebral venous plexus. If necessary, spinal stabilization can be performed after tumor removal. After this approach in patients with significant ED components, it may be necessary to resect residual tumor with an additional anterior approach or a more lateral posterior approach.

### Spinal Meningiomas

The majority of meningiomas may be approached through a standard midline approach with sectioning of the dentate to facilitate resection of more ventral tumors without excessive spinal cord retraction. After internally debulking, a dissection plane is developed and the tumor is rolled away from the spinal cord and toward its dural attachment. The tumor is removed from its dural attachment. Dura with remaining tumor is either coagulated using bipolar cauterization or resected; this decision is based on the patient's age and risk of recurrence and ability to obtain a watertight dural closure. In general, the dural attachment may not be resected in cases involving an anterior dural attachment due to difficulties in reconstructing the dura. The dura is closed primarily or in cases with an extensive dural resection with a dural graft. Also, in some cases it is possible to separate the dura into an outer and inner layer and to resect the tumor with the inner layer, leaving the outer layer available for closure.

## Postsurgical Management

The primary treatment for spinal schwannomas and meningiomas is surgical resection; gross total resection is the goal. Complete resection of spinal schwannomas and meningiomas conveys an excellent prognosis. In general, the rate of gross total resection for these tumors is over 85%. For schwannomas, it may be more difficult to achieve a gross total resection of tumors with extensive ED involvement and those occurring in patients with neurofibromatosis type 2. For meningiomas, potential challenges for total resection include anterior location, en plaque meningiomas, recurrent tumors with arachnoid scarring, tumors with epidural components, and calcified meningiomas. Recurrences are rare when a gross total resection has been achieved, and range from 5% to 10%. Thus the benefit of complete resection needs to always be considered in terms of risk of spinal cord damage, given that these are benign lesions. For IDEM tumors, complications are rare and typically occur in less than 5% of cases. Surgical morbidity is related to cerebrospinal fluid leakage, wound healing, postoperative hematomas, and instability. In general, 80% of patients demonstrate neurological improvement postoperatively, and neurological deterioration is seen in less than 10%. New motor and sensory deficits usually improve over time. The most common late symptoms are mild or intermittent radiating pain, cystic myelopathy, spinal deformities, and arachnoiditis. Although the optimal treatment for spinal meningioma is total microsurgical resection, some authors advocate adjunctive radiotherapy in cases of recurrent tumors.

## EXTRADURAL SPINAL CORD TUMORS

### General Information, Clinical Presentation, and Imaging

Primary tumors of the vertebral column are relatively infrequent, with the vast majority of extradural tumors being spinal column metastases. Metastatic tumors are the most common neoplastic lesions of the spine, and the vertebral column is the most common site of bone metastasis, but metastasis to the cervical spine (10%) occurs less often than to the thoracic (70%) and lumbar regions (20%). Nearly 5% to 10% of patients with systemic cancer suffer spinal metastases, and approximately 30% to 70% of patients with solid tumors have spinal metastatic disease on autopsy. Breast, lung, prostate, and renal cell carcinomas; lymphoma; and sarcoma account for 70% of all sources of spinal metastasis. The metastases occur in the vertebral body (60%), posterior elements (30%), or both (10%). The most common symptom is neck pain (90%); the pain is usually local with tenderness on palpation, but there can also be a radicular component. More than 50% of patients who present with symptomatic epidural spinal cord compression may be nonambulatory, may have bowel or bladder dysfunction, and may present with severe deficits, including acute weakness that may progress to quadriplegia. It is important to assess for mechanical pain secondary to instability, as this is common in the cervical spine, specifically with tumors with significant bone destruction associated with pathological fractures and deformity.

Although epidural spinal cord compression occurs in only 5% to 10% of patients with metastasis, it has a great impact on the quality of a patient's remaining life and his or her overall survival. There has been an increased trend with epidural compression to prolong neurological function, ability to ambulate, and survival with more aggressive surgical management, including circumferential decompression with or without spondylectomy and stabilization with spinal reconstruction followed by radiotherapy. Studies like the one by Patchell and colleagues have demonstrated that direct decompressive surgery plus postoperative radiotherapy is superior to treatment with radiotherapy alone for patients with spinal cord compression caused by metastatic cancer. For example, they demonstrated that surgical resection followed by radiotherapy compared to radiotherapy alone for treatment of spinal cord compression resulted in significantly more patients retaining the ability to ambulate after treatment (84% compared to 57%), and for significantly longer periods of time (122 compared to 13 days).

With respect to primary spinal cord tumors, the cervical region is unique in that malignant lesions are more common than benign. Primary benign tumors of the spinal column include osteoid osteomas, osteoblastomas, osteochondromas, giant cell tumor, aneurysmal bone cyst, and hemangiomas, and primary malignant tumors of the spinal column include plasmacytoma/multiple myeloma (most common), osteosarcomas, chondrosarcomas, chordoma, lymphoma, and malignant fibrous histiocytoma. Generally, benign primary spine tumors are more common in younger individuals, 35% have a neurological deficit on presentation, and they often involve the posterior elements. Malignant primary spinal tumors are far more common in middle-aged individuals (40 to 60 years), more often result in neurological deficit or spinal canal compression (55%), and more often involve the vertebral body (80%).

Imaging modalities used for identification and evaluation of epidural spinal column tumors including primary and metastatic lesions are plain x-ray, CT, and MRI. Interestingly, 80% to 90% of patients with symptomatic spinal metastasis have abnormalities on plain radiograph including osteolytic, or less often, osteoblastic changes of the pedicle or body. Plain x-rays are helpful in determining the stability of the spine and clearly delineate pathological fractures, abnormal alignment, and deformities. CT further demonstrates bony involvement, including the extent of osseous destruction, and is also useful in evaluating spinal stability. As with all types of tumors of the spine, an MRI of the entire neuroaxis is vital to evaluate for tumors at other sites and other levels of epidural compression. MRI with contrast clearly demonstrates the extent of tumor and its relation to the spinal canal and other relevant anatomy including the lower cervical roots, important for arm function, and the VA. If there is tumor involvement extending to vascular structures, a dedicated vascular imaging study is indicated. Bone or PET scans may be helpful to evaluate for other sites of skeletal or systemic involvement.

Biopsy for histological diagnosis of the tumor is performed once the lesion has been fully investigated with imaging studies. In the absence of known diagnosis of primary tumors, a clear diagnosis based on characteristic imaging, a more accessible primary or metastatic lesion, or catastrophic neurological deficit, we perform a CT-guided biopsy of the spinal tumor for diagnosis and for surgical decision-making. During biopsy, it is very important to provide meticulous attention to prevent the seeding of neoplastic cells to healthy tissue. Thus, the route taken during the biopsy should coincide with a region that can be adequately excised during the surgical resection, and imaging studies help dictate the biopsy approach. This detail is very important for tumors in which an en bloc resection provides superior local control or a surgery-related cure or impacts survival, including chordomas and sarcomas. Finally, diagnosis of a radiosensitive tumor may eliminate the need for surgical decompression. After tissue diagnosis, highly vascular tumors including renal cell carcinoma, melanoma, and thyroid carcinoma may be treated with preoperative embolization to limit operative blood loss.

It is beyond the scope of this chapter to discuss the surgical management of every type of primary and metastatic spine tumor, and thus we provide a general overview of this topic. Also, as benign spinal tumors are rarer in adults, we limit any further discussion to malignant ones, which are relevant to the adult and aging population. Below, we discuss the specific management of a primary malignant tumor, a cervical chordoma.

## Operative and Postoperative Management
### Spinal Metastatic Tumors

Generally, indications for surgery include focal spinal metastasis with cord compression, failed radiotherapy, unknown pathology, pathological fracture with or without deformity, or progressive or rapid neurological decline. Surgery may not be indicated if there has been paralysis for over 24 to 48 hours; with anticipated survival of less than 3 months; with radiosensitive tumors including lymphoma, multiple myeloma, or prostate; if there is diffuse metastatic involvement or diffuse epidural compression; or in the presence of significant comorbidities.

The goals of a surgical intervention should be clearly identified before surgery, based on knowledge of the patient's pathology, predicted survival, extent of spinal disease and other systemic metastasis, control of the primary tumor, associated comorbidities, stability created by the tumor or by potential resection, and the tumor's ability to respond to other modalities including chemotherapy and radiation. Generally, the treatment options for cervical metastasis vary from laminectomy with or without stabilization for a mostly dorsal tumor compressing the cord, anterior cervical decompression with corpectomy and reconstruction for tumors involving mostly the vertebral body, to a two-staged anterior and posterior decompression with reconstruction. It is far more difficult to achieve a complete spondylectomy in the cervical spine than in the thoracic and lumbar regions, due to the need to preserve the lower cervical roots for arm function as well as the vertebral arteries. Although it may be possible to perform a complete intralesional resection or an en bloc spondylectomy, both with circumferential spinal reconstruction, these procedures, specifically the latter, have high morbidity and mortality and are rarely associated with increased long-term survival. En bloc spondylectomy requires extensive instrumentation to achieve difficult fusions, and requires extensive exposure of neurovascular structures that poses additional risk of nerve root and vascular injury; thus more limited resections in the cervical spine may reduce these risks. A curative surgery may only be useful and justified with an isolated metastasis to the spine, particularly one of breast or renal cell origin, in patients who have proven themselves fit for long-term survival. Generally, palliative treatment is indicated for cervical spinal metastasis, for treatment of pain and to promote neurological function. In addition to decompression and stabilization, other palliative treatment options may include balloon kyphoplasty; however, it is used far less often in the cervical spine due to its pedicles being smaller and more difficult to approach.

As most metastatic lesions originate in the vertebral body, an anterior cervical corpectomy offers the most direct approach for tumor excision, neurological decompression, and effective reconstruction of the weight-bearing vertebral column. This approach is especially appropriate in patients with significant vertebral body destruction resulting in neck pain or symptomatic spinal cord compression. When choosing spinal reconstructive materials and techniques, multiple biomechanical factors must be considered to achieve anatomical restoration of sagittal and coronal plane deformity and physiological load bearing. Stabilization and reconstruction of the cervical vertebral body defect after corpectomy can be performed with bone allograft, cement, pins or Silastic tubes, or titanium or PEEK interbody spacers and cages. Stabilization is then achieved with anterior instrumentation with cervical plate fixation, to prevent distraction failure and to provide increased rigidity. Additionally, posterior instrumentation with or without bone grafting may be necessary to supplement the anterior construct. As mentioned above, some tumors can also be addressed with anterior followed by posterior decompression or posterior decompression alone with laminectomy or more extensive bony decompression, with stabilization with lateral mass or pedicle screws.

Generally, surgery is followed by standard radiotherapy. As mentioned previously, some tumors, such as those of lymphoreticular origin, are very radiosensitive, and some cervical tumors with epidural spinal compression and even instability can be effectively treated with radiotherapy without surgical intervention. For example, a plasmacytoma with pathological fracture will reossify and regain stability after radiotherapy treatment. Some tumors are radioresistant, including renal cell, melanoma, and sarcoma, but even these often show some response to radiation treatment. There is also an increased primary role of radiosurgery for some of these typically radioresistant tumors. It may result in less neurological complications, and improve local tumor control by delivering a high dose of radiation in a single fraction to a focal area. Also, radiosurgery may be used in addition to standard radiotherapy. Although a variety of treatments are employed based on tumor histology and location, a common spine tumor radiotherapy dose is 3000 rads over 10 fractionated treatments 24 hours apart. The target volume usually encompasses 1 or 2 vertebral bodies above and below the lesion, including paravertebral and epidural disease.

Overall, effective treatment is surgery that decompresses the spinal cord circumferentially, reconstruction and immediate stabilization, followed by radiation therapy. Patient's who undergo this treatment are 1.3 times more likely to be ambulatory after treatment compared to radiation alone and twice as likely to regain ambulatory function. Also, 70% to 90% of patients have significant relief of pain, and 60% to 100% improve or retain ambulatory status. Primary pathology is the principal factor determining survival — some primary tumors including breast and renal cell carcinoma have longer survival after diagnosis of spinal metastasis — and overall, the median survival with metastatic spine disease is 10 months. Patients with preoperative and postoperative ambulatory function have significantly longer survival than nonambulatory patients.

### Primary Malignant Tumors

A CT-guided biopsy is invaluable in the surgical planning for cervical primary tumors. There are classification scales employed for primary spinal tumors for oncologic staging (Enneking) or for planning surgical treatment (Weinstein, Boriani, and Biagini: WBB). For example, malignant lesions in the Enneking system are divided into low-grade (I), high-grade (II), or high-grade with distant metastases (III). Low-grade lesions are further subdivided into those confined to vertebra (IA) or those with extension into paravertebral compartment (IB). These tumors are treated by a wide en bloc resection followed by radiation therapy. High-grade lesions (II) are further subdivided into intracompartmental without capsule (IIA) or invasion of surrounding structures with extensive bone destruction or fracture (IIB). The treatment of high-grade lesions is usually with multiple treatment modalities including wide resection, chemotherapy, and radiation therapy; results are still poor.

In the WBB system, the vertebra, surrounding soft tissue, and spinal canal are divided into 12 zones to allow accurate staging and surgical decision-making regarding operative approach. Tumors can extend to involve soft tissue, bone, spinal canal, epidural space, dura or neural elements, or the VA. The highest chance of curing a primary spine tumor is with wide resection with negative margins, and conversely, the presence of positive margins increases the probability of local recurrence and disease progression. A decision is made based on tumor location, involvement of adjacent structures, size of the tumor, and response to other treatment modalities to determine whether it is necessary or possible to perform an en bloc resection compared to an intralesional resection (with or without negative margins). For some malignant primary spine tumors, en bloc spondylectomy with or without wide margins is not always feasible or necessary for oncological control. For example, the senior author (ZG) effectively treated a C6 primary osteogenic sarcoma with a total cervical spondylectomy with intralesional resection followed by neoadjuvant chemotherapy. Overall, en bloc procedures can be divided into intralesional, wide, and marginal.

### En Bloc Resection and Treatment of Cervical Chordoma (See Figures 32-3 through 32-5)

Chordomas are one of the most common primary malignant tumors of the mobile spine; only plasmacytomas occur at a higher incidence. They account for 2% to 4% of primary malignant bone tumors and arise from the notochord remnants from the clivus to the coccyx. The majority of lesions occur in the sacrum, but 10% to 15% of cases occur in the mobile spine with the cervical region most common among these (50%). C2 and C3 are the most common cervical locations, and there may be significant epidural spread and extensions to the retropharyngeal space. They are slow-growing but locally aggressive and have significant propensity for local bone destruction, neural compression, and recurrence. The extension of the disease to the surrounding vital anatomy may ultimately result in neurological compromise, instability, and death. They arise in the vertebral body and may grow posteriorly to compress the spinal canal or extend anteriorly into the paraspinal muscles. Metastases are initially infrequent, but with later stage disease, they occur in up to 65% of cases.

The median age at diagnosis is 58 years, and 80% occur in patients over 40 years. They occur almost twice as frequently in men. The mean duration of symptoms is 14 months, and patients initially present with local pain. Patients with chordomas of the spine are more likely to present with neurological deficit including weakness, sensory change, or bowel and bladder dysfunction compared to those in the sacrum, which affords more room for tumor growth prior to neurological compromise. Cervical chordomas may result in dysphagia, airway obstruction, or an oropharyngeal mass.

On CT, there is lytic bone destruction as well as a large soft tissue mass, and frequently calcifications. On MRI, it is often possible to see extension or infiltration of tumor across the intervertebral disc space. On T1-weighted images, chordomas are isointense or slightly hypointense compared with muscle, and on T2-weighted images, they are hyperintense. They enhance with contrast, and have foci of low signal in areas of calcifications. A vascular study is performed if there is involvement of the VA or, if there is any concern that one of them must be sacrificed for tumor resection, to confirm patency of the opposite VA. Bone scan may show low or normal isotope uptake. The entire spine and body should be evaluated for other lesions. As mentioned previously, it is very important for treatment of chordomas to select a biopsy tract that does not traverse a major cavity which could seed the area with tumor cells, and that the tract can be clearly defined/marked for future resection.

Chordomas are generally considered poor responders to standard radiation therapy and chemotherapy, and intralesional resection is associated with a high local recurrence. Currently, the best initial treatment includes radical en bloc resection with or without high energy photon or proton beam radiation. Protons allow improved sparing of critical structures because the dose deposition of protons is limited mainly by the Bragg peak, where the dose is low, but the treatment is extremely conformal to the target volume. Residual or recurrent disease is treated with surgical resection followed by these radiation modalities. Mobile spine chordomas treated with intralesional resection and radiation have a high recurrence rate (approximately 66% at 37 months). Overall, 5-year and 10-year survival are 50% to 68% and 28% to 40%, respectively.

Thus, en bloc spondylectomy is an ideal treatment for chordomas, but it is very difficult in the cervical and upper cervical spine because of difficulties with adequate exposure, the need to preserve the VAs and cervical nerve roots, and difficulties with cutting the cervical pedicles. Following is a description of the senior author's (ZG) en bloc resection and reconstruction of a multilevel cervical spine chordoma involving C2 with total spondylectomy of C2-4 and sacrifice of the right C2-4 nerve roots and a segment of the right VA. The patient, a 54-year-old man, presented with 2 years of progressive dysphagia, numbness in hands, and unsteadiness. Imaging revealed a large retropharyngeal mass extending from C2-4 involving the C2-4 vertebra with epidural extension and encasement of the right VA. The treatment of cervical chordomas often involves a multidisciplinary approach with otolaryngologists and plastic surgeons to assist in access and exposure.

The operation was performed in two stages. The first stage, in the prone position, involved the resection of the posterior elements of the involved vertebrae, freeing neural elements that could be spared, completing the dissection around the VAs and the posterior margins of the tumor, and stabilizing the spine. After a tracheostomy was placed, the patient was placed in the prone position with head fixation, and lateral films confirmed the neutral position of the head and neck. Bilateral laminectomies and facetectomies of C2-4 (and a partial C1 right laminectomy) were performed to allow wide exposure of the exiting nerve roots. The right C2-4 roots were ligated and transected as they entered the tumor mass. Next, the right VA was exposed from C2-4 with drilling both rostral and caudal to the tumor. An initial

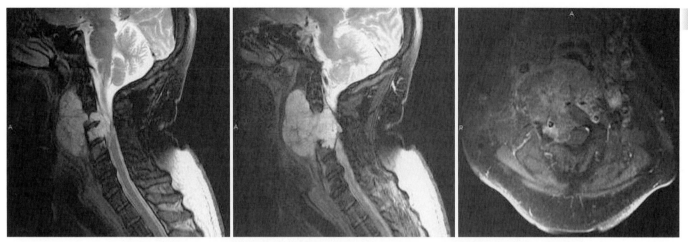

■ **FIGURE 32-3**   Sagittal and axial MR images of the cervical spine. *Left* and *Center,* Sagittal T2-weighted images demonstrating a chordoma involving the C-2, C-3, and C-4 vertebral bodies with retropharyngeal and epidural extension. *Right,* Axial contrast T1-weighted image revealing an extensive soft-tissue mass with encasement of the right VA and displacement of the posterior pharyngeal wall. *(From J Neurosurg Spine 2:199-205, 2005.)*

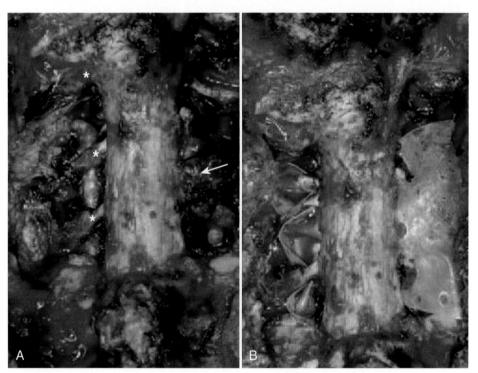

■ **FIGURE 32-4**   Serial intraoperative photographs showing the steps involved in the initial (posterior) stage of the surgery. **A,** Close-up view of the occipitocervical region showing partial C1 and bilateral C2–4 laminectomies and facetectomies, epidural tumor on the right *(arrow),* left C2, C3, and C4 nerve roots *(asterisks),* and skeletonized VA on the left. Also see the proximal portion of the right VA as it enters the tumor. **B,** Dorsal view of the thecal sac after placement of Silastic sheet between ventral dura and the tumor mass. The right C2, C3, and C4 nerve roots have been transected. *(From J Neurosurg Spine 2:199-205, 2005.)*

plane of dissection was created on the right lateral side of the tumor, and a Silastic sheet was placed between the tumor and the ventral thecal sac to protect the neural structures during the subsequent anterior procedure. Occipito-cervicothoracic fixation was performed. At this point, prior to the second stage, MRA was performed to evaluate patency of the left VA to ensure safe sacrifice of the right VA for tumor resection.

Next, the patient was positioned in the supine position. The second stage, an anterior approach, was designed to complete the en bloc resection and stabilize the ventral spinal defect. A right lateral neck dissection accompanied by a transmandibular, circumglossal, retropharyngeal exposure was performed. Subsequently, a C4-5 discectomy was performed, the uncovertebral joints were drilled, and the posterior longitudinal ligament was resected for visualization of the ventral dura. Soft tissue free of tumor was freed from the anterior arch of C1.

On the left, the longus colli insertion on the transverse process of C2-4 was released to allow the transverse process to be drilled away, completing the circumferential exposure of the left VA from C2-5. The surgical margin on the left was thus freed from all structures. On the right, the longus colli muscles were mobilized above and below the tumor and the VA was dissected above C2 and below C4 so as not to violate the tumor. Additional dissection was performed around the lateral aspect of the tumor, medial to the carotid sheath, until this met with the dissection plane from the posterior approach. Temporary aneurysm clips were placed on the right VA and SSEPs were noted to remain stable for 30 minutes. The vessel was ligated and transected at both ends beyond the tumor, freeing the specimen along the right lateral aspect. Finally, a high-speed drill was used to cut across the base of the dens, and rongeurs were used to resect the ligamentous complex behind the dens. This established a superior margin for the resection. The

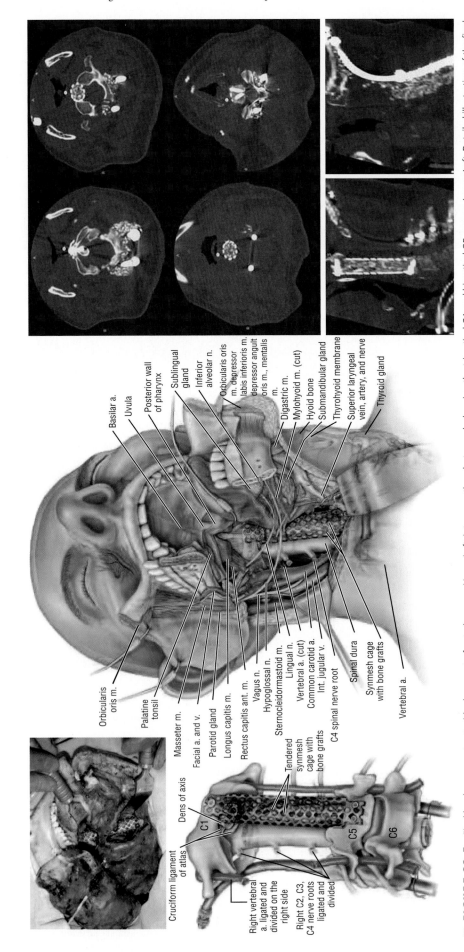

■ **FIGURE 32-5** Final hardware construct with placement of anterior cage. *Upper Left,* Intraoperative photograph showing the tricortical C1 and bicortical C5 screws. *Lower Left,* Detailed illustration of the final construct. The cage functions as a strut and plating device. *Center,* Artist's depiction showing the complete exposure with transmandibular access and tailored cage reconstruction in situ. *Right,* Postoperative axial CT images with bone windows and sagittal reconstructed images revealing the final hardware position. *(From J Neurosurg Spine 2:199-205, 2005.)*

Labels (center illustration):
Basilar a.
Uvula
Posterior wall of pharynx
Sublingual gland
Inferior alveolar n.
Orbicularis oris m. depressor labis inferioris m. depressor anguit oris m., mentalis m.
Digastric m.
Mylohyoid m. (cut)
Hyoid bone
Submandibular gland
Thyrohyoid membrane
Superior laryngeal vein, artery, and nerve
Thyroid gland

Orbicularis oris m.
Palatine tonsil
Masseter m.
Facial a. and v.
Parotid gland
Longus capitis m.
Rectus capitis ant. m.
Vagus n.
Hypoglossal n.
Sternocleidormastoid m.
Lingual n.
Vertebral a. (cut)
Common carotid a.
Int. jugular v.
C4 spinal nerve root
Spinal dura
Synmesh cage with bone grafts
Vertebral a.

Tendered synmesh cage with bone grafts

Labels (lower left illustration):
Dens of axis
C1
C5
C6
Cruciform ligament of atlas
Right vertebral a. ligated and divided on the right side
Right C2, C3, C4 nerve roots ligated and divided

entire tumor mass, including the C2-4 vertebral bodies, the right VA segment, and the right C2-4 nerve roots were removed en bloc, but the resection was marginal at the dura.

A fibular allograft was then cut to size and fashioned to form a sharp spike that could be embedded into the residual dens. The inferior end of the graft rested firmly against the superior endplate of the first remaining vertebra. A cervical plate was then fashioned to C1 and the most superior remaining vertebra (C5) The screws fixing the plate superiorly were placed with tricortical purchase, penetrating the anterior arch of C1 and engaging the residual dens. The posterior pharyngeal nerve was evaluated to determine if it is still intact (if it is not, a free flap should be placed from an external location that has remained prepped during the surgery).

The patient required several weeks of ventilatory support and needed a gastrostomy tube for difficulties with swallowing. Common complications after resection of cervical primary malignant tumors include failure of stabilization, swallowing difficulties, hoarseness, Horner syndrome, and hypoglossal injury; often tracheostomy and gastrostomy tubes are required after surgery. At a year from surgery, the patient is fully ambulatory, is able to swallow a regular diet, had his tracheostomy and gastrostomy tubes removed, his spinal construct remains stable, and he has no clinical or radiologic evidence of tumor recurrence. Radiation therapy has not been administered.

## CONCLUSIONS

In this chapter, we describe the demographics, presentation, physical exam, imaging, surgical planning and techniques including decompression and spine stabilization, postoperative management, and adjuvant treatment of tumors of the cervical spine. We describe tumors of the intramedullary, intradural-extramedullary, and extradural regions with a specific emphasis on more common cervical spine tumors found in adults, including ependymomas, schwannomas, metastases, and chordomas. In summary, the majority of these tumors are ideally managed with complete surgical decompression.

## References

1. Z. Cohen, D. Fourney, R. Marco, L. Rhines, Z. Gokaslan, Total cervical spondylectomy for primary osteogenic sarcoma, J. Neurosurg. Spine 97 (2002) 386–392.
2. O. Gottfried, W. Gluf, Quinones-Hinojosa, Kan P, Schmidt M: Spinal meningiomas: surgical management and outcome, Neurosurg. Focus 14 (2003) 1–7.
3. O. Gottfried, M. Binning, M. Schmidt, Surgical approaches to spinal schwannomas, Contemp. Neurosurg. 27 (2005) 1–8.
4. F. Hanbali, D. Fourney, E. Marmor, D. Suki, L. Rhines, J. Weinberg, I. McCutcheon, I. Suk, Z. Gokaslan, Spinal cord ependymoma: radical surgical resection and outcome, Neurosurgery 51 (2002) 1162–1174.
5. M. McGirt, I. Goldstein, K. Chaichana, M. Tobias, K. Kothbauer, G. Jallo, Extent of surgical resection of malignant astrocytomas of the spinal cord: outcome analysis of 35 patients, Neurosurgery 63 (2008) 55–60.
6. R. Patchell, P. Tibbs, W. Regine, R. Payne, S. Saris, R. Kryscio, M. Mohiuddin, B. Young, Direct decompressive surgical resection in the treatment of spinal cord compression caused by metastatic cancer: a randomized trial, Lancet 366 (2005) 643–648.
7. L. Rhines, D. Fourney, A. Siadati, I. Suk, Z. Gokaslan, En bloc resection of multilevel cervical chordoma with C-2 involvement, J. Neurosurg. Spine 2 (2005) 199–205.
8. D. Sciubba, J. Chi, L. Rhines, Z. Gokaslan, Chordoma of the spinal column, Neurosurg. Clin. N. Am. 19 (2008) 5–15.
9. F. Vincent, M. Fehlings, Spinal column tumors, in: M. Bernstein, M. Berger (Eds.), Neuro-oncology: the essentials, ed 2, Thieme Medical Publishers, New York, 2008.

# 33

# Role of Minimally Invasive Cervical Spine Surgery in the Aging Spine

*Woo-Kyung Kim*

**KEY POINTS**

- The anatomic and pathophysiologic changes of the aging spine are discussed.
- Techniques of various minimally invasive surgical procedures in the cervical spine include anterior cervical microforaminotomy, percutaneous cervical discectomy, microendoscopic discectomy, and percutaneous cervical nucleoplasty.
- The controversies of current minimally invasive surgical procedures are presented.

## INTRODUCTION

The aging of the population in industrialized nations appears to be an inevitable situation. It does not simply mean an increase in life expectancy owing to the improvement of medical science and health care, but additionally a significant decrease in birth rates has led to this situation. Back and neck pain are most frequently occurred presentations of older people, and the unique nature of the spine makes those problems highly complex to evaluate and to manage. The spine is a very specific anatomic and functional unit. The findings of radiological degenerative changes of the cervical spine in aging population are common. By the fourth decade of life, 30% of asymptomatic subjects show degenerative changes of the intervertebral discs, whereas by the seventh decade, up to 90% have developed degenerative alterations.[1,2] Thus, it is always important to interpret such radiological features in the light of the clinical presentation. If symptoms and findings are not correlated, the presence of a different pathology should be suspected, and appropriate evaluations are required. In order to assess the spine unit of patients (clinical, radiological; and laboratory findings; neurophysiology, etc.), cooperation between the orthopedic surgeon, the neurosurgeon, and the neurologisted is needed. Based on the present illness and physical examinations, a proper neurological workup should be performed. In addition to the neurological assessment, additional laboratory evaluations and other studies may be helpful in the differential diagnosis, including electromyography (EMG), electroneurography (ENG), sensory evoked potentials (SEP), and motor evoked potentials (MEP).

The aging of the spine induces considerable alterations in anatomical structures: discs, facet joints, ligaments, muscles, and bones. The degeneration of some of these structures can be responsible for the injury to the neural structures by herniated disc, spinal stenosis, and other degenerative disease.[1]

Although various surgical treatments for spinal disorders have been proposed for years, the current concept in the evolution of all spinal surgical procedure is mostly concerned with minimally invasive techniques. The advantages of minimally invasive procedures include less postoperative pain, shorter hospital stays with faster recovery, and decreased surgical morbidity, mortality, and long-term sequelae. These benefits are the result of reduced damage to surrounding spinal structures.

## BASIC SCIENCE

As a flexible, multisegmental column, the functional role of the spine is to provide stabilization and upright position. The spine is composed of a static, changeless component, the vertebral bodies, and an elastic mobile component, the three joint complexes, consisting of the intervertebral disc and the two posterior facet joints. As mentioned earlier, the aging spine experiences considerable changes in anatomy (the structural components, biomechanics, etc.).[2]

The quantity of water present in the nucleus pulposus (contains a high proportion of hydrophilic glycosaminoglycans) decreases and both spinal height and the cushioning effect are reduced with aging. Gaps and fissures may develop in the discs, and with the time they may become desiccated and even ossified. As the disc height decreases, there may be a buckling of both anterior and posterior longitudinal ligaments. The buckling posterior ligaments may project into the spinal canal, reducing the space available for the spinal cord. Bony osteophytes may develop in the region of the vertebral bodies; endplate osteophytes may expand across the disc spaces and merge with osteophytes of adjacent vertebrae to form bridging osteophytes. If the osteophytes involve posterior endplates, they may protrude into the spinal canal, compressing the dural sac. People with congenitally narrowed spinal canals have greater risk for spinal cord compression as a result of these changes. Large bridging osteophytes on the anterior endplates may lead to severe problems in gastrointestinal, respiratory, or vascular systems. The size of the neural foramen, which the spinal nerves pass through, may be decreased both with the loss of spinal length and ossification and hypertrophy of these soft tissues around the vertebral column. Such age-related changes demonstrate the symptomatology in most patients presenting for cervical spine surgery.[1,2]

## SURGICAL INDICATIONS AND PREPARATION

The indications for surgery include (1) persistent or recurrent upper extremity pain or numbness not responsive to a conservative treatments for more than 3 to 6 months, (2) progressive or profound neurological deficit, (3) static neurological deficit associated with radicular pain, and (4) imaging studies confirming pathoanatomic features consistent with clinical features.

All patients should have routine cervical spine radiographs, including dynamic views, computed tomography (CT) scanning, and magnetic resonance imaging (MRI) preoperatively. Intraoperative somatosensory evoked potentials are useful for monitoring the sensory neurological pathway continuously during the surgery and have been very effective for monitoring the dorsal columns of the spinal cord. This decreases the risk of an obstructed blood vessel, accidental removal of the breathing tube, or a patient becoming conscious during the procedure. Also, the patient may be monitored with motor evoked potentials (MEP) and electromyograms (EMG) intraoperatively.

## RADIOLOGICAL EVALUATION

Routine cervical spine radiographs, including anteroposterior, lateral, flexion, extension, and both oblique views, are taken for the evaluation of degenerative disc disease. The narrowing of the intervertebral disc space and neural foramen, formation of osteophytes or bony spurs, subluxation of facet joints, and segmental instability are commonly shown in degenerative cervical diseases. Although cervical radiographs and CT scanning are useful for visualizing bony anatomy and overall alignment of the spine, they are limited in the evaluation of neural structures, such as neural foramen, spinal cord or nerve roots, and the presence or absence of neural compression.

Magnetic resonance imaging provides excellent images of spinal structures, such as discs, neural elements, bony structures, muscles, and ligaments. It is the preferred method for confirmatory diagnosis and is generally recognized in published studies.

## SURGICAL TECHNIQUES

### Anterior Cervical Microforaminotomy

#### Transuncal Approach

Under general anesthesia, the patient is placed in a supine position. Under fluoroscopic guidance, the incision site is marked at the medial border of the sternocleidomastoid (SCM) muscle perpendicular to the disc space angle. A 2-cm transverse skin incision is made from the medial border of the SCM muscle. The surgical trajectory from skin incision to pathologic lesion is perpendicular to the sagittal plane of the cervical spine, so the bone must be opened at the anterolateral spine along the line of the trajectory. In this case, the uncinate process lies along the perpendicular surgical trajectory. Especially in procedures at C4-C5 or C5-C6 level, a skin incision at the upper or mid portion of the neck produces such a perpendicular surgical trajectory. Skin incision to bone exposure is performed as in the previously discussed approach. The medial 1 to 2 mm of the most medial transverse processes at the upper and lower vertebrae are removed, and the vertebral artery is identified. Then, the lateral uncinate process is dissected from the vertebral artery. The most lateral 2-mm portion of the uncinate is drilled just medial

to the vertebral artery toward the posterior longitudinal ligament. Once the posterior longitudinal ligament is exposed, compressive lesions, such as herniated soft disc or bone spurs, are excised. Often the posterior longitudinal ligament is opened to expose the dura mater at the most lateral portion of the spinal cord and proximal nerve root to detect hidden migrated disc fragments. The thin bone wall of the medial uncinate must not be damaged to maintain the integrity of the intervertebral disc.

### Upper Vertebral Transcorporeal Approach

This approach uses bone opening at the most inferolateral portion of the upper vertebral body, because the anteroposterior surgical trajectory is inclined caudally. It is usually used for C6-C7 and C7-T1 cervical surgery, but it is also used for other levels by placing the skin incision more cephalad. The vertebral artery is slightly exposed, and a 2-mm medial portion of the transverse process of the upper vertebra is removed. The bone is opened at the inferolateral 2- to 3-mm portion of the upper vertebra by drilling toward the posterior longitudinal ligament. The intervertebral endplate, at the anterior two thirds of the intervertebral disc, must not be damaged. The surgical trajectory is directed toward the pathological lesion only through the most posterior portion. The rest of the procedure is the same as described previously.

### Lower Vertebral Transcorporeal Approach

This technique refers to the location of the bone opening at the lateral portion of the lower vertebra of the intervertebral disc. When an operation is at a high level such as C3-C4, this surgical technique is required to expose the pathologic lesion, because the surgical trajectory from the skin incision to the target site is inclined cephalad.

The transverse skin incision about 1 to 2 inches then the platysma can be split longitudinally or dissected transversely. Blunt dissection proceeds medially to the sternocleidomastoid muscle and internal carotid artery toward the anterior aspect of the cervical vertebrae.

## Case Studies

A 67-year-old woman had continuous radiating pain into her left arm. During 6 months of conservative treatment and physiotherapy, the symptoms were not relieved. Plain radiographs showed decrease in the height of disc space at the level of C5-C6 (Figure 33-1). Cervical MRI demonstrated narrowing and obstruction of neural foramen at the levels of C5-C6 and C6-C7 (Figure 33-2). The decision was made to perform a microsurgical decompression with anterior foraminotomy at both cervical segments. Transuncal

approach at C5-C6 and upper vertebral transcorporeal approach at C6-C7 were performed, respectively. Plain and dynamic radiographs and three-dimensional (3-D) cervical CT were done postoperatively (Figure 33-3). The radiculopathy was significantly improved after the operation. The patient was symptom free, and 3-D CT and dynamic radiographs showed no instability of operated levels at follow-up.

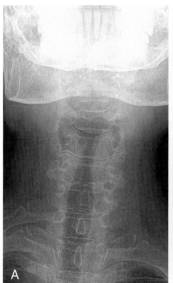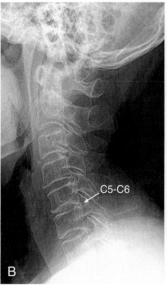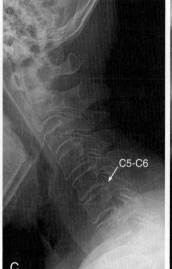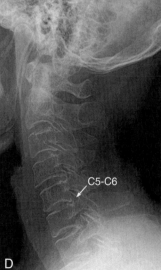

■ **FIGURE 33-1** The plain and dynamic radiographs show decreased disc space at C5-C6 level, preoperatively. A: AP view, B: lateral view, C: flexion view, D: extension view.

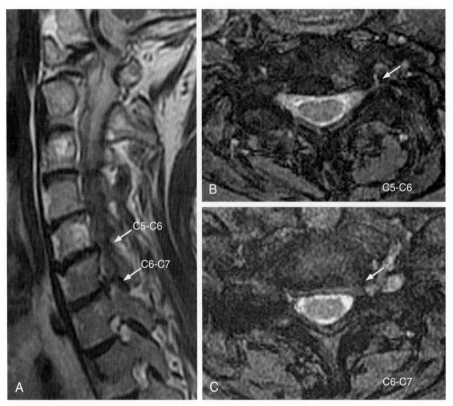

■ **FIGURE 33-2**  A: Cervical MRI sagittal view shows narrowing the neural foramen at C5-C6 and C6-C7 levels. B: Cervical MRI axial view shows narrowing the neural foramen by the compressive pathologic lesion at C5-C6 level. C: C6-C7 level.

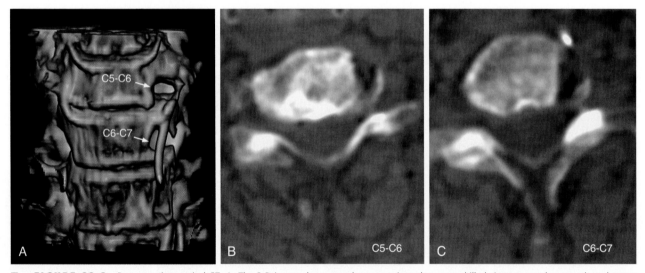

■ **FIGURE 33-3**  Postoperative cervical CT. A: The 3-D image shows two bony openings that were drilled via transuncal approach and upper vertebral transcorporeal approach respectively. B and C: Axial CT images also demonstrate the bone openings and decompression of the pathologic lesion at C5-C6 and C6-C7 levels.

The longus colli muscle is split longitudinally to expose the lateral portion of the cervical spine. An anterior cervical retractor system (e.g., Thompson retractor) is applied before the operating microscope. Endoscopic surgery has been performed for this operation. The medial portion of the transverse process at the rostral and caudal vertebrae are identified. The most medial, upper 1- to 2-mm portion of the transverse process at the lower vertebra is removed, and the vertebral artery is identified. Using a 1- or 2-mm cutting drill bit, the superolateral 2- to 3-mm portion of the lower vertebra is drilled posteriorly just medial to the vertebral artery.

A cephalically inclined surgical trajectory leads the drilling toward the target pathologic lesion posteriorly. Compressive herniated soft disc or bone

spurs are removed with microdissectors and various curettes. The nerve root and most lateral portion of the spinal cord are released. Surgical closure is made as in other anterior cervical surgery.

## Percutaneous Cervical Nucleoplasty

Percutaneous disc decompression, regardless of technique, has been based on the concept that a small reduction of volume in a closed hydraulic space results in a disproportionately large drop of pressure in the intervertebral disc space. Percutaneous cervical discectomy (PCD) has been developed as an effective treatment method for soft cervical disc herniation. Percuta-

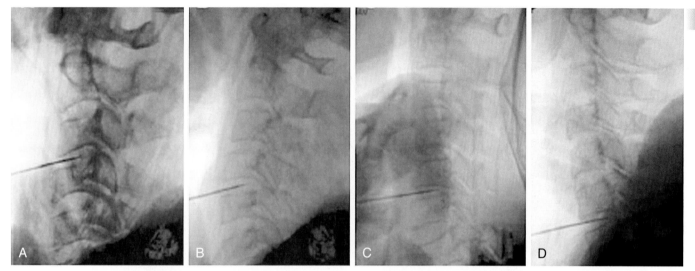

■ **FIGURE 33-4**   Intraoperative PCN procedures in different levels. A: C3-C4, B: C4-C5, C: C5-C6, D: C6-C7.

neous cervical nucleoplasty (PCN) is one of the new minimally invasive techniques that uses radiofrequency energy to ablate the nucleus pulposus (Figure 33-4).

Inclusion criteria are the same as those of other conventional anterior cervical foraminodiscectomy. Exclusion criteria are extruded disc fragment, hemorrhagic diathesis, spondylolisthesis, spinal canal stenosis, ossification of posterior longitudinal ligament (OPLL), previous surgery at the indicated level, and cases of myelopathy.

Under local anesthesia, the patient is placed in a supine position as for other anterior cervical approaches. The anterior cervical spine is palpated with the fingertips, and a spinal needle is used to puncture the right side of the neck and is passed into the indicated disc space under fluoroscopic control. The fiber of the Perc-D SpineWand (ArthroCare Corporation, Austin, Tex.) is inserted through the 18-gauge needle. The wand is connected to the standard ArthroCare power generator. The power for nucleoplasty ablation is set at 3 W with a setting of 1 second for coagulation. If there is no syndrome of pain, the SpineWand is placed in the right space on the disc and then the Coblation device is activated for 14 seconds with fluoroscopic monitoring. When the SpineWand is returned to the annulus, coagulation is applied for 1 second to shrink the surrounding collagen and widen the channel. This process is repeated four to six times during the surgical procedure.

## Percutaneous Endoscopic Discectomy

Under local or general anesthesia, the patient is positioned and other surgical preparations are performed as for other cervical surgery. The exact target level is confirmed fluoroscopically.

A 2- to 3-mm skin incision is made, a spine needle is placed in the target disc using fluoroscopic guidance, and a narrow guide wire is passed through the needle. The needle is removed. A blunt trocar is introduced over the guide wire down to the interspace, followed by the cannula, and the central elements are removed. A trephine is inserted through the cannula and the annulus is cut in a circular fashion. Minicurettes are used to loosen and remove disc material before a suction-irrigation system is introduced and the discectomy is performed with a guillotine cutting blade. The instruments included a probe, grasper forceps, and laser fiber. Movement in a fan sweep maneuver is critical; a 25-degree rocking excursion of the cannula hub from side to side increases the removal up to a 50-degree cone-shaped area within the disc space. The procedure is closely monitored with the fluoroscope and endoscope. The holmium:yttrium-aluminum-garnet laser with right angle or side-fire probe facilitates this discectomy. In addition, nonablative levels of holmium laser energy or thermodiscoplasty causes shrinking of the collagen and fibrocartilage; this tightening effect further decompresses and hardens the herniated cervical disc.

## Microendoscopic Discectomy

Microendoscopic discectomy (MED) (Figure 33-5) is used when there is a need to visualize across the spinal canal and an operating microscope is insufficient. Positioning and anesthesia are the same as those for a posterior cervical microendoscopic foraminotomy. Single level and multilevel decompression can be performed with the standard fixed-aperture tubular retractor. For two-level decompression, the tube can be angled rostrally or caudally. The incision should be centered on a point between the two interspaces. For a three-level grated decompression, a longer incision can be used. A longer incision allows better visualization and decreases the amount of soft tissue resection required. For multilevel decompression, an expandable working channel can be used. Generally, it is easiest to begin with the most caudal level first, minimizing the amount of blood running into the field. After the level has been confirmed with fluoroscopy, soft tissues are cleared off the level of interest and the lateral edges of the lamina are defined. To minimize the risk of injury to the spinal cord, a high-speed drill is used to remove the lateral aspect of the lamina. If an ipsilateral foraminotomy is not needed, take care not to injure the facet capsule. Otherwise, the high-speed burr and Kerrison punches can be used to perform foraminotomy. The tube is then angled medially, exposing the base of the spinous process. The high-speed burr is used to drill away the base of the spinous process. It is usually necessary to angle the working channel rostrally to resect the remainder of the spinous process. Fluoroscopy can be used to confirm the rostrocaudal extent of the decompression. The ligamentum flavum is initially left intact to protect the underlying dura mater. But, to get adequate visualization of the contralateral aspect of the spinal canal, the ligamentum flavum is resected with the aid of curettes and Kerrison punches. The undersurface of the contralateral lamina should be drilled away to provide better visualization. Decompression is complete when a nerve hook can be passed along the lateral aspect of the dura mater contralaterally. Once a single level has been decompressed, further levels can be decompressed with a high-speed burr or a Kerrison punch. Bone bleeding should be waxed as soon as possible to reduce the risk of venous air embolism. The operative wound is then repaired in layers like other cervical spine procedures.

## DISCUSSION

In recent years the general trend in spinal surgery has been one of reductionism and minimization. The concept of minimally invasive cervical spine surgery is ideal for the management of cervical aging disease. The extensive muscle dissection required for the traditional posterior approaches leads to significant postoperative pain and the potential for postoperative deformity. By minimizing the extent of muscular dissection and by preserving the contralateral soft tissue, the less invasive

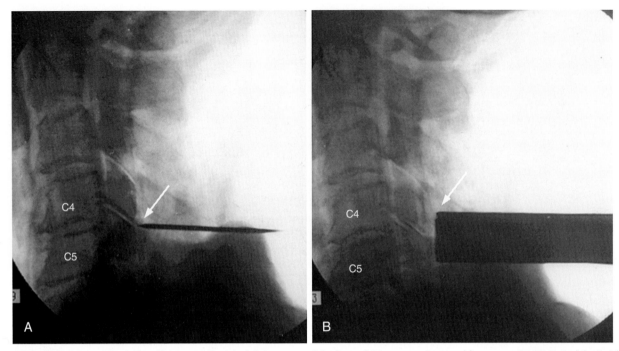

■ **FIGURE 33-5**   A: A guide pin (arrow) is inserted into the inferior aspect of the facet of C4 to access the neural foramen at C4-C5. B: And the Serial dilator (arrow) is docked.

approaches may lead to shortened hospital stays, decreased narcotic use, and better outcomes.

Stookey[3] described the clinical symptoms and anatomic location of cervical disc herniation in 1928. Subsequently, the landmark paper by Mixter and Barr[4] clearly established the relationship between herniated discs and sciatica, and provided evidence that laminectomy and disc excision could successfully relieve pain associated with radiculopathy. Bailey and Badgley[5], Cloward[6], and Robinson and Smith[7] popularized the anterior approach with interbody fusion in the 1950s. Hirsch[8] and Robertson[9] recommended cervical discectomy without fusion. Fukushima[10] introduced the ventriculofiberscope in 1973 and further enhanced the foundation for percutaneous endoscopic cervical discectomy.[3,4]

Minimally invasive treatments aimed at removing nuclear materials and lowering intradiscal pressure through devices inserted percutaneously into the intervertebral disc space have been shown to be safe and effective. A number of techniques have recently been developed that are applicable in the treatment of degenerative disorder on the cervical spine.

## Microsurgical Anterior Cervical Foraminodiscectomy

In the 1930s, Spurling and Scoville[11], and Frykholm[12] pioneered the posterior cervical approach for the treatment of cervical radiculopathy. But the posterior approach was limited in dealing with central compressive pathology and the open approach was associated with significant muscle morbidity. Subsequently, in the 1950s, the anterior approach was described and popularized. Compared to the open posterior approach, the anterior approach is generally associated with shorter recovery times but has a greater potential for complication. Anterior cervical discectomy and fusion (ACDF) results in a loss of mobility at the operated level, and increases rates of degenerative disc disease in adjacent levels. In addition, the compressive pathological factors are located anteriorly, and the immediate surgical outcomes of anterior discectomy are fairly good. However, the consequences of anterior disc-ectomy are obvious. Conventional anterior discectomy and fusion requires complete removal of the remaining disc in the intervertebral disc space, which results in loss of the functional motion unit.[13]

Microsurgical anterior cervical foraminodiscectomy (MACF) is a minimally invasive technique and one that permits anatomic and functional preservation of the functional motion unit of the cervical spine. Therefore this technique was named functional cervical disc surgery. This method

avoids osteoarthrodesis or arthroplasty with disc prosthesis. This technique is efficient with good results and low morbidity, especially in an aging spine.

## Percutaneous Cervical Nucleoplasty(PCN)

Percutaneous disc decompression, regardless of technique, has been based on the principle that a small reduction of volume in a closed hydraulic space, like an intact disc, results in a disproportionately large reduction of pressure. Percutaneous cervical decompression has been developed as an effective treatment option for soft disc herniation. PCN is a minimally invasive technique that uses radiofrequency energy to ablate the nucleus pulposus in a controlled manner for disc decompression.

Treatment of cervical disc hernia with PCN is safe to perform, and the efficacy of this technique is good in patients. The advantage of PCN is that it reduces the volume and pressure of the affected disc without damaging other spinal functional units. Ablation of a relatively small volume of the nucleus pulposus results in a significant reduction in intradisc pressure. Histologic examination revealed no evidence of direct mechanical or thermal damage to the surrounding tissues in human cadavers. Given these radical thermal penetrations, high temperatures and lethal thermal doses do not occur in small regions outside of the nucleus or within the bone endplates in human cadavers.[14]

A small number of complications are associated with PCN. With the approach from the anterior neck to disc space, it is important to monitor the distance from the tip of the needle to the spinal canal. Therefore monitoring of the needle is essential during this procedure. X-ray fluoroscopy is used to confirm the correct position of the needle tip during placement of the needle, permitting accurate nucleoplasty of the intervertebral disc. Vascular injury can occur if the device contacts an artery or a vein. Particular care should be taken to avoid puncture of the anterior annulus. But, according to Chen's study[15] in human cadavers, intradiscal pressure was markedly reduced in the younger, healthy disc cadaver. In the older, degenerative disc cadavers, the change in intradiscal pressure after nucleoplasty was very small. There was an inverse correlation between the degree of disc degeneration and the change in intradiscal pressure. Their conclusion is that pressure reduction through nucleoplasty is highly dependent on the degree of spine degeneration. Nucleoplasty markedly reduced intradiscal pressure in nondegenerative discs, but had a negligible effect on highly degenerative discs.

## Percutaneous Endoscopic Cervical Discectomy

Since the first description of cervical percutaneous discectomy by Tajima and colleagues[16] in 1981, percutaneous endoscopic cervical discectomy (PED) may be considered a good alternative to the standard anterior cervical discectomy and fusion for treating soft cervical disc herniation. The goal of this procedure is to decompress the spinal nerve root through percutaneously removing the herniated mass and shrinking the nucleus pulposus while the patient is under local anesthesia.

Most patients who have cervicobrachial neuralgia caused by disc herniation experience good response to medical treatment. However, symptoms related to perineural cicatricial fibrosis caused by prolonged pressure on the nerve root could become irreversible. Therefore the occurrence or aggravation of a neurologic deficit, even after an adequate period of conservative treatment, requires consideration of surgical decompression. PED is indicated in the surgical treatment of soft cervical disc herniation not contained by the posterior longitudinal ligament, which includes central, lateral, and foraminal disc herniation.

Minimally invasive PED under local anesthesia can prevent such complications as epidural bleeding, perineural fibrosis, graft-related problems, dysphasia, hoarseness, and so on. It also maintains the stability of the intervertebral mobile segment and provides patients with excellent cosmetic effect and early recovery. Moreover, it does not preclude further open procedures even after treatment failure. But PED is contraindicated in patients presenting with a severe neurologic deficit, segmental instability, acute py-ramidal syndrome, progressive myelopathy, and other pathologic conditions, such as tumor, fracture, infection, and nerve entrapment with scar tissue from previous surgery. This procedure is also contraindicated in patients who have migrated discs, calcified disc protrusion, ossification of the posterior longitudinal ligament, marked spondylosis with disc space narrowing, and neurologic or vascular pathologies mimicking disc herniations.[17]

## Microendoscopic Discectomy

Many studies have described the effectiveness of the anterior approach for the treatment of cervical disc prolapse and spondylotic stenosis. Although the anterior approach is more commonly performed for the treatment of cervical disc disease, the posterior approach has distinct advantage in selected cases of foraminal stenosis and posterior-lateral disc herniation.

Frykholm and Scoville described posterior foraminotomy through partial resection of the medial part of the facet joint to relieve the compression of the cervical nerve root in radiculopathy patients. Conventional posterior approaches have the disadvantage of detaching the extensor cervical muscles from the laminae and the spinous process. This operative trauma to the cervical paraspinal muscles is a major cause of postoperative complications in the form of persistent neck and shoulder pain, and sometimes spinal instability may result.[18]

Roh et al[19] described the use of microendoscopic posterior cervical foraminotomy in a cadaveric study, and Burke and Caputy[20] reported on the use of the same technique. The microendoscopic technique has the advantage of providing a minimally invasive approach through transmuscular dilatation. However, the disadvantage of this procedure is that it only allows two-dimensional visualization, and the view often gets blocked by bleeding or obscured by fragments during removal. The main limitation of this procedure is in the treatment of severe bony stenosis that necessitates laminectomy to decompress the spinal cord.

## CONCLUSIONS

These surgical options for the treatment of cervical spinal degenerative disorders in the aging spine provide good relief of the patient's symptoms, such as radiculopathy. It is evident that PCN, MACF, PED, and MED are varied methods of minimally invasive surgery resulting in short-term recovery and return to full functions.

In addition, in MACF there is the special potential for the problems in the long term. First, the disc resection is limited to its lateral part, and the facet joint is not damaged. As a result, the risk of postoperative instability is very low in MACF. No osteoarthrodesis or arthroplasty by disc prosthesis is necessary. Second, the nerve root decompression is perfectly achieved regardless of whether the pathology is soft disc or canal stenosis, and it can be addressed under direct visual control. As with other anterior techniques, however, this procedure is applicable only if the compressive lesion is located anterior to the spinal cord.

Although these microsurgical procedures are technically demanding in executing adequate decompression of the spinal cord, substantial anatomic knowledge is required, and the technique should be mastered thoroughly with cadaveric dissection. This technique can be a favorable anterior surgical procedure in older people with various degenerative pathologies that cannot be treated with other minimally invasive techniques in the aging spine.

## References

1. M. Szpalski, R. Gunzburg, C.M. Mélot, et al., The aging of the population: a growing concern for spine care in the twenty-first century, Eur. Spine J. 12 (Suppl. 2) (2003) S81–83.
2. M. Benoist, Natural history of the aging spine, Eur. Spine J. 12 (Suppl. 2) (2003) S86–S89.
3. B. Stookey, Compression of the spinal cord due to ventral extradural cervical chondromas, Arch. Neurol. Psychiatry 20 (1928) 275–278.
4. W.J. Mixter, J.S. Barr, Rupture of the intervertebral disc with involvement of the spinal canal, N. Engl. J. Med. 211 (1934) 210–215.
5. R.W. Bailey, C.E. Badgley, Stabilization of the cervical spine by anterior fusion, J. Bone. Joint. Surg. Am. 42-A (1967) 565–594.
6. R.B. Cloward, The anterior approach for removal of ruptured cervical disks, J. Neurosurg. 15 (6) (1958) 602–617.
7. G.W. Smith, R.A. Robinson, The treatment of certain cervical-spine disorders by anterior removal of the intervertebral disc and interbody fusion, J. Bone. Joint. Surg .Am. 40-A (3) (1958) 607–624.
8. C. Hirsch, I. Wickbom, A. Lidstroem, K. Rosengren, Cervical-disc resection: A follow-up of myelographic and surgical procedure, J. Bone. Joint. Surg. Am. 46 (1964) 1811–1821.
9. J.T. Robertson, S.D. Johnson, Anterior cervical discectomy without fusion: Long-term results, Clin. Neurosurg. 27 (1980) 440–449.
10. T. Fukushima, B. Ishijima, K. Hirakawa, N. Nakamura, et al., Ventriculofiberscope: a new technique for endoscopic diagnosis and operation, Technical note, J. Neurogurg. 38 (2) (1973) 251–256.
11. R.G. Spurling, W.B. Scoville, Lateral rupture of the cervical intervertebral discs. A common cause of shoulder and arm pain, Surg. Gynecol. Obstet. 78 (1944) 350–358.
12. R. Frykholm, Deformities of dural pouches and strictures of dural sheaths in the cervical region producing nerve root compression, J. Neurosurg. 4 (1947) 403–413.
13. H.D. Jho, Spinal cord decompression via microsurgical anterior foraminotomy for spondylotic cervical myelotomy, Minim. Invasive Neurosurg. 40 (1997) 124–129.
14. G.M. Onik, P. Kambin, M.K. Chang, Minimally invasive disc surgery. Nucleotomy versus fragmentectomy, Spine 22 (1997) 827–828.
15. Y.C. Chen, S.H. Lee, D. Chen, Intradiscal pressure study of percutaneous disc decompression with nucleoplasty in human cadavers, Spine 28 (7) (2003) 661–665
16. T. Tajima, H. Sakamoto, H. Yamakawa, Discectomy cervicale percutanee, Rev. Med. Orthoped. 17 (1989) 7–10.
17. Y. Ahn, S.H. Lee, S.E. Chung, et al., Percutaneous endoscopic cervical discectomy for discogenic cervical headache due to soft disc herniation, Neuroradiology 47 (12) (2005) 924–930.
18. W. Krupp, R. Muke, Clinical results of the foraminotomy as described by Frykholm for the treatment of lateral cervical disc herniation, Acta Neurochir. (Wien) 107 (1990) 22–29.
19. S.W. Roh, D.H. Kim, A.C. Cardoso, R.G. Fessler, Endoscopic foraminotomy using MED system in cadaveric specimens, Spine 25(2) (2000) 260–264.
20. T.G. Burke, A. Caputy, Microendoscopic posterior cervical foraminotomy: a cadaveric model and clinical application for cervical radiculopathy, J. Neurosurg. 93 (Suppl. 1) (2000) 126–129.

# PART 5

# Osteoporotic Surgical Treatment Modalities: Thoracic Spine

# 34

# Kyphoplasty

*Eeric Truumees*

- Kyphoplasty, like vertebroplasty, is a cement augmentation procedure that is used to restore vertebral body strength and stiffness.

- The procedure involves percutaneous placement of balloon tamps that, when inflated, partly restore lost vertebral height after osteoporotic compression fracture. This percutaneous placement requires high-quality fluoroscopic imaging in at least two planes.

- After inflation, the balloons are removed and the cavities created are backfilled with bone cement, typically polymethylmethacrylate.

- The cavities created by the balloon tamps may also decrease the cement leak risk.

- Kyphoplasty is indicated in patients with intractable pain from a compression fracture. Excellent outcomes and rapid pain relief can be seen in patients with focal pain and tenderness over the involved level.

## INTRODUCTION

Kyphoplasty, along with vertebroplasty and newer, related procedures, are forms of vertebral body augmentation (VBA). The procedures employ percutaneous injection of polymethylmethacrylate (PMMA) acrylic cement into a fractured vertebral body to restore strength and stiffness. Other indications, such as pathologic fractures from metastasis, are becoming more common. High energy, bursting, and extension fracture patterns should be avoided because of the increased PMMA extravasation risk.

In appropriately indicated patients, kyphoplasty yields excellent early pain relief and return to activity. Potential disadvantages of kyphoplasty include procedural risks, such as cement leakage and possible fracture of adjacent segment.

## BRIEF DESCRIPTION

Spinal osteoporosis alone is asymptomatic. If allowed to progress, however, it confers increasing risk of fragility fracture. The principal manifestation of osteoporotic vertebral compression fractures (VCFs) is back pain. Some minimally symptomatic patients do not present for medical evaluation.[1] Others require hospital admission for unrelenting pain. Typically, over 3 months, the fracture heals and the back pain subsides.[2] Although the nonunion rate is low, not all VCFs heal.

Back pain can persist after fracture healing. From 33% to 75% of fractures precipitate chronic back pain.[3] The chronic pain has been attributed to hyperkyphosis, leading to excessive muscular strain. Excessive anterior vertebral body loading engendered by this malalignment may propagate stress fractures in the surrounding endplates.[4] Late kyphosis is occasionally associated with myelopathy.[5]

## INDICATIONS AND CONTRAINDICATIONS

The goal of kyphoplasty is to interrupt the cycle of pain and functional decline associated with VCFs. Given the limited data comparing long-term impacts of kyphoplasty relative to nonoperative management, injecting all fractures cannot be justified. Because many patients improve quickly, most patients should try nonoperative management before considering kyphoplasty.

The duration of this nonoperative trial is inversely related to the patient's pain level and functional limitations. Consider early intervention in patients unable to return to ambulation after a few days. Protracted bed rest may be riskier than procedural risks. At least 150,000 VCFs per year are refractory to nonoperative measures and require hospitalization, with bed rest and IV narcotics. Ambulatory patients should undergo 4 to 8 weeks of nonoperative care. In this group, treatment often includes limited contact thoracolumbar bracing, activity limitations, and sparing use of pain medications. For fractures of L2 and above, a CASH or Jewett brace is recommended. Low lumbar fractures may respond to a chairback brace. Fractures above T6 are more frequently related to metastasis than osteoporosis. Fractures less likely to improve with standard medical management include those with the following:

- Thoracolumbar junction (T11-L2)
- Bursting patterns
- Fractures with >30 degrees of sagittal angulation
- Vacuum shadow in fractured body (ischemic necrosis of bone)
- Progressive collapse in office follow-up[6]

Over time, kyphoplasty indications have gradually been expanded to include conditions such as multiple myeloma and osteolytic metastases. Moreover, kyphoplasty has been added to open decompression and internal fixation procedures. Hybrid procedures may be indicated for more complex fracture patterns, significant compression of the neural elements, and neoplastic lesions with cortical destruction.[7] Another hybrid option combines radiosurgery and kyphoplasty. Conventional radiotherapy remains the index treatment in many patients with vertebral body metastasis.[7] Used alone, radiation is associated with delayed pain relief and further vertebral collapse due to both the previous bone erosion and the radiation itself. Newer radiation therapy techniques allow more focused radiation to be applied via intense treatments over a shorter time course.

Absolute contraindications to kyphoplasty include the following:

- Coexisting infection
- Pregnancy
- Young patients
- Nonpainful fractures
- Uncontrolled coagulopathy
- High-velocity fractures
- Fractures with retropulsed bone
- Medical conditions precluding anesthesia or operative intervention[6,8,9]

In this setting, "young" suggests patients younger than 65 years. The stronger the host bone, the less effectively polymethylmethacrylate restores stiffness. Patients with good bone stock fracture only after high energy loading. In this setting, PMMA leakage is more common. Calcium phosphate kyphoplasty (and other resorbable materials) is under study for this indication. Though isolated reports suggest pain improvement with kyphoplasty for sacral fractures, this indication is not widely accepted.

While less common than VCF, osteoporotic burst fractures (senile burst fractures) are not rare. Any fracture precipitating more than 50% height loss will have associated posterior cortical compromise. In many cases, this compromise takes the form of cortical buckling. When the canal occlusion is less than 33%, kyphoplasty can be considered. On the other hand, in the face of cortical comminution, avoid percutaneous kyphoplasty because of the increased risk of cement extravasation. In patients with neurologic injury, open surgery may be required.

Open surgery is indicated in patients with osteoporotic bones who also have progressive neurologic deficit. Unfortunately, in this frail population, operative intervention confers high risk. Similarly, spinal instrumentation systems often fail in osteoporotic bone. PMMA augmentation increases screw pull-out strength. Combination of kyphoplasty with open decompression restores anterior column load bearing and limits the scope of the reconstruction necessary.

## DESCRIPTION OF THE DEVICE

Kyphoplasty requires one or two high quality fluoroscopes and a kyphoplasty kit. The traditional set begins with a modified Jamshidi needle and a guide wire. Other systems remove the guide wire step ("express" and "one step"). Ultimately, each system is used to safely place two working cannulae through which KyphX balloon tamps can be inserted into the vertebral body. Smaller cannulae are available for upper thoracic vertebrae. The balloon tamps are modified angioplasty balloons. Currently, three sizes are available and are selected based on the size of the fractured vertebral body: 10, 15, and 20 mm. The balloons attach to a syringe with an integral pressure gauge. In the operating room, the balloons are prepped at the back table by instilling 10 ml of radiopaque contrast media. As volume is added to the balloon, the balloon pressure (measured in psi) increases. As the tamp displaces bone, the pressure gradually decays.

Kyphon (Sunnyvale, CA) manufactures several specific balloon products thought to assist in challenging clinical scenarios. For example, a bidirectional balloon (KyphX Elevate) emphasizes craniocaudal expansion and limits mediolateral enlargement. Another single-direction balloon (KyphX Exact) is deployed through a metal housing, which is thought to control balloon direction. These tamps confer additional cost to the procedure. There are no data demonstrating improved outcomes or decreased risk with these devices.

The system also includes bone void fillers, each of which holds 1.5 ml of PMMA. The bone void fillers are cannulae with plungers that allow gradual backfilling of the void created by the tamp. A modified bone void filler, the biopsy device, has sharper tips and can be deployed through the working cannula. PMMA with added barium to enhance fluoroscopic visibility and a mixing system are also available in a separate kit.

## BACKGROUND OF SCIENTIFIC TESTING AND CLINICAL OUTCOMES

The source of pain relief after kyphoplasty remains unclear. Currently, most authors suggest that restoration of strength and stiffness to the fractured vertebral body relieves pain. Both cement volume and percentage of the vertebral body filled can predict postaugmentation bone strength and stiffness. Overall, the more PMMA inserted, the higher the postinsertion vertebral strength and stiffness.

Outcomes data include a number of retrospective studies. Very recently prospective data have been reported from the FREE trial.[10] This trial included 21 sites in 8 countries that enrolled 300 patients with acute VCF and randomized them to either kyphoplasty (149) or nonoperative care (151). As of this writing, the complete paper has not been published, but early pain relief seems to be a clear advantage of kyphoplasty. Whether that advantage persists is more difficult. The primary outcome was the difference in the Short Form (SF-36) physical component summary at 1 month. Quality of life measurements and spine radiographs were assessed through 12 months. Kyphoplasty subjects reported greater improvement than controls in their SF-36 physical component (5.2 point difference; $p < 0001$) at one month). By 12 months, the difference declined to 1.5 points and was no longer significant ($p = .2$). Kyphoplasty improved quality of life by the 1-point EuroQol questionnaire at 1 (0.18 points; 95% CI, 0.08–0.28; $p < .001$) and 12 (0.12; 95% CI, 0.01–0.22; $p = .025$) months. Back function, as measured by the 24-point Roland-Morris scale, was improved by 4.0 points by kyphoplasty at 1 month ($p < .001$) and 2.6 points at 12 months

($p = .001$). Kyphoplasty patients reported fewer days with limited activity, less back pain, and less use of analgesics and walking aids.

Of note, the FREE study was funded by the manufacturer and many of its authors are Kyphon consultants. On the other hand, three other small studies comparing kyphoplasty with conventional medical treatment also found that kyphoplasty consistently improved pain and physical function, with results sustained at 6 months.[11-13]

In 2005, Hadjipavlou et al[14] combined the available vertebroplasty and kyphoplasty outcome reports in an effort to compare the procedures. Using meta-regression techniques, the authors found that individual study design had a considerable impact on subsequent analysis. For prospective studies, the rates of success with vertebroplasty and kyphoplasty were not significantly different at 92% and 93% respectively. However, in retrospective studies, kyphoplasty was more successful (95% vs. 86%; $p = .019$)

Aside from pain relief, a major benefit of VBA lies in the restoration of mobility. In one series of 11 wheelchair-bound cancer patients, 73% were able to walk shortly after vertebroplasty.[15] Other studies reported restoration of mobility after kyphoplasty in 84% to 100%.[8,16] In terms of other types of physical functioning, a number of different outcome measures have been used. In a retrospective analysis of patients with painful osteoporotic VCF, 49 patients who were available for follow-up at a mean 9-month interval had an improvement in visual analogue pain scale score of seven points ($p < .05$), and an improvement in Roland-Morris Disability Survey of 11 points ($p < .05$).[17]

In a retrospective analysis of 52 patients with 82 painful osteoporotic VCFs, kyphoplasty restored 4.6 mm and 3.9 mm to the heights of the anterior and medial columns, respectively.[17] The mean Cobb angle increased by 14%. In a meta-analysis, Hadjipavlou et al concluded that, although postural reduction can improve vertebral height following a compression fracture, better reductions are obtained with kyphoplasty than with vertebroplasty.[14] Better reductions may be achieved with earlier treatment.

## CLINICAL PRESENTATION AND EVALUATION

Successful kyphoplasty hinges on distinction of compression fracture pain from other etiologies. Clinical assessment involves an evaluation of the patient's spinal alignment and gait, followed by palpation of the spine, ilium, sacrum, and paravertebral tissues. The importance of local tenderness over the involved spinous process as a principal sign of a painful VCF has been analyzed in two studies. In the first, which comprised 10 patients, Gaughen et al[18] noted that local tenderness was not present despite imaging findings suggestive of an acute fracture. Recently, Gaitanis and coworkers[16] found that spinous process tenderness corresponded to the level of pathology in 100% of osteolytic tumors and in 96% of VCFs when correlated with magnetic resonance imaging (MRI) findings of an acute fracture.

Several imaging techniques are employed in the evaluation of a painful VCF. Recently, flexion and extension or standing and supine lateral radiographs have been used to assess fracture mobility. A number of studies have examined the presence of intravertebral clefts. Although the exact cause of these intraosseous nitrogen pockets has been debated, the so-called Kummel sign may characterize pseudarthrosis. A cone-down lateral view directly perpendicular to the involved level is required in the assessment, because these clefts can easily be missed with standing lateral radiographs alone.[19]

Magnetic resonance imaging is an important technique for detection of osteoporotic compression fractures (Figure 34-1). It is more sensitive than plain radiography, with a reported accuracy of 96%.[19] Fracture acuity (or failure of healing) is also best observed as intense signal on sagittal MRI with short tau inversion recovery (STIR) sequences (Figures 34-2 and 34-3).[20] For patients unable to undergo MRI, the combination of a technetium bone scan with computed tomography (CT) of the scintigraphically active levels can provide useful information on relatively fresh vertebral fractures (Figure 34-4).[21]

There are patients in whom both MRI and CT imaging is useful. For those with questionable endplate erosion, the greater bone–soft tissue contrast of the CT scan often demonstrates erosions more clearly (Figure 34-5). Similarly, a fine-cut (2 mm) CT scan with sagittal reconstructions may demonstrate small lytic lesions not otherwise seen in the fractured vertebral body on MRI (Figure 34-6). Most commonly, however, the CT is ordered as an adjunct to MRI in patients with canal compromise from their fracture.

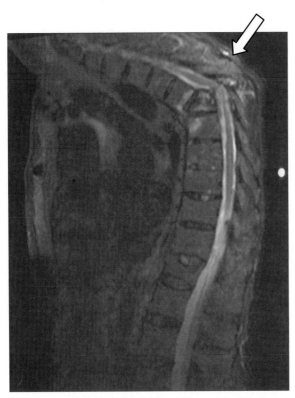

■ **FIGURE 34-1**   In this sagittal MRI, a patient has gradually increased collapse of superior endplate with stress injury to the pars and progressive kyphosis and translation. This patient complained of both a chin on chest deformity and progressive myelopathy. Kyphoplasty is not indicated in this case.

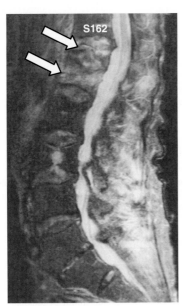

■ **FIGURE 34-2**   Sagittal T2-weighted or STIR MRIs are critical images in the evaluation of a patient with suspected painful osteoporotic vertebral compression fractures. In this STIR image of a patient with a lumbar transitional vertebral, multiple injuries are seen, especially acute L1 and L2 superior endplate injuries. The acute injuries demonstrate marked marrow edema diffusely. In the L1 lesion, a band of edema is seen from anterior to posterior along the fracture line. These bands often reflect "reducible" fractures.

## OPERATIVE TECHNIQUE

Kyphoplasty procedures may be performed in the operating room or in the angiography suite. These procedures can be done under local anesthesia with intravenous sedation or under general anesthesia. There are advantages to both approaches. General anesthesia is associated with more comfortable

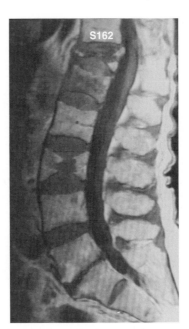

■ **FIGURE 34-3**   The T1-weighted MRI gives better anatomic information than the STIR. Look for evidence of metastatic change such as soft tissue extension or extension of the marrow signal through the pedicle.

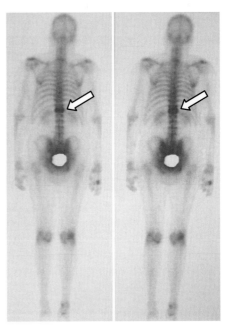

■ **FIGURE 34-4**   For patients unable to have an MRI, a bone scan can be helpful in identifying acute or subacute fractures. In this case, note the marked uptake at the T12 level.

prone positioning and less involuntary motion. On the other hand, rib fractures during positioning can occur.

Kyphoplasty patients are positioned prone on a radiolucent operating table or surgical frame. Lordotic positioning is maintained with bolsters. Lordosis allows a positional reduction. Later, when the balloons are removed, the lordotically positioned patient will be less likely to lose the reduction achieved. With this in mind, the radiolucent Wilson frame often makes lordosis difficult to achieve. A Jackson frame may allow better lordotic placement, but may be less comfortable for awake patients.

Kyphoplasty begins with true anteroposterior (AP) and lateral fluoroscopic images (Figures 34-7 and 34-8). Ensure a true AP with the spinous process in the midline between the pedicles. On the lateral view, the pedicles should line up and yield a clear view of the foramen and the posterior

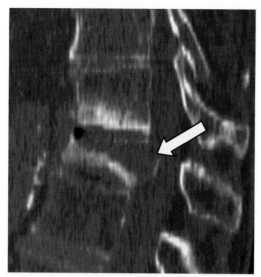

■ **FIGURE 34-5** CT scans are useful for anatomic detail in patients unable to have an MRI. In patients with unusual fracture patterns or in those in whom cortical compromise or metastasis is suspected, order a CT scan for its excellent bone–soft tissue contrast. In this case of a prostate cancer metastasis, note the lytic lesion in the posterior aspect of the vertebral body with the destruction of the posterior cortex. This patient would not be a good candidate for percutaneous kyphoplasty, but mini-open or hybrid procedures could be considered if needed.

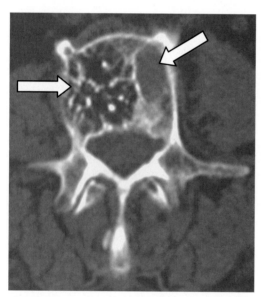

■ **FIGURE 34-6** This axial CT image obtained in a patient noted to have a compression fracture without trauma was found to have both a hemangioma (on the right) and a lytic metastasis (on the left).

vertebral cortex. Both images should show the endplates of the level selected as a single line, not an oval.

When possible, biplanar fluoroscopy should be employed. This saves considerable time when switching from AP to lateral. If only one machine is available, mark the fluoroscope positions achieved, so they are easily reachieved. Most typically, a transpedicular route to the vertebra is selected. In some thoracic cases, the narrow and straight pedicle precludes appropriate medialization and an extrapedicular approach is required. Most authors recommend a bilateral approach.

Beginning with AP fluoroscopy, an 11-gauge Jamshidi needle is placed at the 10 o'clock or 2 o'clock position on the pedicular ring. Unlike pedicle screws, the goal is not to proceed "straight down the barrel," but rather to medialize through the cylinder of the pedicle. Therefore start at the lateral

border and aim medially. Once in bone, verify your trajectory on the lateral image. If the AP and lateral images do not demonstrate a clearly intrapedicular position, an en face or oblique view is useful.

Under lateral fluoroscopic view, advance the Jamshidi to the midway point of the pedicle. Return to the AP view and verify tip position. Until the Jamshidi has passed through the posterior cortical margin of the vertebral body, it must be lateral to the medial pedicle wall on the AP image. If the needle has been medialized appropriately, return to lateral, and advance to 1 to 2 mm past the posterior vertebral body margin. Now the needle should be just barely across the medial pedicle border on the AP. Remove the Jamshidi stylet and place a guide pin.

The osteointroducer instruments are passed over the guide pin. The blunt dissector of the osteointroducer and guide pin are removed, leaving the working cannula in place just anterior to the posterior cortical margin of the vertebral body. Better medialization allows for more aggressive anterior placement. For harder bone, use the provided drill to prepare the path for the bone void filler. Live or pulsed fluoroscopy is recommended when approaching the anterior cortex.

Insert IBT to within 4 mm of the anterior cortex. Inflate the balloon to 50 psi (pounds per square inch) pressure to maintain its position and tamponade the bone. Place instruments through the opposite pedicle in similar fashion. Once the contralateral balloon has been placed, inflate both IBTs in 0.5-ml increments. Once inserted into the vertebral body, the balloons are gradually inflated using visual (radiographic), and volume and pressure controls (via a digital manometer), to reduce the fracture deformity.

Monitor AP, lateral, and oblique images for IBT position in relation to cortices. Sequentially inflate until the following inflation endpoint is reached:

- Realignment of vertebral endplates
- Maximum balloon pressure (>220 psi) without decay
- Maximum balloon volume: 4 ml for the size 15 balloon and 6 ml for the size 20 balloon
- Cortical wall contact

A number of acrylic cements are available. Though the PMMA kits used with total joint arthroplasty can be employed, cement formulations specifically designed for vertebral augmentation may have better handling and setting characteristics. VBA cements also have extra sterile barium added to the polymer powder to increase its radiopacity.

With the balloons removed, bone filler devices are advanced into the distal portion of the cavity. Retrograde fill with PMMA is then undertaken using fluoroscopic monitoring. For kyphoplasty, the PMMA is placed into bone filler devices (BFDs). Then it is left in the device until it reaches a toothpaste consistency. Early implantation with runny PMMA increases leak risk. Operating room temperatures may affect PMMA polymerization times. Occasionally, warm saline solution is useful to accelerate setting of the PMMA.

Using the plunger, apply the PMMA under continuous fluoroscopy. Inject slightly more PMMA than final IBT inflation volume to allow intercalation of the material into surrounding trabeculae. The wound may be closed with a suture or Steri-Strip.

## POSTOPERATIVE CARE

No braces or particular postoperative precautions are needed after kyphoplasty. That said, osteoporotic patients should be restricted in terms of heavy lifting and the carrying of heavy weight away from the body or above shoulder level. Osteoporotic patients should avoid concurrent bending and lifting. Ensure that the patient has been evaluated for and treated for their underlying osteoporosis.

Other postoperative care is fairly straightforward. Many patients will have remaining axial weakness. Consider physical therapy for patients who are weak or have ongoing muscular pain. Wound issues are typically minimal except for those patients taking blood thinners. Address nutritional issues when needed.

## COMPLICATIONS AND AVOIDANCE

Kyphoplasty complications can be categorized: medical, anesthesia related, instrument placement, and PMMA problems. In most cases, failure to improve is due to inappropriate patient selection. The more diffuse the

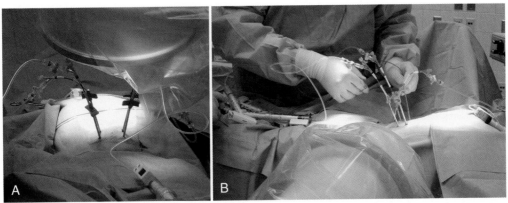

■ **FIGURE 34-7**  These images exhibit craniocaudal and lateral intraoperative views in the operating room during a two-level kyphoplasty. In this case, a single fluoroscopy unit was used and positioning assessed in the AP (**A**) and lateral (**B**) planes. Four working cannulae have been placed. Through the cannulae are seen the inflatable balloon tamps attached to pressure syringes containing contrast medium. Serial inflation is undertaken gradually to effect reduction.

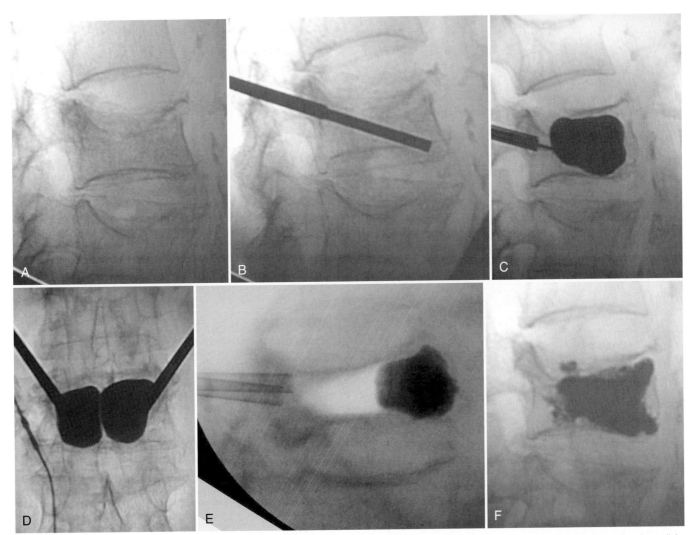

■ **FIGURE 34-8**  This series of fluoroscopic images demonstrates the kyphoplasty procedure beginning with a lateral scout image (**A**). Note that the pedicles line up so that the foramen can be seen clearly. In this case, a biopsy was obtained through the cannula (**B**). The bone void filler or the special biopsy needle can be used for this purpose. A syringe is attached to the needle and mild suction applied. An 8-gauge core is obtained. These cores may obviate open biopsy in cases in which Tru-Cut and Jamshidi biopsies were not diagnostic. In **C** and **D**, balloons have been deployed and an excellent reduction of the superior endplate is noted. On the AP view (**D**), note the medialization of the balloons and the alignment of the spinous process equidistant between the pedicles. In **E**, from another patient, the "air vertebrogram" left when the balloons have been removed is noted. Note the backfilling of the void with PMMA. In the final lateral view (**F**), excellent fill of the void is noted. Additional PMMA has been injected to fill the interstices around the void. Some of the reduction achieved with the balloons was lost, however.

patient's pain, the less likely they are to benefit from VBA. Placement of PMMA into the spine *may* increase the risk of adjacent segment fracture.

Kyphoplasty patients are, by definition, frail. Medical and anesthesia issues are not unusual in this elderly patient population. On the other hand, VBA procedures are not significantly physiologically taxing. When medical problems occur, they can be ascribed to the procedure itself or to preexisting cardiac and pulmonary problems. In markedly functionally limited patients, the risks of activity restriction in terms of deep vein thrombosis, pulmonary embolus (PE), and opiate-related complications are likely underreported and could be riskier than operative treatment.

Many patients in this age group take anticoagulant medications. When possible, reverse these agents before kyphoplasty. In particular, patients with multiple fractures, concomitant rib fractures, and osteoporotic bursting patterns are at higher risk for procedural and medical complications. Biopsies should be performed with kyphoplasty in patients with a history of cancer or an absence of concomitant trauma.

The most devastating technical complication of kyphoplasty arises from PMMA extravasation. Leakage is clinically silent in the vast majority of cases, with symptomatic leaks representing only a small portion of the total.[22] PMMA may extravasate into the vascular tree, disc space, anterior and lateral soft tissues, and spinal canal. Extravasation is most common in metastatic osteolytic tumors or myeloma.[15]

Interestingly, leakage into the central canal is better tolerated in most cases than intraforaminal leak; however, when symptomatic, central canal extravasation leads to more devastating neurological symptoms, such as paraplegia. In most cases, symptoms are transient and respond well to nerve root blocks or oral medication; rarely do they require surgical decompression.[23]

Along with the more viscous cement applied, void creation and bone compacting effects may decrease extravasation rates compared with vertebroplasty. A cadaveric study by Belkoff et al[24] reported reduced rates of PMMA extravasation after kyphoplasty compared with vertebroplasty. In a series of patients with metastatic disease, Fourney et al[25] reported a 9% extravasation rate after vertebroplasty, but no cases of extravasation following kyphoplasty.

Another serious complication of VBA procedures is postoperative infection. Simple wound infections can be identified and treated easily, but deep space infections including those of the cement mantle are serious and difficult to fully eradicate without removal of the cement bolus. Concurrent infection, even in distant organ systems, is a contraindication to kyphoplasty

Improper instrumentation placement most frequently stems from difficulty delineating the bony anatomy in patients in whom poor bone quality coexists with spinal deformity, such as degenerative scoliosis or marked spondylosis. Once the instruments are in place, care must be taken not to apply too much force, because leverage may lead to fractures. Pedicle and transverse process fractures may lead to postoperative pain, irritate local nerve roots, or destabilize the spine. Finally, these breaches create a path for inadvertent leakage of cement into the spinal canal. In one multicenter study, instrument placement problems led to postoperative hematoma in two patients, and a direct injury to the spinal cord when an extrapedicular approach was used on a vertebra with a fractured pedicle.[26]

Methacrylate monomer is toxic. Some recommend that more than 30 ml PMMA be injected per session.[27] The more viscous the cement, the less likely it is that untoward blood pressure or blood gas effects will occur.[14]

Several VBA reports suggest an increased risk of secondary fractures adjacent to the augmented vertebra.[28,29] Two small studies suggest that kyphoplasty decreases adjacent fracture risk. Kasperk and colleagues[11,30] found that at 6-month follow-up, 30% (6 of 20) nonoperatively treated patients developed secondary fractures, whereas only 12.5% of 40 kyphoplasty patients had secondary fractures. Similarly, Komp et al[12] reported that 65% of 17 nonoperatively treated patients had new fractures, whereas only 37% of 19 kyphoplasty patients had additional fractures. In the FREE study, on the other hand, at 12 months, new vertebral fractures were slightly higher but not statistically significantly different between the kyphoplasty (41.8%) and nonsurgical (37.8%) groups ($p = .5$).[10] The exact effects of VBA on adjacent levels probably vary with steroid exposure, spinal level, local spondylosis, and muscular factors; these require further study.

## ADVANTAGES AND DISADVANTAGES

**Advantages**
- Rapid pain relief
- Percutaneous
- Minimal medical impact
- Ability to achieve partial reduction

**Disadvantages**
- Achieving full reduction difficult
- PMMA leakage is possible
- Adjacent segment fractures possible
- Extra cost and time of kyphoplasty has not yet proved advantageous over the simpler, cheaper vertebroplasty

## CONCLUSIONS AND DISCUSSION

Kyphoplasty has been widely available for roughly 10 years. During that time, its popularity as a percutaneous means of stabilizing osteoporotic compression fractures has skyrocketed. Vertebroplasty remains widely popular and highly successful as well. Use of balloon tamps appears to improve fracture reduction and decreases cement leakage rates. But leakage remains problematic in higher energy fractures and those associated with retropulsion. A number of newer procedures are evolving to compete with vertebroplasty and kyphoplasty.

Kyphoplasty should be considered in patients with persistent pain and functional limitation after fracture despite a trial of nonoperative management. Markedly limited and bedridden patients should be offered earlier treatment. In all cases, maximal management of the underlying osteoporosis should be pursued.

A number of controversies remain. Reports conflict as to the degree of reduction achieved and its impact on clinical outcomes. Kyphoplasty adds significant cost, radiation exposure, and operative time over vertebroplasty. So far, clear benefit has not been confirmed.

Though current data suggest that kyphoplasty patients experience marked early pain reduction and return to activity, its impact on long-term outcomes is unclear. As we study these fractures more closely, our ability to predict which fractures are likely to collapse and which may heal uneventfully with observation should improve.

## References

1. A. Guermazi, A. Mohr, M. Grigorian, et al., Identification of vertebral fractures in osteoporosis, Semin. Musculoskelet. Radiol. 6 (2002) 241–252.
2. G.P. Lyritis, B. Mayasis, N. Tsakalakos, et al., The natural history of osteoporotic vertebral fracture, Clin. Rheumatol. 8 (1989) 66–69.
3. S.M. Pluijm, A.M. Tromp, J.H. Smit, et al., C Consequences of vertebral deformities in older men and women, J. Bone Miner. Res. 15 (2000) 1564–1572.
4. M.M. Kayanja, L.A. Ferrara, I.H. Lieberman, Distribution of anterior cortical shear strain after a thoracic wedge compression fracture, Spine J. 4 (2004) 76–87.
5. A.G. Hadjipavlou, P.G. Katonis, M.N. Tzermiadianos, et al., Principles of management of osteometabolic disorders affecting the aging spine, Eur. Spine J. 12 (2003) S113–S131.
6. E. Truumees, A. Hilibrand, A.R. Vaccaro, Percutaneous vertebral augmentation, Spine J. 4 (2004) 218–229.
7. R. Lowe, F. Phillips, Percutaneous vertebral augmentation for malignant disease of the spine, Curr. Opin. Orthop. 16 (2005) 489–493.
8. J.T. Ledlie, M.B. Renfro, Kyphoplasty treatment of vertebral fractures: 2-year outcomes show sustained benefits, Spine 31 (2006) 57–64.
9. I. Lieberman, M.K. Reinhardt, Vertebroplasty and kyphoplasty for osteolytic vertebral collapse, Clin. Orthop. Relat. Res. (Suppl. 415) (2003) S176–S186.
10. C. Muller, D. Wardlaw, L. Bastien, et al., A randomized trial of balloon kyphoplasty and nonsurgical care for patients with acute vertebral compression fractures: one year results, The Internet Journal of Minimally Invasive Spinal Technology, 2008. Supplement I - to IJMIST Vol. 1 No 2. Available at http://www.ispub.com/journal/the_internet_journal_of_minimally_invasive_spinal_technology/volume_2_number_3_1/article/a_randomized_trial_of_balloon_kyphoplasty_and_nonsurgical_care_for_patients_with_acute_vertebral_compression_fractures_one_year_results.html.
11. C. Kasperk, J. Hillmeier, G. Noldge, et al., Treatment of painful vertebral fractures by kyphoplasty in patients with primary osteoporosis: a prospective nonrandomized controlled study, J. Bone Miner. Res. 20 (2005) 604–612.
12. M. Komp, S. Ruetten, G. Godolias, Minimally invasive therapy for functionally unstable osteoporotic vertebral fracture by means of kyphoplasty: a prospective comparative study of 19 surgically and 17 conservatively treated patients, J. Miner. Stoffwechs. 1 (2004) 13–15.

13. M. Weisskopf, S. Herlein, K. Birnbaum, et al., Kyphoplasty—a new minimally invasive treatment for repositioning and stabilizing vertebral bodies, Z. Orthop. Ihre. Grenzgeb. 141 (2003) 406–411.

14. A.G. Hadjipavlou, M.N. Tzermiadianos, P.G. Katonis, et al., Percutaneous vertebroplasty and balloon kyphoplasty for the treatment of osteoporotic vertebral compression fractures and osteolytic tumours, J. Bone Joint Surg. Br. 87 (2005) 1595–1604.

15. L. Alvarez, A. Perez-Higueras, D. Quinones, et al., Vertebroplasty in the treatment of vertebral tumors: postprocedural outcome and quality of life, Eur. Spine J. 12 (2003) 356–360.

16. I.N. Gaitanis, A.G. Hadjipavlou, P.G. Katonis, et al., Balloon kyphoplasty for the treatment of pathological vertebral compressive fractures, Eur. Spine J. 14 (2005) 250–260.

17. A. Rhyne 3rd, D. Banit, E. Laxer, et al., Kyphoplasty: report of eighty-two thoracolumbar osteoporotic vertebral fractures, J. Orthop. Trauma 18 (2004) 294–299.

18. J.R. Gaughen Jr., M.E. Jensen, P.A. Schweickert, et al., Lack of preoperative spinous process tenderness does not affect clinical success of percutaneous vertebroplasty, J. Vasc. Interv. Radiol. 13 (2002) 1135–1138.

19. F. McKiernan, T. Faciszewski, Intravertebral clefts in osteoporotic vertebral compression fractures, Arthritis Rheum. 48 (2003) 1414–1419.

20. M. Qaiyum, P.N. Tyrrell, I.W. McCall, et al., MRI detection of unsuspected vertebral injury in acute spinal trauma: incidence and significance, Skeletal Radiol. 30 (2001) 299–304.

21. A.S. Maynard, M.E. Jensen, P.A. Schweickert, et al., Value of bone scan imaging in predicting pain relief from percutaneous vertebroplasty in osteoporotic vertebral fractures, AJNR Am. J. Neuroradiol. 21 (2000) 1807–1812.

22. J.M. Mathis, A.O. Ortiz, G.H. Zoarski, Vertebroplasty versus kyphoplasty: a comparison and contrast, AJNR Am. J. Neuroradiol. 25 (2004) 840–845.

23. A. Weill, J. Chiras, J.M. Simon, et al., Spinal metastases: indications for and results of percutaneous injection of acrylic surgical cement, Radiology 199 (1996) 241–247.

24. S.M. Belkoff, L.E. Jasper, S.S. Stevens, An ex vivo evaluation of an inflatable bone tamp used to reduce fractures within vertebral bodies under load, Spine 27 (2002) 1640–1643.

25. D.R. Fourney, D.F. Schomer, R. Nader, et al., Percutaneous vertebroplasty and kyphoplasty for painful vertebral body fractures in cancer patients, J. Neurosurg. 98 (2003) 21–30.

26. S.R. Garfin, H.A. Yuan, M.A. Reiley, New technologies in spine: kyphoplasty and vertebroplasty for the treatment of painful osteoporotic compression fractures, Spine 26 (2001) 1511–1515.

27. J.V. Coumans, M.K. Reinhardt, I.H. Lieberman, Kyphoplasty for vertebral compression fractures: 1-year clinical outcomes from a prospective study, J. Neurosurg. 99 (2003) 44–50.

28. I. Legroux-Gerot, C. Lormeau, N. Boutry, et al., Long-term follow-up of vertebral osteoporotic fractures treated by percutaneous vertebroplasty, Clin. Rheumatol. 23 (2004) 310–317.

29. F. Grados, C. Depriester, G. Cayrolle, et al., Long-term observations of vertebral osteoporotic fractures treated by percutaneous vertebroplasty, Rheumatology (Oxford) 39 (2000) 1410–1414.

30. C. Kasperk, J. Hillmeier, G. Noldge, et al., Prospective controlled study of the treatment of painful osteoporotic vertebral fractures by kyphoplasty, Osteoporos. Int. 15 (2004) S108.

# 35

# Vertebroplasty

*Elizabeth Gardner*

**K E Y   P O I N T S**

- Worldwide there are 1.4 million vertebral compression fractures (VCFs) annually. The lifetime incidence in White women is 16%.
- Vertebroplasty is indicated for the treatment of painful acute or subacute vertebral compression fractures due to osteoporosis or neoplasm.
- An acute or subacute osteoporotic VCF typically appears hypointense on T1-weighted and hyperintense on T2-weighted and STIR MRI sequences.
- Complications specifically associated with vertebroplasty include pain localized to the injection site, cement extravasation, paralysis, pulmonary cement/fat embolism, pneumothorax, and even death.
- While a large number of studies have provided anecdotal evidence to support use of vertebroplasty in the treatment of acute/subacute VCFs, Kallmes and Buchbinder published two randomized controlled trials in 2009 doubting the efficacy of the procedure. Though interesting, these studies are plagued with numerous Shortcomings that leave their conclusions in doubt.

## INTRODUCTION

It is estimated that 1.4 million vertebral compression fractures (VCFs) occur annually, causing pain and disability in patients worldwide.[1] The lifetime risk of a vertebral compression fracture in White women is 16%; in men, it is 5%. Historically, treatment of these fractures has been limited to analgesics, bed rest, and bracing. However, recently the development of vertebroplasty and kyphoplasty has provided physicians with additional treatment options for select vertebral compression fractures.

## HISTORY OF VERTEBROPLASTY

Vertebroplasty was initially developed as an open procedure designed to augment the purchase of pedicle screws and to fill large voids from tumor resection. In 1984, however, at the University Hospital of Amiens, France, Galibert and Deramond performed the first documented percutaneous vertebroplasty.[2] The patient presented with severe cervical pain, and imaging demonstrated a large vertebral hemangioma encompassing the entire vertebral body of C2 with extension into the epidural space. After performing a C2 laminectomy to excise the epidural component of the lesion, a 15-gauge needle was inserted into the C2 vertebral body via an anterolateral approach, allowing injection of cement for structural reinforcement. The document of this case, as published in 1987, reports complete pain relief in this patient. Physicians at University Hospital Lyon continued to refine the percutaneous vertebroplasty technique as well as to expand its indications, using 18-gauge needles to inject polymethylmethacrylate(PMMA) into four patients with compression fractures. Since then, its popularity has spread dramatically.

## PATIENT SELECTION/INDICATIONS

As with any procedure, the success of vertebroplasty relies heavily on the selection of appropriate patients and the skill of the operating physician. It is essential to identify patients with pain related to VCF, and exclude the other common sources of back pain in this population, including degenerative disk disease, spinal stenosis, facet arthropathy, or SI joint dysfunction. This process begins, of course, by taking a thorough history of the patient. It is particularly important to ascertain details regarding the timing of the onset of back pain, any known precipitating events, and those activities that worsen and alleviate the pain. Additionally, patients should be questioned regarding previous episodes of similar back pain, and the time until resolution of those symptoms. It is vital to understand the premorbid condition of the patient, as well as the impact of the back pain on activities of daily living. Finally, an assessment for allergies, anticoagulants, and medical problems, especially respiratory compromise, is essential to anticipate potential complications during the procedure. A thorough physical examination seeks to identify pain and tenderness to palpation at the level of radiographic abnormality. During the examination, the operator must pay attention to symptoms that may suggest pain from alternative sources.

Radiographic imaging plays an important role in the screening of patients for vertebroplasty. X-rays are often the first mode of imaging employed, due to their cost-effectiveness and ease of availability. In patients with a VCF, diffuse osteopenia and evidence of one or more compression fractures may be present. With neoplastic compression fractures, it may be possible to see focal lytic lesions or destruction of the bony trabeculae. A CT scan may be obtained for improved visualization of bony details. Used most often with pathologic fractures, CT may demonstrate expansion of the bony contours of the vertebrae and multilevel disease, both of which suggest an underlying malignancy. Preprocedure CT scanning also allows the operator to assess the integrity of the posterior wall of the vertebral body and pedicles, which if destroyed may be a source for significant complication.

MRI is particularly useful in the screening of patients with osteoporotic VCF due to its reported ability to discern the relative age of the fracture. Acute or subacute osteoporotic fractures up to 30 days old typically show evidence of bone marrow edema, with hypointense signal on T1-weighted and hyperintensity on T2-weighted and STIR sequences. At approximately 1 month after fracture, VCFs variably become isointense to normal bone marrow on T1- and T2-weighted sequences. Fully healed fractures are isointense to normal bone elements, or hypointense on T1 and T2 due to significant sclerosis. Recent studies have found a positive correlation between the MRI findings suggestive of a fracture less than 30 days old and clinical pain relief after vertebroplasty.

Interpretation of MRI findings in a patient with a malignant VCF is more challenging. While STIR sequences with fat suppression may be helpful to show edema, there may be heterogeneous or diffuse areas of hyperintensity on STIR or T2-weighted imaging. Some authors have suggested a pattern of hypointensity or isointensity on diffusion-weighted sequences. In any case, evidence of abnormal signal in the posterior elements, an expansion of the contour of the vertebral body or posterior elements, or any associated epidural/extravertebral soft tissue mass suggests an underlying malignancy.

Bone scintigraphy may be employed to detect a relatively recent fracture in patients who cannot tolerate an MRI. Increased radiotracer uptake has been correlated with positive clinical response to vertebroplasty. However, this technique is limited by the fact that the bone scan may show increased tracer uptake for up to 12 months after fracture. Thus this method must be correlated with corresponding anatomic imaging.

After a careful history, physical examination, and assessment of radiographic imaging, the physician must then determine not only that the source of the patient's pain is indeed a VCF, but also that this fracture is amenable to vertebroplasty. The primary indication for vertebroplasty is the alleviation of pain associated with a VCF due to osteoporosis or tumor. Repeated studies have demonstrated superior pain relief with treatment of acute or subacute fractures. Perhaps most notable is the non–industry-sponsored, double-cohort by Alvarez et al[3], which compared vertebroplasty to nonoperative treatment for VCFs. He found statistically significant differences at 3 months follow-up. Wardlaw et al[4] published a randomized controlled trial comparing balloon kyphoplasty with nonsurgical care for VCFs. He too demonstrated a significant improvement in the intervention group at 1 month. Some now advocate the treatment of VCF within days of injury if the pain is so severe as to require parenteral narcotics and hospitalization. Late treatment, 6 months to years after the initial injury, is less likely to completely relieve pain, but symptomatic improvement has been noted in some studies.

## Absolute Contraindications

As the primary indication for vertebroplasty is pain, it follows that an asymptomatic stable vertebral compression fracture is a contraindication for the procedure. Similarly, a painful osteoporotic fracture that is steadily improving with conservative medical treatment should not be treated with vertebroplasty. At this point, as there are no data to suggest that there is a benefit to the stabilization of vertebrae "at high risk of impending fracture" in the osteoporotic patient, a vertebroplasty should not be performed in the absence of radiographic evidence of a VCF. Because a VCF in a young patient with normal bone density should heal without complication, acute traumatic fractures in this population should be treated conservatively. There is evidence to suggest that PMMA may interfere with bone healing in normal bone. Osteomyelitis of the target vertebra, uncorrectable coagulopathy or hemorrhagic diasthesis, and an allergy to any component required for the procedure all also are considered contraindications to vertebroplasty.

## Relative Contraindications

While not an absolute contraindication, patients with radiculopathy localized to the level of the VCF should be warned that vertebroplasty may not improve all their symptoms, and may even worsen the pain. Also, fractures with either significant retropulsion or tumor extension into the epidural space are cases that necessitate significant preoperative planning. A pre-procedure CT scan is indicated to visualize the fracture morphology and potential cord compression. Even a small amount of cement extravasation or displacement of tumor into the spinal canal could worsen symptoms and make decompressive surgery more technically challenging. In these cases, there should at least be consideration for decompression prior to vertebroplasty. VCFs with greater than 70% loss of vertebral body height are technically challenging, and true vertebra plana may be technically impossible. A preoperative CT scan with coronal and sagittal reconstructions may help to identify areas of the vertebra with adequate residual height. Typically height is better preserved along the lateral aspect of the vertebral body; this may be a target for vertebroplasty. Due to the risk of toxicity from PMMA monomers or fat emboli, treatment of more than three levels at a single setting is not suggested. Finally, as evidence suggests poorer outcomes with chronic fractures, a stable, chronic asymptomatic fracture is also a relative contraindication.

## TECHNIQUE

As with any procedure, the process begins with proper patient selection (as discussed earlier) and the procurement of informed consent. A thorough discussion of the risks and benefits of the procedure is not only an ethical necessity, but it also helps to assess and modulate the patient's expectations of clinical results.

Prior to the procedure, a thorough review of the patient's medical history (to allow the identification of potentially complicating disease processes), medications (to assess for anticoagulants), and physical examination allows for necessary procedural modifications to ensure the safety of the patient.

Once optimized, the patient may be brought to the procedure suite. Preoperative antibiotics, typically one gram of cefazolin, should be given 30 minutes prior to the commencement of the procedure.

Anesthesia for vertebroplasty is commonly a combination of conscious sedation and a local anesthetic. It is often advantageous to administer partial doses of sedation prior to positioning to decrease patient discomfort and anxiety. General anesthesia may be used if the patient is unable to tolerate prone positioning with only sedation due to pain or psychological disability; however, this adds risk and substantial cost to the procedure. Once secured in the prone position, radiographic imaging must be properly aligned. Fluoroscopy is the most commonly used modality. While biplanar fluoroscopy machines are now available, allowing fast real-time visualization of the procedure, these are expensive and are not readily available to many physicians. If single-plane imaging is used, it is imperative to obtain orthogonal projections to allow reliable assessment of needle positioning. CT scanning may be used as an adjunct to fluoroscopy: however, alone it does not allow for real-time monitoring of needle placement or cement injection. Also, it may require general anesthesia to limit patient movement. Indications for CT scan use include cervical or high-thoracic fractures necessitating the visualization of the carotid/jugular complex and vertebral vessels, sacral insufficiency fractures, and pathological fractures with risk of tumor displacement. In these cases, if fluoroscopy is not used, then cement must be injected in very small aliquots and scans should be performed frequently to assess for leakage.

The approach should be determined preoperatively based on the location of the lesion and its etiology. Preoperative CT scanning may be employed to help make this assessment.

## Transpedicular Approach

This is the classic approach employed by most physicians for standard thoracic and lumbar fractures, as it provides a discrete anatomic target for needle placement. Also, it has a safe entry point that permits easy compression of overlying soft tissues postoperatively to lessen the chance of hematoma formation. This approach is also effective for biopsy of the lesion, should this be needed as part of a diagnostic workup.

## Parapedicular (Transcostovertebral) Approach

The needle is inserted lateral to the pedicle, and approaches the vertebra from above the transverse process. This approach is useful when the pedicle is deformed, absent, or too small to accept the appropriate needle. Risks associated with this approach include a low incidence of pneumothorax and paraspinal hematoma.

## Posterolateral Approach

This approach is primarily of historical importance. It was used most in patients with small pedicles, in whom a transpedicular approach would be dangerous. Utilizing a more lateral starting point, a small needle traverses the lateral process and thus reaches the vertebral body at a more anterior position than with other approaches. However, as the needle passes below the pedicle, the nerve is placed at risk. In the thoracic region, there is a high potential for pneumothorax if the operator lacerates the pleura.

## Anterolateral Approach

This approach is used for cervical or high-thoracic fractures where small pedicles and the orientation of the pedicles make a transpedicular approach difficult. It is imperative to avoid the carotid/jugular complex, the vertebral arteries, and the esophagus. A right-sided approach, opposite the esophagus, allows the operator to manually push the carotid out of the way. A CT scan may be used to better visualize these structures.

## Procedure

Once the approach has been chosen, local anesthesia should be injected into the skin and subcutaneous tissue along the expected needle tract; The periosteum of the bone at its entry site should also be injected. Next, a small skin incision is made. The trocar and cannula are then introduced through the skin incision and worked through the subcutaneous tissues down to the level of the periosteum. The cannula and trocar should then be passed into the bone. In osteoporotic bone, this can usually be done manually. In neoplastic disease, the normal bone may be dense, necessitating the use of a mallet for appropriate placement. Ultimately the tip of the needle should be positioned beyond the midpoint of the vertebral body as viewed on the lateral projection.

Some operators advocate for the placement of two transpedicular needles in the routine case. This allows for a larger margin of safety, increases the chance of completing filling in a single batch of cement, and minimizes leaks. A single needle may be used, and is successful in most cases. Historically, some operators have utilized venography to identify potential leak sites. However, it was shown to have a low predictive value and has been abandoned.

Once all needles have been properly placed as confirmed by imaging, the cement may be prepared in a sterile vacuum device as recommended by the manufacturer. The cement is then injected through the cannula using small syringes for easy control. Cementing should be conducted either in real time or after injection of small amounts (0.1-0.2 ml aliquots). Any evidence of cement leakage outside of the vertebral body should prompt a pause. After waiting several minutes, reinjection of cement through the same needle may be attempted. If no additional leaks are visualized, continued injection may continue. However, if there is evidence of persistent leakage, a second, contralateral needle should be used for further injection. The amount of cement necessary for optimal results varies in each case. Generally, 50% to 70% of the visualized volume of the compressed vertebra should be filled. A twist of the cannula can help to break the cement at the tip and the cannula may be removed.

To decrease the risk of hematoma formation, local pressure should be applied for 3 to 5 minutes after withdrawing the cannula. The entry site should then be dressed in sterile fashion. Once moved from the procedure table, the patient should remain recumbent for 1 to 2 hours, while being monitored for any neurological changes or other adverse events. If there is no evidence of complication, the patient may be discharged home, but should remain on bed rest, or at least with minimal activity, for 24 hours.

## INJECTION MATERIALS

The ideal filler material for use in vertebroplasty and kyphoplasty must demonstrate good biocompatibility, adequate biomechanical strength and stiffness, and radiopacity for use in fluoroscopically guided procedures. Additionally, the material must be amenable to easy preparation, and possess appropriate flow and polymerization or crystallization characteristics.

In the first vertebroplasty procedures, PMMA bone cement mixed with a contrast agent, typically barium sulfate, was injected into vertebral bodies under image guidance.[5] Since Charnley first reported its use in 1960, PMMA bone cements have been used by orthopedic surgeons for the fixation of both plastic and metal components in joint replacement and, less often, in the stabilization of pathological fracture. Early studies showed maintenance of the bond between the prosthesis and the PMMA with no evidence of harmful systemic effects. Thus, PMMA is now widely used throughout orthopedics.

Advantages to PMMA include its familiarity for operating physicians, its ease of handling, and its cost-effectiveness. Also, PMMA shows good biomechanical strength and stiffness and evidence that it is relatively bioinert. For this reason, as of April 2004, the FDA has approved the labeling of certain brands of PMMA for the treatment of pathological fractures of the vertebral body resulting to osteoporosis and tumor. However, several disadvantages to PMMA have become apparent. Perhaps most notable is PMMA's lack of osteoconductivity. As such, there is no potential for remodeling or integration into the surrounding bone. Histologic studies have reported a thin fibrous membrane surrounding the PMMA injected into vertebral bodies, providing further evidence of the lack of osseous integration. Therefore, PMMA relies solely on the bulk effect of injected cement for strength and stability. Additionally, there have been theoretical concerns regarding the high polymerization temperature of PMMA, though to date there has been no clear evidence to support this. Finally, as is well documented in the arthroplasty literature, PMMA is associated with potential

monomer toxicity. The molecule is known to be arrhythmogenic and cardiotoxic at the volumes used in knee and hip replacement. For this reason, many authors recommend limiting vertebroplasty or kyphoplasty to two or three levels at any surgical setting.

The limitations of PMMA cement have led researchers to seek alternative filler materials. The primary characteristic of these novel products is their osteoconductivity. The best studied of these synthetic bone substitutes is the class of calcium phosphate cements. As osteoconductive agents, these possess the potential for resorption of cement and replacement with new bone, effectively restoring vertebral body bone mass. Studies have shown evidence of osteoclastic resorption of the cement and fragmentation with vascular invasions and bony ingrowth.[6] Histologic results show direct bone apposition suggestive of remodeling. Like PMMA, calcium phosphate fillers initially function as bulk-filling agents. However, due to their osteoconductive capabilities, their strength is gradually reinforced by new bone formation. Biomechanical testing of calcium phosphate cements has verified their ability to restore the mechanical integrity of the vertebral body.

Calcium sulfate, also known as plaster of Paris, has been investigated as a potential filler material. Long used as a bone graft substitute, calcium sulfate is injectable, osteoconductive, and cures with a limited exothermic reaction. Histologic and radiographic analysis has shown progressive resorption of the cement and osteoblastic rimming of the newly woven bone. However, there is concern that the material is too rapidly resorbed, leading to lack of stability during the remodeling process.

Calcium phosphate and calcium sulfate cements share several common problems. Both materials have a low viscosity as well as handling characteristics that are different from PMMA and thus are unfamiliar to most orthopedic surgeons. The cost of these products is also well above that of PMMA. Finally, these products, as ion suspensions, have thixotropic properties. Thus, the material is susceptible to separation within the delivery tube, making injection difficult.

Finally, novel composite materials, such as the cross-linked resin and glass ceramic particles of Cortoss, by Orthovita, have been approved by the FDA as potential alternative fillers. Proposed advantages of these materials include constant flow characteristics, inherent radiopacity, lower polymerization temperature, and mechanical strength properties that exceed those of PMMA. Animal studies have demonstrated its osteoconductive capacity. The potential for these composite fillers is still being defined.

## COMPLICATIONS

In a patient with an osteoporotic VCF treated by percutaneous vertebroplasty, the incidence of complication necessitating surgical intervention is estimated to be less than 1%.[7] In patients with neoplastic VCF, 2.7% to 5.4% will require surgery to manage a complication of vertebroplasty. In this population, less significant complications are estimated to occur in up to 10% of patients. This increased risk is likely due to an increased risk of cement extravasation due to cortical breaks in the vertebral body.

The most common complication of vertebroplasty is approximately 72 hours of mild local tenderness. More severe pain localized to the needle site may be due to hematoma or bruising. This can be minimized with 5 minutes of manual compression after removal of the cannula. More common in patients with an underlying malignancy, is dermatomal or radicular pain. Typically, no specific treatment is needed and NSAIDs are used to treat pain. Occasionally, a brief course of either oral or local steroid injections may be necessary to relieve the pain. Such complications may be monitored and treated conservatively so long as there are no associated motor deficits or bladder or bowel incontinence. The etiology of radicular pain may be from spinal cord or nerve root compression due to retropulsion of tumor fragments or extravasation of cement. At its worst, paraplegia may occur by this mechanism.

Extravasation of cement into the epidural veins can cause a cement embolism to the lung. As in hip and knee arthroplasty, the pressurized injection of cement into the vertebral body can also cause a fat embolism. While the majority of these emboli are asymptomatic, they can be particularly problematic in patients with pre existing pulmonary conditions, such as COPD. Further respiratory complications can be induced by inaccurate placement of the needle, which can cause a pneumothorax. As in all invasive procedures, there is a risk of bleeding, which is more common in the parapedicular approach due to the large paraspinous vessels. Infection is exceedingly rare. Finally, there have been reports of deaths attributed to vertebroplasty and kyphoplasty. These seem to be due to severe cement allergy or pulmonary failure in patients with preoperative pulmonary compromise.

## NEJM RANDOMIZED CONTROLLED TRIALS

The August 6, 2009 issue of the *New England Journal of Medicine* presented two randomized studies seeking to assess the efficacy of vertebroplasty for pain relief in osteoporotic vertebral fractures. In Buchbinder et al,[8] enrolled patients with one or two painful osteoporotic VCFs less than 12 months old and unhealed, as confirmed by MRI, were randomized to either vertebroplasty or a sham procedure. Outcomes were assessed up to 6 months. They concluded that there was "no beneficial effect of vertebroplasty over a sham procedure at 1 week or at 1, 3, or 6 months among patients with painful osteoporotic vertebral fractures." Kallmes et al[9] randomly assigned 131 patients with one, two, or three painful osteoporotic VCFs thought to be less than 1 year old to either vertebroplasty or a similar sham procedure. Outcomes were assessed up to 3 months. Of note, MRI was only employed if the age of the fracture was "unknown." This study concludes that "improvements in pain and pain-related disability associated with osteoporotic compression fractures in patients treated with vertebroplasty were similar to improvements in a control group."

Upon further examination of these studies, several important criticisms have been raised.[10] These are discussed below.

### Fracture Acuity

The natural history of a VCF is approximately 6 to 8 weeks, at which point most fractures will be healed. Buchbinder did use MRI assessment (edema or presence of a fracture line) as part of her inclusion criteria. However, Kallmes only employed MRI if the age of the fracture was unknown, leaving the possibility of enrolled patients with healed or chronic fractures. Only 32% of Buchbinder's cohort consisted of fractures less than 6 weeks old; 44% of Kallmes' group was composed of fractures less than 6 weeks old. Additionally, both groups included fractures up to 12 months old. Again, this extends well beyond the typical natural history of the fracture and therefore may include back pain due to other causes and the most refractory VCFs.

### Enrollment

As in any study, there is an inherent selection bias. Patients with the most severe pain due to VCF are those patients most likely to benefit from vertebroplasty. However, these patients are less likely to enroll in a study where they may receive a sham treatment. Kallmes enrolled only 131 of 1812 patients; the most common reason for not entering was patient refusal. In Buchbinder's group, 141 patients who met all inclusion criteria did not enroll. This has led to an unquantifiable selection bias that limits the applicability of the results.

### Control Group as an "Alternative Intervention"

Both Buchbinder and Kallmes utilized a sham surgery consisting of the injection of an anesthetic into the skin, subcutaneous tissues, and facet capsule/periosteum. In reality, it may not be a placebo at all. This may constitute a plausible mechanism for relief of back pain, albeit not fracture pain, from such common etiologies as facet arthropathy.

### Crossover

Kallmes reported a 12% versus 43% crossover between his treatment and control groups. This difference suggests a patient dissatisfaction with the control procedure that was not fully captured by the reported pain scales. Additionally, the intention-to-treat analysis probably underestimated the true treatment effect.

## CONCLUSION

The introduction of vertebroplasty, and now kyphoplasty, has provided physicians with additional options for the treatment of VCFs. Specifically, vertebroplasty has been shown to be indicated for the acute and subacute treatment of VCFs due to osteoporosis and malignancy. Contraindications to the procedure include asymptomatic VCFs; painful VCFs that are improving with conservative medical treatment; traumatic VCFs in the young, nonosteoporotic patient; and patients with osteomyelitis, an uncorrectable coaguloapthy, or an allergy to any component of the procedure.

While the technique and its indications are continuing to evolve, numerous studies, including Alvarez et al, have suggested that vertebroplasty is a successful and safe procedure to alleviate the pain associated with acute and subacute osteoporotic or neoplastic VCFs. The recent Kallmes and Buchbinder articles do not support the previous robust benefits demonstrated in other studies; however, their efficacy must be questioned in light of the numerous criticisms stated above, most notably the use of a local anesthetic injection as an unproven sham procedure.

## References

1. O. Johnell, J.A. Kanis, An estimate of the worldwide prevalence and disability associated with osteoporotic fractures, Osteoporos. Int. 17 (2006) 1726–1733.
2. P. Galibert, H. Deramond, et al., Preliminary note on the treatment of vertebral hemangioma by percutaneous acrylic vertebroplasty, Neurochirurgie 33 (2) (1987) 166–168.
3. L. Alvarez, M. Alcaraz, et al., Percutaneous vertebroplasty: functional improvement in patients with osteoporotic compression fractures, Spine 31 (10) (2006) 1113–1118.
4. D. Wardlaw, S.R. Cummings, et al., Efficacy and safety of balloon kyphoplasty compared with non-surgical care for vertebral compression fracture: a randomized controlled trial, Lancet 373 (9668) (2009) 1016–1024.
5. I.H. Lieberman, D. Togawa, M.M. Kayanja, Vertebroplasty and kyphoplasty: filler materials, Spine J. 5 (6 Suppl) (2005) 305S–316S.
6. T.M. Turner, et al., Vertebroplasty comparing injectable calcium phosphate cement compared with polymethylmethacrylate in a unique canine vertebral body large defect model, Spine J. 8 (3) (2008) 482–487.
7. J.M. Mathis, H. Deramond, S.M. Belkoff, Percutaneous vertebroplasty and kyphoplasty, ed 2, Springer, New York, 2006.
8. R. Buchbinder, R.H. Osborne, et al., A randomized trial of vertebroplasty for painful osteoporotic vertebral fractures, N. Engl. J. Med. 361 (6) (2009) 557–568.
9. D.F. Kallmes, B.A. Comstock, et al., A randomized trial of vertebroplasty for osteoporotic spinal fractures, N. Engl. J. Med. 361 (6) (2009) 569–579.
10. North American Spine Society: Newly released vertebroplasty RCTs: a tale of two trials: www.spine.org/Documents/NASSComment_on_Vertebroplasty.pdf. Accessed May 5, 2010.

# 36

# Vertebral Body Stenting

*Paul F. Heini*

**KEY POINTS**

- Vertebral body compression fractures are the hallmark of osteoporosis and often represent the starting point for the vicious circle of progressive collapse and further fractures.

- Cement reinforcement for painful osteoporotic compression fractures provides substantial pain relief and can prevent further collapse. However, it does not allow active height restoration and correction of the spinal alignment.

- Vertebral body stenting provides effective and improved height restoration potential in comparison to a kyphoplasty procedure.

- The first clinical application of vertebral body stenting shows its feasibility and safety. Height restoration and maintenance is possible in mobile fractures.

- The impact of height restoration is not clear yet and needs to be assessed further.

## INTRODUCTION

Vertebral body compression fractures (VBCFs) are the hallmark of osteoporosis, and their incidence increases exponentially with increasing age. VBCFs are related to important morbidity and loss of quality of life comparable to that in hip fractures (Figure 36-1).[1,2]

The treatment of painful VBCFs with percutaneous cement reinforcement has a long history and appears very effective in a very high percentage of patients treated. There are many case series published that support this treatment, with the most recent publication also providing encouraging long-term results.[3-5] Furthermore, there is class A evidence based on a large multicenter Randomized Clinical Trial (RCT) comparing percutaneous cement reinforcement after cavity creation with a balloon against conservative treatment. This study clearly shows a superiority of cement reinforcement for pain, activity level, and pain medication in the first year of treatment.[6] Although the study is comparing kyphoplasty as a specific technique of reinforcement against conservative treatment, based on several review articles, there is no clinical advantage of kyphoplasty over vertebroplasty.[7,8] Most recently, two studies were published comparing vertebroplasty with a sham procedure showing no difference in early outcome. Although the studies show a randomized design with independent assessment, there seems to be a selection bias because the inclusion of patients took several years even though a multicenter study design was used.[9,10]

Although cement reinforcement can stabilize a fracture and therefore decrease pain, height restoration remains an issue, that is not solved yet. Kyphoplasty was introduced initially with the idea to restore vertebral body height. However, the amount of height gain remained very modest, and its clinical impact remains obscure. With the inflation of the balloon, excellent height reduction can be achieved, but after deflation a major amount of the reduction gets lost.[11]

The consequences of vertebral height loss and increased kyphosis are reported in several epidemiological studies: impaired quality of life and even an increased mortality are documented (see Figure 36-1).[2,12,13]

The kyphotic deformity leads to a shift of center of gravity and consecutively to an increased load on the anterior column. Consequently, there is an increased risk for new fractures.[14,15] Furthermore the increased kyphosis raises the load of the back muscles enormously (Figure 36-2).[16,17]

## VERTEBRAL BODY STENT

### How to Restore and Maintain Vertebral Height

The concept of the balloon for height restoration appears most reasonable, because it provides optimal, equal force distribution coupled with a growing surface area. Taking advantage of this principle, the combination of a balloon with an expandable stent appears the optimal solution for restoring and maintaining vertebral body height.

### In Vitro Testing

Anatomical data size calculations and Finite Element (FE) modeling allowed the design of a balloon–stent construct strong enough to be expanded and stable enough not to collapse under the elastic load effective in supine position.

Extensive cadaver testing allowed proof of the feasibility of the concept, and in a sophisticated in vitro setup, one could clearly demonstrate the superior potential for height maintenance in comparison to the balloon insertion only with sound significance (Figure 36-3).[18]

### Clinical Application

#### Indications

The use of the vertebral body stent (VBS) is indicated in acute and subacute painful VBCFs with at least 15% of height loss and kyphotic deformity with the potential of reducibility. In consolidated and fixed fractures, the use of a stent is no longer indicated.

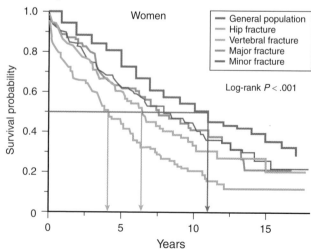

■ **FIGURE 36-1** Survival probability at the age of 75 years for women, comparing the general population with patients after a hip or vertebral fracture. Both groups with fracture show a significant reduction of life expectancy.

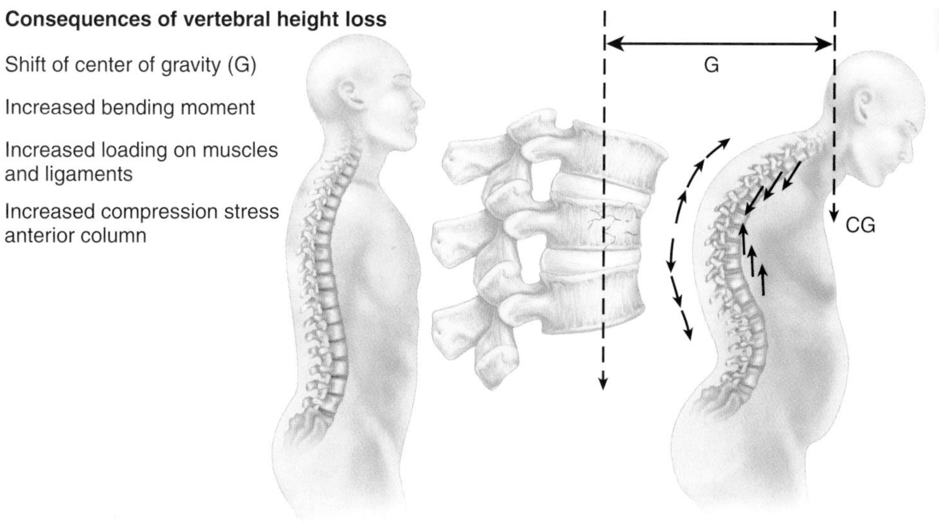

**Consequences of vertebral height loss**

Shift of center of gravity (G)

Increased bending moment

Increased loading on muscles and ligaments

Increased compression stress anterior column

■ **FIGURE 36-2** Vicious circle of vertebral fractures: The increased kyphosis is related to higher stress of the anterior column. There is the risk of new fractures on the one hand, and it increases the load of the back muscles, which further increases loss of posture on the other hand.

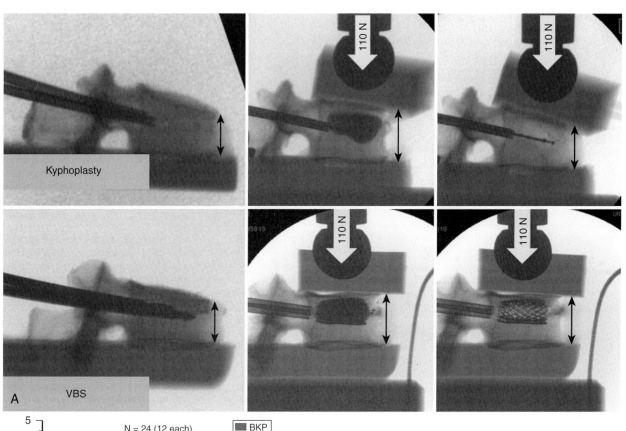

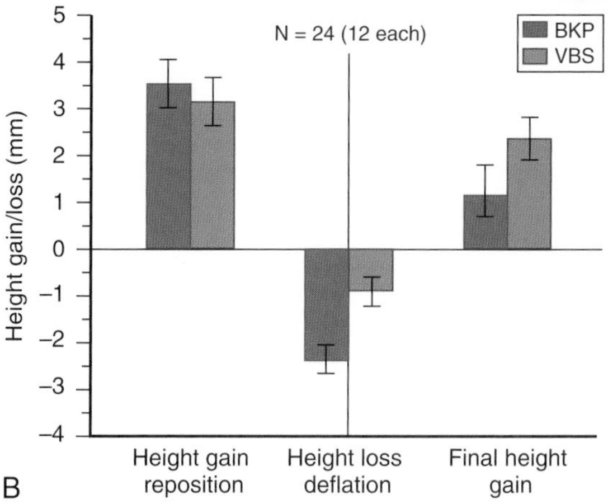

■ **FIGURE 36-3** **A,** Comparison of a kyphoplasty procedure and a vertebral body stenting system as assessed in a cadaver model with a preload of 110 N.[21,22] Initial reduction can be achieved equally well with both systems. After deflation of the balloon there is a significant loss of reduction with the kyphoplasty system (*), whereas the height can be maintained with the VBS (**). **B,** Summary of twelve pairs of vertebrae tested. Initial height gain is similar in both techniques. Loss of height is observed with both systems, but significantly less with VBS ($p = .024$), and consequently the overall height restoration is superior with the VBS system ($p = .035$). (From Wilke HJ, Neef P, Caimi M, Hoogland T, Claes LE. New in vivo measurements of pressures in the intervertebral disc in daily life. Spine 1999;24-8:755-762; and Sato K, Kikuchi S, Yonezawa T. In vivo intradiscal pressure measurement in healthy individuals and in patients with ongoing back problems. Spine 1999;24-23:2468-2474.)

## Surgical Technique

Preferably the procedure is performed under general anesthesia, with the patient placed in hyperextension. Based on the preoperative imaging (either CT scan or MRI and conventional x-rays), the placement of the working cannula and the stent is planned in order to achieve an optimal effect for the fracture reduction (Figure 36-4, *A*). Intraoperatively this placement is navigated by biplanar C-arm control. The crucial landmarks to be respected are the medial border of the pedicle and the posterior wall of the vertebral body. Depending on the individual anatomical situation, the working cannula is placed transpedicular or parapedicular (Figure 36-4, *B*).

Once the working cannula is positioned, the space for the stent is prepared and its size determined and confirmed with the reamer. Then the stents are placed and the appropriate position is monitored in both planes. Make sure that the stents are outside the working cannula but fully inside the vertebral body and that they do not interfere at the tip. Do not start expansion before this check. Then a stepwise symmetrical filling of the balloon stent is performed under pressure, volume, and visual control by imaging. Once the maximal filling or height restoration is achieved, the balloons are deflated and removed. The filling is performed with high viscosity polymethylmethacrylate (PMMA). The cement should fill the void of

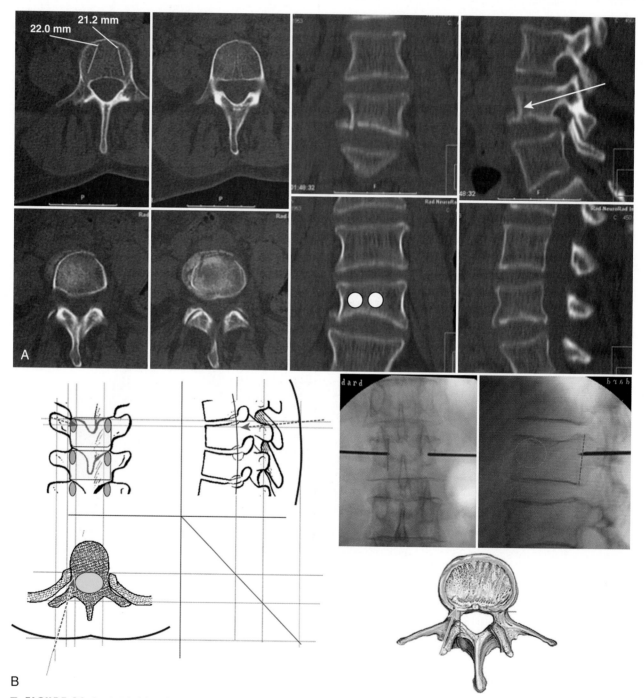

■ **FIGURE 36-4**   **A,** Principles of surgical technique: The optimal placement of the stent is assessed and planned preoperatively based either on a CT scan or MRI investigation. The stents should be located in order to achieve optimal effect, which is about 5 mm below the endplate and in the area of maximal compression. White line are antero posterior vertebral body dimension; arrow is trajectory of trocar placement; white circles are pedicles. **B,** Intraoperative orientation is based on anteroposterior and lateral C-arm projections. The crucial landmarks to be respected are the medial border of the pedicle in the anteroposterior view and the posterior wall of the vertebral body in the lateral view. The tip of the guide wire must not breach the medial border of the pedicle before it reaches the level of the posterior wall. Arrows illustrate angulation (top and bottom left pictures) and inclination (top right picture) of trocar placement; red line is medial border (top left picture) of pedicle and posterior edge (top right and bottom picture) of vertebral body.

the stent and infiltrate the surrounding bone. If there is any leakage, cement injections must be stopped immediately, wait for at least 45 seconds and then cautiously continue with the injection (Figure 36-5). Once the cement is cured remove the filling cannulas.

The after-treatment remains the same as for vertebroplasty. Patients can be mobilized and be active as tolerated immediately after the procedure.

## Clinical Experience

Since conformité européenne (CE) registration of the VBS in November, 2008, we have treated 49 patients with the system and documented these patients in a prospective study. The parameters that were assessed included technical aspects, surgical complications, and potential of height restoration.

## Results

In our series of 49 patients, we treated 32 patients with osteoporotic compression fractures, 12 patients with traumatic fractures of the thoracolumbar spine, and 5 patients with fractures related to myeloma.

The average age was 67 years (range, 27 to 85), and there were 31 women and 18 men.

Technical failures included rupture of the balloon, which was observed in three cases. These failures were observed in cases when the stent showed an eccentric expansion, and the edge of the stent most likely provoked the failure. In one case, a bony spica was the most likely cause. Balloon ruptures were observed at the end of the expansion. These did not lead to further problems, because the balloons could be completely removed with ease and the cementing afterwards was uneventful. In five cases it was not possible to expand the stent because of the already healed fracture. The pressure pump with its built-in peak pressure limit failed at 32 bars in all cases. In two occasions, the stent was removed again with the balloon. In the other cases it remained in place. In all these cases it was possible to inject some cement.

The amount of reduction that was achieved in the cases with still mobile fractures ($n = 40$) was measured by the segmental kyphosis (Figure 36-6, C). The average kyphosis angle preoperatively was 23 degrees

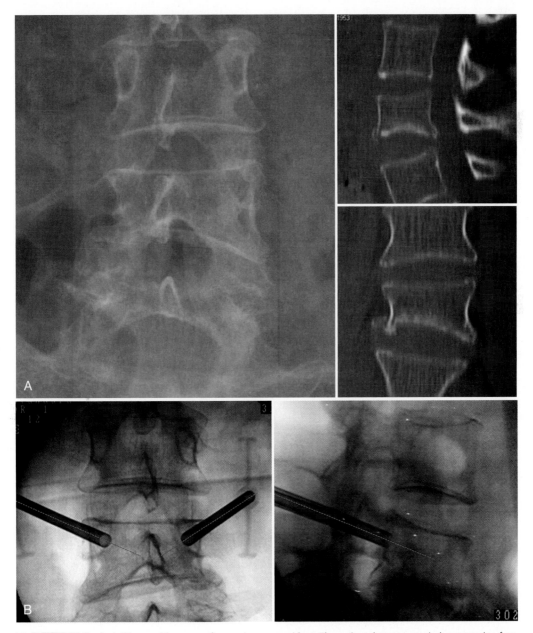

■ **FIGURE 36-5    A,** A 56-year-old woman after a minor car accident. The patient shows an atypical compression fracture of the lower endplate on the right hand side. When standing, the patient complains about L4 nerve root pain. The treatment consisted of a percutaneous reduction with a stent implantation **(B** to **G). B,** The working cannulas are placed bilaterally with slightly increased convergence of the left side. The trajectories give an idea of the final position of the stents The red dotted lines represent trajectory of trocar placement.

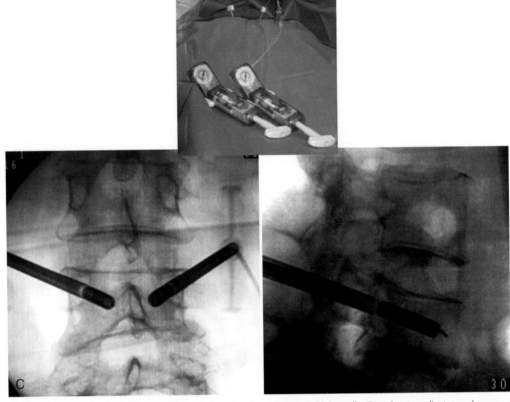

■ **FIGURE 36-5, cont'd    C,** After reaming, the stents are placed bilaterally. Top: Stent applicator and pressure manometer; Top Left: AP view of stent placement prior to stent expansion; Top Right: Lateral view of stent placement prior to stent expansion.

(13 to 32 degrees) and could be corrected to 12 degrees (0 to 16 degrees) postoperatively. Height restoration was assessed semiquantitatively in the cases where the deformity was not mainly the kyphosis. The amount was graded from 0 to 3, where 0 meant no reduction possible and 3 meant complete restoration. There were 9 cases with grade 0. We have seen 18 cases with a reduction of grade 1, which means 50% height gain (see Figure 36-5); 15 cases with grade 2, which is 75% of height gain (Figure 36-7); and 7 cases with complete height restoration (Figure 36-8).

Cement leakage was observed in 9 out of 49 patients. These leaks were observed in the paravertebral tissue in 6 cases; in 2 cases, vascular leaks were present; and in 1 case, leakage into the foramen occurred. None of these leaks were clinically symptomatic.

The best potential for height gain was observed in our series of fresh traumatic fractures (n = 12). The healthy bone provides an optimal counterforce for the application of the reduction forces by the stent.

## DISCUSSION

Vertebral body stents permit restoration and maintenance of vertebral body height in vitro, and clinically it is possible to restore height in acute and subacute fractures. In addition the stent allows the clinician to overcome the limitations of the balloon-only principle. The balloon is optimal in the sense that it provides the best load distribution over the maximum possible area, but it is not able to maintain it after deflation.

So far the feasibility of the system can be demonstrated. Its use and application appears safe and reliable. The surgical procedure is more demanding in comparison to a simple vertebroplasty. Correct stent placement appears crucial in order achieve an optimal effect. For a controlled filling, the use of highly viscous cement with a long working time appears mandatory (i.e., Vertecem).

The clinical impact of height restoration needs to be demonstrated. Based on clinical comparison the impact of the fracture kyphosis seems to

(*Text continues on P. 231*)

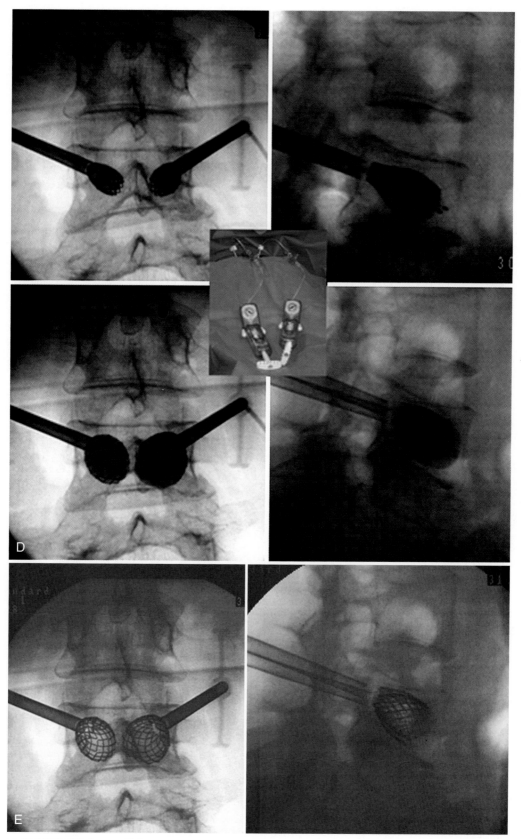

**■ FIGURE 36-5, cont'd    D,** The stent is expanded stepwise until maximal reduction is achieved or the maximal volume has been reached. **E,** After deflation and removal of the balloon, the stents remain expanded and the reduction is maintained. Left side pictures are AP views of stent after expansion and right side pics are lateral views of stent after expansion.

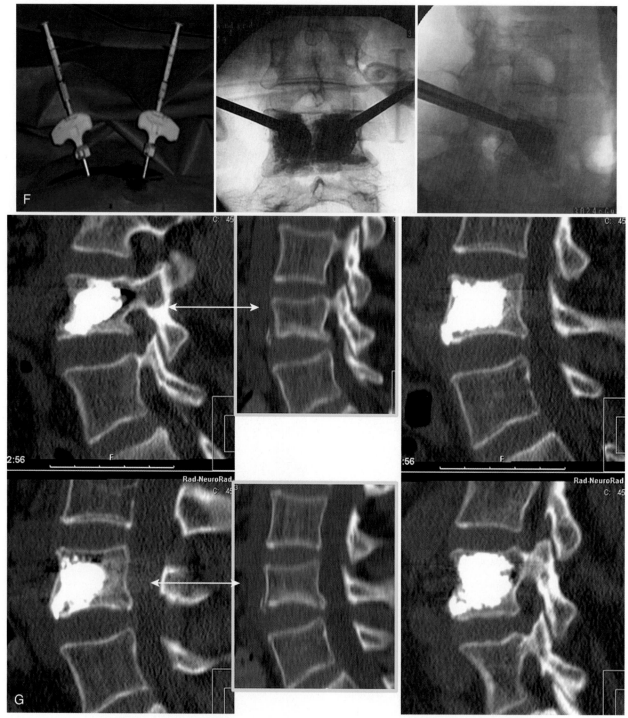

■ **FIGURE 36-5, cont'd**    **F,** Cement reinforcement with PMMA is performed with filling of the stents and infiltration of the surrounding bone. **G, H,** Comparison of the preoperative and postoperative CT scan demonstrating the amount of reduction and the ideal cement filling (left to right).

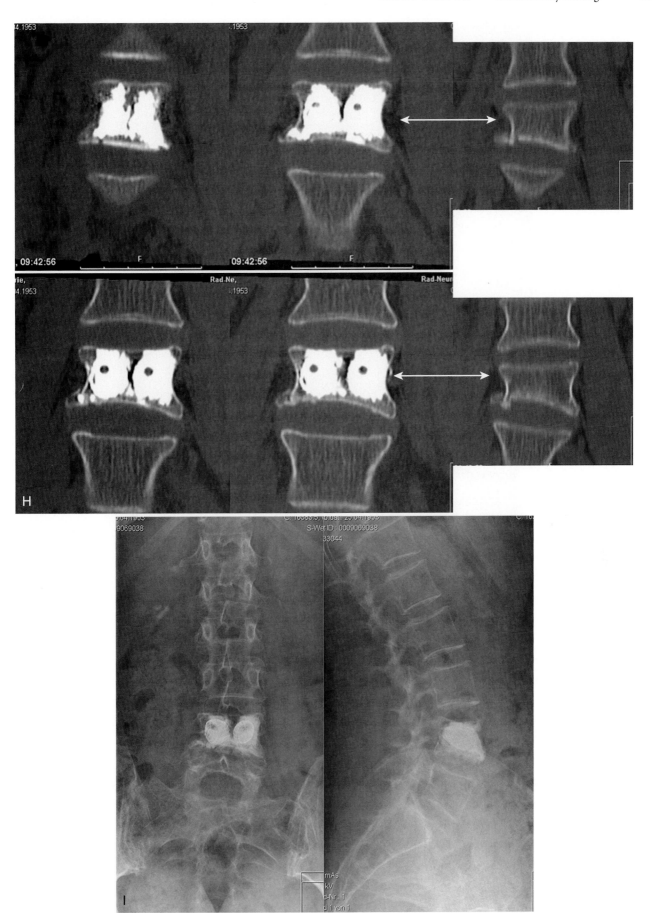

■ **FIGURE 36-5, cont'd**   **I,** Follow-up standing x-ray after 6 months.

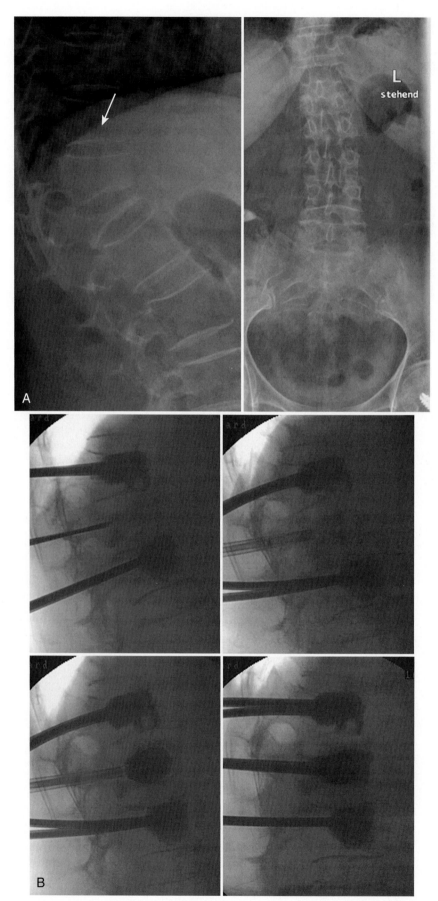

■ **FIGURE 36-6**  **A,** A 72-year-old woman with pain history of 8 weeks. The first x-rays show a complete collapse of L1 with severe kyphosis. **B,** Combining the closed reduction techniques of lordoplasty[23] and VBS allows a nearly complete height restoration. *(From Orler R, Frauchiger LH, Lange U, Heini PF. Lordoplasty: report on early results with a new technique for the treatment of vertebral compression fractures to restore the lordosis. Eur Spine J, 15(2) 1769-1775, 2006.)*

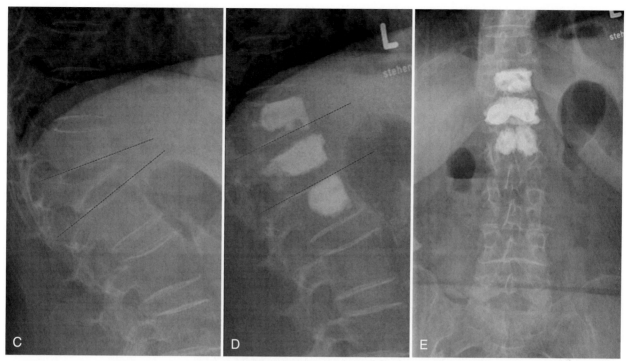

■ **FIGURE 36-6, cont'd    C,** Comparison of preoperative standing film and follow-up x-ray after 6 months. The vertebral height is well restored and maintained and the kyphosis nearly completely corrected (**D** and **E**).

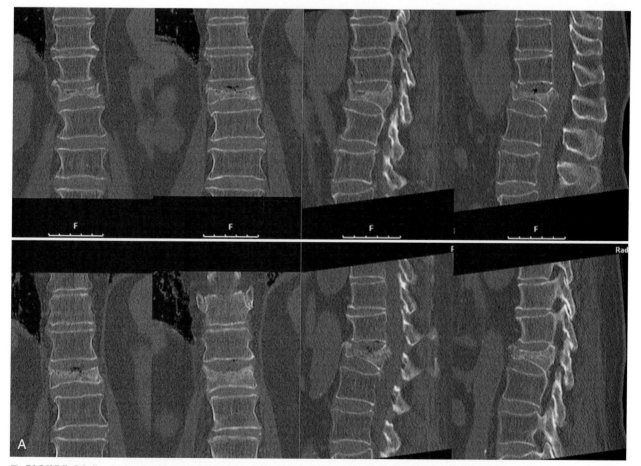

■ **FIGURE 36-7**    A 78-year-old man with severe compression fractures of L1 after simple fall. Known osteoporosis due to steroid medication. Refractory immobilizing pain despite 10 days of hospital stay. **A,** CT scans depict severe vertebral body compression with posterior wall displacement and cleft formation.

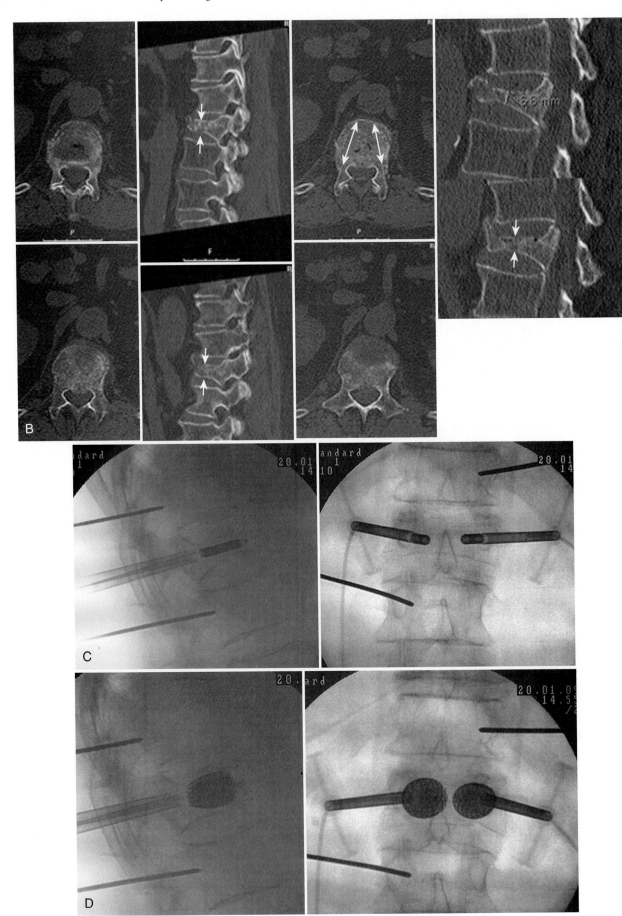

■ **FIGURE 36-7, cont'd    B,** Based on the CT scan, preoperative planning of feasibility and possible stent dimension is performed. The minimal height for stent placement is about 8 mm. **C** to **E,** Intraoperative pictures of the surgical procedure: stent placement, expansion, balloon removal. Arrows in the image indicate the fractures.

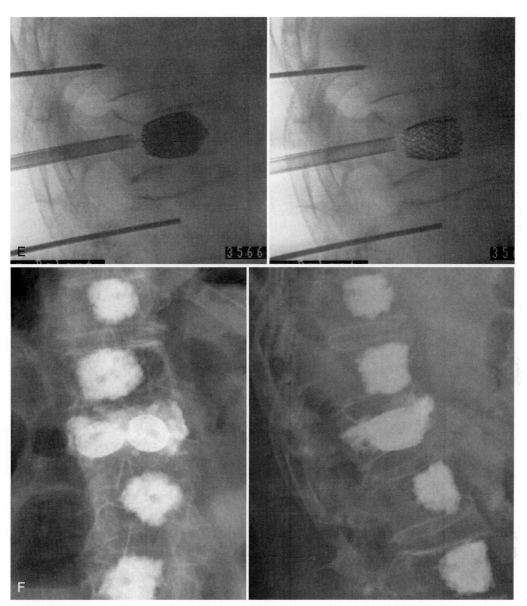

■ **FIGURE 36-7, cont'd    F,** Standing x-ray images at 4 months postoperative with well-maintained vertebral height. The adjacent vertebrae were reinforced in a prophylactic sense.

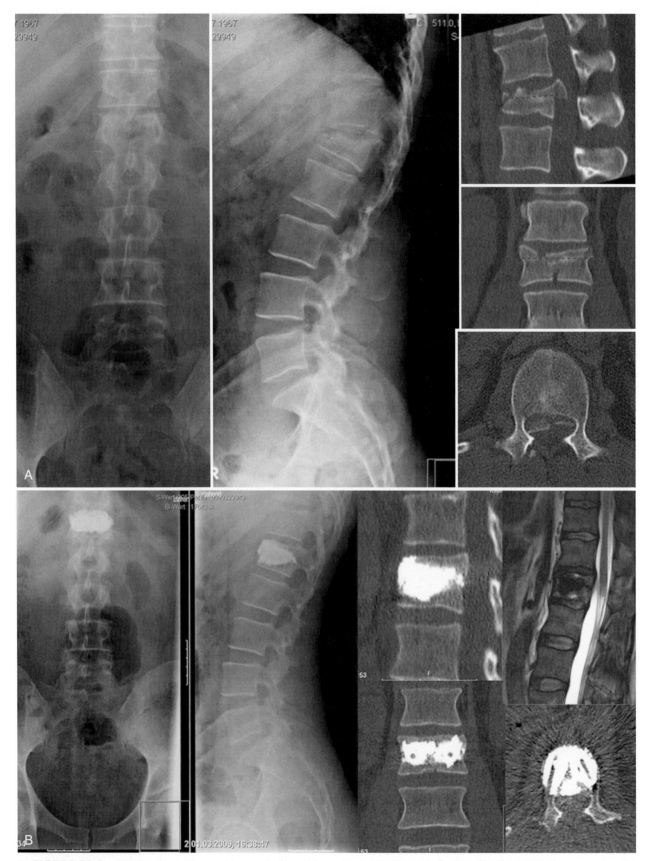

■ **FIGURE 36-8**    **A,** Male patient, 41 years old, presents after a skiing accident with a burst split fracture of L1 (AO 3.2). **B,** The stent restored L1 to its former height. Ligamentotaxis provides realignment of the fragments, the cement then provides stability that allows immediate weight bearing. Reservations against using PMMA in young people are justified; however, alternative material is lacking and histologic workup of a postmortem specimen depicts no adverse effects around the cement, as demonstrated in the MRI taken 1 month after the intervention.[24] *(From Braunstein V, Sprecher CM, Gisep A, Benneker L, Yen K, Schneider E, Heini P, Milz S. Long-term reaction to bone cement in osteoporotic bone: new bone formation in vertebral bodies after vertebroplasty. J Anat 2008;212-5:697-701.)*

## ADVANTAGES AND DISADVANTAGES OF VBS

### Advantages

- Height restoration and maintenance possible
- Controlled expansion with balloon/stent assembly
- Safe filling of void/stent space

### Disadvantages

- Surgical procedure demanding; exact stent placement mandatory
- More expensive

---

be more important than the overall kyphosis regarding balance problems of the spine.[19] Biomechanical calculations suggest that the increase of kyphosis is related to an increase of the pressure on the anterior column on one hand, and, more importantly, a massive increase on the muscle load posteriorly.[14,20] This may be the cause of a vicious circle that ends up in this so-called sagittal plane decompensation.[17] Therefore there is a rationale for height restoration and maintenance of spinal alignment. Further clinical studies are needed to demonstrate how vertebral body stenting is able to contribute to this.

## References

1. Incidence of vertebral fracture in Europe: results from the European Prospective Osteoporosis Study (EPOS), J. Bone Miner. Res. 17–4 (2002) 716–724.
2. D. Bliuc, N.D. Nguyen, V.E. Milch, T.V. Nguyen, J.A. Eisman, J.R. Center, Mortality risk associated with low-trauma osteoporotic fracture and subsequent fracture in men and women, JAMA 301–5 (2009) 513–521.
3. L. Alvarez, M. Alcaraz, A. Perez-Higueras, J.J. Granizo, I. de Miguel, R.E. Rossi, D. Quinones, Percutaneous vertebroplasty: functional improvement in patients with osteoporotic compression fractures, Spine 31–10 (2006) 1113–1118.
4. S.P. Muijs, M.J. Nieuwenhuijse, A.R. Van Erkel, P.D. Dijkstra, Percutaneous vertebroplasty for the treatment of osteoporotic vertebral compression fractures: evaluation after 36 months, J. Bone Joint Surg. Br. 91–3 (2009) 379–384.
5. P.F. Heini, B. Walchli, U. Berlemann, Percutaneous transpedicular vertebroplasty with PMMA: operative technique and early results. A prospective study for the treatment of osteoporotic compression fractures, Eur. Spine J. 9–5 (2000) 445–450.
6. D. Wardlaw, S.R. Cummings, J. Van Meirhaeghe, L. Bastian, J.B. Tillman, J. Ranstam, R. Eastell, P. Shabe, K. Talmadge, S. Boonen, Efficacy and safety of balloon kyphoplasty compared with non-surgical care for vertebral compression fracture (FREE): a randomised controlled trial, Lancet 373–9668 (2009) 1016–1024.
7. P.A. Hulme, S.K. Boyd, P.F. Heini, S.J. Ferguson, Differences in endplate deformation of the adjacent and augmented vertebra following cement augmentation, Eur. Spine J., 2009.
8. J.C. Eck, D. Nachtigall, S.C. Humphreys, S.D. Hodges, Comparison of vertebroplasty and balloon kyphoplasty for treatment of vertebral compression fractures: a meta-analysis of the literature, Spine J. 8–3 (2008) 488–497.
9. D.F. Kallmes, B.A. Comstock, P.J. Heagerty, J.A. Turner, D.J. Wilson, T.H. Diamond, R. Edwards, L.A. Gray, L. Stout, S. Owen, W. Hollingworth, B. Ghdoke, D.J. Annesley-Williams, S.H. Ralston, J.G. Jarvik, A randomized trial of vertebroplasty for osteoporotic spinal fractures, N. Engl. J. Med. 361–6 (2009) 569–579.
10. R. Buchbinder, R.H. Osborne, P.R. Ebeling, J.D. Wark, P. Mitchell, C. Wriedt, S. Graves, M.P. Staples, B. Murphy, A randomized trial of vertebroplasty for painful osteoporotic vertebral fractures, N. Engl. J. Med. 361–6 (2009) 557–568.
11. G. Voggenreiter, Balloon kyphoplasty is effective in deformity correction of osteoporotic vertebral compression fractures, Spine 30–24 (2005) 2806–2812.
12. P.J. Ryan, G. Blake, R. Herd, I. Fogelman, A clinical profile of back pain and disability in patients with spinal osteoporosis, Bone 15–1 (1994) 27–30.
13. C. Cooper, E.J. Atkinson, W.M. O'Fallon, L.J. Melton 3rd, Incidence of clinically diagnosed vertebral fractures: a population-based study in Rochester, Minnesota, 1985-1989, J. Bone Miner. Res. 7-2 (1992) 221–227.
14. M.H. Huang, E. Barrett-Connor, G.A. Greendale, D.M. Kado, Hyperkyphotic posture and risk of future osteoporotic fractures: the Rancho Bernardo study, J. Bone Miner. Res. 21–3 (2006) 419–423.
15. R.P. Heaney, T.M. Zizic, I. Fogelman, W.P. Olszynski, P. Geusens, C. Kasibhatla, N. Alsayed, G. Isaia, M.W. Davie, C.H. Chesnut 3rd, Risedronate reduces the risk of first vertebral fracture in osteoporotic women, Osteoporos. Int. 13–6 (2002) 501–505.
16. A.M. Briggs, A.M. Greig, K.L. Bennell, P.W. Hodges, Paraspinal muscle control in people with osteoporotic vertebral fracture, Eur. Spine J. 16–8 (2007) 1137–1144.
17. A.M. Briggs, A.M. Greig, J.D. Wark, The vertebral fracture cascade in osteoporosis: a review of aetiopathogenesis, Osteoporos. Int. 18–5 (2007) 575–584.
18. R. Rotter, S. Fürderer, P. Heini, Vertebral stenting, a new device for vertebral height restoration, Eur. Spine J. 17 (2008) 1551.
19. A.M. Greig, K.L. Bennell, A.M. Briggs, J.D. Wark, P.W. Hodges, Balance impairment is related to vertebral fracture rather than thoracic kyphosis in individuals with osteoporosis, Osteoporos. Int. 18–4 (2007) 543–551.
20. A.M. Briggs, J.H. van Dieen, T.V. Wrigley, A.M. Greig, B. Phillips, S.K. Lo, K.L. Bennell, Thoracic kyphosis affects spinal loads and trunk muscle force, Phys. Ther. 87–5 (2007) 595–607.
21. H.J. Wilke, P. Neef, M. Caimi, T. Hoogland, L.E. Claes, New in vivo measurements of pressures in the intervertebral disc in daily life, Spine 24–8 (1999) 755–762.
22. K. Sato, S. Kikuchi, T. Yonezawa, In vivo intradiscal pressure measurement in healthy individuals and in patients with ongoing back problems, Spine 24–23 (1999) 2468–2474.
23. R. Orler, L.H. Frauchiger, U. Lange, P.F. Heini, Lordoplasty: report on early results with a new technique for the treatment of vertebral compression fractures to restore the lordosis, Eur. Spine J. 15 (2), 2006 1769–1775.
24. V. Braunstein, C.M. Sprecher, A. Gisep, L. Benneker, K. Yen, E. Schneider, P. Heini, S. Milz, Long-term reaction to bone cement in osteoporotic bone: new bone formation in vertebral bodies after vertebroplasty, J. Anat. 212–5 (2008) 697–701.

# 37

# Structural Osteoplasty: The Treatment of Vertebral Body Compression Fractures Using the OsseoFix Device

*James J. Yue, Hitesh Garg, and Rudolf Bertagnoli*

---

**KEY POINTS**

- Controlled and directional reduction of vertebral compression fractures are not mutually exclusive.
- The OsseoFix device permits directional reduction of fractures with less cement application than in vertebroplasty or kyphoplasty.
- In the laboratory setting, the OsseoFix device offers superior resistance to re-displacement postapplication strength versus kyphoplasty.
- Device is available in 4.5, 5.5, and 7.0 mm sizes.
- In the laboratory setting, less cement is required to produce equivalent strength as compared to kyphoplasty and vertebroplasty.

## INTRODUCTION

The incidence of osteoporosis and osteoporotic vertebral compression fractures (VCFs) increases with advancing age with an estimated incidence of more than 50% in women over the age of 80 years.[1] Adverse anatomical and biomechanical consequences of osteoporotic VCFs contribute substantially to the chronic morbidity and economic impact of osteoporosis.[1] With increasing demand for improved quality of life, immediate pain relief, early mobilization, and preservation of function have become the goals for the management of osteoporotic VCFs.[2]

A single vertebral body compression fracture results in a sagittal plane deformity and greater flexion bending moment around the fractured vertebral body, thereby decreasing the force required to cause further increase in degree and number of additional VCFs with a corresponding increase in kyphosis.[1] Spinal deformity resulting from the loss of vertebral body height also leads to loss of pulmonary capacity, malnutrition, decreased mobility, and depression.[3] Kyphosis secondary to osteoporotic vertebral compression fractures is associated with a two to three times greater incidence of death due to pulmonary causes.[3] Moreover, the pain associated with acute VCFs may be incapacitating and may become chronic in a significant number of cases.[4] Interventions that restore fractured vertebral height and stabilize the fractured segment are presumed to improve spinal biomechanics and thereby mitigate these consequences.[5,6]

Vertebroplasty and kyphoplasty are effective treatment alternatives for osteoporotic VCFs. Disadvantages of vertebroplasty include high injection pressures, inability to correct deformity, and cement extrusion. Similarly, poor directional reduction control, propagation of burst fractures, and cement extrusion are insufficiencies of kyphoplasty. The OsseoFix (Alphatec Spine, San Diego, CA USA) technique and implant permit a hybrid technique that we term *structural osteoplasty*.

Structural osteoplasty is the controlled directional reduction and bone augmentation of VCFs. OsseoFix is a stent-like titanium device that is inserted percutaneously into the fractured vertebral body and is intended to stabilize and restore the height of vertebral compression fractures before the insertion of polymethylmethacrylate (PMMA) cement in a controlled and predictable manner. This implant is designed to overcome the disadvantages associated with vertebroplasty and kyphoplasty.

## CLINICAL INDICATIONS AND CONTRAINDICATIONS

The clinical indications for the OsseoFix device include symptomatic and unhealed osteoporotic VCFs in the thoracic and lumbar spine from T6 to L5. Additional potential indications include its use in tumor and traumatic fractures. Before proceeding with this procedure, it is important to clarify whether the fracture is actually caused by the fractured vertebral body by use of clinical examination and radiographic analysis, which should include radiographs and magnetic resonance imaging (MRI) with short tau inversion recovery (STIR) images. MRI would also confirm any cord or cauda compression necessitating a decompression procedure. It is prudent to obtain a CT scan if a break in the posterior cortex of the involved vertebral body is expected, especially when a traumatic genesis is suspected.

Contraindications to this procedure include titanium allergies, chronic healed fractures, vertebra plana, unstable burst fractures, fractures in the cervical spine, local or systemic infections, elevated white blood cell count, fever, obesity, pregnancy, mental illness, or any other medical condition that would prohibit beneficial surgical outcome apart from general contraindications, such as coagulation disorder, unsuitability for general or local anesthesia, or the inability to lie prone.

## DESCRIPTION OF THE OSSEOFIX DEVICE

The OsseoFix device is a titanium implant composed of surgical grade titanium alloy (Ti-6Al-4V, ASTM F 136) and commercially pure titanium (Ti-CP2, ASTM F 67) with an electrolytic conversion coating. It is a cylindrical-shaped capsule, which expands in the middle after deployment and helps reduce the vertebral fracture and maintains the vertebral body height. Cement is then injected into the deployed implant. The implant is available in various sizes to provide versatility for individual anatomical dimension needs (Figure 37-1; Table 1).

### Biomechanical Studies

The OsseoFix implant has undergone intense in vitro biomechanical testing in terms of stiffness, yield load, and ultimate load after insertion into a fractured vertebral body.[7,8] These studies have evaluated the biomechanical

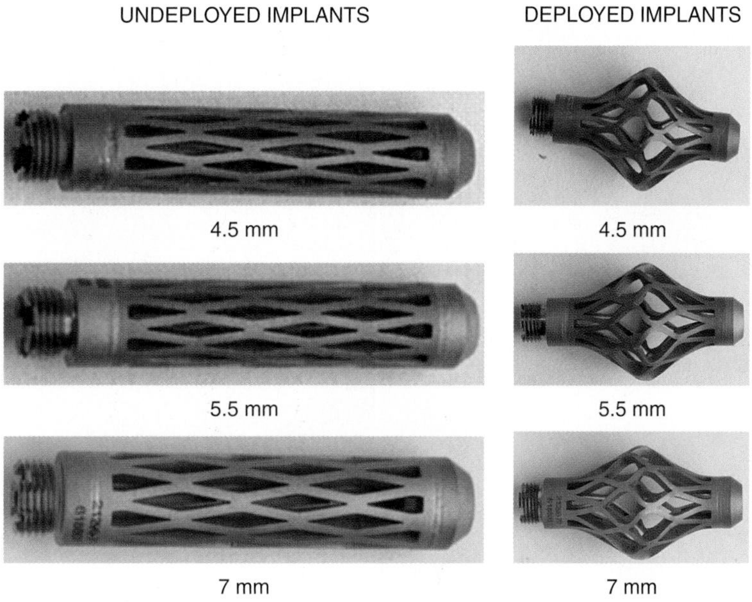

UNDEPLOYED IMPLANTS          DEPLOYED IMPLANTS

4.5 mm                      4.5 mm

5.5 mm                      5.5 mm

7 mm                        7 mm

■ **FIGURE 37-1**   OsseoFix titanium implants.

stability of vertebral compression fractures repaired using kyphoplasty type repair techniques compared to several methods of using the OsseoFix repair technique.[7,8]

In the first reported in vitro biomechanical study evaluating the Osseo-Fix implant, four male human cadaveric (age 68 ± 9 yrs) spines from T2 to L5 were scanned for bone mineral density (BMD) using a 3-D computed tomography (CT) BMD measurement system (average BMD across spines and all levels = 119 ± 44 mg/ml). Individual vertebral bodies were sectioned from each spine and measured for anterior vertebral body height. Once measured, the intact vertebral bodies were mechanically tested using established techniques.[5,6]

To summarize these techniques, the intact vertebral bodies were placed within a test frame with custom fixtures and epoxy resin that conformed to the upper and lower vertebral body endplates (Figure 37-2). Vertebral bodies were then compressed by 25% of the measured intact anterior vertebral body height (30-mm height × 25% = 7.5 mm compression). Following intact testing, data for stiffness (N/mm), yield load (N), and ultimate load (N) were calculated.

Fractured vertebral bodies were then randomly assigned to one of two repair groups: those using standard kyphoplasty or those using the smallest possible OsseoFix device (4.5 mm) (Figures 37-3 and 37-4). Both groups were injected with PMMA cement. Following repair, anterior column heights were remeasured to once again compress the vertebral bodies by 25% of the anterior column heights. The same data were calculated for the repair groups. Data between intact and repaired vertebral bodies as well as data between types of repairs were evaluated using a two-way ANOVA ($p < .05$). In addition, the volume of cement injected and the height maintained following testing of the repaired vertebral bodies were evaluated with a one-way ANOVA ($p < .05$).

## Results – Study 1

Data from this initial study found no differences in anterior column height between repair techniques in the intact or repaired phases. However, there was a statistically greater amount of height *maintained* following mechanical compression of the repaired vertebral bodies for the OsseoFix group compared to the kyphoplasty group (Figure 37-5). In addition, it was found that statistically less cement was injected (1 ml less) for the OsseoFix group compared to the kyphoplasty group.

There were no differences found in any of the mechanical variables between OsseoFix or kyphoplasty repair groups. These data were then normalized to the intact data to evaluate the ability of each repair technique to restore the vertebral body to its intact mechanical strength (Figure 37-6).

| TABLE 37-1 | Implant Deployment Comparison Chart | | |
|---|---|---|---|
| Initial Diameter (mm) | Initial Length (mm) | Maximum Deployment Diameter (mm) | Final Length (mm) |
| 4.5 | 26.4 | 11.4 | 22.8 |
| 5.5 | 30.0 | 13.0 | 26.4 |
| 7 | 35.2 | 14.8 | 31.7 |

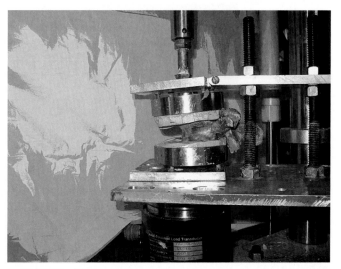

■ **FIGURE 37-2**   Testing configuration setup to compress anterior column by 25% of intact height.

The normalized data were not statistically different between repair groups. The yield load and ultimate load were restored to intact values, but the stiffness did not reach intact values. This result is similar to data previously reported for vertebroplasty or kyphoplasty biomechanical restoration of fractured vertebral bodies.[5,6]

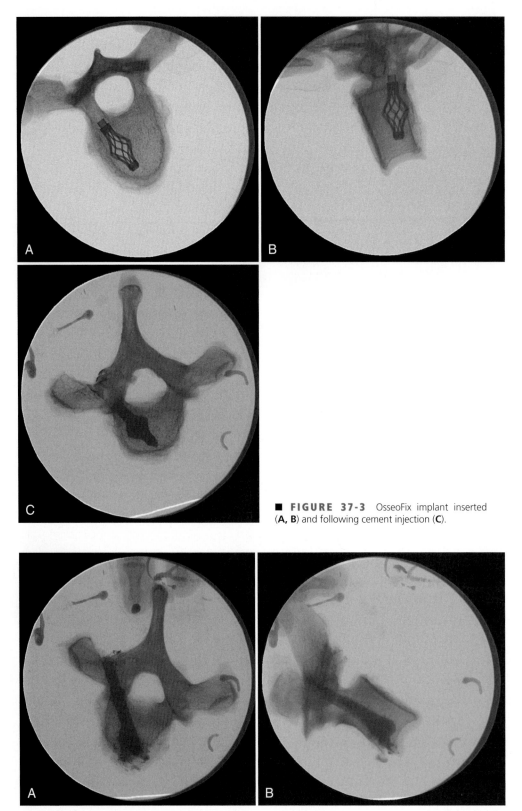

■ **FIGURE 37-3**   OsseoFix implant inserted (**A, B**) and following cement injection (**C**).

■ **FIGURE 37-4**   Kyphoplasty repair **A,** Coronal radiograph with a deployed Ossefix device with cement. **B,** Lateral radiograph with a deployed Ossefix device with cement.

## *Results – Study 2*

Because of the strength provided by the smallest possible implant with the lower injected cement volumes, a second biomechanical study was conducted to evaluate the inherent strength provided by the implant alone when compared to kyphoplasty and OsseoFix implants with cement.[8] This study followed identical specimen preparation as the previous biomechanical study.[7] However, in the second study, the OsseoFix implant repairs were selected based on pedicle width and height and the desired amount of repair height. In addition, the mechanical data were normalized to the BMD of individual vertebral bodies to understand how fractures may be stabilized by eliminating the effect of the inherent bone density.

This study found no mechanical difference for any of the mechanical variables among the kyphoplasty type repair, the OsseoFix with cement repair, and the OsseoFix repair without cement (Table 37-2). Thus an OsseoFix implant alone (without cement) provides biomechanical strength that is equivalent to the other repair techniques evaluated. Whereas the definitive explanation remains unclear, it may be related to the compliance or elasticity of the commercially pure titanium expandable region deforming beneath the superior endplate when loaded. When using the cement, the bolus underneath the superior endplate may not be as elastic and thus causes more directed loading to the endplate and lower stability. Further visualization studies are needed to understand the deformation of the implant in real-time while being loaded. It also may be possible to use alternative injectable materials within the OsseoFix implant, because the implant provides stability and structural support that is not required from the injectable material. Again, further studies are warranted to understand the fracture stabilization provided in this scenario.

## CONCLUSION

Several in vitro biomechanical investigations have found that the OsseoFix implant provides equivalent biomechanical strength compared to standard kyphoplasty type of technique. However, greater height maintenance and lower cement injection volumes were key results in the initial study. The subsequent study found that a stand-alone OsseoFix implant provided strength equivalent to the other repair techniques. From these investigations it can be concluded that the OsseoFix repair technique provides a viable biomechanical alternative to the standard kyphoplasty repair techniques.

## CLINICAL DATA

The first case of vertebral compression fracture reduction and internal fixation using OsseoFix fracture reduction system was done by Dr. Rudolf Bertagnoli on July 21, 2008, at Bogen center in Germany. Several hundred patients have received this treatment since then. The first patient was suffering from acute T12 vertebral compression fracture (Figure 37-7). The surgeon was able to achieve considerable height (Figure 37-8). The patient got immediate pain relief and did not require any external bracing or support. Two such cases have been done to date with good clinical outcomes, and no complications have been reported so far.

## OPERATIVE TECHNIQUE

**Step 1: Positioning.** The patient is carefully placed prone on a Jackson table with all the bony prominences well padded. Fluoroscopic views are taken in the anteroposterior (AP) and lateral projections such that vertebral bodies are clearly visualized. The spinous process should be equidistant from the medial pedicle edges on AP view. The endplates should be superimposed on lateral view. The level of surgical interest is identified and marked.

**Step 2: Creating an access channel into the vertebral body (Figure 37-9).** The transpedicular approach is currently the most commonly used technique to access the vertebral body and is easy to master. An extrapedicular approach may be preferable in the upper and mid thoracic regions, where the size of the pedicle may limit the size of the OsseoFix device that can be used via transpedicular approach.

A 1-cm incision is then made over the bony prominences at the marked level. A targeting Jamshedi cannula with trocar is then placed into the vertebral body via transpedicular or extrapedicular approach. The trocar is then replaced with a guide wire through the Jamshedi cannula. The position of the guide wire must be verified using fluoroscopy at this stage. The Jamshedi cannula is then removed and replaced with a drill sleeve. A pathway

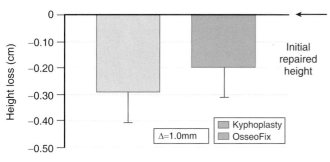

■ **FIGURE 37-5**    Collapse of repaired vertebral bodies following testing.

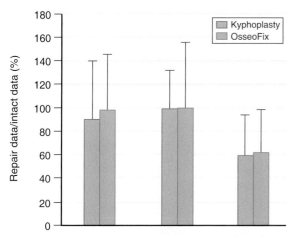

■ **FIGURE 37-6**    Ability of repair to return to intact data.

---

**TABLE 37-2    Normalized Biomechanical Data for Each Treatment Group**

| | Yield Load (N/BMD) | | Ultimate Load (N/BMD) | | Stiffness [(N/mm)/BMD] | |
|---|---|---|---|---|---|---|
| | Intact | Repaired | Intact | Repaired | Intact | Repaired |
| **Kyphoplasty** | | | | | | |
| Mean | 22.2 | 15.8 | 22.9 | 17.0 | 11.0 | 3.9 |
| SD | 17.0 | 9.4 | 16.7 | 9.8 | 10.3 | 2.8 |
| **Implant with Cement** | | | | | | |
| Mean | 23.0 | 16.8 | 23.9 | 18.8 | 11.5 | 4.9 |
| SD | 16.1 | 16.6 | 15.8 | 20.7 | 9.2 | 4.6 |
| **Implant without Cement** | | | | | | |
| Mean | 23.8 | 18.8 | 25.1 | 22.2 | 12.6 | 5.4 |
| SD | 15.5 | 16.1 | 15.5 | 16.9 | 11.3 | 3.4 |

N - Newtons, BMD- Bone Mineral Density, SD- Standard deviation.

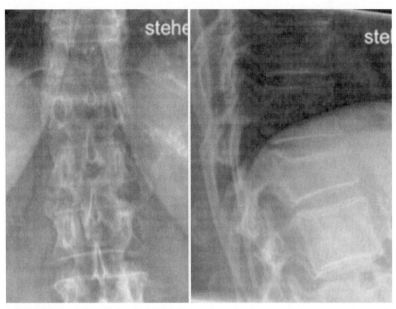

■ **FIGURE 37-7**    Osteoporotic vertebral compression fracture of the T12 vertebral body.

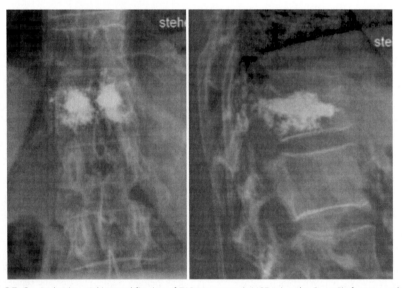

■ **FIGURE 37-8**    Reduction and internal fixation of T12 osteoporotic VCF using the OsseoFix fracture reduction system.

is created into the anterior one third of the vertebral body by drilling over the guide wire through the drill sleeve (Figure 37-10). The pathway should end a few mm posterior to the anterior cortex. Position is reconfirmed with fluoroscopy, and the drill is removed, keeping the guide wire in place.

**Step 3: Insertion and deployment of the implant (Figure 37-11).** The chosen implant size comes preassembled on the inserter. Make sure that the implant is not torqued onto the shaft. The actuator is then positioned perpendicular to and on top of the implant inserter handle. Rotate the fluted metal shaft of the actuator clockwise until a click is heard, indicating locking of the actuator onto the implant inserter handle. If the red band on the top of the actuator is exposed, turn the actuator counterclockwise until it is no longer visible. The color-matched actuation rod is then advanced through the actuator into the implant inserter and is rotated until the end is firmly threaded into the implant. The outer knob of the actuation rod is depressed into the key feature of the actuator and is rotated clockwise until a positive lock is achieved. The tip of the actuation rod should be seen protruding through the distal end of the implant.

The assembled implant inserter instrument with the actuator setup is then inserted over the guide wire. The position of the implant is confirmed with AP and lateral fluoroscopy. The guide wire is then removed, and initial

deployment of the implant is performed by rotating the actuator clockwise under direct visualization using fluoroscopy. If the surgeon is satisfied with the initial deployment of the implant and reduction of the endplates, final deployment of the implant is performed. There is a stop mechanism in the actuator to prevent overdeployment of the implant. The actuator can be turned 3.5 times before the stop mechanism is engaged. After satisfactory deployment of the implant, the implant inserter assembly is disassembled and the actuator rod is removed. The insertion cannula is left behind in the vertebral body. The second implant can be placed in the same vertebral body through the other pedicle, if clinically indicated.

**Step 4: Cement delivery.** The cement powder is mixed with the liquid monomer in the mixing chamber at room temperature. The delivery gun is then loaded with the desired amount of cement. A bone biopsy cannula is inserted through the implant inserter into the most distal portion of the implant. The cement delivery gun is connected to the extension tube. The desired amount of cement is then injected through the bone biopsy cannula into the vertebral body under live AP and lateral fluoroscopy. The cement should never be inserted directly through the implant inserter tube. The cement injection is stopped when a sufficient amount has been placed to stabilize the fracture, if cement reaches cortex or an endplate, or leakage is

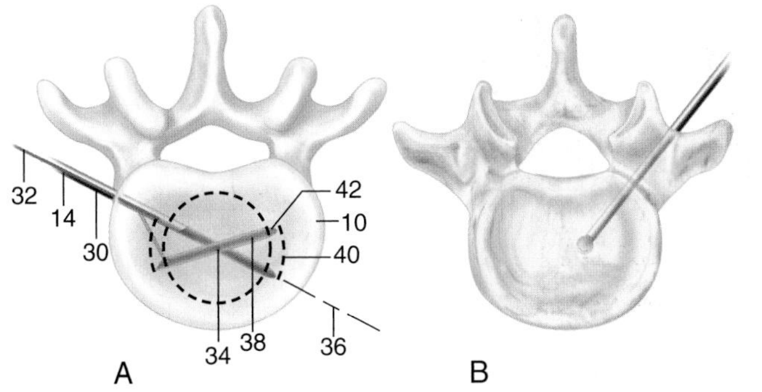

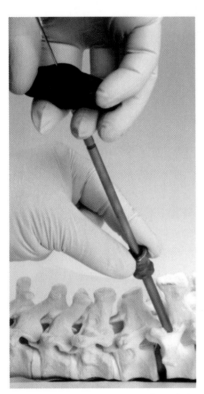

■ **FIGURE 37-9**    An access channel is created into the vertebral body. **A,** Extrapedicular approach. **B,** Transpedicular approach.

■ **FIGURE 37-10**    Creating the pathway in the pedicle and the vertebral body by drilling over the guide wire.

noted. The bone biopsy and the insertion cannula are removed after the cement delivery has been completed. Final fluoroscopic images are taken and the skin is closed.

## PITFALLS AND COMPLICATIONS OF THE PROCEDURE

Besides the usual anesthetic complications that can occur with any procedure, there are certain procedural complications that can occur with OsseoFix. The preoperative radiographs, MRI, and CT scans should be carefully examined for any retropulsed fragments and break in the posterior cortex. The retropulsed fragments may be pushed back into the canal during deployment of the device and can cause adverse neurological outcomes, which may include radiculopathy, paresis, or paralysis. Cement may leak out of the fracture or fissure in the posterior cortex and cause neurological damage. Embolism of fat, thrombus, or other materials can occur during reduction of fracture or delivery of cement and can cause catastrophic clinical sequelae. It is possible, though highly unlikely, that the implant may break, dislocate or get infected and may require revision surgery. Proper patient selection, good fluoroscopic guidance with good quality images, patient compliance, proper surgical training, good understanding of the spinal anatomy to avoid the spinal cord and nerves at all times during insertion of instruments, proper postoperative care and physiotherapy, and treatment of osteoporosis all help to improve the surgical outcome.

## TREATMENT ALTERNATIVES

Vertebroplasty, or augmentation of the vertebral body with cement, was first used in the 1980s for the management of vertebral hemangioma, and later its use was extended to the management of painful osteoporotic VCFs and osteolytic metastasis of spine. The success rate of vertebroplasty for relief of pain is very high as reported in various studies.[9] Cement interdigitates with the trabecular bone of vertebra and thus strengthens the vertebra. However, vertebroplasty does not correct the sagittal alignment, which is important for better biomechanics and to prevent the progression of kyphosis.[10] Moreover, some studies have reported cement leakage and embolism with vertebroplasty, possibly a result of cement injection under high pressure.[11]

Kyphoplasty is a minimally invasive procedure involving the insertion of a bone tamp "pump" via a small cortical window, allowing the low-pressure injection of bone cement (PMMA) into a compression fracture to restore vertebral body height. Kyphoplasty is supposed to correct the vertebral deformity and thus improve the sagittal alignment of spine. It is also argued that cement is injected under low pressure in kyphoplasty, because a cavity is usually created with the bone tamp before the cement is injected. Recent studies have shown that injection pressures depend on the size of the cannula and rate of injection rather than creation of intravertebral cavity. One of the problems with kyphoplasty is that some of the restored height is lost on removal of the balloon tamp before insertion of cement. Also, because

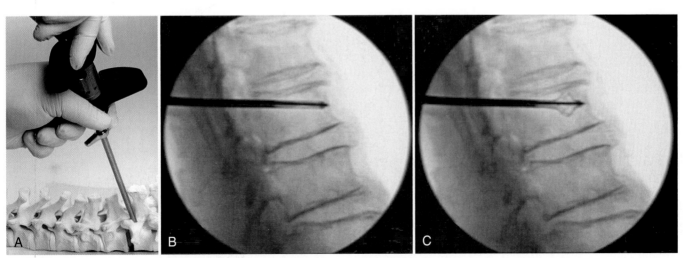

■ **FIGURE 37-11**    **A,** Rotating the metal shaft of the actuator for the deployment of the device. **B,** Fluoroscopic image showing implant insertion in the anterior one third of the vertebral body. **C,** Fluoroscopic images showing deployment of the implant.

the cement bolus does not interdigitate with the cancellous bone in kyphoplasty, it compresses the adjacent cancellous bone with progressive loading and leads to some loss of regained height.

Bed rest, analgesics, bracing, and treatment of osteoporosis remain the mainstay of treatment for stable VCFs. Open decompression, reduction, and fixation by anterior, posterior, or combined approach is warranted whenever there is mechanical compression of the spinal cord or cauda equina with or without neurological deficit.

## DISCUSSION AND CONCLUSION

Early clinical and biomechanical results indicate that the OsseoFix device is successfully able to correct the vertebral deformity and restore the spinal alignment, provide rapid pain relief with dramatic improvement in the quality of life, and also prevent subsequent fractures and progressive kyphosis. Unlike kyphoplasty, OsseoFix allows interdigitation of the cement with the cancellous bone and thus has load-bearing properties. It also uses less cement than kyphoplasty. Moreover, it allows for controlled deployment of the device and reduction of vertebral fracture before injection of cement, delivering predictable and reproducible results. Therefore, positive patient outcomes, improved clinical results, and fewer complications may be expected when using the OsseoFix implant in properly selected patients.

## References

1. D.M. Kado, W.S. Browner, L. Palermo, et al., Vertebral fractures and mortality in older women: a prospective study. Study of Osteoporotic Fractures Research Group, Arch. Intern. Med. 159 (11) (1999) 1215–1220.
2. S.R. Garfin, R.A. Buckley, J. Ledlie, Balloon kyphoplasty for symptomatic vertebral body compression fractures results in rapid, significant, and sustained improvements in back pain, function, and quality of life for elderly patients, Spine 31 (19) (2006) 2213–2220.
3. C. Schlaich, H.W. Minne, T. Bruckner, et al., Reduced pulmonary function in patients with spinal osteoporotic fractures, Osteoporos. Int. 8 (3) (1998) 261–267.
4. S.L. Silverman, M.E. Minshall, W. Shen, et al., The relationship of health-related quality of life to prevalent and incident vertebral fractures in postmenopausal women with osteoporosis: results from the Multiple Outcomes of Raloxifene Evaluation Study, Arthe. Rheum. 44 (11) (2001) 2611–2619.
5. C. Kim, A. Mahar, A. Perry, et al., Biomechanical evaluation of an injectable radiopaque polypropylene fumarate cement for kyphoplasty in a cadaveric osteoporotic vertebral compression fracture model, J. Spinal. Disord. Tech. 20 (8) (2007) 604–609.
6. A. Perry, A. Mahar, J. Massie, et al., Biomechanical evaluation of kyphoplasty with calcium sulfate cement in a cadaveric osteoporotic vertebral compression fracture model, Spine J. 5 (5) (2005) 489–493.
7. V. Upasani, C. Robertson, D. Lee, et al. Biomechanical comparison of kyphoplasty versus a titanium mesh implant for stabilization of vertebral compression fractures. Spine (Accepted, In Press).
8. H. Ghofrani, T. Nunn, C. Robertson, et al., Biomechanical evaluation of a titanium mesh implant compared to kyphoplasty: is bone cement necessary for vertebral body fracture stabilization? Presented: at meeting of North American Spine Society, San Francisco, Calif., 2009.
9. S.R. Garfin, H.A. Yuan, M.A. Reiley, New technologies in spine: kyphoplasty and vertebroplasty for the treatment of painful osteoporotic compression fractures, Spine 26 (14) (2001) 1511–1515.
10. C. Kasperk, J. Hillmeier, G. Noldge, et al., Treatment of painful vertebral fractures by kyphoplasty in patients with primary osteoporosis: a prospective nonrandomized controlled study, J. Bone Miner. Res. 20 (4) (2005) 604–612.
11. M.E. Majd, S. Farley, R.T. Holt, Preliminary outcomes and efficacy of the first 360 consecutive kyphoplasties for the treatment of painful osteoporotic vertebral compression fractures, Spine J. 5 (3) (2005) 244–255.

# 38

# Kiva System in the Treatment of Vertebral Osteoporotic Compression Fractures

*Luis M. Rosales*

---

### KEY POINTS

- The Kiva system is useful for the reduction and the treatment of pathologic compression fractures of the vertebral body that may result from osteoporosis, in segments T10 to L5 of the spine.

- The Kiva system device preserves cancellous architecture using a percutaneously introduced PEEK (Poliether etherKetone) implant in a continuous loop to form a nesting, cylindrical column.

- The implant is delivered over a removable guide wire to provide structural support to the vertebral body. A vertical displacement of the column results in endplate re-elevation and fracture reduction.

- Bone cement is delivered through the lumen of the implant, which provides contained interdigitation into the cancellous bone, thus stabilizing the fracture and minimizing the risk of extravasation.

- The Kiva system achieves an improvement in analog pain scales and Oswestry Disability Index (ODI) and has no adverse effects from components.

## INTRODUCTION

Vertebral compression fractures (VCFs) have a high incidence in the elderly population and are the most common fractures in osteoporotic bones. The majority present without a history of major trauma.[1] The incidence of VCF is increased in patients with a prior vertebral compression fracture, with studies indicating that nearly 20% of patients who have an osteoporotic VCF will develop a second fracture within a year of the first.[2] Not only do these fractures cause significant morbidity in terms of pain, loss of mobility, and kyphosis, but the relative risk of death after a vertebral fracture is nearly nine times greater than in people without a vertebral fracture.[2]

Percutaneous vertebroplasty (PVP) was introduced in France in 1984 by Galibert and Deramond as a treatment for a malignant aggressive hemangioma.[1] It is a therapeutic procedure performed to reduce pain and perhaps to stabilize vertebral lesions. Subsequently PVP was used to treat painful lesions such as hemangiomas, metastasis, multiple myeloma, and osteoporotic fractures. Today most patients undergoing PVP suffer from vertebral osteoporotic compression fractures. PVP is generally seen as a safe and efficient procedure for treatment of painful osteoporotic fractures.

Vertebral augmentation using balloon kyphoplasty and vertebroplasty[3] is traditionally performed with polymethyl methacrylate (PMMA) cement. Clinical studies have demonstrated the efficacy of both methods in reducing fracture-related pain.[2,4] However, there have also been reports of complications: extrusion of cement into surrounding tissue, vascular embolism in the corresponding vascular system, adverse systemic reactions to unpolymerized toxic monomers, and thermal damage to adjacent structures. The two latter complications are specific to PMMA. For this reason, and because PMMA does not become osseointegrated, attempts have been increasingly made in recent years to explore the possibilities of alternative cements by looking into biomaterials based on calcium phosphate (CaP). The properties of such bone cements, however, would have to fit a specific profile that takes into account the following parameters: setting behavior, mechanical fitness, and biological behavior.

There is a new vertebral augmentation device, the Kiva VCF Treatment System (Benvenue Medical, Santa Clara, Calif.), that can be used in the treatment of patients sustaining painful VCFs. Unlike the traditional balloon kyphoplasty procedure that pushes cancellous bone peripherally to form a repository for bone cement, the Kiva device preserves cancellous architecture using a percutaneously introduced Poliether etherKetone implant in a continuous loop to form a nesting, cylindrical column. The implant is delivered over a removable guide wire to provide structural support to the vertebral body, and it is a conduit for bone void filler placement. Vertical displacement by the column results in endplate re-elevation and fracture reduction. Bone cement is delivered through the lumen of the implant, which provides contained interdigitation into the cancellous bone thus stabilizing the fracture and minimizing the risk of extravasation.

## INDICATIONS

The Kiva system is indicated for the management of pathological compression fractures of the vertebral body that may result from osteoporosis, in segments T10 to L5 of the spine. It can also used to treat benign or malignant lesions, by creating a transpedicular channel through which a PEEK implant is inserted into the vertebral body.

## CONTRAINDICATIONS

Contraindications include the following:

- Infection, systemic or local, at the surgical site
- Any medical condition that would preclude the patient from having surgery or would impede the benefit of surgery
- Pathology at the index level(s) (e.g., cancer)
- Neurologic signs or symptoms related to the compression fracture
- Previous surgical treatment for a vertebral body compression fracture
- Index level(s) vertebral body collapse to the degree that access to the vertebral body is not feasible

## PRECAUTIONS

Precautions that should be taken include the following:

- Failure to observe recommendations may contribute to serious patient injuries.
- Avoid contact with the sharp distal tip of the Osteo Coil wire.

- If the device appears damaged, do not use. Discard or return to the manufacturer. This device is intended for single use only.
- This device must be deployed under fluoroscopic guidance. Failure to use fluoroscopic guidance could result in serious patient injuries.

## DESCRIPTION OF THE DEVICE

The Kiva system is packaged as a single-use, sterile device incorporating an implantable PEEK distraction sleeve. It is a surgical instrument designed to provide percutaneous access and channel creation in the cancellous bone of the spine followed by delivery of a PEEK distraction sleeve implant into that channel. The Kiva system consists of five primary components:

1. Nitinol Kiva coil track. (Kiva coil track is a guide wire made of nitinol).
2. Stainless steel deployment with a PEEK liner
3. Polycarbonate deployment handle (Figure 38-1)
4. PEEK distraction sleeve implant made of PEEK-OPTIMA with 15% $BaSO_4$
5. PMMA bone cement delivery needle

The "shape memory" nitinol coil track is preset into a loop shape and it can be temporarily straightened into a cannula for deployment into cancellous bone. Once the cannula is positioned in the cancellous bone, the Kiva coil track is then advanced forward out of the cannula. The surgeon controls the amount of coil track wire deployment with the use of the handle, which allows for 2-mm increments per quarter turn of the coil track deployment knob. Upon exiting the cannula, the coil track regains its loop shape as it channels through the cancellous bone. Once channel creation is complete, the radiopaque PEEK-OPTIMA implant is advanced over the nitinol Kiva coil track and into the channel using the implant deployment knob on the deployment handle.

## CLINICAL PRESENTATION AND EVALUATION

### Material and Methods

Twenty-two patients with radiologically confirmed VCFs between T10 and L5 underwent treatment with the Kiva device for persistent back pain symptoms. Study eligibility required a back pain visual notestyle scale (VAS) score of 5, fracture age less than 6 months, and Oswestry Disability Index (ODI) score of 30%. Patient-reported outcomes (VAS, ODI) were repeated at 3 and 12 months.

## RESULTS

Patients in to the study group ($n = 22$) had a mean age of 70.4 years, and 95.5 % were women. Mean pain scores declined from 7.6 to 2.8 ($p < .0001$). Mean ODI scores declined from 61.0% to 31.7% ($p < .0001$). There were no device-related adverse events.

## OPERATIVE TECHNIQUE

The procedure should be performed under strict aseptic conditions. The treating physician can administer prophylactic antibiotics according to usual practice. The patient is placed on the table in prone position and subjected to sedation according to the ACR Standard for sedation and analgesia in adults. Conscious sedation is induced by intravenous administration of fentanyl and midazolam (Versed) or other medications (e.g., propofol) in accordance with the preference of the treating physician. The patient's vital signs must be monitored during the procedure. If needed, oxygen can be administered by nasal cannula, controlling the breath. Standard fluoroscopy is used to locate the body or the vertebral bodies to be treated and to place the needle to correctly. A 1-inch, 25-gauge needle is used to create a blister to administer subcutaneous bupivacaine 0.25%. Then a 2-inch, 25-gauge needle under fluoroscopic guidance is inserted at the site of the blister and introduced to the periosteum of the pedicle. The periosteum is then infiltrated with 6 to 7 ml bupivacaine 0.25%. A small incision is made in the skin over the pedicle, and the access needle is placed for a transpedicular approach.

The vertebral body is accessed with a cannula, using a standard transpedicular vertebral access technique, always through the right pedicle of the vertebra. With the Kiva handle in the vertebral body, the coil track is advanced using the coil track deployment knob, located on the right hand side of the deployment handle.

1. Using imaging guidance, insert the deployment cannula into the access site and through the cancellous bone. Position the cannula to deploy the Kiva coil track centrally in the anterior column.
2. Rotate the coil track deployment knob on the deployment handle forward slowly to incrementally control to the deployment of the Kiva coil track in the cancellous bone. After one-half turn, check fluoroscopic image for proper orientation of the Kiva coil track exiting the cannula (Figure 38-2).
3. If the Kiva coil track is not oriented in the proper plane or at to the proper position, retract the coil track back into the cannula and reposition the cannula to achieve a more optimal orientation.
4. Repeat steps 2 and 3 until the Kiva coil track is oriented at an optimum plane and position.
5. Using imaging guidance, continue to deploy the Kiva coil track making sure to check the fluoroscope image often (Figure 38-3).
6. Using imaging guidance, continue to deploy the Kiva coil track until the full length of the wire is reached or until the desired number of loops are deployed into a symmetrical stacked toroidal shaped coil.

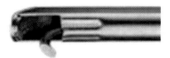

■ **FIGURE 38-2** Percutaneously introduced nitinol Kiva coil (guide wire) advanced through a deployment cannula.

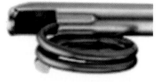

■ **FIGURE 38-3** The nitinol Kiva coil is advanced fully coiled within the cancellous portion of the fractured vertebral body.

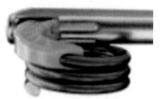

■ **FIGURE 38-4** Radiopaque PEEK-OPTIMA Implant is delivered progressively over the removable Kiva coil.

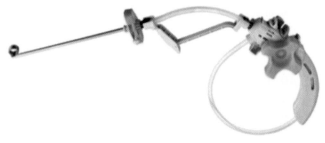

■ **FIGURE 38-1** Kiva handle.

## DEPLOYMENT OF THE DISTRACTION SLEEVE

The radiopaque PEEK-OPTIMA implant is advanced using the distraction sleeve implant deployment knob located on the lefthand side of the deployment handle. The radiopaque PEEK-OPTIMA implant can only be advanced forward, and it may not be retracted once advanced.

1. Once the coil track has been adequately deployed into the cancellous bone, using imaging guidance, advance the radiopaque PEEK-OPTIMA implant over the coil track and into the channel created by the coil track (Figure 38-4).
2. Monitor advancement of the radiopaque PEEK-OPTIMA implant using anteroposterior and lateral fluoroscopy to ensure proper advancement of the distraction sleeve implant.
3. Using imaging guidance, continue advancing the distraction radiopaque PEEK-OPTIMA implant until it reaches the end of the coil track or until resistance is encountered (Figure 38-5).
4. Using imaging guidance assess the position of both the coil and the implant. If any loop of the coil track has opened up to a larger diameter compared to the other coil loops, retract additional lengths of the coil in quarter to half-turn increments until all the loops of the coil track have a uniform diameter.
5. Using imaging guidance, slowly advance the coil in half-turn increments until either the full length of the wire is reached or until or until one of the wire loops begins to open up into a larger diameter than the other loops.
6. Using imaging guidance, advance the distraction implant.
7. Continue to advance the distraction sleeve implant until resistance is encountered or until one of the wire loops beginning to open up to a larger diameter than the other coil track loops.
8. At this point, the implant deployment is complete (Figure 38-6). Remove the coil track completely by rotating the coil track deployment knob backward until the coil track is fully retracted in the deployment handle (Figure 38-7).
9. Retract the distraction sleeve implant pusher completely by rotating the distraction sleeve implant deployment handle backward until the pusher wire is completely retracted into the deployment handle.
10. Disconnect the flexible connector at the end of the deployment handle from the deployment cannula by releasing the tab on the connector switch.

## INJECTING PMMA BONE CEMENT

1. Insert the PMMA bone cement delivery needle through the deployment cannula and advance the needle until the distal tip of the needle engages the lumen of the distraction sleeve implant.
2. Once the tip of the needle has engaged the lumen of the implant, ensure that the bone cement delivery needle is steadily inserted into the implant by rotating the needle back and forth while it is applying gentle forward pressure to the needle.
3. The distraction sleeve implant and vertebral body are now ready for delivery of bone cement. Use bone cement approved for use in the spine (Figure 38-8, *A* and *B*).

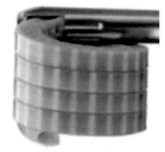

■ **FIGURE 38-5**  A continuous loop forms a nesting, cylindrical column, providing vertical displacement that results in endplate elevation and fracture reduction.

## POSTOPERATIVE CARE

No special postoperative care is needed. After the procedure, the patient can stand up, either the same day or the day after.

## COMPLICATIONS AND AVOIDANCE

This procedure, although performed percutaneously, has the risks of any procedure of vertebroplasty, including infection, bleeding, and neurological complications. With careful technique, these potential complications can be avoided.

## CONCLUSIONS AND DISCUSSION

These findings, albeit short-term, suggest robust and consistent clinical improvement for pain and function outcomes, following this novel vertebral augmentation procedure in patients with painful VCFs. Clinically relevant gains were realized early postoperatively and maintained through follow-up. The device could be deployed and implanted without adverse events, with improvement in VAS pain scores ($p = .0002$) and ODI scores ($p < .0001$),

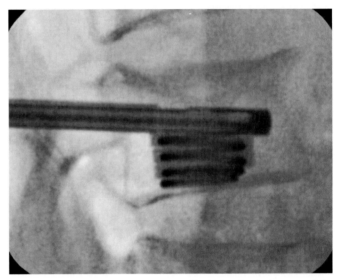

■ **FIGURE 38-6**  Fluoroscopic image illustrating the deployment of the implant over the removable Kiva coil in a continuous loop, properly positioned within the vertebral body.

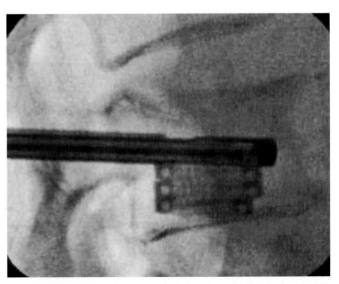

■ **FIGURE 38-7**  After removal of the Kiva coil, the implant is fully deployed and it serves as a conduit for bone cement placement.

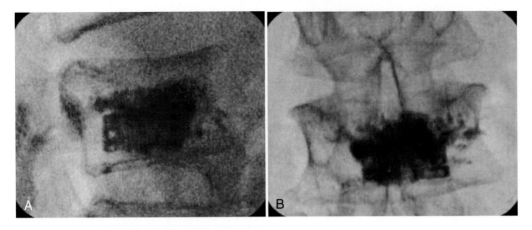

■ **FIGURES 38-8** AP and lateral fluoroscopic images show contained interdigitation of cement into the adjacent cancellous bone, minimizing the risk of cement extravasation, and the fracture is fully stabilized in situ. (A) Lateral and (B) AP view of the fluoroscopic images, show the PEEK implant filled with bone cement in the center of the vertebral body.

with the following overall clinical success criteria: 2-point improvement in VAS and 15-point improvement in ODI. Two cases of cement extravasations occurred without clinical manifestations.

Although the PMMA cement has proved useful in these procedures, biodegradable vertebroplasty materials are being tested. A recent report[5] showed for the first time that there is no difference in clinical and morphologic outcomes after kyphoplasty using either CaP cement (Calcibon) or conventional PMMA material in patients with painful osteoporotic vertebral fractures for at least 3 years of follow-up. There was no significant difference with regard to postoperative pain reduction or the improvement of mobility between the CaP and PMMA groups. Furthermore, there was a comparable height restoration of the fractured vertebral bodies, and no significant difference in the number of vertebral follow-up fractures during the 3-year study period. In daily routine, PMMA is used for the internal stabilization of vertebral fractures by kyphoplasty. However, PMMA is not biodegradable and heals with a fibrous tissue layer around the implant. Therefore CaP cement materials have been developed, which are biodegradable by osteoclastic resorption and allow a direct osseous integration of the entire surface of the implant, whereby a slow replacement by normal bone tissue seems possible.

Vertebroplasty is widely accepted as an effective, minimally invasive procedure, and is becoming the standard of care for the management of painful osteoporotic VCFs. Significant pain relief has been reported in 78% to 95% of patients suffering from osteoporotic VCFs. However, very few articles in the literature have focused on those patients who failed

to respond to the initial PV. Although one study reported that a repeat PVP performed on previously treated vertebral levels for recurrent pain might offer therapeutic benefits (these patients experienced pain relief for 8 to 167 days after the initial PV), we are not aware of any studies on the use of repeat PVs in patients whose pain does not resolve after the initial treatment.[5]

## References

1. R. Rousing, O. Andersen Mikkel, M. Jespersen Stig, K. Thomsen, J. Lauritsen, Percutaneous vertebroplasty compared to conservative treatment in patients with painful acute or subacute osteoporotic vertebral fractures: three-months follow-up in a clinical randomized study, Spine 34 (13) (June 1, 2009) 1349–1354.
2. K. Becky Benz, M. John Gemery, J. John McIntyre, J. Clifford Eskey, Value of immediate pre-procedure magnetic resonance imaging in patients scheduled to undergo vertebroplasty or kyphoplasty, Spine 34 (6) (March 15, 2009) 609–612.
3. R. Blattert Thomas, L. Jestaedt, A. Weckbach, Suitability of a calcium phosphate cement in osteoporotic vertebral body fracture augmentation: a controlled, randomized, clinical trial of balloon kyphoplasty comparing calcium phosphate versus polymethylmethacrylate, Spine 34 (2) (January 15, 2009) 108–114.
4. Shi-Cheng He, Teng, Gao-Jun; Deng, Gang; Fang, Wen; Guo, Jin-He; Zhu, Guang-Yu; Li, Guo-Zhao, Repeat vertebroplasty for unrelieved pain at previously treated vertebral levels with osteoporotic vertebral compression fractures, Spine 33 (6) (March 15, 2008) 640–647.
5. A. Grafe Ingo, M. Baier, G. Nöldge, C. Weiss, K. Da Fonseca, J. Hillmeier, M. Libicher, G. Rudofsky, C. Metzner, P. Nawroth, P.-J. Meeder, C. Kasperk, Calcium-phosphate and polymethylmethacrylate cement in long-term outcome after kyphoplasty of painful osteoporotic vertebral fractures, Spine 33 (11) (May 15, 2008) 1284–1290.

# 39

# Directed Cement Flow Kyphoplasty for Treatment of Osteoporotic Vertebral Compression Fractures

*Kern Singh and Robert Pflugmacher*

> **K E Y   P O I N T S**
>
> - Osteoporotic compression fractures of the thoracic and lumbar spine can be treated successfully from a unilateral approach using the Shield Kyphoplasty System with medium viscosity bone cement.
>
> - Minimally invasive access to the center of the vertebral body is achieved through the use of a novel, curved cavity creation instrument set inserted through a single portal.
>
> - Symmetrical cement augmentation with a low incidence of leakage, particularly in the posterior direction, is facilitated by a cement-directing implant positioned in the center of the vertebral body, which guides cement flow in the anterior, superior, and inferior directions.
>
> - Assessment of vertebral body strength and ability to withstand repeated cyclic compressive loading demonstrates that adequate cement fill, interdigitation, and biomechanical reinforcement is provided by the Shield Kyphoplasty System.
>
> - Treatment of painful osteoporotic compression fractures using the Shield Kyphoplasty System results in immediate pain relief, which is sustained long term, as supported by patient follow-up for up to 2 years.

## INTRODUCTION

Vertebroplasty is one of the most widely used image-guided minimally invasive vertebral augmentation procedures for treating painful vertebral compression fractures. A percutaneous bipedicular approach is typically used to access the vertebral body. Polymethylmethacrylate (PMMA) bone cement is injected directly into the cancellous bone, stabilizing the fracture and providing virtually immediate pain relief. Relatively low viscosity cement is required for this procedure to achieve adequate fill and interdigitation. The cement flow is uncontrolled, however, and leakage into the vascular system, paravertebral space, or disk is commonly reported. Although most cement leaks are asymptomatic, serious leakage-related clinical complications such as compression of neurologic structures or formation of pulmonary embolus have been reported.

In an effort to achieve fracture reduction and restore sagittal balance, balloon kyphoplasty was introduced. This procedure has proven to be safe and efficacious, and its beneficial effects are sustained according to the most recent clinical studies.[1] However, reproducible and clinically significant fracture reduction has not been clearly demonstrated in these same studies.[2,3] The technique involves the use of inflatable bone tamps to create a cavity through compaction of bone and marrow, followed by high viscosity cement injection using bone filling cannulas. The cumulative volume required to fill the large voids requires the use of multiple cannulas, but provides the surgeon greater control of the cement injection rate and volume compared to vertebroplasty. Cement flow and interdigitation are limited to some extent by the compressed bone lining the cavity walls and by the cement viscosity. This technique is generally reliable and safe, provided cement viscosity is high and the operator includes careful fluoroscopic monitoring.

More recently, new devices and procedures have been designed to achieve fracture reduction and reduce leakage rates. The Shield Kyphoplasty System (Soteira, Inc., Natick Mass.) was developed to better contain and control the flow of cement, reduce cement leakage rate and create biomechanically optimized cement augmentation. In this chapter, the components of the Shield Kyphoplasty System and the associated surgical technique will be described in detail. Mechanical testing of fractured osteoporotic vertebral bodies treated with this system under monotonic and cyclic loading conditions will be discussed. Finally, the primary outcomes from long-term clinical evaluations of this system will be presented, including a randomized multicenter study that compared pain relief and cement leakage for the Shield Kyphoplasty System and conventional bipedicular vertebroplasty.

## SYSTEM OVERVIEW

The Shield system features a non–load-bearing, hollow, self-expanding implant that is deployed into a cavity created within the center of the fractured vertebral body. The function of the device is to initially contain injected cement, then to regulate and direct the flow of the cement through engineered openings in the anterior wall of the device. Cement injection into the implant and through the openings creates a mantle of cement in the anterior vertebral body, which spans the endplates and stabilizes the fracture by filling cracks and voids, interdigitating with viable trabecular bone. Placement of the device in a central cavity helps to limit posterior flow of cement via the basivertebral plexus and allows cement to permeate the entire vertebral body using a unipedicular approach.

The Shield system includes a set of single patient use disposable instruments for unipedicular percutaneous access and specially designed instruments for cavity creation, implant deployment, and cement injection, as shown in Figure 39-1. The unique curved design of the cavity creation instrument allows the surgeon to drill a curved path from one pedicle, crossing the sagittal midline, and stopping within the contralateral anterior quadrant of the vertebral body. The cavity creation instrument then converts to a reamer in situ, which is capable of creating a 10-mm diameter cylindrical cavity in the retrograde (proximal) direction that is matched to the implant size. The delivery system subsequently provides a means to insert and deploy the cement directing device within the cavity and facilitates cement injection with a high pressure injection system.

The Shield cement director is an elongated 10-mm diameter hollow structure fabricated from braided nitinol wire and other biocompatible textile and polymeric materials. The device is available in three lengths: 15 mm, 20 mm, and 25 mm, a range selected to approximate the anatomic distance between the medial pedicle borders in the thoracic and lumbar spine in the patient population with osteoporosis. The cylindrical wall of the implant is impermeable to bone cement with the exception of small holes located anteriorly-superiorly and anterior-inferiorly on the device, as shown in Figure 39-2. The implant is supplied preloaded onto a delivery device and

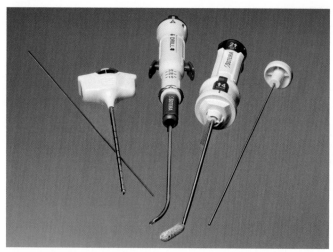

■ **FIGURE 39-1** Components of the Shield Kyphoplasty System. Shown from left to right are the blunt tipped wire, working channel, curved drill/cavity cutter, implant and cement delivery system, and tamp.

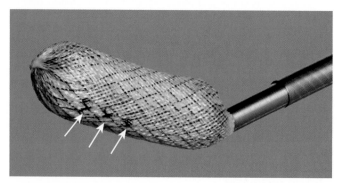

■ **FIGURE 39-2** The Shield implant, shown in the expanded state. The holes (3 of 6 holes shown, arrows) are positioned to direct cement flow in the anterior, superior and inferior directions. There are no holes on the posterior surface of the implant to prevent cement flow in this direction.

collapsed within a sheath to facilitate placement into the cavity through the working channel. After placement, the sheath is retracted to deploy the self-expanding implant in the prepared cavity.

## INDICATIONS

The Shield Kyphoplasty System is intended for use in the treatment of osteoporotic vertebral body compression fractures in the adult spine in levels T4-L5. It is intended to be used with a PMMA bone cement cleared for use in vertebral body fixation. Up to three levels with osteoporotic compression fractures may be treated during one operative session regardless of fracture age, excluding vertebral plana, unstable fractures, or suspected infection.

## CONTRAINDICATIONS

The Shield Kyphoplasty System should not be used when the following conditions are present:

- Previously resected or augmented vertebral body
- Burst fractures
- Spinal canal compromise
- Uncorrectable coagulation disorder or bleeding disorders of any etiology
- Active systemic or local infection
- Pregnancy
- Multiple myeloma
- Vertebral bodies having less than adequate space between endplates for 10-mm cavity creation.

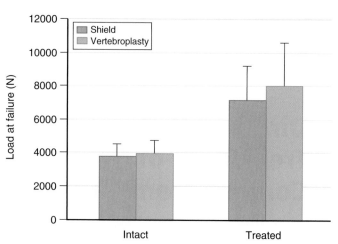

■ **FIGURE 39-3** Comparison of failure loads for intact and treated vertebral body specimens. The vertebral bodies were subjected to uniaxial compression until a 25% reduction in height was achieved. The failure load was defined as the maximum load attained during compression. The mean failure loads were equivalent for both treatments.

- Vertebral bodies with less than adequate space to allow for the creation of a 15-mm long cavity
- Greater than three levels needing treatment
- Inability to intraoperatively visualize anatomy under fluoroscopic guidance

## BIOMECHANICAL TESTING

The mechanical behavior of fractured osteoporotic vertebral bodies treated with the Shield Kyphoplasty System has been studied under monotonic and cyclic loading conditions. Controlled, reproducible compression fractures were created by applying a uniaxial compressive load until the vertebral body experienced a 25% loss in height. The fractured vertebral bodies were subsequently treated with either the Shield Kyphoplasty System or bipedicular vertebroplasty, which was used as a comparative control. The failure strength of intact and treated vertebral bodies is shown in Figure 39-3. There were no statistically significant differences between the intact failure strengths or the treated failure strengths for both groups ($p = .146$). Treatment of vertebral compression fractures with Shield Kyphoplasty System, using a unipedicular approach, resulted in biomechanical performance that was equivalent to conventional bipedicular vertebroplasty. Furthermore, the presence of the cement director appears to have no detectable effect on the ability of the bone cement to interdigitate and reinforce the fractured vertebral body.

Cyclic loading tests were performed to assess the ability of fractured vertebral bodies treated with the Shield Kyphoplasty System to withstand repeated compressive loads and bending moments, as encountered during activities associated with daily living. Stryker SpinePlex PMMA bone cement (Stryker Howmedica, Allendale, N.J.) was used to treat all specimens. Because fresh cadaveric vertebral bodies cannot be tested in a 37° C saline bath for long periods of time without experiencing biological degradation, the cyclic loading tests were accelerated by increasing the compressive load stepwise until the treated vertebral body failed.

Treated vertebral bodies either failed during cyclic loading at the first load level (6 of 15 specimens), or they required multiple loading levels to fail (9 of 15 specimens). A compilation of all of the results from the cyclic testing of treated vertebral bodies is provided in Figure 39-4. For 6 of 8 specimen pairs, the specimen treated with the Shield Kyphoplasty System withstood a greater number of loading cycles and failed at a higher load than the specimen treated with conventional vertebroplasty. These results demonstrate that directed cement flow using the unipedicular Shield Kyphoplasty System can provide biomechanical reinforcement to fractured osteoporotic vertebral bodies that is equivalent to or better than conventional vertebroplasty, while reducing the risk of posterior leakage.

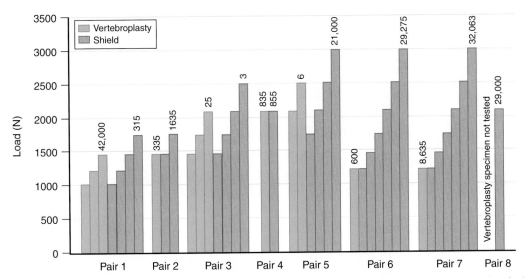

■ **FIGURE 39-4**    Summary of cyclic testing results for treated vertebral body specimens. Testing was performed on specimen pairs, obtained from adjacent levels from the same donor spine. For 6 of 8 pairs, vertebral bodies treated with the Shield Kyphoplasty System withstood a greater number of loading cycles and failed at higher load levels as compared to specimens treated with vertebroplasty.

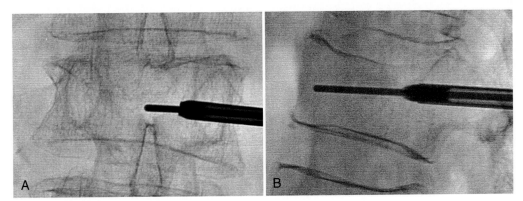

■ **FIGURE 39-5**    Blunt tip wire verifies medial needle placement in A/P (**A**) and lateral (**B**) fluoroscopic images. *(Images provided by Dr. G. C. Anselmetti, Institute for Cancer Research and Treatment, Torino, Italy.)*

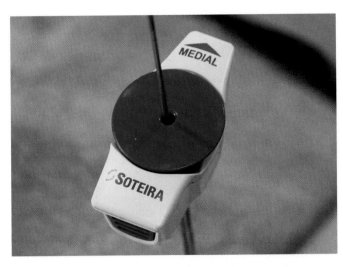

■ **FIGURE 39-6**    The working channel cannula is placed over the wire and advanced into the vertebral body 3 to 5 mm beyond the posterior cortical wall. Medial marking is oriented toward the patient's spine.

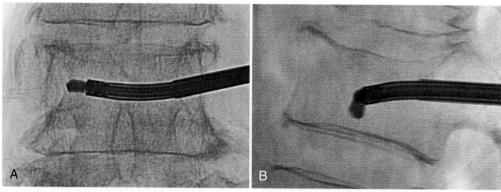

■ **FIGURE 39-7** Fluoroscopic images of the drill advancing along a curved path (**A,** AP view). Drilling is complete when the contralateral pedicle is reached. The blade is deflected and a 10-mm diameter cavity is created as the instrument is counterrotated (**B,** lateral view). *(Images provided by Dr. G. C. Anselmetti, Institute for Cancer Research and Treatment, Torino, Italy.)*

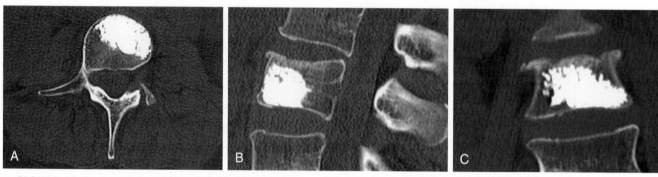

■ **FIGURE 39-8** Axial (**A**), lateral (**B**), and AP (**C**) CT images of the cement mantle created by the Shield implant. Cement fills the implant, flows through the holes and is directed to the anterior, superior and inferior regions of the vertebral body. Flow in the posterior direction is limited, reducing the risk of posterior leakage. *(Images provided by Dr. G. Stender, Groenemeyer-Institute, Bochum, Germany)*

## THE SHIELD KYPHOPLASTY SYSTEM SURGICAL TECHNIQUE

The percutaneous needle approach used for the Shield Kyphoplasty System is similar to the original kyphoplasty procedure widely used to treat vertebral compression fractures. However, only a single needle placement targeting the anterior sagittal midline is required for the Shield system for all levels of the spine. The approach angle and needle position is verified with anteroposterior (AP) and lateral fluoroscopy, as shown in Figure 39-5. Once angular orientation has been established, the needle is advanced into the vertebral body beyond the posterior cortical wall. The stylet of the needle is removed and replaced with a blunt tipped wire. The needle is then retracted leaving the wire in place. A 4-mm outer diameter working channel cannula is then placed over the wire to a depth of 5 mm anterior to the posterior cortical wall, as depicted in Figure 39-6. Proper placement of the working channel cannula includes orienting the key slot in the medial direction. This ensures that all subsequent invasive steps in the procedure involving bone cutting will have the proper medial orientation.

The Shield Kyphoplasty System cavity cutter is inserted within and locked to the working channel. The cutting device is designed to drill along a curved path projecting anteriorly and medially from the end of the working channel. The surgeon advances the drill by manually rotating in the clockwise direction while stabilizing the working channel with the other hand. It is recommended that drilling be ceased once the blade tip has reached the medial border of the contralateral pedicle, as shown in Figure 39-7. Once the path is complete, the blade is deflected to 10 mm. A cylindrical cavity is created as the blade rotates and translates along the original path in the proximal direction. After several turns, the blade is retracted at a predetermined point on the proximal end of the path to create a cavity that is the same length as the selected implant: 15 mm, 20 mm, or 25 mm.

The appropriate size delivery system with a preloaded Shield implant is then inserted into the working channel. The delivery system is curved, allowing the Shield implant to be deployed precisely within the central cavity. Removal of an internal wire exposes a luer connector, which is the

cement fill portal. The Shield Kyphoplasty System includes a bone cement mixing and injection device that mates with the delivery system. The injection system is capable of injecting high viscosity cement. Cement injection should be performed under biplanar fluoroscopic imaging. The materials used in the construction of the Shield cement director allow visualization of the cement while it fills the implant and flows into the anterior, superior, and inferior regions of the cancellous bone, as shown in Figure 39-8.

Postoperatively, patients treated with the Shield Kyphoplasty System require the same care as given following standard vertebroplasty and kyphoplasty procedures. Potential complications are also similar to these procedures and include possible cement leakage, pulmonary embolus, neuropathy, and endplate fracture.

## CLINICAL OUTCOMES

The clinical performance of the Shield Kyphoplasty System has been evaluated in a 1-year, multicenter, prospective, 2:1 randomized controlled study comparing pain relief, cement leakage rates, and leak locations for the Shield and conventional percutaneous vertebroplasty.[4] The patient population for this study consisted of adults at least 50 years old with osteoporosis and painful benign vertebral compression fractures at one to three levels between T4 and L5. A total of 77 patients and 104 levels were treated, 49 patients (65 levels) with the Shield Kyphoplasty System and 28 patients (39 levels) with conventional vertebroplasty. The Shield procedure was performed using a unilateral transpedicular or extrapedicular approach, whereas the vertebroplasty procedure was performed using a standard bipedicular approach.

Pain was assessed using a 10-point visual analog scale (VAS) at 24 hours postoperatively, 3 months, and again at 1 year. To evaluate and compare cement leakage rates, plain radiographs (AP and lateral) and CT scans were obtained within 24 hours of the procedure. Cement leakage was assessed by the operating surgeon (radiographs) and an independent reviewer (CT images). The increased resolution of the CT images allowed small leaks to be identified that would have been overlooked on radiographic images.

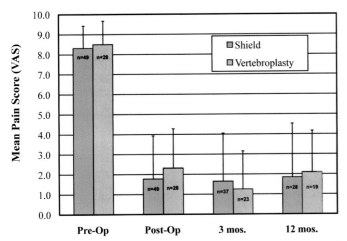

■ **FIGURE 39-9**    Pain scores for multicenter randomized 1-year clinical study comparing treatment of painful osteoporotic compression fractures with the Shield Kyphoplasty System and conventional vertebroplasty. Pain scores dropped substantially 24 hours postoperatively, and pain relief was sustained through the 12-month follow-up period.

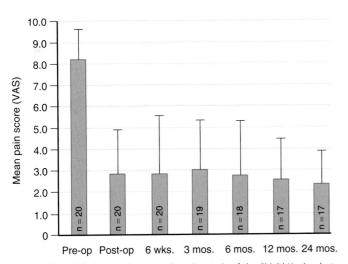

■ **FIGURE 39-10**    Pain scores for pilot study of the Shield Kyphoplasty System. Pain relief was maintained throughout the 2-year follow-up period.

Cement leaks were classified as follows: Type B—through the basivertebral vein, Type C—through a cortical bone defect (including endplates), and Type S—through a segmental vein.[5]

Significant pain relief was achieved immediately following treatment with both the Shield Kyphoplasty System and conventional vertebroplasty, as shown in Figure 39-9. Mean preoperative pain scores were $8.31 \pm 1.12$ and $8.49 \pm 1.18$ for the Shield and vertebroplasty groups, respectively. The mean pain scores decreased by more than 6 points for both groups at 24 hours post-op, and pain relief was sustained during the 12-month follow-up period. The results of a single arm, two-year pilot study (20 patients) further demonstrate that long-term pain relief is achieved in patients treated with the Shield Kyphoplasty System, as shown in Figure 39-10.

In the randomized clinical study, cement leaks were identified and classified from both plain radiographic images and CT reconstructions. Leakage rates reported in the literature are highly variable, ranging from 7% to 90% for vertebroplasty and 0% to 33% for kyphoplasty.[6] This data is often difficult to interpret because different methods are used to assess leak rates, and the resolution can vary among the methods and among institutions. In general, studies that use CT imaging to quantify cement leaks report much greater leakage rates than studies that rely on routine radiographic interpretation. The overall leakage rate for patients treated with the Shield Kyphoplasty System was substantially lower than the leakage rate for patients treated

**TABLE 39-1    Cement Leakage Rates (Leaks/Treated Levels)**[*]

|  | Radiographs | CT Images |
| --- | --- | --- |
| Shield Kyphoplasty System | 8/65 (12.3%) | 42/65 (64.6%) |
| Vertebroplasty | 10/39 (25.6%) | 54/39 (138.5%) |

[*]Some levels exhibited multiple leaks.

**TABLE 39-2    Leak Classification (Leaks/Treated Levels)**[*]

|  | Type B | Type C | Type S |
| --- | --- | --- | --- |
| Shield Kyphoplasty System | 8/65 (12.3%) | 15/65 (23.1%) | 19/65 (29.2%) |
| Vertebroplasty | 12/39 (30.8%) | 22/39 (56.4%) | 20/39 (51.3%) |

[*]Some levels exhibited multiple leaks.

with conventional vertebroplasty, as shown in Table 39-1. Eight levels in the Shield group and 14 levels in the control group exhibited multiple leaks and in these instances, each leak was counted and classified separately. The leakage rate for all types of leaks was decreased for the Shield treatment group, as compared to the vertebroplasty treatment group shown in Table 39-2. The Type B leakage rate, involving cement leakage into the basivertebral vein, was markedly decreased for patients treated with the Shield system and was the lowest leakage rate observed overall. This result confirms that anteriorly directed cement flow is effectively achieved by using the Shield implant.

## CONCLUSIONS

The Shield Kyphoplasty System provides new direction and control capabilities for treatment of osteoporotic vertebral compression fractures. This system can be used to effectively treat painful fractures of the thoracic and lumbar spine from a unilateral approach. The unique curved cavity creation instrument provides minimally invasive access to the center of the vertebral body, allowing the Shield cement-directing implant to be reproducibly positioned and oriented. Bone cement is injected into the implant, which guides cement flow in the anterior, superior and inferior directions. Mechanical testing demonstrates that the cement mantle formed by the Shield implant interdigitates with the intact bone structure, stabilizes the fracture, and provides enduring biomechanical reinforcement. Good long-term clinical outcomes have been obtained for the Shield system, as compared to bipedicular vertebroplasty. Pain relief is immediate and sustained for at least 2 years postoperatively. Directed cement flow additionally reduces leakage rates and the risk of leakage-related complications, potentially improving the safety of the procedure.

## References

1. D. Wardlaw, S.R. Cummings, J. Van Meirhaeghe, L. Bastian, J.B. Tillman, J. Ranstam, R. Eastell, P. Shabe, K. Talmadge, S. Boonen, Efficacy and safety of balloon kyphoplasty compared with non-surgical care for vertebral compression fracture (FREE): a randomised controlled trial, Lancet 373 (9668) (2009 Mar 21) 1016–1024.
2. A. Hiwatashi, R. Sidhu, R.K. Lee, R.R. deGuzman, D.T. Piekut, P.L. Westesson, Kyphoplasty versus vertebroplasty to increase vertebral body height: a cadaveric study, Radiology 237 (3) (2005) 1115–1119.
3. B.B. Pradhan, H.W. Bae, M.A. Kropf, V.V. Patel, R.B. Delamarter, Kyphoplasty reduction of osteoporotic vertebral compression fractures: correction of local kyphosis versus overall sagittal alignment, Spine 31 (4) (2006 Feb 15) 435–441.
4. R. Pflugmacher, J. Hierholzer, G. Stender, R. Hammerstingl, E. Truumees, A.K. Wakhloo, M.J. Gounis, T.J. Vogl, Evaluation of leakage rates for a cement directing kyphoplasty system, Presented at the 25th Annual Meeting of the North American Spine Society, San Francisco CA, Nov. 10-14, 2009.
5. J.S. Yeom, W.J. Kim, W.S. Choy, C.K. Lee, B.S. Chang, J.W. Kang, Leakage of cement in percutaneous transpedicular vertebroplasty for painful osteoporotic compression fractures, J. Bone Joint. Surg. Br. 85 (1) (2003 Jan) 83–89.
6. P.A. Hulme, J. Krebs, S.J. Ferguson, U. Berlemann, Vertebroplasty and kyphoplasty: a systematic review of 69 clinical studies, Spine 31 (17) (2006 Aug 1) 1983–2001.

# 40

# Radiofrequency Kyphoplasty: A Novel Approach to Minimally Invasive Treatment of Vertebral Compression Fractures

*Kieran Murphy*

---

**K E Y   P O I N T S**

- In-line use of radiofrequency (RF) energy to warm cement immediately before being delivered permits extended working time for consistent delivery of an ultra-high viscosity cement.

- A navigational osteotome device permits site- and size-specific cavity creation before cement augmentation, increasing the potential for uniportal treatment of vertebral compression fractures.

- Remote-controlled cement delivery system provides potential for reduced radiation exposure.

- RF kyphoplasty provides pain relief and reduction in vertebral compression fracture–related disability similar to that reported for conventional balloon kyphoplasty and vertebroplasty.

---

## INTRODUCTION

Percutaneous treatment of vertebral compression fractures (VCFs) was first performed in France in 1984 by Galibert and Deramond.[1] The two most commonly performed minimally invasive VCF procedures are known as vertebroplasty and kyphoplasty. The primary difference is that in kyphoplasty, commonly referred to as percutaneous vertebral augmentation, a cavity using a mechanical device is created before cement delivery.* Both procedures have been shown to provide dramatic pain relief in vertebral body fractures associated with underlying osteoporosis or malignancy, and have been successfully applied in cases in which conservative management has failed and surgery is undesirable.[1-7,10-14] Because they have a higher incidence of osteoporosis, most patients referred for this procedure are women. However, men with vertebral body fractures from osteoporosis also present for treatment. Many of the characteristics of the male population with osteoporotic vertebral body fractures have recently been described.[4,7] Vertebral body fractures are the most common osteoporotic fractures in men. Like those in women, they are associated with significant morbidity and restriction of activities of daily living.[8] The economic impact of osteoporotic fractures was estimated at nearly $2.7 billion in 1995 for men alone,[9] making this a substantial health care problem from the standpoint of both cost and morbidity.

Minimally invasive treatment of vertebral compression fractures requires the image-guided insertion of a needle or working cannula through or adjacent to the pedicle into the vertebral body. Acrylic or calcium phosphate bone cement is then injected into the vertebral body (either with or without performing cavity creation) where it solidifies, providing structural support and preventing the movement associated with pain.[3,14]

In 2002 there were approximately 38,000 vertebroplasties and 16,000 kyphoplasties performed in the United States. By 2007 this grew to approximately 80,000 vertebroplasties and 50,000 kyphoplasties in 2007. As the use of both modalities for the treatment of vertebral compression fractures has increased, so have questions regarding safety and efficacy and the need for greater control of cement delivery. A desire for restoration of height (in mobile fractures) and a minimalist approach to the procedure has lead to interest in convergence and evolution in the field of minimally invasive treatment of VCF, just as the Montgolfier brothers and the Wright brothers competed in some ways. Although both procedures are largely safe, U.S. Food and drug Administration (FDA) data have highlighted two main concerns: venous extravasation resulting in cord compression and pulmonary emboli leading in some cases to paralysis.

Although both vertebroplasty and kyphoplasty are largely safe and provide similar rates of pain relief, the added complexity and possible radiation exposure of multiple steps associated with conventional (balloon-assisted) kyphoplasty have been considered by some as warranted because it offers the possibility of restoring vertebral height and it carries lower rates of cement leakage than vertebroplasty. The value of controlling cement delivery and potential for height restoration, when possible, are universally accepted. Cement control in a clinical environment can be modified in two ways—the viscosity at the time of delivery and the amount of time (working time) the cement can be delivered. Numerous emerging technologies are focused on providing physicians promising new therapies for managing vertebral compression fractures of the spine in a minimalist, safe way, while providing patients with much needed pain relief. Since 2006, technology has evolved so extensively that the traditional use of the procedural term kyphoplasty has been expanded to incorporate the use of other technologies. Initially, kyphoplasty was defined as the "balloon procedure." Today there are additional technologies designed for minimally invasive, cavity creating VCF treatment. Consequently, procedure terminology has evolved, as evidenced by Centers for Medicare and Medicaid Services (CMS) 2009 fiscal year International Classification of Diseases (ICD-9) code title for "Kyphoplasty" being replaced with "Percutaneous Vertebral Augmentation," and "conventional" balloon-assisted procedures being listed as an example of vertebral augmentation procedures.

The StabiliT Vertebral Augmentation System (DFine Inc., San Jose, CA, USA) is a novel product intended for the treatment of VCFs associated with osteoporotic fractures and tumors of the spine in a procedure known as radiofrequency (RF) kyphoplasty. RF kyphoplasty is designed

---

*AMA Current Procedural Terminology (CPT) 2009 for Vertebral Augmentation Procedures reads: "Percutaneous vertebral augmentation, including cavity creation (fracture reduction and bone biopsy included when performed) using mechanical device, one vertebral body, unilateral or bilateral cannulation (e.g., kyphoplasty)". ICD-9-CM procedure code addendum (ICD-9 CM 2009 Volumes 1 & 2) for Percutaneous Vertebral Augmentation reads: Insertion of inflatable balloon, bone tamp, or other device displacing (removing) (compacting) bone to create a space (cavity) (void) prior to the injection of bone void filler (cement) (polymethylmethacrylate) (PMMA) or other substance.

to minimize leakage, enable height restoration of mobile fractures, and provide pain relief through fracture stabilization by way of site- and size-specific cavity creation and extended, controlled delivery of an ultra-high viscosity cement. This new percutaneous vertebral augmentation system combines the following unique attributes: navigational cavity creation device; RF energy modulated, ultra-high viscosity cement; unique, hydraulic delivery system; and a remotely controlled delivery mechanism to offer additional control to the physician in treatment of a VCF. The use of RF energy to modulate bone cement polymerization immediately before entering the patient permits the system to maintain cement in a reservoir at ambient temperature with a very long working time, yet deliver cement of a viscosity many times higher than conventionally delivered polymethyl methacrylate (PMMA) cement. This control during the cement delivery results in the potential for reduced venous extravasation and yet retains the ability to move bone fragments and restore height.

This chapter reviews the novel StabiliT Vertebral Augmentation System and the initial cadaver and clinical experience in which the system was used to perform the RF kyphoplasty. The potential ability of the StabiliT Vertebral Augmentation System in performing RF kyphoplasty to restore vertebral height is comparable to that of conventional vertebroplasty and conventional balloon kyphoplasty procedures in a cadaver model. The early clinical experience, generated by interventional neuroradiologists, orthopedic surgeons, and neurosurgeons, is compared with clinical results previously reported for conventional vertebroplasty and balloon kyphoplasty. To date, over 1200 patients have been treated with the StabiliT Vertebral Augmentation System without symptomatic cement extravasation.

## MATERIALS AND METHODS

### The StabiliT Vertebral Augmentation System

The StabiliT Vertebral Augmentation System is a unique RF controlled cement delivery system for the treatment of vertebral compression fractures. It has been cleared for use in the United States for percutaneous delivery of StabiliT ER (Energy Responsive) Bone Cement in kyphoplasty procedures in the treatment of painful vertebral compression fractures, which may result

from osteoporosis, benign lesions (hemangioma), and malignant lesions (metastatic cancers, myeloma). It contains the following components: a proprietary energy-responsive PMMA bone cement (StabiliT ER Bone Cement); a unique vacuum saturation cement mixing system (Saturate Mixing System); a controller (Mulitplex Controller) that contains both a radiofrequency generator and a hydraulic drive; introducer/working cannulae for access to the vertebral body; straight and navigational cavity creation devices to permit specificity of the site and size of the cavity; a PFA (Teflon-like)-lined heating element (Activation Element) and delivery cannulae to permit the delivery of uniquely high viscosity PMMA cement; and a 3-m-long cable to permit remote-control delivery of the cement, thereby controlling the operator's radiation exposure (Figure 40-1). Following cavity creation using the articulated arm of the Mid-Line Osteotome, the StabiliT System (DFine Inc., San Jose, CA, USA) preferentially delivers cement to the cavity but further permits interdigitation of the ultra-high viscosity cement into the adjacent trabecular beds (Figure 40-2).

## In Vitro Evaluation of Height Restoration and Intravertebral Pressure in Three Minimally Invasive Procedures Using an Osteoporotic Cadaver Bone Model

The potential to restore height in mobile vertebral compression fractures and the possible impact on intravertebral pressure have been reported in various studies.[17,18] Cadaver spines obtained from women between 66 and 87 years of age were used. The specimens in each study had bone mineral densities (BMDs) of $0.687 \pm 0.136 \text{ g/cm}^3$ and $0.707 \pm 0.136 \text{ g/cm}^3$ respectively. Individual vertebral bodies (VBs) were prepared by transecting the pedicles and removing all disc material from the endplates. Cephalac and caudal surfaces of each vertebral body were rigidly embedded in a urethane potting compound (Smooth ON, Easton, Penn.).

Each vertebral body was mounted in a custom semiconstrained fixture and rigidly attached to a servohydraulic load frame (8521S, Instron Corp, Canton, Mass.). A 500-N offset load was applied to the specimen and a radiograph taken to determine prefracture anterior vertebral body height (GE OEC Diasonics Model 9000, Fairfield, Conn.). Offset loads were applied at a displacement rate of 5 mm/min with a data acquisition rate of 20 Hz. Monotonic testing was performed until the height of the vertebral body had been

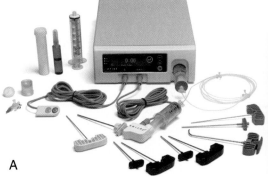
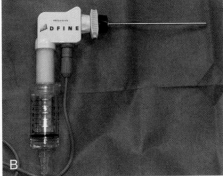

■ **FIGURE 40-1**  **A,** StabiliT Vertebral Augmentation System for radiofrequency kyphoplasty. **B,** Cement in the reservoir before passing through the Activation Element and delivery cannula has extended working time.

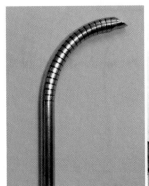
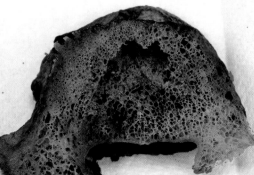
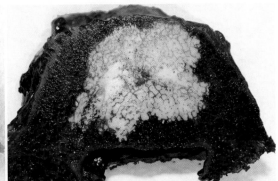

■ **FIGURE 40-2**  Navigational Osteotome permits site-specific cavity creation and interdigitation of ultra-high viscosity cement.

reduced by 30%. Postfracture height was determined using radiographic images under a 500-N compressive offset loads. Each treatment, conventional balloon kyphoplasty (BKP) (KyphX, Medtronic Inc., Memphis, Tenn.) , RF kyphoplasty (RFK) (StabiliT Vertebral Augmentation System) and vertebroplasty (Vertebroplastic, DePuy Spine Inc., Raynham, Mass.), was performed on randomly assigned vertebral bodies.

All three procedures (BKP, RFK, and vertebroplasty) were utilized by physicians skilled in these minimally invasive techniques. Standard bipedicular technique was used in the BKP specimen. RFK was performed using a unipedicular technique and the MidLine Osteotome. A total of 6 ml bone cement was used in all specimens. After each treatment, vertebral bodies were incubated in a 37° C water bath for a minimum of 2 hours before posttreatment radiographic evaluation. Posttreatment radiographs were taken while a 500-N offset load was applied to the specimen. Anterior height was measured from the prefracture, postfracture, and posttreatment radiographs using Photoshop (Adobe Systems, Inc., San Jose, Calif.). Each measurement was done by five different individuals blinded to the treatment performed on the specimens (Figure 40-3). Statistical comparisons between the treatment groups were performed, and statistical significance was defined as $p < .05$. In one of the studies, a pressure transducer was placed into the venous plexus through the posterior cortex to measure the intravertebral pressure during cement delivery.

## RESULTS

A significant difference in height was found between the prefracture and postfracture specimens for all three groups. Mechanical VCF height elevation equivalent to that observed in BKP was achieved using RFK. In contrast, conventional vertebroplasty procedure, in which cement simply fills existing VCF voids before extravasation via the path of least resistance, was unable to restore comparable height. The mean anterior height restorations for the conventional BKP, RFK, and vertebroplasty systems were 74.8 ± 9.4%, 83.7 ± 17.5%, and 32.8 ± 8.1%, respectively.[17] There was no significant difference between the BKP and RFK groups ($p = .40$). The BKP and RFK procedures both restored significantly more height than that achieved with the vertebroplasty procedure ($p \leq .001$ and $p \leq .002$ respectively). The mean maximum intravertebral pressures recorded during RFK, BKP, and vertebroplasty were 9.8 ± 0.1 kPa, 9.8 ± 0.0 kPa, and 14.7 ± 9.7 kPa, respectively. Wilcoxon signed rank tests did not yield any significant differences between the RF kyphoplasty and vertebroplasty ($p = .5$), balloon kyphoplasty, and vertebroplasty ($p = 1.0$) or RF kyphoplasty and balloon kyphoplasty ($p = 1.0$) treatment groups.[16] These data demonstrate that the use of an ultra-high viscosity cement and an appropriate delivery system can provide an alternative to currently available methods to restore height in a VCF without adverse increases in intravertebral pressure.

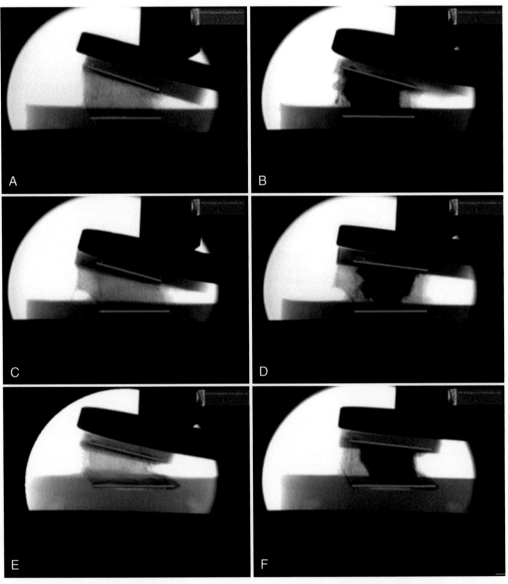

■ **FIGURE 40-3**    Images of postfracture (on left) and posttreatment (on right) vertebral bodies vertebroplasty (**A, B**), conventional balloon kyphoplasty (**C, D**), and radiofrequency kyphoplasty (**E, F**).

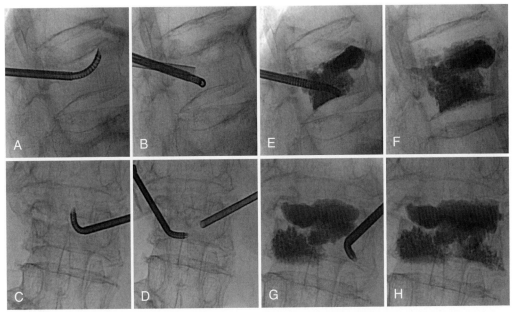

**■ FIGURE 40-4** Intraoperative images demonstrating site-specific cavity creation and ultra-high viscosity cement augmentation. Pre injection xrays: with single cannula (A and B) and double cannulas (C and D); Post injection xrays (E, F, G and H). *(Courtesy of Dr. Florian Elgeti, Charité-Universitätsmedizin Berlin.)*

## RF KYPHOPLASTY CLINICAL EXPERIENCE WITH THE StabiliT VERTEBRAL AUGMENTATION SYSTEM

To date, over 2000 vertebral levels and 1200 RF kyphoplasty cases have been performed using the StabiliT Vertebral Augmentation System. No cement-related symptomatic adverse events have been reported to date. The procedure involves a site-specific cavity creation using the MidLine Osteotome under fluoroscopic guidance, followed by controlled delivery of an ultra high viscosity cement (Figure 40-4). The ultra-high viscosity cement preferentially fills the site-specific cavity before driving into the fracture planes and interdigitating into the adjacent trabeculae. Because only the cement that is delivered into the patient is exposed to RF energy, cement delivery can be delayed for extended periods of time if need be to minimize extravasation in cases of large fractures planes or lytic lesions. The initial clinical experience included a prospective controlled clinical trial performed under an Ethics Committee–approved protocol at three sites in two countries (Hungary and Austria) and performed by physicians of three disciplines: neurosurgery, interventional radiology, and orthopedic surgery. Patients in this study (SPACE—Spinal Augmentation with Cement and Energy) were eligible for enrollment if they had one to three vertebral fractures from T7 through L5. Clinical results of the first 104 fractures in 73 patients treated to date with the StabiliT system were reported in the 2009 Scientific Meeting of the Society for Interventional Radiology.[17] The study demonstrated pain relief (measured by visual analogue scale [VAS]) and improved function (measured by Oswestry Disability Index [ODI]) consistent with published data for conventional balloon kyphoplasty and vertebroplasty (Table 40-1). As has been reported for conventional balloon kyphoplasty and vertebroplasty, RF kyphoplasty reduced pain scores greater than 50% when measured by the VAS, a validated instrument.

Additionally, in a series of 20 VCFs in 14 patients, Elgeti reported height restoration and kyphosis correction in 50% of the fractures, with an average height restoration of 4 mm and kyphosis correction of 5.6 degrees (Figure 40-5).[18]

## DISCUSSION

The StabiliT Vertebral Augmentation System has been cleared for use in the United States for percutaneous delivery of StabiliT ER Bone Cement in kyphoplasty procedures in the treatment of pathological fractures of the vertebrae. Painful vertebral compression fractures may result from osteoporosis, benign lesions (hemangioma), and malignant lesions (metastatic cancers, myeloma).

**TABLE 40-1    Clinical Results from the European Prospective Clinical Trial with the StabiliT Vertebral Augmentation System Compare Favorably with Previously Documented Pain Relief and Functional Scores for Conventional Balloon Kyphoplasty and Vertebroplasty**

| Procedure | VAS score (n) | | ODI Score (n) | | |
|---|---|---|---|---|---|
| | Pre | 3 mo | Pre | 1 mo | 3 mo |
| Balloon kyphoplasty*,† | 6.2 | 2.8 | 46 | 30 | ND |
| Vertebroplasty‡,§ | 7.5 | 3.5 | 75 | ND | 38.7 |
| RF kyphoplasty | 7.2 | 2.4 | 55 | 33 | 26 |

*ND*, Not done.
*I. Lieberman and M.K. Reinhardt. CORR 415S (2003) s176–s186.
†From S. Garfin et al. SPINE vol. 31 19(2006) 2213–2220.
‡F. McKiernan, T. Faciszewski, R. Jensen. JBJS vol. 86A 12 (2004) 2600–2606.
§K.-Y. Ha et al. JBJS (Br), 88 (B) (2006) 629–633

Site-specific cavity creation and ultra-high viscosity cement delivery with a unique hydraulic delivery system has been shown to enable mechanical VCF height elevation equivalent to that observed in balloon-assisted kyphoplasty without committing the physician to filling large cavities created by balloon inflation. Control in where and how much cement is used to augment VCFs may prove invaluable in providing the physician with a new means of stabilizing fractures and, in mobile fractures, reducing the height without long-term fear of stress shielding.

Since 1984, technology has converged in a way that impacts the traditional use of the term kyphoplasty. Initially kyphoplasty was defined as the "balloon procedure." Today, there are additional technologies designed for minimally invasive, cavity creating VCF treatment. Consequently, procedure terminology has evolved, as evidenced by CMS recently replacing the ICD-9 code title of "Kyphoplasty" with "Percutaneous Vertebral Augmentation," with examples of this procedure category including conventional kyphoplasty and other various technologies commercially available at the time of publishing, included in the description. High viscosity cement has the ability to combine the minimalism of vertebroplasty with the mechanical potential benefits of a vertebral implant or balloon. Our data show an ability to deliver

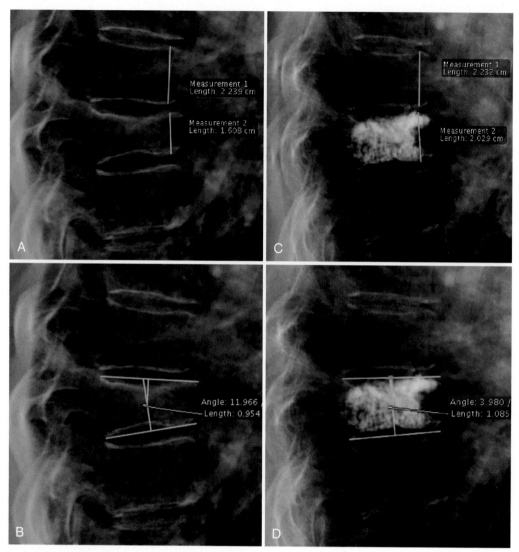

■ **FIGURE 40-5** Preoperative (**A** and **B**) and postoperative (**C** and **D**) radiographs of a 3-week-old T9 osteoporotic vertebral compression fracture demonstrating 4-mm height restoration (19% reduction in compression) and 8-degree correction of kyphotic angle (12 degrees preoperative vs 4 degrees postoperative) following radiofrequency kyphoplasty. *(Courtesy of Dr. Florian Elgeti, Charité-Universitätsmedizin, Berlin).*

cement in a more controlled manner and to create height-restorative forces based on location and the cohesive properties of the cement. Ultimately this new method will find its place in a modern buffet of options for repair of these VCFs with benefits for the patient and simplicity for the physician.

## References

1. P. Galibert, H. Deramond, P. Rosat, et al., Preliminary note on the treatment of vertebral angioma by percutaneous acrylic vertebroplasty, Neurochirurgie 33 (2) (1987) 166–168. French.
2. G.H. Zoarski, P. Snow, W.J. Olan, et al., Percutaneous vertebroplasty for osteoporotic compression fractures: quantitative prospective evaluation of long-term outcomes, J. Vasc. Interv. Radiol. 13 (2002) 139–148.
3. A. Weill, J. Chiras, J.M. Simon, et al., Spinal metastases: indications for and results of percutaneous injection of acrylic surgical cement, Radiology 199 (1996) 241–247.
4. A. Cotton, F. Dewatre, B. Cortet, et al., Percutaneous vertebroplasty for osteolytic metastases and myeloma: effects of the percentage of lesion filling and the leakage of methyl methacrylate at clinical follow-up, Radiology 200 (1996) 525–530.
5. J.K. McGraw, J.A. Lippert, K.D. Minkus, et al., Prospective evaluation of pain relief in 100 patients undergoing percutaneous vertebroplasty: results and follow-up, J. Vasc. Interv. Radiol. 13 (2002) 883–886.
6. A.J. Evans, M.E. Jensen, K.E. Kip, et al., Vertebral compression fractures: pain reduction and improvement in functional mobility after percutaneous polymethylmethacrylate vertebroplasty retrospective report of 245 cases, Radiology 226 (2) (2003) 366–372.
7. C. Vasconcelos, P. Gailloud, N.J. Beauchamp, et al., Is percutaneous vertebroplasty without pretreatment venography safe? Evaluation of 205 consecutive procedures, AJNR Am. J. Neuroradiol. 23 (6) (2002) 913–917.
8. T.W. O'Neill, D. Felsenberg, J. Varlow, et al., The prevalence of vertebral deformity in European men and women: the European vertebral osteoporosis study, J. Bone Miner. Res. 11 (1996) 1010–1018.
9. N.F. Ray, J.K. Chan, M. Thamer, et al., Medical expenditures for the treatment of osteoporotic fractures in the United States in 1995: report from the National Osteoporosis Foundation, J. Bone Miner. Res. 12 (1997) 24–35.
10. M.J. McGirt, S.L. Parker, et al., Vertebroplasty and kyphoplasty for the treatment of vertebral compression fractures: an evidenced-based review of the literature. Spine J. 9 (2009) 501–508.
11. I.H. Lieberman, S. Dudeney, M.K. Reinhardt, et al., Initial outcome and efficacy of "kyphoplasty" in the treatment of painful osteoporotic vertebral compression fractures, Spine 26 (14) (2001) 1631–1638.
12. S.R. Garfin, H.A. Yuan, M.A. Reiley, Kyphoplasty and vertebroplasty for the treatment of painful osteoporotic compression fractures, Spine 26 (2001) 1511–1515.
13. E. Truumees, A. Hilibrand, A.R. Vaccaro, Percutaneous vertebral augmentation, Spine J. 4 (2004) 218–229.
14. D.K. Resnick, S.R. Garfin, Vertebroplasty and kyphoplasty, Thieme, New York, 2005.
15. K. Murphy, E.Wong, R. Poser, et al., Comparison of intravertebral pressure and height restoration in three minimally invasive treatments of vertebral compression fractures. 2009 SIR Annual Scientific Meeting, Abstract #34.
16. T. Raley, R. Poser, A. Kohm. Comparative Height restoration of three vertebral augmentation systems for treatment of vertebral compression fractures. 55th Annual Meeting of the Orthopedic Research Society (2009), 0639.
17. L. Miko, I. Szikora, J. Grohs, et al., Initial clinical experience with radio-frequency based vertebral augmentation in treatment of vertebral compression fractures. 2009 SIR Annual Scientific Meeting, Abstract #35.
18. Fourth Symposium Vertebroplastie/Kyphoplastie. 26 September 2009. Potsdam, Germany.

# 41

# Structural Kyphoplasty: The StaXx FX System

*Harvinder S. Sandhu and Wayne J. Olan*

### KEY POINTS

- The StaXx FX system is an alternative to balloon kyphoplasty or vertebroplasty for the treatment of vertebral compression fractures.

- The StaXx FX system involves the progressive application of permanent individual Polyetheretherketone (PEEK) wafers to reduce the fracture and provide sustained support to the endplate. After implantation into the vertebral body, the wafers are embedded in bone cement.

- The amount of cement used with the StaXx system is less than with either kyphoplasty or vertebroplasty, thereby reducing the risk of cement-related complications.

- Preliminary biomechanical data collected on the StaXx FX device suggest a substantial restoration of normal disc pressure and lower stresses on the anterior cortical shell of the treated vertebral body.

- Although clinical data are required to confirm this, the restoration of normal disc pressure may reduce the rate of adjacent level fractures after treatment with the StaXx FX device.

## INTRODUCTION

The goal of percutaneous vertebroplasty and kyphoplasty is to provide relief to patients presenting with painful osteoporotic vertebral compression fractures. Vertebroplasty was introduced as a means of stabilizing these insufficiency fractures by injecting high-pressure, low-viscosity cement directly into the fractured vertebra. The short-term effect of the intervention is to also alleviate the disabling pain associated with the vertebral injury. There are a number of drawbacks associated with traditional vertebroplasty. These include extravasation of cement from the vertebral body and an inability to correct the deformity or reduce the fracture. Balloon kyphoplasty was developed as an attempt to address these issues. In balloon kyphoplasty, an inflatable bone tamp is used to create a void in the fractured vertebra, which is then filled with cement.

Hadjipavlou et al[1] provided a thorough review of the existing literature for these procedures. The reported success rates for these procedures is consistently above 80% (defined as patient-reported good to excellent pain response) with risk for certain complications. These complications include a transient increase in pain, infection, leakage of cement, and secondary vertebral compression fractures. With kyphoplasty, there have been a small number of reports of balloon rupture, but the failed balloons were withdrawn without incident. Cement leakage is the most common cause of pulmonary or neurological complications. The comparison of cement leakage risk between kyphoplasty and vertebroplasty remains controversial. Some reports suggest a clinically insignificant difference in risk, whereas others suggest that kyphoplasty is associated with less leakage.

Both vertebroplasty and kyphoplasty may increase the risk of subsequent vertebral fractures, particularly at the adjacent level. Some have hypothesized that this may be due to changes in load distribution across the endplate that occur when disc is pressure lost after endplate fracture. Fracture of the endplate increases the volume for the nucleus pulposus and reduces its ability to hydrostatically resist compressive load. In flexion, the reduced load on the nucleus causes greater load on the annulus and the anterior cortex of the vertebral body adjacent to the fractured endplate. This mechanism is being investigated by Patwardhan et al.[2] Some have speculated that the addition of cement to the vertebral body increases the stiffness of the vertebral body and that this may play a role in subsequent fractures. The effect of cement on the treated and adjacent levels is still being studied, but it appears that this effect is small compared to bone mineral density.[3]

Advocates of kyphoplasty believe that the procedure actually reduces the rate of adjacent level fractures, compared to vertebroplasty, because it more effectively reduces the fracture. However, no randomized studies have been conducted to compare the two techniques, and the natural history of adjacent level fractures has been difficult to quantify. Frankel and Vandergrift[4] reviewed the results of 2,000 patients enrolled in a trial evaluating bisphosphonate in patients with vertebral compression fractures. The authors noted that the rates of new fractures were 7.9% and 15% in patients treated with bisphosphonate and placebo, respectively. Moreover, in the bisphosphonate group, only 3.4% of new vertebral compression fractures were at the adjacent level, compared to 7.1% in the placebo group.[4] Frankel and vandergrift review of the literature found the rates of subsequent adjacent level fractures following kyphoplasty to be 13% compared to 10% with vertebroplasty, suggesting that cement implantation with both of these techniques increased the risk of subsequent fractures compared to natural history.[4]

Frankel et al[5] compared outcomes in a series of 17 patients (20 fractures) undergoing kyphoplasty and 19 patients (26 fractures) undergoing vertebroplasty. The authors reported an average of 4.65 ml and 3.78 ml of cement per vertebral body with kyphoplasty and vertebroplasty, respectively. There were five adjacent level fractures in three kyphoplasty patients (3/17 [18%]) and none in the vertebroplasty group.[5] Fribourg et al[6] published a retrospective review of 38 patients (47 fractures) treated with kyphoplasty. Patients received between 1.5 and 6.0 ml cement per vertebral body. The authors reported that 10 patients (26%) had a subsequent fracture during the follow-up period (average 8 months), and 8 of those patients had a subsequent fracture within 2 months. The 8 patients with early "new fractures" all had a fracture at the adjacent level and the 2 patients with later "new fractures" all had fractures that were not adjacent to the index fracture.[6]

A larger study was performed by Harrop et al[6] in which 115 patients were treated with kyphoplasty. All patients had at least 3 months follow-up. In this group, 26 patients (22.6%) developed 34 new compression fractures. The authors then classified patients as having primary osteoporosis (80 patients) or secondary steroid-induced osteoporosis (35 patients) and calculated at the rate of subsequent fractures in each group. They reported that the incidence of postkyphoplasty compression factures in primary osteoporosis patients was 11%, and the incidence in the steroid-induced osteoporosis group was 49% ($p < .00001$).[7] There was no mention of the use of bisphosphonates in these patients.

The Frankel[4,5] and Harrop[7] papers demonstrate that both bisphosphonates and steroids have a significant effect on bone quality and should be considered in any analysis of adjacent-level fractures following vertebroplasty or kyphoplasty. Each of these papers reported subsequent fractures in 18% to 26% of patients, with the best case being 11% in patients specifically with primary osteoporosis. Because the natural history of adjacent level fractures is likely between 8% and 15%, standard vertebroplasty and balloon kyphoplasty may actually increase the risk of subsequent compression fractures, despite the success in reducing a patient's pain from the index fracture.[4-7]

Cadaver testing has been used to test the hypothesis that kyphoplasty is more efficacious for deformity correction than standard vertebroplasty. Belkoff et al[8] experimentally created compression fractures in 16 osteoporotic vertebral bodies and treated them with either balloon kyphoplasty or vertebroplasty. The vertebral bodies were compressed to 25% of their initial height; however, there was an initial elastic recovery of about 15%. The authors measured the change in height with the application of cement and then subjected those vertebral bodies to compressive failure. The authors reported that 97% of the height loss was regained with kyphoplasty, whereas only 30% of height loss was regained with vertebroplasty.[8] These results may not reflect the in vivo situation, because muscle forces and body weight will resist height restoration, as measured clinically by Voggenreiter.[8] The vertebral bodies in both groups were found to be stronger after the application of cement. However, those treated with kyphoplasty were found to return to their initial stiffness, whereas those treated with vertebroplasty did not.[9] Kim et al[10] performed a similar cadaver evaluation with the addition of cyclic loading to determine how vertebral fracture correction was maintained over time. They reported that balloon kyphoplasty was able to restore vertebral height, but there was significant loss of height over 100,000 cycles of compressive load. Vertebroplasty was better able to maintain height under dynamic loading. Ultimately, after the cyclic testing regimen, the vertebrae treated with kyphoplasty had less height than those treated with vertebroplasty.[10] In contrast to Belkoff,[8] the vertebral bodies treated with vertebroplasty were more stiff than with kyphoplasty.

Cadaver studies of isolated vertebral bodies cannot capture the interaction between vertebral bodies or in vivo loads. Clinical data are necessary to realistically measure the ability to achieve reduction of a vertebral compression fracture. Pradham et al[11] evaluated a series of 65 consecutive patients treated with kyphoplasty between 1 to 3 levels. Kyphoplasty reduced the local kyphotic deformity by an average of 7.3 degrees (63% of preoperative kyphosis), but this did not translate into a similar correction of overall sagittal alignment. Angular correction decreased to 2.4 degrees when measured from the level above to the level below. Similarly, the reductions decreased to 1.5 and 1.0 degree at spans of 2 and 3 levels above and below the index level, respectively. The authors concluded that it was unrealistic to expect a 1- or 2-level kyphoplasty to significantly improve sagittal alignment after vertebral compression fracture.[11]

The StaXx FX Structural Kyphoplasty System (Spine Wave, Inc., Shelton, Conn.) was introduced to allow the physician to reduce the vertebral fracture and to correct the kyphotic deformity with a system of progressively stacked wavers made from PEEK (Figure 41-1). The permanent implant system allows controlled vertical expansion in situ and eliminates the intraoperative height loss that may occur after deflation of a balloon. Pradhan et al[11] remarked that using balloons to reduce the fracture is not ideal, because the balloon and subsequently inserted cement follow a path of least resistance, resulting in localized stresses on the endplate. These localized stresses compromise the endplate's ability to maintain an improvement in the spine's overall sagittal alignment. The geometry of the StaXx system includes a wide, flat surface to support the endplate, which encourages hydrostatic compression of the nucleus and normalization of load across the disc. This endplate support may enable the system to reduce the number of adjacent level fractures following treatment of an initial compression fracture. Tactile feedback and manual wafer implantation provide greater physician control and directed axial expansion to reduce the fractured endplate.

The StaXx FX Structural Kyphoplasty System requires only a small amount of cement, because the PEEK wafers occupy much of the volume created during reduction. This may reduce the incidence of cement-related pulmonary complications compared to kyphoplasty. The device itself impedes the flow of cement when placed anteriorly, thereby reducing the risk of posterior cement extravasation.

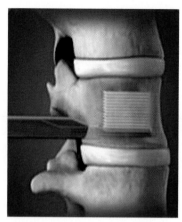

**■ FIGURE 41-1** Stackable PEEK wafers of the StaXx FX Structural Kyphoplasty device allow the physician to have controlled repair of a vertebral compression fracture.

## INDICATIONS AND CONTRAINDICATIONS

The intended use of The StaXx FX Structural Kyphoplasty System is for the reduction of spinal fractures. The device is contraindicated in patients presenting with markedly displaced bony fragments or retropulsion of one or more fragments that compromise the spinal canal. The physician should also evaluate the patient's medical history for such conditions as inability to tolerate anesthesia, morbid obesity, active infections, fever, leukocytosis, or factors inhibiting proper claudication. Attention should also be given to the spinal anatomy and morphology. Safe surgical access and appropriate size implant components are paramount for a successful procedure.

## DESCRIPTION OF THE DEVICE

The StaXx FX Structural Kyphoplasty System is a novel device to be used in kyphoplasty procedures. Unlike traditional balloon kyphoplasty, structural kyphoplasty allows for physician-controlled fracture reduction. This device is implanted in the fractured vertebra via a percutaneous, peripedicular surgical approach. StaXx wafers are 1 mm thick and made from PEEK Optima. Wafers are inserted one at a time, using a wedge action to create vertical lift and reduce the fractured vertebral body. The first wafer, or base wafer, acts as a terminus for subsequently inserted wafers and is the foundation of the wafer stack. Once the StaXx wafers are inserted, bone cement is injected into the vertebral body for further stabilization. A small volume of cement is injected anteriorly at the base of the wafer stack, securing the anterior column. Interventional radiologists, neurosurgeons, and orthopedists may perform this procedure.

## BACKGROUND OF SCIENTIFIC TESTING AND CLINICAL OUTCOMES

The StaXx FX Structural Kyphoplasty System was introduced to the European market in 2006. It was cleared for the U.S. market via the 510(k) pathway in April 2007, and the first surgery was in August of that year. Although clinical experience thus far is limited to only a few hundred cases, results are very promising. No neurological complications related to the device or surgical procedure have been reported. Cement use is greatly decreased, averaging 2.5 ml per level in preliminary registries of patients. In relatively acute fractures, physicians have reported extreme satisfaction in the ability of the StaXx FX Structural Kyphoplasty System to correct endplate deformities.

Cadaveric testing by Dr. Stephen M. Belkoff has shown similarities in both strength and stiffness between balloon kyphoplasty and structural kyphoplasty (presented at the Annual Meeting of Congress of Neurological Surgeons, September 15-20, 2007).[12] The study methods compared bilateral Kyphon Bone Tamp (KyphX) and unilateral StaXx FX Structural Kyphoplasty (Spine Wave Shelton, CT USA). Vertebral bodies were preconditioned with a preload of 89 N and then subjected to compressive loading at a displacement rate of 5 mm/min until the body had lost half its height. The fractures were then put under a preload of 144 N to simulate a recumbent position during surgery and treated with either KyphX or StaXx. The average cement volume when using StaXx was 2.50 ml, compared with 7.25 ml with KyphX. Restoration of vertebral body height was greatest in the anterior portion of the body and only observed when using the StaXx device. The amount of height restoration was 5 to 10 mm. The authors observed that the inflatable bone tamps were able to restore height until they were deflated and removed. At this time, the compressive preload caused the vertebral body to lose all height restoration. Treated vertebral bodies were crushed again, and there were no significant differences in strength or stiffness between the two devices.[11]

Patwardhan performed cadaver testing to determine if the StaXx FX device could restore the vertebral disc pressure adjacent to the fractured endplate to its prefracture values (unpublished company sponsored research). Restoration of adjacent level disc pressure is believed to decrease anterior cortical strain and thus reduce the rate of subsequent fractures. Vertebral height restoration and the reduction in endplate deformity were also studied. Patwardhan used pressure sensors to measure the vertebral disc pressure before fracture, postfracture and posttreatment. Though the results are still being analyzed, the author's preliminary report describes that the disc pressure adjacent to the fractured endplate reduced with StaXx is substantially restored to prefracture values. Clinical data are necessary to determine if this finding translates to a decrease in the rate of subsequent fractures.

## CLINICAL PRESENTATION AND EVALUATION

Patients with vertebral compression fractures typically present with pain that can be localized to a specific area of the spine. Often, the pain is severe enough to functionally completely disable the patient. Antiinflammatory and other pain medication often fail to provide adequate pain relief. A comprehensive evaluation should include sensory, tactile, and reflex assessment. The physician should also question the patient to determine when the pain was noticed and the patient's activity at that time. A comprehensive medical history will also give insight as to the nature of the pain source. Patients with known osteoporosis; long-term corticoid steroid use, such as with asthma inhalers; or a history of cancer are at greater risk for suffering a vertebral compression fracture. Patients with a history of vertebral compression fractures are likely to present with subsequent fractures.

A standing scoliosis radiographic series should be performed, but at minimum a standing lateral view and a standing anteroposterior (AP) view are required. Magnetic resonance imaging (MRI) is imperative visualization to help pinpoint and confirm the location of the pain and visualize the fracture and it's configuration. It is important to be aware that radiographs are of limited utility in determining if the fracture is acute or chronic. Ideally, a previous radiograph will be available so that a new vertebral fracture can be distinguished from an existing deformity of the vertebral body. MRI is particularly well suited for determining if the compression fracture is acute, because edema will accompany an acute fracture. A T2-weighted image will show this edema as a brighter area. The specificity of the film can be optimized with an imaging sequence altered to suppress the appearance of fat in the vertebral body, which also tends to show bright on FSE (fast spin echo) T2 images (Figure 41-2). The clinician should be aware that outside MRIs may not be collected with fat suppression and the diagnostic value of the film may be decreased. Alternatively in those cases, T1-weighted images will show an edema as a darker area (Figure 41-3). Computed tomography (CT) scans performed during the initial evaluation provide a better view of the fractured vertebra and the location of any resulting fragments. If the patient is not a suitable candidate for an MRI, then the CT scan in conjunction with nuclear medicine bone scan can also be used to establish fracture age. With any vertebroplasty or kyphoplasty procedure, endplate restoration and vertebral height augmentation are more readily achieved on active fractures. Typically, chronic fractures do not have a great deal of mobility and this may interfere with the ability to restore the endplate or augment the height of the vertebral body. In fact, reduction may not be possible on a chronic fracture.

All results should be compared with the patient-reported location, to determine if the pain is a result of the fractured body. A T-score determination is useful in determining if a patient has osteoporosis or not, especially with a first-time fracture, and requires bisphosphonate medications to help prevent further bone loss.

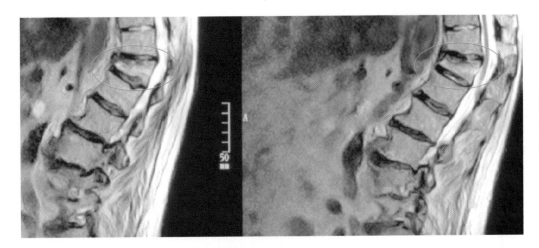

■ **FIGURE 41-2**  A T2-weighted MRI sequence with bright edema, indicating an active fracture. *(Images courtesy of Orlando Ortiz, MD.)*

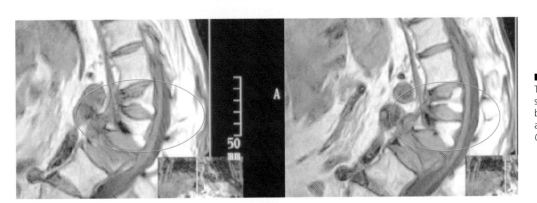

■ **FIGURE 41-3**  A T1-weighted MRI sequence demonstrates decreased signal in the vertebral body consistent with edema and active fracture. *(Images courtesy of Orlando Ortiz, MD.)*

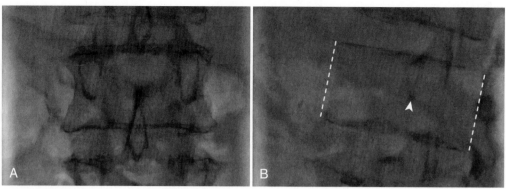

■ **FIGURE 41-4**   Initial set-up. **A,** The StaXx structural kyphoplasty procedure begins with the initial fluoroscopy image in the AP view. The vertebral body is correctly aligned once the inferior endplate is perpendicular to the image, and the spinous process bisects the pedicles. **B,** After the initial setup image is properly aligned, then the view is rotated to an en face view or to an oblique view that aligns the anterior aspect of the pedicle to the midline of the vertebra. (Arrow is pedicle and dotted lines are the margins of the vertebra). *(Images courtesy of Wayne Olan, MD.)*

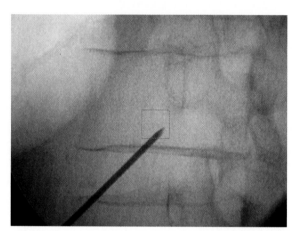

■ **FIGURE 41-5**   The red box indicates the peripedicular area targeted during needle placement. *(Image courtesy of Wayne Olan, MD.)*

## OPERATIVE TECHNIQUE

### Anesthesia

Structural kyphoplasty procedures are suitable for both general anesthesia and conscious sedation. Choice of anesthesia is at the discretion of the physician performing the procedure. Regardless, proper assessment to the patient's medical history and any preexisting conditions should be considered when selecting the mode of anesthesia.

### Position

The patient should be placed in the standard prone position. Placement of the StaXx Structural Kyphoplasty device is performed under fluoroscopy using a peripedicular approach. First, the vertebral body is viewed en face in both AP and lateral images. It's important that the AP image be square to the vertebral body and not the patient; thus the C-arm must be rotated to account for the lateral curvature of the spine. Once the C-arm is properly oriented for the AP view, the arm should be rotated until the lateral aspect of the pedicle has moved over about 50% of the vertebral body (Figure 41-4). A perpendicular line should be dropped from the lateral aspect of the pedicle toward the inferior endplate (Figure 41-5). The target is on this perpendicular line, 3 to 5 mm superior to the inferior endplate. The targeting needle should be coincident with the C-arm, similar to looking down a rifle barrel. This trajectory ensures that the needle will be placed above Kambin's triangle, which is a safe area avoiding the exiting nerve roots below.

The procedure is slightly modified in the thoracic spine because the rib head must be used as an additional landmark. The targeting needle should

be placed medial to the rib head, to ensure that the pleural space is not violated, and lateral to the pedicle, to give clearance to the nerve root. Although the target is smaller in thoracic cases, the landmarks are better defined. The peripendicular approach is ideal for thoracic cases, in contrast with the transpedicular approach, because it is parallel to the endplates and facilitates fracture reduction.

Confirmation of needle placement is observed in the AP and lateral views (Figure 41-6). The needle stylet is removed, and a Steinmann pin is advanced to the midline in both the AP and lateral views. This confirms the proper trajectory and subsequent positioning of the stack in the center of the vertebral body.

### Procedure

A mini-incision (no more than 1.5 cm) is made, and the introducer and access port assembly is placed over the Steinmann pin and advanced 5 to 10 mm into the vertebral body.

The C-arm is then rotated perpendicular (90 degrees) to the instrumentation and fluoroscopy is used to confirm that the introducer and access port assembly are inserted in the vertebral body, allowing the Steinmann pin to be removed. The access port assembly is advanced until sufficiently secured in the cortical wall (Figure 41-7). The introducer is then removed, leaving the access port. Under perpendicular and lateral fluoroscopic guidance, a depth gauge is used to determine the length across the vertebral body (Figure 41-8).

After the wafer length is selected, the wafer cartridge is inserted into the implant delivery gun. The gun and cartridge assembly is primed and inserted into the access port under perpendicular fluoroscopic guidance (Figure 41-9). Using lateral fluoroscopic guidance, 1-mm interlocking stackable PEEK wafers are inserted sequentially, allowing for direct control of the fracture reduction (Figure 41-10).

Fracture reduction, tactile feedback, superior endplate deformation, or inferior cartridge track deflection are stopping points for wafer insertion. Once the gun has been removed from the access port, still in the lateral view, a port seal is used to guide the cement needle along the anterior side of the wafer stack. Bone cement, mixed to a toothpaste consistency, is injected anterior to the wafer stack for stabilization. The cement advances up the wafer stack, filling the anterior aspect of the vertebral body. If the cement does not flow across midline, in the AP view, additional cement may be placed posterior to the wafer stack (Figure 41-11).

## POSTOPERATIVE CARE

The structural kyphoplasty procedure is generally performed in the outpatient setting, as is the case with vertebroplasty or balloon kyphoplasty. The patient is typically discharged home after standard postprocedure recovery care. Standing radiographs may be obtained before patient discharge.

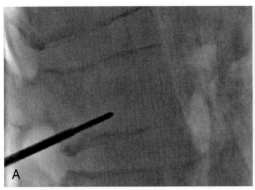 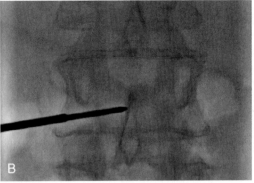

■ **FIGURE 41-6** En face. **A,** When performing en face, the lateral view is used to confirm the targeting needle insertion point. **B,** Once targeting has been confirmed in both the AP and lateral views, the Steinmann pin is advanced. *(Images courtesy of Wayne Olan, MD.)*

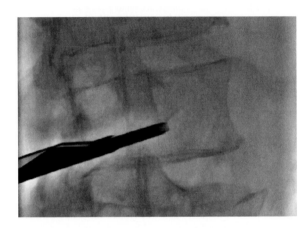

■ **FIGURE 41-7** Seating of the access port. Once the introducer and access port are securely fixed in the vertebra, the Steinmann pin is removed. *(Image courtesy of Wayne Olan, MD.)*

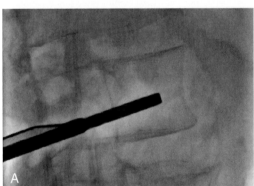 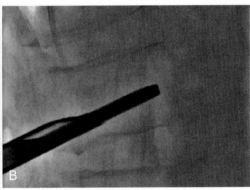

■ **FIGURE 41-8** Advancement of the sizer. **A,** Through the access port, the sizer is advanced into the vertebral body. **B,** The advancement of the sizer near the far cortex is monitored in an oblique view. This determines the size of the implant to be used. *(Images courtesy of Wayne Olan, MD.)*

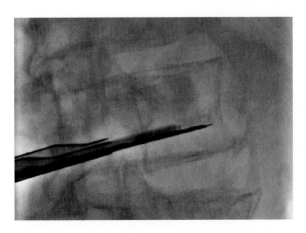

■ **FIGURE 41-9** Wafer Insertion. PEEK wafers are sequentially inserted until endplate fracture reduction is achieved, or endplate deformation occurs, or deflection of the track to the inferior endplate or tactile feedback from the insertion gun demonstrates excessive resistance. *(Image courtesy of Wayne Olan, MD.)*

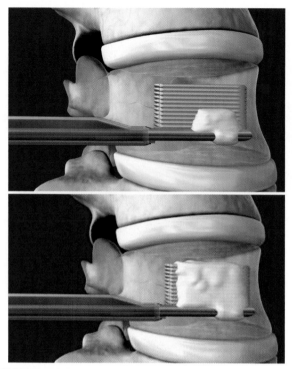

**FIGURE 41-10**   A small amount of cement is used to secure the StaXx implant following implantation.

## COMPLICATIONS AND AVOIDANCE

Kyphoplasty is a relatively safe procedure. Many complications that arise are a result of the use of bone cement rather than from the actual procedure. Neurologic injury may occur from malposition of implants in any vertebroplasty or kyphoplasty procedure but are uncommon. The most common,

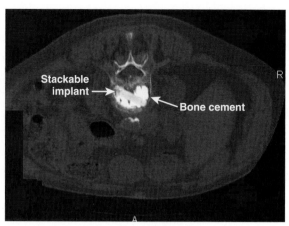

**FIGURE 41-11**   A CT image shows the cement placed in the anterior aspect of the vertebral body after the implantation of the StaXx device. (*Image courtesy of Kent Remley, MD.*)

nonfatal complications to be anticipated include a transitory fall in blood pressure, hemorrhage, hematoma, or short-term cardiac conduction irregularities. Increased pain, rib or vertebra fracture, bone cement allergy, hematuria, dysuria bladder fistula, and infection are other reported complications. As with any kyphoplasty procedure, users of the StaXx Structural Kyphoplasty device should monitor for bone cement related events including myocardial infarction, respiratory and cardiac failure, pneumothorax, abdominal intrusions or ileus, and pulmonary embolism. Care should be given to assess patients closely for these events, because they are potentially fatal. The operative suite should have the capacity to immediately treat these events.

Although structural kyphoplasty uses less cement than the traditional balloon kyphoplasty, there is still the potential for cement to leak outside of the vertebral body. Patients should be monitored for signs and symptoms of soft tissue damage, nerve root pain, cord compression, and neurological

## *Case Studies*

Two case studies are provided. The first is shown in Figure 41-12. This demonstrates a compression fracture with almost complete loss of anterior height. The inferior and superior endplates form an angle of 45 degrees. Following the application of StaXx and cement, much of the anterior height is restored, and the endplates form an angle of 30 degrees. The reduction required 11 wafers and 3 ml cement. The second case study is shown in Figure 41-13. This demonstrates reduction of a two-adjacent-vertebrale compression fracture. Following reduction, the kyphotic angle had improved from 38 degrees to just 21 degrees. The cement shows good diffusion through the both vertebral bodies.

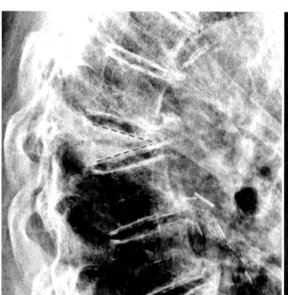

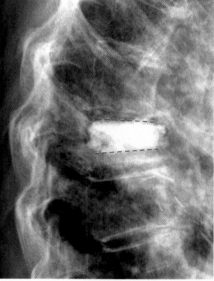

**FIGURE 41-12**   Case 1. Red dotted lines illustrates height restoration (*Images courtesy of Kent Remley, MD.*)

Pre-op

Post-op

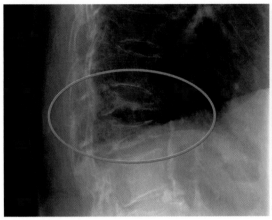
Pre-op

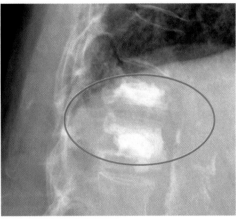
Post-op

■ **FIGURE 41-13** Case 2. Circles indicate fractures. *(Images courtesy of Kent Remley, M.D.)*

impairment. These complications may not always be evident immediately following the procedures. The physician should assess for these events at follow-up either in the office or via the phone.

Consideration should be given to prevent complications from a malpositioned or misaligned percutaneous spinal device. Care should be taken to ensure the structural kyphoplasty device in positioned and implanted correctly to ensure the best possible clinical outcome. Also, as with implantation of any spinal hardware, failure to properly position and implant the structural kyphoplasty device may result in damage to adjacent neurovascular structures.

## CONCLUSIONS AND DISCUSSION

Vertebroplasty and subsequently balloon kyphoplasty were innovative technologies that enabled physicians to treat a previously untreatable but disabling condition of the spine. In fact, insufficiency fractures of the spinal vertebra are still a leading cause of progressive morbidity in the elderly population. Structural kyphoplasty using the StaXx stackable wafer system provides the latest iteration in therapy and solves many of the problems associated with the previous technologies. The system enables the physician to have precise control of corrective technology. The positioning of the wafer stack determines the exact location where the corrective loads will be applied. The individual 1-mm wafers allow precision in the degree of correction. The use of the stack as a permanent implant reduces the risk of subsequent loss of correction. Finally, the wafer stack permits the physician to control the placement and distribution of the cement.

Ex vivo mechanical testing indicates that injury and deformity of the endplate is responsible for increasing the risk of fracture of the vertebra adjacent to the index fracture. Similar testing suggests that the wafer stack concept provides a more ideal footprint for the correction of endplate deformities. Ultimately, clinical data will be required to prove this point. However, the very promising early experience with this device validates formal clinical examination in larger series.

## References

1. A.G. Hadjipavlou, M.N. Tzermiadianos, P.G. Katonis, et al., Percutaneous vertebroplasty and balloon kyphoplasty for the treatment of osteoporotic vertebral compression fractures and osteolytic tumors, JBJS 87-B (12) (2005) 1595–1604.
2. M. Tzermiadianos, A. Hadjipavlou, S. Renner, et al., Altered disc properties after an osteoporotic vertebral fracture. Is it a risk factor for adjacent fractures? Journal of Bone and Joint Surgery - British, Vol. 91-B, Issue (Suppl. 1), 108-109.
3. J. Luo, D.M. Skrzypiec, P. Pollintine, et al., Mechanical efficacy of vertebroplasty: influence of cement type, BMD, fracture severity, and disc degeneration, Bone 40 (4) (2007) 1110–1119.
4. Frankel B and Vandergrift A. The natural history of subsequent adjacent level vertebral compression fractures. Paper #13. Presented at the North American Spine Society 22nd Annual Meeting, October 23-27, Austin, Texas.
5. B.M. Frankel, T. Monroe, C. Wang, Percutaneous vertebral augmentation: an elevation in adjacent-level fracture risk in kyphoplasty as compared with vertebroplasty, Spine J. 7 (2007) 575–582.
6. D. Fribourg, C. Tang, P. Sra, et al., Incidence of subsequent vertebral fractures after kyphoplasty, Spine 29 (20) (2004) 2270–2276.
7. J.S. Harrop, B. Prpa, M.K. Reinhardt, et al., Primary and secondary osteoporosis incidence of subsequent vertebral compression fractures after kyphoplasty, Spine 29 (19) (2004) 2120–2125.
8. S.M. Belkoff, J.M. Mathis, D.C. Fenton, et al., An ex vivo biomechanical evaluation of an inflatable bone tamp used in the treatment of compression fracture, Spine 26 (2) (2001) 151–156.
9. G. Voggenreiter, Balloon kyphoplasty is effective in deformity correction of osteoporotic vertebral compression fractures, Spine 30 (24) (2005) 2806–2812.
10. M.J. Kim, D.P. Lindsey, M. Hannibal, et al., Vertebroplasty versus kyphoplasty: biomechanical behavior under repetitive loading conditions, Spine 31 (18) (2006) 2079–2084.
11. B.B. Pradhan, H.W. Bae, M.A. Kropt, et al., Kyphoplasty reduction of osteoporotic vertebral compression fractures: correction of local kyphosis versus overall sagittal alignment, Spine 31 (4) (2006) 435–441.
12. S.M. Belkoff, R. Manzi, R.D. Paxson, Mechanical comparison of vertebral body compression fracture reduction: StaXx FX versus Kyphoplasty. Annual Meeting of Congress of Neurological Surgeons, September 15-20, 2007.

## ADVANTAGES AND DISADVANTAGES

**Advantages**
- Directional and controlled correction
- Endplate restoration
- Permanent implant with sustainable correction
- Less cement
- Barrier to contain cement

**Disadvantages**
- Requires surgical or radiological expertise
- Requires an understanding of anatomy

# 42

# Crosstrees Percutaneous Vertebral Augmentation

*Philip S. Yuan, Huilin Yang and Dewei Zou*

| K E Y   P O I N T S |
| --- |
| • Osteoporosis is typically a silent disease that can first manifest with vertebral compression fractures (VCFs). |
| • VCFs can lead to kyphosis and functional decline. |
| • Treatment of VCFs with bedrest, bracing, and narcotic medications is often not effective. |
| • The Crosstrees system for percutaneous vertebral augmentation uses a removable pod to initially contain the polymethylmethacrylate, allowing for safer injection and preventing complications from cement extravasation. |
| • The Crosstrees pod also allows for more controlled height restoration and fracture reduction than that possible with kyphoplasty or vertebroplasty. |

## INTRODUCTION

Osteoporosis is a major public health problem affecting an estimated 55% of people over 50 years of age. Every year in the United States more than 700,000 people suffer from vertebral compression fractures (VCFs), with osteoporosis being the main cause. Osteoporosis, the most common metabolic bone disorder, is typically a silent disease, but has the potential to cause debilitating back pain when VCFs occur. Other causes of vertebral fracture include trauma, benign lesions (e.g., hemangioma), and malignant lesions (e.g., multiple myeloma and metastatic cancer). Osteoporosis is characterized by decreased bone mineral density.

In a normal person, the vertebral bodies are composed of a porous structure, called trabecular or cancellous bone, encapsulated within a thin external cap of cortical (dense) bone. In a person with osteoporosis, the trabeculae that form the central porous bone become thinner and weaker. When this occurs, the vertebra can fracture and become deformed. This deformation of the vertebral bodies is classified into three types according to the shape: wedge, biconcave, and crush. As the vertebral bodies collapse, the natural curvature of the spinal column changes. These changes have mechanical effects on the paraspinal musculature and nerves, resulting in a wide range of symptoms, including pain, decreased sensitivity, tingling, and weakness. Multiple VCFs can produce kyphotic deformity, pulmonary dysfunction, loss of appetite, depression, and functional decline.

Until recently, the options for treatment of vertebral fractures were limited. Patients were confined to bed for prolonged periods and were given large doses of analgesics. Bracing was used but was usually not well tolerated by these typically elderly patients and has fallen out of favor. These palliative treatments do not restore the anatomy of the patient's vertebral column to the alignment and morphology it had before the fracture. Treatment success, defined as relief of pain symptoms, depended on the individual's capacity to heal the fracture. This physical change, along with forward angulation, can cause persistent deformity.

The traditional surgical techniques used to treat vertebral fractures or to maintain spinal stabilization are not as effective in the setting of osteoporosis, because the weakened bone is often not strong enough to support the metallic rods and screws. Because of the debilitating nature of the disease, many different procedures have been attempted. Among these, the procedure that has been the most successful is the injection of polymethyl methacrylate (PMMA) bone cement into the vertebral body to stabilize it. This procedure, known as vertebroplasty or kyphoplasty (when a balloon is first used to create a space in the vertebra) is performed in patients with painful fractures that fail to respond to conservative treatment.

A potentially devastating complication of vertebroplasty is the accidental escape (or leakage) of PMMA from the vertebral body, a problem known as cement extravasation. This problem can damage the vital structures, such as the spinal cord, or can contribute to the formation of emboli as a result of the flow of cement to the venous plexus. This can result in serious neurological complications or even death. Kyphoplasty was developed to help minimize cement extravasation by first introducing a balloon tamp to create a space for the cement and compact the surrounding bone. However, cement leakage is still possible with kyphoplasty, because the cement is only injected after removal of the balloon.

The Crosstrees PVA (percutaneous vertebral augmentation) pod is a device designed to percutaneously provide well-controlled delivery of PMMA during vertebral augmentation. The Crosstrees PVA System (Crosstrees Medical, Boulder, Colo.) is designed for use with Mendec Spine PMMA manufactured by Tecres S.p.a. (Verona, Italy), which is marketed with approved indications for use in the treatment of pathologic vertebral fracture. The pod device consists of a catheter for administering the cement into a releasable closed fabric barrier. Following delivery of a known volume of PMMA and expansion of the pod to a defined size, the fabric barrier is opened and removed from the vertebral body, leaving only the PMMA within the bony structure. A final volume of highly viscous PMMA can be added to the center of the initial bolus to provide additional interdigitation of PMMA to the cancellous bone. The system is novel in providing the ability to control the delivery of PMMA to the vertebral body and maintaining fracture reduction without the need for a permanent implant to remain within the patient.

## INDICATIONS AND CONTRAINDICATIONS

Surgical treatment of VCFs with the Crosstrees PVA pod is indicated when debilitating back pain persists despite nonsurgical therapies (Table 42-1). MRI, the imaging study of choice for diagnosing VCF, typically shows increased signal on short T1 inversion recovery (STIR) sequences when a VCF is acute/subacute or if there is residual bony edema indicating incomplete healing. A nuclear medicine study (bone scan) is particularly useful when a MRI cannot be performed (e.g., when pacemaker is present).

In cases of chronic fracture, vertebral augmentation is not indicated. Other absolute contraindications to Crosstrees or any other PVA technique include pregnancy, coagulopathy, osteomyelitis, spinal instability, known allergy to PMMA, and previous augmentation with PMMA (Table 42-2).

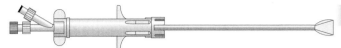

■ **FIGURE 42-1**    Crosstrees pod device.

## TABLE 42-1    Relative Indications

1. Confirmed acute pain and tenderness over the spine at or near the level of x-ray compression deformity and positive MRI or bone scan evaluation

2. Not more than three vertebral compression fractures located between T4 and L5

3. Painful fracture with a loss of 0% to 60% of the height of the vertebral body compared with the height of an adjacent vertebral body that is normal, as determined by the radiological evaluation

4. Confirmation of fracture by MRI including T1-, T2-, and STIR-weighted sequences to determine the type and presence of fracture(s); or nuclear medicine study (bone scan) when MRI cannot be performed (e.g., because of pacemaker)

5. Adequate vertebral body height and geometry for insertion of the access instruments of 5.2 mm outside diameter

6. Minimum vertebral body anterior height of 6.0 mm

## TABLE 42-2    Absolute Contraindications

1. Chronic fracture

2. Spinal instability

3. Known or suspected allergy to PMMA

4. Pregnancy

5. Irreversible coagulopathy or bleeding disorder

6. Active or local infection

7. Previous cement injection or augmentation at the fractured level

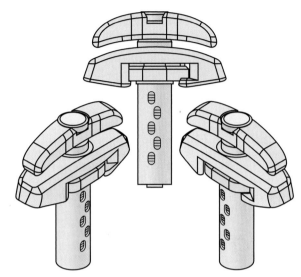

■ **FIGURE 42-2**    Crosstrees CDrive cement dispenser.

## TABLE 42-3    Relative Contraindications

1. Comminuted or high-energy fracture with extension to posterior wall

2. Burst fracture or pedicle fracture

3. Vertebra plana or significant vertebral collapse, defined as >60% of the original height of the vertebral body, as measured against the nearest normal vertebral body

4. Significantly compromised spinal canal or bony retropulsion, especially in setting of neurologic injury

5. Spinal stenosis

6. Pathologic fractures, both benign and malignant (e.g., myeloma, metastatic lesions)

7. Presence of more than three acute VCFs

Relative contraindications (Table 42-3) include neurologic deficit (i.e., burst fracture with significant bony retropulsion, or fracture extending to the posterior cortical wall) and pathologic vertebral fracture related to primary or metastatic cancer; however, because the Crosstrees pod fully contains the cement during implantation and has a defined shape, it may be used more safely in these cases than current vertebroplasty or kyphoplasty techniques. Another relative contraindication is vertebra plana or greater than 60% loss of height.

## DESCRIPTION OF THE DEVICE

The Crosstrees pod device (Figure 42-1) was developed to provide a percutaneous method of delivering a specific volume of bone cement to the surgical site in orthopedic procedures. The device is designed such that the woven fabric pod is inserted into the intravertebral space, and a predetermined volume of bone cement is delivered into it, thus reducing the likelihood of extravertebral cement leakage. The pod expands to a defined shape with a broad surface area as the cement is injected, elevating the endplates and restoring height to the fractured vertebra. Following delivery of the bone cement, the pod is opened and withdrawn from the vertebra. Additional cement can be delivered to the center of the cement bolus, to provide interdigitation with the bone. PMMA is delivered to the pod by a threaded injection syringe, the Crosstrees CDrive cement dispenser (Figure 42-2), designed to measure and deliver the volume required for the selected pod.

## PRINCIPLES OF PROCEDURE

The Crosstrees pod device is composed of a woven fabric mounted on the end of a stainless steel cement delivery shaft. The cement delivery shaft is housed within an additional stainless steel insertion sleeve which can be positioned along the axial length of the cement delivery shaft and pod such that the pod is contained within the insertion sleeve or exposed before PMMA fill. The proximal end of the delivery shaft is bonded to a Y-adaptor with Luer connector fittings on each arm of the Y-adaptor.

The pod is designed with a nylon release cord that is attached with a conventional stitch to the pod. The release cord runs the length of the device within the delivery shaft and through the straight leg of the Y-adaptor, providing access to the release cord at the proximal end of the device. A polymer cap is bonded to the proximal end of the release cord and secured by Luer thread to the Y-adaptor. The cap can be removed from the Y-adaptor and used to apply tension to the release cord. Following delivery of a defined volume of PMMA to the pod, tension is applied by the user to the release cord, pulling the stitch from the wall of the pod, opening the distal pod end.

Using a stylet and 5.2-mm-diameter access cannula, the paraspinal musculature is traversed to access the vertebral body via the pedicle. Either a transpedicular or extrapedicular approach can be used. The stylet and cannula can be advanced to the bony site and withdrawn slightly to create a location for placement of the Crosstrees pod within the bony site. As an alternative method, the stylet can be withdrawn from the cannula and a bone drill advanced through the access cannula into the vertebra and then withdrawn creating a space for placement of the Crosstrees pod within the bony site. Often bone fragments that remain on the drill can be sent for pathologic examination.

The Crosstrees pod is advanced through the lumen of the access cannula and, under fluoroscopic guidance, placed at the desired location within the vertebral body. Placement in the bone is confirmed by radiographic imaging. On confirmation of positioning, the insertion sleeve is withdrawn to expose the pod. The fabric component of the pod will fill to a known and predictable cubic geometry, aligned such that the maximum surface area is oriented parallel to the vertebral endplate. This geometry will provide the optimal surface area for lifting of the compressed bone and restoring vertebral body height.

Mendec Spine cement (PMMA) is prepared according to manufacturers instructions. The PMMA is loaded into the Crosstrees CDrive and attached to the pod by Luer taper distal connection fitting. Using fluoroscopic guidance, PMMA is advanced from the CDrive cement dispenser to the delivery shaft and injected into the pod. PMMA delivery continues until a maximum pod capacity is contained within the pod located in the bone. After filling to maximum pod capacity, the release cord cap is removed from the straight leg of the Y-adaptor and tension applied to the release cord. The release cord is withdrawn from the Crosstrees pod, removing the stitch from the distal pod end. The release cord is fully withdrawn from the Crosstrees pod assembly. Following removal of the release cord and opening of the distal pod end, the Crosstrees pod is withdrawn from the access cannula. The open pod is removed from the patient, leaving no implant other than the specific PMMA. Withdrawal is controlled by rotation of the threaded extractor mechanism at the proximal end of the pod assembly, resulting in linear proximal movement of the fabric pod component to a position within the access cannula. Withdrawal of the pod will decrease the pod fabric diameter on entry to the access cannula, leaving the PMMA within the bone. Following removal of the Crosstrees pod, the access cannula may be used for further access to the bone to deliver a final PMMA bolus, and it is removed from the patient on completion of the surgical procedure.

## BACKGROUND OF SCIENTIFIC TESTING AND CLINICAL OUTCOMES

It is well established in the published medical literature that the effectiveness of vertebral augmentation is evident almost immediately after the procedure. Numerous authors have reported significant pain relief within 24 to 48 hours, with stable results preserved at subsequent follow-up in a majority of patients.[1] Studies in vertebral augmentation have generally evaluated efficacy principally based on pain relief, because pain is typically the reason patients seek treatment. Pain relief assessment by VAS is widely reported, with patients reporting significant relief at 24 hours and later following the procedure. Functional outcomes have also been reported using multiple assessment methods, but is typically secondary to evaluation based on pain relief.[2-4] Ledlie et al[5] showed the stability of outcomes with respect to pain relief post procedure. The study included 117 consecutive subjects undergoing vertebral augmentation procedures. The authors observed rapid relief in pain, with substantial improvement within 1 week postprocedure and relatively stable results from 1 through 24 months postoperative.

In a 2006 review, Hulme et al[4] reported that complication rates are in the range of 1% to 2% for osteoporotic fractures and 5% to 10% for metastatic lesions.[6] Complications specifically related to cement leakage can include increased local pain, symptomatic pulmonary embolus, radiculopathy, and cord compression and are estimated to occur in approximately 1% to 3% of cases.[7] Of the complications potentially associated with vertebroplasty and kyphoplasty, all but new vertebral fractures occur during or immediately following the procedure. Thus the majority of complications can be identified within a very short period following the procedure.

Clinical literature in vertebral augmentation reports on the incidence of additional fractures as the primary focus of longer term follow-up. Leakage of PMMA from the vertebra has been associated with incidence of new fracture, with average time to new fracture of 48 days for levels adjacent to PMMA extravasation and 98 days absent PMMA extravasation.[8] There are reports of the incidence of fracture adjacent to and remote from treated levels with half of new fractures occurring adjacent to treated levels within

3 months follow-up. A majority of subsequent vertebral fractures appear to occur within the first 30 days following a vertebroplasty procedure. Lin et al[9] reported that in a series of 38 patients treated with vertebroplasty, new fractures occurred in 14 patients. When cement leakage occurred, the average time to new fracture was 48 days. It was 98 days in patients who did not have any cement leakage.

The time to observation of cement leakage occurrence is similar across studies. The existence of cement leakage is generally identified during or soon after the vertebroplasty procedure. Thus, although cement leakage appears to be the most commonly occurring complication of vertebroplasty, the existence of such an event would be identified well within a 30-day follow-up period.

In addition to evaluation of safety and pain relief, vertebral augmentation studies reported in the literature have often included an assessment of vertebral body morphology. There is disagreement in the literature on the efficacy of current treatments in the restoration of vertebral height and the clinical importance of vertebral height restoration.[4,7]

Procedural characteristics including the volume of cement used are also reported in the literature. Clinical literature reports variability in the volume of PMMA required for procedure success.[8,10] The Crosstrees system delivers an initial bolus of known volume of PMMA, with device size selection determined by the investigator, based on vertebral level, degree of vertebral collapse, and physician assessment of device placement strategy. Pain relief is often immediate and sustained as noted in the literature review noted previously. If complications occur, they should become apparent early in the postoperative period.

## OPERATIVE TECHNIQUE

### Anesthesia

General anesthesia is usually preferred, because it prevents the patient from feeling any discomfort and allows a controlled environment for safe passage of the cannulas down the pedicles. The procedure can be safely performed using local anesthesia if the patient is medically too unstable to undergo general anesthesia.

### Position

The procedure is always performed with the patient prone on a radiolucent frame, such as the Jackson table. All attempts should be made to extend the spine, in an attempt to restore height to the fractured vertebra using ligamentotaxis.

### Surgical Procedure for the Crosstrees System

Position the patient prone on a radiolucent table. Drape and prep according to standard surgical technique. Position two C-arms to achieve biplanar fluoroscopy capability as shown. If only one C-arm is available, the radiolucent table used must allow the C-arm to freely complete its arc as it moves from the anteroposterior (AP) to the lateral imaging position and back again.

#### Transpedicular Approach

Make a skin incision slightly lateral and superior (varies per level) to the intersection of the superior and lateral edges of the pedicle as determined under fluoroscopic guidance. Insert the 11-gauge needle into the incision and anchor it in bone, gently tapping it with a mallet if necessary. Confirm its location with fluoroscopy (AP view). Continue tapping the 11-gauge needle into place, confirming the location of the tip periodically with both AP and lateral fluoroscopic views. To avoid the spinal canal, make sure the tip of the needle does not pass medial to the medial border of the pedicle before entering the posterior vertebral cortex. Once the 11-gauge needle has crossed the posterior wall of the vertebral body, remove the inner stylet and replace it with the Indexed Guide Pin. Advance the guide pin anteriorly and medially into the vertebral body. Use the proximal most visible sizing indicator to select the appropriate size pod. With the guide pin approximately halfway across the vertebral body on the lateral view, remove the 11-gauge needle cannula and insert the blunt cannulated assembly over the guide pin.

Attach the strike plate to the strike plate extension. Insert the tines of the strike plate into the mating feature of the blunt cannulated stylet and use the mallet to gently tap the stylet until its tip is just past the posterior vertebral wall on the lateral view.

Remove the inner stylet and guide pin and leave the access cannula in place. Note: The wings of the access cannula should be oriented in a cephalad-caudad position at this point if the primary geometry of the pod is being used. For an alternate geometry, the cannula wings should be parallel to the vertebral endplates. Under fluoroscopic guidance, use the cannulated drill to create a space in the bone before the placement of the pod and injection of PMMA into the pod. Advance the cannulated drill under fluoroscopic observation, avoiding contact with the anterior wall of the vertebra.

### Extrapedicular Approach (Usually Recommended in Thoracic Spine)

Make a skin incision a few centimeters lateral and slightly superior to the intersection of the superior and lateral edges of the pedicle. Insert the 11-gauge needle into the incision and anchor it in bone, gently tapping it with a mallet if necessary. The correct entry point to the vertebral body is the costovertebral junction. Confirm the location with fluoroscopy (AP view). Under fluoroscopic guidance, use the cannulated drill to create a space in the bone before the placement of the pod and injection of PMMA into the pod. Advance the cannulated drill under fluoroscopic observation, avoiding contact with the anterior wall of the vertebra.

Use the laser markings on the drill shaft to confirm drill depth relative to the distal end of the access cannula. Do not drill more than 20 mm beyond the distal end of the access cannula. Under fluoroscopic guidance, insert the pod through the access cannula, and slide the extractor collar connector over the cannula wings to seat. The Y-adaptor will be oriented laterally and parallel to the vertebral endplates if the primary pod geometry is being used.

### Delivery of PMMA

Remove the insertion sleeve lock from the pod assembly and set aside. Expose the pod membrane by pulling back on the wings of the device assembly. Repeat this process on the contralateral side. Under fluoroscopic guidance, turn the handle on the CDrive to inject spine resin into the pod membrane. Inject the entire contents of the CDrive by rotating the handle until it is flush with the CDrive sleeve. Repeat this process on the contralateral side. Confirm PMMA delivery to the pod with fluoroscopy in AP and lateral views. Remove the luer cap and release cord by withdrawal proximal from the pod assembly, opening the distal end of the pod fabric. Withdraw the pod from the vertebra by rotation of the extractor nut wings clockwise to the limit of the thread travel length. Withdraw the pod assembly from the cannula. Repeat this process on the contralateral side.

Insert the filler placement cannula (FPC) through the access cannula, advancing just far enough to place the tip of the FPC into the center of the cement bolus. Use fluoroscopy and the marks on the FPC cannula to confirm position. Manually dispense additional PMMA under continuous fluoroscopic guidance to achieve interdigitation (Table 42-4).

## POSTOPERATIVE CARE

Patients usually notice immediate relief of back pain and often do not require any narcotic medication postoperatively. Patients can be discharged home the same day or monitored overnight to watch for other medical comorbidities if necessary. Often these patients are weak because they have been bedridden and may benefit from the overnight stay and a session with a physical therapist.

## CONCLUSIONS AND DISCUSSIONS

In 2005, osteoporosis-related fractures were responsible for an estimated $19 billion in costs. Osteoporosis is a disease characterized by low bone mass, leading to bone fragility and an increased susceptibility to fractures, especially of the spine, hip, and wrist, although any bone can be affected. VCFs are a frequent cause of pain and disability among the elderly population.

**TABLE 42-4** Timing for the Preparation and Application of the PMMA (Mendec Spine Resin, 68° F)

| Operation (Mendec) | Definition | Function (Crosstrees pod) | Phase Duration (sec) |
|---|---|---|---|
| Mixing | Mixing of the components | | 60 |
| Delivery device filling | The dough is transferred into the delivery device | The dough is transferred to the CDrive | 60 |
| Waiting | The cement cannot be used | | 300 |
| Working | The cement can be delivered | Cement delivery, release cord removal, pod withdrawal | 600 |
| Hardening | The cement hardens and increases in viscosity and cannot be delivered anymore; exothermic reaction takes place | Manual cement delivery and interdigitation via filler placement cannula | 360 |

### ADVANTAGES AND DISADVANTAGES

The Crosstrees device enables controlled implantation of PMMA into a fractured vertebra, while filling to a known shape and minimizing the chance of cement leakage. It does not require insertion and removal of a balloon tamp before the insertion of cement, rather the pod is inserted, reduces the fracture, and is removed after cement injection and reduction.

Despite the advantages, the Crosstrees procedure may be more technically challenging, because placement of the pod is essential for a good result. The pods need to be placed near the center of the vertebral body because they will not necessarily seek the path of least resistance, as in balloon procedures for VCF. The cement will only fill the pod in a defined shape. With that being said, once the pod is removed, there is the possibility of back filling additional cement if so desired, but the risk of leakage is possible if that path is chosen.

Both vertebroplasty and kyphoplasty have proved to be effective in relieving pain related to VCF. A potentially serious complication of these procedures is cement extravasation. The Crosstrees Medical PVA System for percutaneous vertebral augmentation consists of instruments designed to deliver the cement to the vertebral body in a controlled manner preventing extravasation without the requirement for an implant device. This device is designed to decrease the risk of leakage of bone cement (PMMA) into the spinal canal and the venous plexus, thereby preventing the complications associated with extravasation. The Crosstrees pod also has the added benefit of achieving and maintaining fracture reduction during cement injection, whereas in kyphoplasty the balloon tamp can achieve reduction but is then removed before cement insertion, and reduction is lost in many cases. The Crosstrees pod adds to the surgeon's armamentarium for treatment of VCFs.

### References

1. C. Bono, C.P. Kauffman, S. Garfin, in: H. Herkowitz (Ed.), Surgical options and indications: kyphoplasty and vertebroplasty in the lumbar spine, Lippincott Williams & Wilkins , 2004.
2. J.M. Mathis, Percutaneous vertebroplasty or kyphoplasty: which one do I choose? Skel. Radiol. 35 (2006) 629–631.
3. J.B. Gill, Comparing pain reduction following kyphoplasty and vertebroplasty for osteoporotic vertebral compression fractures, Pain Physician 10 (4) (2007 Jul) 583–590.

4. P. A. Hulme, Vertebroplasty and kyphoplasty: a systematic review of 69 clinical studies, Spine 31 (17) (2001), 1983.

5. J.T. Ledlie, Kyphoplasty treatment of vertebral fractures: 2-year outcomes show sustained benefits, Spine 31 (1) (2006) 57–64.

6. K.M. Eicholz, J.E. O'Toole, S.D. Christie, R.G. Fessler, Vertebroplasty and kyphoplasty, Neurosurg Clin N Am 17 (2006) 507–518.

7. K. Talmadge, Vertebral compression fracture treatments, in: S.M. Kurtz, A.A. Edidin (Eds.), Spine technology handbook, Elsevier Academic Press, 2006, pp. 371–396.

8. E.P. Lin, Vertebroplasty: cement leakage into the disc increases the risk of new fracture of adjacent vertebral body, AJNR Am J Neuroradiol 25 (2) (2004 Feb) 166–167.

9. E.P. Lin, S. Ekholm, A. Hiwatashi, P.L. Westesson, Vertebroplasty: cement leakage into the disc increases the risk of new fracture of adjacent vertebral body, AJNR Am J Neuroradiol 25 (2004) 175–180.

10. B.M. Frankel, Percutaneous vertebral augmentation: an elevation in adjacent level fracture risk in kyphoplasty as compared with vertebroplasty, Spine J 7 (5) (2007 Sept-Oct) 575–582.

# 43

# Biologic Treatment of Osteoporotic Compression Fractures: OptiMesh

*Karl D. Schultz, Jr.*

**K E Y   P O I N T S**

- Goals of treating osteoporotic vertebral compression fractures
- Current treatment options with polymethyl methacrylate (complications: extravasation, higher number of adjacent level vertebral fractures)
- New biologic option (porous mesh filled with bone allograft)
- Surgical procedure (cavity creation, mesh filling)
- Fracture stabilization and graft incorporation

## INTRODUCTION

The Centers for Disease Control and Prevention (CDC) reports that there were 36.8 million U.S. residents older than 65 years in 2005. That number is predicted to grow to over 70 million by 2030.[1] Presently, it is estimated that 25% of women older than 50 years, 40% of women older than 80 years, and 33% of men reaching 75 years of age will sustain an osteoporotic compression vertebral fracture (OCVF).[2] Although many OCVFs appear to go clinically undetected, up to 30% of symptomatic fractures remain unresponsive to conservative management and are considered candidates for surgical intervention.[3,4] Considering these statistics along with the general effectiveness of vertebral augmentation in treating chronic pain from OCVFs, it is easy to understand the expected steady increase in frequency of procedures performed to treat this disease process.

Originally developed in France during the mid-1980s to treat vertebral hemangiomas and later introduced in the United States in 1994 in the treatment of symptomatic OCVFs, the percutaneous injection of bone cement, polymethyl methacylate (PMMA), has gained widespread use by physicians who treat OCVFs. Vertebroplasty and kyphoplasty have consistently demonstrated the ability to improve patient function and quality of life through excellent pain control and rapid mobilization for this "at risk" group of patients.[5] However, risks pertaining to cement toxicity, exothermic reactions and tissue damage, embolism, and the potential neurologically devastating complication of cement extravasation outside the vertebral body (spinal canal, neuroforamen) remain.[2,6] Furthermore, concerns have been raised and debated about whether vertebral bodies augmented with PMMA (with or without intradiscal extravasation) are associated with a higher adjacent-level vertebral fracture (ALF) rate than would be expected because of the natural risk of additional fractures. Investigators have challenged the direct causal relationship between PMMA-augmented vertebral bodies and ALF, arguing that ALFs may simply be the result of the natural history of the underlying disease (osteoporosis). However, it is generally agreed that when fractures occur following PMMA augmentation, it is more common to see them occur within the first 3 months after the procedure, and they are more likely to occur at an adjacent level than elsewhere in the spinal column.[7] In contrast, people with osteoporotic bones with compression fractures who have not had PMMA vertebral augmentation have subsequent vertebral fractures that are distributed more randomly throughout

the spine and will occur sporadically throughout the following year. Data such as these do suggest that PMMA augmentation of vertebral bodies at least predisposes adjacent vertebral levels to fracture.[8-12]

It has been proposed that the ideal bone cement for vertebral augmentation should be biodegradable and nontoxic, have a low setting temperature, and have a biomechanical profile close to that of human bone.[13] To avoid some of the drawbacks of PMMA noted previously, and to provide an "ideal" biological cement for vertebral augmentation, a new option was developed that involves the minimally invasive injection of morselized allograft bone into a polyester expandable mesh container (OptiMesh, Spineology Inc., Minneapolis, Minn.). The bone injection procedure generates lifting force for potential fracture reduction, and the resultant bone graft strut is immediately load sharing and has a modulus of elasticity closely approximating that of native bone.

## INDICATIONS AND CONTRAINDICATIONS

The primary indications for use of this mesh–bone construct include painful osteoporotic, traumatic, or steroid-induced Vertebral compression fractures (VCFs) from T4 to L5, with or without secondary kyphosis, that has not responded to a reasonable trial of conservative therapy. An additional indication is for benign but symptomatic vertebral hemangiomas. Pain and tenderness should be localized to the fracture level identified on x-ray, CT, MRI, or technetium Tc 99m bone scan. Patients should be medically stable to at least tolerate a percutaneous procedure and be able to assume a prone position for the procedure.

The main contraindication, as with all vertebral augmentation procedures, is the presence of an unstable vertebral fracture with retropulsed fragments causing more than 20% canal compromise (i.e., true burst fracture pattern) or any fracture pattern with neurologic deficit. The author has successfully and safely used this technique to treat compression fractures with "bowing" of the posterior cortex (posterior longitudinal ligament intact) along with fractures demonstrating minimal retropulsion of the superior or inferior endplate into the canal causing less than 20% canal compromise. Of interest, the use of this device as a minimally invasive option to treat true burst fractures with the AO classification of A1 has even been shown effective when combined with short-segment pedicle screw fixation.[14]

Because of issues of healing in the presence of adjuvant therapy as well as the inherent biologic aggressiveness of metastatic tumor leading to compression fractures, this device should not be used, when used with allograft bone as a filler material. Other absolute contraindications include comorbid conditions such as uncorrected coagulation or bleeding disorders, osteomyelitis, epidural abscess, and vertebra plana. Finally, the efficacy of prophylactic treatment in patients at high risk for VCFs has not been proved.

## DESCRIPTION OF THE DEVICE

The basic concept behind this technology is that a cavity within a fractured vertebra is created percutaneously through a relatively small access portal via a fluoroscopically guided unilateral, extrapedicular approach. A deflated

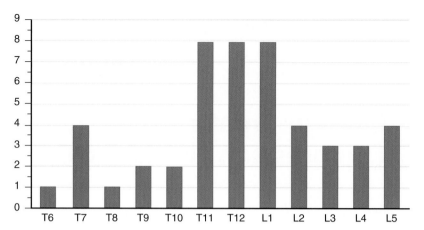

**FIGURE 43-1** Distribution of fracture levels among patients treated with OptiMesh.

porous polyester mesh bag (OptiMesh) is inserted and subsequently filled with allograft morsels, allowing a large load-sharing graft and strut to be built within the vertebral body. OptiMesh is designed to contain and reinforce morselized bone graft. The pore size of the mesh is nominally 1500 μm, allowing the mesh to effectively constrain the morselized allograft while also allowing ingrowth of vessels and native bone elements for ultimate graft incorporation and remodeling.

Using the principles of granular mechanics, impaction of bone granules into the mesh bag generates a distractive force, producing the capability for reduction (i.e., height restoration) of the fractured vertebra. Because the bone granules are tightly packed, force chains develop between the bone chips, thus creating a strut capable of supporting the axial loads of the spine.

The bone allograft (Musculoskeletal Transplant Foundation [MTF], Edison, N.J.) is a mixture of lyophilized corticocancellous chips and demineralized bone matrix (DBM), providing both osteoconductive and osteoinductive properties for graft incorporation.

## BACKGROUND OF SCIENTIFIC TESTING AND CLINICAL OUTCOMES

The nonresorbable mesh is knitted from yarn made of polyethylene terephthalate (PET) thread. Animal studies have shown that the mesh does not produce an adverse tissue reaction or create a barrier to bone growth from the host into the graft pack.[15] In vitro biomechanical testing has shown that the mesh filled with bone graft restores intact vertebral body strength in compression. The final construct's restored strength and stiffness is less than PMMA-augmented vertebral bodies, which may have a desired protective effect to reduce the potential for adjacent level fractures. As the reduction of the fracture (i.e., height restoration) occurs while the device is being deployed and filled, the author has found that this procedure more reliably restored and maintained vertebral body height. This is in contrast to loss of almost two thirds of potential restored height that occurs upon deflation of the kyphoplasty balloon in treating similar "mobile" compression fractures.[16] Finally, the MTF bone mixture has been shown to generate new bone formation equivalent to autograft when placed in the vertebral bodies of sheep.[17]

To assess clinical efficacy, the author conducted an INVESTIGATIONAL REVIEW BOARD (IRB)-approved retrospective study to review consecutive patients treated with OptiMesh from March, 2004, to December, 2007. Forty patients were enrolled under the protocol. There were 32 women and 8 men with an average age of 73.4 years (range: 44 to 95 years). Of the 40 patients, 29 patients had osteoporotic compression fractures, 10 patients had trauma, and 1 patient had breast cancer. A total of 48 levels were implanted. More than 50% of the fractures occurred at the thoracolumbar junction (Figure 43-1). Average follow-up was 16 months. There were 27 patients (67.5%) who had greater than 6-month follow-up, with an average of 23 months. Of the patients treated for osteoporotic VCFs, 19 patients had preoperative DUAL X-RAY ABSORPTIOMETRY(DEXA) scores with an average T-score of −2.4.

Pain and function were assessed using the four-point Odom score (excellent, good, fair, poor). This scale allows the treating physician to combine clinical observations and physical examination with the patient's global

assessment. Only two patients (5%) rated a poor score in the early postoperative period. All of the patients with longer than 6-month follow-up expressed satisfaction with the procedure and were rated an excellent or good Odom score.

Postoperative x-rays were evaluated for new vertebral body fractures and maintenance of restored vertebral body height. Six patients (15%) suffered new fractures, but only two patients (5%) had ALF. The postoperative CT scan on one patient identified a fracture of the medial pedicle wall, without sequelae. One patient with a recurrent glioblastoma was treated for an osteoporotic VCF, but at 3-month follow-up had significant loss of restored vertebral body height on x-ray, although this was asymptomatic. All patients who had a CT scan beyond 12 months postoperatively showed good evidence of graft incorporation within the mesh.

## CLINICAL PRESENTATION AND EVALUATION

Patent MW: A 69-year-old woman with osteoporosis who suffered T7 and T8 VCFs (T-score: −2.5) secondary to a fall. Fractures were demonstrated by plain x-rays and MRI, and she had severe pain and disability unresponsive to conservative therapy. She underwent a T7 and T8 biologic vertebral augmentation procedure with OptiMesh and morselized allograft during a single session under IV conscious sedation. She reported complete pain relief at 24 hours, and within 48 hours was able to ambulate and perform activities of daily living without assistance. At the 3-year postoperative visit, she continued to be pain free and her 3-year follow-up CT scan showed osseous integration of the graft pack (Figure 43-2).

## OPERATIVE TECHNIQUE

These procedures are performed most commonly with monitored anesthesia control on a radiolucent table. Because the procedure uses a unilateral, parapedicular approach into the vertebral body, biplanar fluoroscopic imaging is required to guide instrument placement, reduce the risk of neural injury, and size and fill the mesh.

Guide pin (i.e., Steinmann pin) placement determines instrument trajectory throughout the entire procedure and is thus the most critical portion of the procedure to perform correctly. The guide pin is passed percutaneously from a paramedian approach (approximately 7 cm from midline, depending on the level being treated). It is ultimately docked and then allowed to penetrate the lateral base of the pedicle at the pedicle–vertebral body junction. The pin is then advanced into the center of the vertebral body with a trajectory that ultimately positions its tip halfway across the silhouette of the vertebral body on both anteroposterior (AP) and lateral fluoroscopic images. Once an appropriate trajectory is obtained, a dilator is introduced over the guide pin and docked onto the pedicle vertebral body junction. The access portal (i.e., working channel), in turn, is passed over the dilator tube and similarly docked onto the vertebral body. The guide pin and dilator tube are then removed.

A cavity is then created within the vertebral body by first drilling obliquely across the vertebral body to within 5 to 6 mm of the contralateral vertebral body cortex with a 6-mm hand drill. An expandable shaper is then used to core out a cavity that leaves 2 to 3 mm of bone between the cavity and the endplates.

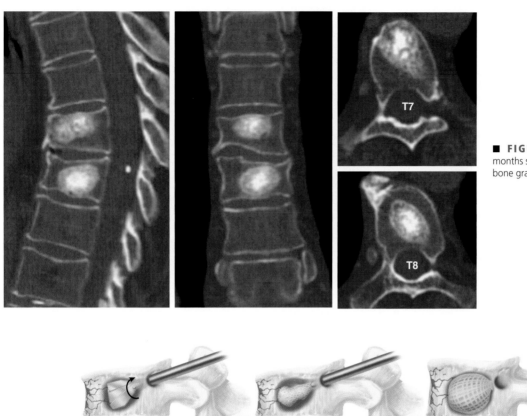

■ **FIGURE 43-2** CT scans at 36 months showing good osseous integration of bone graft.

■ **FIGURE 43-3**  **A,** A cavity is created. **B,** Mesh is inserted empty. **C,** Mesh is filled and released.

Based on the drill depth, shaper usage, neighboring normal vertebral body height, and the stiffness of the fracture (i.e., acute vs subacute), the appropriate size of mesh bag is determined. An acute fracture may require a larger construct to restore vertebral body height, whereas in a nonmobile fracture, the goal may only be to fill the cavity created without height restoration. Each size mesh has a maximum fill volume, and this should never be exceeded to avoid potential rupture and loss of containment of the allograft. Chronic fractures may allow little expansion of the mesh if a cavity is inappropriately undersized. In this situation, the graft pack may achieve load-bearing capabilities at fill volumes less than recommended.

The mesh bag is attached to a mesh holder and passed into the cavity. The mesh is then filled using prefilled tubes prepared and provided by Musculoskeletal Transplant Foundation. The mesh bag is filled circumferentially utilizing initially the diverted (i.e., angled tip) tubes to fill the bag peripherally followed by a straight (i.e non-angled tip) tube which fills the mesh bag centrally ensuring an even packing of allograft throughout the construct. Upon completion of filling, the mesh is detached from its crimp tip, and then all instruments are removed from the patient (Figure 43-3).

## POSTOPERATIVE CARE

These procedures are often done on an outpatient basis with the patients allowed to ambulate following clearance by the anesthesia team. No bracing is necessary and patients can return to light to moderate levels of activity immediately. In patients with osteoporosis, treatment of the underlying disease with best medical management is essential.

## COMPLICATIONS AND AVOIDANCE

This procedure involves placement of an actual implant in the vertebral body, so prophylactic antibiotics should always be used to avoid the development of spondylitis. As with all percutaneous spinal procedures, adequate

visualization with biplanar fluoroscopy and surgeon experience with interpreting these images are mandatory. Though the extrapedicular approach reduces the likelihood of canal violation, nerve root injury, pedicle fracture, spinal cord injury, and misplacement of the device outside the confines of the fractured vertebral body can occur if the landmarks for guide pin placement and trajectory are not well visualized or interpreted.

The potential for retroperitoneal bleeding (for lumbar fracture repair) and for hemothorax or pneumothorax (with thoracic fracture repair) are valid concerns but in the author's experience rarely occur. To avoid violating the pleural space in treating thoracic fractures, the guide pin should be walked along the dorsal side of the rib cage as it is guided from lateral to medial to the costovertebral junction, and then more ventrally along the lateral aspect of pedicle. Ipsilateral exiting nerve root injury at any level can be avoided by always keeping the guide pin (which defines the subsequent trajectory of all additional instrumentation) within the shadow of the pedicle on lateral fluoroscopic imaging.

### ADVANTAGES AND DISADVANTAGES

The primary advantage of using a biologic material for VCF treatment is avoidance of complications associated with cement, which include containment, toxicity, and stiffness of final construct. With the biologic vertebral augmentation with OptiMesh and bone graft, the chances for extravasation and embolism of PMMA can be all but eliminated. The porous construct designed is entirely biocompatible and yet is strong enough to bear weight and provide equivalent pain relief. The final result may be that with biologic vertebral augmentation, a less stiff construct is less likely to cause or predispose to adjacent level fractures. Our early experience has demonstrated only a 5% rate of ALFs compared with the quoted literature average for new adjacent level fractures after treatment with vertebroplasty and kyphoplasty of 15% to 20%.[18] Confirmation of these rates by other investigators will need to be performed to confirm these results.

## CONCLUSIONS AND DISCUSSION

The clinical study indicates that placement of a load-sharing mesh and bone graft strut into the anterior column creates structural stability and is effective in reducing pain and increasing function in patients with VCFs. Long-term radiographic follow-up shows a low incidence of ALFs, and osseous integration of the graft occurs even in osteoporotic patients. New advancements of this technology currently being developed include new biologic graft materials and a smaller (5.5-mm outside diameter) access portal with fewer steps to the implant procedure.

## References

1. Health, United States, 2007, Table 1. Retrieved 11/3/08 from http://www.cdc.gov/nchs/fastats/older_americans.htm.
2. M. Eicholz, J.E. O'Toole, S.D. Christie, et al., Vertebroplasty and kyphoplasty, Neurosurg Clin. N. Am. 17 (2006) 507–518.
3. D.M. Kado, T. Duong, K.L. Stone, et al., Vertebral fractures and mortality in older women, Arch. Intern. Med. 159 (1999) 1215–1220.
4. T. Jalava, S. Sarna, L. Pylkkanen, et al., Association between vertebral fracture and increased mortality in osteoporotic patients, J. Bone Miner. Res. 18 (2003) 1254–1276.
5. R.S. Taylor, P. Fritzell, R.J. Taylor, Balloon kyphoplasty in the management of vertebral compression fractures: an updated systematic review and meta-analysis, Eur. Spine J. 16 (2007) 1085–1100.
6. A.A. Patel, A.R. Vaccaro, G.G. Martyak, et al., Neurologic deficit following percutaneous vertebral stabilization, Spine 32 (16) (2007) 1728–1734.
7. D. Fribourg, C. Tang, P. Sra, R. Delamarter, H. Bae, Incidence of subsequent vertebral fracture after kyphoplasty. Clinical Case Series, Spine 29 (20) (October 15, 2004) 2270–2276.
8. T. Faciszewski, F. Kiernan, R. Rao, Treatment of osteoporotic vertebral compression fractures, in: J.M. Spivak, P.J. Connolly (Eds.), Orthopedic Knowledge Update, Spine 3, American Academy of Orthopedic Surgeons, Rosemont, IL, 2006.
9. F. Grados, N. Hardy, Treatment of vertebral compression fractures by vertebroplasty [abstract], Rev. Rheum. 64 (1997) 38.
10. Carlson SD, Smith JS, Gordon CD. Is there an increased risk of adjacent segment compression fracture after kyphoplasty. Poster presentation, Annual Meeting of the American Academy of Orthopaedic Surgeons, Feb 13-17, 2002, Dallas, TX.
11. Anselmetti GC. Long-term data confirm benefit of vertebroplasty for back pain relief after osteoporotic vertebral collapse. Presented at Society of Interventional Radiology 33rd Annual Scientific Meeting: Abstract 182, March 18, 2008, Washington, DC.
12. E.P. Lin, S. Ekholm, A. Hiwatashi, P.L. Westesson, Vertebroplasty:cement leakage into the disc increases the risk of new fracture of adjacent vertebral body, AJNR Am. J. Neuroradiol. 25 (2004) 175–180.
13. U. Berlemann, S.J. Ferguson, L.P. Nolte, P.F. Heini, Adjacent vertebral failure after vertebroplasty. A biomechanical investigation, J. Bone Joint Surg. Br. 84 (2002) 748–752.
14. J. Inamasu, B.H. Guiot, J.S. Uribe, Flexion-distraction injury of the L1 vertebra treated with short-segment posterior fixation and OptiMesh, J. Clin. Neurosci. 15 (2008) 214–218.
15. B.W. Cunningham, S.D. Kuslich, J.C. Sefter, et al., Interbody arthrodesis using a polyester surgical mesh (the BAG™ surgical mesh): an in-vivo and in-vitro assessment. Presented at the 3rd Annual Meeting of the Spine Society of Europe, Gotenburg, Sweden, Sept. 4-8, 2001.
16. L. Beckman, D. Giannitsios, T. Steffen, An evaluation of the height restoration performance of three vertebral body fracture repair procedures, ex-vivo. Presented at the 8th Annual Meeting of the Spine Society of Europe, Istanbul, Turkey, Oct. 25-28, 2006.
17. T. Fujishiro, T.W. Bauer, N. Kobayashi, et al., Histological evaluation of an impacted bone graft substitute composed of a combination of mineralized and demineralized allograft in a sheep vertebral bone defect. J Biomed Mat Res, published online 16 February 2007 in Wiley Inter-Science (www.interscience.wiley.com). DOI: 10.1002/jbm.a.31056.
18. R. Lindsay, S. Silverman, C. Cooper, et al., Risk of new vertebral fracture in the year following a fracture, JAMA 285 (3) 320–323, 2001.

# 44

# Vessel-X

*Darwono A. Bambang*

## KEY POINTS

- The Vessel-X is designed to restore the height of symptomatic vertebral compression fractures and to prevent the leakage of the injected bone filler material (BFM).
- The device is made of double-layer nonstretchable polyethylene terephthalate with 100 μm pores, the anterior titanium marker, and titanium nozzle.
- When the BFM is injected inside, the Vessel-X acts as an implant body expander, combining the advantages of both balloon and vertebroplasty yet preventing the leakage.
- Injection of the BFMs inside a container creates a pressure that will be distributed equally to all directions, and it is followed in the same distribution when the interdigitation of BFMs through the pores occurred, thus preventing the leakage.[1]

## INTRODUCTION

Since vertebroplasty was introduced by Herve and Deramond in 1984, many methods of percutaneous osteoplasty (molding the bone) evolved to treat symptomatic vertebral compression fractures (VCFs), by injection of bone filler material (BFM): polymethylmethacrylate (PMMA), other kinds of bone cement, and bone grafts (autografts and allografts), or different kinds of osteoinductive or osteoconductive materials. The same risk in performing the previously mentioned techniques is the leakage of BFM, because the injected pressure will go to the fracture's weakest area and lead to a leakage. Vesselplasty is an osteoplasty technique using the Vessel-X, which acts as an implant body expander to restore vertebral height in VCFs but prevents the potential risk of leakage.[1,2]

## INDICATIONS AND CONTRAINDICATIONS

### Indications

The procedure is indicated for symptomatic VCFs in the thoracic or lumbar vertebrae stemming from[2]:

- Primary osteoporosis
- Secondary osteoporosis
- High energy trauma
- Lesion from multiple myeloma or bone metastasis
- Painful vertebral hemangioma

### Contraindications

Contraindications include the following[2]:

- Pregnancy
- Uncorrected coagulopathy
- Pain unrelated to vertebral compression fractures
- Technically not possible (e.g., vertebra plana)
- Osteolytic tumor
- Allergy to components used
- Fractures with posterior wall interrupted

## DESCRIPTION OF THE DEVICE

The idea behind the prototype originated in Taiwan, in February 2002 (Figure 44-1). The cadaveric study using the prototype was done by the author in Jakarta, Indonesia, in July 2003. The first generation used in the clinic was named threadplasty, because the connection used was thread (Figure 44-2).

A clinical trial was done in Jakarta, Indonesia, by the author from July 2004 until July 2005. As a preliminary report the first three cases were presented at the Asia Pacific Orthopaedic Association (APOA) Triennial Meeting in Kuala Lumpur on September 5-10, 2004. After the ten first-generation vesselplasty devices (Threadplasty) were made and during the clinical trial, major improvements and developments were made to formulate the last-generation instruments available for clinical use (Figure 44-3).[1-6]

Vessel-X is a bone filler container made of polyethylene terephthalate (PET), a nonstretchable material. In deflated condition its shape is long, and when it is inflated the shape becomes short and bigger until a certain size is reached. When the pressure inside the container is equal to the surrounding resistance, the final size is achieved and the size will remain constant. This mechanical device is used to lift the vertebral endplate, acting like an implant body expander (Figure 44-4).

The Vessel-X container is a PET mesh and has 100-μm porosity. When the pressure inside the container is greater than the surrounding resistance, the BFM starts to interdigitate through the pores; some pressure is then relieved and the endplate is lifted further (Figures 44-5 and 44-6).

The Variations in technical concepts in percutaneous osteoplasty have led to the differences in techniques and results for the numerous methods: vesselplasty (KYPHON INC. CA), vertebroplasty, kyphoplasty, VEX-3000 (Taeyeon Medical CO., LTD, South Korea), Sky Expander (DISC-O-TECH MEDICAL TECHNOLOGIES, LTD., IS), arcuplasty (Warsaw Orthopedic, Inc, IN), and the Optimesh system (Spineology, Inc., MN) (Figure 44-7). Vertebroplasty is not used to restore the vertebral body height (VBH), whereas the other techniques are accomplishing the same goal by first creating a void. The other concepts do restore VBH and create a void by mechanical or hydrostatic pressure. The difference between the restoring VBH group is based on the technical methods and instruments to lift the vertebral endplate. To restore VBH, all techniques except vesselplasty need to first create a void by mechanical or hydrostatic pressure, followed by filling the void with PMMA or other BFM. All the previously mentioned techniques carry different risks of leakage, because if the BFM is injected directly into the bone or void, it will go to the weakest fracture area. The vesselplasty technique requires only that a hole be drilled into the vertebral body as a place to be occupied by the deflated PET container (almost like screw insertion into the bone). Then the container is inflated by injecting viscous PMMA or other BFM, and the hydrostatic pressure lifts the vertebral endplate, acting as an implanted vertebral body expander.[1,6-16]

Sequential injection of BFM into a nonstretchable container will prevent leakage, because inside the container the pressure will be distributed equally to all direction. Under a continuous sequential injection the pressure is released outside the Vessel-X through the pores sequentially, because the container size is constant, and starting the interdigitation works like vertebroplasty. The sequential pressure release and the interdigitation will further lift the endplate yet still preventing leakage, because the pressure is equally distributed in all directions. The most

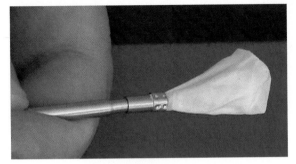

■ **FIGURE 44-1**    The prototype.

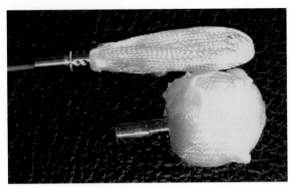

■ **FIGURE 44-4**    Vessel-X, the PET container.

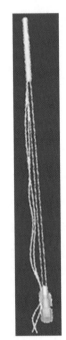

■ **FIGURE 44-2**    The threadplasty.

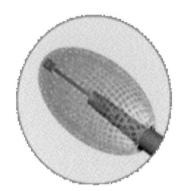

■ **FIGURE 44-5**    Mesh container.

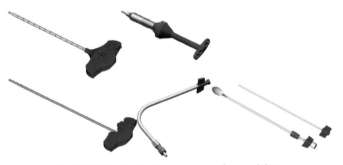

■ **FIGURE 44-3**    The instruments for vesselplasty.

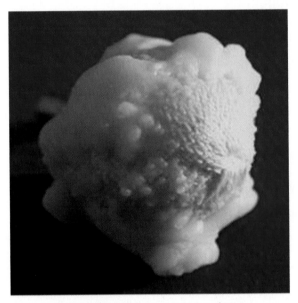

■ **FIGURE 44-6**    Interdigitation of BFMs.

important point is the experienced surgeon's judgment of when to end the procedure, which is related to the individual patient's condition (Figures 44-8 and 44-9).

## BACKGROUND OF SCIENTIFIC TESTING AND CLINICAL OUTCOMES

A nonrandomized 3-year prospective follow-up study on 103 patients who had single- or multiple-level stable VCFs from T5 to L5, involving a total of 117 vertebrae (Figure 44-10). In 86 cases, fractures were in osteoporotic vertebrae, compared to 17 cases where the fractures were due to high energy trauma. The number of females, 69 cases, was twice the number of males, at 34 cases. The average patient age was 70.3 years, with the youngest 34 years old and the oldest 98 years old. Fracture age ranged from 1 day to 70 days after the trauma.

All cases were treated with 20-mm Vessel-X through transpedicular or extrapedicular routes, using either unilateral or bilateral containers. The minimum follow-up was 3 months, and the outcomes were measured with Visual Analoq Scale (VAS), SF-36, and Oswestry Disability Index (ODI).

One day after treatment, all patients gained significant pain relief, as determined from the VAS, which dropped from 9.9 to 1.7 ($p < .001$), and

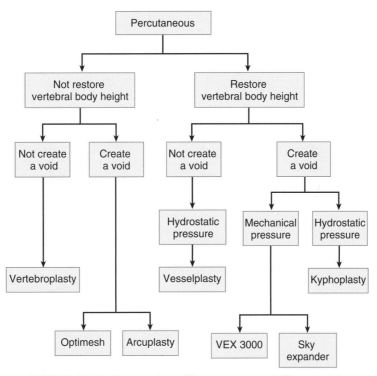

■ **FIGURE 44-7**  The osteoplasty: different concepts and different techniques.

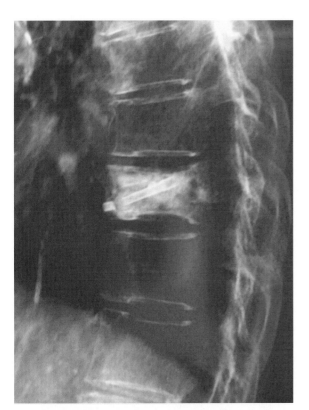

■ **FIGURE 44-8**  Vesselplasty's x-ray shows 100% correction.

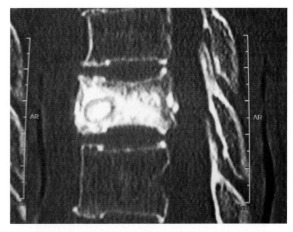

■ **FIGURE 44-9**  Vesselplasty's CT scan shows container size is constant.

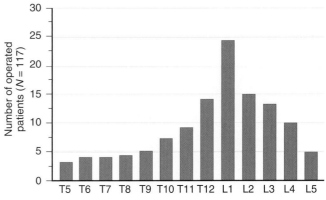

■ **FIGURE 44-10**  Distribution of level of the affected vertebrae relief (T5-L5;) .

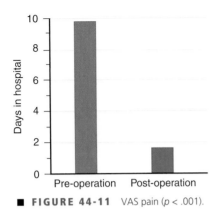

**■ FIGURE 44-11**    VAS pain (*p* < .001).

the average hospital stay was 2.2 days (Figure 44-11). The average vertebral height restoration was 96.4% (range, 100% to 50%) related to the variable bone density from old to young patients, fracture type, and fracture age. A variable amount of BFM was injected into the small 20-mm Vessel-X, from 2.5 ml to 10.25 ml, without any leakage, bleeding, or neurologic deficits, and only two adjacent level fractures were detected 1 year after treatment on the eldest patients, who were older than 90 years.

## OPERATIVE TECHNIQUE

### Anesthesia

During the procedure both local anesthesia and conscious sedation to make the patient comfortable and relaxed are recommended rather than general anesthesia. The combination of conscious sedation and local anesthesia could reduce the risk of injuring the nerve root because the patient can feel the radiating pain caused by the procedure, which is not possible with general anesthesia. The local anesthetic preparation should involve the skin and subcutaneous tissues along the expected needle tract, and the periosteum of the bone at the bone entry site must be thoroughly infiltrated. Once this is accomplished, the patient will experience only mild discomfort while the bone needle is being placed, and the patient will become more relaxed if conscious sedation is used. The local anesthesia being used is a mixture of 0.5% lidocaine and 1:200,000 epinephrine, because it allows the use of a more generous volume locally with less risk of toxicity.[4]

### Position

Patient positioning should be prone on a beanbag or just supported by pillows located under the chest and the hip. If hyperextension is needed to promote some reduction of the fractured vertebra, additional pillows can be added under the hip and the legs of the patient. This position allows a clear visualization during fluoroscopy using the C-arm in both the anteroposterior and lateral views because there is no metal in between.[2]

## *Case Studies*

### CASE 1 (2005) (Figures 44-12 and 44-13)

The patient was a 77-year-old woman with VCFs at T11 and T12 that occurred during a fall 2 days earlier. Vesselplasty was done on two levels on day 3 using a 20-mm container, unilaterally through the extrapedicular route. Bone cement of 3.5 ml was injected, without leakage, and 100% restoration was achieved. One day after treatment the patient was able to sit and walk, and was discharged on day 4. Follow-up was done for 3 years, and the patient remained in good condition.

### CASE 2 (2006) (Figures 44-14 and 44-15)

The patient was a 67-year-old woman with a VCF at L3 that occurred during a fall 1 week earlier. Vesselplasty was performed with a 20-mm container, 6.75 ml cement was injected through a unilateral extrapedicular route, with no leakage. Height restoration of 100% was achieved, and the patient was discharged the day after in good condition. After 2 years of follow-up, the patient remained in good condition.

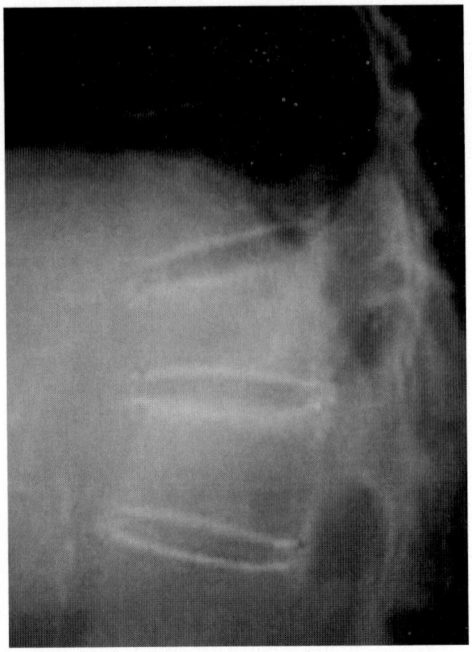

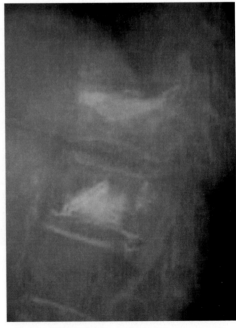

**■ FIGURE. 44-12**    Case 1: Before vesselplasty.

**■ FIGURE 44-13**    Case 1: After vesselplasty.

**CASE 3 (2007)** (Figures 44-16 and 44-17)

The patient was a 77-year-old woman with VCFs at T12 and L1 that occurred 2 weeks earlier. Two levels of vesselplasty using 20-mm containers were performed using a unilateral extrapedicular route. Complete height restoration (100%) was achieved in both vertebrae. Different amounts of cement were injected in each vertebra, with 9 ml in one and 7.25 ml in the other without any leakage. The patient was discharged the day after in good condition.

**CASE 4 (2005)** (Figures 44-18 and 44-19)

The patient was a 98-year-old woman with a VCF of T12 that occurred 2 weeks previous. Single level and bilateral vesselplasty using 20-mm containers was performed through a transpedicular route; 3.5 ml cement was injected into each Vessel-X for a total of 7 ml, and 100% restoration was achieved. The patient was discharged 1 day after. She still had good quality of life 4 years later at the age of 102 years.

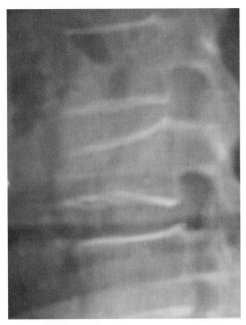

■ **FIGURE 44-14**   Case 2: Before vesselplasty.

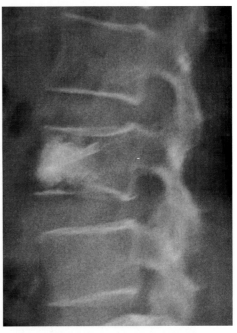

■ **FIGURE 44-15**   Case 2: After vesselplasty.

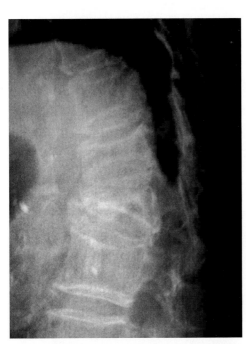

■ **FIGURE 44-16**   Case 3: Before vesselplasty.

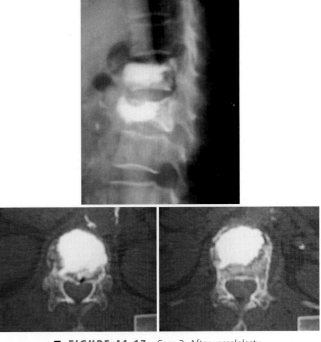

■ **FIGURE 44-17**   Case 3: After vesselplasty.

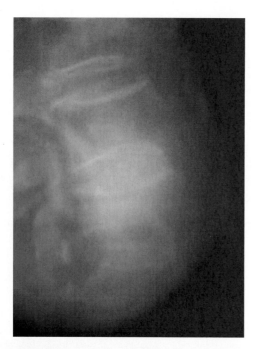

■ **FIGURE 44-18**   Case 4: Before vesselplasty.

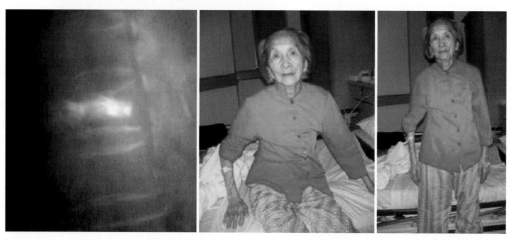

■ **FIGURE 44-19**   Case 4: After vesselplasty.

### CASE 5 (2006) (Figure 44-20)

The patient was an 81-year-old woman with a VCF at L1 that occurred 1 month earlier. Vesselplasty was performed with a 20-mm container. A unilateral extrapedicular approach was used. A total of 10.25 ml cement was injected, but because of the fracture's age (1 month), the maximum height restoration was only 90%. The advantage was that no leakage occurred, and the patient was discharged the day after with good quality of daily living.

### CASE 6 (2005) (Figure 44-21)

The patient was a 70-year-old woman with a 2-month-old VCF (vertebra plana) at T9. Vesselplasty was performed using a 20-mm container. A unilateral, extrapedicular route was used and 4 ml cement was injected. The height restoration was 90% yet no leakage occurred, and the patient was discharged the day after.

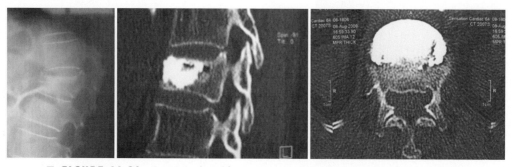

■ **FIGURE 44-20**   Case 5: Neglected fracture at 1 month, 90% height restoration, no leakage.

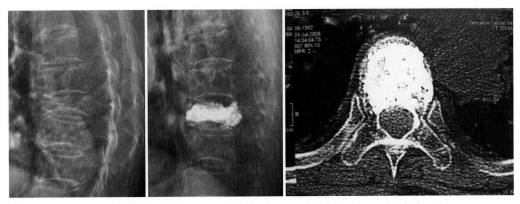

**■ FIGURE 44-21**   Case 6: Vertebra plana, 90% height restoration, no leakage.

## PROCEDURE

Related to the biomechanical theory of VCFs, the restoration of VBH could be achieved by delivering enough pressure inside the vertebral body to counteract the resistance of the surrounding bone density and the large bending moment due to the shift of the center of body gravity toward the anterior vertebral body side (Figures 44-22 and 44-23).[1-8,9,17-19] The restoration is more related to the amount of pressure that can be created, rather than the amount of BFM to be injected. The BFM being delivered with pressure into a vertebral body tends to fill the cavity or void, going toward the weakest area of the fracture, which is its side, and leads to a leakage risk. A nonstretchable container can be used to control the leakage risk because the delivered BFM will be distributed equally in all directions inside the container, and the created pressure inside the container can be used to lift the vertebral endplate toward its normal position accordingly.[1-4]

The Vessel-X container (A-Spine Holding Taipei, Taiwan) was designed to meet this purpose. It is made of polyethylene terephthalate (PET), a biocompatible material that is ordinarily used for blood vessel grafts and mesh grafts in herniorrhaphy. The PET mesh container has multipores of 100-μm diameter and is available in one or two layer containers. The number of layers, the pore diameter, and size of a nonstretchable PET container are used to control the amount of the pressure created and the volume of BFM. The relatively weakest area of the container is the posterior part, where the pressure is applied. A titanium nozzle (also a biocompatible material) is used to facilitate the pressure delivery and also to counteract the rebound pressure (Figure 44-24).[1,2,6]

Because the Vessel-X is strongly connected to the inserter by a six-turn clockwise-threaded surface, the inserter should be turned six times counterclockwise to release it (Figure 44-25).

An anterior titanium marker is available for intraoperative confirmation after inserting the Vessel-X container. A preloaded 1.2-mm guidewire is positioned within the inserter, engaged together with the anterior marker in maintaining the overall length of the Vessel-X during insertion (Figure 44-26).

A bone access needle and precision drill are used to facilitate the delivery of the Vessel-X into the vertebral body through a transpedicular or

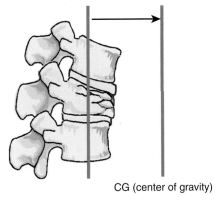

CG (center of gravity)

**■ FIGURE 44-22**   Center of gravity shift toward anterior.

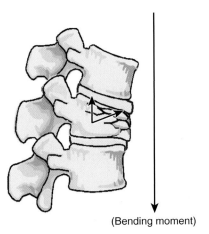

(Bending moment)

**■ FIGURE 44-23**   Pressure inside vertebra to counteract the resistance and bending moment.

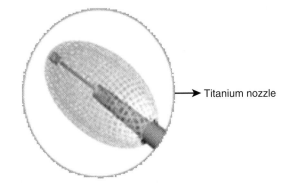

→ Titanium nozzle

**■ FIGURE 44-24**   Layer, pore diameter, and titanium nozzle of Vessel-X.

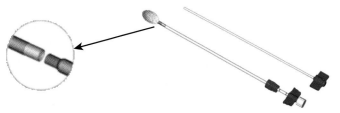

**■ FIGURE 44-25**   Threaded connection between nozzle and inserter.

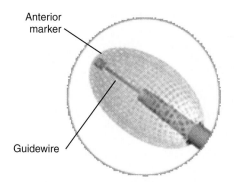

■ **FIGURE 44-26**    Anterior marker and guidewire.

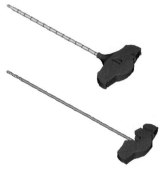

■ **FIGURE 44-27**    Bone access needle and precision drill.

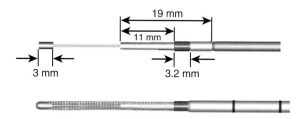

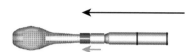

■ **FIGURE 44-28**    Pushing a few millimeters anterior, facilitating the inflation.

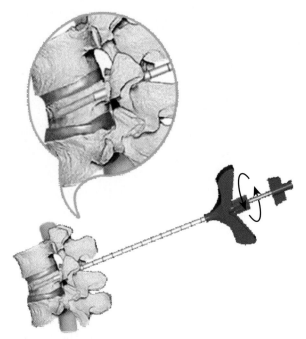

■ **FIGURE 44-29**    Tightening the Luer connector

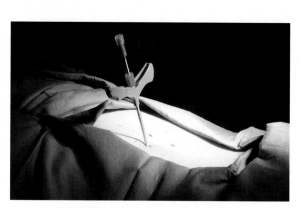

■ **FIGURE 44-30**    Final position of the inserter

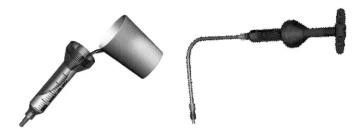

■ **FIGURE 44-31**    Controllable cement delivery and extension tube.

extrapedicular approach (similar to screw delivery into the bone) (Figure 44-27.) Once the Vessel-X is in its proper position inside the vertebral body, the guidewire is removed, and the inserter is pushed a few mm anterior to facilitate the inflation of the nonstretchable container (Figure 44-28).[1,3]

To prevent inserter migration, the position of the inserter is secured by tightening the Luer connector of the lock knob of the inserter to the working cannula tube before removing the guidewire (Figure 44-29). The final position of the Vessel-X and the inserter before the delivery of BFM is shown in Figure 44-30.[1,3]

A proper viscosity of the BFM is important to create the hydrostatic pressure to lift the vertebral endplate. (Note: Powder has no hydrostatic pressure, whereas paste has some.) When the proper viscosity is reached, the BFM is delivered through the controllable cement delivery (CCD) system and extension tube (Figure 44-31). The extension tube is connected to the CCD, and the BFM is slowly injected until it comes out from the distal tip of the extension tube. Then by turning the handle of the CCD 180 degrees, amount of 0.25 ml of BFM will be ejected.[1,3,5,6]

The extension tube is connected to the Vessel-X inserter by tightening the Luer-lock connector to prevent the disengagement of the extension tube. The final setting is achieved and it is now ready for the injection of the BFM (Figure 44-32).[1,3]

The maximum volume of BFM to be added to the respective Vessel-X container outside the bone is:

- 2 ml for 20-mm Vessel-X
- 2.5 ml for 25-mm Vessel-X
- 3 ml for 30-mm Vessel-X

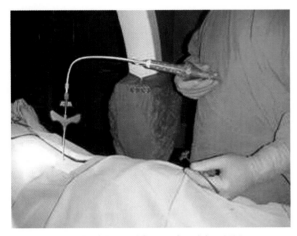

**FIGURE 44-32**　Ready to inject BFMs.

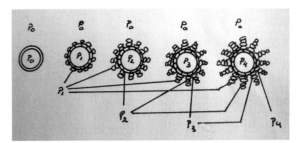

**FIGURE 44-34**　Gradual pressure release. The central core is the highest ($P_4 > P_3 > P_2 > P_1 > P_0$).

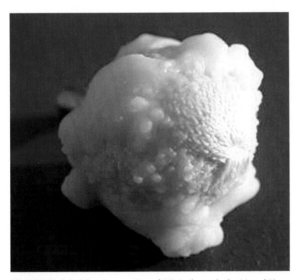

**FIGURE 44-33**　Penetration of BFMs through the Vessel-X pores.

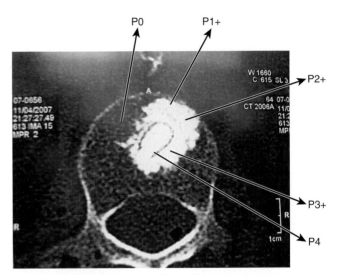

**FIGURE 44-35**　Gradual stiffness of bone plus BFMs ($P_4 > P_3 > P_2 > P_1 > P_0$).

The injected volume of BFM inflates the Vessel-X into its final shape, and the pressure inside the container will be equal to the air resistance: 1 atm. As more BFM is injected inside, the pressure will increase above 1 atm, the BFM starts to penetrate the pores, and the released pressure will lift the vertebral endplate (Figure 44-33).[1,3,6]

Inside the bone, the resistance is above 1 atm depending on the variable bone density (fracture's age, osteoporosis, bone age) and the large bending moment due to kyphotic deformity. Restoring the VBH requires a different pressure to counteract the different bone resistance and the kyphotic bending moment. For example, if the bone resistance is $P_0$ ($P_0 > 1$ atm), the volume of BFM to be injected into a 20-mm container will be over 2 ml until the pressure inside the container is equal to $P_0$, then the final shape of the container is achieved and constant. The final shape of the container, which is bigger than before, allows some restoration of the vertebral body height. As more BFMs are injected inside the container, the pressure will increase until $P_1$ ($P_1 > P_0$) and the BFM starts to penetrate the pores to the surrounding bone.[1,3]

The surrounding bone resistance is affected by the penetrated BFMs; it changes from $P_0$ to $P_1$, from the center toward the periphery of the container. The released pressure $P_1$ will lift the endplate further and more restoration of the VBH is achieved. When the penetrated BFM contacts body fluid and temperature of the surrounding bone, it hardens faster than inside the container. The bone resistance changes from $P_0$ to $P_1+$ ($P_1+ > P_1$), while the inside container is still $P_1$.

To counteract the $P_1+$ bone resistance, more BFM should be injected inside the constant shape of the nonstretchable container to increase the pressure until it reaches $P_2$ ($P_2 > P_1+$); then it starts to penetrate again, and the released pressure $P_2$ will lift the endplate higher.

By doing the procedure step by step, gradual pressure lifts the endplate until the desired restoration of VBH is achieved. The final outcome is a creation of gradual resistance or stiffness of the bone plus BFM; the central core of the container has the highest pressure, and this might prevent fractures at the adjacent or same level (Figures 44-34 and 44-35).[1,4-6]

The first 1.25 ml of BFM to be injected fills the inserter, and the following gradual injections will fill the container. After each 0.25 ml injection of BFM, the procedure should be stopped to perform a fluoroscopy check and to achieve some hardening of the penetrated BFM. Then injection is repeated until the properly desired volume is injected. Once the desired restoration of VBH is properly achieved, based on surgeon's judgment under fluoroscopic control, the injection is stopped (Figures 44-36 and 44-37).[1,3]

The next step is to detach the extension tube and use a pusher to push the 1.25 ml BFM inside the inserter into Vessel-X to achieve the final interdigitation through the 100-μm pores. The gradual interdigitation and stiffness of BFM could stabilize the Vessel-X in the surrounding bone and might prevent later fractures of the adjacent or same level.[7] When the BFM starts to change from viscous to paste condition, the Vessel-X container should be detached from the inserter by loosening the Luer connector, turning the handle counterclockwise for six full turns, and pulling the inserter out (the working cannula should always stay in position without moving). The needle is inserted into the cannula and they are removed together, leaving the Vessel-X as an implant (Figure 44-38).[1,3]

It is critically important that the vesselplasty procedure be performed under fluoroscopic imaging control (Figure 44-39).[1,3,7,8]

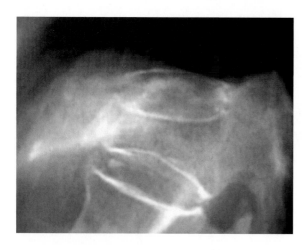

■ **FIGURE 44-36** Before treatment. A 67-year-old woman with fracture of L2 vertebra.

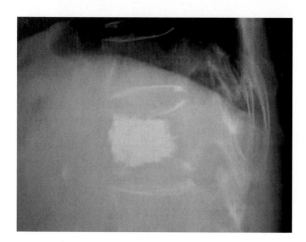

■ **FIGURE 44-37** After treatment. 20-mm vessel. Extrapedicular approach. 5.25 ml of BFMs. No leakage.

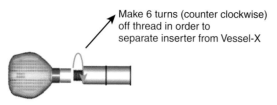

Make 6 turns (counter clockwise) off thread in order to separate inserter from Vessel-X

■ **FIGURE 44-38** Detaching Vessel-X.

## POSTOPERATIVE CARE

When the conscious sedation anesthesia has worn off, the patient is allowed to sit and walk. Patient activity should be adjusted to the healing process of the bone, which will take around 3 months. Two activities in particular should be restricted: bending forward and lifting. The patient is discharged from the hospital the same day or one day after vesselplasty, and assessments by x-ray are done every month until the bone heals.[2,3]

## COMPLICATIONS AND CAUTIONS

The complications are related to errors in patient selection and improper handling of the procedure. The indications should be restricted only for stable fractures and the symptomatic levels only, because the nonfusion technique will not stabilize the instability. Injection of the viscous BFMs should be done slowly, because the delivery of this material needs time to reach the Vessel-X inside the bone, because the viscosity is greater than water. If the injection is done too quickly, it will suddenly elevate the pressure

inside the inserter very high and cause the system to fail, which will break the delivery system. Selection of the proper viscosity of BFM with a setting time of at least 10 minutes is very important. A fast-setting cement could force the procedure to end too soon. The container should be delivered gently, because a rough insertion could break the predeployment mesh container; an improper positioning of the Vessel-X inside the vertebral body, such as too close to the vertebral body wall, spinal canal, or partially outside the bone, could cause the BFM to leak outside the vertebral body.[2,3]

## CONCLUSION

In comparison to the other osteoplasty techniques, the advantage of Vessel-plasty is its ability to control the leakage of BFM, by injecting the BFM into a nonstretchable PET container previously inserted inside the vertebral body. The hydrostatic pressure is created by the resistance of the PET container related to the pore diameter of 100 μm, PET layers, and the container size (20, 25, or 30 mm). The viscosity of BFM also plays an important role in achieving the optimum hydrostatic pressure, because the paste condition of BFM provides a lower hydrostatic pressure.[1,3]

The maximum pressure can be created inside the container, and it is related to the relative resistance of the surrounding individual bone density. The density of the bone is totally different between fresh and old fractures, or between young and osteoporotic bone. Once the created pressure exceeds the resistance of the surrounding bone density, the BFM starts to penetrate the 100-μm pore, interdigitating and stabilizing the container, and the increased pressure can lift the vertebral endplate. Injecting more BFM increases interdigitation and pressure. Once the penetrated BFM contacts body fluids and their higher temperature, it becomes harder than the BFM inside the container, and it increases the surrounding bone density. When

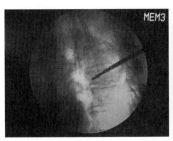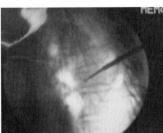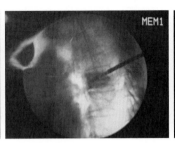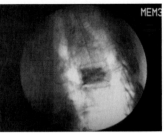

■ **FIGURE 44-39** Vesselplasty procedure under fluoroscopic imaging (C-arm).

## ADVANTAGES AND DISADVANTAGES

The Vessel-X system is designed to prevent the leakage of BFM, but it should be done properly. The amount of BFM to be injected is related to the pressure created, and the end restoration of vertebral body height is different for each case. Every patient has different bone density, different fracture type, and different fracture age and stage of healing. A wise surgeon's judgment of when to end the procedure is very important; it plays the key role in achieving the best results for the patient and prevents leakage of the BFM outside the bone.[1-3]

this procedure is done step by step, injecting BFM and releasing pressure, the end result is a restoration of vertebral body height and a gradual stiffness of the bone plus BFM from periphery to the central container. This gradual stiffness theoretically might prevent fractures in the same and adjacent levels. In vivo studies showed that up to 9.5 ml BFM can be injected into a 20-mm Vessel-X container without leakage, and restore vertebral height 100%.[1,2,4-6]

## References

1. B. Darwono, Vesselplasty: a novel concept of percutaneous treatment for stabilization and height restoration of vertebral compression fractures. J. Musculoskelet. Res. 11 (2008) 71–79.
2. A.B. Darwono, Vesselplasty as an alternative to kyphoplasty: a preliminary report, Triennial APOA meeting, Kuala Lumpur, Malaysia, 2004; September 5-10 Abstract not published.
3. A.B. Darwono, Surgical technique of vertebroplasty and vesselplasty, 13th APOA Spine Surgery Course, Coimbatore, India, 2007; March 8–11 Abstract not published.
4. A.B. Darwono, Vesselplasty as an alternative to Kyphoplasty: a new concept, 2nd CAMISS congress, Changsha, Hunan, PRChina, 2007; June 17 Abstract not published.
5. A.B. Darwono, Vesselplasty as an alternative to kyphoplasty: 2 years follow-up study, 7th PASMISS Congress, Qeongju, SouthKorea, 2007; August 17 Abstract not published.
6. A.B. Darwono Vesselplasty, A new concept to treat vertebral compression fractures: 3 years follow-up study, 1st Panhellenic Congress, Athens, Greece, 2007; September 21 Abstract not published.
7. P. Galibert, H. Deramond, P. Rosat, et al., Preliminary note on the treatment of vertebral angioma by percutaneous acrylic vertebroplasty, Neurochirurgie 33 (1987) 166–168.
8. A. Gangi, S. Guth, J.P. Imbert, et al., Percutaneous vertebroplasty: indications, technique, and results, Radiographics 23 (2003) 10.
9. O. Johnell, J. Kanis, A. Oden, et al., Mortality after osteoporotic fractures, Osteoporos. Int. 15 (2001) 35–42.
10. D.M. Kado, M.H. Huang, A.S. Karlamangla, et al., Hyperkyphotic posture predicts mortality in older community-dwelling men and women: a prospective study, J. Am. Geriatr. Soc. 52 (2004) 1662–1667.
11. C. Kasperk, J. Hillmeier, G. Noldge, et al., Treatment of painful vertebral fractures by kyphoplasty in patients with primary osteoporosis: a prospective nonrandomized controlled study, J. Bone Miner. Res. 20 (2005) 604–612.
12. J.T. Ledlie, M.B. Renfro, Kyphoplasty treatment of vertebral fractures: 2-year outcomes show sustained benefits, Spine 31 (2006) 57–64.
13. I.H. Lieberman, S. Dudeney, M.K. Reinhardt, et al., Initial outcome and efficacy of "kyphoplasty" in the treatment of painful osteoporotic vertebral compression fractures, Spine 26 (2001) 1631–1638.
14. M.E. Majd, S. Farley, R.T. Holt, Preliminary outcomes and efficacy of the first 360 consecutive kyphoplasties for the treatment of painful osteoporotic vertebral compression fractures, Spine J. 5 (2005) 244–255.
15. D.B. Moreland, M.K. Landi, W. Grand, Vertebroplasty: techniques to avoid complications, Spine J. 1 (2001) 66–71.
16. D.A. Nussbaum, P. Gailloud, K. Murphy, A review of complications associated with vertebroplasty and kyphoplasty as reported to the Food and Drug Administration medical device related website, J. Vasc. Interv. Radiol. 15 (2004) 1185–1192.
17. R.D. Rao, M.D. Singrakhia, Painful osteoporotic vertebral fracture. Pathogenesis, evaluation, and roles of vertebroplasty and kyphoplasty in its management, J. Bone Joint Surg. Am. 85-A (2003) 2010–2022.
18. J. Cauley, D. Thompson, K. Ensrud, et al., Risk of mortality following clinical fractures, Osteoporos. Int. 11 (2000) 556–561.
19. W. Cockerill, M. Lunt, A. Silman, et al., Health-related quality of life and radiographic vertebral fracture, Osteoporos. Int. 15 (2004) 113–119.

# PART 6

# Other Surgical Treatment Modalities: Thoracic Spine

# Treatment of Thoracic Vertebral Fractures

45

*Samer Ghostine, Kamal Woods, Shoshanna Vaynman, Ali Shirzadi, Stephen Scibelli,*
*Srinath Samudrala, and J. Patrick Johnson*

## KEY POINTS

- Stable thoracic vertebral fractures may be treated conservatively with external bracing and pain management.

- When patients with stable vertebral compression fractures have persistent back pain despite conservative measures, they may benefit from kyphoplasty, vertebroplasty, StaXx, or percutaneous instrumentation.

- Unstable thoracic vertebral fractures necessitate stabilization with instrumentation and fusion. A variety of surgical approaches are available either as stand-alone procedures or in combination, including anterior, posterior, and/or lateral approaches.

- Neurologic deficit is present in about 10% of thoracic fractures, and urgent spinal decompression with thoracic laminectomies is necessary.

- Fractures that cause thoracic deformity, with or without myelopathy, may require deformity correction using pedicle subtraction osteotomy, Smith-Peterson osteotomy, pedicle screw instrumentation, and/or arthrodesis.

## INTRODUCTION

Thoracic fractures account for approximately 16% of all spinal fractures.[4] Multiple classification systems have been developed in an attempt to characterize thoracic fractures as stable or unstable. While it is important to realize that no classification is perfect, these classification systems aid in making sound clinical decisions. They range in simplicity from the Denis three-column classification to the complicated Magerl (AO) classification.[7] Regardless of the type of classification system employed, the presence of neurologic deficits, ligamentous injury, and a significant loss of height, angulation, translation, distraction, and/or rotation at the level of the vertebral injury must always increase suspicion for spinal instability.[5]

## BASIC SCIENCE

The thoracic spine is unique because of its articulations with the rib cage, which serves as an internal brace. The intact rib cage is thought to increase fourfold the capacity of the thoracic spinal region to resist axial load. As the ribs also limit thoracic rotation and ***, most thoracic vertebral fractures are caused by flexion or compression forces.

The thoracic spine has a natural kyphotic curvature between 20 and 45 degrees. This curvature partly results from the thoracic vertebral bodies being shorter ventrally than they are dorsally. In turn, this kyphotic position places the thoracic vertebral bodies at an increased risk of sustaining compression fractures during axial loading. When the compressive force exceeds the strength of the ventral vertebral body, a compression fracture develops. If the axial force is sufficiently great, it will also exceed the strength of the dorsal vertebral body and ligamentous elements to produce a burst fracture.

The incidence of neurological deficits from thoracic fractures is about 10% or greater; this occurs for several reasons. First, the diameter of the thoracic spinal canal is smaller than the canal of the cervical or lumbar region, being narrowest at T3-T9.[9] Second, the midthoracic cord is located in a watershed region between the blood supply to the cervicothoracic and thoracolumbar spines. Last, the high-energy mechanism of injury required for most thoracic fractures is transferred to the underlying cord and spinal nerve roots.

## CLINICAL PRACTICE GUIDELINES

### Stable Thoracic Vertebral Fractures

Stable thoracic vertebral fractures are amenable to bracing with thoracolumbar spinal orthosis, accompanied by pain management. Spinal stability in the orthosis may be confirmed radiographically with upright anteroposterior (AP) and lateral x-ray films, which assess the alignment and the sagittal and coronal balance of the thoracic spine. The presence of any acute neurological deficit or persistent significant back pain should prompt further workup to reassess the degree of stability.

Stable vertebral fractures may be very painful. If conservative management fails to control the patient's pain, a kyphoplasty, vertebroplasty, StaXx placement or percutaneous pedicle screw placement can be considered. Vertebroplasty and kyphoplasty have the advantage of possibly being performed under local anesthesia. In addition, kyphoplasty may restore greater vertebral height. StaXx allows vertebral restoration in the absence of an intact posterior vertebral wall. Percutaneous pedicle screw placement may provide additional support at the level of the fracture when used to supplement a vertebroplasty, kyphoplasty, or StaXx. Some authors believe that injecting cement in the vertebroplasty, kyphoplasty, and StaXx may not only help in partially restoring vertebral height and subsequently sagittal spinal balance, but also function in alleviating the patient's pain by killing the responsible nerve endings in the vertebrae.

A significant percentage of thoracic compression fractures fail to heal within 3 to 6 weeks. Such fractures are prone to a progression in the kyphotic deformity and may cause severe back pain. In some instances, the pain is so debilitating that patients remain sedentary, placing them at increased risk for deep vein thrombosis, pneumonia, and bone resorption. Initially developed to treat painful vertebral hemangiomas, vertebroplasty and kyphoplasty offer marked to complete pain relief in 63% to 90% of nonhealing thoracic compression fractures.[8]

Careful patient selection is essential to successful outcomes with vertebroplasty and kyphoplasty. Especially in osteoporotic patients, there may be multiple vertebral compression fractures. Point tenderness that localizes to the radiographic location of the fracture is a reliable method of selecting the appropriate level for intervention. However, the absence of such tenderness does not preclude a nonhealing fracture, and performing a T2-weighted MRI sequence with fat suppression (such as short T1 inversion recovery [STIR]) is useful. Apart from showing increased T2 signal in acute, nonhealing fractures, MRI allows for the evaluation of the integrity of the posterior longitudinal ligament, exclusion of spinal canal stenosis, and identification of underlying neoplasms with gadolinium enhancement. X-rays are also useful for preoperative planning, as well as for comparison with older x-rays to detect new fractures or progression of deformity.

While there are few absolute contraindications to vertebroplasty and kyphoplasty, these interventions are strongly discouraged in the presence of

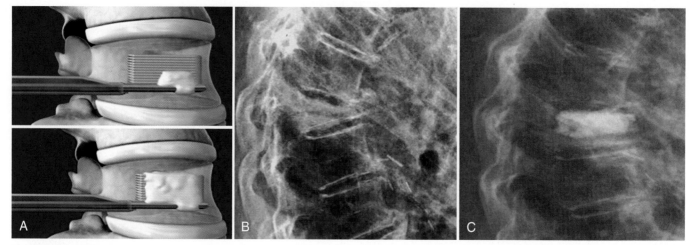

■ **FIGURE 45-1** **A,** cartoon illustrating PEEK wafers stacked at the level of a vertebral body fracture with the addition of PMMA. **B,** Lateral x-ray of T10 compression fracture with angulation and focal kyphosis. **C,** Lateral x-ray after StaXx and PMMA placement with satisfactory reduction of the focal kyphosis and height restoration.

systemic infection, bleeding diathesis, and spinal canal or neural foraminal stenosis leading to myelopathy or radiculopathy, respectively. Patients with pathologic compression fracture resultant from an underlying neoplasm are also candidates for vertebroplasty or for kyphoplasty; however, surgery must be coordinated with chemotherapy and/or irradiation.

For both vertebroplasty and kyphoplasty, the needle may be placed via a transpedicular or parapedicular approach. The transpedicular approach minimizes the risk of injury to the postganglionic nerve root and minimizes the leakage of cement because it entails a longer intraosseous path to the vertebral body. The parapedicular route enables the trajectory of the needle to be more medialized, especially in the upper to midthoracic spine, where the usual axis of the pedicles is directed more lateral.

Once the cannulated needle is satisfactorily positioned in the vertebral body using radiographic guidance, polymethyl methacrylate (PMMA) cement is instilled. In the case of kyphoplasty, a balloon is first inflated through the cannulated needle to create a cavity for the cement. This maneuver enables a 50% restoration in vertebral body height and alignment in two thirds of patients undergoing kyphoplasty.[6]

The StaXx kyphoplasty is a newer system that allows the firing of a series of PEEK wafers into the vertebral body through a device secured just inferior to the pedicle and at its lateral edge (Figure 45-1). This is performed under fluoroscopic guidance. The number of PEEK wafers required in the fractured vertebral body is determined once endplate reduction is obtained and appropriate vertebral body height correction is established. The wafers

*Text Continued on p.7*

## CLINICAL CASE EXAMPLES

### Case 1: Kyphoplasty

An 80-year-old male with steroid-induced osteoporosis presented with mid-back pain of 10 week's duration. X-rays of the thoracic spine showed T7, T8, and T9 compression fractures with significant height loss and mild kyphotic deformity (Figure 45-2A). MRI showed a T2 hyperintensity at T8 consistent with acute fracture, while the other two fractures appeared chronic. Despite undergoing thorough conservative management, the

patient continued to experience back pain that significantly limited both function and mobility.

He underwent a kyphoplasty of the T8 with satisfactory restoration of height and reduction of his kyphotic deformity (Figure 45-2B). Postoperatively, the patient had no significant residual back pain and returned to his premorbid function.

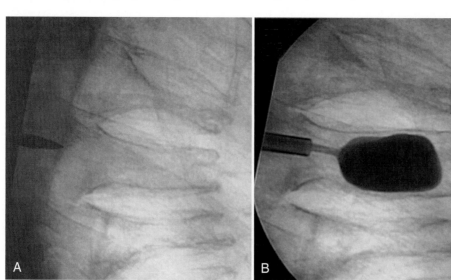

■ **FIGURE 45-2** **A,** Lateral thoracic x-ray showing T7, T8, and T9 compression fractures. **B,** Intraoperative fluoroscopy after PMMA injection at T8 level with height restoration.

## Case 2: Percutaneous Instrumentation

An 84-year-old female presented 1 month after she was involved in a motor vehicle accident in which she sustained a T9 Chance fracture (Figure 45-3A). Thoracic MRI performed hours after the accident showed a spinal epidural hematoma at the level of the fracture and an intact posterior ligamentous complex. The patient underwent multilevel thoracic laminectomies and evacuation of the epidural hematoma. Subsequent MRI showed no residual spinal cord compression; however, she had persistent spinal cord injury and was unable to lift the lower extremities against gravity. She also had severe back pain, which limited her mobility and rehabilitation. We opted to perform percutaneous T6-12 instrumentation (Figure 45-3B). Two months later, the patient was tolerating rehabilitation well, and her lower extremity strength was markedly improved.

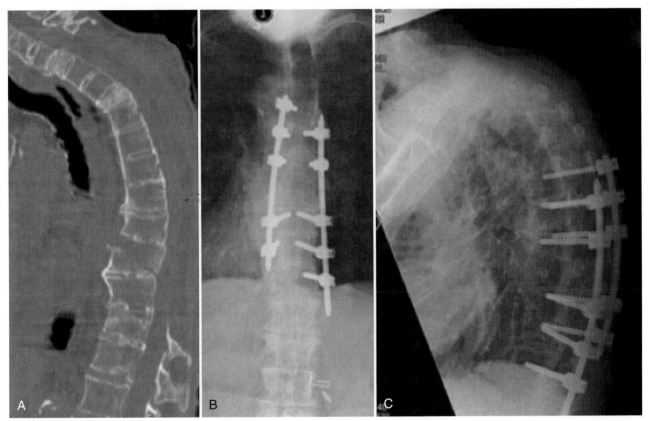

■ **FIGURE 45-3** **A,** Preoperative CT demonstrating T9 Chance fracture. Postoperative AP **(B)** and lateral **(C)** x-rays showing bilateral T6-8 and T10-12 pedicle screw and rod fixation.

## Case 3: Pedicle Subtraction Osteotomy

A 57-year-old male presented with progressive myelopathy, including gait disturbance due to spasticity progressing over a 5-year period. Bowel and bladder control had been compromised, and the lower extremities were diffusely weak to resistance. He reported severe paresthesias in his lower extremities. Bilateral Babinski signs and bilateral ankle and knee clonus were present. He also had a palpable nontender gibbus in the upper thoracic spine.

MRI and CT scans revealed severe compression of the ventral spinal cord due to a 30-degree focal kyphotic deformity at the level of T3-T4. A T2 signal change was detected within the spinal cord at the same level, consistent with advanced spinal cord injury (Figure 45-4A and B).

A posterior transpedicular osteotomy was performed using biplane fluoroscopy, which guided the resection of a wedge of the superior T4 vertebra (Figure 45-5A-C). Rib osteotomies were completed at the level of T4, and lateral wall osteotomies with preservation of the pleura were accomplished. After a spontaneous partial reduction of the osteotomy, the Mayfield head holder was elevated to reduce the gibbus and correct the alignment of the upper thoracic spine. Longitudinal rods were contoured and placed at the level of T1, T2, and T3 after reduction was completed manually, with biplane fluoroscopy and intraoperative evoked potentials, by closing the bony defect created by the vertebral osteotomy (Figure 45-5 C-D). The longitudinal rods were placed into a reduced position, achieving complete reduction of the kyphotic and sagittal plane deformity and annihilating the gibbus deformity (Figure 45-5E). Biplane fluoroscopy confirmed alignment of the sagittal and coronal plane at the instrumented levels with complete resolution of the gibbus, and evoked potentials remained unchanged (Figure 45-5E and F).

Two days after the surgery, the patient was transferred from the intensive care unit to the floor, where he quickly recuperated his baseline strength and was discharged home ambulating independently with the use of a cane. Postoperative CT scans confirmed the established correction of the sagittal plane deformity (Figure 45-6A and B).

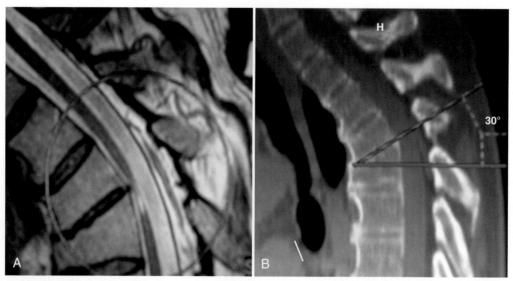

■ **FIGURE 45-4  A,** T2-weighted MRI sequence sagittal view, showing the ventral spinal cord compression and stretching resulting from the posttraumatic focal kyphosis at the level of T4. At the T4 level, the spinal cord is markedly atrophied and shows a significantly increased signal consistent with spinal cord injury. **B,** Sagittal thoracic CT scan showing a healed compression fracture at T4 the level with a resultant focal kyphosis of approximately 30 degrees.

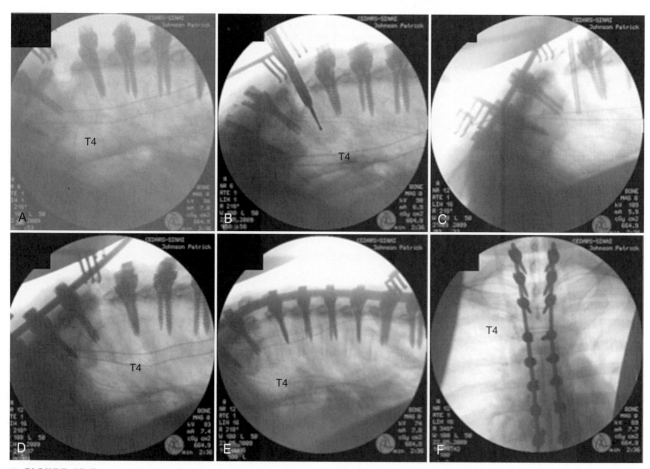

■ **FIGURE 45-5  A,** Intraoperative fluoroscopy showing placement of bilateral 5.5-mm and 6.5-mm pedicle screws from T1 to T10. The inferior part of the spinous process and laminae of T3 are resected, as well as the inferior facets of T3 bilaterally. The superior facets of T4 and the pedicles of T4 are resected, creating a giant foramen containing both T3 and T4 nerve roots. Rib heads at the level of T4 are osteomized along with the transverse processes. **B,** Under fluoroscopic guidance, a wedge of the vertebral body of T4 is removed with different sizes of curettes and an electric drill. Rongeurs are used to osteomize the lateral edges of the vertebral body. **C,** Placement of the contoured rods at T1, T2, and T3 allows manual reduction of the focal kyphosis at the level of T3 with the guidance of biplane fluoroscopy and intraoperative evoked potentials **(D)** by closing the bony defect created by the vertebral oste-otomy. **E,** The longitudinal rods were placed into a reduced position, where a complete reduction of the kyphotic and sagittal plane deformity was achieved, annihilating the gibbus deformity and closing the bony wedge defect created by the PSO. **F,** Biplane fluoroscopy confirmed alignment of the coronal plane at the instrumented levels.

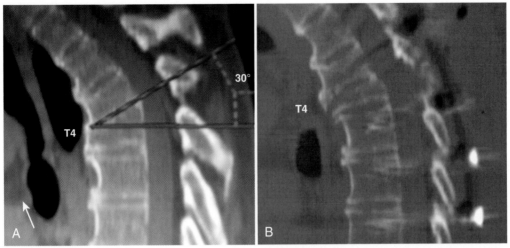

■ **FIGURE 45-6**  **A,** Preoperative sagittal CT scan of the thoracic spine showing the wedge resection planning. **B,** Postoperative sagittal CT scan of the thoracic spine showing the "closing" of the wedge resected by the PSO, and subsequent "shortening" of the spine at T4.

provide structural support to the vertebral body. A smaller amount of PMMA is then injected through the same channel around the PEEK construct, as compared to both vertebroplasty and kyphoplasty. The StaXx kyphoplasty system potentially offers an advantage over kyphoplasty alone, in which the space opened by the balloon may undergo some collapse before the PMMA is injected. In vertebroplasty, the PMMA simply flows to the spaces of least resistance, but does not offer height restoration.

## Thoracic Stabilization

Surgical approaches for the treatment of unstable thoracic vertebral fractures include anterior, posterior, and combined anterior and posterior stabilization methods. Minimally invasive percutaneous pedicle screws may be placed if the fracture involves mostly bony elements and the ligaments are intact. If ligamentous injury is present, pedicle screw placement with joint arthrodesis is advised.

## Spinal Cord or Nerve Decompression

Thoracic vertebral fractures associated with cord or nerve compression require decompression. Spinal cord decompression may be accomplished with laminectomy alone (when the compressive pathology is dorsal to the cord), although removal of a bone fragment ventral to the spinal cord may be necessary. This can be done from a posterior approach using a facet-sparing transpedicular approach or a far lateral approach. If the bone fragment compressing the spinal cord is in a central and ventral location, an anterior approach may then be required. Instrumentation and fusion are generally needed.

## Deformity Correction

To treat spinal deformity (kyphosis and/or scoliosis), with or without myelopathic symptoms, several surgical techniques may be used, including pedicle subtraction osteotomy (PSO), Smith-Peterson osteotomy, pedicle screw instrumentation, and arthrodesis. The use of PSO and Smith-Peterson osteotomy in a posterior approach is a good alternative to a combined anterior and posterior approach.

The abnormal focal concavity, which results from the kyphotic deformity caused by a compression fracture, stretches the spinal cord. The spinal cord moves ventrally in an attempt to minimize the stretching effect. Myelopathic deficits ensue once the ventral compression becomes significant, requiring ventral compression of the bony elements and removal of the upper thoracic concavity to reestablish the normal three-dimensional conformation of the spinal cord. The distinct anatomy of the upper thoracic spine renders the spinal cord more vulnerable to ventral compression.

Anterior approaches to treat a spinal deformity can also be performed. However, any multisegment anterior fusion construct is subject to sustaining increased mechanical stress, which can thereby result in the failure of

the anterior spinal fusion.[3] In addition, the upper thoracic spine is a difficult region to access anteriorly due to the presence of major vascular elements as well as vital structures ventral to the spine.[2] Moreover, Boockvar et al reported that anterior reconstruction alone might not meet the biomechanical needs of the upper thoracic spine. Recent advances in anesthesia, neural monitoring, and posterior instrumentation have made a posterior approach to the upper thoracic spine possible and treatment of the upper thoracic spine achievable.[1]

In some cases, PSO may be safely used to correct abnormal severe focal kyphotic deformities, which result in spinal cord stretching and ventral compression, because it allows for significant correction through one spinal segment by shortening the spinal column and reestablishing sagittal alignment. When PSO is performed, instrumented fusions are usually necessary, and dural buckling needs to be ruled out with thoracic laminectomies at the osteotomy sites.

## CONCLUSIONS/DISCUSSION

The management of thoracic fractures is challenging because of the complex anatomic variations in this region. In addition, most spinal surgeons are less comfortable with dealing with the thoracic area than with the cervical vor lumbar regions. Nevertheless, with current technical and technologic advances, the spinal surgeon is equipped with a wide variety of available resources and methods to treat thoracic fractures according to severity, presenting symptoms, and impact on patient function.

## References

1. K. Abumi, Y. Shono, M. Ito, H. Taneichi, Y. Kotani, K. Kaneda, Complications of pedicle screw fixation in reconstructive surgery of the cervical spine, Spine 25 (2000) 962–969.
2. J.A. Boockvar, M.F. Philips, A.E. Telfeian, D.M. O'Rourke, P.J. Marcotte, Results and risk factors for anterior cervicothoracic junction surgery, J. Neurosurg. 94 (2001) 12–17.
3. H.F. Defino, A.E. Rodriquez-Fuentes, F.P. Piola, Surgical treatment of pathological kyphosis [in Spanish], Acta Ortoped. Bras. 10 (2002) 10–16.
4. S.D. Gertzbein, Scoliosis Research Society: multicenter spine fracture study, Spine 17 (1992) 528.
5. J.Y. Lee, A.R. Vacarro, M.R. Lim, et al., Thoracolumbar injury classification and severity score: a new paradigm for the treatment of thoracolumbar spine trauma, J. Orthop. Sci. 10 (2005) 671–675.
6. I.H. Lieberman, S. Dudeney, M.K. Reinhardt, et al., Initial outcome and efficacy of "kyphoplasty" in the treatment of painful osteoporotic vertebral compression fractures, Spine 26 (2001) 1631–1638.
7. F. Magerl, M. Aebi, S.D. Gertzbein, et al., A comprehensive classificaton of thoracic and lumbar injuries,, Eur. Spine J. 3 (1994) 184–201.
8. J.B. Martin, B. Jean, K. Sugui, et al., Vertebroplasty: clinical experience and follow-up results, Bone 25 (1999) 11S–15S.
9. M.M. Panjabi, K. Takata, V. Goal, et al., Thoracic human vertebrae: quantitative three-dimensional anatomy, Spine 26 (1991) 888–901.

# 46

# Tumors of the Thoracic Spine

*Timothy F. Witham, Vivek A. Mehta, and Ziya L. Gokaslan*

**KEY POINTS**

- Surgical decompression followed by radiotherapy has replaced radiotherapy alone as the gold standard for treatment of spinal cord compression caused by metastatic cancer.

- Tumor histology, location, and anterior column compromise should dictate the surgical approach.

- Anterior, posterior, combined, or en bloc approaches should be considered in a disease-directed fashion for the treatment of thoracic spinal column neoplasms.

- Instability must be considered, particularly when there is anterior column compromise.

- The clinical goals of surgical intervention should be local disease control, preservation or restoration of neurological function, stabilization of the spinal column, and pain control.

## INTRODUCTION

Nearly 1.4 million new cases of cancer are diagnosed in the United States per year.[1] In a majority of the approximately 724,000 cancer-related deaths per year, patients ultimately succumb to complications related to metastatic disease. Approximately 30% to 90% of cancer patients will have evidence of metastases to the spinal column at autopsy, and 5% to 10% of cancer patients develop symptomatic metastatic epidural spinal cord compression (MESCC), an oncologic emergency.[1] There are approximately 25,000 cases of symptomatic MESCC in the united states each year.[1] The thoracic spine is the most common site of metastatic disease involvement in the vertebral column and the most common site of primary vertebral column tumors. Because symptomatic degenerative disease is less common in the thoracic spine relative to the cervical or lumbar spine, thoracic region pain in a middle-aged or elderly patient should be considered a red flag symptom. Imaging should be considered expeditiously, particularly if the patient has a history of primary cancer. Nonetheless, delay in the diagnosis of thoracic region tumors is common. Surgical intervention for thoracic spinal cord and spinal column neoplasms continues to present significant challenges. Lesions in the thoracic spine can be subdivided into four major categories: metastatic disease, intradural extramedullary tumors, intramedullary spinal cord tumors, and primary neoplasms involving skeletal elements.

### Metastatic Tumors

Approximately 70% of metastatic disease to the vertebral column involves the thoracic spine, making it the most common site of spinal metastases.[2] As increased survival due to improved treatment strategies for primary neoplasms becomes a trend, the incidence of bone metastases to the spine will also increase. The unique venous drainage of visceral organs through the Batson plexus is one explanation for this anatomical phenomenon, along with the close proximity of the thoracic spine to thoracic and abdominal viscera.[2] Eighty percent of metastases involve the vertebral body, while 20% involve the posterior elements.[2] Of the four subtypes of tumors of the tho-

racic spine, metastatic tumors are by far the most common. Cancers that have a propensity to spread to the thoracic spine include breast, lung, leukemia/lymphoma, prostate, and renal cell.[2] Surgical management requires consideration of the need for decompression of the neural elements, for restoration of spinal stability, and for pain relief. With tumors of breast, prostate, or renal origin, aggressive resection is indicated, as this has been shown to have a favorable impact on ambulatory function and may have a favorable impact on survival.[3]

### Intradural Extramedullary Tumors

Intradural extramedullary (IDEM) tumors account for two thirds of intradural spinal tumors.[4] The most common IDEM tumors of the thoracic spine are meningiomas, neurofibromas and schwannomas, which account for over 80% of tumors in this location.[5] Meningiomas arise from arachnoid cap cells; 75% of spinal meningiomas are contained within the thoracic spine, and they show a strong predilection for women (80%).[5] Meningiomas have a benign biological behavior in the spinal column and management should be directed toward gross total resection to achieve a cure. This may not be feasible with anteriorly situated, calcified tumors, and the risk of neurological injury must be weighed against the indolent growth rates usually observed after subtotal resection. Radiotherapy is thus reserved for recurrent tumors that cannot be completely resected.

Schwannomas arise from Schwann cells of the posterior nerve roots and are most common in the thoracic and upper lumbar spine. The location, in 13% of cases, may be both extradural and intradural. Spinal schwannomas have an increased frequency in certain genetic disorders, such as neurofibromatosis type 2 (NF2).

Neurofibromas of spinal nerve root origin may be seen sporadically or in patients with neurofibromatosis. These tumors will have an extradural component in 30% of cases.[5] The surgical goal in the treatment of thoracic schwannomas and neurofibromas is complete surgical resection. If the tumor cannot be separated from the nerve root of origin, then sacrifice of that root may be necessary. Fortunately, this is usually of little consequence in the thoracic spine.

IDEM tumors of the thoracic spine most often manifest with long tract signs, and the corticospinal tracts are particularly vulnerable. Stiffness and muscle fatigue are often primary signs with spasticity frequently occurring secondarily. In patients presenting with myelopathy, surgical indications are straightforward. It is the incidentally found meningioma or nerve sheath tumor that may present a dilemma. Patient age, medical comorbidities, and tumor growth observed with serial imaging help direct the necessity and timing of surgical intervention.

### Intramedullary Spinal Cord Tumors

Intramedullary spinal cord tumors (IMSCTs) make up 2% to 8.5% of all central nervous system(CNS) tumors and approximately one third of primary spinal column tumors.[6] Approximately 90% are of glial origin.[4] The major types observed in the thoracic spine are astrocytomas and ependymomas, which are seen with almost equal frequency in adults. Hemangioblastomas, which are less commonly observed, may be sporadic or a part of von Hippel-Lindau syndrome. Astrocytomas are most often seen at the cervicothoracic junction and in the lower thoracic spinal cord. In adults, ependymomas are the most common IMSCT. However, the majority of these occur in the cervical spine or arise from the filum terminale (myxopapillary ependymoma). Treatment of ependymomas is focused on gross total resection. Patients who have incompletely-removed tumors should be considered for re-resection or followed closely with serial imaging and considered for reoperation if growth is documented. Radiation therapy is often reserved for incomplete resection after reoperation. Astrocytomas in adults tend to be infiltrative and blend imperceptibly with the spinal cord at the margins of the tumor. For this reason, total removal may not be possible. Most commonly, infiltrative tumors treated with subtotal resection will undergo radiation therapy. For high-grade infiltrative lesions, biopsy or subtotal resection is also often followed by radiation therapy. For some low-grade lesions treated with subtotal resection, postoperative radiation therapy remains controversial.[6]

Pain is the most common presentation of IMSCT in the thoracic spine; it usually localizes to the level of the tumor and is either regional back pain or radicular.[4] Up to one third of patients may also experience sensory or motor complaints and spasticity. The most common sign of an IMSCT within the thoracic spine is a mild scoliosis with spasticity and sensory disturbance.[6] Until recently, it was believed that posterior decompression and radiation therapy were the limits of therapy, but aggressive gross total resection, with the aid of microsurgical tools and intraoperative monitoring, has been shown to be safe and to improve functional recovery and reduce tumor recurrence.

## Primary Vertebral Column Tumors

Primary tumors of the vertebral column are rare, making up less than 10% of all tumors involving the spinal column.[7] It should be emphasized that when patients present with a vertebral column mass in the absence of impending neurological compromise, minimally invasive, image-guided biopsy should be performed prior to definitive treatment planning. Many of the primary neoplasms of the thoracic spinal column are best treated via radical en bloc surgical resection. These types of surgical approaches require careful and detailed preoperative surgical planning by an experienced surgical team. Therefore, knowing the tumor histology up front is critical to the surgical plan.

Primary osseous tumors can be divided into three categories: benign, benign but locally aggressive, and malignant. Benign tumors include hemangiomas, osteoid osteomas/osteoblastomas, chondroma/osteochondromas, aneurysmal bone cysts, and eosinophilic granulomas. Hemangiomas are the most common primary neoplasm affecting the thoracic spine and have been seen in approximately 11% of all postmortem examinations.[7] Infrequently, hemangiomas can behave in an atypical or locally aggressive fashion and can cause spinal cord compression. In this situation, aggressive surgical resection is advocated. Giant cell tumors have a variable biological behavior and may act in a locally aggressive fashion. Because of this, the authors often recommend radical en bloc excision of tumors exhibiting this pathology and will strongly consider adjuvant radiation therapy postoperatively. Chordomas occurring in the thoracic spine are almost uniformly locally aggressive and recurrences are common after intralesional resection, including gross total resection. Similarly, we recommend radical en bloc resection techniques for thoracic chordomas. Chemotherapy protocols for chordomas have not been promising to date, nor have conventional radiation therapy modalities. Proton beam irradiation therapy has been shown to be the most promising radiation modality and patients are evaluated postoperatively for this modality on an individual basis. However, it is our belief that the most effective treatment modality for achieving long term local disease control is aggressive en bloc resection with negative margins, including resection of the biopsy tract if possible. Proton beam irradiation should not be relied on for cases where gross total resection cannot be achieved. However, it may be employed even in cases of en bloc resection with negative margins.

Malignant types include plasmacytomas, chondrosarcomas, and osteosarcomas. Plasmacytomas make up nearly 30% of all primary tumors and have a propensity to occur in the thoracic spine.[8] While these tumors are radiation-sensitive lesions, surgery may be necessary for failure of radiation therapy, acute neurological decline from spinal cord compression, and overt instability of the spinal column. Sarcomas present a specific treatment challenge. Biopsy is recommended to assess the specific histology and grade.

Systemic workup for metastases is important prior to embarking on treatment. High-grade lesions that are large or those tumors associated with metastatic disease may be treated with neoadjuvant chemotherapy protocols to shrink the local disease and address metatstatic disease prior to surgical resection. En bloc resection is the technique that gives the patient the best opportunity for a longer-term survival with these tumor types, particularly when metastatic disease is not present.

Thoracic spinal column neoplasms present a host of treatment challenges. Knowing the tumor histology through a biopsy is ideal prior to embarking on a formal surgical plan. In the setting of impending neurological decline, a biopsy may not be possible and urgent decompression may be necessary. However, surgical planning is best determined when the histology, systemic disease status, patient age, and medical comorbidities are known.

## BASIC SCIENCE

Research related to the molecular biology and genetics of specific tumor types that affect the spinal column either as primary or metastatic lesions is beyond the scope of this text. However, several animal models of spinal column neoplasia and the translational research related to these animal models are worth discussion. Recently, animal models for metastatic disease to the spine and intramedullary spinal cord gliomas have been developed that will allow for more rigorous preclinical analysis of novel therapies. Mantha et al have established a reproducible model of metastatic breast adenocarcinoma to the vertebral column in rats.[9] The establishment of this model represents the first of its kind and has allowed for the study of multiple treatment modalities focused on treating spinal metastatic disease, including surgery, radiation therapy, and the novel use of locally delivered chemotherapeutic agents.

Using the metastatic model developed by Mantha et al, Bagley et al have shown that radiation reliably delays paraparesis and death in this model, as does local delivery of paclitaxel.[10,11] The combination of these two modalities has been shown to be more effective than either treatment alone.[11] Additionally, Gok et al. have shown that the combination of decompressive surgery, local chemotherapy, and radiation has the most profound results in terms of preservation of neurological function and prolongation of survival in this animal model of with metastatic epidural spinal cord compression.[12] The hope is that this experimental data may translate into useful clinical trials designed to improve neurological morbidity and, potentially, survival in patients with MESCC due to metastatic breast cancer and other tumor histologies.

Pennant et al. have examined the efficacy of microsurgical excision in a rat model of intramedullary spinal cord tumor. The established model mimics the behavior of IMSCTS, both functionally and histopathologically.[13] Following tumor implantation, animals were randomized into a treatment group (microsurgical resection) or to no treatment. The animals that underwent resection had a significant delay in the onset of functional paraplegia as compared to the controls and these results were highly reproducible. This new model allows for the study of new treatment options for high-grade intramedullary tumors.

Schuster et al have developed a novel model of spine metastasis using human osteoblasts implanted in immune incompetent (SCID) mice that has shown to be highly reproducible.[14] This model allows for the study of bone-tumor interaction in metastatic disease, as well as the basic biology of bone metastases. Chordoma models have been difficult to establish, but through human cell culture, nude animal models have been conceptualized. Laboratory study of this extremely aggressive local tumor is much needed given the limited options for treatment outside of aggressive radical resection.

## CLINICAL PRACTICE GUIDELINES

Surgical intervention has a clear and proven role in the treatment of patients with metastatic disease involving the thoracic spine that results in spinal cord compression. Surgical treatment, followed by radiation therapy, not only extends ambulatory status but also results in a trend toward longer survival and reduces the need for steroids and pain medications.[3]

The indications for surgical intervention include the need to establish a diagnosis, the treatment of spinal instability, and the restoration or preservation of neurological function in the setting of epidural spinal cord compression. Additional indications include the treatment of radioresistant tumors, and the treatment of tumor recurrence following radiation therapy or the treatment of neurological decline during radiation therapy. A systemic approach for treatment of thoracic metastases has been developed and may aid in designing the optimal surgical strategy.[15] The mnemonic "MAPS" stands for (1) method of resection; (2) anatomy of spinal disease; (3) patient's level of fitness; and (4) stabilization.

Surgical approaches to the spine can be generally categorized as either anterior, posterior, or combined. Posterior approaches may include laminectomy alone, or laminectomy combined with transpedicular, costotransversectomy, or lateral extracavitary resection techniques and stabilization. Anterior approaches in the upper thoracic spine include cervicothoracic and trap door exposure. Anterior access to the lower thoracic spine can be accomplished by a thoracotomy or thoracoabdominal approach.

The vascular anatomy is particularly important when designing an anterior approach as well as the tumor laterality. For example, above T6 or T7 a right-sided thoracotomy is preferred, because the aortic arch often complicates a left-sided approach to the mid/upper thoracic spine. Similarly, tumors situated between T1 and T4 are a unique challenge from the perspective of an anterior approach. With metastatic lesions in the upper thoracic spine, the authors will often consider a posterior approach. If anterior column resection or reconstruction is necessary, it is often done with a transpedicular, costotransversectomy, or lateral extracavitary technique.

The method of resection may be en bloc (wide or marginal) or intralesional resection of various degrees ranging from open biopsy to gross total resection. En bloc resection may be considered with a solitary spinal metastatic lesion, in the absence of visceral metastatic disease and with a favorable histological tumor type (breast, prostate, renal cell carcinoma, thyroid carcinoma). In addition, the feasibility of such an approach should be considered with respect to surgical staging and medical fitness of the patient. En bloc spondylectomy in the thoracic spine may be performed through an all-posterior approach or a combined posterior approach first and a second staged anterior approach. En bloc spondylectomy through a posterior-only approach requires laminectomy above and below the vertebral segment of interest. Then while protecting the spinal cord and nerve roots, the pedicles are cut at the junction with the vertebral body using a chisel or saw. This allows the posterior elements to be removed in one piece after the facets are disrupted on each side. A wide costotransversectomy is performed on each side to allow for dissection around the entire vertebral body, so that the aorta and venous structures may be dissected off of the spinal column. Radical discectomies are performed above and below the segment of interest to mobilize the entire vertebral body. With the pleura completely exposed, the vertebral body may be rotated, carefully translated

posteriorly around the side of the spinal cord, and resected in one piece. Staged posterior followed by anterior en bloc spondylectomy is similar, but after the radical discectomies, a Silastic sheath is placed between the posterior vertebral body and the anterior dura. Subsequent staged thoracotomy is performed to remove the mobilized vertebral segment in one piece. Special care is taken not to injure the anterior vasculature. The spinal cord is relatively protected with this technique because the Silastic sheath was placed during the first stage to clearly identify the plane between the spinal cord dura and the vertebral body.

The majority of metastases within the thoracic spinal column will affect the vertebral body, which favors an anterior approach. A disease-directed approach to the thoracic spine provides the most direct access for resection of tumors contained within the vertebral body and allows for the most effective reconstruction of the anterior aspects of the weight-bearing spine. A consideration of patient fitness is essential in the choice of surgical approach. Previously irradiated tissue increases the risk of wound dehiscence and thus may favor an anterior approach. Additionally, the possibility of high intraoperative blood loss, nutritional depletion, corticosteroid use, advanced age, comorbidity, and paraparesis are significant risk factors that should be considered.

Though the thoracic spine is well supported by the rib cage, additional stabilization should be considered in the case of significant disease or removal of the vertebral bodies, facet joints or pedicles. Anterior stabilization is always indicated following vertebrectomy, and the need for additional posterior stabilization should be considered. Supplementary posterior stabilization following vertebrectomy and vertebral body reconstruction might be considered in a variety of situations, including the case of a posterolateral approach, in patients with a significant kyphosis or deformity, in patients with junctional zone disease, significant adjacent chest wall reconstruction, a greater than two-level corpectomy, spondylectomy, or in the case of poor bone quality. The authors do not recommend laminectomy alone for the treatment of thoracic tumors, except in the setting of IMSCTs. Often laminoplasty is an attractive option for IMSCTs. Typically with posterior reconstruction for metastatic tumors, we will place pedicle screws two to three levels above and two or three levels below the area of the laminectomy, particularly if a posterior approach is used for anterior column reconstruction.

Finally, metastatic spread from lymphomas, multiple myeloma, and small cell lung carcinoma represent tumors that are particularly radiosensitive; therefore radiation modalities may be considered as a first-line treatment and the need for surgery may be obviated or withheld until radiotherapy has been implemented and failed.

## CLINICAL CASE EXAMPLES

### *Case 1: Posterolateral Approach for Metastatic Spine Disease*

#### PATIENT PRESENTATION

A 70-year-old female with a history of diabetes and osteoarthritis of the hips presented to an outside emergency department with shortness of breath and dyspnea. Work-up included a chest CT scan and an incidental lesion was found in the T3 vertebral body. Formal imaging of the spine was done via a dedicated MRI and CT scan. Initially the lesion was thought to represent metastatic disease. The patient initially had no neurological symptoms and the lesion was felt to be incidentally found. A systemic metastatic work-up was negative. Given the lack of neurological symptoms despite evidence of epidural spinal cord compression on the MRI scan, CT-guided biopsy was recommended. The results were nondiagnostic on two occasions despite thorough review by an experienced neuropathologist. The pathology sample did show rare plasma cells, but serum protein electrophoresis and urine protein electrophoresis were negative. The patient was referred to our institution for further care when she began to develop mild lower extremity weakness, subtle gait difficulty, lower extremity paresthesias, and long tract findings on exam.

MRI of the thoracic spine and CT scan of the thoracic spine are shown in Figure 46-1. We felt that despite the negative biopsy, the imaging was most characteristic of an atypical vertebral hemangioma with epidural

spinal cord compression. Imaging features that  support this diagnosis include the appearance of vascular channels on the MRI and the "polka-dot" appearance with vascular channels also present on the CT scan. Also included in the differential diagnosis was plasmacytoma/multiple myeloma.

Because of impending neurological deterioration and the lack of a diagnosis, a surgical approach was recommended. Given the possibility of a highly vascular lesion such as a vertebral hemangioma, preoperative embolization by an interventional neuroradiologist was recommended and successfully carried out through glue embolization via the right T3 intercostal artery feeding an arteriovenous fistula to the T3 vertebral body and tumor blush. The following day the patient was taken to surgery.

Approaches to this lesion were discussed, with several considerations in mind. First, the epidural compression was noted to occur from an anterolateral direction at one segment, making an anterior approach appealing. However, at the T3 level, anterior approaches are more complicated and involve splitting the sternum to gain access to this location and working around the great vessels. We recommended a posterolateral approach to allow for decompression, resection of tumor, and both anterior column and posterior reconstruction.

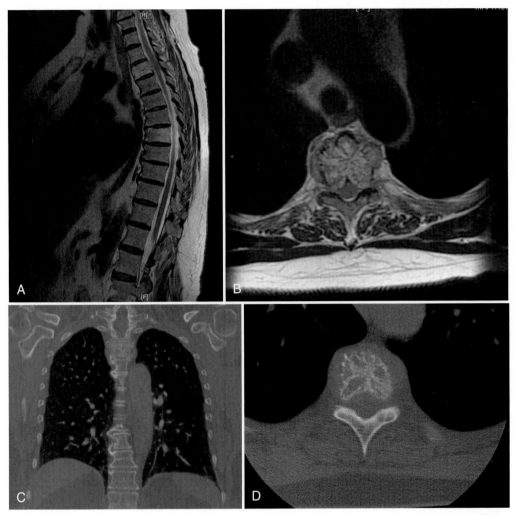

■ **FIGURE 46-1**   **A,** Sagittal and **B,** Axial T2-weighted MRI of the thoracic spine demonstrating a T3 lesion with epidural spinal cord compression. Also of note is a lesion at T7 consistent with a typical hemangioma on all sequences. **C,** Coronal and CT scan of the thoracic spine demonstrated a "polka-dot" type lesion at T3 with the appearance of vascular channels. This lesion was felt to be consistent with an atypical hemangioma.

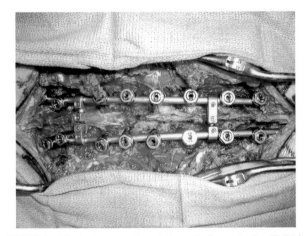

■ **FIGURE 46-2**   Intraoperative photograph demonstrating T2-T4 laminectomies and posterior spinal instrumentation extending from T1-T9.

## SURGICAL TECHNIQUE

With the patient in a prone position on the Jackson table with neurological monitoring, T2-T4 laminectomies, T3 costotransversectomy, transpedicular decompression of the spinal canal, and T3 corpectomy with intralesional resection of the tumor were performed. Reconstruction was achieved with an expandable cage placed from T2 to T4 and supplemented with pedicle screw instrumentation extending from T1 to T9. An intraoperative photo is shown in Figure 46-2. We elected to extend the construct multiple levels below the site of tumor resection because we did not want to stop our instrumentation just above or at the site of the apex of the thoracic kyphosis for fear of inferior construct failure. Bone grafting was performed with allograft and demineralized bone matrix. In the setting of potential malignant disease affecting the bone marrow and with spinal tumor surgery in general, we tend to avoid the use of autograft bone or BMP.

## POSTOPERATIVE COURSE

The patient tolerated the procedure well and spent one night in the neuro intensive care unit. The patient had no new neurological deficits. Postoperative CT scan demonstrating the cage reconstruction and pedicle screw instrumentation is shown in Figure 46-3. Pathological analysis confirmed the tumor to be a hemangioma. The patient was discharged to rehab and is being followed with serial imaging and clinical evaluation to assess for tumor recurrence. However, given the benign nature of the histopathology despite aggressive local behavior, it is suspected that the patient is cured of her disease, and adjuvant therapy has not been recommended.

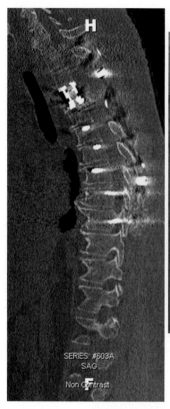

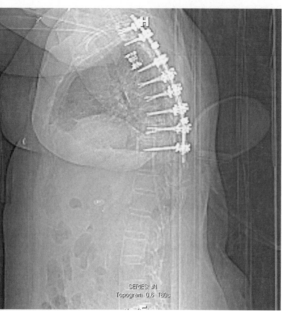

■ **FIGURE 46-3** Postoperative sagittal CT scan and lateral scout view showing cage reconstruction of T3 and pedicle screw instrumentation construct.

## Case 2: Anterior Approach

### PATIENT PRESENTATION

A 61-year-old male with a history of pheochromocytoma presented with progressive midthoracic pain. Nineteen years prior to presentation the patient was diagnosed with a pheochromocytoma and was treated successfully with left adrenalectomy. Six years prior to presentation the patient developed midthoracic region pain and was treated conservatively with physical therapy and NSAIDs. The patient developed myelopathic signs and symptoms to include lower extremity weakness and gait dysfunction. And an MRI of the thoracic spine disclosed a lesion at T5 with significant epidural spinal cord compression. He was then treated with radiation therapy and his pain and neurological dysfunction improved. Several years following the radiation therapy, the patient developed worsening and severe midthoracic pain that had a mechanical component to it. Associated symptoms included bilateral thoracic radicular pain and subjective lower extremity weakness. He described dragging his feet, but denied sphincter dysfunction. On exam he had 4/5 strength of the iliopsoas and dorsiflexors bilaterally. He was also noted to be hyperreflexic in his lower extremities. MRI of the thoracic spine (Figure 46-4) showed partial collapse of the T5 vertebral body with kyphosis and epidural spinal cord compression. T2 signal change was noted in the spinal cord at this level, consistent with myelomalacia. Surgery was recommended, given evidence of spinal cord compression, clinical myelopathy, anterior vertebral column compromise and kyphosis. An all-posterior approach with transpedicular corpectomy and reconstruction of the anterior column was considered. However, it was felt that an anterior approach would be the best approach to resect the anterior compressive tumor, correct the kyphosis, and reconstruct the anterior column without having to perform a multilevel instrumented fusion that would be required with an all-posterior approach.

### SURGICAL TECHNIQUE

Given the history of pheochromocytoma, the patient was seen by endocrinology and anesthesia preoperatively and was premedicated with phenoxybenzaprine for alpha blockade. Pheochromocytomas are highly vascular tumors and preoperative embolization was also recommended. The right and left T5 intercostal vessels were entered and the tumor was successfully embolized with embospheres. A right-sided, high posterolateral thoracotomy approach was selected to allow for access to the anterolateral vertebral column, because of the prominence of the aortic arch on the left side. The high posterolateral thoracotomy requires mobilization of the scapula, and in this case, partial resection of the right 5th rib. A T5 corpectomy was performed with opening of the posterior longitudinal ligament for complete decompression of the spinal cord (Figure 46-5). Reconstruction of the anterior column was achieved with a distractible cage and plate. Bone grafting was performed using allograft bone. Autograft bone was avoided to limit the rest of metastatic spread of tumor potentially present in the bone marrow of the adjacent rib.

### POSTOPERATIVE COURSE

The patient was observed in the neuro intensive care unit overnight. A chest tube was placed at the time of surgery and removed 72 hours postoperatively. He remained at his baseline neurological exam. He was discharged to home, fully ambulatory, on postoperative day number 8. Postoperative x-rays demonstrated excellent position of the cage and plate (Figure 46-6). At 1-year follow-up the patient had excellent pain control and stable postoperative imaging.

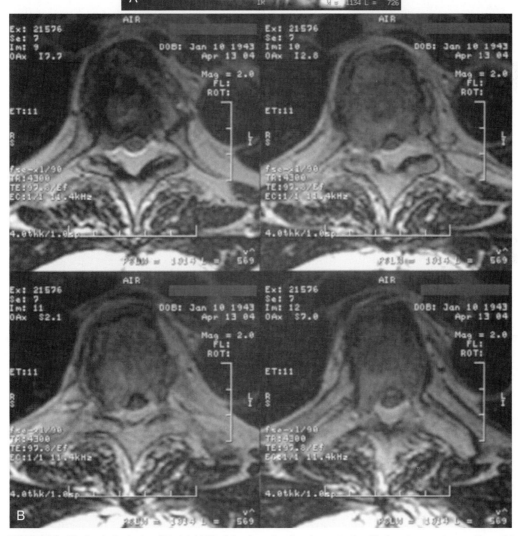

■**FIGURE 46-4    A,** Sagittal and **B,** Axial MRI of the thoracic spine demonstrating T5 pheochromocytoma with partial anterior column collapse and epidural spinal cord compression with T2 signal change in the spinal cord.

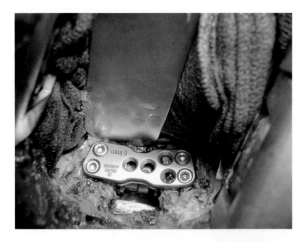

■ **FIGURE 46-5** Intraoperative photograph demonstrating right thoracotomy approach, T5 corpectomy with decompression of the spinal cord, and reconstruction with expandable cage and plating from T4-T6.

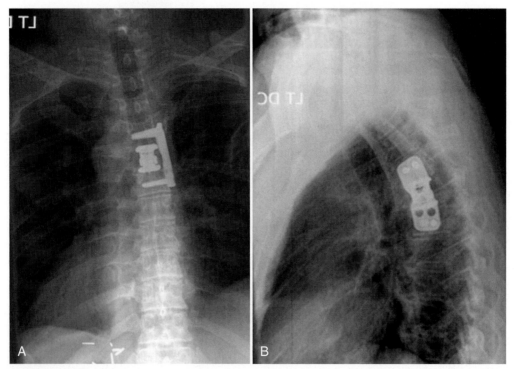

■ **FIGURE 46-6** Postoperative AP and lateral thoracic spine x-rays demonstrating stable position of the cage and plate.

## Case 3: Anterior/-Posterior Combined Approach

### PATIENT PRESENTATION

A 52-year-old male with a history of hypertension presented with a 1-year history of progressive right-sided abdominal and flank region pain. His pain subsequently progressed to include axial back pain that was most severe at night when recumbent in bed. A CT scan (Figure 46-7) of the thoracic spine revealed a lytic/destructive lesion at T9-T10 with associated large paraspinal posterior pleural-based mass on the right side. MRI (Figure 46-8) disclosed significant epidural extension and spinal cord compression. The patient denied lower extremity sensory changes, weakness, or bowel or bladder dysfunction. He had no history of systemic cancer. Neurological exam was significant for 5/5 strength in his lower extremities, and a normal sensory exam except for dermatomal sensory loss in the right T9-T10 location. He was also noted to have hyperreflexia in his lower extremities and two to three beats of bilateral ankle clonus. Given the prolonged history, it was felt that this lesion might represent a relatively slow-growing histopathological entity. Considerations were sarcoma,

plasmacytoma/multiple myeloma, and possibly metastatic carcinoma. Given his preserved motor function, an expedited CT-guided biopsy of the lesion was recommended. The pathology proved the lesion to be a plasmacytoma/multiple myeloma. Further staging disclosed this to be stage 1A IgG kappa multiple myeloma. Despite the lytic appearance of this tumor, the patient initially did not have mechanical pain and the anterior column height was preserved without pathological fracture or deformity. Given the high radiation sensitivity of multiple myeloma, radiation therapy was recommended with close follow-up. The patient failed to respond to radiation therapy and developed mild gait dysfunction. Surgical resection was recommended. The lack of response to radiation called into question the diagnosis of multiple myeloma. Concomitant thoracotomy and posterior approach was planned. In any situation when an anterior approach is planned and a greater than 1 level corpectomy is performed, we recommend supplemental posterior stabilization. In this case, we felt as well that a combined posterior approach would also assist with the tumor resection and decompression.

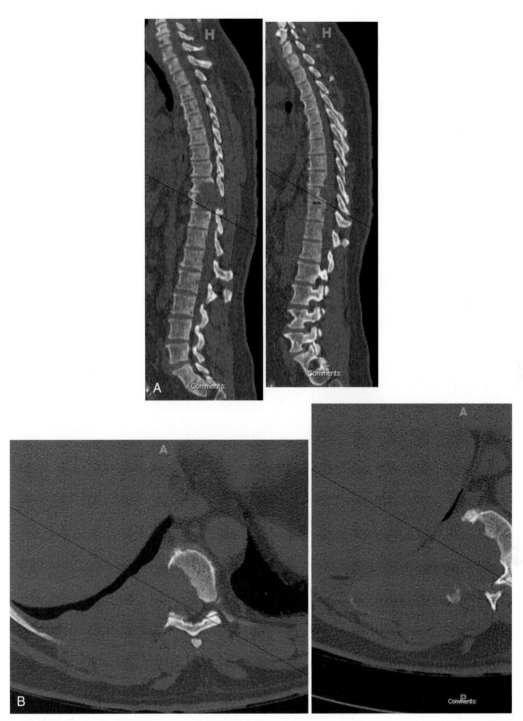

**■ FIGURE 46-7**   Sagittal **(A)** and Axial **(B)** CT images of the spine demonstrating a lytic destructive process at T9-10, with associated large right paraspinal mass (myeloma). Note that despite the significant destruction of the bone, there is no deformity of the spine.

## SURGICAL TECHNIQUE

The patient was placed in the left lateral decubitus position to allow access to the right thoracoabdominal region and the posterior thoracolumbar spine. The posterior thoracolumbar spine was exposed from T7 to L2. Pedicle screws were placed at T7 to T8, and T11-L1. Only one screw could be placed at L2, and in the lateral position, screws could not be successfully placed at T6. A temporary rod was placed on the left side of the spine to stabilize the spine during the decompression. T9 and T10 laminectomies were fashioned and tumor in the epidural space was resected. A right thoracotomy incision was fashioned over the 9th and 10th ribs and connected to the thoracolumbar incision dorsally. A portion of the 9th and 10th ribs distal to the tumor was resected. This allowed access to the pleural cavity. The 9th and 10th ribs were disarticulated from the spine to allow the paraspinal component of the tumor to be resected with the chest wall. Corpectomies of T9 and T10 were performed to resect the remaining tumor. The segment was reconstructed with an expandable cage encompassing T8 to T11. A lateral plate was also placed from T8 to T11. Final rods were placed posteriorly and bone grafting was performed with allograft. Plastic surgery assisted with the closure and reconstruction of the chest wall.

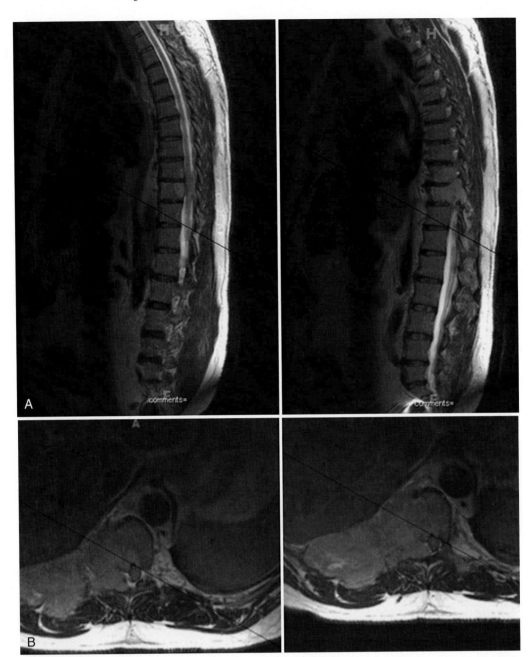

■**FIGURE 46-8**   **A,** Sagittal and **B,** Axial T2-weighted images, demonstrating a mass (myeloma) at T9-10 with epidural spinal cord compression. Note the extensive paraspinal component of the mass.

## POSTOPERATIVE COURSE

The patient remained at his neurological baseline postoperatively. His pathology again confirmed the diagnosis of multiple myeloma. His postoperative course was complicated by a prolonged air leak requiring a chest tube. He was discharged on postoperative day 17. Postoperative imaging showed good position of the instrumentation (Figure 46-9). At 2.5 years post surgery he remains neurologically intact with an intact construct. He has had skeletal progression of the myeloma to stage III.

## DISCUSSION

Metasatic tumors are the most common neoplasms affecting the thoracic spine. Based on the work of Patchell et al surgery followed by radiation therapy has replaced radiation therapy alone as the gold standard for treatment of MESCC. Extremely radiation-sensitive tumors include small cell lung carcinoma, lymphoma, and multiple myeloma. For these lesions, radiation therapy may still be employed as a first-line treatment modality for MESCC. The surgical approach may be anterior, posterior, or combined anterior/posterior. En bloc spondylectomy may be employed specifically for certain locally aggressive primary spinal column neoplasms. Prior to embarking on treatment, it is important to know the tumor histology. Therefore, CT-guided biopsy is recommended in patients who have stable or preserved neurological function. Tumor history, tumor location, anatomy of spinal disease, extent of systemic disease/medical comorbidities, and vertebral column compromise are factors that dictate the surgical approach. Thoracic spinal column neoplasms require reconstruction with instrumentation, with the exception of IMSCTs and some IDEM tumors. The clinical goals of surgery for thoracic spinal column neoplasms include local disease control, preservation or restoration of neurological function, stabilization of the spinal column, and pain control.

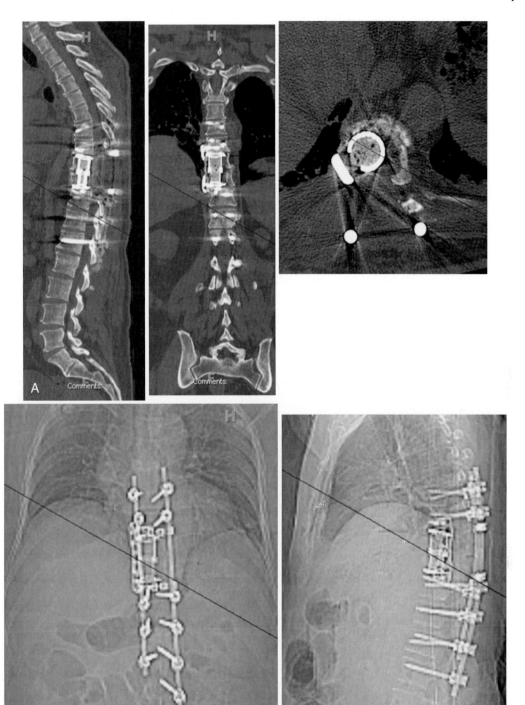

■**FIGURE 46-9**   Sagittal, coronal, axial, and scouts views, status post resection and reconstruction with instrumentation via a combined anterior and posterior approach.

## Case 4: En Bloc

### PATIENT PRESENTATION

A 67-year-old male with a history of prostate cancer treated with resection and thought to be in remission presented with upper lumbar/lower thoracic and right paraspinal pain. Associated symptoms included local numbness and paresthesias and more recent numbness and paresthesias in his feet. An MRI of the thoracic and lumbar spine (Figure 46-10) was performed with and without contrast as well as plain films. The plain films did not demonstrate evidence of bony changes; however, MRI showed a T2-hyperintense and contrast-enhancing lesion at T10 with epidural extension and spinal cord compression. Although the patient had some mild myelopathic signs on exam (hyperreflexia), his motor exam was normal and his gait and sphincter function were both normal. The differential diagnosis included chordoma, given the T2 hyperintensity that is typical of this lesion. Also included on the list was metastatic disease, with prostate being the highest possibility on the list given his previous history. Because chordoma was on the list, representing a locally aggressive tumor that is rarely cured with intralesional resection alone, a CT-guided biopsy was recommended through a posterior approach to confirm the pathology prior to recommending further treatment. The report confirmed a chordoma. An en bloc surgical resection was recommended. An all-posterior approach was recommended with the caveat that if en bloc resection could not be achieved in this fashion, the posterior resection of the posterior elements at T10 would be followed by a thoracotomy with anterior en bloc vertebral body resection.

### SURGICAL TECHNIQUE

The patient was positioned prone on the Jackson table. The posterior spine was exposed from T7 to T12. The surgical plan was to stop the construct at T12/the thoracolumbar (TL) junction. Although stopping a construct at a junctional level may not be ideal, the authors feel that when this is done with a construct ending on the superior side of the TL junction, it is better tolerated than ending on the inferior side of the TL junction. However, there is no solid data to support this clinical belief. We also felt that ending at T7 was high enough above the apex of the patient's thoracic kyphosis, which we estimated to be at T8-9 or T9-10 based on the imaging. Pedicle screws were therefore placed at T7-T9 and T11-T12 bilaterally. Laminectomies at T9 and T11 were subsequently fashioned. Two Tomita saws were then placed between the lamina of T10 and the dura at the junction with the facet joint. Using the Tomita saws, the spinous process and bilateral lamina of T10 were removed in en bloc fashion. Using silk ligatures to prevent a CSF leak, the bilateral T9 and T10 nerve

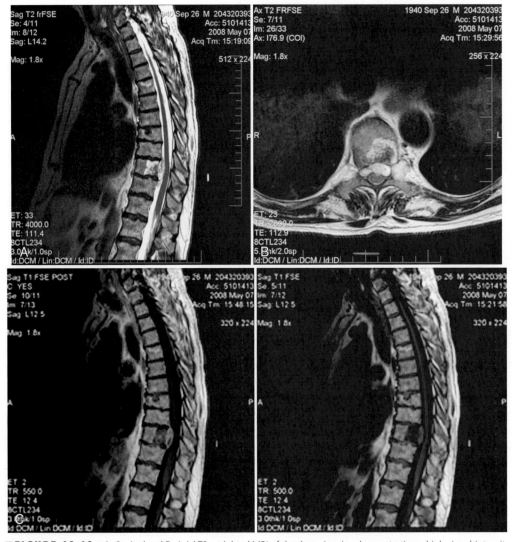

**■ FIGURE 46-10    A,** Sagittal and **B,** Axial T2-weighted MRI of the thoracic spine demonstrating a high-signal-intensity lesion at T10 (chordoma) with epidural spinal cord compression. T1-weighted postcontrast and precontrast images **(c)** demonstrate enhancement of the lesion.

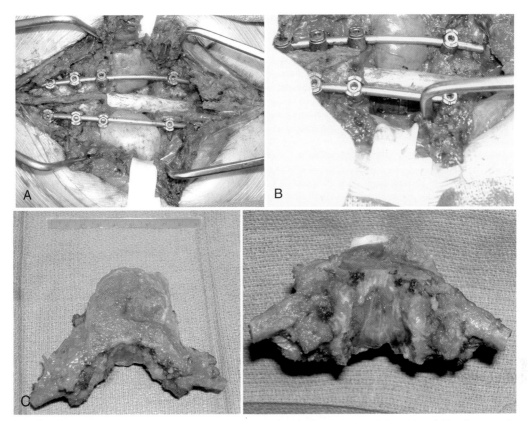

■**FIGURE 46-11**  Intraoperative photographs. **A,** Posterior spinal hardware and the bilateral lung fields adjacent to the spinal cord at the spondylectomy site. **B,** Anteriorly-placed distractible cage at the site of the en bloc spondylectomy. **C,** Gross pathological specimen of the T10 en bloc spondylectomy. Note the epidural tumor capsule posterior to the vertebral body.

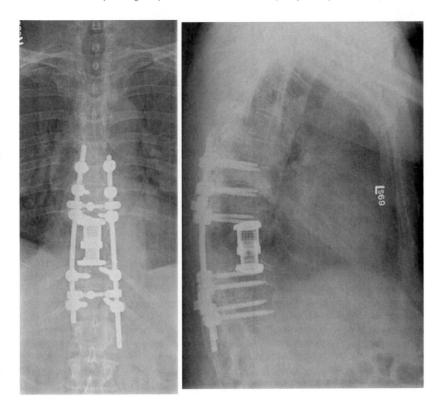

■ **FIGURE 46-12**  Postoperative AP and lateral x-rays of the thoracic spine demonstrating the reconstruction.

roots were ligated proximal to the dorsal root ganglion. The nerve roots typically have to be sectioned at one or two levels to deliver the vertebral body posteriorly in an en bloc spondylectomy. It is felt that sectioning the roots proximal to the dorsal root ganglion decreases the possibility of postoperative neuropathic radicular pain. The thecal sac was carefully dissected from the anterolaterally situated epidural tumor. The paraspinal muscles were dissected off of the rib cage and retracted medially with Penrose drains. The bilateral T10 ribs were then resected from 1 cm distal to the costotransverse junction to 5 cm distal to that point. The pleura was opened and a chest spreader was placed, first on the left and then on the right. The lung was retracted away from the field and the vessels (aorta and vena cava) were dissected off the pleura and T9 and T10 vertebral bodies in a circumferential fashion. Both T9 and T10 segmental vessels were ligated bilaterally. Rods were then attached to the screw heads from T7 through T12. Using Tomita saws, the midvertebral body of T9 was transected, as was the T10-T11 disc space. This completely mobilized the specimen. The specimen was then removed posterolaterally in en bloc fashion (Figure 46-11). A distractible cage was placed from T9 to T11. Bone grafting was done with allograft. Neurological monitoring remained stable throughout the case.

## POSTOPERATIVE COURSE

The patient was taken to the intensive care unit with preserved lower extremity neurological function. He remained intubated until postoperative day 1 when he was successfully extubated. Postoperative imaging disclosed good position of his cage and posterior screws (Figure 46-12). His postoperative course was complicated by new-onset atrial fibrillation. His chest tubes were discontinued on postoperative days 5 and 6 respectively. He was discharged on postoperative day 8. At 3 months after surgery, he was off narcotics and returned to work. Proton beam irradiation was scheduled.

## References

1. T.F. Witham, et al., Surgery insight: current management of epidural spinal cord compression from metastatic spine disease, Nat. Clin. Pract. Neurol. 2 (2) (2006) 87–94.
2. M. Bilsky, Metastatic tumors of the spine and spinal cord, in: C.A. Dickman, M.G. Fehlings, Z.L. Gokaslan (Eds.), Spinal Cord and Spinal Column Tumors, Thieme, New York, 2005.
3. R.A. Patchell, et al., Direct decompressive surgical resection in the treatment of spinal cord compression caused by metastatic cancer: a randomised trial, Lancet 366 (9486) (2005) 643–648.
4. P.C. McCormick, BB: Spinal tumors, in:  L.C., R.G. Grossman (Eds.), Principles of neurosurgery, Lippincott-Raven, Philadelphia, 1999.
5. S.J. Hentschel, M.I., Intradural extramedullary spinal tumors, in: M.G. Fehlings, C.A. Dickman, Z.L. Gokaslan (Eds.), Spinal cord and spinal column tumors, Thieme, New York, 2005.
6. P.R. Cooper, H.K, Intramedullary spinal cord tumors, in:M.G. Fehlings, C.A. Dickman, Z.L. Gokaslan (Eds.), Spinal cord and spinal column tumors, Thieme, New York, 2005.
7. W.B. Jacobs,  F.M, Primary vertebral column tumors, in: M.G. Fehlings, C.A. Dickman, Z.L. Gokaslan (Eds.), Spinal cord and spinal column tumors, Thieme, New York, 2005.
8. J.H. Chi, et al., Epidemiology and demographics for primary vertebral tumors, Neurosurg. Clin. N. Am. 19 (1) (2008) 1–4.
9. A. Mantha, et al., A novel rat model for the study of intraosseous metastatic spine cancer, J Neurosurg. Spine 2 (3) (2005) 303–307.
10. C.A. Bagley, et al., Fractionated, single-port radiotherapy delays paresis in a metastatic spinal tumor model in rats, J. Neurosurg. Spine 7 (3) (2007) 323–327.
11. C.A. Bagley, et al., Local delivery of oncogel delays paresis in rat metastatic spinal tumor model, J. Neurosurg. Spine 7 (2) (2007) 194–198.
12. B. Gok, et al., Surgical resection plus adjuvant radiotherapy is superior to surgery or radiotherapy alone in the prevention of neurological decline in a rat metastatic spinal tumor model, Neurosurgery 63 (2) (2008) 346–351.
13. W.A. Pennant, et al., Microsurgical removal of intramedullary spinal cord gliomas in a rat spinal cord decreases onset to paresis, an animal model for intramedullary tumor treatment, Childs Nerv. Syst. 24 (8) (2008) 901–907.
14. J. Schuster, J. Zhang, M. Longo, A novel human osteoblast-derived severe combined immunodeficiency mouse model of bone metastasis, J Neurosurg. Spine 4 (5) (2006) 388–391.
15. D.R. Fourney, Z.L. Gokaslan, Use of "MAPs" for determining the optimal surgical approach to metastatic disease of the thoracolumbar spine: anterior, posterior, or combined: invited submission from the Joint Section Meeting on Disorders of the Spine and Peripheral Nerves, March 2004, J. Neurosurg. Spine 2 (1) (2005) 40–49.

# Infections of the Thoracic Spine

*47*

*Daniel J. Hoh and Michael Y. Wang*

### K E Y   P O I N T S

- The incidence of reported spinal infections is increasing, which is likely to be related to a growing elderly population that is living longer with chronic disease and undergoing more spinal procedures.

- Spinal infections are of significant concern, as they can cause pathologic fractures, instability, loss of spinal alignment, and neural compression resulting in pain, deformity, and neurological deficit.

- Improved diagnostic and therapeutic modalities are available that make possible earlier identification of the pathologic organism, initiation of appropriate pharmacotherapy, and better eradication of infection with less recurrence.

- The indications for surgical intervention are to identify the pathologic organism, prevent neurological deterioration, restore spinal alignment, maintain stability, and treat disabling pain. A variety of surgical approaches are available including anterior, posterior, and circumferential techniques. Decision-making regarding surgical approach is dependent on extent of disease, need for spinal reconstruction and stabilization, and the patient's overall surgical risk.

- Advances in surgical technique, instrumentation, and biomedical technology are improving operative treatment of spinal infections. Recent developments include the increasingly safe use of titanium-based implants, alternative graft options, and the introduction of minimally invasive spinal surgery. Prognosis for patients with spinal infections is improving as a result of these advances in diagnostic, medical, and surgical modalities.

## INTRODUCTION

The last several decades have witnessed a rise in reported spinal infections. This increase has largely been attributed to factors associated with a growing elderly population. Improvements in medical care have directly resulted in prolonged life expectancy with more individuals living longer with chronic diseases. As a result, various medical conditions associated with advanced age, such as diabetes or illnesses that lead to immunocompromise, predispose patients to developing spinal infections. Additionally, as individuals are living longer, more elderly patients are seeking to undergo spinal procedures for degenerative conditions that otherwise, left untreated, result in debilitating pain. Both minor procedures such as discography and epidural injections and extensive spinal fusion surgeries pose the risk of direct bacterial inoculation of the spine.

Infections of the spine are characterized either by their microbiology or by the location of pathology. From a microbiology standpoint, spinal infections are differentiated by pyogenic or granulomatous etiologies. Pyogenic infections are generally of bacterial origin. Granulomatous spinal infections encompass fungal etiologies, but include some bacterial sources, and refer primarily to the histologic course of the infection. Spinal tuberculosis is by far the most common of the granulomatous spinal infections worldwide.

Spinal infections are also classified by the primary location of pathogenesis. Sole involvement of the disc space is referred to as discitis. Osteomyelitis is an infection of the bony spine (Figure 47-1). Osteodiscitis or spondylodiscitis is combined involvement of the intervertebral disc and the vertebra. Abscess or granulation formation can occur in a subdural, epidural, or paravertebral location (Figure 47-2). Frequently, spinal infections invade all compartments of the spinal column, including the soft tissues, bony spine, and within the spinal canal.

Spinal osteomyelitis is estimated to occur in 1 in 100,000 to 250,000, and accounts for 2% to 7% of all cases of osteomyelitis. Spinal osteomyelitis occurs more commonly among older individuals, with approximately one half of all patients being over 50 years of age. Similarly, epidural abscesses occur in adults and are estimated to occur in 0.2 to 1.2 per 10,000 hospital admissions annually. When bacterial spinal infections occur in younger individuals, they are more commonly seen in intravenous drug users. Both osteomyelitis and epidural abscesses generally occur in the thoracic and lumbar spine, with thoracic infections representing over a third to half of all cases, and lumbar infections accounting for a majority of the remainder. Cervical spine infections are estimated to account for only 5% to 14% of all cases.

Outside the United States, spinal tuberculosis still represents a considerable health care problem. Tuberculosis is relatively common in underdeveloped countries where malnutrition and overcrowding are present. It is estimated that 2 billion people have tuberculosis worldwide, with 9 million new cases each year. Approximately 5% of these patients have spinal involvement. Spinal tuberculosis is a major source of morbidity, representing the most common cause of nontraumatic paraplegia in underdeveloped countries.

While the incidence of spinal infections is increasing, management of these conditions is also dramatically evolving. Earlier detection, better screening and surveillance, and advanced imaging modalities have improved diagnosis of spinal infections and identification of pathogenic organisms. More effective antimicrobial pharmacotherapy has led to better medical treatment with clearance of infection and less recurrence. Surgical treatment options have incorporated advances in surgical technique, instrumentation, and biomedical technology to increase eradication of infection, preservation of neurological function, restoration of spinal alignment, and prevention of deformity and chronic pain.

## PATHOPHYSIOLOGY

The pathophysiology of spinal infection ultimately begins with the individual's underlying predisposing risk factors. Advanced age, diabetes, and multiple medical comorbidities are associated with increased risk for spinal infection. Additionally, spinal surgery, intravenous drug use, and immunocompromise contribute to further risk. Infection generally metastasizes hematogenously to the spine from extraspinal sources such as the urinary tract, respiratory system, skin or soft tissue infections, or cardiac vegetations. Direct inoculation from surgery, percutaneous procedures, or penetrating trauma is an additional modality for bacterial seeding. Local invasion to the spine also occurs from infected adjacent or contiguous sources such as the retroperitoneal, abdominopelvic, pleural, or retropharyngeal spaces. Spread of infection can also occur within the spinal column by direct extension from the bony or soft tissue elements to the epidural space.

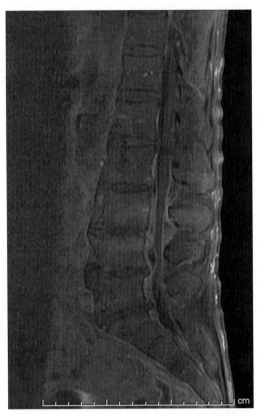

**■ FIGURE 47-1** T1-weighted sagittal MRI after administration of intravenous gadolinium in the same patient, demonstrating abnormal enhancement. The osteodiscitis at the lower thoracic region has an associated epidural abscess causing ventral spinal cord compression.

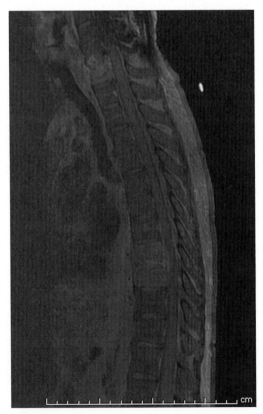

**■ FIGURE 47-2** T1-weighted sagittal MRI with gadolinium of the lumbar spine in a different patient, demonstrating the ring-enhancing contrast pattern of an epidural abscess.

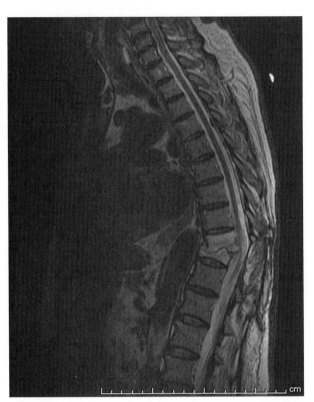

**■ FIGURE 47-3** T2-weighted sagittal MRI in a 64-year-old male with subacute osteodiscitis. Advanced bone loss and significant subchondral destruction has created a severe local kyphosis at the affected level.

## Bacterial Pathogenesis

Hematogenous seeding of the spine may occur via either arterial or venous pathways. The venous plexi that drain from within the spinal canal communicate with plexi that form a venous ring around each vertebral body. This venous system communicates with the venous drainage of the pelvis. Batson demonstrated that this venous pathway is a valveless system in which microorganisms may circulate and lodge in the low-flow end-organ vasculature surrounding the vertebral body. Alternatively, direct bacterial seeding of the vertebral body may occur from ascending and descending arterial branches that send penetrating vessels to the vertebral body.

Pathologic sequelae of spinal infection include loss of spinal alignment with progressive deformity, and risk of neurological compromise. Bacterial involvement of the spinal column with subsequent inflammatory infiltration causes bony destruction and eventually erodes the subchondral plate to involve the relatively avascular disc space (Figure 47-3). Advanced bone loss, particularly across multiple adjacent segments, combined with disc space narrowing, leads to progressive kyphotic deformity. neurological compromise may result from severe bony destruction, resulting in pathologic fracture with retropulsed bony fragments into the canal. Epidural abscess formation or extension of inflammatory granulation tissue into the canal can cause direct compression of the spinal cord or nerve roots. Additionally, septic thrombosis of veins within the epidural space or the arteriolar supply can cause ischemic injury. Particularly, in a spinal cord already compromised by mechanical compression from either an abscess or fracture, hypoperfusion from thrombosed feeding arteries or draining veins may lead to rapid neurological deterioration.

Gram-positive cocci are the most prevalent inciting organism, representing 50% to 67% of all causative organisms. *Staphylococcus aureus* is the most prevalent bacteria identified, accounting for 80% of all gram-positive infections, and 55% of all spinal infections. In a meta-analysis of 915 patients with epidural abscess, *S. aureus* was identified as the causative organism in 73.2% of cases. Gram-negative bacteria, particularly *Escherichia coli* and *Proteus*, are more frequently identified in patients with pre-existing urinary tract infections. *Pseudomonas aeruginosa* is most common

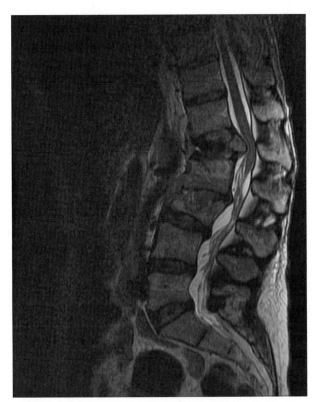

**■ FIGURE 47-4** T2-weighted sagittal MRI of the lumbar spine in a 58-year-old woman with spinal tuberculosis, showing fracture of L1, retropulsed fragments in the canal, and neural compression.

among immunocompromised patients or intravenous drug users. Indolent infections are more likely to occur with low-virulence organisms such as *Streptococcus viridans* or *Staphylococcus epidermisdis*.

## Pathogenesis of Tuberculosis

Tuberculosis of the spine results from hematogenous spread of *Mycobacterium tuberculosis* from well-established extraspinal foci, primarily originating from the respiratory or genitourinary tract. Unlike pyogenic osteomyelitis, spinal tuberculosis may begin in the paradiscal area and spread under the anterior longitudinal ligament to involve adjacent vertebral bodies, while relatively preserving the disc space. Additionally, spinal tuberculosis frequently involves the posterior spinal arch, whereas pyogenic osteomyelitis is primarily a disease of only the anterior spinal column. Because spinal tuberculosis often causes widespread destruction of a spinal segment, vertebral collapse with pathologic subluxation, kyphosis, and retropulsion occur in severe cases and present greater risk for acute neurological compromise than bacterial osteomyelitis (Figure 47-4). Delayed chronic paresis also occurs with progressive deformity or in the setting of epidural granulomas that result from longstanding tuberculous infection.

## CLINICAL PRESENTATION

The clinical presentation of bacterial spinal infections often depends on the virulence of the organism, the duration of infection, and the overall integrity of the patient's immune system. Improved diagnostic modalities have led to earlier detection of disease, with initiation of appropriate medical therapy often before patients develop systemic illness or potentially irreversible neurological compromise. Over 90% of patients with pyogenic osteomyelitis present with axial neck or back pain as the primary complaint. The pain is generally characterized as insidious and nonmechanical in nature, and unrelieved by recumbency. Patients frequently note local spine tenderness with limited range of motion. Constitutional symptoms associated with infection such as fevers, chills, and malaise may also be present: however, an elevated temperature is only found in 52% of patients at time of presentation.

Neurological findings are less common with pyogenic osteomyelitis. A review of the literature reveals that only 17% of patients with bacterial osteomyelitis have neurological signs or symptoms on initial presentation. Alternatively, neurological complaints are frequently associated with acute bacterial epidural abscess, with 56% of patients presenting with motor deficits, and 36% with radicular pain. The clinical triad of localized spine pain, fever, and progressive neurological deficit is seen, however, in only 36% of patients with epidural abscess.

Spinal tuberculosis has a similar presentation to bacterial osteomyelitis, with most presenting with spine pain and localized tenderness. Unlike bacterial osteomyelitis, however, patients with tuberculosis present with a more insidious course. A mean duration of symptoms prior to diagnosis is 6.1 months. neurological deficits at the time of presentation are also more prevalent with tuberculosis, with 44.9% of patients having neurological findings. Motor function abnormalities are present in 34.6% of patients with spinal tuberculosis, with 6.4% being paraplegic at time of presentation.

## DIAGNOSTIC EVALUATION

The initial evaluation of a patient suspected of spinal infection includes standard serologic markers for infection or inflammation. A basic panel includes peripheral white blood cell count (WBC), erythrocyte sedimentation rate (ESR), and C-reactive protein (CRP). WBC is elevated at time of presentation, however, in only 42% of cases, and often normalizes in patients with chronic infection. ESR and CRP are markers of inflammation and demonstrate high sensitivity for spinal infection. CRP, an acute phase protein, increases within 4 to 6 hours of infection. ESR begins to increase only several days after the onset of infection and peaks at 7 to 8 days. ESR is elevated in over 90% of patients with spinal infection; however, ESR and CRP lack specificity, and may be increased in patients either with infection or with other inflammatory disorders. Individuals suspected of tuberculosis are assessed with a PPD and subsequently sputum staining for acid-fast bacilli.

Definitive diagnosis of spinal infection is made upon identifying the causative organism from positive culture. Prompt blood and urine cultures are obtained immediately on presentation, as infection commonly spreads to the spine either from the genitourinary tract or hematogenously. Positive blood cultures identify the inciting organism in 25% to 59% of cases. Ideally, cultures are obtained prior to initiating antimicrobial therapy to obviate the potential of a sterile nondiagnostic culture.

Biopsy of an abnormal spinal lesion can confirm the diagnosis of infection as well as isolate the inciting organism. Percutaneous closed biopsy is performed using computed tomography (CT) or fluoroscopic guidance. Closed biopsy demonstrates a reported accuracy of 70% to 100% in identifying the causative organism. Open surgical biopsy is indicated in the setting of a nondiagnostic closed biopsy in a patient with persistent clinical infection or deterioration despite broad-spectrum medical therapy, or for lesions inaccessible percutaneously. Open biopsy is diagnostic in over 80% of patients, likely due to a larger bony sample. A high concordance rate is observed in patients with both positive blood and biopsy specimens, reinforcing the importance of early blood culture sampling prior to initiating antimicrobial pharmacotherapy.

## Imaging

Plain spine x-rays may demonstrate characteristic findings associated with osteomyelitis or osteodiscitis, and often serve as a rapid method for surveying the full spinal axis for potential infection. Disc space narrowing is the earliest and most consistent radiographic finding, occurring in 74% of cases, generally after approximately 2 to 4 weeks. Enlargement of the paravertebral shadow may indirectly suggest a thoracic paravertebral abscess. After 3 to 6 weeks, leukocyte infiltration into the subchondral bone and vertebral body leads to bony destructive changes, appearing as a lytic area in the anterior aspect of the vertebral body adjacent to the disc, or blurring of the endplates. With advanced bone loss, the vertebral body collapses. Thirty-six inch standing x-rays are essential for assessing progression of sagittal and coronal plane deformity in severe cases. With chronic disease (after 8 to 12 weeks), reactive bone formation and endplate sclerosis occurs. Ultimately, the reparative process results in new bone formation and hypertrophic changes.

Eventually, 50% of cases lead to spontaneous fusion; however, it may require several years for this to take place. The remaining cases likely form a fibrous ankylosis which may similarly effectively immobilize the involved segment.

Radionuclide studies are capable of detecting and localizing infection before abnormal findings are observed on plain radiographs. Gallium scanning demonstrates 89% sensitivity, 85% specificity, and 86% accuracy for diagnosing disc space infections. Technetium scanning is 90% sensitive, 78% specific, and 94% accurate. Combined gallium and technetium scanning is reported to have 94% accuracy. SPECT is a sensitive bone scintigraphic modality for early detection of osteomyelitis and is often performed in conjunction with technetium and gallium scanning.

CT imaging is beneficial for evaluating the extent of bony destruction. Axial CT imaging demonstrates the presence of retropulsed fragments and the degree of canal compromise in the setting of pathologic fracture. Sagittal reconstructed CT imaging may reveal endplate osteopenia as an early finding of infection. Superb detailing of bony anatomy may be useful for preoperative planning in cases necessitating surgical intervention. Also, CT imaging can delineate adjacent soft tissue abscess or granulation tissue that may require operative debridement.

Magnetic resonance imaging (MRI) is the gold standard for radiologic evaluation of spinal infection. MRI demonstrates high sensitivity (96%), specificity (92%), and accuracy (94%). Intravenous gadolinium further delineates areas of abnormal enhancement and facilitates localization of infection to the vertebral body, intervertebral disc, or epidural space. Optimal visualization of the neural elements allows for evaluation of canal compromise or spinal cord compression. MRI is readily capable of delineating paravertebral abscesses. Multiplanar imaging allows for full evaluation of the complete spinal column in sagittal and axial planes to assess for the extent of involvement.

## MANAGEMENT

Management of spinal infections has dramatically evolved over the last several decades. Advances in imaging allow for prompt diagnosis with initiation of appropriate antimicrobial pharmacotherapy, often early in the clinical course. Improved surgical technique combined with developments in spinal instrumentation has resulted in decreased surgical morbidity and better long-term clinical outcomes. The general principles of treatment for spinal infections, regardless of medical or surgical intervention, are fundamentally the same. The primary objectives are to eradicate infection, preserve neurological function, maintain spinal alignment, and prevent pain.

## Medical Therapy

Medical therapy for spinal infection consists primarily of antimicrobial pharmacotherapy. Most patients with vertebral osteomyelitis respond successfully to nonsurgical treatment. The main tenet of medical therapy is identification of the inciting organism with either a positive blood or biopsy specimen, and initiation of an appropriate antimicrobial agent. The selection of either a single or multi-drug regimen is dictated by the virulence and resistance of the causative organism. Therefore, optimal treatment is entirely dependent on isolating an organism. As a result, antimicrobial treatment is withheld in patients that are neurologicalally and clinical stable until definitive cultures are obtained. Patients presenting with sepsis or progressive deterioration may necessitate empirical broad-spectrum coverage until an organism is identified.

Antimicrobial therapy is generally delivered parenterally for a minimum of 6 weeks. A 25% failure rate is observed in patients treated with antibiotics for less than 4 weeks. Serial serologic evaluation of ESR is an effective measure of therapeutic response. After 6 weeks of intravenous antibiotics, some advocate continuing oral therapy until the ESR has diminished by a minimum of one half the pretreatment level to prevent relapse. A two-thirds reduction in ESR from pretreatment levels is an indication of complete eradication of infection. In addition to antimicrobial pharmacotherapy, immobilization with an external orthosis is recommended for patients with severe pain, greater than 50% vertebral height loss, or involvement of the thoracolumbar junction.

Medical treatment for spinal tuberculosis is primarily reserved for patients without any neurological involvement. The Medical Research Council Committee for Research on Tuberculosis in the Tropics concluded that treatment for spinal tuberculosis in developing countries consists of ambulatory pharmacotherapy with 6- or 9-month regimens of isoniazid or rifampin. In Western countries, drug therapy for spinal tuberculosis is 6 months of isoniazid, rifampin, and pyrazinamide. Others advocate a more aggressive approach to spinal tuberculosis with 12 months of treatment, beginning with isoniazid, ethambutol, rifampin, and pyrazinamide for the first 2 months, followed by tailoring of the therapy based on sensitivities. Multimodal therapy is often necessary due to potential drug resistance, as well as the decreased accessibility of certain agents to different involved organ systems. Unfortunately, many of these agents have potential side effects, with the risk of liver failure among the more clinically significant.

## Indications for Surgical Intervention

There are several indications for surgical intervention for spinal infection. Open surgical biopsy to determine the bacteriologic diagnosis is recommended in patients with nondiagnostic cultures or closed biopsy. Patients in sepsis refractory to medical treatment may require abscess drainage or debridement of necrotic tissue to facilitate penetration of antimicrobial therapy to sites of active infection. Individuals presenting with acute neurological deficit resulting from spinal cord compression require emergent decompression. Delaying surgical intervention in neurologicalally compromised patients may be cautiously reserved in those who are too significantly medically compromised to undergo surgery, and those who present with over 72 hours of neurological deficit. Chronic pain and significant deformity are relative indications for surgical intervention.

Patients with spinal tuberculosis and neurological deficit generally are require radical debridement with bone grafting and stabilization. There are data to suggest that patients with tuberculosis and mild neurological deficits may respond to medical therapy alone. In a study of 200 cases of patients with spinal tuberculosis and neurological impairment, 38% of patients recovered with only medical therapy. Sixty-two percent, however, ultimately required surgery, with 69% of surgically treated patients having a complete neurological recovery. A direct correlation between duration of neurological symptoms prior to surgery and time for recovery from paraplegia supports early operative intervention in patients with neurological impairment. With prompt surgical treatment, better neurological outcomes and prevention of deformity can be expected.

## Surgical Management

Several important issues require consideration once it is determined that a patient requires surgical intervention. The primary issue is deciding upon an appropriate surgical approach and fusion technique, from a broad spectrum of operative modalities previously described. Anterior approaches include anterior debridement and fusion with or without instrumentation. Posterior approaches involve a posterior decompression, debridement, and instrumented fusion. Circumferential approaches include anterior debridement with strut grafting and instrumentation with posterior supplemental fixation in a single-stage or delayed fashion. Ultimately, surgical decision-making is dependent upon whether the primary pathology is ventral, dorsal, or circumferential, and whether the infected tissue requires complete or partial debridement. Additional factors include the degree of preexisting deformity, determining the optimal technique for restoring spinal alignment, and whether spinal reconstruction and stabilization are necessary. Last, given the propensity for significant medical comorbidities in this patient population, serious consideration must be given toward selecting a surgical approach that the patient can tolerate with minimized morbidity.

Timing of surgical intervention is also a critical factor. Patients with acute neurologicalal deficits secondary to spinal cord compression require emergent decompression to prevent irreversible injury. Persistent sepsis despite medical therapy, with significant abscesses and infected or necrotic tissue, may necessitate urgent drainage or debridement to decrease the overall infectious burden and facilitate antimicrobial penetration. Acute instability that threatens neurological structures demands immediate immobilization and may require urgent operative stabilization. Delayed surgical intervention is indicated for patients that are stable neurologically and clinically, but have disabling pain or evidence of chronic progressive deformity. Generally, in these instances, surgical instrumented stabilization and arthrodesis is performed after the acute infection is cleared.

The use of instrumentation and certain grafting techniques in an acutely infected wound is controversial. Instrumented spinal fusion surgery is associated with increased risk of infection compared to nonfusion surgery. However, there are growing laboratory and clinical data to suggest that titanium-based implants may have improved resistance to bacterial colonization than traditional stainless steel, and may be appropriate for spinal stabilization even in the setting of acute infection. Selection of appropriate graft material to promote arthrodesis without serving as a host environment for further bacterial seeding is also critical. Last, various minimally invasive techniques for surgical debridement, instrumented stabilization, and fusion have become available that may serve to improve clinical outcomes and reduce surgical morbidity compared to conventional open surgical modalities.

### Posterior Approach

Posterior decompression for spinal infection is primarily reserved for evacuation of isolated epidural abscesses without involvement of the bony anterior spinal column or intervertebral discs. Epidural abscesses, particularly in the thoracic and lumbar spine, preferentially occur dorsal to the thecal sac, and therefore are amenable to laminectomy for decompression and drainage. The extent of the laminectomy ideally does not involve the facet joints, so as to prevent iatrogenic destabilization. Reports of limited interlaminar decompression with epidural abscess fenestration have been described; however, the benefit of this minimal approach over standard laminectomy has not been demonstrated. The additional insertion of an epidural suction-irrigation catheter at the time of surgery, for postoperative continuous washout, has also been reported to have beneficial results.

Posterior decompression alone is not recommended in the setting of osteomyelitis, discitis, or osteodiscitis. Laminectomy with removal of the posterior tension band further destabilizes the spine in patients with already impaired anterior column support. Posterior decompression in the setting of vertebral osteomyelitis has resulted in unfavorable outcomes related to deformity progression, increased instability, and neurological deterioration.

With the advent of pedicle screw-rod fixation, a single-stage posterior approach for decompression, debridement, and instrumented stabilization may be an appropriate alternative surgical modality (Figure 47-5 A-C). Various posterior approaches for accessing anterior thoracic and lumbar pathology are available. Costotransversectomy, lateral extracavitary, and transpedicular techniques allow access to the anterior spinal column via a posteriorly based approach. With these techniques, debridement of varying degrees of the anterior column may be performed, although complete vertebrectomy via a solely posterior approach is technically challenging, given limited visualization of the anterior aspect of the thecal sac.

After debridement of infected, necrotic tissue, anterior column reconstruction may be achieved using either stackable or expandable interbody devices that are designed to be inserted from a posterior approach (Figure 47-6 A-B). Particularly in the thoracic spine, a unilateral single nerve root may be ligated to facilitate insertion of an interbody cage. Again, however, limited exposure via a posterior approach may restrict the size of interbody graft that can be inserted, thereby presenting potential risk for graft subsidence, kyphosis, or nonunion. Supplemental posterior fixation with a pedicle screw-rod construct provides instrumented stabilization, and thereby prevents progressive sagittal deformity as well as facilitates arthrodesis. A single-stage posterior approach for debridement, decompression, and stabilization may be particularly suited for medically compromised patients with osteomyelitis who may not tolerate a thoracotomy for anterior exposure.

### Anterior Approach

Anterior procedures to surgically treat osteomyelitis have become increasingly popular since Hodgson first reported anterior debridement and fusion for spinal tuberculosis in 1960, and have since become the standard treatment for pyogenic osteomyelitis as well. Because the pathology is generally ventral, an anterior approach allows for thorough debridement of infected and necrotic tissue, and drainage of psoas or paravertebral abscesses. With an anterior approach, it is possible to completely remove all necrotic tissue until bleeding, well-vascularized bone is encountered, and to decompress the ventral thecal sac. Anterior spinal column reconstruction with an interbody graft for arthrodesis, anterior column support, and restoration of sagittal alignment is also best attained from an anterior approach. Spinal fixation

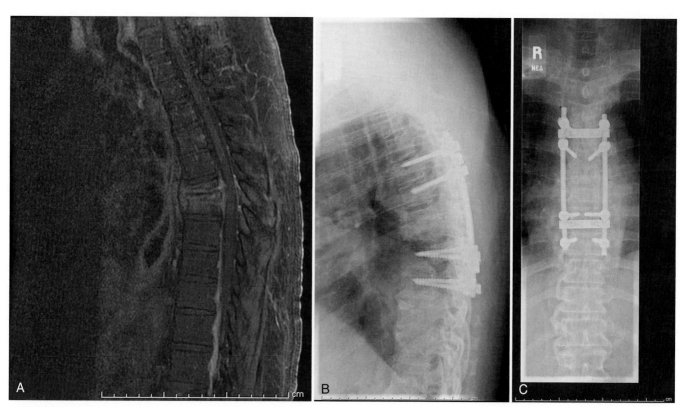

■ **FIGURE 47-5**    A-C. **A,** T1-weighted sagittal MRI with gadolinium of the same patient, demonstrating abnormal enhancement in the vertebral bodies and an associated epidural abscess. **B,** Lateral x-ray of the same patient revealing the pedicle screw-rod instrumentation and sagittal alignment. **C,** Anteroposterior x-ray after posterior decompression and instrumented stabilization with a pedicle screw-rod construct.

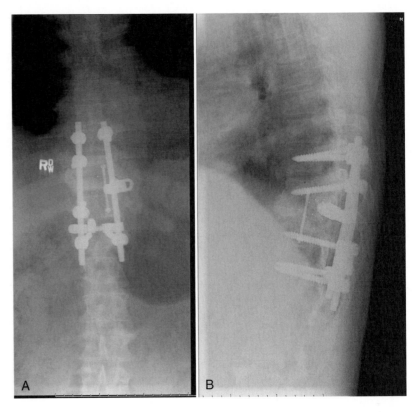

■ **FIGURE 47-6** A-B. Anteroposterior **(A)** and lateral **(B)** x-rays in a 50-year-old male with T10-11 osteomyelitis. The patient underwent a left costotransversectomy approach for T10-11 partial corpectomy and debridement. Through the same posterior approach, a stackable cage was inserted for anterior column reconstruction, and pedicle screw-rod stabilization was performed.

for stabilization and to facilitate arthrodesis can also be performed from an anterior approach (Figure 47-7 A-D).

Various techniques for anterior debridement, vertebral column reconstruction, and instrumented stabilization have been described. Hodgson's original description of an anterior procedure to treat spinal tuberculosis involved anterior debridement and autologous strut grafting without instrumentation. While initial reports demonstrated successful clinical outcomes, subsequent studies have observed loss of correction, progressive deformity, and pseudarthrosis without the use of instrumentation. As a result, various developments in device technology for spinal reconstruction and stabilization have been made to improve upon these findings. The uses of anterior instrumentation with or without posterior supplemental fixation in single-stage or two-stage procedure have evolved as modern modalities for the treatment of vertebral osteomyelitis.

### Anterior Approach with Anterior Fixation

An anterior approach allows for a single-stage, single-approach surgical treatment for debridement, decompression, arthrodesis, and stabilization. Initially, anterior procedures incorporated autologous strut grafting without instrumented stabilization, because of concern about placing a foreign body in a contaminated wound. As a result, patients were immobilized and maintained on prolonged bed rest postoperatively. Recently, however, numerous reports have described successful use of titanium-based implants in the setting of spinal infection without evidence of persistent infection or relapse. The use of anterior spinal fixation in combination with anterior debridement and grafting allows for early patient mobilization, thereby reducing the risk of complications associated with prolonged recumbency such as pneumonia, pulmonary embolism, decubitus ulcer, and muscle atrophy.

Dai et al reported on 22 patients treated with an anterior-only approach for the treatment of thoracic and lumbar osteomyelitis.[1] Patients underwent an anterior debridement, interbody fusion with autologous graft, and anterior instrumented stabilization. Follow-up was for a minimum of 3 years, and there were no cases of residual or recurrent infection. ESR and CRP returned to normal levels within 4 to 10 weeks postoperatively.

With anterior column reconstruction, the investigators observed an improvement in kyphosis, with an average correction rate of 93.1%. Solid arthrodesis was achieved in all patients within 6 months, with only two patients requiring immobilization with an external orthosis. Significantly,

there were no cases of implant failure and only three instances of mild graft subsidence.

Patients also demonstrated significant functional and neurological recovery. Eighteen patients were standing and ambulating within 1 week postoperatively. The remaining 3 patients were walking within 4 weeks. There were no cases of postoperative neurological deterioration. All patients with preoperative neurological deficits had complete recovery within 6 months except for one Frankel grade C patient who improved to a Frankel grade D.

The anterior-only approach provides the benefit of thorough debridement, reconstruction, fusion and stabilization in a single-stage, single approach. With a single surgical procedure, there is less morbidity associated with prolonged anesthesia, lengthy operative time, blood loss, and potential tissue injury in patients who are generally medically compromised and may be predisposed to poor wound healing. The addition of supplemental posterior fixation may result in longer constructs with further loss of spinal motion segments. Others are concerned that placing instrumentation in a contaminated wound results in formation of a biofilm on the implant surface layer that harbors bacteria and is poorly penetrable by antibiotics. Therefore, additional posterior spinal instrumentation may present an increased risk for persistent infection or recurrence.

### Single-Stage Anterior and Posterior Procedure

A combined anterior and posterior procedure to treat vertebral osteomyelitis provides several benefits over a single anterior approach. Circumferential access to the spinal canal allows for complete neural decompression in patients who may have both ventral compression from retropulsed bone fragments and dorsal compression from epidural abscess or posterior spinal arch involvement.

Korovessis et al studied 24 patients with osteomyelitis treated with a single-stage anterior debridement, partial vertebrectomy, mesh cage and autologous bone graft, and supplemental pedicle screw fixation.[2] Follow-up was for an average of 56 months, with all patients demonstrating complete resolution of infection. While three patients who were ASIA A on presentation remained ASIA A postoperatively, patients with incomplete spinal cord injuries improved an average of 1.4 Frankel grades postoperatively. Six patients with incomplete injuries preoperatively had full recovery of neurological function within 1 year of surgery. Eleven patients who were neurologically intact preoperatively returned to full premorbid functional and

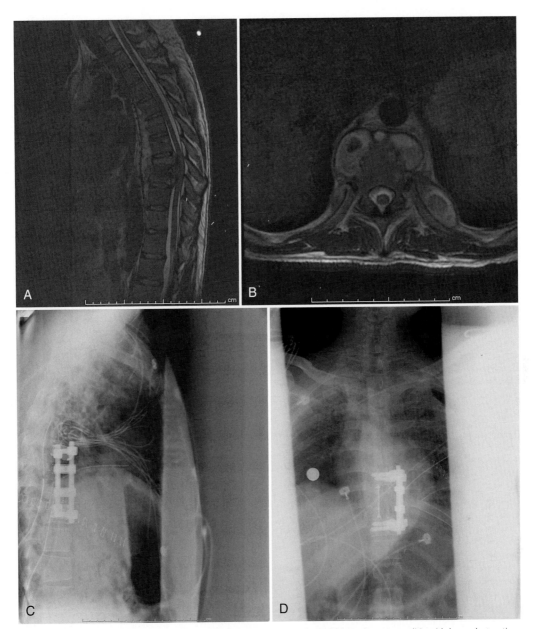

■ **FIGURE 47-7**    A-D. **A,** Sagittal T2-weighted MRI demonstrating midthoracic osteomyelitis with bony destruction, kyphosis, retropulsed fragments, and cord compression. **B,** Axial T2-weighted MRI showing multiple loculated paravertebral abscesses at a level adjacent to the pathologic fracture. **C,** Postoperative lateral x-ray revealing the cage and anterolateral instrumented stabilization. **D,** Postoperative anteroposterior x-ray demonstrating an anterior debridement, corpectomy, cage placement, and anterolateral instrumentation.

activity levels within 4 to 6 months after surgery. Visual analog pain scores improved postoperatively as well.

Combined anterior and posterior instrumentation provides an idealized biomechanical construct to treat advanced bony destruction, spinal instability, and deformity secondary to vertebral osteomyelitis. Anterior removal of necrotic tissue with anterior column reconstruction provides optimal load sharing and restoration of sagittal alignment in cases of vertebral height loss. Posterior supplemental fixation recreates the posterior tension band to restrict potential for long-term loss of sagittal plane correction.

An anterior-only procedure presents concern regarding long-term stability. Some have observed that an anterior procedure without posterior supplemental fixation results in poor sagittal correction and long-term increase in kyphosis. An anterior fusion alone may be appropriate for a single-level corpectomy with an intact posterior tension band. However, patients with multilevel involvement, significant bony endplate destruction, or disease that crosses the thoracolumbar junction may be predisposed to failure with an anterior-only construct. Particularly, patients with loss of

the posterior tension band, either through extensive posterior spinal arch involvement such as in spinal tuberculosis, or from iatrogenic destabilization via laminectomy, may also require supplemental posterior instrumentation. Alternatively, excellent restoration of sagittal alignment with long-term maintenance of correction has been demonstrated with a combined anterior-posterior procedure.

A combined anterior-posterior procedure also creates an optimal mechanical environment for arthrodesis. With an anterior interbody fusion, the graft is placed under compressive rather than tensile forces, which facilitates arthrodesis. Posteriorly placed transpedicular instrumentation provides rigid immobilization in all three planes of rotation to effectively stabilize the spine and improve fusion.

### Two-Staged Anterior-Posterior Procedure

Circumferential treatment of vertebral osteomyelitis can be performed as a single-stage procedure or in a two-staged fashion, with initial anterior debridement and then delayed posterior fixation. Staged spinal surgery has gained popularity for the treatment of various other complex spinal disorders such as deformity, trauma, and oncologic and rheumatologic conditions. The benefit of staged surgery is a shorter operative time and less blood loss for each individual procedure, which may be particularly relevant for patients with worse overall general health. A two-staged surgery allows for a convalescent period to bridge between the two procedures, in which the patients may have an opportunity to recover clinically and neurologicalally. Also, performing supplemental posterior instrumentation in a delayed manner allows for a longer course of antimicrobial therapy to further reduce the infected environment prior to implantation of hardware.

Dimar et al reported on 42 patients with osteomyelitis treated with anterior debridement and strut grafting, followed by delayed instrumented posterior spinal fusion at an average of 14.4 days after the initial procedure.[3] Many patients were acutely ill at presentation requiring urgent treatment, but were in poor overall clinical status to undergo an extensive circumferential operation. Most were significantly debilitated from inadequate nutrition as well. For these patients, Dimar et al performed anterior debridement and anterior strut grafting urgently to thoroughly remove the infection and restore anterior column support. Patients were then immobilized in an external orthosis, continued on intravenous antibiotics, aggressively resuscitated nutritionally, and initiated on physical therapy. Delayed posterior spinal fusion was then performed on a semi-elective basis when patients were clinically stable to undergo a second procedure.

All patients had complete resolution of their infection with no evidence of recurrence. Patients with preoperative neurological deficits improved postoperatively. No significant deterioration in patients' overall medical condition was observed as a result of the interoperative period. The average length of hospitalization, however, was prolonged in this series, with a mean length of stay of 24 days and range of 14 to 53 days.

## Use of Instrumentation

The use of instrumentation in patients with spinal infection remains a controversial issue. Hardware placement for fusion operations in uninfected patients has been shown to increase postoperative infection rates. As a result, historically, there has been concern regarding placement of instrumentation in a known contaminated field. This is particularly an issue in complex spinal reconstructive procedures, which often represent longer operations with extensive muscle exposure and tissue devitalization. This is further compounded by a patient population who are typically older with multiple medical comorbidities, and who may be predisposed to poor wound healing and infection.

Concern for use of instrumentation in the setting of infection arises from the risk of bacterial colonization of the implant. With traditional stainless steel implants, a biofilm harboring bacteria develops around the material. This colonized surface layer is poorly penetrated by antibiotics, resulting in persistent infection. Laboratory studies, however, suggest that titanium implants may be less susceptible to bacterial seeding than stainless steel. Titanium, especially when smooth polished, may be more resistant to bacterial adherence than other materials.

As a result, recently there has been increasing use of titanium-based spinal instrumentation in the surgical treatment of spinal osteomyelitis. The growing popularity of spinal instrumentation stems from an improved ability to restore sagittal alignment, maintain spinal stability, protect neurological function, and relieve pain. Spinal instrumentation also serves to reduce the risk of graft extrusion and to facilitate arthrodesis through rigid immobilization. Additionally, with internal spinal fixation, early patient mobilization is possible, thereby reducing the risk of complications associated with prolonged bed rest and use of external orthoses. Because of the general concern for increased infection with instrumentation, however, the indications for instrumented spinal stabilization in the setting of spinal infection must be clearly established prior to use.

Spinal instrumentation to treat vertebral osteomyelitis has evolved dramatically. Pedicle screw-rod fixation has become a standard method for supplemental posterior stabilization. More recently, device technology has developed titanium cages as a method for rigid anterior column support. Titanium cages offer several significant advantages over traditional anterior strut grafting with either tricortical iliac crest or rib autograft. Titanium cages provide immediate stability, and because of their rigidity can tolerate compressive forces. Titanium cages can be tailored for size and

shape, and have a broad contact area for load distribution. They also have significant interface strength between the implant and the vertebral endplates to prevent extrusion or displacement. Newer expandable cages are designed to be inserted and then increased longitudinally in situ, thereby exerting corrective forces to restore sagittal alignment. Titanium cages also are engineered with a hollow mesh design to allow for packing of morselized bone graft within the cage and for bony ingrowth during the healing and fusion process.

Ruf et al examined 88 patients with vertebral osteomyelitis treated with anterior column reconstruction with a titanium mesh cage.[4] Thirty-four cases involved placement of the cage in a single disc space. Twenty-eight cases replaced a single vertebral level. Twenty-three cases were two-level vertebral body replacements, and three cases involved three-level reconstructions. Kyphosis angles at the affected levels improved a mean 11.2° after surgery, with a minimal loss of correction of only 1.4°. Four patients with osteoporosis had evidence of cage settling, with three cases requiring revision surgery and additional posterior instrumentation. All patients demonstrated solid arthrodesis at last follow-up, with no recurrent infection.

Pee et al retrospectively reviewed 60 patients who underwent anterior debridement, posterior stabilization, and anterior column reconstruction with either tricortical iliac strut, titanium cage, or polyether ether ketone (PEEK) cage.[5] The titanium and PEEK cages were packed either with allograft bone chips, with autograft, or with mixed autograft/allograft for arthrodesis. Pee et al observed that the tricortical iliac strut group had an average 200 ml increase in operative blood loss compared to the titanium or PEEK cage groups. While there was no significant difference in postoperative fusion rate between iliac strut and cage groups, there was a significantly higher subsidence rate in the iliac strut group. Also, the mean time interval until subsidence was shorter in the autograft group compared to the cage group. They secondarily observed that patients with subsidence (regardless of graft type) had more pain and disability than those without subsidence. Therefore, the authors inferred that use of a cage may decrease the risk of this adverse outcome, although this was not proven to statistical significance in their series. Most relevant, however, was that all patients, regardless of iliac strut or cage, had normalization of ESR and CRP postoperatively, with complete resolution of infection at final follow-up.

While some may still have concern about the use of instrumentation in the setting of spinal infection, there is clearly a growing body of evidence that titanium-based implants can be reasonably used with safety. Particularly, given the benefits of instrumentation with regards to spinal reconstruction, sagittal plane correction, stabilization, and early patient mobilization, a serious recommendation for use of instrumentation to treat vertebral osteomyelitis in select cases can be made.

## Graft Type

The selection of graft type for arthrodesis in the setting of spinal infection is also controversial. The gold standard remains autologous bone graft, due to its ideal osteobiologic properties. Fresh autologous tissue also may allow rapid vascular ingrowth for effective antimicrobial delivery to the affected site and prevent the risk of persistent bacterial colonization. For this reason, vascularized grafts such as rotational rib grafts or free vascularized fibular grafts may be necessary for complicated revisions due to persistent infection or pseudarthrosis, although obtaining these grafts is technically demanding and time-consuming. Because of the morbidity associated with harvesting autologous bone graft, an alternative option is the use of allograft. Although allograft represents a devascularized foreign body, more recent studies have found that use of allograft struts in patients treated for vertebral osteomyelitis is otherwise safe and can be effective for arthrodesis.

A potentially exciting option is the use of bone morphogenetic protein (BMP) to promote fusion. Recombinant human BMP (InFuse, Medtronic, Memphis, TN, USA; OP-1, Stryker Biotech, Hopkinton, MA, USA) is a synthetic osteoinductive agent that has been demonstrated in both animal and clinical models to result in increased fusion rates. The use of BMP in the setting of spinal infection, however, has not been widely clinically explored and currently represents an off-label and contraindicated use of the product. Laboratory studies in animal models, however, show that BMP retains its osteoinductive properties even in the setting of acute or chronic infection. Interestingly, in experimental models, BMP in combination with antibiotics results in more rapid healing than BMP alone. This may be secondary to increased angiogenesis caused by BMP-stimulated osteoblast-derived vascular endothelial growth factor. Therefore increased vascular ingrowth not only facilitates osteogenesis, but also leads to increased local antibiotic delivery to better eliminate infection.

Limited clinical studies have investigated the use of BMP to promote fusion in patients with vertebral osteomyelitis. However, a handful of studies evaluating the use of BMP placed either in structural allograft or in a titanium cage with supplemental spinal fixation demonstrate successful bony fusion, without recurrence of infection or evidence of complication related to BMP use. While the use of BMP in the setting of spinal infection is still not FDA approved, there is a small body of preclinical and clinical evidence to suggest that BMP may be beneficial in promoting early fusion in vertebral osteomyelitis. Certainly, further testing is warranted prior to any recommendation for the clinical use of BMP for spinal infection can be made.

### Minimally Invasive Surgery

In many instances, spinal infections are successfully treated with conservative medical therapy. When surgical intervention is required, however, operative treatment often requires extensive procedures consisting of radical debridement with spinal reconstruction and stabilization. Perioperative morbidity in the elderly population or in patients with significant medical comorbidities is of particular concern. Significant complications after complex spinal instrumentation procedures in patients with spinal infections are reported to be as high as 47%. Recently, minimally invasive surgical techniques have been developed as an alternative surgical modality for the treatment of a variety of spinal disorders. These techniques, coupled with novel device technology, have provided measures for performing many of the same types of open decompressive and fusion procedures, albeit through tissue-sparing approaches. As a result, decreased blood loss, less postoperative pain, shorter hospitalization, and earlier return to function have been observed.

### Thoracoscopic Spinal Surgery

An anterior approach for vertebral osteomyelitis allows for direct visualization and access to the primary pathology. Anterior exposure of the thoracic and thoracolumbar spine via a conventional open approach, however, requires a thoracotomy and potential splitting of the diaphragm. Significant morbidity is associated with a standard thoracotomy, including chronic postoperative pain and respiratory compromise. To circumvent this issue, video-assisted thoracoscopic surgical techniques have been applied for minimally invasive treatment of thoracic spinal disease. While thoracoscopic spinal surgery is already widely used for basic procedures such as thoracic discectomy and sympathectomy, more recently this technique is being incorporated in operations to treat more complex pathology like scoliosis, trauma, tumors, and infection. Through multiple ports, exposure of the thoracic and thoracolumbar junction as well as anterior debridement, partial corpectomy, interbody cage placement, and spinal stabilization are possible.

The literature reporting thoracoscopic treatment of vertebral osteomyelitis is limited. Muckely et al described three patients with thoracic osteomyelitis that underwent thoracoscopic partial corpectomy, anterior reconstruction, and anterior spinal fixation.[6] The improvement in kyphotic angle among the three patients ranged from 6° to 15° with no evidence of loss of correction at a minimum of 22 months of follow-up. There were no cases of recurrence and no instances of graft or hardware failure. Of note, one patient in the series was ambulating as early as postoperative day one. Amini et al presented a case report of a 70-year-old patient who developed osteodiscitis after a T11-12 discectomy.[7] The patient was treated with a thoracoscopic vertebrectomy, allograft strut, and anterior instrumentation. At 1-year follow-up, the patient demonstrated solid fusion without evidence of recurrent disease.

### Percutaneous Technology

Open posterior exposure of the spine consists of a midline incision with dissection of the musculature away from the bony elements. This approach allows for access to the dorsal spine for decompression as well as the necessary anatomy for placement of instrumentation and fusion bed preparation. Extensive muscle dissection and prolonged retraction, however, can result in tissue ischemia, denervation, scarring, and postsurgical dead space with increased risk of blood loss, infection, chronic pain, and delay to functional recovery.

Recently, percutaneous technology has been developed to perform a variety of spinal procedures including discectomy, spinal decompression, interbody fusion, and instrumented stabilization. These minimally invasive techniques have been incorporated in the treatment of spinal infections as well. Nagata et al applied a technique for percutaneous excision of lumbar disc herniations as a method for aspiration and drainage of pyogenic spondylodiscitis.[8] Under local anesthesia, a percutaneous trocar that is 5.4 mm in diameter is inserted under intraoperative fluoroscopy into the affected level. Through this trocar, specialized forceps and a motor-driven shaver are used to curette the infected disc and endplate, which are then removed piecemeal. After debridement, large volume irrigation is flushed through the trocar. Finally, a small suction drainage tube is left in the disc space and the trocar is removed to allow for postoperative continuous antibiotic suction-irrigation.

Nagata et al performed this procedure in 23 patients with spondylodiscitis.[8] The causative organism was identified through cultured tissue removed during curettage in 53% of patients. Ninety-one percent of patients had immediate relief of back pain after surgery, with 43% ambulating without pain within 3 days of surgery. All patients were followed for a minimum of 2 years with only one patient requiring a repeat operation for recurrent infection. No vascular or neurological complications were encountered as a result of the procedure. Three of 6 patients with preoperative neurological deficits, however, continued to have mild sensory impairment at last follow-up, and therefore, this procedure is not recommended for patients with significant bony destruction, epidural abscess, or neurological compromise.

Instrumentation for spinal fixation of unstable pathologic fractures and deformity correction has also been advanced by percutaneous technology. Standard open placement of pedicle screws requires extensive dissection of the posterior musculature to expose the necessary anatomic landmarks for screw insertion and connecting rod placement. Cannulated pedicle screws, however, have been introduced that allow for placement of screws over a guidewire percutaneously inserted under fluoroscopic imaging. With this technique, multilevel fixation can be performed with multiple separate stab incisions for each screw placement (Figure 47-8 A-E). Novel technology has been developed to allow for introducing a connecting rod through the screw heads via an additional separate stab incision. Due to its low operative morbidity, percutaneous stabilization may have a particularly beneficial role as supplemental posterior fixation for patients undergoing primary anterior debridement and spinal reconstruction.

## PROGNOSIS

With earlier diagnosis and better medical and surgical intervention, clinical outcomes and prognosis from spinal infection are improving. Mortality rates from pyogenic osteomyelitis were once as high as 25% to 71%. Depending on patient age and comorbidities, mortality rates for treated pyogenic osteomyelitis are now as low as 5% to 16%. Ninety-one percent of patients are estimated to recover uneventfully with either medical therapy or combined medical and surgical intervention. Similar improvement in mortality has been observed for patients with epidural abscesses. Dandy in 1926 reported a mortality rate of 83% for patients with spinal epidural abscesses. Now, with prompt surgical intervention and improved antibiotic therapy, the mortality rate ranges from 5% to 32%.

The prognosis for neurological recovery generally depends on the duration and severity of neurological impairment prior to intervention. Patients with epidural abscesses that are treated within 24 hours of onset of deficits have a better prognosis for recovery of function. Rigamonti et al observed that only 10% of patients with severe neurological deficits who were treated within 24 hours of onset of symptoms had poor neurologic outcomes, compared to 47% of patients treated more than 24 hours after onset of symptoms having a poor neurological outcome.[9] Additionally, patients with complete paralysis, especially if present for more than 36 hours, do not generally recover, despite any intervention.

Chronic pain is a potential long-term complication associated with osteomyelitis, and may be multifactorial. Some studies have found that

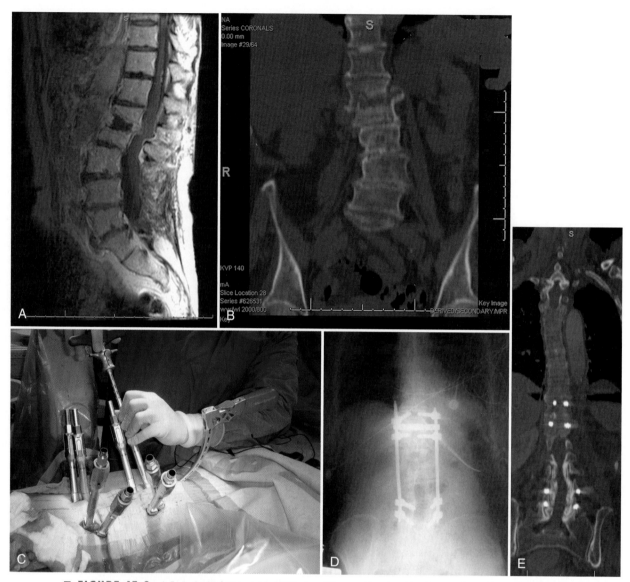

■ **FIGURE 47-8** A-E. **A,** Sagittal T1-weighted MRI of an 83-year-old male with a history of *Mycobacterium abscessus* and debilitating pain related to instability from bone loss and progressive deformity. **B,** Coronal CT reconstruction of the same patient demonstrating significant bony destruction and coronal plane deformity. Given the patient's advanced age, significant medical comorbidities, and poor nutritional status, he underwent minimally invasive percutaneous spinal stabilization. **C,** Intraoperative photograph after percutaneous placement of multilevel cannulated pedicle screws, and demonstrating securing the locking nuts after percutaneous insertion of the connecting rod. **D,** Postoperative AP radiograph demonstrating the final construct with restoration of the coronal plane deformity. The connecting cross-link was also placed percutaneously. **E,** Postoperative coronal CT reconstruction demonstrating correction of the coronal plane deformity.

patients that underwent surgical intervention are actually less likely to have chronic back pain than those treated with antibiotics alone. Better restoration of sagittal alignment and spinal stabilization with surgery may account for this difference in outcome. However, 36% of patients treated only with medical therapy do recover without any long-term disabling back pain. This observation may be due to less severe bony destruction in patients treated nonsurgically, or to spontaneous fusion that occurs from the inflammatory response. Spontaneous bony ankylosis forms in 35% of patients; this, however, may require 6 to 24 months to occur. Deformity is another potential complication that may contribute to pain and long-term dysfunction. Deformity is more common with spinal tuberculosis, especially when occurring at the thoracic or thoracolumbar spine, or when involving more than 50% of one or more vertebral bodies. Good clinical outcomes, however, are demonstrated with surgical intervention. With an anterior decompression and fusion, 94% of patients with spinal tuberculosis recover normal neurological function, with a fusion rate of 92% at 5 years.

## CONCLUSION

The reportedly growing number of spinal infections may become an increasingly significant health care problem. Spinal infections are predisposed to occur in the elderly and those who are medically compromised. As a result, spinal infections are often a complex medical condition with multiple contributing factors, and are therefore challenging to manage. The importance of successfully treating spinal infections is all the more relevant given the potential for significant associated medical complications, neurological compromise, functional impairment, and chronic disability.

Spinal infections represent a wide-ranging spectrum of pathologic involvement and therefore are not amenable to simple treatment algorithms or protocols. General principles dictate that early diagnosis with identification of the pathogenic organism is critical for successful medical therapy with eradication of infection and minimized complications. Patients who are neurologically intact and clinically stable can generally be managed nonsurgically. Patients who present with neurological deficits, clinical deterioration despite medical therapy, or evidence of spinal instability, deformity, or chronic pain may necessitate surgical intervention. Currently, a variety of surgical treatment options are available ranging from minimally-invasive techniques to radical debridement with complex spinal reconstruction and instrumented stabilization.

Developments in diagnostic imaging, antimicrobial therapy, and surgical techniques are advancing our therapeutic capabilities and improving clinical outcomes. Better understanding of the disease response to surgical interventions, particularly the use of instrumentation and osteobiologic agents, are reshaping current treatment paradigms. As a result, we are witnessing greatly reduced morbidity and mortality. With a multidisciplinary approach committed to early and aggressive management of spinal infections, we can continue to expect even better patient outcomes.

## References

1. L.Y. Dai, W.H. Chen, L.S. Jiang, Anterior instrumentation for the treatment of pyogenic vertebral osteomyelitis of thoracic and lumbar spine, Eur. Spine J. 17 (8) (2008) 1027–1034.
2. P. Korovessis, T. Repantis, P. Iliopoulos, A. Hadjipavlou, Beneficial influence of titanium mesh cage on infection healing and spinal reconstruction in hematogenous septic spondylitis: a retrospective analysis of surgical outcome of twenty-five consecutive cases and review of literature, Spine 33 (21) (2008) E759–E767.
3. J.R. Dimar, L.Y. Carreon, S.D. Glassman, M.J. Campbell, M.J. Hartman, J.R. Johnson, Treatment of pyogenic vertebral osteomyelitis with anterior debridement and fusion followed by delayed posterior spinal fusion, Spine 29 (3) (2004) 326–332. discussion 32.
4. M. Ruf, D. Stoltze, H.R. Merk, M. Ames, J. Harms, Treatment of vertebral osteomyelitis by radical debridement and stabilization using titanium mesh cages, Spine 32 (9) (2007) E275–E280.
5. Y.H. Pee, J.D. Park, Y.G. Choi, S.H. Lee, Anterior debridement and fusion followed by posterior pedicle screw fixation in pyogenic spondylodiscitis: autologous iliac bone strut versus cage, J. Neurosurg. Spine 8 (5) (2008) 405–412.
6. T. Muckley, T. Schutz, M.H. Schmidt, M. Potulski, V. Buhren, R. Beisse, The role of thoracoscopic spinal surgery in the management of pyogenic vertebral osteomyelitis, Spine 29 (11) (2004) E227–E233.
7. A. Amini, R. Beisse, M.H. Schmidt, Thoracoscopic debridement and stabilization of pyogenic vertebral osteomyelitis, Surg. Laparosc. Endosc. Percutan. Tech. 17 (4) (2007) 354–357.
8. K. Nagata, T. Ohashi, M. Ariyoshi, K. Sonoda, H. Imoto, A. Inoue, Percutaneous suction aspiration and drainage for pyogenic spondylitis, Spine 23 (14) (1998) 1600–1606.
9. D. Rigamonti, L. Liem, P. Sampath, et al., Spinal epidural abscess: contemporary trends in etiology, evaluation, and management, Surg. Neurol. 52 (2) (1999) 189–196. discussion 97.

# 48

# Thoracic Spinal Stenosis

*Josef B. Simon and Eric J. Woodard*

**KEY POINTS**

- Thoracic myelopathy can be caused by numerous pathologies such as tumor, disc herniation, and ossification of the ligamentum flavum (OLF) and/or posterior longitudinal ligament (OPLL).
- Cultural differences exist in the etiology of thoracic myelopathy.
- The thoracic spinal cord takes up 40% of the space available for the spinal cord. Due to this anatomical difference, space-occupying lesions in the thoracic spine may cause more rapid and profound impingement and impairment of the spinal cord.
- Multiple imaging modalities should be utilized to assess patients with signs and symptoms of thoracic myelopathy.
- When surgery is indicated, the approach should be dictated by the location and type of pathology. Patients with OLF or OPLL or neoplasm will most likely require both surgical decompression and fusion. Circumferential decompression carries a high risk of neurological deterioration.

## INTRODUCTION

Stenosis of the thoracic spine is a relatively rare condition when compared to stenosis of the cervical or lumbar spine. Because it is unusual, a full understanding of the condition's epidemiology and clinical presentation is limited, yet like stenosis in other spinal regions, its causes are numerous. These include ossification of the ligamentum flavum (OLF) (Figure 48-1) or posterior longitudinal ligament (OPLL) (Figures 48-2 and 48-3), herniation of intervertebral discs (Figures 48-4 and 48-5), and spondylosis. Other causes include neoplastic lesions, facet cysts, vascular malformations, and fracture. Stenosis of the thoracic spine typically presents with a variable combination of three main symptoms: back pain, radiculopathy, and myelopathy.

Much of what is known about thoracic stenosis has been derived from the experience of Japanese practitioners. OLF is cited as the most common cause of thoracic spinal stenosis. Although case reports of OLF with thoracic myelopathy in whites and North Americans have been published,[12] patients of Asian descent are most frequently affected. Up to 20% of Asians older than 65 years of age have some degree of thoracic stenosis due to OLF.[3] Aizawa et al, in a retrospective study of 265 Japanese patients, found OLF to account for more than half of all cases of thoracic myelopathy.[4] Middle-aged men had the condition more frequently than women. It is not yet clear why this condition has a gender discrepancy and why it tends to occur in younger patients than those with cervical or lumbar stenosis.

Because OLF and OPLL are unusual among Westerners, much of the European and North American literature focuses on thoracic intervertebral disc disease as the primary etiology of thoracic spinal stenosis. As with OLF and OPLL, thoracic disc herniation is overall an unusual cause of thoracic back pain, radiculopathy, and myelopathy. Studies suggest than it affects males most frequently and tends to occur between the fourth and sixth decades.[4]

## PATHOLOGY

A number of anatomical features make the thoracic spinal cord particularly vulnerable to injury. Unlike the cervical region, where the spinal cord takes up approximately 25% of the cross-sectional area of the canal, the thoracic cord constitutes 40% of the canal. Due to this anatomical difference, space-occupying lesions in the thoracic spine may cause more rapid and profound impingement and impairment of the cord. The thoracic kyphosis also creates a relative "bowstring" effect with the spinal cord draped across the posterior longitudinal ligament, the intervertebral discs, and the vertebral bodies. This positions the ventral cord in close apposition to compressive pathology of these structures.

The thoracic spinal cord has a more tenuous blood supply than the lumbar and cervical neurological segments. Ventral perfusion derives from the main feeding vessel, the artery of Adamkiewicz, which variably supplies the thoracic spinal cord. Intrinsic blood supply comes from the midline anterior spinal artery and two posterior vessels that are smaller than their counterparts in other regions of the spine. Intercostal arteries make up the extrinsic blood supply and are smaller and fewer in number than those in the cervical and lumbar spine. This vascular arrangement creates a relative watershed area between T4 and T9 that makes the region vulnerable to ischemic injury.

OLF occurs as a normal part of the aging process and rarely leads to stenosis. Histologically, the normal ligamentum flavum is composed of significant amounts of elastin that, with aging and degeneration, is progressively replaced by collagen, fragments of bone, cartilage, and fibrous tissue.[5] Pathologic ossification is characterized by extreme progression of these processes leading to overgrowth and, ultimately, canal and foraminal stenosis. The precise mechanisms of pathologic OLF have not yet been clearly determined. It has been suggested that high mechanical stress of the thoracolumbar junction leads to degeneration of the facets and intervertebral discs, initiating progressive injury of the ligamentum flavum in this region.[6] Ossification then proceeds in response to repetitive injury. This may explain why OLF occurs more frequently in the lower thoracic spine. Although plausible, this theory has been questioned because the cervical and lumbar spinal regions are more mobile than the thoracic spine, yet ossification in these locations is less common.[7] It is also rare for OLF lesions to extend across multiple levels. Medical comorbidities such as diabetes mellitus, abnormalities in calcium metabolism, hypoparathyroidism, and Paget disease may play a significant role and have been associated with pathologic OLF.[8,9] The higher incidence of OLF in the Japanese population clearly suggests a genetic etiology.

OLF associated with thoracic myelopathy most typically occurs in the lower thoracic spine.[10] In their epidemiologic study, Aizawa et al found that T11-12 was the most common site of compression, followed by T10-11 and T9-10. When OPLL was the cause, T1-2 was affected most commonly, followed by T2-3 and T3-4.[11]

As with OLF and OPLL, isolated traumatic injury to thoracic intervertebral discs is rare. The splinting effect of the rib cage as well as the vertical orientation of the thoracic facets serves to reduce the forces on thoracic discs compared to those in the lumbar spine. This is thought to decrease the incidence of discal injury in the thoracic area. Degeneration of thoracic discs

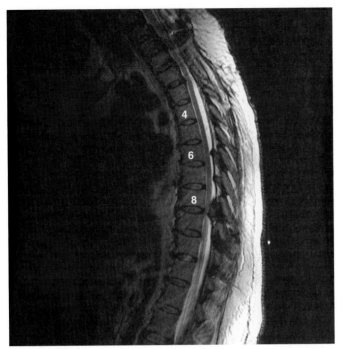

■ **FIGURE 48-1** Ossification of the ligamentum flavum (OLF) of T8-9 with severe cord compression and progressive paraparesis in a 61-year-old male. OLF is more common in Asian males and in the lower segments of the thoracic spine.

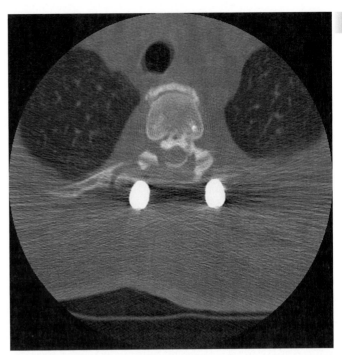

■ **FIGURE 48-3** Multisegment laminectomy, fusion, and instrumentation was required for cord decompression and junctional stabilization. The dorsal dura is extensively ossified.

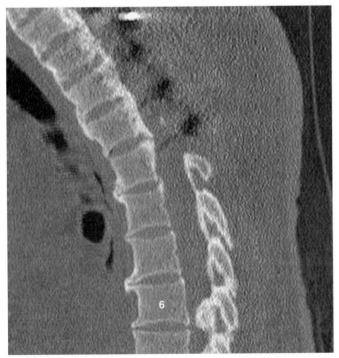

■ **FIGURE 48-2** Sagittal plain CT scan demonstrating ossification of the posterior longitudinal ligament (OPLL) of the upper thoracic segments extending to the cervicothoracic junction in a 56-year-old female.

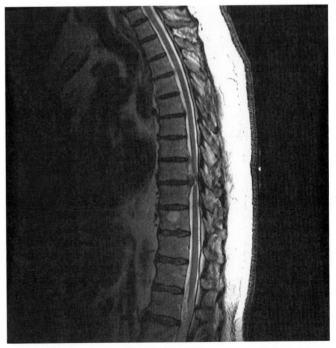

■ **FIGURE 48-4** Thoracic disc herniation, T8-9, with symptomatic cord compression and T2 signal change of the cord.

demonstrated that, often, thoracic disc herniations exist without symptoms.[13] An additional study by Wood et al showed that these herniations do not frequently progress.[14]

## CLINICAL PRESENTATION

The clinical presentation of thoracic stenosis ranges from simple back pain to frank myelopathy. Thoracic back pain is the most common presentation of a disc herniation, with patients describing the pain as "passing through

due to aging can occur as well, being most common in the fourth through the sixth decades of life, with males affected more frequently than females. Thoracic disc herniation tends to occur in the midline or just lateral to the midline, and predominates in the lower thoracic levels (Figures 48-6 and 48-7).[12] Wood et al reviewed 90 MRI scans of asymptomatic patients and

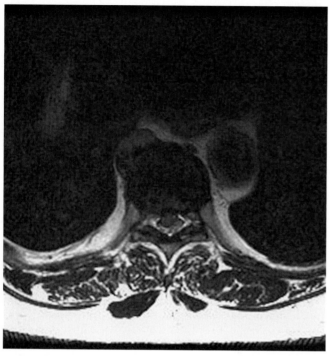

■ **FIGURE 48-5** Axial view demonstrates significant midline cord compression. This lesion requires a direct, ventral approach and was resected by costotransversectomy.

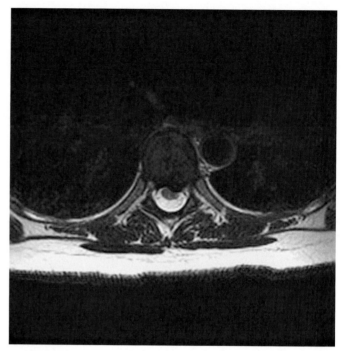

■ **FIGURE 48-7** Minimal cord displacement and lateral lesion position make this situation optimal for transpedicular or transfacet discectomy.

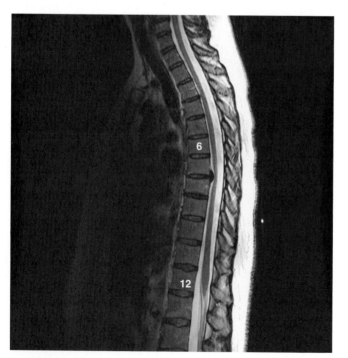

■ **FIGURE 48-6** Left-sided T7-8 HNP with predominantly radicular symptoms, refractory to conservative care.

their chest." When lower thoracic discs are affected, the pain may radiate to the abdomen, flank, or groin. Paresthesias, numbness, intercostal neuralgias, unsteady gait, and fatigue while walking may also be present. When myelopathy occurs, it often presents itself as trunk and lower extremity weakness (especially of proximal musculature), spasticity, and sensory loss. The upper extremities should be spared. Alterations in bladder control can occur. Because of the similarities in presentation, and the infrequency of thoracic spinal stenosis, thoracic myelopathy can often be confused with lumbar and/or cervical stenosis, leading to delays in diagnosis.

## DIAGNOSIS

Physical findings of patients with thoracic myelopathy are similar to those seen in lumbar and cervical stenosis. Lower extremity weakness, hyperreflexia, decreased sensation, sphincter malfunction, loss of abdominal reflexes, and gait instability can be present. In addition, patients may localize their pain and hypesthesia in a thoracic distribution. Complete paraplegia due to thoracic spinal cord compression has also been documented.[15]

Patients with symptoms of thoracic spinal stenosis often may have findings on plain x-rays that suggest the etiology of the condition. Destructive lesions such as tumors and vascular malformations may be directly visualized, as can some fractures. When there is OLF, beak-like bony densities are characteristically seen projecting into the posterior aspect of the spinal canal on the lateral x-ray.[16] Asymptomatic disc herniations are poorly visualized with plain x-ray, unless there is a significant amount of ossification.[17] Unless there is an underlying metabolic abnormality, laboratory studies are typically normal.

Studies have compared the utility of CT and MRI in the diagnosis of thoracic spinal cord compression due to ossification of spinal ligaments.[18] Both CT and MRI scanning may play a role in the diagnosis of thoracic spinal cord compression. Plain CT provides detailed information regarding the bony anatomy and degree of ossification of the spinal ligaments, as well as ossification of intervertebral discs and facet hypertrophy. MRI, on the other hand, helps to define the extent of spinal cord injury and identify facet cysts. In the setting of OLF, CT myelography is unnecessary, as it adds little to the data collected by MRI, and the contrast injection occasionally exacerbates symptoms of stenosis. If MRI is contraindicated in a patient, such as with a pacemaker, CT myelography is the study of choice.

## TREATMENT

Thoracic myelopathy due to OLF or OPLL is not well treated by conservative methods such as nonsteroidal antiinflammatory medications and physical therapy. Surgical decompression is often required when stenosis results in myelopathy or debilitating radiculopathy. The best mode of surgical treatment for stenosing OLF is not well defined in the literature. Depending on the extent of compression, laminoplasty, partial or total laminectomy, circumferential decompression, and decompression with fusion have been proposed. The proponents of laminoplasty suggest that this procedure may produce less instability than other modes of decompression.[19]

Prognosis after surgery depends on the extent of compression and neurological deficit. Recurrent stenosis has been documented, making routine follow-up necessary.[20]

For thoracic stenosis due to OPLL, multiple treatment options have been described, including laminectomy, laminoplasty, resection of the PLL, anterior decompression and fusion via thoracotomy, and posterior decompression and fusion.[21,22] Anterior decompression with fusion has been supported by a recent long-term study.[23] Fujimura et al reviewed the data of 33 patients followed for more than 5 years after anterior decompression and fusion was performed for myelopathy in the thoracic spine due to ossification of the PLL. Their results suggested that anterior decompression with fusion can lead to favorable long-term results. They indicated, however, that patients with OPLL that affects multiple levels and those with concurrent OLF may not do as well in long-term follow-up.

Posterior surgical approaches provide an alternative treatment option for myelopathy due to OPLL, particularly when there is also OLF. It is suggested that, for OPLL, posterior decompression alone may not be sufficient due to draping of the spinal cord over the kyphotic thoracic spine. Some advocate a circumferential decompression through an isolated posterior approach.[24] High complication rates have been documented with this treatment, however, particularly when more than five levels are decompressed. In a study by Masahiko et al, as many as 33% of patients had deterioration in their neurological status following surgery. Both the relatively avascular nature of the thoracic spinal cord and adhesion of dural sac to the PLL are thought to contribute to these complications. Even higher rates of neurological deterioration have been seen with laminectomy alone, while lower rates have been reported with posterior decompression and fusion.[25] In theory, performing a laminectomy without fusion further destabilizes the spine and subjects the injured spinal cord to additional stresses that lead to a further decline in neurological function. Masashi et al suggested that in the neurologically intact patient, resection of the PLL is an acceptable treatment, but for patients with preoperative spinal cord injury, removal of the PLL increases the risk of paralysis.[26]

Many patients with thoracic disc herniations are asymptomatic. When symptoms do exist, unlike patients with OPLL and OLF, conservative treatment and time can be sufficient to treat the majority of herniations. Modification of activities, physical therapy, and the careful use of nonsteroidal antiinflammatory drugs are the mainstays of conservative care. The literature suggests that less than 2% of thoracic discs require surgical treatment.[27] When conservative care fails to alleviate symptoms after 4 to 6 weeks, a neurological deficit progresses, or there is evidence of worsening myelopathy, surgical treatment is warranted.

Operative care of patients with thoracic disc herniations requires assessing several factors to determine operative risk and approach. Depending on the location and nature of the disc herniation, anterior, thoracoscopic, lateral, or posterior approaches may be used, the details of which are largely beyond the scope of this chapter. In general, anteriorlyoriented lesions require a direct ventral approach such as a transthoracic, thoracoscopic, or posterolateral (e.g., costotransversectomy, extracavitary) technique for safe resection that avoids cord manipulation, with bony reconstruction as necessary. Pulmonary function tests should be performed on patients with questionable pulmonary reserve if thoracotomy is considered. Discal calcifications, which are more common in the thoracic spine,[28] are associated with a greater degree of dural adhesion or associated dural calcification. Such information is important for the treating surgeon in deciding how much disc to remove from the dura, and whether concomitant dural resection needs to be considered. Once in the operating room, it is essential to identify the correct disc for resection. Sagittal CT reconstructions or MR images are essential to determine the appropriate level, and plain radiography or fluoroscopy in the operating room is standard practice for localization.

For most lateral soft disc herniations, the preferred approach is posterior and usually involves a pediculofacetectomy, typically perfomed by transpedicular or transfacet technique rather than laminectomy. Significant complications have been reported with posterior laminectomy alone,[29] including cord contusion and lack of improvement of symptoms. The need for fusion following thoracic disc removal remains controversial but generally depends on the assessed degree of stability of the region following decompression. It may be beneficial to resect a significant amount of vertebral body in cases of multilevel disc disease, or when the disc is in the lower thoracic spine, which may render the spine unstable and require secondary fusion.

## OTHER CAUSES FOR THORACIC SPINAL STENOSIS

### Neoplasms

Both intramedullary and extramedullary spinal cord tumors can lead to thoracic myelopathy and must be considered as a possible etiology in every older patient with thoracic spinal stenosis. In their experience treating 78 patients with intramedullary spinal cord tumors, Sandalcioglu et al found that 32% of the tumors were located in the thoracic spine. Low-grade neuroepithelial tumors, ependymomas, astrocytomas, vascular tumors, and metastatic lesions were identified. The most important predictor of postoperative neurological status was a patient's preoperative neurological function.[30] Compared to patients with intramedullary tumors in the cervical or lumbar spine, these authors found that those with thoracic lesions had a higher surgical morbidity. This most likely reflects the regional vulnerability of the thoracic cord due to tenuous blood supply, constricted canal anatomy, and kyphosis. When intramedullary spinal cord tumors are identified, decompression and tumor removal can be performed by laminectomy or laminoplasty.

Metastatic disease to the thoracic spine is more common than metastasis to the cervical or lumbar spine, due to the greater relative size and bony blood supply of the thoracic region. Lesions from lung, breast, prostate, and gastrointestinal carcinomas, as well as other tumor types, are known to metastasize to the thoracic spine. Until recently, many authors could not define the best mode of treatment for extramedullary spinal cord tumors with cord compression causing neurological symptoms. Earlier studies looking at laminectomy alone or laminectomy in combination with radiotherapy did not show surgery to be beneficial.[31-33] The importance of surgical decompression, however, was shown in a randomized multicenter trial by Patchell et al, who compared the outcomes of 101 patients treated with either radiotherapy alone or a combination of radiotherapy and decompressive surgery.[34] All but 13 of the patients had tumors in the thoracic spine. The median age of their study group was 60. The authors found that patients treated with a combination of postoperative radiotherapy and decompressive surgery were significantly better in terms of ambulatory status, functionality, maintenance of urinary continence, strength, and overall survival than those treated with radiation alone. Their data also suggested that laminectomy may not always be the best mode of treatment. Rather, approaching the lesion directly: anterior tumors anteriorly, posterior tumors posteriorly, and lateral tumors laterally may offer the best results for decompression (see Figure 48-6).

### Synovial Cysts

Rare cases of synovial cysts leading to thoracic myelopathy have been reported. Graham et al outlined a case in which a 54-year-old woman developed right lower extremity weakness secondary to a cyst at T11-12.[35] The cyst was successfully excised via a laminectomy and the patient had a full recovery. Aspiration has been used as a treatment for synovial cysts in the lumbar spine and might prove to be a useful treatment option in the thoracic spine.

## PROGNOSIS

An understanding of the long-term results of surgical treatment of thoracic spinal stenosis due to OLF is limited due to the lack of sufficient study. The literature suggests that a number of factors may make surgical outcomes less favorable. These include a longer duration of symptoms prior to decompression,[36] the presence of a proximal stenotic lesion,[37] and a greater degree of stenosis.[38] Another study looking at OLF did not show an association between preoperative symptom duration and results of surgery, although only 24 patients were evaluated.[39] As with the importance of the duration of symptoms, the data are also not clear on how preoperative neurological status affects surgical outcome. A meta-analysis by J. Anamasu et al suggests that the larger, more recent studies indicate a positive association between preoperative neurological function and surgical outcomes.[40] Other studies have highlighted some of the long-term complications of thoracic decompressive surgery, including the development of late kyphotic deformities and spondylosis.[41,42]

Treatment of thoracic stenosis due to disc herniation has poorer outcomes for those patients with advanced age, extended preoperative duration of the condition, and greater degrees of myelopathy. Studies of patients with nonligamentous causes of thoracic stenosis have questioned the long-term prognosis following surgical decompression. Palumbo et al reviewed 12 patients with thoracic stenosis.[43] In 11 of the patients, stenosis was due to spondylosis. Their results showed that 5 of 12 patients had initial improvement that later declined. They suggested that deterioration was due to development of delayed stenosis, instability, or deformity.

## CONCLUSIONS

Although thoracic spinal stenosis is a relatively rare condition as compared to stenosis of the cervical or lumbar spine, the treating physician must consider it in the differential diagnosis of the older patient with thoracic back pain or symptoms or signs of myelopathy. This awareness may prevent delay in the diagnosis of this condition due to its similarity to the presentation of lumbar stenosis. Most patients with a discogenic etiology for their pain can be treated conservatively. Both CT and MRI aid in defining the pathology and determining the most appropriate treatment. CT myelography should be avoided when possible in patients with OLF, as it can exacerbate myelopathy. When surgery is indicated, the approach should be dictated by the location of the disc. Patients with OLF or posterior longitudinal ligament or neoplasm will most likely require both surgical decompression and fusion.

Circumferential decompression carries a high risk of neurological deterioration. Patients with neurological complications due to metastatic lesions in the thoracic spine benefit from surgical decompression in addition to radiation. Larger, longer-term studies need to be performed to better define the importance of preoperative duration of symptoms, neurological status, and mode of decompression to overall prognosis. This task is made difficult by the relative rarity of thoracic spinal stenosis.

## References

1. R. Van Oostenbrugge, Spinal cord compression caused by unusual location and extension of ossified ligamenta flava in a Caucasian male: a case report and literature review, Spine 24 (1999) 486–488.
2. J. Kruse, Ossification of the ligamentum flavum as a cause of myelopathy in North America: report of three cases, J. Spinal Disord. 13 (1) (2009) 22-25.
3. T. Shiraishi, Thoracic myelopathy due to isolated ossification of the ligamentum flavum, J. Bone Joint Surg. Br. 77 (1995) 131–133.
4. T. Aizawa: Thoracic myelopathy in Japan: epidemiological retrospective study in Miyagi prefecture during 15 years, Tohoku J Exp Med., 210 (3) (2006) 199-208.
5. P.S.P. Ho, Ligamentum flavum: appearance on sagittal and coronal MR images, Radiology 168 (1988) 469–472.
6. M. Payer, Thoracic myelopathy due to enlarged ossified yellow ligaments, J. Neurosurg. Spine 92 (1) (2000) 105-108.
7. N.E. Epstein, Ossification of the yellow ligament and spondylosis and/or ossification of the posterior longitudinal ligament of the thoracic and lumbar spine, J. Spinal Disord. 12 (1999) 250–256.
8. C.L. Vera, Paraplegia due to ossification of the ligamenta flava in x-linked hypophosphatemia: a case report, Spine 22 (1997) 710–715.
9. D. Resnick, Calcification and ossification of the posterior spinal ligaments and tissues, in: D. Resnick, D. Niwayama (Eds.), Diagnosis of bone and joint disorders, ed 2, WB Saunders, Philadelphia, 1988.
10. K. Yonenobu et al: Thoracic myelopathy secondary to ossification of the spinal ligament, J. Neurosurg. 66 (1987) 511-518.
11. T. Aizawa, Thoracic myelopathy in Japan: epidemiological retrospective study in Miyagi prefecture during 15 years.
12. M.A. Rogers, Surgical treatment of the symptomatic herniated thoracic disc, Clin. Orthop. 300 (1994) 70–78.
13. K.B. Wood, Magnetic resonance imaging of the thoracic spine: evaluation of asymptomatic individuals, J. Bone Joint Surg. Am. 77 (1995) 1631–1638.
14. K.B. Wood, The natural history of asymptomatic thoracic disc herniations, Spine 22 (1997) 525–530.
15. M. Takahata, Clinical results and complications of circumferential spinal cord decompression through a single posterior approach for thoracic myelopathy caused by ossification of posterior longitudinal ligament, Spine 33 (11) (2008) 1199–1208.
16. Xiong, et al., CT and MRI characteristics of ossification of the ligamenta flava in the thoracic spine, Eur. Radiol. 11 (2001) 1798–1802.
17. M.A. Rogers, Surgical treatment of the symptomatic herniated thoracic disc, Clin. Orthop. 300 (1994) 70–78.
18. Xiong, et al., CT and MRI characteristics of ossification of the ligamenta flava in the thoracic spine, Eur. Radiol. 11 (2001) 1798–1802.
19. O.S. Okadak, Thoracic myelopathy caused by ossification of the ligamentum flavum: clinicopathologic study and surgical treatment, Spine 16 (1991) 280–287.
20. K. Yonenobu, Thoracic myelopathy secondary to ossification of the spinal ligament, J. Neurosurg. 66 (1987) 511–518.
21. Y. Fujimura, Long-term follow-up study of anterior decompression and fusion for thoracic myelopathy resulting from ossification of the posterior longitudinal ligament, Spine 22 (3) (1997) 305–311.
22. M. Yamazaki, Clinical results of surgery for thoracic myelopathy caused by ossification of the posterior longitudinal ligament: operative indication of posterior decompression with instrumented fusion, Spine 31 (13) (2006) 1452–1460.
23. M. Takahata, Clinical results and complications of circumfrential spinal cord decompression through a single posterior approach for thoracic myelopathy caused by ossification of posterior longitudinal ligament, Spine 33 (11): 1199–1208
24. M. Yamazaki, Clinical results of surgery for thoracic myelopathy caused by ossification of the posterior longitudinal ligament: operative indication of posterior decompression with instrumented fusion, Spine 31 (13) (2006) 1452–1460.
25. Masashi, Clinical results of surgery for thoracic myelopathy caused by ossification of the posterior longitudinal ligament, operative indication of posterior decompression with instrumented fusion, Spine 31 (13) (2006) 1452–1460.
26. C.B. Stillman, Management of thoracic disc disease, Clin. Neurosurg. 38 (1992) 325–352.
27. P. Severi, Multiple calcified thoracic disc herniations: a case report, Spine 17 (4) (1992) 449–451.
28. C.A. Arce, Thoracic disc herniation: improved diagnosis with computed tomographic scanning and a review of the literature, Surg. Neurol. 23 (1985) 356–361.
29. I.E. Sandalcioglu, T. Gasser, S. Asgari, Functional outcome after surgical treatment of intramedullary spinal cord tumors. Experience with 78 patients. Spinal Cord 43 (2005) 34-41.
30. P.S. Sorensen, Metastatic epidural spinal cord compression: results of treatment and survival, Cancer 65 (1990) 1502–1508.
31. R.F. Young, Treatment of spinal epidural metastases: randomized prospective comparison of laminectomy and radiotherapy, J. Neurosurg. 53 (1980) 741–748.
32. G.F.G. Findley, Adverse effects of the management of malignant spinal cord compression, J. Neurol. Neurosurg. Psych. 47 (1984) 761–768.
33. R.A. Patchell, Direct decompressive surgical resection in the treatment of spinal cord compression caused by metastatic cancer: a randomized trial, Lancet 366 (2005) 643–648.
34. E. Graham, Myelopathy induced by a thoracic intraspinal synovial cyst: case report and review of the literature, Spine 26(17): E392–394.
35. N. Miyakoshi, Factors related to long-term outcome after decompressive surgery for ossification of the ligamentum flavum of the thoracic spine, J. Neurosurg. Spine 99 (2003) 251–256.
36. C.J. Chen, Intramedullary high signal intensity on T2-weighted MR images in cervical spondylitic myelopathy: prediction of prognosis with type of intensity, Radiology 221 (2001) 789–794.
37. K. Shiokawa, Clinical analysis and prognostic study of ossified ligamentum flavum of the thoracic spine, J. Neurosurg. Spine 94 (2001) 221–226.
38. L. Cheng-Chin, Surgical experience with symptomatic thoracic ossification of the ligamentum flavum, J. Neurosurg. Spine 2 (2005) 34–39.
39. J. Inamasu, A review of factors predictive of surgical outcome for ossification of the ligamentum flavum of the thoracic spine, J. Neurosurg. Spine 5 (2006) 133–139.
40. L. Cheng-Chin, Surgical experience with symptomatic thoracic ossification of the ligamentum flavum, J. Neurosurg. Spine 2 (2005) 34–39.
41. M.A. Palumbo, Surgical treatment of thoracic spinal stenosis: a 2- to 9- year follow-up. Spine 26 (5) (2001) 558–566.
42. M.A. Palumbo, Surgical treatment of thoracic spinal stenosis: a 2- to 9- year follow-up. Spine 5 26 (2001) 558–566.

# 49

# Stereotactic Radiosurgery for Spine Tumors

*Carmina F. Angeles, Robert E. Lieberson, and Jon Park*

---

**K E Y   P O I N T S**

- The CyberKnife system is a frameless stereotactic radiosurgery (SRS) instrument that consists of a six megavolt linear accelerator (LINAC) mounted on an industrial robot, a repositionable treatment couch, orthogonally placed digital x-ray cameras, and a computerized targeting system, used to treat spine tumors.

- The overall accuracy of image-guided spinal SRS is ± 0.5 to 1.0 mm.

- Lesions amenable to spinal SRS mainly include metastatic tumors, intradural extramedullary tumors, select intramedullary tumors, and vascular malformations.

- Spinal instability and severe or progressive neurological deficits from mass effect are contraindications for SRS unless decompression and stabilization have been performed first.

- Radiation-induced myelopathy is the most feared complication of SRS, but is uncommon.

---

## INTRODUCTION

Stereotactic radiosurgery (SRS) for the spine is a noninvasive technique that accurately delivers large doses of radiation to small targets, through the use of numerous highly collimated cross-fired beams. Spinal SRS has proved effective in treating most metastases, many benign intradural tumors, some intramedullary tumors, and compact intramedullary arteriovenous malformations. It can be used for the older patient or in patients with widely metastatic disease, when open surgery might be contraindicated.

Radiosurgery was developed in 1949 by Lars Leksell and Bjorn Larsson at the Karolinska Institute in Stockholm. Their first system used orthovoltage x-rays, and a subsequent variant used a proton beam generated by a cyclotron. Leksell's Gamma Knife was introduced in 1967, as a lower cost and more efficient system. Gamma Knife treatments provided a steeper dose gradient outside the target region. Embedded in a cast-iron enclosure, the device contained 201 radioactive cobalt sources focused at a single point or isocenter. During treatment, the patient's head was secured to a rigid frame with pins and then inserted into the cast-iron device with the lesion positioned at the isocenter. In the mid-1980s, to make radiosurgery more accessible and less costly, Betti and Colombo modified conventional radiotherapy linear accelerator-based (LINAC) systems to deliver frame-based radiosurgery. Although both the Gamma Knife and LINAC systems were powerful tools for intracranial disease, they could not be easily adapted for extracranial cases, primarily because of the necessity for frame-based target localization.

In 1991, the frameless CyberKnife system was developed by Adler at Stanford University. From its inception, this device was intended to treat both cranial and extracranial lesions with sub-millimeter accuracy. Since the installation of the first clinical unit in 1994, over 8000 spinal lesions have been treated at more than 180 worldwide CyberKnife sites. As in cranial radiosurgery, spinal SRS delivers large but precise doses of radiation to a target while sparing adjacent healthy tissues. In comparison, conventional radiotherapy doses are limited by the sensitivity of the spinal cord.

## RADIOSURGERY

Ionizing radiation damages DNA, protein, and lipids by creating free radicals and causing either mitotic or apoptotic cell death. Larger doses, while more effective in killing neoplastic tissues, endanger normal structures. Conventional radiotherapy, which uses small numbers of broad and relatively inaccurate beams, addresses the problem by dividing the dose over many daily treatments. In contrast, SRS instruments can deliver scores of small, precisely collimated beams. As a consequence, large radiation doses can be directed at irregularly shaped lesions while avoiding adjacent radiosensitive tissue. The target's location and shape are delineated using computed tomography (CT) or magnetic resonance (MR) images, and processed using dedicated treatment-planning software. Current radiosurgery systems capable of treating spinal lesions include the CyberKnife, the Tomoscan (a CT-like device) and various modified linear accelerators (LINACs). The Gamma Knife is currently able to treat only select upper cervical lesions.

The CyberKnife system is a completely frameless, image-guided, robotic radiosurgery system which consists, in part, of a lightweight, six megavolt

## *Clinical Case Examples*

### CASE 1

MC, a 66-year-old woman with medical contraindications to open surgery, was treated with SRS for a spinal schwannoma. She initially presented with a chronic cough and generalized weakness. Routine laboratory studies showed pancytopenia, and flow cytometry was consistent with acute lymphocytic leukemia. The diagnosis was confirmed by bone marrow biopsy. While undergoing chemotherapy in December 2008, she developed lower back pain with subjective right leg weakness. A 10-by 7-mm epidural lesion, compressing the S1 nerve root, was seen on MRI (Figure 49-1). A CT-guided biopsy was consistent with schwannoma, but definitive treatment was postponed because of her leukemia. By July 2009, the pain became intolerable. She had 4/5 gastrocnemius weakness, numbness in the S1 distribution, and loss of the ankle reflex. A repeat MRI confirmed an increase in the size of the schwannoma. Open surgery remained high risk, so in September 2009, the patient underwent CyberKnife treatment. She received 16 Gray (Gy) in a single session. Pain complaints improved, and all examination findings resolved over 2 months.

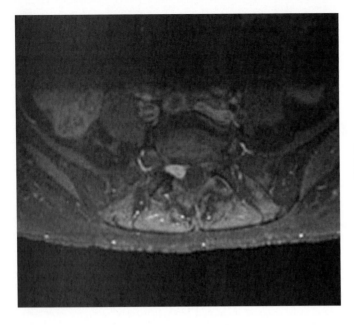

**■ FIGURE 49-1** Gadolinium-enhanced T1-weighted axial image demonstrating a 10- by 7-mm intradural extramedullary lesion compressing the S1 nerve root. A CT-guided biopsy was consistent with schwannoma.

## CASE 2

WF is a 68-year-old man with melanoma who received SRS treatment for a recurrent spinal metastasis in a previously irradiated field. The patient was initially seen with a melanoma of the back in 1999 and another of the neck in 2003. Following local resections, he remained disease-free until March 2007, when, after complaining of low back pain, he was found to have a 4 × 3 cm lesion of the L3 vertebral body. There was significant compression of the cauda equina due to epidural extension. A PET-CT showed hypermetabolic areas in the lung, bone, and brain. He received conventional radiotherapy of 37.5 Gy to the brain and 37.5 Gy to the lumbar spine. In September 2009, the patient returned with increasing back pain, associated with weakness. His strength was 4/5 in the right leg but his sensation was intact. A follow-up PET-CT and MRI showed multiple new lesions and enlargement of the previously treated L3 mass (Figure 49-2). Additional conventional radiotherapy was not an option and a surgical decompression was contraindicated based on his other medical problems. The L3 lesion was treated with CyberKnife SRS, 24 Gy in three sessions. His symptoms improved.

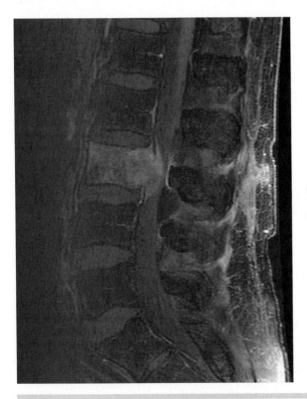

**■ FIGURE 49-2** Sagittal T1-weighted image with contrast, demonstrating enlargement of the previously treated L3 vertebral body metastasis with epidural extension causing central canal stenosis.

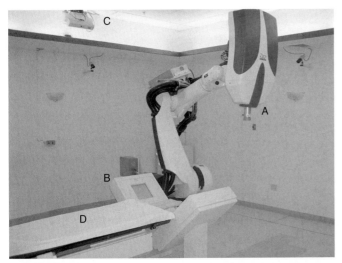

■ **FIGURE 49-3**   CyberKnife frameless stereotactic radiosurgery suite. A modified 6-MV X-band LINAC designed specifically for radiosurgery is mounted on a highlymaneuverable robotic manipulator (KUKA Roboter GmbH, Augsburg, Germany) (A). Two high-resolution x-ray cameras are mounted orthogonally to the headrest (B). One of the two x-ray sources is mounted in the ceiling projecting onto the camera (C). The treatment couch is mobile, allowing the x-ray sources to image targets at any point along the neuraxis (D).

### TABLE 49-1    Indications for Spinal SRS

Tumors that are highly radiosensitive.

Post-resection cavity

Post-radiation therapy local irradiation

Recurrent disease post surgery and/or irradiation

Inoperable lesion

High-risk location of lesion

Slowly progressive but minimal neurological deficits

Patient with medical comorbidities that preclude surgery

Patient declines surgery.

### TABLE 49-2    Contraindications for Spinal SRS

Spinal instability

Neurological deficit due to physical spinal cord or nerve root compression

Adjacent cord previously irradiated to the maximum dosage

Generalized metastatic involvement of the axial skeleton

Epidural carcinomatosis

### TABLE 49-3    Lesions Treatable with CyberKnife Radiosurgery

**Tumors**
**Benign**
   Neurofibroma, schwannoma, meningioma, hemangioblastoma, chordoma, paraganglioma, ependymoma, epidermoid
**Malignant/metastatic**
   Breast, renal, non-small cell lung, colon, gastric and prostate metastases; squamous cell (laryngeal, esophageal, and lung) tumors; osteosarcoma; carcinoid; multiple myeloma; clear cell carcinoma; adenoid cystic carcinoma; malignant nerve sheath tumor; endometrial carcinoma; malignant neuroendocrine tumor

**Vascular Malformations**
   Arteriovenous malformation (types 2 and 3)

linear accelerator attached to an industrial robot (Figure 49-3). The robotic arm is unconstrained, using six degrees of freedom to deliver beams to virtually any part of the body from a wide range of angles. During treatment, real-time orthogonal images of the patient are obtained frequently, enabling the system to identify and automatically correct for small changes in patient position.

Several conventional radiation therapy systems have been modified to provide spinal SRS. The BrainLab Novalis and TX systems both use floor- and ceiling-mounted x-ray cameras to verify patient position during therapy. In contrast, the Varian Trilogy and Elektra Synergy systems utilize cone-beam CT scanners mounted on the gantry of the LINAC. The cone CT scanners acquire images before treatment, but do not do so regularly during each session, and cannot always accommodate for changes in patient movement during therapy.

## INDICATIONS FOR SPINAL RADIOSURGERY

Indications for spinal SRS continue to evolve (Tables 49-1 and 49-2). The most commonly treated spinal lesions are metastatic (Table 49-3). A biopsy may not be necessary prior to treatment if the diagnosis is clear from the clinical history and imaging. Ideally, lesions should be less than 5 cm in maximal diameter, well demarcated, and clearly seen on CT and/or MRI. For most tumors, local control rates are equivalent or superior to conventional radiation and complications are generally lower than with open surgery. In some particular cases, spinal SRS may be useful for ablating the more radioresistant tumors.[1] However, in those previously irradiated patients where the adjacent spinal cord has already received the maximum tolerated radiation dosage, the efficacy of spinal radiosurgery may be compromised because of the need to lower the radiosurgical dose.

Spinal SRS is contraindicated in several situations. When there is significant cord or nerve root compression resulting in severe or progressive neurological deficits, surgery may yield the best outcome. This is especially true for bony or benign lesions, which involute slowly following treatment. In the presence of spinal instability, SRS should only be performed as an adjuvant therapy after decompression and stabilization or vertebroplasty has been performed first. In cases in which there is no known systemic disease and pathology cannot be reasonably ascertained by radiographic studies, radiosurgery is contraindicated without first establishing a diagnosis. Some large tumors are best treated with a debulking procedure followed by SRS.

## TREATMENT DETAILS

Image-guided systems do not require rigid immobilization or invasive frames. Instead, noninvasive custom masks or cradles are made for each patient and used during image acquisition and radiosurgery. These devices improve comfort, expedite alignment, and limit movement. For upper cervical lesions, a thermoplastic mask is made for each patient (Aquaplast, WFR Corp., Wyckoff, NJ; Figure 49-4A). For thoracic and lumbar lesions a custom vacuum-molded body cradle is used (AlphaCradle, Smithers Medical Products, Inc., Akron, OH; Figure 49-4B). For some cervicothoracic lesions, both devices are utilized.

Bony landmarks of the spine are used to target cervical, thoracic, and lumbar lesions, as well as some pelvic lesions, scapular and rib head masses, and paravertebral soft tissue tumors. The presence of spinal stabilization hardware does not interfere with target localization. Digitally-reconstructed radiographs (DRRs) are created as part of the treatment plan and are used to establish the relationship of the target to regional bony landmarks. The accuracy of CyberKnife using bony landmarks approaches ±0.5 mm$^2$.

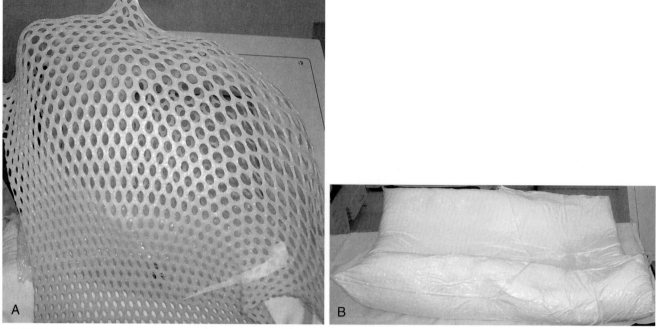

■ **FIGURE 49-4**   The Aquaplast mask is used as an immobilization device in cervical spine patients during CyberKnife treatment **(A)**. AlphaCradle custom body mold is used in thoracic, lumbar, and sacral lesions during CyberKnife treatment **(B)**.

Synthetic image A            Camera image A            Overlay of images A

Synthetic image B            Camera image B            Overlay of images B

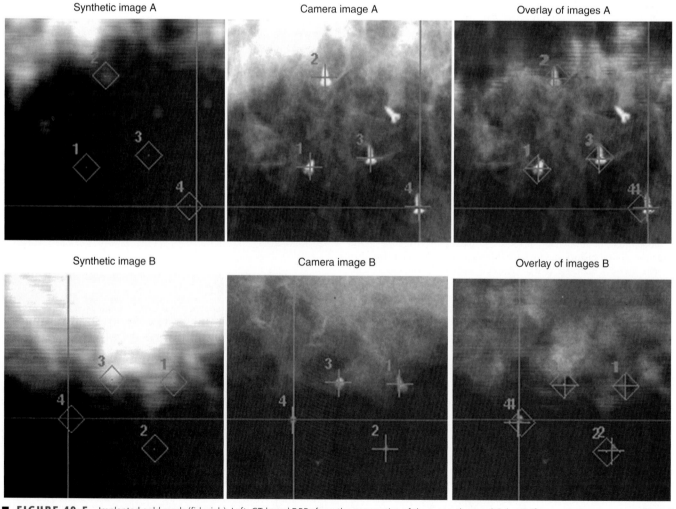

■ **FIGURE 49-5**   Implanted gold seeds (fiducials). Left: CT-based DRRs from the perspective of the two orthogonal CyberKnife mounted x-ray cameras **(A and B)**. Center: Real time x-ray images from the two x-ray cameras. Right: Superimposed DRRs and actual radiographic images.

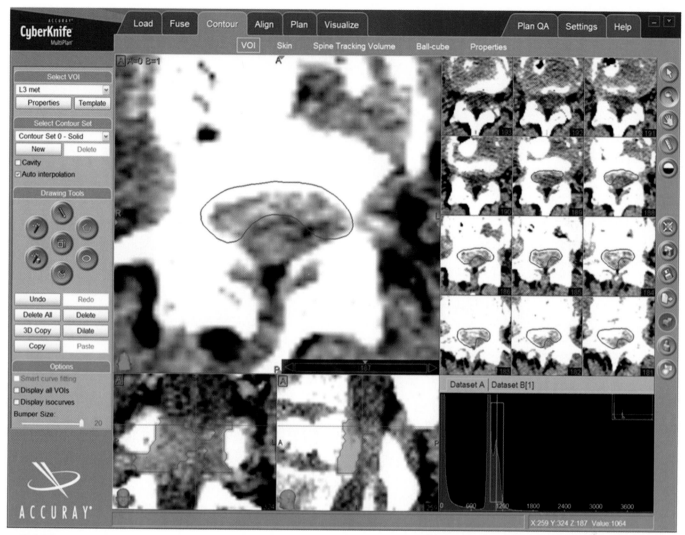

■ **FIGURE 49-6**    Fine-cut CT is used in delineating the lesion to be treated. Contour of L3 metastasis in axial, sagittal, and coronal projections is drawn. The epidural metastasis is in red.

For lesions not associated with bony landmarks, or where there is severe osteoporosis, localization may be based on implanted fiducials. Stainless steel screws in adjacent bone, or "gold seeds" adjacent to or within the lesion, can be inserted prior to imaging (Figure 49-5). A minimum of three clearly visible, non-collinear fiducials is needed. Ideally, they are placed in bone or firm tissue, surround the target lesion, and do not overlap in 45° oblique images. Prior to treatment delivery, the tumor location relative to the implants or bony landmarks is established based on DRRs. The accuracy using implanted fiducials may be lower than with bony landmarks and depends on the number and location of the implants.[2]

Most patients are imaged and treated supine. Treatment planning begins with a fine cut CT scan, (1.25-mm slices). The CT has the special resolution of available technologies and is required to delineate the lesion (Figure 49-6) and create the DRRs used for localization (Figure 49-7). MRIs, positron emission tomography (PET) scans, or three-dimensional (3-D) angiograms are commonly used in addition. Treatment plans for CyberKnife are designed using the Accuray Multiplan System (Figure 49-8). The various stereotactic image sets needed for target definition are transferred to the planning computer and aligned to one another using a semi-automatic process. Utilizing a graphic interface, the surgeon outlines the target lesion and adjacent radiation-sensitive structures, such as the spinal cord, esophagus, or kidneys, creating a 3-D representation of relevant anatomy (Figure 49-9). A dose and treatment schedule is specified by the surgeon and the radiation oncologist. A radiation physicist computes treatment plans, seeking an optimal dose conformation and a corresponding array of treatment beams.

Physical parameters are adjusted and refined iteratively until an optimal plan is obtained. Ideally, the beams are evenly distributed over the surface of the target, the target receives at least the prescribed dose, and the dose to adjacent structures is minimized.

Spinal SRS is an outpatient procedure. At the time of treatment, patients are positioned so that the lesion is near the center of an imaginary 80 cm diameter sphere. Orthogonal images are obtained by the digital x-ray cameras and compared with precalculated DRRs. The couch position is adjusted and the location of the target is confirmed. The robotic arm then moves the LINAC to each of the individual beam positions, and each beam's dose is delivered. During treatment, images are repeated frequently and the couch position is adjusted to preserve accuracy. The process is automatic, but is monitored closely by a radiation therapist.

## TREATMENT OF SPINAL METASTASES

In older populations, the majority of spinal tumors are metastatic (see Case 2). Forty percent of cancer patients develop at least one spinal metastasis. SRS is perhaps the least invasive of available treatments, and can deliver much higher doses than conventional radiotherapy while limiting cord exposure. SRS generally takes 1 to 3 days, while conventional radiotherapy may require 4 to 6 weeks. Multiple lesions can be treated safely and, because of the shorter treatment schedules, the treatment of asynchronous metastases is more convenient. SRS is appropriate as an adjuvant following a debulking procedure or in conjunction with a stabilization procedure such as fusion or

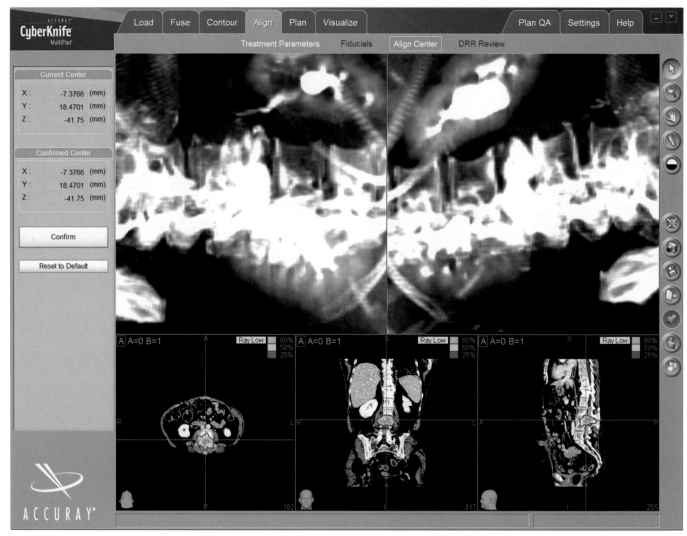

■ **FIGURE 49-7**    Contour of L3 metastasis and spinal roots with superimposed isodose lines from the treatment plan, in axial, sagittal, and coronal projections. The epidural metastasis is in red, the spinal roots are blue, and the 80% isodose line is the smaller green line.

vertebroplasty. SRS can be a good treatment modality for those with limited life expectancies, or those undergoing other concurrent treatments. Spinal radiosurgery can be highly effective in controlling pain, such as in Case 1, with up to 100% of patients reporting relief in some series.[3]

Debate continues regarding the most appropriate treatment margins. Some centers radiate only tumor seen on MRI, while others recommend treating the entire affected vertebral body including pedicles. Up to 18% of local failures are due to recurrences in the pedicles.[4] Amdur et al[5] advocate treating visible tumor plus a 1-cm margin in bone or a 2-mm volume beyond the cortex. We typically treat only the volume of tumor seen on CT or MRI. There are no studies that clearly demonstrate a benefit of one approach over the other. Dose recommendations are variable, with single session prescriptions ranging from 8 to 24 Gy in the published literature.[5] We use 16 to 25 Gy in one to three fractions, depending on tumor type. Local control is achieved in 77% to 100% of cases, and control rates are independent of histopathology (Table 49-4).

## TREATMENT OF INTRADURAL EXTRAMEDULLARY LESIONS

Most intradural extramedullary lesions are benign. Surgical resection is most commonly recommended since it provides immediate decompression, yields a tissue diagnosis, and is usually curative. Intracranial lesions of similar histology have been shown to respond well to SRS. SRS for these benign spinal lesions is appropriate for inaccessible tumors, syndromic lesions that are multiple, for patients with significant medical comorbidities, or for those who decline open surgery. In older patients, the risks associated with open surgery are greater, so SRS may be appropriate for most intradural extramedullary lesions in this population.

In our institution, we have treated 110 patients with 117 lesions[6] (unpublished data). Fifty-six percent of schwannomas (see Case 1) and meningiomas have stabilized after SRS and 44% have regressed radiographically. Neurofibromas did less well, with 11% enlarging, and up to 80% of patients reporting progressive neurological deficits. We have observed that most myelopathies and radiculopathies improve after SRS treatment. Two of our SRS-treated patients required open resection for tumor enlargement. Three needed surgery for persistent or progressing symptoms. One patient developed a radiation-induced myelopathy.

## TREATMENT OF INTRAMEDULLARY LESIONS

Sixteen of the 92 hemangioblastomas treated in our institution were spinal intramedullary tumors. These were treated with a median radiosurgical dose of 23 Gy. After a median follow-up of 34 months, 15 of the 16 spinal hemangioblastomas either decreased or remained the same in size. Intramedullary hemangioblastomas associated with significant edema or

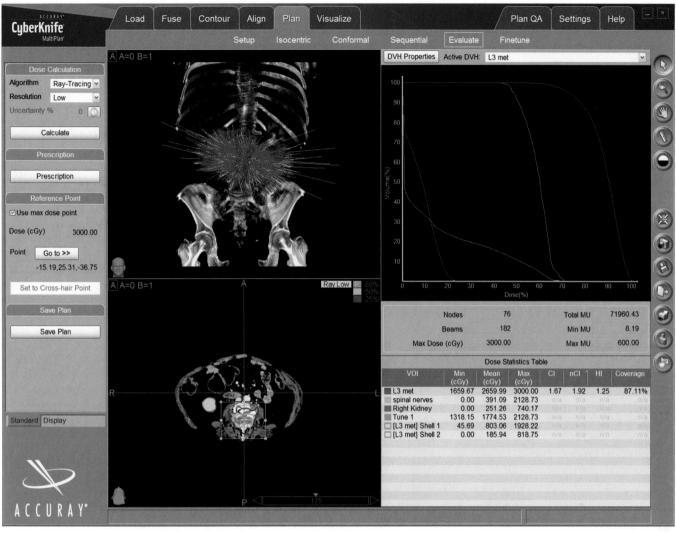

■ **FIGURE 49-8**   Treatment plan for L3 metastasis is designed using the Accuray Multiplan System.

cysts might do less well, based on our experience with similar intracranial lesions.

Although the data for ependymomas are limited, a few published studies have shown SRS to be efficacious.[7] We know less about SRS for spinal astrocytomas, but for those which are well circumscribed, spinal SRS may be an appropriate alternative to surgery.

Intramedullary spinal cord metastases are rarely seen. They constitute only 8.5% of central nervous system metastases,[8] but their frequency will likely increase with longer patient survival and as the population ages. Wowra et al[9] reported that 96% of spinal metastases were well controlled with spinal SRS and that the risk of radiation myelopathy was less than 1%.

## COMPLICATIONS

SRS treatment failures can be categorized as "in-field failures" and "marginal failures." "In-field failures" involve tumor regrowth within the treated volume and may be related to inadequate dosing. "Marginal failures" involve regrowth at the edges of the treated volume and may be related to poor imaging, an underestimation of the tumor volume, or inaccuracies in the position or set-up. "Distant failures," which involve new lesions in untreated portions of the spine, occur in 5% of patients, and are due to the underlying disease and not to a failure of technique.

Neurological complications of SRS are categorized by their time of onset. Acute complications occur within a month and are usually transient. They are related to edema and can be treated with steroids. Subacute complications occur 3 to 6 months after treatment and are usually secondary to demyelination. The prognosis for recovery is good. Radiation-induced myelopathy, the most feared side effect of SRS, is a late effect, occurs after 6 months, and is usually irreversible. In 1000 patients treated with CyberKnife for spinal lesions, six developed myelopathy (0.6%).[10] To prevent radiation-induced myelopathy, we avoid exposing more than one cubic centimeter of spinal cord to more than 8 Gy in single session plans.

Other less severe side effects of spinal SRS include local skin reactions, which are occasionally seen when the posterior elements are treated, and gastrointestinal complaints such as nausea, pharyngitis, esophagitis, or diarrhea. Renal complications are rare even after thoracolumbar treatments.

## CONCLUSION

The successes of intracranial radiosurgery inspired the development of spinal SRS. Many spinal lesions may not be amenable to complete surgical resection. SRS is both safe and effective treatment for metastatic lesions of the spine and for some intradural extramedullary tumors. Early results in treating intramedullary lesions are encouraging. Spinal SRS, a completely noninvasive treatment, is particularly suited for older patients and those with significant concomitant medical problems.

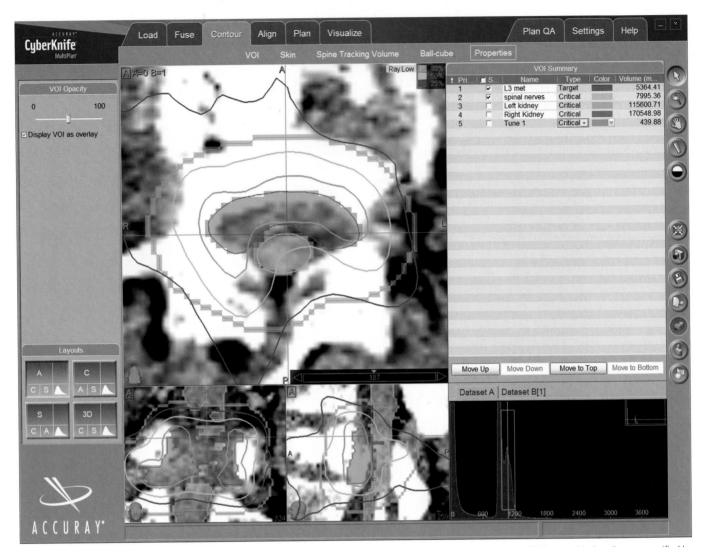

■ **FIGURE 49-9** Outlines of the target lesion and adjacent radiation-sensitive structures, such as the spinal nerves and kidneys, with dose lines as specified by the surgeon and the radiation oncologist.

**TABLE 49-4   SRS for Spinal Vertebral Metastases**

| Site | Lesions / Patients | Tumor Type | Modality | Dose / Fractions | Contouring | Complications | Pain Reduced | Local Control | Overall Survival |
|------|--------------------|-----------|----------|------------------|------------|---------------|--------------|---------------|------------------|
| Amdur, et al., 2009[11] | 25 / 21 | Various | LINAC / IMRT | 15 Gy / 1 | Lesion with margin | No neurological toxicity | 43% | 95% | 25% at 1 year |
| Wowra, et al., 2009[15] | 134 / 102 | Various | CyberKnife | 15 to 24 Gy / 1 | Not specified | No SRS-related neurological deficits | 86% | 88% | Median survival 1.4 years |
| Yamada, et al., 2008[14] | 103 / 93 | Various | LINAC / IMRT | 18 to 24 Gy / 1 | Entire vertebral body | No neurological toxicity | Not reported | 90% | 36% at 3 years |
| Gibbs, et al., 2007[6] | 102 / 74 | Various | CyberKnife | 14 to 25 Gy / 1 to 5 | Lesion only | Three cases myelopathy | 84% | No symptom progression | 46% at 1 year |
| Chang, et al., 2007[7] | 74 / 63 | Various | LINAC / IMRT | 27 to 30 Gy / 3 to 5 | Entire vertebral body | No neurological toxicity | 60% | 77% | 70% at 1 year |
| Ryu, et al., 2007[16] | 230 / 177 | Various | LINAC / IMRT | 8 to 18 Gy / 1 | Entire body with pedicles | 1% risk of myelopathy | 85% | 96% | 49% at 1 year |
| Gerszten, et al., 2005[17] | 68 / 50 | Breast | CyberKnife | 12.5 to 22.5 Gy / 1 | Entire vertebral body | No neurological toxicity | 96% | 100% | Not reported |
| Milker-Zabel, et al., 2003[18] | 19 / 18 | Various | LINAC / IMRT or FCRT | 24 to 45 / variable | Entire vertebral body | No neurological toxicity | 81% | 95% | 65% at 1 year |

# References

1. F.C. Henderson, K. McCool, J. Seigle, W. Jean, W. Harter, G.J. Gagnon, Treatment of chordomas with CyberKnife: Georgetown University experience and treatment recommendations, Neurosurgery 64 (Suppl. 2) (2009) A44–A53.
2. S. Ryu, F. Fang Yin, J. Rock, J. Zhu, A. Chu, E. Kagan, L. Rogers, M. Ajlouni, M. Rosenblum, J.H. Kim, Image-guided and intensity-modulated radiosurgery for patients with spinal metastasis, Cancer 97 (2003) 2013–2018.
3. P.C. Gerszten, S.A. Burton, W.C. Welch, A.M. Brufsky, B.C. Lembersky, C. Ozhasoglu, W.J. Vogel, Single-fraction radiosurgery for the treatment of spinal breast metastases, Cancer 104 (2005) 2244–2254.
4. E.L. Chang, A.S. Shiu, E. Mendel, L.A. Mathews, A. Mahajan, P.K. Allen, J.S. Weinberg, B.W. Brown, X.S. Wang, S.Y. Woo, C. Cleeland, M.H. Maor, L.D. Rhines, Phase I/II study of stereotactic body radiotherapy for spinal metastasis and its pattern of failure, J. Neurosurg. Spine 7 (2007) 151–160.
5. R.J. Amdur, J. Bennett, K. Olivier, A. Wallace, C.G. Morris, C. Liu, W.M. Mendenhall, A prospective phase II study demonstrating the potential value and limitation of radiosurgery for spine metastases, Am. J. Clin. Onc. 32 (2009) 1–6.
6. R.L. Dodd, M.R. Ryu, P. Kamnerdsupaphon, I.C. Gibbs, S.D. Chang, J.R. Adler, CyberKnife radiosurgery for benign intradural extramedullary spinal tumors, Neurosurgery 58 (2006) 674–685.
7. S.I. Ryu, D.H. Kim, S.D. Chang, Stereotactic radiosurgery for hemangiomas and ependymomas of the spinal cord, Neurosurg. Focus 15 (15(5)) (2003) E10.
8. S. Parikh, D.E. Heron, Fractionated radiosurgical management of intramedullary spinal cord metastasis: a case report and review of the literature, Clin. Neurol. Neurosurg. 111 (2009) 858–861.
9. B. Wowra, S. Zausinger, C. Drexler, M. Kufeld, A. Muacevic, M. Staehler, J.C. Tonn, CyberKnife radiosurgery for malignant spinal tumors: characterization of well-suited patients, Spine 33 (2008) 2929–2934.
10. I.C. Gibbs, C. Patil, P.C. Gerszten, J.R. Adler Jr., S.A. Burton, Delayed radiation-induced myelopathy after spinal radiosurgery, Neurosurgery 64 (2009) A67–A72.

# PART 7

# Surgical Treatment Modalities:
# Lumbar Spine

# 50

# The Role of Spinal Fusion and the Aging Spine: Stenosis without Deformity

*Nelson S. Saldua, Chukwuka Okafor, Eric B. Harris, and Alexander R. Vaccaro*

### KEY POINTS

- The incidence of spinal stenosis is increasing secondary to the growing size of the elderly patient population.

- Because these patients lead more physically demanding lives and participate more in physical leisure activities than was common for the elderly in the past, demand for aggressive treatment of stenosis symptoms is likely.

- Most of these patients can be managed nonoperatively and, of those that require decompressive surgery, only a minority will also require fusion.

- Instability is the primary indication for including fusion in operative treatment of stenosis; it may be subtle and present prior to surgery or may be expected secondary to the extent of decompression required.

- Careful patient selection and limited use of fusion in appropriate cases results in excellent long-term results for patients with spinal stenosis.

## INTRODUCTION

Spinal stenosis is defined as any condition that results in a narrowing of the spinal canal, nerve root canal, or intervertebral foramina. This narrowing can occur at several locations at the same spinal level, or it can affect multiple levels at similar locations at each level. Spinal stenosis may be due to soft tissue impingement from a herniated intervertebral disc or an infolded ligamentum flavum, from bony processes such as osteophytes or hypertrophied facet joints, or from a combination of these.

Spinal stenosis usually involves the lumbar spine and tends to affect patients in the sixth or seventh decade of life. With an increase in the average age of the patient population, the incidence of patients seeking medical care for symptomatic spinal stenosis is also increasing. Not only are patients living longer, but also they are remaining more active in their older years, thereby making symptoms of neurogenic claudication more apparent. Additionally, surgeries such as total hip and knee arthroplasties are helping patients remain very active further into their lives. Patients with lumbar spinal stenosis often complain of symptoms consistent with neurogenic claudication, including pain, numbness, and paresthesias in the posterolateral portions of the legs and thighs. These symptoms are improved by activities in which the lumbar spine is held in flexion, such as leaning over a walker or shopping cart or riding a bicycle. Spinal stenosis also occurs in the cervical and thoracic spine. The clinical presentations are different, as is the decision-making process for treatment options.

The initial treatment for symptomatic spinal stenosis is nonoperative and consists of activity modification, oral medications, epidural steroid injections, and physical therapy. For those cases recalcitrant to nonoperative treatment, surgery is considered. Surgical options include decompression alone, decompression with a noninstrumented fusion, decompression with an instrumented fusion, and, recently, decompression followed by posterior pedicle-based dynamic stabilization. Newer technologies involving minimally-invasive approaches to the spine have been developed that indirectly improve the dimensions of the spinal canal and neuroforamina in select cases of moderate spinal canal stenosis (interspinous process spacers). Minimally invasive surgical (MIS) techniques have also been developed for spinal decompression as well as fusion.

Fusion in the aging spine can be problematic, due to poor bone quality. Spinal arthrodesis should be incorporated in the surgical treatment of spinal stenosis, either when potentially significant instability is present preoperatively, or if postoperative instability is expected secondary to the extent of decompression performed. The indications for spinal arthrodesis for spinal stenosis will be discussed in this chapter, as well as the arguments both for and against fusion. Outcomes and potential complications of spinal arthrodesis for stenosis will also be discussed.

## Basic Science

As with other segments of the spine, the etiology and specific location of the narrowing is important when treating cervical spinal stenosis. Cervical spinal stenosis can occur from a herniated cervical disc, an ossified posterior longitudinal ligament, a redundant ligamentum flavum, an ossified ligamentum flavum, a hypertrophied facet joint, or from any combination of these potentially compressive pathologies.

Stenosis in the cervical spine is of particular importance, due to the relatively small canal diameter as compared to the caliber of the spinal cord. Some surgeons now recommend surgical treatment for severe asymptomatic cervical spinal stenosis for prophylaxis against paralysis, while others recommend observation.

The clinical presentation of stenosis in the cervical spine can be that of myelopathy, radiculopathy, or both. Patients with compressive pathology secondary to a herniated disc pressing on the spinal cord may report symptoms of myelopathy, including loss of hand dexterity and gait abnormalities. Physical exam will show signs of upper motor neuron pathology, which can be manifested as hyperactive deep tendon reflexes, a positive Hoffmann sign, or as a Babinski sign. If, instead, this herniated disc places pressure on an exiting nerve root, or if the loss of intervertebral disc height causes a loss of cross-sectional area of the neuroforamen, then the patient may exhibit signs and symptoms of a particular nerve root radiculopathy. This will result in motor weakness, paresthesias, and loss of deep tendon reflexes (if applicable) for that particular cervical nerve root.

Radiographically, cervical stenosis is often diagnosed using a radiographic measurement called the Pavlov ratio. This ratio is defined as the ratio between the sagittal diameter of the spinal canal and the sagittal diameter of the vertebral body, as measured on a lateral radiograph. A ratio of greater than 1 is considered normal, while a ratio of less than 0.8 is considered to be diagnostic for spinal stenosis. A cervical MRI can help determine the etiology of the compression if the source is a herniated disc or a redundant ligamentum flavum. Additionally, an MRI can show any evidence of spinal cord compression, such as a lack of cerebrospinal fluid around the spinal cord and/or myelomalacia within the cord itself. A CT scan can be used to diagnose bony abnormalities such as osteophytes or hypertrophied facet joints.

## Stenosis in the Cervical Spine

### CASE 1

A 63-year-old female presented to clinic with an 8-year history of worsening neck pain radiating to her bilateral shoulders and scapulae. The pain radiated primarily down her bilateral biceps and radial forearms into the thumb and index fingers of both hands. Additionally, she had noted a gradually worsening weakness in her legs, with loss of balance, worsening handwriting, and difficulty buttoning buttons and manipulating small objects with her hands. She had no bowel or bladder dysfunction. Despite nonoperative management that included activity modification, physical therapy, and nerve root and trigger point injections, her symptoms persisted and seemed to be worsening.

Physical examination revealed tenderness to palpation in the cervical paraspinal musculature as well as in the midline. She had an unsteady gait with a positive Romberg sign. Range of motion was limited by pain, and neck extension reproduced the pain, numbness, and tingling in her arms. She had weakness in her right greater than left biceps, wrist extensors, and hand intrinsics, but intact sensation throughout all dermatomes. Reflex testing was significant for global hyperreflexia and a positive Hoffmann sign bilaterally.

Radiographs, seen in Figure 50-1A and B, demonstrate loss of normal cervical lordosis, severe spondylosis, and a spondylolisthesis of C4 on C5. Sagittal and coronal MRI cuts, seen in Figure 50-2A and B, demonstrate significant spinal stenosis, loss of normal disc height, and severe spinal cord compression with myelomalacia.

The patient was taken to the operating room for a combined anterior and posterior cervical decompression and fusion. Discectomies and interbody fusion were performed with allograft spacers and an anterior plate at C4-5, C5-6, and C6-7. This portion of the procedure restored normal lordosis and addressed the anterior pathology, including reduction of the spondylolisthesis at C4-5. The posterior procedure included laminectomy from C3 to C7 with screw and rod fixation from C3 to C7 as well (Figure 50-3A and B).

Postoperatively, the patient did well, with complete resolution of her arm pain. At last visit, her gait and balance were steadily improving, with overall improved function compared to preoperatively.

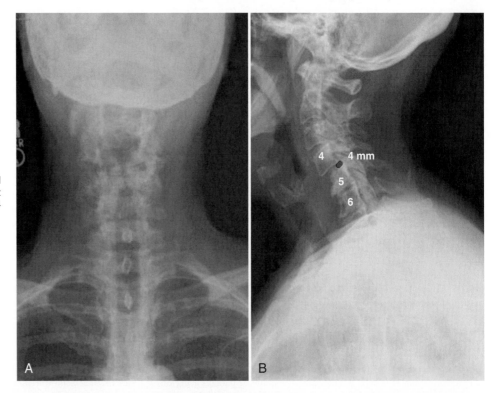

■ **FIGURE 50-1** **A and B**. AP and lateral radiographs demonstrating severe spondylotic changes and a 4 mm anterolisthesis of C4 on C5.

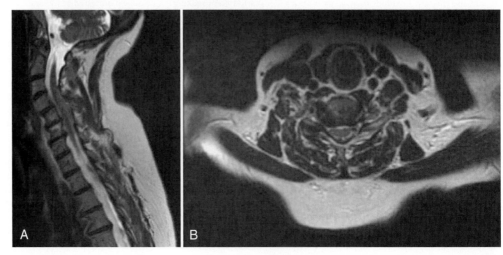

■ **FIGURE 50-2** **A and B**. MRI showing severe stenosis from C3 to C7 with cord compression at multiple levels and signal change within the spinal cord.

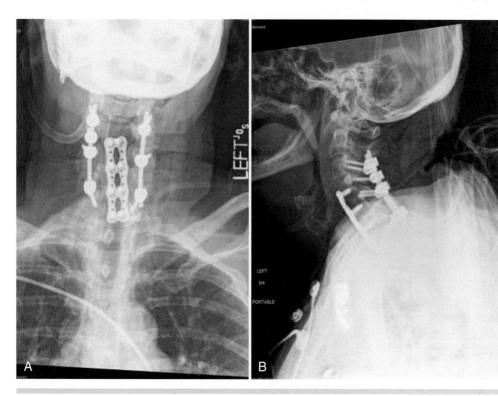

■ **FIGURE 50-3  A and B.** AP and lateral postoperative radiographs. Note the restoration of natural cervical lordosis accomplished through multiple anterior discectomies. Posterior decompression and fusion creates additional space for the spinal cord and provides increased stability for fusion.

## Clinical Practice Guidlines

Cervical radiculopathy can be successfully treated nonoperatively with activity modification, oral medications, and selective nerve root block injections. Operative indications include symptoms that are recalcitrant to nonoperative treatment as well as development of myelopathy. The natural history of cervical myelopathy is that of a stepwise progression of symptoms alternating with periods of nonprogressive neurological symptoms.

The location of the compressive pathology in cervical stenosis is important, as it dictates the operative approach. Cervical stenosis due to a central or moderate-sized posterolateral cervical herniated nucleus pulposus is best treated with an anterior approach, in order to adequately remove the compressive pathology. This anterior cervical discectomy is typically combined with a fusion. Fusion is achieved with or without instrumentation, consisting of an anterior plate and screws. Anterior cervical discectomy and fusion (ACDF) has been described with good results without the use of instrumentation. An anterior cervical discectomy (ACD) without fusion is rarely performed today, and is almost never performed for multilevel disease. Discectomy without fusion has been reported in a prospective, randomized trial to be equivalent to ACDF for the treatment of cervical radiculopathy.[1] For the treatment of myelopathy, ACD without fusion has been reported to result in good relief of neck and arm pain as well as a 76% rate of return to work.[2] However, ACD without fusion has been shown in other case series to be associated with worsening of preexisting cervical myelopathy in 3.3% of cases.[3] Worsening of symptoms after ACD without fusion was also reported by Nandoe Tewarie et al in a retrospective review of 102 patients evaluated up to 18 years after surgery.[4] While ACD alone has been shown to be successful in the treatment of cervical myeloradiculopathy, the possibility of worsening of symptoms, combined with the difficulty of revision of anterior cervical surgery, makes this a possible yet unattractive surgical option.

If the compressive pathology is secondary to redundant ligamentum flavum, hypertrophied facet joints, or other posterior pathology, then a posterior approach allows the surgeon to directly decompress the offending agent. A posterior-only approach is only indicated if neutral or lordotic alignment of the cervical spine is maintained. A kyphotic deformity in the cervical spine often mandates an anterior approach to restore the normal cervical sagittal alignment. Decompression from a posterior approach consists of laminotomy, laminectomy, or laminoplasty. Removal of significant portions of the facet joints should be avoided in order to avoid causing iatrogenic postlaminectomy cervical kyphosis. Raynor et al reported a cadaveric study comparing the potential degrees of instability on biomechanical testing of intact specimens, and following 50% facetectomy, and 70% facetectomy. The conclusion of this study was the recommendation that a facetectomy should involve less than 50% of the facet joint in the absence of fusion, in order to avoid spinal instability.[5] Postlaminectomy kyphosis after posterior cervical decompression alone is common when there is evidence of hypermobility on preoperative flexion-extension radiographs. A cervical fusion should be considered after posterior decompression if:

- A neutral plain lateral radiograph demonstrates a kyphotic cervical alignment.
- The decompression involves removal of more than 50% of the facet joint.
- The supraspinous and interspinous ligaments are incompetent or iatrogenically injured.
- Instability is seen on preoperative static radiographs or dynamic flexion-extension radiographs.

For multiple-level posterior cervical spinal cord compression, laminoplasty is another option. In this procedure, the space available for the spinal cord is increased by cutting the affected lamina on one side and scoring the contralateral lamina. The posterior elements are then "booked" open, utilizing the scored side as a hinge, and held open with suture, structural grafts/spacers, or plate and screws. With the newly increased space available for the spinal cord, the spinal cord can float away from the vertebral body. This treatment plan only works in cases in which a neutral or lordotic curve of the cervical spine is maintained. In a kyphotic cervical spine, the spinal cord will remain draped over the vertebral bodies regardless of the increased space posterior to the cord.

A combined anterior and posterior approach may be needed for kyphotic deformities with spinal stenosis and for multiple level disease. Posterior instrumentation and fusion is usually warranted when performing three or more cervical corpectomies or when doing four or more cervical discectomies.

## Basic Science

Thoracic stenosis is encountered by the surgeon much less frequently than stenosis of the cervical or lumbar spine. As in the cervical spine, thoracic stenosis is defined when the canal diameter is less than 10 mm. The compressive pathology is most often a herniated intervertebral disc, with the majority of the disc herniations being paracentral. Other etiologies, such as tumors, are possible. Thoracic stenosis can occur from a progressive kyphosis seen with multiple adjacent insufficiency fractures.

Thoracic stenosis presents with some similar signs and symptoms to cervical stenosis. Since the brachial plexus has already exited the spinal cord,

the patients with thoracic stenosis do not complain of the hand dexterity problems associated with cervical stenosis. They can exhibit signs and symptoms of thoracic level radiculopathy, lower extremity upper motor neuron dysfunction, or gait abnormalities.

## Clinical Practice Guidelines

Operative indications for stenosis in the thoracic spine are similar to those in the cervical spine: symptoms recalcitrant to nonoperative measures and cases in which myelopathy develops.

## *Stenosis in the Thoracic Spine*

### CASE 2

A 58-year-old woman with no significant past medical history presented to an outside hospital with progressive bilateral lower extremity weakness, right greater than left, and decreased sensation below the nipple line. In addition, she reported 5 out of 10 pain in the midthoracic area, urinary retention, mild constipation, and an inability to bear weight. Emergency department records indicated that she had twisted her back one week prior to admission and complained of subsequent onset of these progressive symptoms. Of note, several months prior to presentation, the patient noted irritation and a possible mass in the upper outer quadrant of her right breast. Radiographs obtained at an outside hospital demonstrated a pathologic fracture of her sixth thoracic vertebrae. She was transferred to our facility for evaluation and for further radiologic and immunopathic workup for presumed metastatic breast cancer to the thoracic spine.

Physical exam at the time of admission was notable for a 2 × 2 cm purple nodule on her right breast with induration and no discharge. Tenderness to palpation over the cervical spine was noted. Neurological exam demonstrated weakness in bilateral lower extremities with 2/5 hip flexors, 4/5 quadriceps, 1/5 tibialis anterior, 1/5 extensor hallucis longus, and 2.5 gastrocnemius; upper extremity strength was 5/5. Sensation was

decreased bilaterally; clonus was present, particularly on the right; Babinski sign was absent; and rectal tone was decreased. The patient was afebrile with stable vital signs, and admission labs were within normal limits.

The patient had a CT scan of her spine that demonstrated pathologic fractures of T5 and T6 and lytic lesions at multiple spinal levels with bony destruction, predominantly from T3 to T6, with encroachment upon the adjacent central canal and neural foramen (Figure 50-4). These findings were most suggestive of metastatic lesions. MRI of her spine demonstrated metastatic disease with multilevel involvement and posterior epidural extension in T5 and T6 resulting in spinal cord compression (Figure 50-5).

The patient underwent a T3 to T6 laminectomy for extradural tumor, posterolateral fusion of T2 to T10, and open biopsy of the presumed metastatic lesion. Pathologic examination was consistent with metaplastic breast cancer (Figure 50-6). The patient tolerated the procedure well without complication. At the time of discharge from inpatient rehabilitation, lower extremity motor strength had improved to 3/5, and sensation had improved as well. Bladder function did not return and a Foley catheter was maintained. The neurogenic bowel responded well to enema, Dulcolax, Colace, and senna.

The patient was transferred to the oncology service for further evaluation and treatment of her metastatic breast cancer.

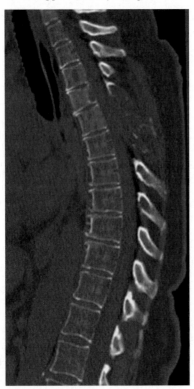

■ **FIGURE 50-4** CT scan of the thoracic spine showing multilevel lytic lesions with bony destruction, predominantly from T3 to T6, with encroachment of the adjacent central canal and neural foramen. These are most suggestive of metastatic lesions.

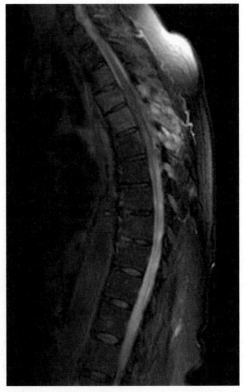

■ **FIGURE 50-5** MRI scan of the thoracic spine showing extensive multilevel metastatic involvement, most prominent in the upper thoracic spine, with posterior epidural extension at T5 and T6 compressing the spinal cord.

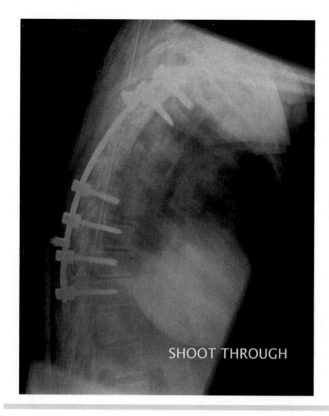

■ **FIGURE 50-6**   Lateral x-ray of thoracic spine, status post T3-T6 laminectomy and T2-T10 fusion, with pedicle screws and rods in stable positioning.

Treatment for thoracic stenosis is usually limited to decompression alone. The decision on whether to use an anterior, posterior, or transthoracic approach depends on the source of the compressive pathology. Fusion, historically, has rarely been indicated due to the greater inherent stability of the thoracic spine afforded by the rib cage and sternum. Palumbo et al described a retrospective review of 12 patients treated for thoracic stenosis. All were treated with a decompression alone, without fusion. Although the majority of their patients improved with regard to pain, ambulation, and neurological function, five patients exhibited early deterioration of symptoms due to recurrent stenosis, deformity/instability, or both. The authors imply that a decompression at the thoracolumbar junction was more prone to instability.[6]

When surgically treating spinal stenosis in the thoracic spine, fusion should be considered in cases where:

- Anterior column support is lost, such as in severe compression or burst fractures or with tumor resections.
- The decompression involves the thoracolumbar junction.
- Instability is seen on preoperative static radiographs or dynamic flexion-extension radiographs.

## Basic Science

Spinal stenosis is most frequently encountered in the lumbar spine. It typically affects patients in their sixth or seventh decade of life. As a normal age-related change of the intervertebral disc, the nucleus pulposus itself loses water content, which in turn leads to a loss of disc height. This loss of water may result in increased motion at the vertebral body–disc interface, leading to increased motion at the level of the facet joint. This excess motion at the facet joint may lead to facet joint arthrosis and hypertrophy. Finally, the loss of intervertebral disc height translates to decreased cross-sectional area of the neural foramina as well as redundancy of the ligamentum flavum. All of these age-related changes contribute to lumbar spinal stenosis.

The clinical syndrome of lumbar spinal stenosis is that of neurogenic claudication. Patients often report lower extremity pain that is worsened with activity, but lessened when the patient is allowed to assume a position in which the lumbar spine is flexed. Activities such as riding a bicycle or leaning over a shopping cart are better tolerated by patients with lumbar stenosis, because they are performed with the lumbar spine in a flexed position.

The radiographic workup of lumbar stenosis begins with plain radiographs of the lumbar spine. Radiographs should be scrutinized for osteophytes, malalignment, facet hypertrophy or any other abnormalities that could potentially decrease the space available for the neural elements. Flexion-extension radiographs are needed to determine the presence of instability. The presence of any preoperative instability necessitates a spinal fusion. A MRI can be useful in determining the specific location (paracentral, lateral recess, or foraminal) of the stenosis. A CT myelogram is useful in localizing the specific area of the compressive lesion, but this has been largely supplanted by MRI.

## Clinical Practice Guidelines

Controversy exists in the literature with regard to whether a spinal fusion should be added to decompression. Decompression alone without fusion has been reported to treat lumbar spinal stenosis with good results. However, other reports in the literature, primarily those including patients with instability, report better clinical outcomes with addition of spinal fusion. Yone et al reported on a group of 34 patients with lumbar spinal stenosis.[7] Of this group, 17 patients had radiographic spinal instability as described by Posner. Ten patients underwent decompression and fusion, and the remaining seven underwent decompression alone. The decompression-alone patients had significantly worse Japanese Orthopaedic Association back scores. Still others report no difference in clinical outcomes for patients treated with decompression alone and decompression plus fusion.[8, 9]

Expansive laminoplasty has been reported as an alternative to lumbar decompression and fusion, with good results.[10] This procedure shares the technical demands present in cervical laminoplasty.

## *Stenosis in the Lumbar Spine*

### CASE 3

An active 90-year-old man was referred to the spine surgery clinic with a long history of worsening bilateral buttock pain and decreased walking tolerance. He was otherwise in excellent health, but noted a burning pain in his buttocks with radiation down the posterior and lateral thighs after ambulating more than about 50 yards. The pain quickly improved with rest, and would not occur if he had a shopping cart to lean on while ambulating. Descending stairs or inclines would aggravate symptoms but ascending stairs would not. He had been evaluated by the vascular surgery service and was not found to have vascular insufficiency. Despite an intensive program of physical therapy focusing on core strengthening, flexibility, and cardiovascular fitness his symptoms persisted. Interventions by the pain management service, including epidural steroid injections, had been unsuccessful.

Physical examination was relatively unremarkable, with normal strength throughout all muscle groups and intact sensation in all dermatomes. Gait was steady and neurological testing was unremarkable.

Radiographs, seen in Figures 50-7A and B, demonstrate advanced degenerative changes, with significant disc height loss, large disc osteophyte complexes, and facet hypertrophy from L2 to L5. Sagittal and coronal MR images seen in Figure 50-8A and B show severe central, lateral recess, and foraminal stenosis, with increased fluid in the zygapophyseal joints and buckling of the ligamentum flavum.

The patient was taken to the operating room for a L2 to L5 decompression and posterolateral instrumented fusion. Postoperative images are shown in Figure 50-9A and B. At last follow-up, the patient had returned to his premorbid level of functioning, with complete resolution of his claudication symptoms and no postoperative pain.

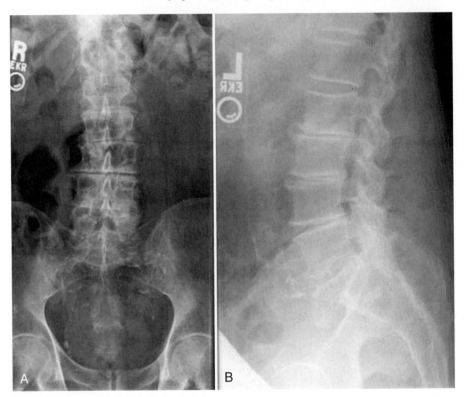

■ **FIGURE 50-7  A,** AP x-ray of lumbar spine showing multilevel spondylosis with a degenerative scoliosis and mild lateral listhesis at multiple levels. **B,** Lateral view showing severe disc collapse and listhesis at multiple levels.

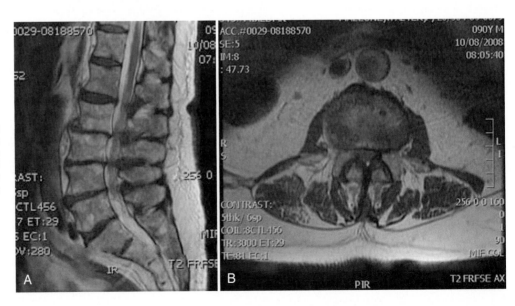

■ **FIGURE 50-8  A,** Sagittal MR image depicting moderate to severe central stenosis from L2 to S1. **B,** Coronal MRI cut showing lateral recess and foraminal stenosis accompanied by facet hypertrophy and broad-based disc bulging.

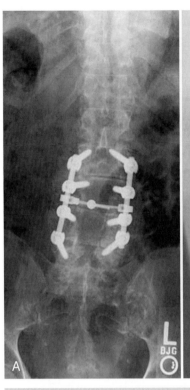
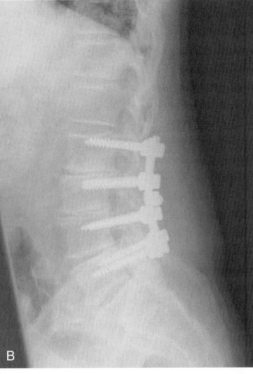

■ **FIGURE 50-9 A,** Postoperative AP radiograph showing instrumented fusion from L2 to L5 with wide laminectomy from L2 to the sacrum. **B,** Postoperative lateral radiograph showing stabilization of the lumbar spine with screw fixation and restoration of normal lumbar lordosis.

As with stenosis found elsewhere, successful surgical management of lumbar stenosis depends on adequate decompression of the neural elements. Fusion should be considered in cases in which:

- An inherently unstable degenerative pattern is present in which a stenotic canal is found to have rotational and translational deformity resulting in either degenerative spondylolisthesis or scoliosis.
- Greater than 50% of the facet joint is removed in the process of the decompression.
- Instability is seen on preoperative static radiographs or dynamic flexion-extension radiographs.
- The restoration of normal disc height will result in increased foraminal area as well as return the ligamentum flavum back to its normal length and tension .
- Stenosis exists after prior lumbar decompression surgery.

The addition of a lumbar interbody fusion to the spinal decompression can restore the disc space back to its normal height. This helps treat the stenosis by reducing any buckling of the ligamentum flavum as well as restoring the native cross-sectional area of the neural foramina. This interbody lumbar fusion can be done from a variety of approaches: anterior (anterior lumbar interbody fusion or ALIF), retroperitoneal (extreme or direct lateral lumbar interbody fusion or XLIF/DLIF), or posterior (transforaminal lumbar interbody fusion or TLIF). ALIF and XLIF/DLIF can be used as a standalone procedure for a spinal fusion, while TLIF must be augmented with posterior pedicle screw instrumentation. Each of these approaches has its pros and cons. An ALIF allows for excellent visualization of the intervertebral disc, but it often requires an access surgeon to mobilize the great vessels off the spinal column. Additionally, since this is done in a supine patient, the patient must be turned prone if posterior decompression and/ or instrumentation is needed. An XLIF/DLIF also requires repositioning for a posterior approach. The TLIF allows for 360-degree fusion from a posterior-alone approach. No access surgeon is needed, and no repositioning is required. This approach may require some manipulation of the neural elements, thereby putting those structures at risk.

## CONCLUSIONS

Spinal stenosis is primarily a condition occurring in elderly patients. It most commonly affects the lumbar spine of patients in their sixth or seventh decade of life. With the increasing average age of the general population as well as the increasing levels of activity of these elderly patients, the incidence of symptomatic spinal stenosis is increasing. Nonoperative management can be successful, but some cases are recalcitrant to nonoperative treatment. Successful surgical treatment of spinal stenosis depends on properly locating the area of compression, completely decompressing that area, and fusing the spinal segment if there is instability seen preoperatively or after decompression.

## References

1. J. Hauerberg, et al., Anterior cervical discectomy with or without fusion with ray titanium cage: a prospective randomized clinical study, Spine 33 (5) (2008) 58–64.
2. P.J. Rao, et al., Clinical and functional outcomes of anterior cervical discectomy without fusion, J. Clin. Neurosci. 15 (12) (2008) 1354–1359.
3. H. Bertalanffy, H.R. Eggert, Complications of anterior cervical discectomy without fusion in 450 consecutive patients, Acta Neurochir. (Wien) 99 (1-2) (1989) 41–50.
4. R.D. Nandoe Tewarie, R.H. Bartels, W.C. Peul, Long-term outcome after anterior cervical discectomy without fusion, Eur. Spine J. 16 (9) (2007) 1411–1416.
5. R.B. Raynor, J. Pugh, I. Shapiro, Cervical facetectomy and its effect on spine strength, J. Neurosurg. 63 (2) (1985) 278–282.
6. M.A. Palumbo, et al., Surgical treatment of thoracic spinal stenosis: a 2- to 9-year follow-up, Spine 26 (5) (2001) 558–566.
7. K. Yone, et al., Indication of fusion for lumbar spinal stenosis in elderly patients and its significance, Spine 21 (2) (1996) 242–248.
8. M. Cornefjord, et al., A long-term (4- to 12-year) follow-up study of surgical treatment of lumbar spinal stenosis, Eur. Spine J. 9 (6) (2000) 563–570.
9. D. Grob, T. Humke, J. Dvorak, Degenerative lumbar spinal stenosis: decompression with and without arthrodesis, J. Bone Joint Surg. Am. 77 (7) (1995) 1036–1041.
10. K. Adachi, et al., Spinal canal enlargement procedure by restorative laminoplasty for the treatment of lumbar canal stenosis, Spine J. 3 (6) (2003) 471–478.

# 51

# The Role of Spinal Fusion and the Aging Spine: Stenosis with Deformity

*Barton L. Sachs*

| K E Y   P O I N T S |
|---|
| • Adult scoliosis with spinal stenosis is a progressive condition that has a significant effect on the aging U.S. population. |
| • Management is complicated by the general medical conditions associated with aging and by metabolic bone disease. |
| • The goal of surgery is to perform the least aggressive procedure, usually a decompression, to treat the compressed neural elements. |
| • The aim of surgery is to leave a patient with a balanced stable spine in the coronal and sagittal planes. Fusion should not stop at an adjacent degenerative level. |
| • Adult scoliosis classification systems help establish the most appropriate type of surgery and the appropriate anatomic levels to maximize clinical and reconstructive outcome. |

## INTRODUCTION

Adult scoliosis is a common and sometimes disabling degenerative condition of the spine, with an overall prevalence reported in up to 60% of the elderly population.[1] Adult scoliosis has a marked impact on patients' general medical health and well-being; it has been shown that scoliotic patients have a significantly depressed perception of their mental and physical health in comparison with the general U.S. population. Even when individuals are compared with those having additional comorbidities, the adult scoliosis patients rate lower in clinical health assessment. In addition to the subjective considerations of this progressive disease, severe pain and disability occur in this population.[2]

The management of patients with symptomatic spinal deformity and spinal stenosis is controversial. The greatest challenge confronting contemporary spine surgeons in management of the aging patient population is patient selection; the surgeon must balance benefits, risks, complicatios, and the durability of various interventions. Analysis and application of these is difficult because of the limited number of prospective outcome studies and because there is a wide array of different interventions used in this patient population. The spine surgeon is increasingly confronted with the older patient and must decide on a suitable yet realistic treatment plan while considering the social and psychological factors affecting this unique patient population.

## PATHOANATOMIC CHANGES

Aging of the spine is similar to the degenerative process throughout the body. The physiologic aging cascade affects the anatomic structures and creates progressive changes that are biomechanical, biochemical, and physiologic. Changing pathophysiology affects the structure and function of the spine, which becomes relatively important because of the spine's role as the central foundation for the human upright posture.

Degenerative adult scoliosis occurs as result of both macroinstability and microinstability. There is segmental instability and translation of adjacent vertebral aligment in the lumbar spine, acquired secondary to years of chronic disc disease and progressive facet incompetence. Disc degeneration leads to disc collapse and bulging of the annulus fibrosus and posterior longitudinal ligament, thus triggering subperiosteal osteophyte formation. Additionally, articulating facets undergo degenerative changes that result in hypertrophy, calcification, and thickening of the ligamentum flavum. These changes eventually result in forward and translational displacement of the posterior elements that, in combination with degenerative disc changes, result in severe narrowing of the spinal canal and neural foramen (spinal stenosis) to cause symptoms of neurogenic claudication and radiculopathy.

## DEFINITION OF STENOTIC DEGENERATIVE DISEASE IN DEFORMITY

Lumbar spinal stenosis is defined as a narrowing of the spinal canal that produces compression of the neural elements before their exit from the neural foramen. The narrowing may be limited to a single motion segment (two adjacent vertebrae and the intervening intervertebral disc, facet joints, and supporting ligaments) or it may be more diffuse, spanning two motion segments or more.

Adult deformity of the spine with degenerative disease can be a major contributing factor in the narrowing of the spinal canal. Adult degenerative scoliosis occurs on the right and left sides with equal frequency. Adult degenerative scoliosis develops as a result of asymmetrical narrowing of the disc space and vertebral rotation secondary to the instability caused by degeneration of the disc.

Neural compression associated with adult lumbar scoliosis is commonly manifested as a radicular pain that may be related to physical activity. As the apex of a curve rotates, there is associated hypertrophy and subluxation of the facet joints in the concavity of the curve. Additionally, collapse in the concavity results in narrowing of a neural foramen between adjacent pedicles. As a result, symptoms occur in the anterior portion of the thigh and leg (resulting from compression of the cephalic and middle lumbar nerve roots). Radiating pain in the posterior portion of the lower extremity is more common on the side of the convexity of the lumbar curve; such pain is due to compression of the caudal lumbar nerve roots and the sacral nerve roots, well caudad to the apex, as the spine curves back to meet the pelvis.[2]

## CLINICAL COMPLEX OF SYMPTOM PRESENTATION

The degenerative aging spine with deformity creates the complex of four major categories of clinical symptom presentation:

- Neurologic pain (both peripheral and radicular)
- Back pain
- Activity-related limitations of lifestyle
- Deformity-related issues

Neurologic pain occurs with activity-related claudication caused by diminished blood flow to the nerves. It is incumbent upon the healthcare

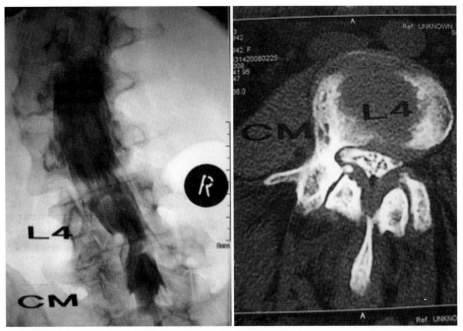

**■ FIGURE 51-1** A 66-year-old woman with an AO type 1 de novo scoliosis curve pattern. Myelogram and intrathecal CT scan demonstrate typical pathoanatomic changes consistent with severe spinal stenosis at the L4 vertebral level. Note the facet hypertrophy, facet malalignment, ligament flavum hypertrophy, thecal sac compression, disc degeneration, and vertebral olisthesis.

provider to rule out common causes of leg pain such as peripheral vascular disease, cardiac disease, arteriosclerotic vascular disease, and/or primary neurologic disease. Compressive radicular pain occurs on the concave collapsing side of a degenerative scoliosis, from direct compression of the nerve at the exiting foramen or subarticular space. Nerve stretch radicular pain occurs on the convex nerve roots that are exiting from the stenotic collapsing scoliotic spine. Therefore, a patient may present with either convex radicular pain or concave nerve root pain, or both.

Back pain may be caused by arthrosis and normal aging body changes of the discs, facets, or other structures. Another cause of back pain may occur from abnormal restricted segmental spine motion, as referred to by the term "mechanical pain." Also, back pain may occur secondary to nerve root compressive pain, which is secondary to decreased circulation and/or nerve compression.

Activity-related complaints from the aging spine patient generally involve lifestyle changes. Often the patient will present to the healthcare provider with statements describing restriction of normal activities of living. The patient may state that she or he cannot participate in dance, golf, normal work, recreational activities of hunting and fishing, or normal walking and exercise.

Deformity-related issues include complaint of a cosmetic changing appearance to the body, with or without a rib producing pressure on the pelvis. The patient may be twisting and leaning more on one side relative to the other side of his or her body. Less often, the patient will describe a shortness of breath secondary to restrictive lung capacity from scoliotic collapse and degenerative changes around the chest. The final and probably the most daunting problem is when the patient presents with complaints of balance and instability that affect normal ambulation. The patient may have a spine deformity that is so significant that he or she is not able to maintain normal balance, and requires orthotic spine supports such as a cane or walker to ambulate through daily activities.

## ADULT SCOLIOSIS CLASSIFICATION

Adult Scoliosis is classified by Aebi[3] using an AO system based on a pathoanatomic etiology and on a temporal onset of deformity. His classification defines adult scoliosis as spinal deformity in a skeletally mature patient with a Cobb angle of more than 10 degrees in the coronal plane. Aebi separates adult scoliosis into four types:

- Type I: Primary Degenerative Scoliosis ("de novo" form), mostly located in the thoracolumbar or lumbar spine. This occurs on basis of a disc and/or facet joint arthritis, affecting structures asymmetrically, and presents with back pain symptoms, often with or without signs of spinal stenosis (central and/or lateral stenosis) (Figures 51-1 and 51-2).
- Type II: Idiopathic Adolescent Scoliosis of the thoracic and/or lumbar spine, which progresses in adult life and is usually combined with secondary degeneration and/or imbalance.
- Type III: Secondary Adult Curves:
  a) In the context of an oblique pelvis (i.e., due to a leg length discrepancy or hip pathology), or as a secondary curve in idiopathic, neuromuscular, and congenital scoliosis or asymmetrical anomalies at the lumbosacral junction.
  b) In the context of metabolic bone disease (mostly osteoporosis combined with symmetric arthritic disease and/or vertebral fractures).[3]

Schwab et al.[4] proposed a three-tier classification system for adult scoliosis based on parameters of coronal and sagittal plane. These radiographic criteria include lumbar lordosis, location of coronal curve apex, olisthesis of vertebra segments relative to each other, and sagittal balance on x-ray (Figures 51-3 through 51-6). The classification system has accurately correlated radiographs with clinical significance, in an attempt at suggesting the most appropriate successful treatment in the adult patient. The rate of disease progression is influenced by the magnitude of the curve, the degree of lateral listhesis, the quality of the bone and the severity of associated spondylotic disease. Table 51-1 shows two classification schemes.

## CONSIDERATIONS FOR NONSURGICAL OR SURGICAL MANAGEMENT

Nonoperative treatment should always be the initial form of management. However, attempts to alleviate symptoms, including physical therapy and steroid injections, oral medications, diet and protein supplements, orthotics, and active muscle training, rarely yield satisfactory long-term results because the underlying pathology remains unchanged.

Surgical management of spinal disorders in the elderly poses challenges not faced in younger patients. Poor bone quality, the possibility of extensive spinal degenerative changes, and changes in sagittal alignment with increased thoracic

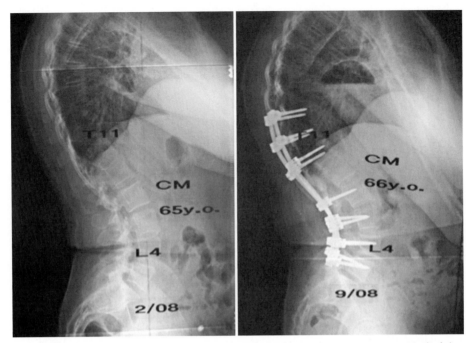

■ **FIGURE 51-2**    A 66-year-old woman with an AO type 1 de novo scoliosis curve pattern. Sagittal view shows postoperative fusion from T10 to L5 with maintenance of lumbar lordosis for standing balance.

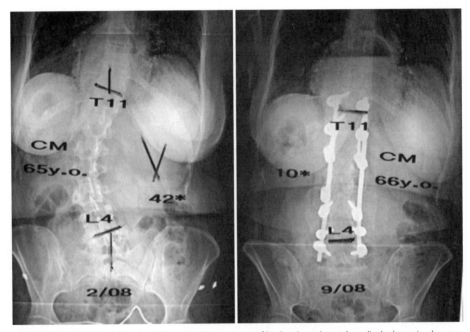

■ **FIGURE 51-3**    A 66-year-old female with symptoms of back pain and pseudo-radicular leg pain plus neurogenic claudication. She had an AO (Aebi) type 1 de novo scoliosis curve pattern, also categorized as a Schwab type 5, A+ pattern. After work-up and failure of extended nonoperative treatment, she underwent a posterior multilevel spine decompression /laminectomy and stabilization reconstruction / realignment with fusion and segmental pedicle screw implant instrumentation. Follow-up evaluation demonstrated excellent clinical improvement with resolution of symptoms and an excellent radiographic result, similar to that demonstrated in Figure 51-6.

kyphosis and loss of lumbar lordosis all complicate surgical management. The presence of multiple coexisting medical conditions, reduced wound-healing potential, and malnutrition can markedly increase the risk of complications for extensive surgical procedures. Osteoporosis and osteopenia complicate fixation options. The option of harvesting large quantities of autogenous iliac crest bone graft is not practical in patients with poor bone stock and osteopenia. Additionally, complications of fusion procedures in the elderly may lead to adjacent segment degeneration and the development of junctional kyphosis.

## GOALS OF TREATMENT (See Table 51-2)

The accepted and basic general goals of surgical management of the spine should include:

- Decreased pain
- Improved neurologic symptoms
- Improved activity status

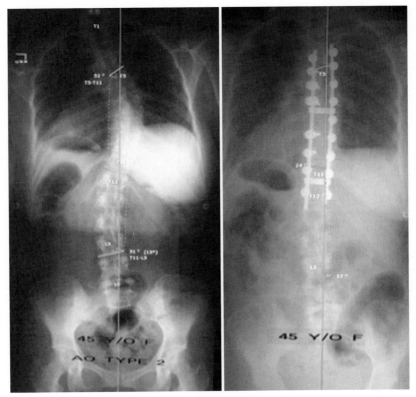

■ **FIGURE 51-4**   A 45-year-old female with AO (Aebi) type 2 adult scoliosis curve. She met the Schwab criteria of type II, A0. Therefore, she was treated with a limited thoracic (T3-T12) posterior spine reconstruction fusion with segmental pedicle screw instrumentation; she had an excellent result with improvement of clinical pain and correction of deformity.

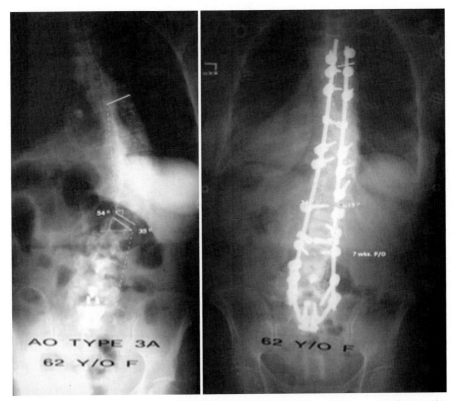

■ **FIGURE 51-5**   62-year-old female with AO (Aebi) type 3a adult scoliosis curve classification. This patient was also categorized as a type IV, B+ according to the Schwab criteria. She was treated with an anterior spinal release with implant interbody arthrodesis reconstruction followed by a posterior multilevel laminectomy /foraminotomy and long reconstruction / realignment fusion from T4 to sacrum using segmental pedicle screw fixation and implant stabilization. She had an excellent clinical and radiographic outcome.

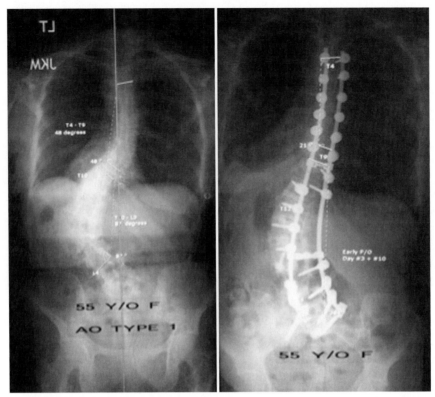

■ **FIGURE 51-6**  55-year-old female with AO (Aebi) type 1 de novo adult scoliosis classified as type IV, B++ by Schwab criteria. Patient was treated with anterior and posterior spine reconstruction and realignment with implant segmental pedicle screw instrumentation from T4 to sacrum. Also, she had multilevel posterior laminectomy /foraminotomy of the lumbar spine to complete the neurologic decompression. She showed excellent clinical and radiographic outcome.

- Improvement of balance and stability in both the coronal and sagittal plane deformity
- Prevention of further deformity
- Improvement of cosmetic appearance and body image

In essence, surgery for these patients should primarily address improvement of the spinal stenosis that is causing clinical and lifestyle issues. Stabilization, realignment, and/or reconstruction of the deformity is a secondary surgical consideration.

## SURGICAL PROCEDURES

The types of surgical procedures include:

- Decompression operation alone (generally epitomized by the laminectomy bone removal)
- A stabilization procedure (rarely performed alone and usually performed with implant instrumentation)
- A decompression and stabilization procedure with arthrodesis
  - Rarely, an in situ procedure with bone alone, without metal implants
  - Typically, with metal implant instrumentation
- Realignment and reconstruction
  - A decompression (either direct or indirect) with implant instrumentation for stabilization and fusion
- Anterior versus posterior versus combined anterior and posterior approaches

## OUTCOMES ASSOCIATED WITH SPINAL DEFORMITY TREATED WITH SURGICAL DECOMPRESSION

Frazier, Lipson, Fossel, and Catz[5] published their report in 1997, of a series of 90 patients with preoperative scoliosis associated with back pain, who were treated surgically and followed at 6 months and

### TABLE 51-1    Adult Spine Deformity Classifications

| Aebi – *Eur. Spine J*, 2005 | Schwab et al. – *Spine*, 2006 |
|---|---|
| **Type 1:** "De novo" scoliosis<br>Primary degenerative scoliosis<br>Disc and/or facet joint arthritis | Type<br>• I Thoracic curve only<br>• II Upper thoracic major (T4-T8)<br>• III Lower thoracic major (T9-T10)<br>• IV Thoracolumbar major (T11-L1)<br>• V Lumbar major curve (L2-L4) |
| **Type 2:** Idiopathic scoliosis<br>Progresses in adult life<br>Combines with degenerative imbalance | Lumbar Lordosis Modifier<br>• A Marked lordosis (>40°)<br>• B Moderate lordosis (0° to 40°)<br>• C No lordosis present (Cobb <0°) |
| **Type 3:** Secondary adult curves<br>a) Related to oblique pelvis, leg length discrepancy, or hip pathology<br>b) Related to metabolic bone disease (mostly osteoporosis) | Subluxation Modifier<br>• + Maximum measured subluxation (1-6 mm)<br>• ++ Maximum subluxation (>7 mm) |

24 months after surgery. These authors show that there was an increase in olisthesis, but this fact was associated with greater improvement in walking capacity at 6 months and at 24 months after surgery. Their data indicated that minor increases in the olisthesis after surgery for spinal stenosis generally were well tolerated by the patients. These authors showed that results support that preoperative scoliosis is associated with less favorable outcomes in patients who undergo decompression alone for spinal stenosis.

### TABLE 51-2   Surgical Planning Goals

- Decompression of neurologic structures
- Stabilization of spinal segmental anatomy
  - Fusion
    - In situ without implant instrumentation
    - With implant instrumentation
  - Sagittal balance (*imperative*)
- Deformity correction (*as indicated*)
  - Realignment/reconstruction
- Minimizing complications
- Maximizing:
  - Function
  - Quality of life

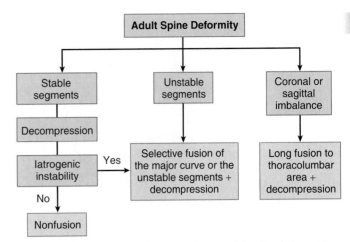

■ **FIGURE 51-7** Algorithm for adult spine deformity. *(Adapted from Ploumis A, Transfeldt EE, Denis F: degenerative lumbar scoliosis associated with spinal stenosis, Spine J 7(4):428-36, 2007.)*

## OPERATIVE TREATMENT OF DEGENERATIVE LUMBAR SCOLIOSIS ASSOCIATED WITH SPINAL STENOSIS

Patients who present with symptoms of spinal stenosis and who have degenerative scoliosis less than 20 degrees and without instability may be treated with spinal decompression only. Male patients with large vertebral structures and stabilizing osteophytes can tolerate more than two-level laminectomy without fusion. Otherwise, patients with degenerative scoliosis more than 15 to 20 degrees, lateral subluxation, or dynamic instability should be treated with decompression and fusion. Simmons[6] selects different fusion strategies according to his classification types of degenerative scoliosis; pedicle screws are considered the most appropriate fixation method for the aging osteoporotic bone with absent posterior elements after decompression. It is often imperative to extend the fusion to the sacrum with the addition of multiple fixation points in the sacrum and the pelvis to reduce increased strains to the implants and help healing of the fusion.

In referencing an article published by Poloumis, Transfeldt, and Denis,[7] a modification of their proposed treatment algorithm for patients can be established (shown in Figure 51-7). An extensive study of their patients was made, for which treatment was determined by using their algorithm, which included statistical significant improvement outcomes measured by SF 36, Oswestry, and VAS scores postoperatively.

The important consideration for surgery is whether or not the spinal segments are:

- Stable (less than 2 mm motion in dynamic x-rays),
- Unstable (greater than 2 mm of motion in dynamic x-rays), or
- If there is coronal or sagittal imbalance preoperatively.

If the initial spine is stable, then a decompressive operation is indicated. The decompression alone would be sufficient unless iatrogenic instability is produced at the time of surgery. If iatrogenic instability is produced, then a selective fusion of the major curve should be performed over the area of decompression. If the spine shows instability of the segments prior to commencing surgery, then a selected fusion of the major curve with decompression should be planned and carried out. In contrast, if the preoperative analysis of the patient shows a coronal or sagittal plane imbalance, then a long fusion from the thoracolumbar area, along with decompression of the lumbar area, is planned and carried out (see Figure 51-7).

## PRINCIPLES FOR SELECTING FUSION LEVELS IN ADULT SPINAL DEFORMITY WITH LUMBAR CURVES

An article by Kuklo[8] suggested some key points for consideration of surgical levels. Kuklo stated that sagittal imbalance is poorly tolerated in the adult scoliosis patient (Figure 51-8). Surgery should leave the patient with a good sagittal alignment; preoperative workup should include evaluation of adjacent segment disease with discographic evaluation of the degenerated discs as well as pain provocative injection tests of the facet joints in determining fusion levels.

Kuklo stated that a fusion should not be stopped adjacent to a degenerated segment. Additionally, he suggested that stopping long fusions at L5

would frequently lead to subsequent degeneration. Lastly, Kuklo stated that fusion to the sacrum was associated with increased complications and pseudoarthrosis at the lumbosacral junction.

## SPINAL STENOSIS WITH SCOLIOSIS

In 1992, Simmons and Simmons[6] published in *Spine* their retrospective review of a series of 40 patients who had lumbar scoliosis associated with spinal stenosis and symptoms of neurogenic claudication and were treated with posterior decompression and pedicle screw fixation techniques. In follow-up at an average of 44 months, 38 patients (93%) reported mild or no pain. These workers reported no deaths and no instrumentation-related failures or pseudoarthrosis in their series.

With regard to correction and stabilization with fusion, they recommended that pedicle screw instrumentation systems offered the most advantageous method of handling the difficult problems after removal of posterior elements. Simmons and Simmons believed that long fusions incorporating the entire scoliotic curve were necessary in most patients, because a fusion from the lower portion of the thoracic spine down to the sacrum would often be required. They felt that it was important to end the fusion at a disc space that appeared level. (Table 51-3 *shows the operative treatment guidelines and principles described by Simmons and Kuklo.*)

## RATE OF COMPLICATIONS IN SCOLIOSIS SURGERY

Weiss and Goodall[9] published a report in *Scoliosis* in August 2008 that stated that a meta-analysis review of scoliosis surgery checking for complications revealed 2590 titled articles. Although the rates varied, scoliosis surgery had a very high rate of complications, averaging 44% for adults (range 10% to 78%) as published in 11 different studies. (Table 51-4 *summarizes surgical complications in treatment of adult scoliosis.*)

Guigui and Blamoutier[10] published a treatise in French in 2005 in the review of orthopedic surgery. Their review of 3311 patients during a 12-month period who underwent surgical treatment of spine deformity found that 704 patients (21.3%) had one or more complications (850 complications) during or shortly after the index operation. The categories of complications were listed as:

- General
- Infectious
- Neurologic
- Mechanical

Older patients have an overall higher rate of complications. Ocular blindness is a serious complication that requires special note. A review by Myers and Stevens implies a relationship of blindness to operative time, blood loss, and operative hypotension, as well as an association with direct compression of the eye.

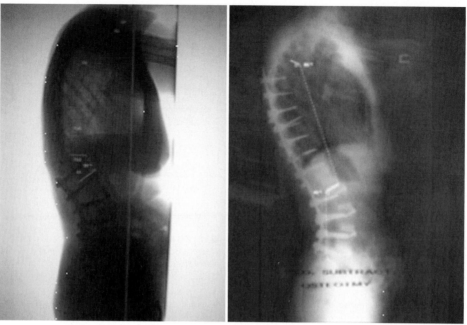

■ **FIGURE 51-8**   A 68-year-old woman treated with anterior and posterior four-level spine fusion in 2005. No pain-free interval. She developed kyphotic sagittal imbalance and T12 fracture collapse and vertebral angular instability, with inability to stand and function upright. She was treated with posterior pedicle subtraction osteotomy at T12 and sagittal realignment and extension of fusion with implant instrumentation to T5. She had excellent clinical and radiographic outcome.

### TABLE 51-3    Operative Treatment Guidelines and Principles

**Indications for Surgery**

*Pain*
- How much do symptoms affect lifestyle?

*Progressive neurologic deficit*
- Increasing leg weakness
- Paresthesias (nonvascular)

Consider *metabolic bone quality*

**Key Considerations** (*Kuklo – 2006*)

Don't stop fusion adjacent to degenerated segment.
- Fusion to L5 leads to further degeneration.
- Fusion to sacrum is associated with increased complication rate and pseudarthrosis at L/S junction.

**Simmons et al.**

*Spinal decompression only*
- Scoliosis <20%
- Without instability
- Lumbar lordosis maintained

*Decompression and fusion*
- Scoliosis 15-20 degrees
- Lateral subluxation
- Dynamic instability

*If fusion performed*
- Use implant instrumentation with pedicle screws

### TABLE 51-4    Surgical Complications: Rate and Categories

Adult Scoliosis**: 11 published studies

- Average rate ~44% (SD 24) (Range 10%-78%)
- **Weiss and Goodall: Meta-analysis review, *Scoliosis*, 2008.
- 2590 references reviewed, 287 rated complications

Categories of Complications

(Guigui et al., *Revue de Chirurgie Ortho*, 2005: 3311 patients over 12 months for deformity; 704 patients [21.3%] had one or more complication [850 complications])
- General
- Infectious
- Neurological
- Mechanical

of surgery is to decompress the compromised neural elements, in cases of symptomatic spinal stenosis, and to end with a balanced and stable spine in the coronal and sagittal plane, when there is imbalance. The idea is to proceed with the least aggressive procedure, usually posterior only, that would involve both decompression and stabilization of the spine. The important points are that fusions should not be stopped adjacent to a degenerated level and that sagittal imbalance is not tolerated by the elderly patient. The operative surgeon must make a decision as to whether the fusion should be stopped at L5, which may necessitate future surgery, or carry the fusion to the sacrum, which would in turn lead to greater risk for perioperative complications.

## SUMMARY

Scoliosis is a progressive disease that is associated with significant back pain and decreased bone mass in most patients. Because both problems complicate the management of the neurogenic claudication, decompression is indicated for the symptoms of spinal stenosis, along with adequate stabilization and fusion. A correction of deformity can also be attempted, but it is technically very difficult and fraught with great hazard. The aim

## References

1. A.S. Kanter, A.R. Asthagiri, C.I. Shaffrey, Aging spine: challenges & emerging techniques: chap. 3, Clin. Neurol. 54 (2007) 10–18.
2. J.M. Spivak, Current concepts review: degenerative lumbar spinal stenosis, J. Bone Joint Surg. Am. 80 (1998) 1053–1066.
3. M. Aebi, The adult scoliosis, Eur. Spine J. 14 (2005) 925–948.
4. F. Schwab, J.P. Farcy, K. Bridwell, S. Berven, S. Glassman, J. Harrast, W. Horton, A clinical impact classification of scoliosis in the adult [deformity], Spine 31 (18) (2006) 2109–2114.

5. D.D. Frazier, S.J. Lipson, A.H. Fossel, J.N. Katz, Associations between spinal deformity and outcomes after decompression for spinal stenosis, Spine 22 (17) (1997) 2025–2029.

6. E.D. Simmons, Surgical treatment of patients with lumbar spinal stenosis with associated scoliosis , Clin. Orthop. Relat. Res. (348) (2001) 45–53.

7. A. Ploumis, E.E. Transfeldt, F. Denis, Degenerative lumbar scoliosis associated with spinal stenosis, Spine J. 7 (4) (2007) 428–436.

8. T.R. Kuklo, Principles for selecting fusion levels in adult spinal deformity with particular attention to lumbar curves and double major curves, Spine 31 (19 Suppl.) (2006) S132–S138.

9. R.R. Weiss, D. Goodall, Rate of Complications in Scoliosis Surgery-A Systematic Review of the Pub Med Literature. Scoliosis. 3(9)(2008) 1-18.

10. P. Guigui, A. Blamoutier. Complications of Surgical Treatment of Spinal Deformities: A Prospective Multicentric Study of 3311 Patients. Rev. Chir. Orthop. Reparatrice. Appar. Mot. (Groupe d'Etude de la Scoliose), 91(4)(2005) 314-327.

# 52

# A Case Study Approach to the Role of Spinal Deformity Correction in the Aging Spine

*Oheneba Boachie -Adjei and Satyajit Marawar*

**K E Y   P O I N T S**

- *Primary adult scoliosis:* De novo appearance of deformity in a previously straight adult spine resulting from degenerative disc disease, osteoporosis, or both.

- *Secondary adult scoliosis:* An untreated adolescent scoliotic curve that either continues to progress in adulthood or worsens because of superimposed degenerative changes.

- *Thoracic idiopathic curves* progress at 1° per year, thoracolumbar at 0.5° per year. Factors associated with curve progression include Cobb angle more than 30°, apical vertebral rotation more than 30%, presence of lateral olisthesis, and a poorly seated L5 vertebra over S1 in lumbar curves.

- Risk factors for progression of degenerative curves include lateral olisthesis, a high Harrington factor (Cobb angle divided by the number of vertebrae involved in the curve), and the disc index.

- Surgical indications and techniques vary and are patient-to-patient dependent. Relative indications include: (1) younger patients less than 50 years old who present with mostly untreated idiopathic curves that have progressed to greater than 50° to 60° and are painful and symptomatic, and (2) patients over the age of 50 with mostly degenerative curves or idiopathic curves worsened by superimposed degenerative changes. In these patients, surgery is most likely indicated for progressive deformities with sagittal or coronal plane imbalance, or refractory back or radicular pain with or without symptoms of spinal stenosis.

## INTRODUCTION

Adult scoliosis, by definition, is spinal deformity presenting in adult life. Adult scoliosis may be untreated adolescent idiopathic scoliosis that presents after skeletal maturity, or it may be a de novo spinal deformity in an adult. Thus adult thoracic or lumbar scoliosis can be classified as:

**Primary adult scoliosis:** de novo appearance of deformity in a previously straight adult spine resulting from degenerative disc disease, osteoporosis, or both.

**Secondary adult scoliosis:** an untreated adolescent scoliotic curve that either continues to progress in adulthood or worsens because of superimposed degenerative changes (Figure 52-1).

The incidence of adult scoliosis increases with age. In adults, right- and left-sided curves are equally prevalent. Unlike in adolescent scoliosis where cosmesis is the major issue, in adults, pain and disability present as significant problems in addition to the deformity. With increasing longevity and increasing expectations regarding physical activity and quality of life in older patients, increasing number of adult patients with symptomatic thoracolumbar deformity seek surgical treatment.

Adult degenerative deformity usually presents as a mild curve, which is rarely greater than 30 degrees unless it is superimposed on an adolescent-onset curve. Symptomatic lumbar curves tend to be larger in the idiopathic group than in the degenerative group.[1] Degenerative disc disease and osteoporosis are major contributing factors in adult-onset deformity. In these adult deformities, vertebral structural changes with lateral olisthesis are typically associated with degenerative disc and facet joint arthrosis. Adult deformity may also present as a sequela after a decompression for spinal stenosis or spinal fusion for degenerative disc disease. In primary as well as secondary deformities, the degenerative process plays a central role and leads to loss of lumbar lordosis, not infrequently progressing to thoracolumbar kyphosis.

## NATURAL HISTORY

### Idiopathic Curves

Untreated adolescent idiopathic curves are known to progress after skeletal maturity [2-4]. On long-term follow-up of patients with adolescent scoliosis at the University of Iowa, Weinstein et al reported that 68% of the curves progressed after maturity. Thoracic curves progressed at 1 degree per year, thoracolumbar at 0.5 degree per year. Factors associated with curve progression were Cobb angle greater than 30 degrees, apical vertebral rotation more than 30%, presence of lateral olisthesis, and a poorly seated L5 vertebra over S1 in lumbar curves [4].

### Degenerative Curves

Pritchett and Bortell reported on the natural history of degenerative scoliosis in 200 patients. The number of vertebrae involved in the curve were from 3 to 6 (mean 3), with the apex commonly located between L2 and L3, and with 68% of the curves being left-sided. While degenerative spondylolisthesis was noted in half the patients, lateral listhesis was even more common (78%). They found that all the curves with the intercrestal line passing through L5 or the L4-5 interspace with vertebral rotation of 2 or more on the Nash and Moe scale progressed, as did curves greater than 30 degrees with lateral listhesis of 6 mm or more [5].

Korovessis et al. followed up 91 adults with de novo spinal deformity for a period of 3.7 years. The average curve size was 16.5 degrees (range 10° to 36°). Risk factors for progression were lateral olisthesis, a high Harrington factor (the Cobb angle divided by the number of vertebrae involved in the curve), and the disc index [6]. In a similar study, Perennou et al. also reported a curve progression of 10 degrees or more in 73% of their patients over a follow-up period of 10 to 30 years, at an average of 3 degrees per year [7].

## IMAGING EVALUATION

Radiographic studies for diagnosis and evaluation of adult scoliosis include full-length standing radiographs, bending films, hyperextension films, CT myelograms, and MRI. Assessment of bone mineral density will provide information regarding the presence and severity of osteporosis.

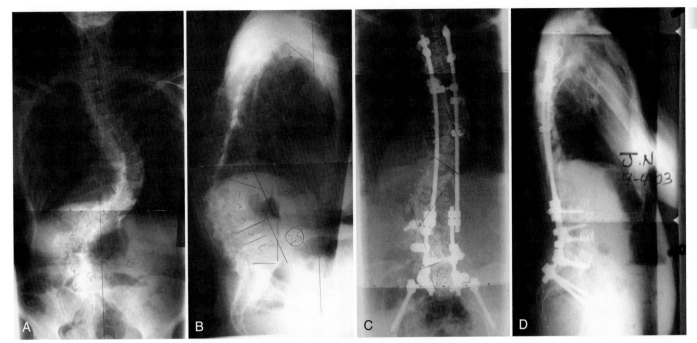

■ **FIGURE 52-1    A,** Preoperative standing AP radiograph of 63-year-old woman with progressive thoracic and lumbar scoliosis. **B,** Preoperative standing lateral image showing the loss of sagittal balance with thoracolumbar kyphosis. **C,** Postoperative standing AP image following anterior and posterior thoracolumbar sacral and pelvic fixation. Normal coronal balance. **D,** Postoperative standing lateral view shows restoration of sagittal balance and normal lumbar lordosis.

Standing radiographs with hips and knees in extension are necessary to evaluate the extent of the deformity and to assess sagittal and coronal balance. Supine side-bending radiographs may not be useful in degenerative scoliosis, but are useful in idiopathic scoliosis to assess curve rigidity and flexibility. Other options include traction views and fulcrum-bending views.[8] Curve location, curve magnitude, number of levels involved, curve direction, and rotation should be evaluated on the radiographs. The presence of anterolisthesis, the maximum lateral olisthesis, the height of the residual disc spaces, and the presence of osteoporotic compression fractures are the radiographic factors that impact curve progression.

Achievement of coronal and sagittal balance is more important in adults than correction of deformity. Coronal balance is defined by the distance of the C7 plumb line from the central sacral vertical line (CSVL) on standing radiographs. Lateral trunk shift (LTS) measurement is also useful in thoracolumbar curves and is defined as the distance between the midpoint of the horizontal line drawn to the edges of the ribs at the apex of the deformity and the CSVL. (Figure 52-2)

Global sagittal balance evaluation is essential, as this may have a major role in causation of symptoms in adult deformity. In adult scoliosis, the sagittal contour may vary from hyperlordosis to frank kyphosis. Sagittal vertical axis (SVA) measurement quantifies the global sagittal balance and is the distance of the C7 plumb line from the posterosuperior corner of the lumbosacral disc. The SVA usually falls anterior to the thoracic spine and passes posterior to the apex of the lumbar lordosis. Sagittal balance is considered positive when SVA falls anterior to the S1 body and negative when it falls posterior to the S1 body.

It is found that as lumbar lordosis reduces with progressive disc degeneration, the sacropelvis rotates posteriorly, leading to a vertical sacral inclination with hip extension. In the presence of hip flexion contractures, this compensatory mechanism may be compromised, leading to worsening of sagittal imbalance.

Patients with radiculopathy, with or without neurological deficit, and patients with neurogenic claudication should be evaluated with an MRI or a postmyelogram computed tomography scan. MRI can provide detailed information about central, lateral recess, and foraminal stenosis. The extent of disc degeneration can be assessed on MRI, which may be helpful with decision-making regarding the extent of fusion.

CT myelogram with sagittal and coronal reconstructions provides better bony details in cases of severe rotational deformity or in the presence of metal implants. Diskography is usually not beneficial in adult scoliosis for determining levels of fusion.

## THE ROLE OF CONSERVATIVE MANAGEMENT

A commonly described prerequisite to surgical intervention is the lack of response to conservative care. Even though multiple nonsurgical options are advocated for adult scoliosis, there is currently a lack of evidence in the literature regarding the efficacy of these treatment options. Everett et al reviewed the literature on nonsurgical treatment options for adult scoliosis. They concluded that in the conservative treatment of adult deformity, there is level IV evidence for the role of physical therapy, bracing, and chiropractic care, while there is level III evidence for injections.[9]

Still, most surgeons would attempt nonsurgical treatment as the first option. The goal of conservative treatment is pain relief, and any safe conservative care option that a patient can use to obtain relief reasonable. At the least, this is likely to improve the conditioning of the patient and promote weight loss, which may eventually improve the surgical outcome.

## INDICATIONS FOR SURGERY

Adult scoliosis patients fall into two broad categories when they present as surgical candidates. The first category is that of younger patients less than 50 years old, who mostly present with untreated idiopathic curves that have progressed to greater than 50 to 60 degrees and have become painful and symptomatic. Chronic, disabling pain refractory to conservative management and/or significant and cosmetically unacceptable deformity are indications for surgery.

The second category is that of patients over the age of 50, who present mostly with degenerative curves or with idiopathic curves worsened by superimposed degenerative changes. In these patients, surgery is most likely to be indicated for progressive deformities with sagittal or coronal plane imbalance, or for refractory back or radicular pain with or without symptoms of spinal stenosis. Although compromised pulmonary function has also been suggested as an indication, Korvessis et al did not find any difference in pulmonary function in adult scoliosis patients compared with age-related changes in normal persons at an average of 23 years follow-up.[6]

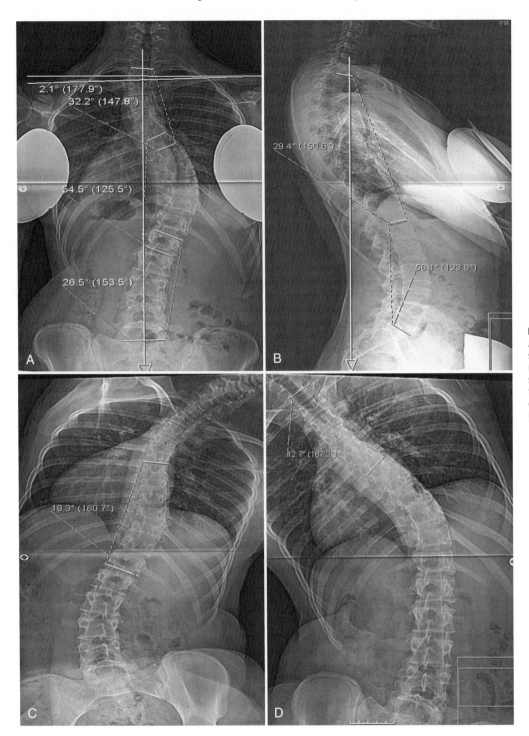

■ **FIGURE 52-2** **A,** Preoperative AP radiograph of single thoracic scoliosis. **B,** Preoperative lateral image with no obvious sagittal deformity. **C,** Right side-bend. Moderate thoracic curve flexibility. **D,** Left side-bend shows complete improvement in lumbar compensatory curve.

## SURGICAL PLANNING

A multitude of factors impact surgical decision-making in this patient population. Achievement of coronal and sagittal balance is the most important goal for many patients. A balanced spine orients the skull so that it is placed over the pelvis. This reduces paraspinal muscle fatigue and pain, improves patient satisfaction, improves cosmesis, and reduces the risk of complications associated with persistent decompensation in the sagittal or coronal plane. A well-balanced spine in the sagittal plane has been found to correlate with a better self-image score in adult deformity patients.[10] While extensive surgery might be required to achieve an adequately decompressed and well-balanced spine, the individual surgical plan needs to be matched with the overall health, medical fitness, and expectations from surgery for every patient. Medical and social factors that are known to correlate with poor

outcome are nutritional deficiency,[11] chronic respiratory conditions,[12] diabetes,[13] smoking,[14,15] coronary or cerebrovascular artery disease, and osteoporosis.[16] Osteopenia is a major concern, especially if significant deformity correction is one of the goals. Segmental fixation can create a large surface area for force transmission and possibly prevent fixation failure. Medical treatment of osteoporosis with daily subcutaneous injections of parathyroid hormone for 2 to 6 weeks has been shown to enhance spinal fusion, in animal models.[17,18]

If an anterior and posterior fusion is planned, a same-day procedure is preferable to a staged procedure, as nutritional status has been found to take 6 to 12 weeks to return to the baseline after posterior surgery.[19] Use of parenteral nutrition has been advocated if a staged procedure is planned, to improve the nutritional status before the second stage.[20]

## The Role of Decompression Only in Adult Scoliosis Surgery

In carefully selected patients with degenerative scoliosis, performing a decompression alone without an instrumented fusion may be an option. If the patient presents with symptoms of neurogenic claudication and minimal back pain, it is possible that the patient will get relief with a trial of epidural steroids. If such patients have collapsed disc spaces without any evidence of anterolisthesis or lateral listhesis, they can be treated with decompression alone or decompression with an in situ fusion without instrumentation. Frazier et al. assessed the relationship between preoperative scoliosis and clinical outcome after a decompression only procedure for spinal stenosis in 90 patients with degenerative scoliosis. They inferred that the presence of preoperative scoliosis was associated with less improvement in back pain in these patients postoperatively; however, there was no correlation between preoperative scoliosis and satisfaction or improvement in leg pain and walking capacity after a decompression-only procedure [21].

## The Role of Deformity Correction and Fusion

The natural history of adult deformity has been detailed earlier. The role of deformity in the causation of symptoms is not entirely clear. However, it is important to understand these issues to analyze the role of deformity correction in the treatment of adult scoliosis.

## The Role of Deformity in the Clinical Presentation

Early studies indicated that the incidence of back pain in adult scoliosis patients is about the same as in age-matched controls. Kostuik found a 60% incidence of back pain in adult patients with scoliosis, which was similar to that noted in patients without spinal deformity [22]. In other studies, patients with adult scoliosis were found to have more severe back pain as compared to controls, especially if the curve progressed beyond 45 degrees [23]. In more recent studies, Weinstein et al. have reported that chronic back pain was present in 61% of the scoliotic patients as compared to 35% of the controls [24]. Schwab et al. found a highly significant correlation between the severity of pain in adult scoliosis patients and the presence of lateral olisthesis and obliquity of L3 and L4 endplates on plain radiographs [1]. Jackson et al. had found the fractional lumbosacral curves most disabling and painful. They reported that while scoliosis greater than 40 degrees and kyphosis greater than 50 degrees correlated with pain, rotational deformity had the highest correlation with pain [25]. More recently, Buttermann et al. analyzed the correlation between degenerative disc findings on MRI with pain in scoliosis patients. In adult scoliosis patients, they found that the pain typically corresponded to the apex of the curve or to the lumbosacral junction. They found a higher incidence of disc degeneration and inflammatory end plate changes in adult scoliotics than asymptomatic controls. When compared with symptomatic patients with disc degeneration without a deformity, adults with scoliosis had a higher incidence of disc degeneration and inflammatory end plate changes at proximal lumbar levels (T12 – L3) [26].

The role of osteoporosis in the causation of adult deformity is well known. Osteoporotic fractures may cause pain, in addition to their contribution to the deformity. Radicular pain in the lower extremities is caused by degenerative changes in adult scoliosis. Root entrapment is more common in the concavity of the curve [7,25]. In 200 patients with adult scoliosis, Pritchett et al. had found a 72% incidence of neurogenic claudication and a 45% incidence of neurological symptoms in the lower limbs, most commonly paresthesias [5].

Spinal balance in sagittal and coronal plane can be adversely affected in adult scoliosis. Poor spinal balance is known to worsen the functional status in these patients, and can be quite disabling. Pain in adult scoliosis may arise from muscle fatigue due to abnormal biomechanics caused by the deformed and poorly balanced spine. Glassman et al studied the impact of spinal balance on clinical symptoms in 298 adult scoliosis patients with or without prior surgery. They reported that positive sagittal balance led to greater pain, poor function, and poor self image in patients with or without prior surgery while coronal balance of more than 4 cm correlated with greater pain and poor function. Additionally, the severity of symptoms was found to increase linearly with worsening sagittal imbalance. In terms of location, thoracic curves were better tolerated than thoracolumbar or lumbar curves; however, the magnitude of the curve had a poor correlation with functional status [27,28]. In patients with adult degenerative lumbar or thoracolumbar scoliosis, Ploumis et al. reported that coronal imbalance more than 5 cm affected bodily function and moderate to severe lateral olisthesis (more than 6 mm) correlated with higher bodily pain, while sagittal balance did not show a good correlation with functional results [29]. In another study, positive sagittal balance (C7 plumbline more than 6 cm) in patients with adult scoliosis has been correlated with worse Oswestry Disability Index scores (ODI), while there was no correlation found between ODI and coronal imbalance. However none of the patients in this study had coronal imbalance worse than 4 cm [30]. Loss of lumbar lordosis and thoracolumbar kyphosis have also been found to have a positive correlation with self-reported pain scores in adult scoliosis patients [1].

In addition to pain and spinal balance abnormalities, adult deformity can lead to significant body image and cosmesis issues. Deformity has been known to promote a negative body image, which can lead to difficulties in physical functioning and social interaction. Body image is known to be a significant issue with scoliosis patients [31,32] Psychosocial studies in adult scoliosis patients have reveled difficulties in social and intimate relationships due to physical difficulties in participation, fear of injury, or self-consciousness [33-35] . Attempts have been made to correlate radiographic deformity parameters with health-related quality of life (HRQL) and body image score in adult deformity patients. Except for the sagittal profile, other radiographic measures are found to correlate poorly with HRQL and body image scores in adults [1,27,33]. Walter Reed Visual Assessment Score (WRVAS) is a visual scale for patients' assessment of deformity. It has been suggested that, in adults, the WRVAS is a more accurate reflection of the impact of scoliosis deformity on patient body image and HRQL than radiographic indicators. Tones et al. reported that the items of the WRVAS shared a consistent negative correlation with the Physical Functioning, Vitality, and General Health subscales of the SF-36v2, and the Physical Component Summary score in adult scoliosis patients. They also reported that older participants perceived their deformities as more severe than younger participants [26,36].

The importance of these issues from the patients' perspective is exemplified by postoperative outcome studies in patients who have surgical correction of the deformity. Bridwell et al. had used SRS 22, ODI and SF-12 to assess outcome after surgery in 56 adult scoliosis patients at 1- and 2-year follow-up. They concluded based on these scores that surgical treatment significantly improved pain, self image, and function. They found that the greatest responsiveness to the change after surgery was demonstrated by self image domain, then the SRS total score and pain scores [37].

## SURGICAL TECHNIQUES

### Posterior Instrumentation

Posterior fusion and instrumentation is the most common method used in adult deformity correction. Most surgeons are familiar with the approach and comfortable with the procedure. It allows decompression of the stenotic levels and correction of deformity in all three planes. Usually, segmental instrumentation using pedicle screws and hooks or all screws is preferred, as this creates a large area of force transmission during correction of the deformity [38]. Traditionally sublaminar wires, hooks, and pedicle screws have been used for deformity correction and segmental fixation either individually or in different combinations. All–pedicle-screw constructs are becoming more popular for deformity correction. Although some studies have found that sublaminar wires with hooks provide similar or sometimes better coronal plane correction, [39,40] multiple studies have found that pedicle screw constructs offer better correction, better long-term durability of correction, better rotational correction, improved pulmonary function values, and lesser blood loss than hybrid constructs [39,41,42]. Additionally, pedicle screws provide three column fixation, have better pullout strength, [43] and improve the ability to maintain and enhance lumbar lordosis. [44] Pedicle screw constructs are, however, significantly costlier [42]. (Figure 52-3)

### Anterior Release or Anterior-Only Surgery

Many studies have documented that anterior release is not necessary in most patients with adolescent idiopathic scoliosis even if the curves are larger than 70 degrees, especially when adequate posterior release is

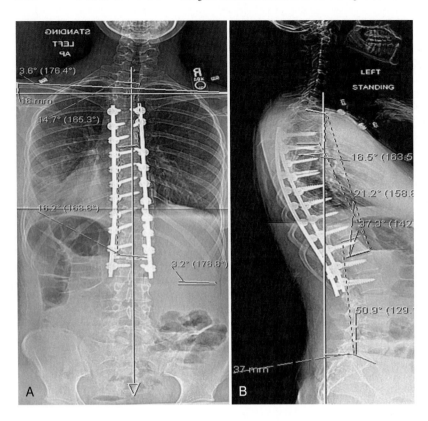

■ **FIGURE 52-3   A,** Postoperative AP radiograph after posterior spine fusion and segmental instrumentation with pedicle screw construct. **B,** Postoperative lateral image. Normal sagittal alignment.

performed and posterior instrumentation using an all–pedicle-screw construct is utilized.[45-47] However, adult scoliosis is a pathologically different entity. Due to superimposition of the degenerative process, curves are more rigid, and the presence of rotatory olisthesis at multiple levels compounds the coronal plane deformity. Additionally, the presence of thoracolumbar kyphosis may make it difficult to achieve sagittal and coronal balance with a posterior-only procedure. So, traditionally, an anterior spinal release has been proposed for the treatment of adult lumbar spinal deformities,[48-51] which is to be followed by posterior instrumentation and fusion.

Anterior release would aid deformity correction by release of the anterior longitudinal ligament and an adequate diskectomy. Also, the addition of interbody structural grafts after diskectomy could improve the sagittal alignment. The addition of anterior release could also provide a 360° fusion. These benefits come at the cost of an additional thoracolumbar procedure or a retroperitoneal procedure, which has its own set of complications in this patient population, as has been reported recently.[52] This has led to questioning the necessity of anterior release in all patients with adult scoliosis and the suitability of using a posterior-only procedure in well-selected cases based on flexibility of the curves and sagittal balance. With successful reports of use of posterior-only procedures in larger curves in adolescents, there are also reports of the use of segmental third-generation instrumentation to correct adult deformities in posterior-only procedures. Earlier reports indicate use of posterior-only procedure in flexible adult curves.[53] More recently, Kim et al reported a retrospective, comparative study of radiographic and functional outcomes with and without an anterior apical release of the lumbar curve in adult scoliosis patients. On comparing the two groups, it was found that the surgeons chose to do an anterior procedure in curves with larger Cobb angles and less flexibility. At follow-up, there was no significant difference in the two groups in terms of correction achieved, lumbar lordosis, thoracic kyphosis, coronal balance, and sagittal balance. The clinical outcome as measured by SRS-22 scores was better in the posterior-only group.[54] Use of minimally invasive techniques like extreme lateral interbody fusion[55] may reduce the morbidity of a multilevel anterior procedure and may increase the acceptability of an anterior procedure in this patient population. Even though this procedure has been performed in some institutes for anterior diskectomy fusion in adult scoliosis, as yet there are no reports in the literature (Figure 52-4).

Another option in these patients with flexible double major or thoracolumbar curves can be a hybrid fusion where partially overlapping anterior and posterior instrumentation is used. This has been tried in our institute in recent years. In this procedure, anterior instrumentation is placed in the form of vertebral body screws with either one or two rods extending from the lower thoracic spine to either the L3 or L4 level. Anterior diskectomy is performed and structural grafts or cages are used in the lumbar region. Following this, the thoracolumbar portion of the curve is corrected using a rod rotation maneuver while at the same time putting the rod into lordosis. The anterior procedure is completed by segmental compression, going away from the apex proximally and distally. The posterior procedure involves only a posterior fusion extending from either L3 or L4 to S1, so as to overlap the levels of the anterior fusion. This instrumentation design may spare the proximal spinal fusion levels and does not require instrumentation or fusion to the pelvis. In an initial cohort of 10 patients, it has been shown to provide similar correction with similar complication rates to a posterior-only or a traditional anterior and posterior procedure.[56]

## Extent of Fusion

The possibility of coronal and sagittal imbalance in adults is high because curves are stiffer. The extent of fusion needs to be decided carefully after considering the extent of the curves, the flexibility of the curves, and the sagittal and coronal balance.

In case of lumbar or thoracolumbar curves, the ideal construct length remains unclear. However, there are a few well-recognized rules. It is useful preoperatively to identify which segments contribute to the patient's pain. The apex of the deformity with any areas of lateral listhesis should be included. There is no general consensus about where the construct should end rostrally. Usually, the upper instrumented vertebra should be a stable one. The construct should not terminate at the apex of a kyphosis or apex of a curve in the coronal plane. Some earlier studies had recommended avoiding L1 or L2 as proximal fusion levels and considering extension to the thoracic spine, to avoid termination of fusion at the thoracolumbar junction with possible junctional failure.[57,58] However, more recently, Kim et al. reported a retrospective study comparing the prevalence of revision surgeries and proximal junctional change after instrumented fusion from T9, T11, or L1 to L5 or S1. They reported a significantly high incidence of

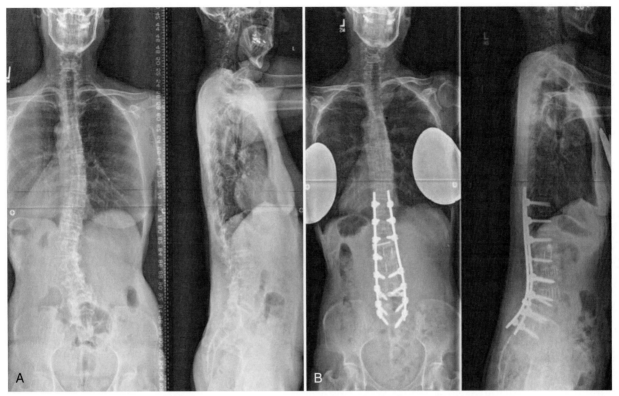

■ **FIGURE 52-4** **A,** Preoperative AP and lateral radiographs of a 62-year-old woman with degenerative scoliosis. **B,** Postoperative AP and lateral images after anterior interbody fusion using minimally invasive lateral approach technique and posterior segmental instrumentation.

proximal junctional kyphosis; however, there was no significant difference in the proximal junctional angulation or revision rates in the three groups based on the proximal extent of fusion.[59] They opined that a more distal proximal fusion level at a neutral and stable vertebra, regardless of whether the construct ends at the distal thoracic spine or proximal lumbar spine should be used as the radiographic outcome, and revision rates are similar.

It has been suggested before that in selected cases of lumbar degenerative scoliosis, fusion can be performed within the scoliotic curve restricted to the levels that are decompressed instead of fusing to the end vertebrae proximally. Kyu et al reported that such short fusion within the curve might be sufficient for curves with a smaller Cobb angle and good spinal balance. They reported a significantly lower value for average Cobb correction and average correction of coronal imbalance and a higher incidence of proximal junctional failure in the patients with short fusion. The rate of early complications and distal junctional failure was higher in patients with longer fusions. They reported that the clinical outcome as measured by improvement in the ODI was similar between the two groups.[60]

In cases of double thoracic and lumbar curve, the goal of surgery is to achieve global balance and provide pain relief by obtaining a good fusion. Achieving sagittal balance is the most important goal, followed by correction of coronal imbalance, rotational deformities, rib hump, and shoulder asymmetry for cosmetic concerns. The extent of instrumentation should include the whole of thoracic curve proximally, as adult thoracic deformities tend to be stiff. In case of severe and stiff deformities, an anterior diskectomy and fusion procedure preceding posterior instrumentation may be required to achieve adequate sagittal and coronal balance.

## Extension of Fusion to the Sacrum

The distal extent of fusion in adult deformity is most commonly near the lumbosacral junction. The surgeon needs to answer the question of whether the need for fusion to sacrum is worth the risk of complications that have been found to be associated with ending a long fusion at S1. The current literature does not provide any definitive answers. It is generally recommended that fusion to S1 should be considered when there is significant degeneration at L5-S1, obliquity of the L5-S1 disc (greater than 15°), stenosis at L5-S1

requiring decompression, previous decompression at L5-S1, and spondylolisthesis at L5-S1.[61] However, long fusions to the sacrum may require longer time, involve more blood loss, and have been found more likely to develop complications and require more additional surgical procedures.[62,63] Especially, the risk of pseudarthrosis at L5-S1 in long fusions has been reported to be as high as 24%.[64,65] Kim et al. reported that factors that increased the risk of pseudarthrosis at L5-S1 were thoracolumbar kyphosis (T10-L2 > 20° vs. < 20°), osteoarthritis of hip joints, thoracoabdominal approach, positive sagittal balance greater than or equal to 5 cm postoperatively, age at surgery older than 55 years, and incomplete sacropelvic fixation.[64] Additionally, there is a small but real risk of development of sacral insufficiency fractures after long fusions to the sacrum.[66]

Recently, there have been reports comparing the complications and outcome in adult deformity patients with fusion to L5 to those with fusion to S1. Edwards et al compared complications, radiographic parameters, and functional outcomes in matched cohorts of patients with adult deformity that underwent long fusions from the thoracic spine to either L5 or the sacrum at a minimum 2-year follow-up. They found that the correction of sagittal imbalance was superior for patients fused to the sacrum (C7 plumb line: L5 0.9 cm, sacrum 3.2 cm, P = 0.03), and, on follow-up, they tend to maintain sagittal balance better than those with fusion to L5. At latest follow-up, 67% of patients with fusion to L5 had radiographic evidence of advanced L5-S1 disc degeneration, which may explain the worsening of sagittal balance in these patients. The sacrum cohort, however, required more surgical procedures and experienced a greater frequency of major complications (L5 22%, sacrum 75%, P = 0.02), including nonunion (L5 4%, sacrum 42%, P = 0.006) and medical morbidity (L5 0%, sacrum 33%, P = 0.001). SRS-24 scores reflected a similar patient assessment of outcome and function for the two cohorts.[67] Cho et al compared the results of fusion to L5 to those for fusion to the sacrum in patients with adult degenerative scoliosis. They found that the duration of surgery and blood loss was not significantly different in the two groups. The correction of lumbar lordosis was better in patients fused to the sacrum; however, the ultimate change in sagittal and coronal balance was similar in both groups. On follow-up, 58% of the patients with fusion to L5 developed advanced disc degeneration at L5-S1. They found that patients with preoperative sagittal imbalance

(C7 plumb line greater than 5 cm) and lumbar hypolordosis (lordosis less than 30°) are more likely to develop symptomatic L5-S1 disc degeneration when fusion to L5 is performed. [68] Kuhns et al specifically evaluated the fate of the L5-S1 disc at a minimum follow-up of 5 years in patients with long deformity fusions to L5. They found that advanced disc degeneration developed in 69% of the patients who had healthy L5-S1 discs before surgery, with 23% requiring extension of fusion to the sacrum later, while a further 19% had indications for extension of fusion to the sacrum but either had comorbidities precluding surgery or declined further surgery. They reported that the risk factors of development of advanced disc degeneration at L5-S1 were long fusion extending to the upper thoracic spine and having a circumferential lumbar fusion [69] (Figures 52-5, 52-6).

## The Role of Osteotomies and Spinal Column Shortening in Adult Deformity Patients

Osteotomies are required to achieve sagittal and coronal balance in severe adult deformities when the flexibility of the deformity would not allow acceptable correction with instrumentation alone. More commonly, osteotomies are used to correct sagittal imbalance. The osteotomies utilized commonly are the Smith-Peterson osteotomy (SPO) and the pedicle subtraction osteotomy (PSO). Smith-Peterson described the osteotomy in which a chevron-shaped wedge of bone is removed from the posterior elements. [70] Correction is achieved by closing this wedge and opening the disc space anteriorly. The axis of rotation is located at the posterior disc space.

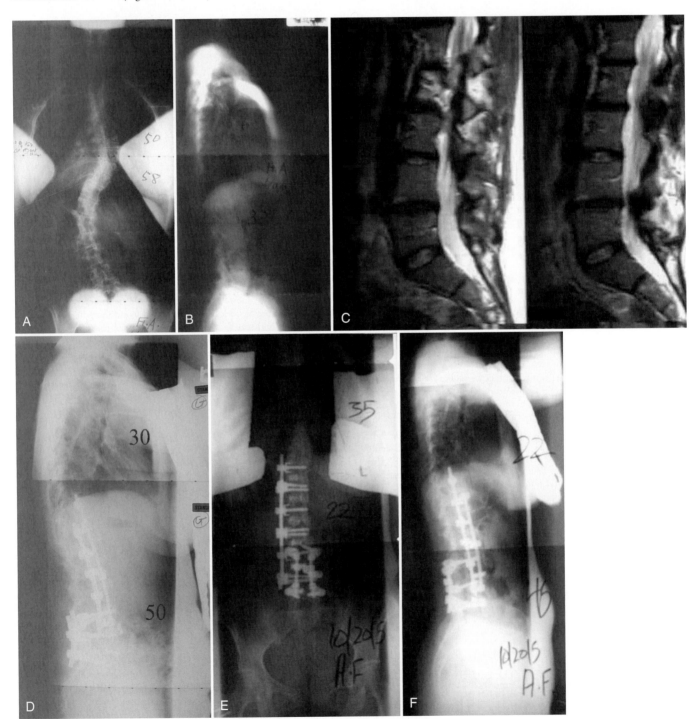

■ **FIGURE 52-5**   **A, B,** Preoperative AP and lateral radiographs of 53-year-old woman with progressive painful lumbar scoliosis. Loss of lumbar lordosis is present in the lateral radiograph. **C,** MRI shows degenerative disc disease and normal appearing L5-S1 discs. **D – F,** Postoperative standing AP and lateral radiographs following anterior fusion and instrumentation of the lumbar curve and short posterior overlapping fixation. Note restoration of lumbar lordosis.

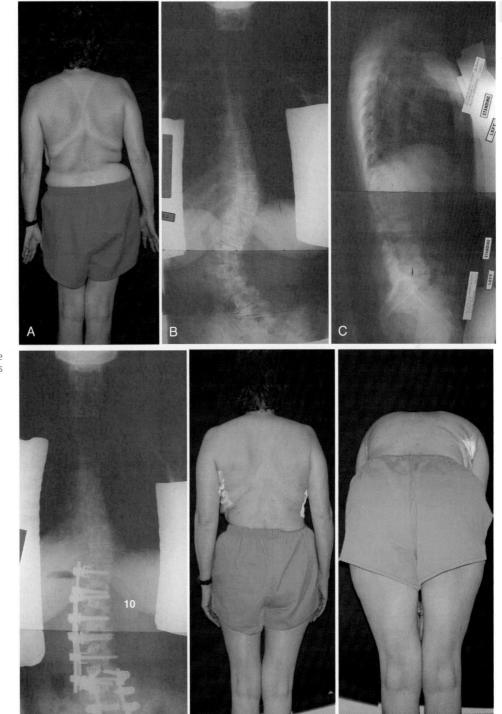

■ **FIGURE 52-6   A-E,** Preoperative and postoperative clinical photographs show balance correction and fusion.

Sagittal correction up to 15 degrees per level can be achieved with SPO. However, the lengthening of the anterior column is associated with the risk of vascular and neurologic complications.[71-73] Also, it may create an anterior bony defect that may make arthrodesis difficult.

PSO is a V-shaped wedge resection of the vertebral body along with the pedicles and posterior elements. It was described by Thomasen for treating kyphotic deformities in ankylosing spondylitis.[74] This osteotomy hinges about an axis at the anterior vertebral body. It enables shortening of the vertebral column posteriorly and causes no lengthening anteriorly, reducing the risk of vascular injuries. It provides a more stable correction, as closure of the osteotomy closes the gap posteriorly. This osteotomy can achieve an average correction of 30 to 40 degrees at a single segment and is useful for correcting high-grade fixed sagittal deformities.[75-77] Kim et al reported on the outcome of 35 consecutive patients who underwent pedicle subtraction osteotomies at a minimum 5-year follow-up. They reported 76% improvement in self-image scores, 66% improvement in pain scores, and 69% improvement in function scores at ultimate follow-up. Patients who maintained a sagittal vertical axis of less than 8 cm continued to have good SRS scores, while those with a sagittal vertical axis greater than or equal to 8 cm had worsening of self-image and function scores.[78] Cho et al compared the clinical and radiographic outcome in patients who underwent SPO to those who underwent a PSO. They reported that the mean correction of the kyphotic angle at the osteotomy site after an SPO was 10.7 degrees. They compared the radiographic outcome after three or more SPOs to that

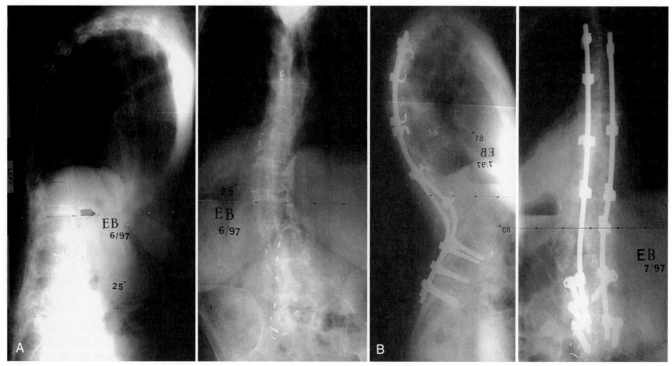

■ **FIGURE 52-7** **A,** Preoperative AP and lateral radiographs of 56-year-old with sagittal imbalance after multiple spine procedures. **B,** Postoperative AP and lateral films following pedicle subtraction osteotomy and instrumentation with restoration of sagittal balance.

after a single-level PSO to evaluate whether they were comparable. They found that even though the average correction in both groups was close to 30 degrees, the improvement in sagittal balance was, statistically, significantly less with three or more SPOs (5.5 ± 4.5 cm) than with a single-level PSO (11.2 ± 7.2 cm). Also, patients with multiple SPOs showed significantly more decompensation toward concavity. The mean estimated blood loss was significantly higher in patients with a PSO than with multiple SPOs.[79] Rose et al analyzed the role of pelvic incidence (PI) and thoracic kyphosis (TK) in predicting the ideal lumbar lordosis (LL) required to achieve sagittal balance in patients undergoing a PSO. They found that the formula PI + LL + TK ≤ 45° showed 91% sensitivity in predicting ideal sagittal balance. They also reported that patients with fusion to the upper thoracic spine after a PSO preserved correction better than those with fusion to the thoracolumbar region.[80] (Figure 52-7).

## SUMMARY

Patients with adult scoliosis more commonly present with pain and worsening balance as major issues, unlike adolescent scoliosis patients who present with cosmesis as the major concern. Conservative treatment has not been shown to be of any reliable long-term benefit in adult patients with symptomatic scoliosis. There are multiple surgical options for these patients; however, surgical planning should be customized to the patient based on clinical presentation, sagittal and coronal profile, curve flexibility, and medical comorbidities. Requirement for anterior release, extent of fusion proximally, inclusion of the sacrum in the construct, and the requirement for osteotomies are some of the major questions that need to be answered during surgical planning. Based on the current literature, restoration of sagittal and coronal balance is the most important factor for predicting a good surgical outcome in these patients.

## References

1. F.J. Schwab, V.A. Smith, M. Biserni, L. Gamez, J.P. Farcy, M. Pagala, Adult scoliosis: a quantitative radiographic and clinical analysis, Spine 27 (4) (2002) 387–392.
2. S.L. Chuah, B.A. Kareem, K. Selvakumar, K.S. Oh, A. Borhan Tan, S. Harwant, The natural history of scoliosis: curve progression of untreated curves of different aetiology, with early (mean 2 year) follow up in surgically treated curves, Med. J. Malaysia 56 (Suppl C) (2001) 37–40.
3. E. Ascani, P. Bartolozzi, C.A. Logroscino, et al., Natural history of untreated idiopathic scoliosis after skeletal maturity, Spine 11 (8) (1986) 784–789.
4. S.L. Weinstein, I.V. Ponseti, Curve progression in idiopathic scoliosis, J. Bone Joint Surg. Am. 65 (4) (1983) 447–455.
5. J.W. Pritchett, D.T. Bortel, Degenerative symptomatic lumbar scoliosis, Spine 18 (6) (1993) 700–703.
6. P. Korovessis, G. Piperos, P. Sidiropoulos, A. Dimas, Adult idiopathic lumbar scoliosis. A formula for prediction of progression and review of the literature, Spine 19 (17) (1994) 1926–1932.
7. D. Perennou, C. Marcelli, C. Herisson, L. Simon, Adult lumbar scoliosis. Epidemiologic aspects in a low-back pain population, Spine 19 (2) (1994) 123–128.
8. K.D. Luk, K.M. Cheung, D.S. Lu, J.C. Leong, Assessment of scoliosis correction in relation to flexibility using the fulcrum bending correction index, Spine 23 (21) (1998) 2303–2307.
9. C.R. Everett, R.K. Patel, A systematic literature review of nonsurgical treatment in adult scoliosis, Spine 32 (Suppl. 19) (2007) S130–S134.
10. Y. Kim, K. Bridwell, L. Lenke, O. Boachie-Adjei, S. Marawar, What radiographic sagittal parameters correlate with improved SRS self-image scores postoperatively in patients with sagittal imbalance? Analysis of 102 lumbar pedicle subtraction osteotomy patients, Spine J. 8 (5), (Suppl. 1) (2008) 29S–30S.
11. J.D. Klein, L.A. Hey, C.S. Yu, et al., Perioperative nutrition and postoperative complications in patients undergoing spinal surgery, Spine 21 (22) (1996) 2676–2682.
12. G.W. Smetana, Preoperative pulmonary evaluation [see comment], N. Engl. J. Med. 340 (12) (1999) 937–944.
13. V.K. Moitra, S.E. Meiler, The diabetic surgical patient, Curr. Opin. Anaesthesiol. 19 (3) (2006) 339–345.
14. M.A. Warner, K.P. Offord, M.E. Warner, R.L. Lennon, M.A. Conover, U. Jansson-Schumacher, Role of preoperative cessation of smoking and other factors in postoperative pulmonary complications: a blinded prospective study of coronary artery bypass patients, Mayo. Clin. Proc. 64 (6) (1989) 609–616.
15. J.M. Mok, J.M. Cloyd, D.S. Bradford, S.S. Hu, V.S. Deviren, A. Jason, B.B. Tay, H. Sigurd, Reoperation after primary fusion for adult spinal deformity: rate, reason, and timing, Spine 34 (8) (2009) 832–839.
16. J.T. Lin, J.M. Lane, Osteoporosis: a review, Clin Orthop (425) (2004) 126–134.
17. P.F. O'Loughlin, M.E. Cunningham, S.V. Bukata, et al., Parathyroid hormone (1-34) augments spinal fusion, fusion mass volume, and fusion mass quality in a rabbit spinal fusion model, Spine 34 (2) (2009) 121–130.
18. Y. Abe, M. Takahata, M. Ito, K. Irie, K. Abumi, A. Minami, Enhancement of graft bone healing by intermittent administration of human parathyroid hormone (1-34) in a rat spinal arthrodesis model, Bone 41 (5) (2007) 775–785.
19. L.G. Lenke, K.H. Bridwell, K. Blanke, C. Baldus, Prospective analysis of nutritional status normalization after spinal reconstructive surgery, Spine 20 (12) (1995) 1359–1367.
20. S.S. Hu, F. Fontaine, B. Kelly, D.S. Bradford, Nutritional depletion in staged spinal reconstructive surgery. The effect of total parenteral nutrition, Spine 23 (12) (1998) 1401–1405.
21. D.D. Frazier, S.J. Lipson, A.H. Fossel, J.N. Katz, Associations between spinal deformity and outcomes after decompression for spinal stenosis, Spine 22 (17) (1997) 2025–2029.
22. J.P. Kostuik, J. Bentivoglio, The incidence of low-back pain in adult scoliosis, Spine 6 (3) (1981) 268–273.

23. J.L. Briard, D. Jegou, J. Cauchoix, Adult lumbar scoliosis, Spine 4 (6) (1979) 526–532.

24. S.L. Weinstein, L.A. Dolan, K.F. Spratt, K.K. Peterson, M.J. Spoonamore, Health and function of patients with untreated idiopathic scoliosis: a 50-year natural history study, JAMA 289 (5) (2003) 559–567.

25. R.P. Jackson, E.H. Simmons, D. Stripinis, Coronal and sagittal plane spinal deformities correlating with back pain and pulmonary function in adult idiopathic scoliosis, Spine 14 (12) (1989) 1391–1397.

26. G.R. Buttermann, W.J. Mullin, Pain and disability correlated with disc degeneration via magnetic resonance imaging in scoliosis patients, Eur. Spine J. 17 (2) (2008) 240–249.

27. S.D. Glassman, S. Berven, K. Bridwell, W. Horton, J.R. Dimar, Correlation of radiographic parameters and clinical symptoms in adult scoliosis, Spine 30 (6) (2005) 682–688.

28. S.D. Glassman, K. Bridwell, J.R. Dimar, W. Horton, S. Berven, F. Schwab, The impact of positive sagittal balance in adult spinal deformity, Spine 30 (18) (2005) 2024–2029.

29. A. Ploumis, H. Liu, A.A. Mehbod, E.E. Transfeldt, R.B. Winter, A correlation of radiographic and functional measurements in adult degenerative scoliosis, Spine 34 (15) (2009) 1581–1584.

30. J.T. Mac-Thiong, E. Ensor, A.A. Mehbod, J.H. Perra, et al., Can C7 plumbline and gravity line predict health related quality of life in adult scoliosis?[miscellaneous article], Spine 34 (15) (2009) E519–E527.

31. N. Rumsey, D. Harcourt, Body image and disfigurement: issues and interventions, Body Image 1 (2004) 83–97.

32. M.A. Asher, D.C. Burton, Adolescent idiopathic scoliosis: natural history and long term treatment effects, Scoliosis 1 (1) (2006) 2.

33. S.L. Weinstein, L.A. Dolan, K.F. Spratt, K.K. Peterson, M.J. Spoonamore, I.V. Ponseti, Health and function of patients with untreated idiopathic scoliosis: a 50-year natural history study, JAMA 289 (5) (2003) 559–567.

34. A.J. Danielsson, A.L. Nachemson, Childbearing, curve progression, and sexual function in women 22 years after treatment for adolescent idiopathic scoliosis: a case-control study, Spine 26 (13) (2001) 1449–1456.

35. A.J. Danielsson, I. Wiklund, K. Pehrsson, A.L. Nachemson, Health-related quality of life in patients with adolescent idiopathic scoliosis: a matched follow-up at least 20 years after treatment with brace or surgery, Eur. Spine J. 10 (4) (2001) 278–288.

36. M. Tones, N. Moss, The impact of patient self assessment of deformity on HRQL in adults with scoliosis, Scoliosis 2 (2007) 14.

37. K.H. Bridwell, S. Berven, S. Glassman, et al., Is the SRS-22 instrument responsive to change in adult scoliosis patients having primary spinal deformity surgery? Spine 32 (20) (2007) 2220–2225.

38. D.S. Bradford, B.K. Tay, S.S. Hu, Adult scoliosis: surgical indications, operative management, complications, and outcomes, Spine 24 (24) (1999) 2617–2629.

39. O. Karatoprak, K. Unay, M. Tezer, C. Ozturk, M. Aydogan, C. Mirzanli, Comparative analysis of pedicle screw versus hybrid instrumentation in adolescent idiopathic scoliosis surgery, Int. Orthop. 32 (4) (2008) 523–528.

40. I. Cheng, Y. Kim, M.C. Gupta, et al., Apical sublaminar wires versus pedicle screws—which provides better results for surgical correction of adolescent idiopathic scoliosis? Spine 30 (18) (2005) 2104–2112.

41. Y.J. Kim, L.G. Lenke, S.K. Cho, K.H. Bridwell, B. Sides, K. Blanke, Comparative analysis of pedicle screw versus hook instrumentation in posterior spinal fusion of adolescent idiopathic scoliosis, Spine 29 (18) (2004) 2040–2048.

42. Y.J. Kim, L.G. Lenke, J. Kim, et al., Comparative analysis of pedicle screw versus hybrid instrumentation in posterior spinal fusion of adolescent idiopathic scoliosis, Spine 31 (3) (2006) 291–298.

43. P.W. Hitchon, M.D. Brenton, A.G. Black, et al., In vitro biomechanical comparison of pedicle screws, sublaminar hooks, and sublaminar cables, J Neurosurg 99 (Suppl. 1) 2003) 104–109.

44. J.A. Smith, Adult deformity:management of sagittal plane deformity in revision adult spine surgery, Curr. Opin. Orthop. 12 (3) (2001) 206–215.

45. S.J. Luhmann, L.G. Lenke, Y.J. Kim, K.H. Bridwell, M. Schootman, Thoracic adolescent idiopathic scoliosis curves between 70 degrees and 100 degrees: is anterior release necessary? Spine 30 (18) (2005) 2061–2067.

46. D.C. Burton, A.A. Sama, M.A. Asher, et al., The treatment of large (>70 degrees) thoracic idiopathic scoliosis curves with posterior instrumentation and arthrodesis: when is anterior release indicated? Spine 30 (17) (2005) 1979–1984.

47. V. Arlet, L. Jiang, J. Ouellet, Is there a need for anterior release for 70-90 degrees masculine thoracic curves in adolescent scoliosis? Eur. Spine J. 13 (8) (2004) 740–745.

48. J.A. Byrd 3rd, P.V. Scoles, R.B. Winter, D.S. Bradford, J.E. Lonstein, J.H. Moe, Adult idiopathic scoliosis treated by anterior and posterior spinal fusion, J. Bone Joint Surg. Am. 69 (6) (1987) 843–850.

49. J. Dick, O. Boachie-Adjei, M. Wilson, One-stage versus two-stage anterior and posterior spinal reconstruction in adults. Comparison of outcomes including nutritional status, complications rates, hospital costs, and other factors, Spine 17 (Suppl. 8) (1992) S310–6.

50. S. Swank, J.E. Lonstein, J.H. Moe, R.B. Winter, D.S. Bradford, Surgical treatment of adult scoliosis. A review of two hundred and twenty-two cases, J. Bone Joint Surg. Am. 63 (2) (1981) 268–287.

51. G.S. Shapiro, G.B. Taira, O. Boachie-Adjei, Results of surgical treatment of adult idiopathic scoliosis with low back pain and spinal stenosis: a study of long-term clinical radiographic outcomes, Spine 28 (4) (2003) 358–363.

52. Y.B. Kim, L.G. Lenke, Y.J. Kim, Y.W. Kim, K. Blanke, G. Stobbs, K.H. Bridwell, The morbidity of an anterior thoracolumbar approach: adult spinal deformity patients with greater than five-year follow-up, Spine 34 (8) (2009) 822–826.

53. R.M. Ali, O. Boachie-Adjei, B.A. Rawlins, Functional and radiographic outcomes after surgery for adult scoliosis using third-generation instrumentation techniques, Spine 28 (11) (2003) 1163–1169.

54. Y.B. Kim, L.G. Lenke, Y.J. Kim, Y.W. Kim, K.H. Bridwell, G. Stobbs, Surgical treatment of adult scoliosis: is anterior apical release and fusion necessary for the lumbar curve? Spine 33 (10) (2008) 1125–1132.

55. B.M. Ozgur, H.E. Aryan, L. Pimenta, W.R. Taylor, Extreme Lateral Interbody Fusion (XLIF): a novel surgical technique for anterior lumbar interbody fusion, Spine J. 6 (4) (2006) 435–443.

56. O. Boachie-Adjei, G. Charles, M.E. Cunningham, Partially overlapping limited anterior and posterior instrumentation for adult thoracolumbar and lumbar scoliosis: a description of novel spinal instrumentation,"the hybrid technique,", HSS J 1 (2007) 93–98.

57. Swank ML: Adjacent segment failure above lumbosacral fusions instrumented to L1 or L2.

58. Suk SI, Kim JH, Lee SM: Incidence of proximal adjacent failure in adult lumbar deformity correction.

59. Y.J. Kim, K.H. Bridwell, L.G. Lenke, S. Rhim, Y.W. Kim, Is the T9, T11, or L1 the more reliable proximal level after adult lumbar or lumbosacral instrumented fusion to L5 or S1? Spine 32 (24) (2007) 2653–2661.

60. K.J. Cho, S.I. Suk, S.R. Park, et al., Short fusion versus long fusion for degenerative lumbar scoliosis, Eur Spine J 17 (5) (2008) 650–656.

61. K.H. Bridwell, C.C. Edwards 2nd, L.G. Lenke, The pros and cons to saving the L5-S1 motion segment in a long scoliosis fusion construct, Spine 28 (20) (2003) S234–42.

62. F.J. Schwab, V. Lafage, J.P. Farcy, K.H. Bridwell, S. Glassman, M.R. Shainline, Predicting outcome and complications in the surgical treatment of adult scoliosis, Spine 33 (20) (2008) 2243–2247.

63. J.P. Kostuik, B.B. Hall, Spinal fusions to the sacrum in adults with scoliosis, Spine 8 (5) (1983) 489–500.

64. Y.J. Kim, K.H. Bridwell, L.G. Lenke, S. Rhim, G. Cheh, Pseudarthrosis in long adult spinal deformity instrumentation and fusion to the sacrum: prevalence and risk factor analysis of 144 cases, Spine 31 (20) (2006) 2329–2336.

65. J.K. Weistroffer, J.H. Perra, J.E. Lonstein, et al., Complications in long fusions to the sacrum for adult scoliosis: minimum five-year analysis of fifty patients, Spine 33 (13) (2008) 1478–1483.

66. P. Vavken, P. Krepler, Sacral fractures after multi-segmental lumbosacral fusion: a series of four cases and systematic review of literature, Eur. Spine J. 17 (Suppl. 2) (2008) S285–90.

67. C.C. Edwards 2nd, K.H. Bridwell, A. Patel, A.S. Rinella, A. Berra, L.G. Lenke, Long adult deformity fusions to L5 and the sacrum. A matched cohort analysis, Spine 29 (18) (2004) 1996–2005.

68. K.J. Cho, S.I. Suk, S.R. Park, et al., Arthrodesis to L5 versus S1 in long instrumentation and fusion for degenerative lumbar scoliosis, Eur. Spine J. 18 (4) (2009) 531–537.

69. C.A. Kuhns, K.H. Bridwell, L.G. Lenke, et al., Thoracolumbar deformity arthrodesis stopping at L5: fate of the L5-S1 disc, minimum 5-year follow-up, Spine 32 (24) (2007) 2771–2776.

70. M.N. Smith-Petersen, C.B. Larson, O.E. Aufranc, Osteotomy of the spine for correction of flexion deformity in rheumatoid arthritis, J. Bone Joint Surg. Am. 27 (1945) 1–11.

71. J.C. Adams, Technique, dangers and safeguards in osteotomy of the spine, J Bone Joint Surg Br 34-B (2) (1952) 226–232.

72. C. Weatherley, D. Jaffray, A. Terry, Vascular complications associated with osteotomy in ankylosing spondylitis: a report of two cases, Spine 13 (1) (1988) 43–46.

73. F. Li, H.C. Sagi, B. Liu, H.A. Yuan, Comparative evaluation of single-level closing-wedge vertebral osteotomies for the correction of fixed kyphotic deformity of the lumbar spine: a cadaveric study, Spine 26 (21) (2001) 2385–2391.

74. E. Thomasen, Vertebral osteotomy for correction of kyphosis in ankylosing spondylitis, Clin. Orthop. (1985) 142–152.

75. K.H. Bridwell, S.J. Lewis, L.G. Lenke, C. Baldus, K. Blanke, Pedicle subtraction osteotomy for the treatment of fixed sagittal imbalance, J. Bone Joint Surg. Am. 85-A (3) (2003) 454–463.

76. N. Thiranont, P. Netrawichien, Transpedicular decancellation closed wedge vertebral osteotomy for treatment of fixed flexion deformity of spine in ankylosing spondylitis, Spine 18 (16) (1993) 2517–2522.

77. B.J. van Royen, G.H. Slot, Closing-wedge posterior osteotomy for ankylosing spondylitis. Partial corporectomy and transpedicular fixation in 22 cases, J. Bone Joint Surg. Br. 77 (1) (1995) 117–121.

78. Y.J. Kim, K.H. Bridwell, L.G. Lenke, G. Cheh, C. Baldus, Results of lumbar pedicle subtraction osteotomies for fixed sagittal imbalance: a minimum 5-year follow-up study, Spine 32 (20) (2007) 2189–2197.

79. K.J. Cho, K.H. Bridwell, L.G. Lenke, A. Berra, C. Baldus, Comparison of Smith-Petersen versus pedicle subtraction osteotomy for the correction of fixed sagittal imbalance, Spine 30 (18) (2005) 2030–2037.

80. P.S. Rose, K.H. Bridwell, L.G. Lenke, et al., Role of pelvic incidence, thoracic kyphosis, and patient factors on sagittal plane correction following pedicle subtraction osteotomy, Spine 34 (8) (2009) 785–791.

# 53

# Assessment and Avoiding Complications in the Scoliotic Elderly Patient

*Kirkham B. Wood and Charles S. Carrier*

**KEY POINTS**

- Functional improvement following surgery in the elderly can be equal to or greater than that seen in younger individuals.
- Pain relief is the number one indication for surgery.
- Restoration of sagittal balance is the most important surgical goal.
- Because so many elderly patients suffer from osteoporosis, additional forms of fixation (e.g., iliac fixation, wires) are often indicated.
- The complication rate is significant and ranges from 30% to 80%.

## INTRODUCTION

Scoliosis — defined as a curvature of the spine in the coronal plane measuring over 10 degrees — can be found in the adult population and can be a significant source of disability, especially in the elderly.[1,2] There are three principal forms of scoliotic spinal deformity that can be described: idiopathic, i.e., that whose development can be found during the juvenile or adolescent growing years of life and which persists into adulthood; de novo, which involves the development of a new scoliosis later in life as a result of degenerative changes in the lumbar spine; and osteoporotic scoliosis, a less common form of spine curvature secondary to osteopenic collapse of vertebral bodies.

In the adolescent with scoliosis, the primary focus of treatment is the deformity and concerns of curve progression. In the older patient, it is much more common that pain is the primary complaint.[3,4] In the later decades of life, curve progression becomes less and less of a concern, primarily because of the restraint provided by the degenerating and ossifying disc spaces and the arthritic facet joints. Being out of balance, especially in the sagittal plane, adds an element of posturally related fatiguing pain that limits patients' ability to perform upright activities.[5] Older adults are most commonly symptomatic in the lower thoracolumbar or lumbar region, due to the age-related disc degeneration and osteoarthritis associated with the deformity.

## PATIENT EVALUATION

Clinically, the evaluation of the elderly patient with scoliosis begins with an appreciation of the overall coronal and sagittal balance. There are many reasons other than spinal deformity for the patient to have difficulty standing upright: hip and knee degeneration, spinal stenosis, lumbosacral or thoracolumbar kyphosis, trunk muscle weakness, or flatback pathology. The last entity — flatback syndrome — typically due to some form of loss of the normal lumbar lordosis, can result in a loss of trunk strength and difficulty fully extending the hips. All patients should thus have a careful examination of the hip range of motion, including assessment of their ability to extend completely when in the supine examining position. Hips that have become locked into contracture may well require some form of release before considering any corrective surgery on the spine. On occasion, degenerative arthritis

of the hips can be treated with arthroplasty first before proceeding with spinal surgery.

Routine radiographs are obtained in the upright position and should include standing, full-length, anterior-posterior, and lateral films to assess not only the dimensions of the curve, but the overall alignment in both the coronal and sagittal planes. It is important to obtain the images with the patient's hips and knees as extended as possible in order to appreciate the true sagittal profile. In addition, side-bending or hyperextension lateral films are quite helpful in determining the flexibility of the curve, and, if considering surgery, whether some form of anterior release or posterior osteotomy is necessary.

Because the majority of patients present with pain, magnetic resonance imaging is often obtained. MRI can assess the quality of the distal intervertebral discs, and as many patients will complain of varying degrees of leg pain from stenosis, axial MRI imaging is useful to study the spinal canal and foramen and determine levels of decompression if necessary. MRI can also be used to study the most caudal intervertebral discs of the spine, as a fusion may on occasion stop short of the sacrum if distal painful pathology does not appear to exist, although this is somewhat less common in the elderly compared with younger patients. MRI is also very helpful in ruling out malignancies or infections.

Computerized tomography is helpful during the planning stages for studying the bony anatomy; in the setting of previous fusions, the quality and extent of the previous arthrodesis can be best obtained with CT imaging. CT is also quite helpful in analyzing the size of the pedicles, the width of the ilium, and the morphology of the vertebrae themselves.

## TREATMENT

Elderly patients with painful scoliosis can be considered candidates for nonoperative treatment modalities, just as their younger counterparts are. As the majority of the patients present with symptomatic curves in the lumbar or thoracolumbar region, simple education and an understanding that the curvature does not present an immediate threat to their cardiac or pulmonary systems (as did primary thoracic curves left untreated) may be reassuring enough to many. Combinations of the judicious use of nonsteroidal antiinflammatory medications, activity modifications, and physical therapy are often helpful. Physical therapy will tend to be more successful when it is low-impact and focused on aerobic conditioning rather than vigorous activity. Water-based conditioning is also quite helpful in many. Use of orthotics is not typically well tolerated by the elderly, but an occasional patient may find the use of a brace supportive and helpful in his or her daily activities.

## SURGERY

Patients are considered candidates for surgical intervention if their symptoms have remained significant despite attempts at nonoperative care or, less commonly, if there is problematic curve progression.

Elderly patients undergoing surgery for scoliosis face the prospect of increased morbidity and mortality compared with their younger counterparts, primarily because they enter into the surgery much more disabled and with worse health status.[6-8] In the preoperative assessment, careful attention should be paid to their cardiac and pulmonary systems, as many patients have become quite sedentary and the stress of surgery may thus become problematic. If patients smoke, they should be encouraged to quit at least a number of weeks before the operation, not only to improve the chances of bone healing but to lessen the likelihood of pulmonary and wound complications, which are already elevated in the elderly population. If there is a suspicion of respiratory compromise, a history of smoking, or planned procedures about the diaphragm, preoperative pulmonary function should be assessed.

Similarly, if elderly patients have a history of cardiac or ischemic disease, they should undergo preoperative stress testing and formal cardiac evaluation. It is recommended that the elderly who have concomitant diagnoses of either hypertension, hypercholesterolemia, or diabetes be considered for perioperative beta-blockers.[9]

Elderly patients may have become relatively malnourished and the associated risks of sepsis, wound breakdown, etc., are well established.[9] Total parenteral nutrition should be considered in staged surgical treatments, as it has been shown to diminish the rate of nutritional depletion and postoperative infections.

## SURGICAL TECHNIQUES

A multitude of issues need to be assessed in each elderly surgical patient, including sagittal balance, coronal alignment, any complicating spinal or nerve root stenosis, disc degeneration, listhesis either anterior or lateral, osteoporosis, and any complicating medical comorbidities.

Unlike in the adolescent, where maximal safe correction of the coronal plane curvature is sought, in the elderly, aside from obtaining a solid arthrodesis, much more critical than Cobb angle correction is the obtaining and maintenance of appropriate balance in both the coronal and sagittal planes. A stable and balanced spine is the principal goal of deformity surgery in the elderly, and this often involves accepting less curvature correction. Numerous studies have emphasized that the component of postoperative radiography most closely tied to overall clinical success is the achievement of adequate balance, especially in the sagittal plane. Glassman and other members of the Spine Deformity Study Group, in a review of nearly 300 patients, have suggested that restoration of the normal sagittal balance is the most critical goal for any reconstructive spine surgery.[5] A plumbline dropped from C7 should fall in the middle of the sacrum in the coronal plane and within the disc space of the lumbosacral articulation in the lateral view. Older adults have typically developed pronounced disc degeneration and narrowing, which leads to a loss of the normal lumbar lordosis and a forward drift of the sagittal plumbline. Osteopenic compression-type fractures can worsen the sagittal alignment, as can any thoracolumbar kyphosis.[10] For these reasons, fusions of primarily lumbar pathology may well need to be extended proximally into the upper thoracic spine.

With the increased use of pedicle-screw fixation and advancing techniques such as vertebral resections, the majority of surgery in the elderly is performed through the posterior approach.[11] This would even include access to the anterior column, e.g., the intervertebral discs via posterior or transforaminal lumbar interbody fusion (PLIF or TLIF, respectively). Interbody support at the lumbosacral junction within at least the lower two spaces, L4-5 and L5-S1, is biomechanically mandatory for successful fusion rates.[12-14] Support here lessens the strain seen on the posterior instrumentation and protects to a certain degree against pull-out failure. As a general rule, but especially in the elderly, instrumentation should be used to maintain correction, not obtain correction.

In the case of previous decompressive surgery, scarring within the spinal canal may, however, make these PLIF and TLIF approaches somewhat more difficult. Direct anterior access to the lumbosacral junction can be successfully accomplished via a midline or paramedian incision, retraction of the peritoneal contents, and direct visualization via the retroperitoneum of the disc spaces from L3 to the sacrum with little morbidity and low risk of complications. Through this approach, more extensive removal of disc material and direct placement of femoral rings or specialized cages packed with bone fusion material can be realized.

Osteotomies have become increasingly popular and have become a part of the armamentarium of most adult deformity spine surgeons for effecting corrective change in the sagittal balance. Especially in the elderly, they have become vehicles for avoiding the time and morbidity of separate anterior approaches. Smith-Peterson osteotomy, a V-shaped resection of the posterior arch through the facets bilaterally, can effect moderate corrections per level; however, if multiple resections are combined, the overall effect on sagittal balance can be significant. The success for Smith-Peterson osteotomy, however, depends on the integrity of the anterior intervertebral disc, which must retain a certain degree of flexibility, as the correction hinges posteriorly. In other words, a disc space that is severely narrowed or even ankylosed, as can be seen in many older individuals, may not have enough residual motion and the ability to correct may be lost.

Pedicle subtraction osteotomies (PSOs) are very powerful tools for obtaining sagittal plane correction at single levels — up to 35 or more degrees per level. However, as the procedure involves a wedge-shaped resection of the laminae, the pedicles, and the posterior vertebral body itself, the blood loss can be significant, and may not be well tolerated by the aged patient . PSOs are also most efficient when performed in a previously fused spine, especially anteriorly, as the hinge is at the anterior vertebral body wall. It may be difficult to obtain the same degree of correction in spines without previous fusions. Also, as the success of maintaining the correction depends on a rigid anterior aspect of the vertebral body, significant osteoporosis, as seen in many elderly patients, can be a potential contraindication, for if the remaining vertebral body is not sufficiently strong, the bone may collapse, lessening the degree of correction.

Adequate fixation of the thoracolumbar spine with surgical implants can be problematic in the elderly patient for a number of reasons. Obviously, the quality of the bone of the spine is less than that in a younger age group, and the spine itself is typically much stiffer. In addition, many patients have had prior surgery including fusions and decompressions, which can obscure the typical landmarks for fixation and actually limit the number of possibilities for obtaining purchase, especially in the setting of previous decompressions. Use of fluoroscopy can aid in finding the pedicles, especially in the thoracic spine.

Pedicle screws have become the primary method of fixation in deformity surgery, including the elderly, although their bone quality still remains a concern. Pull-out strength of pedicle screws in patients with normal bone density is typically about 1400 N; however, in patients with osteoporosis, the strength can be as low as 200 N.[15] Fixation strength of pedicle screws has been correlated with insertional torque. Hence, it is recommended that, in order to obtain some purchase with the inner cortical wall of the osteopenic pedicle, the largest-sized screw that can comfortably be placed be chosen. This is another reason for careful assessment of preoperative computed tomography with measurement of the inner diameters of the pedicles. In settings of reduced purchase quality, many surgeons treating the elderly may reinforce pedicle screws with adjacent laminar hooks or sublaminar wires. Of note, in the elderly spine, compared with younger adolescent patients treated for scoliosis, the transverse processes are typically quite brittle, and, with few exceptions, are not commonly recommended as points of principal fixation for instrumentation such as hooks.

In some setting of robust previous fusions, however, especially when extending down the ilium or sacrum, hooks can still be used when pedicle screws are not possible or practical. Hook site placement can be performed with small power burrs into the fusion mass — typically in multiple claw formations — and connected to the rods extending down to the more distal spine.

Fixation into the sacrum is a particular problem as the quality of the bone is probably the poorest here, and the risk of fusion failure (pseudarthrosis) may be one of the highest.[16, 17] This is another reason why combined anterior and posterior surgery is recommended for long fusions down to the sacrum or the ilium: at a minimum, L4-5 and L5-S1 require strong structural support. In addition, because of the risk of osteopenic fracture of the sacrum when long fusions extend distally, supplemental iliac fixation is highly recommended (Figure 53-1).[18]

Screws fixed into the sacrum can be directed down the S1 pedicle to the anterior cortex or the sacral promontory where the bone is most dense.

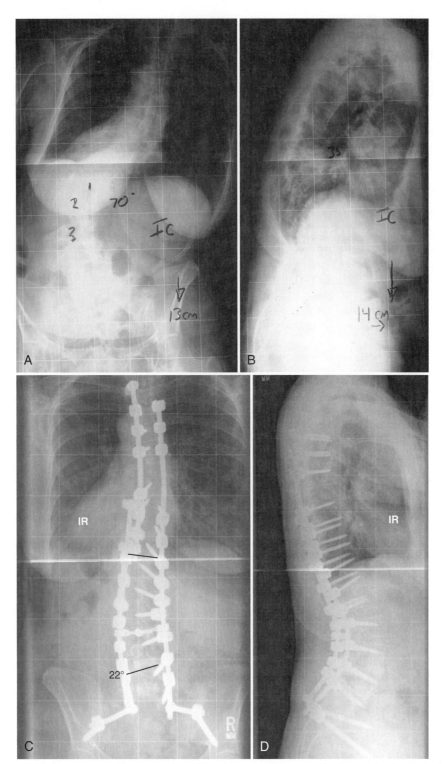

■ **FIGURE 53-1**  A 73-year-old woman with painful scoliosis, osteoporosis, and both coronal and sagittal imbalance. **A, B,** Preoperative anterior-posterior and lateral radiographs. **C, D,** Postoperative radiographs showing restoration of normal sagittal and coronal alignment. **C,** Anterior-posterior view shows bilateral fixation to support distal fixation. **D,** Lateral radiographs show normal lumbar lordosis. Interbody structural fusions can be seen at the lower two levels

Alternatively, they can be directed 30 degrees laterally out into the thickest part of the sacral ala. Either way, it is important to try to perforate and actually gain purchase into the anterior cortex with the screw threads, which will increase the holding power of the screw significantly.[19] Cancellous screws are preferred over cortical ones as the strength of purchase correlates directly with the amount of bone found between the screw threads.

## OSTEOPOROSIS AND SCOLIOSIS

There exists a known association between scoliosis and osteoporosis.[20,21] Two studies of osteoporotic women have described an incidence of scoliosis between 35% and 45%.[9,22,23] The majority of these curves will progress somewhat because of a combination of disc degeneration and facet overloading as well as compression of the osteopenic bones within the apices of the curves.[20,22]

It is important to have an appreciation for the quality of the elderly patient's bone before planning deformity correction that involves the implantation of instrumentation; it is difficult to accurately quantify the degree of osteopenia with plain radiographs before significant quantities of bone are lost.[24] Accurate assessment of bone mineral content includes quantitative computerd tomography (QCT), dual-photon absorptiometry (DPA), or dual-energy radiography (DXA).

Multiple surgical techniques have been suggested to improve fixation strength in the elderly osteopenic spine including supplemental sublaminar wiring, increasing fixation points, cement augmentation of pedicle screws, cement kyphoplasty of adjacent uninstrumented vertebrae, hydroxyapatite-coated screws, and expandable screws. Instrumentation-related complications still remain a principal concern in the elderly, however. In a review of 47 deformity procedures in 38 patients over the age of 65, DeWald and Stanley[20] reported a 13% early and 11% late instrumentation-related complication rate. Early complications included compression fractures of the most cephalic instrumented vertebrae as well as the superior adjacent body, and fractures of the pedicle. Late complications included loose or painful pedicle or iliac screws. Ten of 38 patients (26%) developed junctional kyphosis at the superior end of the construct, including late compression fractures.

## COMPLICATIONS

Elderly patients who undergo surgery for spinal deformity are at a much greater risk for complications than adolescents and even younger adults.[18,25,26] A wide range of complication rates have been reported, from 30% to 80%.

The risk of pseudarthrosis has been detailed above; it is mildly elevated from that of younger age groups, largely due to issues with fixation adequacy. Vascular injury can take place during anterior exposures of the thoracolumbar spine; however, again, A specific age-related difference has not been shown. What has been shown to be statistically age-related is the development of nutritional depletion perioperatively and hence an increased risk for infection following major reconstructive spine surgery. Patients at risk should be screened preoperatively with serum albumin and prealbumin values and supplemented as necessary before embarking on a surgical course. For patients undergoing staged procedures, again, at-risk patients should be considered for nutritional supplementation between and after the two stages, either with total parenteral nutrition, or the more frequently recommended gastric tube feedings.

Another complication of correction of sagittal imbalance or kyphotic deformities is the development of junctional kyphosis just proximal to the cephalic ends of the instrumentation. This is a known problem with overcorrection of kyphotic thoracic spines, even in the younger age groups, but it can be especially worrisome in the elderly with long instrumented fusions and correction of sagittal imbalance. Overcorrection of kyphosis or dramatic improvement of a longstanding sagittal malalignment can impart a large kyphosing force to the adjacent uninstrumented proximal levels — as the spine attempts to return to its longstanding alignment — with the development of a painful angulation, instrumentation failure, or vertebral fracture. Care in contouring the proximal instrumentation and sparing the adjacent level ligaments and facet joints can also reduce the incidence of this complication.

## OUTCOMES

Because of improved medical screening, advanced surgical techniques, and specialized anesthesia training, patient-related outcomes following extensive reconstructive surgery for scoliosis in the elderly have dramatically improved from a generation ago. Li et al, [2] using SRS-22, SF-12, and ODI instruments, reported that adults over the age of 65 treated operatively had significantly less pain; better health-related quality of life, self-image, and mental health; and were overall more satisfied than age-related counterparts treated nonoperatively or simply observed. In fact, compared with younger age groups undergoing similar surgeries, it is the elderly who typically report similar, and in many cases, statistically superior improvements in pain and function, often because of extensive preoperative disability.[3, 7, 8] Radiographically, however, despite such significant functional and pain-related improvements, maintaining correction remains challenging in an age-dependent manner.

## References

1. S.D. Glassman, G.M. Alegre, Adult spinal deformity in the osteoporotic spine: options and pitfalls, Instr. Course Lect. 52 (2003) 579–588.
2. G. Li, P. Passias, M. Kozanek, E. Fu, S. Wang, Q. Xia, et al., Adult scoliosis in patients over sixty-five years of age: outcomes of operative versus nonoperative treatment at a minimum two-year follow-up, Spine 34 (20) (2009) 2165–2170.
3. S. Takahashi, J. Delecrin, N. Passuti, Surgical treatment of idiopathic scoliosis in adults: an age-related analysis of outcome, Spine 27 (16) (2002) 1742–1748.
4. V. Deviren, S. Berven, F. Kleinstueck, J. Antinnes, J.A. Smith, S.S. Hu, Predictors of flexibility and pain patterns in thoracolumbar and lumbar idiopathic scoliosis, Spine 27 (21) (2002) 2346–2349.
5. S.D. Glassman, S. Berven, K. Bridwell, W. Horton, J.R. Dimar, Correlation of radiographic parameters and clinical symptoms in adult scoliosis, Spine 30 (6) (2005) 682–688.
6. B.E. van Dam, D.S. Bradford, J.E. Lonstein, J.H. Moe, J.W. Ogilvie, R.B. Winter, Adult idiopathic scoliosis treated by posterior spinal fusion and Harrington instrumentation, Spine 12 (1) (1987) 32–36.
7. J.S. Smith, Risk-benefit assessment of surgery for adult scoliosis: an analysis based on patient age, Scoliosis Research Society 44th Annual Meeting and Course Final Program 2009:66–7, September, 2009.
8. B.A. O'Shaughnessy, Is there a difference in outcome between patients under and over age 60 who have long fusions to the sacrum for the primary treatment of adult scoliosis, Scoliosis Research Society 44th Annual Meeting and Course: Final Program 2009:67–8, September, 2009.
9. S.S. Hu, S.H. Berven, Preparing the adult deformity patient for spinal surgery, Spine 31 (19 Suppl) (2006) S126–S131.
10. E.M. Hammerberg, K.B. Wood, Sagittal profile of the elderly, J. Spinal Disord. Tech. 16 (1) (2003) 44–50.
11. P.S. Rose, L.G. Lenke, K.H. Bridwell, D.S. Mulconrey, G.A. Cronen, J.M. Buchowski, et al., Pedicle screw instrumentation for adult idiopathic scoliosis: an improvement over hook/hybrid fixation, Spine 34 (8) (2009) 852–857.
12. I.B. McPhee, C.E. Swanson, The surgical management of degenerative lumbar scoliosis. Posterior instrumentation alone versus two stage surgery,, Bull. Hosp. Jt. Dis. 57 (1) (1998) 16–22.
13. K.H. Bridwell, L.G. Lenke, K.W. McEnery, C. Baldus, K. Blanke, Anterior fresh frozen structural allografts in the thoracic and lumbar spine. Do they work if combined with posterior fusion and instrumentation in adult patients with kyphosis or anterior column defects? Spine 20 (12) (1995) 1410–1418.
14. J.P. Kostuik, Treatment of scoliosis in the adult thoracolumbar spine with special reference to fusion to the sacrum, Orthop. Clin. North Am. 19 (2) (1988) 371–381.
15. T.L. Halvorson, L.A. Kelley, K.A. Thomas, T.S. Whitecloud 3rd, S.D. Cook, Effects of bone mineral density on pedicle screw fixation, Spine 19 (21) (1994) 2415–2420.
16. K.R. Eck, K.H. Bridwell, F.F. Ungacta, K.D. Riew, M.A. Lapp, L.G. Lenke, et al., Complications and results of long adult deformity fusions down to L4, L5, and the sacrum, Spine 26 (9) (2001) E182–E192.
17. V.J. Devlin, O. Boachie-Adjei, D.S. Bradford, J.W. Ogilvie, E.E. Transfeldt, Treatment of adult spinal deformity with fusion to the sacrum using CD instrumentation, J. Spinal Disord. 4 (1) (1991) 1–14.
18. S.S.B. Hu, H. Sigurd, D.S. Bradford, Adult spinal deformity, in: J.W. Frymoyer, SWW (Eds.), The adult and pediatric, third ed., spine, Lippincott Williams and Wilkins, Philadelphia, 2004, pp. 465–477.
19. J.P.H. Kostuik, MH, Indications for surgery of the osteoporotic spine, in: J.Y. Margulies, FY, J.C. Farcy, M.G. Neuwirth (Eds.), Lumbosacral and spinopelvic fixation, Lippincott-Raven, Philadelphia, 1996.
20. C.J. DeWald, T. Stanley, Instrumentation-related complications of multilevel fusions for adult spinal deformity patients over age 65: surgical considerations and treatment options in patients with poor bone quality, Spine 31 (Suppl. 19) (2006) S144–S151.
21. S. Jaovisidha, J.K. Kim, D.J. Sartoris, E. Bosch, S. Edelstein, E. Barrett-Connor, et al., Scoliosis in elderly and age-related bone loss: a population-based study, J. Clin. Densitom. 1 (3) (1998) 227–233.
22. D.W. Vanderpool, J.I. James, R. Wynne-Davies, Scoliosis in the elderly, J. Bone Joint Surg. Am. 51 (3) (1969) 446–455.
23. J.H. Healey, J.M. Lane, Structural scoliosis in osteoporotic women, Clin. Orthop. Relat. Res. (195) (1985) 216–223.
24. D.N. Resnick, G, Osteoporosis, bone and joint imaging, WB Saunders, Philadelphia, 1989.
25. S.D. Glassman, C.L. Hamill, K.H. Bridwell, F.J. Schwab, J.R. Dimar, T.G. Lowe, The impact of perioperative complications on clinical outcome in adult deformity surgery, Spine 32 (24) (2007) 2764–2770.
26. T. Faciszewski, R.B. Winter, J.E. Lonstein, F. Denis, L. Johnson, The surgical and medical perioperative complications of anterior spinal fusion surgery in the thoracic and lumbar spine in adults. A review of 1223 procedures, Spine 20 (14) (1995) 1592–1599.

# 54

# Interspinous Spacers for Minimally Invasive Treatment of Dynamic Spinal Stenosis and Low Back Pain

*H. Michael Mayer*

| K E Y   P O I N T S |
| --- |

- Interspinous distraction of a motion segment of the lumbar spine has different biomechanical effects:

  ○ It increases the size and areas of the spinal canal as well as of the subarticular zones and the foramen and thus has an indirect "decompression" effect on neural structure.

  ○ It unloads the facet joints as well as the posterior part of the disc and thus has a potential effect on low back pain arising from pathologic load pattern on these anatomical structures. The different implants that are currently on the market or in clinical studies provide these biomechanical effects. They can be categorized in two groups:

    ■ Nonstabilizing devices used for primary treatment of dynamic spinal stenosis and low back pain ("extension stoppers")

    ■ Dynamic/rigid interspinous stabilizers, i.e., stabilizing devices used as an adjunct to open decompression procedures as a substitute for fusion or to promote fusion (dynamic or rigid fixation devices)

- All devices are characterized by their less-invasive (as compared to open decompression procedures or fusion) application and low complication rates that make them attractive for use in an elderly patient population. They are, however, most probably, devices with a temporary clinical effect, which makes their acceptance strongly dependent on their degree of invasiveness.

## INTRODUCTION: INTERSPINOUS SPACERS – HOW DO THEY WORK?

Indirect enlargement of the spinal canal through interspinous distraction devices has become popular for the treatment of dynamic spinal canal stenosis of the lumbar spine.[1-5] Biomechanical data acquired with the first implant on the market (X-Stop, Medtronic, Memphis, TN, USA), could show that interspinous distraction induces segmental slight flexion, reduces segmental lordosis, and limits extension.[6] Thus, the spinal canal and neural foramen areas and diameters are enlarged.[7] These findings are considered to be the most important primary effects that justify the clinical use of the device for the treatment of dynamic spinal stenosis. Randomized controlled trials could confirm the therapeutic efficiency and proved that the implantation of an interspinous spacer leads to clinical results superior to conservative treatment.[5]

In ex vivo experiments it could also be demonstrated that interspinous distraction can lead to a significant unloading of the facet joints[8,9] and the posterior annulus fibrosus, as well as the nucleus pulposus in neutral position and predominantly in extension.[8,10,11] Kinematics of the adjacent segments seem not to be affected.[6,12]

## THE "EXTENSION STOPPERS"

A variety of these implant types are currently either in routine clinical use or in clinical application studies. Their purpose is to achieve interspinous segmental distraction and to limit extension. They are promoted mainly for the primary treatment of dynamic degenerative lumbar spinal stenosis, as a substitute for open decompression. The main therapeutic goal is to increase the diameter of the spinal canal and foramen as well as to unload the facet joints and the disc.

### X - Stop (Medtronic) (Figure 54-1)

The X-Stop has been the prototype of this class of implants. The implant body is made of titanium, and the spacer of PEEK (polyether ether ketone). It has both a fixed and an adjustable wing. The latter is mounted after implantation.

The main indication is neurogenic claudication with leg/buttock pain due to dynamic degenerative lumbar spinal stenosis, which is relieved upon flexion of the lumbar spine.[5]

#### Surgical Technique

It is implanted through a posterior approach. The patient is in a prone position. The dorsolumbar fascia is split on both sides of the spinous processes, the paravertebral muscles are retracted, and the interspinous ligament is pierced. The spinous processes are then actively distracted with a distraction forceps and the X-Stop is implanted from one side. The wing on the contralateral side is then attached (Figure 54-2).

#### Results

In a randomized controlled trial, it could be shown that the results of the treatment of dynamic spinal stenosis are superior to those in conservative therapy .[1,5,13] Whereas in initial reports its usefulness was also documented for degenerative spondylolisthesis not greater than grade I, recent data could not confirm this.[14]

#### Summary

Although the implantation of the X-Stop device is claimed to be minimally invasive, it occasionally requires a larger skin incision and a wider bilateral muscular dissection as compared to modern microsurgical direct decompression techniques.[15,16] Due to the iatrogenic alteration of the dorsolumbar fascia and the paraspinal muscles, it also cannot be considered as a treatment option for discogenic or arthrogenic low back pain. Moreover, bisegmental or multilevel implantations require larger surgical approaches.

### InSpace (Synthes, Paoli, PA, USA) (Figure 54-3)

In order to solve the problem of invasiveness, a new cylindrically shaped PEEK interspinous implant with a central titanium screw and four wings that can be deployed once the implant is placed into the interspinous space,

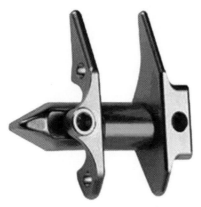

■ **FIGURE 54-1**   The X-Stop device (CF).

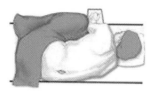

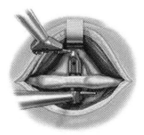

■ **FIGURE 54-2**   Implantation technique of the X-Stop.

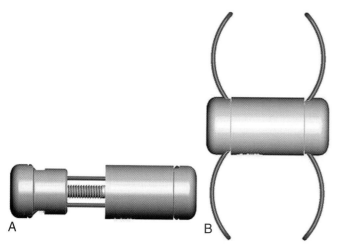

■ **FIGURE 54-3**   The InSpace implant. **A,** Wings undeployed. **B,** Wings deployed.

has been presented recently. Biomechanical tests have shown that the implant effectively reduces extension without affecting lateral bending of the segment.[17,18] Cyclic loading tests have shown that the functionality of the implant is preserved and that the integrity of anatomic structures is not impaired through 15,000 loading cycles.[19,20] The effects are thus comparable to the ones described for the X-Stop implant.

The indications are also identical with those described for X-Stop. There are preliminary reports on its potential usefulness for the treatment of discogenic and/or arthrogenic low back pain.[21,22]

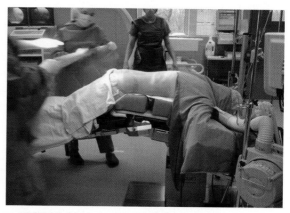

■ **FIGURE 54-4**   Patient positioning for InSpace implantation.

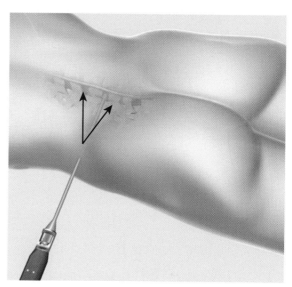

■ **FIGURE 54-5**   Lateral percutaneous approach.

## Surgical Technique

The surgical procedure can be performed under local or general anesthesia. The patient is placed in a prone position on a flat soft-frame on an adjustable operating table or on a Wilson frame. Passive distraction of the interspinous space is achieved and adjusted by tilting the foot end of the surgical table until maximum "opening" of the interspinous space is reached (Figure 54-4). The implant is placed through a lateral percutaneous approach (Figure 54-5). Piercing of the interspinous ligament is performed with a K-wire; enlargement of the interspinous space is achieved with blunt distractors of increasing sizes. After removal of the distractors, the implant can be introduced through an application sleeve and the implant wings are deployed under AP fluoroscopic control. Once the wings are deployed completely, the implant is uncoupled from the implant holder, which, together with the application sleeve, is then removed en bloc, leaving the implant in place (Figure 54-6).

## Results

The first operation worldwide was performed on March 15, 2006. Preliminary results in 41 patients show a good reduction of pain level as well as of the Oswestry Disability Index in patients with low back pain as well as in patients with dynamic degenerative lumbar spinal stenosis.[22]

## Summary

InSpace is significantly less invasive as compared to all other extension stoppers currently on the market. The average intraoperative blood loss was less than 5 cc. Surgical time for a single level is usually less than 15 minutes in uncomplicated cases. There were no clinically relevant intraoperative

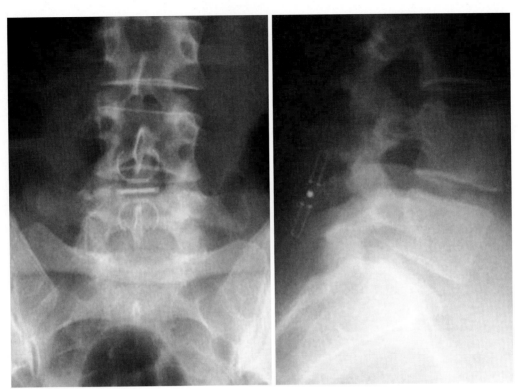

■ **FIGURE 54-6**   AP and lateral postoperative x-rays showing the InSpace implant correctly in place.

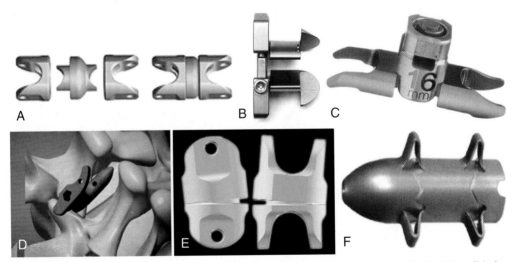

■ **FIGURE 54-7**   Other "extension stoppers." **A,** Flexis (Lindare Medical, Smarden, UK). **B,** Spinos (Privelop, Neunkirchen, Germany). **C,** Superion (Vertiflex, San Clemente, CA, USA). **D,** Retain (Globus Medical, Audubon, PA, USA). **E,** RODD (Novaspine, Amiens, France). **F,** Aperius (Medtronic, Minneapolis, MN, USA).

complications. Other advantages of this lateral approach are the short learning curve and no significant blood loss. It can be performed as an outpatient procedure. Postoperative magnetic resonance imaging does not show any evidence of muscular damage or hematoma. The technical limitations are at L5-S1 or in patients with a high iliac crest, due to the angulation required to access the interspinous space. There are still few clinical data available. The implant is currently used in a prospective randomized controlled IDE trial in the United States for the treatment of dynamic lumbar spinal stenosis.

## Other Implant Types (Figure 54-7)

There are a variety of other implants with comparable biomechanical effects. Most of them are implanted through a posterior midline approach.

## Coflex (Paradigm Spine, New York, NY, USA) (Figure 54-8)

This is a U-shaped titanium implant with two bendable wings on its cranial and caudal parts. The Coflex is a dynamic extension stopper that acts like a spring in such a way that extension leads to an elastic compression of the "U" (Figure 54-9). It is either used as an adjunct to open decompression in spinal stenosis cases to unload the facet joints and to "keep the spinal canal open," or following discectomy to "protect" the disc from excessive load. It thus represents a low back pain treatment concept, i.e., a dynamic stabilization to reduce the load on the facet joints and/or the disc space, and/or to keep the spinal canal "open" by interspinous distraction following decompression procedures.

## Surgical Technique

The patient positioning is the same as for open decompression (knee-chest or prone). After segmental decompression the surfaces of the spinous processes are "shaped" to achieve a good press fit of the implant (Figure 54-10). The interspinous ligament is completely resected, and the supraspinous ligament is detached from the spinous processes and reattached with transosseous sutures after the implantation. The size of the implant is determined with templates. The implant is inserted and press fit between the spinous processes as far anterior as possible, leaving 2 to 3 mm space between the dura and the bottom of the U.

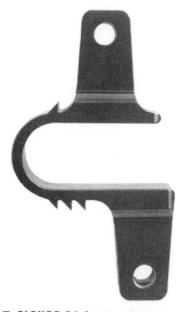

■ **FIGURE 54-8**   The Coflex implant.

## Results

First results have been presented by Adelt et al.[23] The implant was used as an adjunct to open decompression in a series of more than 200 patients with spinal stenosis. After a follow-up period of an average of 2 years, more than 90% of the patients reported subjective satisfaction. In 429 patients followed for 1 year postoperatively, the authors found an improvement in low back pain in 75%, an improvement in leg pain in 87%, and an improvement in intermittent neurogenic claudication in 87%. Ninety-three percent answered "yes" when asked whether they would again decide to have this type of operation if they were in the same situation. The complication rate in their series was 6%. Satisfactory results were also published recently by Brussee et al in a series of 65 patients with degenerative lumbar spinal stenosis, 74.2% of whom were very or moderately satisfied.[24] However, considering all domains of the Zurich Claudication Questionnaire, an overall good result could only be achieved in 30.6% of the patients.[24] In a prospective study, the Coflex was used in 18 patients with segmental lumbar instability and compared to 24 patients in whom a PLIF procedure was applied.[25] After 1 year follow-up, both groups showed significant improvement on the Visual Analog Scale (VAS); however, the range of motion in the segment above the index level increased significantly following the fusion procedure as compared to the dynamic stabilization with Coflex. The authors conclude that Coflex can be a good alternative to fusion, posing less stress in the adjacent level.

## Summary

The Coflex implant seems to be a valuable alternative to segmental fusion following open decompression in patients with lumbar spinal stenosis and low back pain. Considering the fact that the patient population is old and usually multimorbid, the low complication rates of the Coflex device as compared to fusion procedures, as well as the high subjective satisfaction rates, seem to justify its application. However, evidence-based data are lacking. The implant is currently in an FDA-IDE trial in the United States.

## DYNAMIC/RIGID INTERSPINOUS STABILIZERS

The rationale behind this second group of interspinous distraction devices is to achieve an interspinous stabilization to avoid or to augment fusion. Whereas the extension stoppers described above do not provide

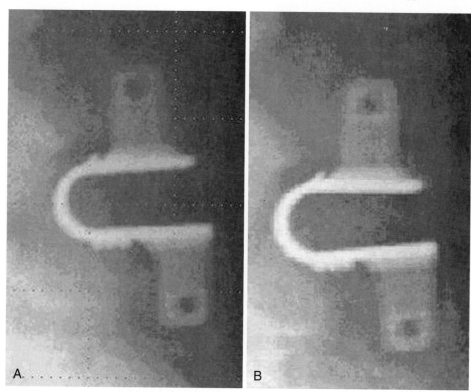

Flexion                                   Extension

■ **FIGURE 54-9**   Coflex implant behavior in **(A)** extension and **(B)** flexion.

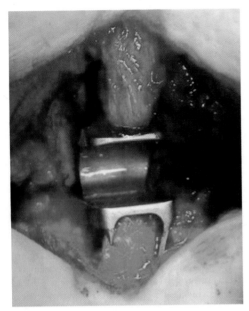

■ **FIGURE 54-10** Intraoperative picture showing the Coflex implant in place.

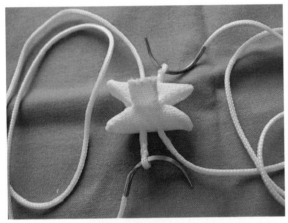

■ **FIGURE 54-11** The DIAM implant.

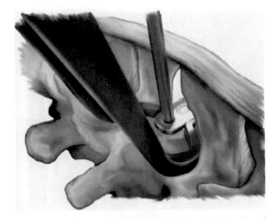

■ **FIGURE 54-12** Determination of the DIAM implant size.

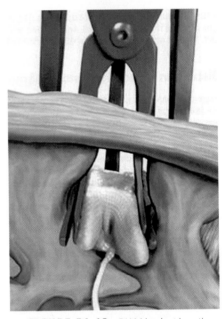

■ **FIGURE 54-13** DIAM implant insertion.

stabilization, these implants can achieve an interspinous distraction as well as an increased dynamic or rigid stability. They are thus nearly exclusively promoted to be used as an adjunct to open decompression procedures in patients with spinal stenosis or as an alternative to other types of lumbar fusion in cases of low back pain. The indications thus do not overlap with most of the extension stoppers, with perhaps the exception of the Coflex.

### The DIAM Implant (Medtronic, Minneapolis, MN, USA) (Figure 54-11)

The DIAM is a soft implant that consists of an H-shaped silicone core covered by a polyethylene sheath (Figure 54-11). It can be fixed to the spinous processes with two synthetic ligaments. The biomechanical effect, aside from interspinous distraction, is shock absorption, as well as dynamic neutralization of the motion segment.[26,27] The indications promoted by the protagonists are facet joint pain, for postdiscectomy patients, and spinal and foraminal stenosis with low back pain.[28-30] The product has been mainly used as an alternative to rigid fixation with pedicle screws.

### Surgical Technique

The implantation can be performed with or without resection of the supraspinous ligament. The interspinous ligament is resected and the implant size is determined with a template after interspinous distraction with a

distraction forceps (Figure 54-12). Within a special implant holder, the elastic implant is "folded" and inserted into the interspinous space. The ligaments are passed around the spinous processes and fixed (Figure 54-13).

### Results

First results were reported by Mariottini et al,[31] who reported satisfactory outcomes in 97 % of 43 patients. In an Italian multicenter trial, high rates of satisfaction as well as low complication rates were reported by Guizzardi in 2005.[32] Results with the DIAM implant have been reported by Taylor et al.[28] in a multicenter series of 104 patients with herniated discs, and foraminal or central spinal canal stenosis. The median follow-up was 18.1 months. There was significant pain relief in 83.8 % of patients.

Kim et al. used the implant in patients suffering from disc herniations. They compared the results of simple microdiscectomy with microdiscectomy followed by the implantation of DIAM in patients suffering from radicular as well as low back pain symptoms.[29]

After a mean postoperative follow-up of 12 months, they saw a significant improvement in both treatment groups; however, there were no differences referred to the disc space height or VAS values between the DIAM and the non-DIAM group.

### Summary

DIAM is a stabilizing interspinous implant that provides soft interspinous distraction and tension banding. The biomechanical behavior leads to a dynamic neutralization of the motion segment. Although the technique

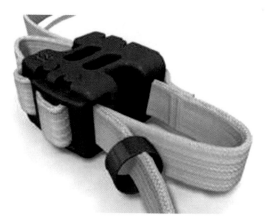

■ **FIGURE 54-14**    The Wallis implant.

seems to be less aggressive as compared to lumbar fusion techniques, good clinical data are lacking, and the evidence is still poor. The implant is currently in an FDA-IDE trial in the United States.

### The Wallis Implant (Abbott Spine, Austin, TX, USA) (Figure 54-14)

The Wallis implant was invented by Senegas in the mid-1980s.[33,34] It is an H-shaped interspinous spacer made from PEEK. It can be fixed at the spinous processes with woven Dacron bands that contain radiodense tantalum markers (Figure 54-14). The spacer blocks extension and the bands limit flexion of the motion segment. It is mainly used to increase intersegmental stability after decompression procedures.[35] Thus the main indication is low back pain that accompanies disc herniation, spinal stenosis, recurrent disc herniation, degenerative disc disease with or without Modic type I changes, as well as degenerative disc disease in a level adjacent to fusion.[34]

### Surgical Technique

The patient is usually placed in a prone position. After the decompression operation or discectomy procedure, the supraspinous ligament is detached from the spinous processes and the interspinous ligament is resected (Figure 54-15). The size of the interspinous spacer is determined with a template, after the surfaces of the spinous processes are trimmed. The concave surface of the superior spinous process is flattened, as is the junctional zone between the spinous process and the laminae. The spacer is inserted and the bands are passed around the superior and inferior spinous process (Figure 54-16). They are then passed through a clip that is snapped into the spacer. Next, the tightness of the band can finally be adjusted (Figure 54-17) to achieve a good compression. Finally, the supraspinous ligament is reattached and fixed.

### Results

In 2007, Senegas first reported a long-term survivorship of the implant in a series of 241 patients who had been treated between 1987 and 1995.[34] The survivorships were 75.9% for "any subsequent lumbar operation," and 81.3% for "implant removal."

Overall reoperation rate was 21.1%. In 2007 Floman et al reported a series of 37 patients who underwent lumbar discectomy followed by fixation with the Wallis implant.[35] The follow-up was 16 months. The indication included patients with low back pain and patients with large voluminous disc herniations. The intention was to "protect" the segment from collapse and thus to prevent recurrent disc herniation and/or low back pain postdiscectomy.

There was a significant improvement in Oswestry Disability Index (ODI) values, and in VAS for back and leg pain. However, reherniation occurred in 13% of patients. The authors thus concluded that, although the implant had a good effect on VAS and ODI values, it is probably not capable of reducing the incidence of recurrent disc herniation.

### Summary

The Wallis implant is probably the strongest interspinous implant and the one with the greatest capability to "stabilize" the segment. It is, likewise, the implant that requires the most aggressive surgical approach and is thus no less invasive than lumbar fusion techniques. Its protective effect for the disc has

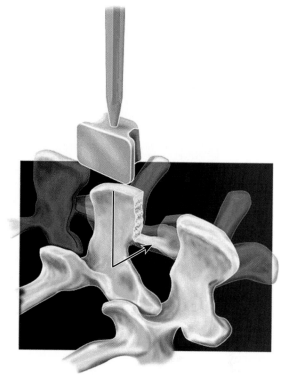

■ **FIGURE 54-15**    Preparation of the interspinous space for Wallis implantation.

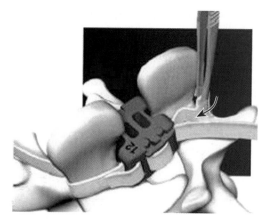

■ **FIGURE 54-16**    After the Wallis has been implanted, the ligaments are passed around the adjacent spinous processes.

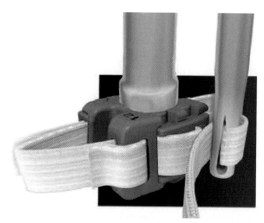

■ **FIGURE 54-17**    Final tightening of the tension bands.

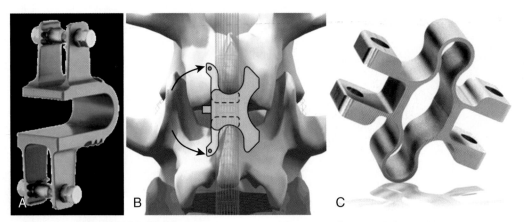

■ **FIGURE 54-18**   Other interspinous stabilizers. **A,** Coflex F. **B,** InSwing. **C,** ISS.

not been proven yet, and whether it can be an alternative to other less invasive interspinous spacers or to fusion procedures remains to be determined.

## Other Implants (Figure 54-18)

There are other interspinous spacers with stabilizing properties that are currently in clinical trials around the world, such as the Coflex F (Paradigm Spine, New York), the InSwing (Orthofix, Verona, Italy), and the ISS (Biomet, Dordrecht, Netherlands). They all follow more or less the same clinical and biomechanical principles.

## CONCLUSION

Interspinous distraction or fixation has become a new trend in spinal surgery. As with all new trends in medicine, we are currently facing a situation with an increasing number of implant and procedure concepts and a lack of empirical as well as evidence-based data for most of these implants. The mode of action and the rationale behind the clinical application of all of these interspinous spacers seems to be clear. The biomechanical studies support the expected or already proven clinical effects. There seems to be a population of patients which will probably be good candidates for these new surgical concepts. For the extension stoppers, these are mainly older patients with dynamic or early stage lumbar spinal stenosis who would otherwise be candidates for more invasive procedures such as open decompression. These patients can potentially, at least temporarily, profit from minimally invasive interspinous distraction with implant types such as Inspace or X-Stop. The other group could be younger patients with discogenic and/or arthrogenic low back pain due to degenerative disc disease (DDD) and/or facet joint osteoarthritis who would, in case of failed or unsuccessful conservative treatment, be candidates for either spinal fusion or total disc replacement.

The third main group of patients who might profit from stabilizing interspinous devices are patients who definitely require an open decompression or discectomy, who may benefit from a fusion because of segmental instability and low back pain. These patients might well profit from implants such as Coflex, DIAM, Wallis, or InSwing. The big advantages, which seem to be obvious from the short-term outcomes at the low complication rates and the reduced invasiveness as compared to fusion procedures. In a clinical setting, this lowers the application threshold, especially in a subpopulation of patients with severe comorbidities, old age, or other contraindications for fusion procedures.

Considering that all the interspinous implant techniques described in this chapter are most probably surgical solutions with an only temporary clinical effect, the level of invasiveness as well as the requirement of not "burning bridges" for further surgical procedures becomes paramount.

These aspects are addressed in most of the current clinical trials. The usefulness, clinical efficacy, and average time this clinical efficacy lasts is still to be determined for the majority of the implants. This is also true for a clearer definition of indications and contraindications. However, it seems to be obvious that there will be a place in clinical routine for at least some of the presented concepts.

## References

1. P.A. Anderson, C.B. Tribus, S.H. Kitchel C.A. Hartjen: Treatment of neurogenic claudication by interspinous decompression: application of the X-Stop device in patients with lumbar degenerative spondylolisthesis, J. Neurosurg. Spine 4 (2006) 463–471.
2. K.Y. Hsu, J.F. Zucherman, T.F. Mehalik, D.A. Implicito, M.J. Martin, D.R. Johnson, G.A. Skidmore, P.P. Vessa, J.W. Dwyer, J.C. Cauthen, R.M. Ozuna, Quality of life of lumbar stenosis-treated patients in whom the X-Stop interspinous device was implanted, J. Neurosurg. Spine 5 (2006) 500–507.
3. D.G. Kondrashov, M. Hannibal, K.Y. Hsu, J.F. Zucherman, Interspinous process decompression with the X-Stop device for lumbar spinal stenosis: a 4-year follow-up study, J. Spinal Disord. Tech. 19 (2006) 323–327.
4. C. Lauryssen, Appropriate selection of patients with lumbar spinal stenosis for interspinous process decompression, Neurosurg. Focus 22 (2007) 121–126.
5. J.F. Zucherman, K.Y. Hus, C.A. Hartjen, T.F. Mehalic, D.A. Implicito, M.J. Martin, D.R. Johnson, G.A. Skidmore, P.P. Vessa, J.W. Dwyer, S.T. Puccio, J.C. Cauthen, R.M. Ozuna, A multicenter, prospective randomized controlled trial evaluating the X-Stop interspinous process decompression system for the treatment of neurogenic intermittend claudication, Spine 30 (2005) 1351–1358.
6. D.P. Lindsey, K.E. Swanson, P. Fuchs, K.Y. Hsu, J.F. Zucherman, S.A. Yerby, The effects of an interspinous implant on the kinematics of the instrumented and adjacent levels in the lumbar spine, Spine 28 (2003) 2192–2197.
7. J.C. Richards, S. Majumbar, D.P. Lindsey, G.S. Beaupré, S.A. Yerby, The treatment mechanism of an interspinous process implant for lumbar neurogenic intermittend claudication, Spine 30 (2005) 744–749.
8. M. Siddiqui, M. Nicol, E. Karadimas, F. Smith, D. Wardlaw, The positional magnetic resonance imaging changes in the lumbar spine following insertion of a novel interspinous process distraction device, Spine 30 (2005) 2677–2682.
9. C.M. Wiseman, D.P. Lindsey, A.D. Fredrick, D, S.A. Yerby The effect of an interspinous process implant on facet loading during extension,, Spine 30 (2005) 903–907.
10. M. Siddiqui, E. Karadimas, M. Nicol, F.W. Smith, D. Wardlaw, Influence of X-Stop on neural foramina and spinal canal area in spinal stenosis, Spine 31 (2006) 2958–2962.
11. K.E. Swanson, D.P. Lindsey, K.Y. Hsu, J.F. Zucherman, S.A. Yerby, The effect of an interspinous implant on intervertebral disc pressures, Spine 28 (2003) 26–32.
12. M. Siddiqui, E. Karadimas, M. Nicol, F.W. Smith, D. Wardlaw, Effects of X-Stop device on sagittal lumbar spine kinematics in spinal stenosis, J. Spinal Disord. Tech. 19 (2006) 328–333.
13. C. Idler, J.F. Zucherman, S. Yerby, K.Y. Hsu, M. Hannibal, D. Kondrashov, A novel technique of intra-spinous process injection of PMMA to augment the strength of an interspinous process device such as the X-Stop, Spine 33 (2008) 452–456.
14. O.J. Verhoof, J.L. Bron, F.H. Wapstra, B.J. van Royen, High failure rate of the interspinous distraction device (X-Stop) for the treatment of lumbar spinal stenosis caused by degenerative spondylolisthesis, Eur. Spine J. 17 (2008) 188–192.
15. H.M. Mayer, Microsurgical decompression for acquired central and lateral spinal canal stenosis, in: H.M. Mayer (Ed.), Minimally invasive spine surgery, second ed., Springer-Verlag, Berlin – Heidelberg - New York, 2005.
16. A. McCulloch, Microsurgery for lumbar spinal canal stenosis, in: J.A. McCulloch, P.H. Young (Eds.), Essentials of spinal microsurgery, Lippincott-Raven, Philadelphia, PA, 1998.
17. J. Lim, J. Park, Biomechanical study of InSpace interspinous device, Spine Arthroplasty Society, Annual Meeting 08, Miami Poster 162, 2008.
18. L.I. Voronov, R.M. Havey, S.M. Renner, G. Carandang, C. Abjornson, A.G. Parwadhan, Biomechanics of novel posterior dynamic stabilization device (InSpace), Spine Arthroplasty Society, Annual Meeting 08, Miami Poster 148, 2008.
19. G.A. Goel, V.K. Goel, A. Mehta, D. Dick, A. Khere, C. Abjornson, Cyclic loading does not compromise functionality of interspinous spacer or any damage to the segment, Spine Arthroplasty Society, Annual Meeting 08, Miami Poster 212, 2008.
20. B. Kelly, E. Sander, N. Zufelt, D. DiAngelo, Low endurance testing of a novel spinous process spacer under coupled loading conditions, Spine Arthroplasty Society, Annual Meeting 08, Miami Poster 197, 2008.
21. H.M. Mayer, C. Mehren, G. Skidmore, et al., A new percutaneous lateral approach for the insertion of an interspinous spacer, Annual Meeting of the American Academy of Neurological Surgeons (AANS), San Diego, May 2-4, 2009.

22. H.M. Mayer, C. Mehren, C. Siepe, et al: A new interspinous spacer for minimally invasive treatment of dynamic lumbar spinal stenosis and low back pain Annual Meeting of the American Academy of Neurological Surgeons (AANS), San Diego, May 2-4, 2009.

23. D. Adelt, J. Samani, W.K. Kim, M. Eif, G. Lowery, R.J. Chomiak, Coflex interspinous stabilization: clinical and radiographic results from an international multicenter retrospective study, Paradigm Spine J. 1 (2007) 1–4.

24. P. Brussee, J. Hauth, R.D. Donk, A.L.M. Verbeek, R.H.M. Bartels, Self-rated evaluation of outcome of the implantation of interspinous process distraction (X-Stop) for neurogenic claudication, Eur. Spine J. 17 (2) (2008) 200–203.

25. D.S. Kong, E.S. Kim, W. Eoh, One-year outcome evaluation after interspinous implantation for degenerative spinal stenosis with segmental instability, J. Korean Med. Sci. 22 (2007) 330–335.

26. J.F. Schmoelz, T. Nydegger, L. Claes, H.J. Wilke, Dynamic stabilization of the lumbar spine: an in vitro experiment, J. Spinal Disord. Tech. 16 (2003) 418–423.

27. F.M. Phillips, L.I. Voronov, I.N. Gaitanis, G. Carandang, et al., Biomechanics of posterior dynamic stabilization device (DIAM) after facetectomy and discectomy, Spine J. 6 (2006) 714–722.

28. J. Taylor, P. Pupin, S. Delajoux, S. Palmer, Device for intervertebral assisted motion: technique and initial results, Neurosurg. Focus 22 (1) (2007) E6.

29. K.A. Kim, M. McDional, J.H.T. Pik, P. Khoueir, Dynamic intraspinous spacer technology for posterior stabilization: clinical safety, sagittal angulation, and pain outcome at 1-year follow-up evaluation, Neurosurg. Focus 22, 2007.

30. D. Kim, T. Albert: Interspinous process spacers, J. Am.Acad. Orthop. Sur. 15 (2007) 200–207.

31. A. Mariottini, S. Pieri, S. Giachi, et al., Preliminary results of a soft novel lumbar intervertebral prosthesis (DIAM) in the degenerative spinal pathology, Acta Neurochir. Suppl. 92 (2005) 129–131.

33. G. Guizzardi, P. Petrioni, A.P. Fabrizi, et al., The use of DIAM (interspinous stress-breaker device) for the DDD: Italian multicenter experience, Spine Arthroplasty Society Meeting, 2005.

34. J. Senegas, Mechanical supplementation by non-rigid fixation in degenerative intervertebral lumbar segments: the Wallis system, Eur. Spine J. 11 (Suppl. 2) (2002) S164–S169.

35. J. Senegas, J.M. Vital, V. Pointillard, P. Mangione, Long-term survivorship analysis of an interspinous stabilization system, Eur. Spine J. 16 (2007) 1279–1287.

36. Y. Floman, M.A. Millgram, Y. Smorgick, N. Rand, E. Ashkenazi, Failure of the Wallis Interspinous Implant to lower the incidence of recurrent lumbar disc herniations in patients undergoing primary disc excision, J. Spinal Disord. Tech. 20 (2007) 337–341.

# 55

# Lumbar Disc Arthroplasty: Indications and Contraindications

*Jessica Shellock and Richard D. Guyer*

**K E Y   P O I N T S**

- Lumbar total disc replacement (TDR) is a motion-preserving alternative to lumbar fusion.

- The established indication for TDR is chronic low back pain from single-level degenerative disc disease that has failed extensive conservative treatment.

- Patient selection is of significant importance to optimize surgical outcome from TDR.

- Patients should have minimal or no facet disease if undergoing TDR.

- In patients with osteoporosis, spinal instability, significant scoliosis, morbid obesity, or infection, TDR is contraindicated.

## INTRODUCTION

Total disc replacement (TDR) surgery began in Europe over 20 years ago and migrated to the United States in 2000 with the first TDR Food and Drug Administration (FDA) Investigational Device Exemption (IDE) trial of the Charité III disc. Results based on the long-term follow-up from European literature have been promising so far, as have the early results from our U.S. experience.[1-5] Some of the first 5-year follow-up data from the FDA IDE trial comparing the Charité disc to lumbar fusion are now available.[6] The results show no statistically significant differences in outcome measures (visual analog scales (VAS) assessing pain and the Oswestry Disability Index) between the groups at the five-year mark, substantiating the noninferiority of the disc arthroplasty group. Additionally, the Charité patients had a statistically greater rate of part-time and full-time employment and a lower rate of long-term disability at 5 years. Furthermore, the range of motion of the prosthesis, as evaluated by radiographic criteria, remained the same at 5-years compared with the 2-year data, showing preservation of motion at the surgical level.

At the time of writing of this chapter, a recently published systematic review analyzing the association of symptomatic adjacent segment disease (as distinguished from asymptomatic adjacent segment degeneration) in lumbar arthroplasty compared to arthrodesis showed that 14% of arthrodesis patients developed adjacent segment disease, compared with 1% of arthroplasty patients.[7] Given this positive trend for arthroplasty, it is reasonable to assume that disc replacement surgery will remain a valid tool in the spine surgeon's armamentarium and will likely become more prevalent in years to come.

There are a number of factors that influence the outcome following total disc replacement, including meticulous surgical technique and appropriate implant selection. However, as with any surgical procedure, patient selection is of utmost importance for ultimate success and reproducible results. A thorough knowledge of appropriate indications and contraindications for spinal disc arthroplasty is the key to maximizing patient safety and surgical outcome. It is the goal of this chapter to discuss these various indications and contraindications as they pertain to disc arthroplasty in the lumbar spine, with particular emphasis on older patients. It is not our intention to simply reiterate the various indications and contraindications for the multiple devices as previously published for the FDA studies. Rather, we will examine this topic from a practical standpoint, considering some of the intrinsic patient factors, surgical factors, radiographic factors, and device-specific factors that would make a patient either a favorable candidate for total disc replacement or an unfavorable one. It is still important to realize that the strict criteria set forth by the FDA for the initial studies on disc replacement were intended to maximize the expected benefit from the procedure and minimize any possible complications. Additionally, one should keep in mind that the participating surgeons for the trials were chosen in large part because of their many years of surgical experience. These surgeons were poised to climb the necessary learning curve more readily than many other surgeons who were still early in their training. Therefore, the aforementioned strict inclusion and exclusion criteria for the clinical trials should be viewed as a beacon for those surgeons embarking on the first part of the learning curve with artificial disc replacement.

When we focus our attention specifically on the aging spine, we must consider a few different scenarios. The first scenario is that of the chronologically-young patient with a physiologically aged and degenerative disc, who meets the requirements for disc arthroplasty. In this case, the prosthesis will be subjected to the normal physiologic aging process and it will be the longevity of the prosthesis that poses the ultimate challenge. One must be aware of the likely need for some type of revision procedure in the future and weigh this risk with the anticipated benefit from the surgery. Furthermore, the question must be asked whether a motion-preserving implant such as a disc arthroplasty will still provide any motion in 20 years, and what the relevance of this might be. These are questions that should be answered once more long-term data are available. The second scenario is that of the patient of more advanced age who presents for consideration of a disc arthroplasty. This scenario, as would be expected, poses a completely different set of diagnostic and treatment challenges for the spine surgeon. With advanced age, the likelihood of medical comorbidities or other physiologic contraindications to disc replacement is increased. Moreover, what happens when a disc arthroplasty is implanted in an older patient who meets all the inclusion criteria at the time of surgery, but in the years to follow develops osteoporosis or significant osteopenia? Will this have an impact on the performance of the prosthesis or dramatically increase the risk of subsidence? In this chapter, we will make a specific effort to touch upon some of the special challenges of the aging spine. It is becoming more prevalent to have patients that remain highly active well into their sixth and seventh decades and who want to be evaluated as candidates for the new technology of motion preservation.

## CLINICAL PRACTICE GUIDELINES

### Indications

The established indication initially set forth by the FDA IDE studies for lumbar disc arthroplasty is severe unremitting low back pain resulting from single-level degenerative disc disease that has failed to respond to a prolonged course of conservative measures. The trial period for conservative treatment is usually defined as a minimum of 6 months, although the exact time frame itself is less important than the extent to which nonoperative management has been attempted. Nonoperative treatments should incorporate the use of various antiinflammatory, nonnarcotic, and even narcotic medications if necessary; physical therapy, including active exercise and core stabilization; chiropractic modalities; and a trial of spinal injections, including epidural injections and facet injections as appropriate. The purpose of these conservative efforts is to ensure that the patient has been afforded every opportunity to obtain a satisfactory result without surgery. We know that MRI alone is not a reliable indicator in predicting whether a degenerative-appearing disc is truly symptomatic.[8, 9] In some cases, discography may be helpful in delineating whether the disc is responsible for the patient's clinical symptoms. The exact role for discography as part of the clinical work-up for potential surgical candidates is not clearly established, and is still an issue of significant controversy. That being said, at our institution we incorporate the use of discography in all patients that we feel might be appropriate candidates for total disc replacement. Because the interpretation of results from discography can heavily depend on the skill of the technician performing the procedure, the established relationship between the surgeon and the physician performing the test cannot be overemphasized. In our opinion, a poorly-done discogram is worse than no discogram at all.

A patient must be skeletally mature to undergo disc replacement. While many of the studies have cited an age range from 18 to 60 years of age in the inclusion criteria, the actual chronological age itself is simply a number

for reference. It must be taken into account with more relevant factors such as appropriate vertebral body size to accommodate the prosthesis and adequate bone quality to support the implant, which often, but not always, can be correlated with the patient's age. It is also the authors' belief that disc arthroplasty technology should be reserved for those patients over the age of 25 years until further long-term data becomes available. We have been proponents of recommending bone density scans in all females older than 40 years of age and all males over 50 years of age unless other risk factors are present. The acceptable bone quality is to have a T-score of more than −1.0, based on World Health Organization criteria, meaning that there is no evidence of osteopenia. Some patients with an advanced chronological age remain physiologically young and could still be a legitimate candidate for disc arthroplasty. In fact, these are important patients to identify when we are considering the issue of the 'aging spine.' On the contrary, some patients with a younger chronological age can have medical comorbidities or poor bone quality that effectively removes them from surgical consideration. It also becomes important, particularly in the elderly population, to carefully evaluate whether motion preservation is justified compared to the alternative of fusion surgery. We do not yet have enough long-term data to make resolute conclusions regarding the proposed advantages of motion preservation in comparison with fusion as it pertains to adjacent segment disease; however, with the knowledge currently available, we can feel fairly justified in our desire to preserve motion in young patients with isolated discogenic pain. The more elderly candidates may not ultimately see the benefit of disc

## Clinical Case Examples

### CASE 1

A 54-year-old woman presents to your clinic with complaints of severe low back pain that has progressed over the past 2 years. She has been through physical therapy focusing on core muscle strengthening and has had a trial of epidural steroid injections and various facet injections that did not improve her symptoms. She denies any radicular leg pain, but states that her low back pain is constant and is aggravated by prolonged standing, sitting, or walking. She has been on NSAIDs for the past few years, and has

recently started to take narcotics because of increased pain. A complete neurological examination reveals no motor or sensory deficits. She has pain and limited motion with forward flexion of her lumbar spine. Her radiographs (Figures 55-1A and B) show normal spinal alignment with decreased disc space height at the L4-5 and L5-S1 level. No instability is present on flexion-extension views. A T2-weighted MRI (Figures 55-2A and B) reveals a dessicated L4-5 disc with preservation of hydration in the remaining lumbar discs. Given this scenario, what treatment option(s) would you discuss with this patient?

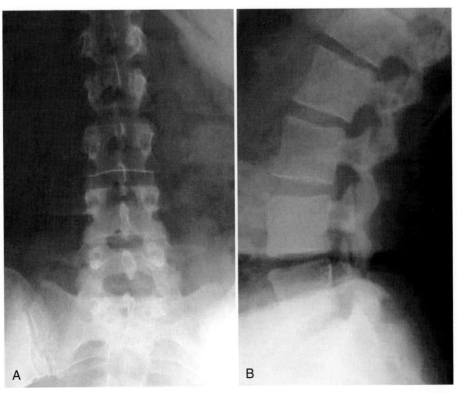

■ FIGURE 55-1   A and B. AP **(A)** and lateral **(B)** radiographs showing disc space narrowing at L4-5 and L5-S1.

## CASE 2

A 56-year-old male presents to your clinic for evaluation of debilitating low back pain over the last 6 years. He reports daily pain that radiates across his low back, worse on the right side. His primary care physician sent him to physical therapy for 6 weeks, but he did not see any symptomatic improvement. He has been taking hydrocodone for the past 6 months in order to bring his pain to a tolerable level but is frustrated by the need to be on narcotic medications and wishes for something to be done surgically to address his pain. His physical examination is fairly unremarkable and he has normal motor and sensory function. His plain radiographs reveal only minimal narrowing at the L4-5 and L5-S1 levels (Figure 55-3A and B). A T2-weighted MRI reveals pronounced desiccation with a small posterior bulge, along with minimal disc desiccation at the L4-5 level (Figure 55-4). On axial MRI views, the facet joints at both levels appear normal or with minimal degenerative changes. He asks whether he is a candidate for the disc replacement surgery. What do you tell him?

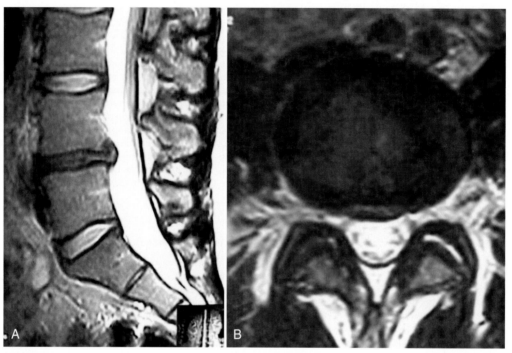

■ **FIGURE 55-2**   Sagittal **(A)** and axial **(B)** T2-weighted MRI views showing disc dehydration and posterior bulge at the L4-5 level.

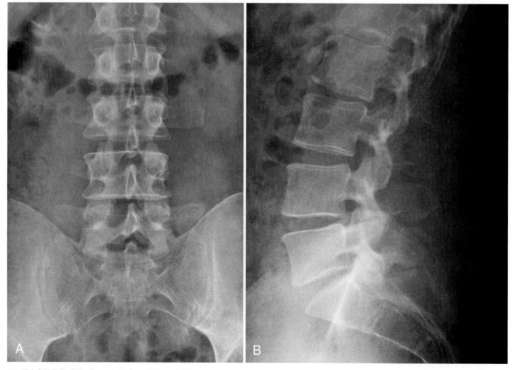

■ **FIGURE 55-3**   AP **(A)** and lateral **(B)** radiographs showing only minimal disc space narrowing at L4-5 and L5-S1.

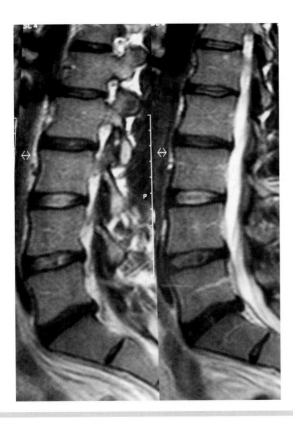

■ **FIGURE 55-4**    Sagittal T2-weighted MRI showing significant disc dessication at L5-S1 and slight desiccation at the L4-5 level.

replacement, particularly if further studies suggest that adjacent-level disease is borne out over periods of 10 years or greater.

Bertagnoli and Kumar stratified indications for disc arthroplasty into four categories based on remaining disc height, status of the facet joints, adjacent level degeneration, and stability of the posterior elements.[10] The prime candidate for a disc replacement, based on their evaluation of clinical outcome in 108 patients who underwent implantation of a ProDisc II prosthesis, had at least 4 mm of remaining disc space height, no radiographic changes suggestive of facet arthritis, no adjacent level disc degeneration, and intact posterior elements.

Certainly, having competent, nondegenerative facets and posterior element stability are important inclusion criteria for a patient to be considered appropriate to undergo TDR. We will discuss the issue of facet arthrosis further as a part of contraindications to disc arthroplasty, but as far as a clinical evaluation is concerned, facets should be assessed with direct palpation and by having the patient demonstrate whether spinal extension (i.e., facet loading) reproduces pain. Radiographically, the facets should be evaluated by examining their appearance on plain films, CT scans, and/or axial MR images. There exist a few grading systems for facet joints, although none has gained universal acceptance. The first, proposed by Pathria, assigned a grade of 0 to 3, depending on the extent of facet joint narrowing.[11] A "normal" facet joint is given a grade of 0, whereas a grade 1 is assigned for mild narrowing, 2 for moderate, and 3 for severe narrowing. Patients with grade 3 facets in this grading system should be excluded as candidates for disc arthroplasty. Fujiwara also proposed a grading system based on evaluation of the facet joints as they appear on axial MR images.[12] In this system, a grade of 0 is again assigned to "normal" facets, grade 1 for moderately compressed facets with small osteophytes, grade 2 for facets with subchondral sclerosis and moderate osteophytes, and grade 3 for facets lacking articular joint space and with large osteophytes. Again, patients who meet the criteria for grade 3 facets in this classification system are not indicated for total disc arthroplasty.

Since the facets transmit nearly 20% of the load-bearing forces in the lumbar spine in the normal state, but can increase this number to 50% in the degenerative state when a patient is standing, they must not be a contributing pain generator if a patient is to expect maximal benefit from a motion-preserving procedure. As for the importance of the posterior elements, a prosthetic disc alone cannot substitute for lack of stability in a given spinal motion segment. This is certainly true in the case of the less constrained prostheses.

A patient must also have no more than 3 mm of anterolisthesis at the level under consideration to be considered appropriate for disc replacement.

Concern over the relationship between preoperative disc height and clinical outcome in disc arthroplasty with severely collapsed disc space (i.e., less than 4 mm) is somewhat controversial. Despite speculation that TDR is not appropriate for severely collapsed discs, there exist few data to support or refute this. At our institution, we set out to determine if there was a relationship between preoperative and/or postoperative disc height and clinical outcome at 2 years (Li, Guyer, et al., International Meeting on Advanced Spinal Techniques, 2008).[13] For 117 patients (42 Charité and 75 ProDisc-L) undergoing a single-level TDR, we recorded disc height as a ratio of vertebral body height, thereby accounting for variation in individual size and radiographic magnification. Patients were categorized into four groups based on these ratios (most collapsed, second most collapsed, second least collapsed, least collapsed). For all groups, the mean VAS pain score improved significantly from preoperative values, but there were no statistically significant differences among the groups. We therefore concluded that there is no relationship between preoperative disc height and clinical outcome. If patients with severely collapsed discs otherwise meet the strict selection criteria for TDR, they can expect as favorable an outcome from the surgery as patients with discs that are not as collapsed.

In addition to the aforementioned clinical criteria, it is also important to ensure that the patient is capable of completely understanding the various risks related to the surgery itself and the realistic expectations following the procedure. Based on the accumulated VAS and Oswestry scores from the various IDE studies of disc arthroplasty, including data from the Charité, ProDisc-L, Maverick, Flexicore, and Kineflex studies, patients can be counseled that 80% of people undergoing lumbar TDR can expect to achieve a 50% reduction in their pain and a 50% improvement in their functional ability. They must be willing to comply with any postoperative restrictions imposed on them by the surgical procedure and must also be willing participants in the postoperative rehabilitation protocol.

## Contraindications

It is often easier to define patients who are not good candidates for a given procedure than to accurately define those who would be suitable. To some extent, the same can be said for lumbar disc arthroplasty. In recent years, much attention has turned toward defining and understanding the established contraindications for TDR, and this, in turn, has generated some controversy. In an epidemiological study to investigate the contraindications to lumbar total disc arthroplasty in their patient population (that of an academic medical center), Huang et al reported that 95% of patients had at least one of ten contraindications to surgery.[13] This finding was further substantiated in a recent publication by Wong et al,[14] who retrospectively reviewed 100 consecutive lumbar spine surgery patients with specific analysis of facet arthrosis and noted that all patients had one or more of the aforementioned ten contraindications to the procedure. In their population (a private medical center), they found that 97% of patients had facet arthrosis as the contraindication against TDR, followed by spondylolisthesis (75%), and central spinal stenosis (72%).

For the purpose of our discussion, we will group contraindications into two categories: absolute or "hard" contraindications, and relative or "soft" contraindications. Absolute contraindications include osteopenia and osteoporosis, history of previous disc infection or ongoing infection, prior fusion at the level of consideration, severe posterior element pathology, instability at the operative segment, vertebral fracture, malignancy, curves of greater than 11 degrees, metal allergy, and a psychosocial state that places a given patient at increased risk for poor surgical outcome. Additionally, as this is entirely an elective procedure, pregnancy should be viewed as an absolute contraindication. Relative contraindications include history of prior abdominal surgery, and obesity. To better appreciate the reasons behind the various contraindications, we will discuss a number of them in further detail. The reader may also refer to Table 55-1, which gives a summary of the contraindications that will be discussed in the chapter.

### Osteopenia and Osteoporosis

Osteopenia with a T-score between −1.0 and −2.5 and osteoporosis (T-score < −2.5) are absolute contraindications for lumbar total disc arthroplasty. During some of the initial FDA IDE studies, the exclusion criteria for T-scores was not quite as stringent; however, early investigator experience with endplate fractures and prosthesis subsidence resulted in a revision of the exclusion criteria. On that note, in the case of an intraoperative endplate fracture for any reason, the only salvage option is to proceed with a fusion procedure. A motion-sparing device cannot function appropriately and maintain rigid fixation in the face of an endplate fracture.

Although normal bone quality does not guarantee against an endplate fracture, lack of adequate bone mineral density greatly increases the risk that vertebral bodies could be fractured during placement of the device or sustain a fracture in the postoperative period, particularly if the placement of the prosthesis is anything less than perfect. Additionally, even in ideally positioned devices, osteoporotic bone has a greater chance of allowing implant subsidence secondary to deficiency of endplate structural integrity, which could lead to a need for revision surgery.

If a patient has any risk factors for osteoporosis, a DEXA scan should be ordered. In our institution, all women over age 40 and men over age 50 who are being considered for a disc arthroplasty receive a preoperative DEXA scan as part of the screening process. If the results of the study reveal osteopenia or osteoporosis, we do not proceed with arthroplasty and make sure that the patient's primary care physician is made aware of the results so that appropriate medical treatment can be initiated. One caveat, however, is that if the T-score is −1.1 to −1.5, the authors will refer the patient for medical treatment and then follow up with repeat DEXA scans to see if there has

been interval improvement that would perhaps allow for proceeding with arthroplasty.

### Infection or Malignancy

Any patient with a history of active local or systemic infection or prior disc infection is not a candidate for TDR. This is also true for patients with active malignancy. Disc arthroplasty is an elective surgical procedure aimed at improving a patient's pain and restoring functional capacity. Health issues that put a patient at increased risk for a poor outcome from surgery should be viewed as absolute contraindications.

### Facet Joints

An appreciation of the status of the facet joints is vital in evaluating a patient for a TDR. Yet, this is arguably the area of greatest controversy in discussions of disc arthroplasty candidates. The question of "how much is too much?" remains to be answered definitively. In an earlier section of this chapter, we discussed that any patient under consideration for TDR should have no or minimal degenerative changes of the facet joints. Clearly, facet arthrosis follows a spectrum of degenerative processes, and there exists no reliable and universally accepted grading system by which to categorize the various stages of disease. Despite attempts by various authors at defining such stages, as was discussed earlier in the chapter,[12, 15] it remains unclear what the clinical implications of these stratifications are. Eventually, with more long-term data, it is likely that the issue will unfold more clearly; however, for the time being, we are left with many opinions and few hard data.

Fortunately, there are a few situations that are fairly straightforward and should be viewed as absolute contraindications to disc arthroplasty. The first situation is when a patient with presumed discogenic pain undergoes isolated facet injections that completely render that patient asymptomatic, even if for a brief time period. In that case, the facet joints are a proven pain generator and disc replacement is clearly not the solution to improving the patient's pain. Even in cases where the relief is not complete, but is greater than 50%, one should consider that TDR may not be the appropriate procedure.

### Scoliosis

Many elderly patients eventually develop some degree of degenerative scoliosis that may or may not be symptomatic. Scoliotic curves of greater than 11 degrees have traditionally been considered a deformity beyond the scope of artificial disc replacement. The senior author's experience is that 5 degrees is a safer set point because, with the original 11-degree cut-off, there have been cases of progression. However, with future prostheses that may provide increased stability, cases of mild scoliosis may not be an exclusion criterion for disc arthroplasty. The issue is simply that of inability to position the prosthesis in such a way that early loosening or failure would not be of particular concern.

### Spondylolysis and Spondylolisthesis

Bilateral spondylolysis is an absolute contraindication to total disc arthroplasty. This presents a situation of posterior instability that cannot be compensated for by the prosthesis. In the FDA studies, most cited exclusion criteria of greater than 3 mm of listhesis. Again, this is an area where controversy exists. Is there an "absolute" measurement of listhesis beyond which a total disc replacement should be contraindicated? What about the variability inherent in the grouping of "Grade I" spondylolisthesis? Many spine surgeons have observed a trend for slight retrolisthesis of the cranial vertebral body at a degenerative level because of the loss of disc space height alone. The authors do not consider retrolisthesis or relative retrolisthesis as a contraindication, especially at L5-S1, where it is extremely common. Ultimately, the issue comes down to that of instability. If, on flexion-extension radiographs of the lumbar spine (which we routinely get in patients we evaluate for surgery), there is any instability greater than a few millimeters, the patient should undergo a fusion procedure, not a disc replacement.

### Prior Abdominal Surgery

Because the standard surgical approach to the disc space for TDR is through an anterior retroperitoneal approach, a history of prior abdominal surgery is a relative contraindication, since the patient is likely to have adhesions that can make the subsequent surgical approach fraught with difficulty and

---

**TABLE 55-1    Contraindications to TDR**

Central or lateral recess stenosis
Facet arthrosis
Bilateral spondylolysis
Spondylolisthesis
Scoliosis with curves > 5°
Osteoporosis or osteopenia (T-score < −1.0)
Posterior element deficiency
Active systemic infection or malignancy
Morbid obesity
Psychosocial "red flags"

possible complications. Prior retroperitoneal surgical approach is an absolute contraindication, due to scarring of the great vessels. It is vital to have good communication with the approach surgeon who will be assisting in the case, and the ultimate decision as to whether the approach can be safely navigated should be his or hers.

## Obesity

Morbid obesity (defined as a body mass index > 40) is an absolute contraindication for lumbar disc replacement. From the standpoint of the prosthesis, obesity theoretically results in increased stress across the disc space, possibly resulting in implant subsidence or increased wear, although this has not yet been proven. Furthermore, from the standpoint of the surgical approach alone, access to the disc space is much more difficult in an excessively large patient. Should any intraoperative vascular complication arise, the patient would be at increased risk of morbidity or mortality because of size alone. Many of the required surgical instruments are simply not long enough to be easily used in obese patients. In questionable cases due to patient size, it is helpful to again recruit the opinion of the approach surgeon to determine whether the procedure can be done safely for the patient. At our institution, we counsel morbidly obese patients regarding the necessity of weight loss, including the possibility of lap-band surgery, prior to consideration of TDR.

## Metal Allergy

Most spinal disc arthroplasty prostheses are composed of a cobalt-chromium-molybdenum alloy and/or polyethylene. Any patient with a history of allergy to cobalt-chromium should be considered an inappropriate candidate for total disc arthroplasty. Some spinal arthroplasty devices have a titanium coating in addition, so titanium allergy should also be a contraindication. To date, we are aware of the existence of four cases of spinal disc arthroplasty (three lumbar and one cervical) in which the patients developed early prosthetic failure and subsequent mass effect from presumptive metal hypersensitivity to various metal-on-metal prostheses. All patients ultimately required removal of their prostheses and salvage fusion procedures.

Although metal sensitivity has long been recognized as an entity in the orthopedic world, specifically in reference to total joint prostheses, little has been published to date regarding effects seen from spinal implants. Metal ions released with metal-on-metal bearings have not resulted in any reported adverse clinical sequelae, but numerous reports exist of local soft-tissue masses and early prosthetic failure resulting from this situation. The reported prevalence of metal allergy in the hip literature is approximately 1%. From the limited data available with metal-on-metal spinal prostheses, it seems that a similar prevalence may exist, although many more studies are needed in this area.

## Anatomic and Vascular Considerations

In particular regard to the aging population, there are certain vascular considerations that must be accounted for prior to undergoing disc replacement surgery. Significant calcification of the abdominal aorta, especially circumferential calcification, at the disc level of interest should be a contraindication to the procedure, as necessary surgical retraction of the vessel during the procedure can increase the chance of a calcific plaque embolizing distally to the extremities. This becomes particularly risky at the L4-5 level, which is often subject to the greatest amount of aortic retraction to gain exposure to the disc space. Calcifications in the vessel that exist at levels cranial or caudal to the disc space of interest may not be as serious an issue, but consideration should be given to these in all circumstances. The lateral radiograph of the lumbar spine is often the best and most reliable indicator of the presence of significant aortic calcifications, and a CT scan will give accurate information as to the degree.

## Discussion of Clinical Case Examples

### CASE 1

In our first case example, the patient is a middle-aged woman who has been through appropriate conservative management but has persistence of severe back pain. She has imaging studies suggestive of single-disc disease at the L4-5 level. If she is insistent upon having surgery, it is a reasonable option to discuss a one-level fusion at the suspected symptomatic L4-5 level. However, concern might exist that by fusing the L4-5 level, an increased amount of stress would be placed upon the L5-S1 level, possibly causing it to become symptomatic sooner than it otherwise would have done. She is also a very reasonable candidate to undergo total disc replacement, and given the aforementioned concern, we would likely be in favor of TDR over fusion. She ultimately decided to undergo TDR and had complete resolution of her back pain (Figure 55-5 A and B).

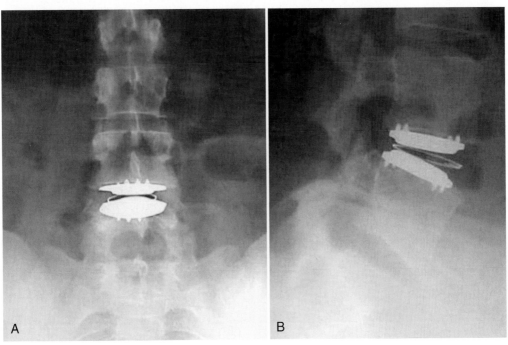

■ **FIGURE 55-5**  Postoperative AP **(A)** and lateral **(B)** films showing a Charité TDR at the L4-5 level.

## CASE 2

The gentleman presented in the second case represents more of a diagnostic and treatment challenge. He has two disc levels that could be symptomatic, with the L5-S1 level appearing the worst, based solely on imaging studies. However, knowing that imaging studies alone can be misleading, it would be helpful to ensure that the suspected level is truly the pain generator and determine whether the L4-5 level is also a contributing factor. We used discography to help with our decision-making (Figure 55-6). Both the L5-S1 and L4-5 levels reproduced concordant pain of 10/10 and 8/10 respectively, and the L3-4 level was completely asymptomatic. The options discussed with him included either fusion at both levels or consideration of fusion at the more caudal level and a disc replacement at the cranial level. At this point, two-level lumbar total disc replacement has not been FDA-approved. He decided to undergo a hybrid procedure, with L5-S1 fusion and an artificial disc at the L4-5 level (Figure 55-7 A and B). Within 6 weeks following surgery, he was able to discontinue use of all narcotic medications.

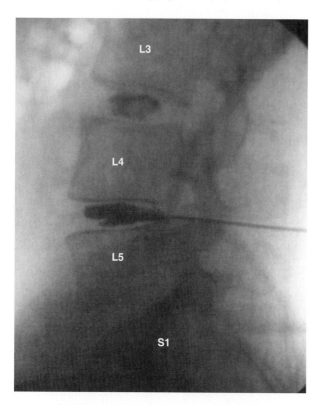

■ **FIGURE 55-6** Discography was utilized to evaluate the L3-S1 levels. This figure shows the normal L3-4 disc and the injection at L4-5.

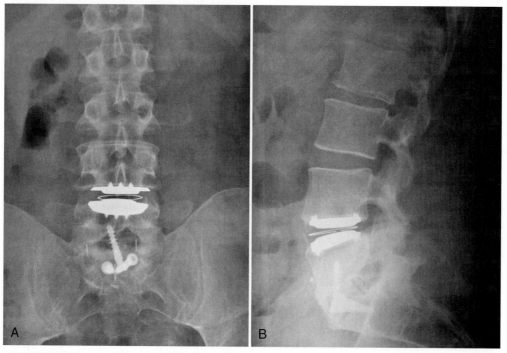

■ **FIGURE 55-7** Postoperative AP **(A)** and lateral **(B)** films showing fusion at the L5-S1 level and TDR at the L4-5 level.

Another anatomical consideration that may preclude disc arthroplasty is the slight anatomical variations that exist at the more cranial lumbar levels with regard to the kidneys and the renal vasculature. At the L2-3 level, it may sometimes not be possible or safe to implant an artificial disc because of the inability to mobilize the renal artery or vein, or even the kidneys themselves.

## Psychosocial Factors

Last, but certainly not least, we must discuss psychosocial factors as a potential contraindication to total disc arthroplasty. Much work has been done with regard to evaluating the effect of a patient's psychological state in relation to predicting surgical outcome. Even the most perfectly executed surgical procedure will fail to alleviate pain in patients with serious psychological overlay. The concept of presurgical psychological screening (PPS) has been advocated to objectively identify psychosocial risk factors that can lead to poor results from surgery, even when the physical pathology causing pain has been eliminated. The screening process takes many things into consideration, including personality and emotional factors, behavioral and environmental factors, and even historical factors for a given patient.

One of the strongest risk factors for poor surgical outcome relates to excessive pain sensitivity as assessed by the hysteria and hypochondriasis scales of the MMPI. Elevations in these scales have been shown to be associated with poor spine surgery outcome in numerous studies.[16] Other studies have determined that patients who abuse narcotic medications and/or alcohol also have a high failure rate following spine surgery. Recently the use of PPS, specifically in lumbar TDR patients, was reported (Block et al, North American Spine Society, 2008). The authors found that the results of screening were significantly related to clinical outcome. In cases where the spine surgeon has suspicion that multiple psychosocial factors may exist and compromise outcome from the proposed surgery, it can be quite helpful to incorporate the use of PPS as part of the preoperative work-up.

## CONCLUSIONS

Technological advances in materials and design, coupled with a greater biomechanical appreciation for motion, have spawned a new age in spine surgery. Total disc replacement has yet to see the pinnacle of its day, but has generated enough press that patients often present to clinics with the expectation and desire to be recipients of this procedure. Our excitement to participate in the wave of this emerging technology must be met with great caution as we evaluate potential candidates for disc replacement. Strict adherence to inclusion and exclusion criteria benefits everybody involved in the process. Most importantly, this ensures that patients have the greatest chance of expecting a positive outcome and surgical success. Positive outcomes help to ensure that the technology will become more widely appreciated and accepted, whether by our patients, by the federal agencies funding the procedure, or by private insurers.

As the population continues to age and remain active, the demand from our patients has moved toward expectations of maintaining function. Patients who are chronologically aged but remain physiologically young may be appropriate candidates for disc replacement. Age alone may not be an appropriate exclusion criterion in isolation, but should be taken in context with the many other factors we have discussed in the chapter. In other words, the "aging spine" may still be deserving of this new technology. In fact, data on patients enrolled in the IDE study of the Charité Artificial Disc were analyzed based on age, with groupings of patients aged 18 to 45 years compared with those aged 46 to 60 years.[16] At 2-year follow-up, there was no significant difference between the groups with respect to changes in ODI scores, VAS scores, or SF-36 component scores compared to baseline values. Patient satisfaction was equivalent in both groups (87% and 85%, respectively), and no significant differences were noted as far as adverse events or reoperation. This reflects the fact that, given judicious application of inclusion and exclusion criteria, patients who are chronologically older can still expect equivalent outcomes to their younger counterparts. Bertagnoli et al

prospectively evaluated a series of patients aged 60 years or older (range 61 to 71 years) who underwent TDR for discogenic low back pain.[17] They noted statistically significant improvement in patient satisfaction and ODI scores by 3 months after surgery and maintenance of these improvements throughout the 24-month follow-up. Although the authors recommend cautious use of TDR in this population, their results suggest that if patients otherwise meet indications for TDR, with particular attention to spinal stenosis and bone quality, age greater than 60 years alone is not a factor that should preclude them from having this procedure.

There are many questions for which we do not yet have answers. What happens to the patient with a TDR who develops osteoporosis? Will the prosthesis subside or will Wolff's law protect the endplates? Will the prostheses function for the 40 years for which they have been biomechanically tested or will the TDRs give way to a slow fusion? With more time and with the accumulation of more long-term data from the population of total disc arthroplasty patients, these questions and others will be answered, and more stringent inclusion and exclusion criteria will be defined. Until that point, it is our hope that the discussion presented in this chapter will provide enough of a framework for surgeons who are currently performing disc replacements or those who are interested in pursuing this procedure to be able to provide the best possible outcomes for our patients, with consideration of their safety as our primary goal.

## References

1. T. David, Long-term results of one-level lumbar arthroplasty: minimum 10-year follow-up of the CHARITÉ artificial disc in 106 patients, Spine 32 (2007) 661–666.
2. J.P. Lemaire, H. Carrier, H. Sariali el, W. Skalli, F. Lavaste, Clinical and radiological outcomes with the Charite artificial disc: a 10-year minimum follow-up, J. Spinal Disord. Tech. 18 (2005) 353–359.
3. P. Tropiano, R.C. Huang, F.P. Girardi, F.P. Cammisa, T. Marnay, Lumbar total disc replacement: seven to eleven-year follow-up, J. Bone Joint Surg. Am. 87 (2005) 490–496.
4. S. Blumenthal, P.C. McAfee, R.D. Guyer, S.H. Hochschuler, F.H. Geisler, R.T. Holt, et al., A prospective, randomized, multicenter Food and Drug Administration investigational device exemptions study of lumbar total disc replacement with the CHARITÉ artificial disc versus lumbar fusion: part I: evaluation of clinical outcomes,, Spine 30 (2005) 1565–1575.
5. J. Zigler, R. Delamarter, J.M. Spivak, R.J. Linovitz, G.O. Danielson, T.T. Haider, et al., Results of the prospective, randomized, multicenter Food and Drug Administration investigational device exemption study of the ProDisc-L total disc replacement versus circumferential fusion for the treatment of 1-level degenerative disc disease, Spine 32 (2007) 1155–1162.
6. R.D. Guyer, P.C. McAfee, R.J. Banco, F.D. Bitan, A. Cappuccino, F.H. Geisler, et al., Prospective, randomized, multicenter Food and Drug Administration investigational device exemption study of lumbar total disc replacement with the CHARITÉ Artificial Disc versus lumbar fusion: five-year follow-up, Spine J., in press.
7. J.S. Harrop, J.A. Youssef, M. Maltenfort, P. Vorwald, P. Jabbour, C.M. Bono, et al., Lumbar adjacent segment degeneration and disease after arthrodesis and total disc arthroplasty, Spine 33 (2008) 1701–1707.
8. S.D. Boden, D.O. Davis, T.S. Dina, N.J. Patronas, S.W. Wiesel, Abnormal magnetic-resonance scans of the lumbar spine in asymptomatic subjects: a prospective investigation, J. Bone Joint Surg. Am. 72 (1990) 403–408.
9. N. Boos, R. Rieder, V. Schade, K.F. Spratt, N. Semmer, M. Aebi, 1995 Volvo Award in clinical sciences. The diagnostic accuracy of magnetic resonance imaging, work perception, and psychosocial factors in identifying symptomatic disc herniations, Spine 20 (1995) 2613–2625.
10. R. Bertagnoli, S. Kumar, Indications for full prosthetic disc arthroplasty: a correlation of clinical outcome against a variety of indications, Eur. Spine J. 11 Suppl 2 (2002) S131–S136.
11. M. Pathria, D.J. Sartoris, D. Resnick, Osteoarthritis of the facet joints: accuracy of oblique radiographic assessment, Radiology 164 (1987) 227–230.
12. A. Fujiwara, K. Tamai, H.S. An, T.H. Lim, H. Yoshida, A. Kurihashi, et al., Orientation and osteoarthritis of the lumbar facet joint, Clin. Orthop. Relat. Res. 385 (2001) 88–94.
13. R.C. Huang, M.R. Lim, F.P. Girardi, F.P. Cammisa, The prevalence of contraindications to total disc replacement in a cohort of lumbar surgical patients, Spine 29 (2004) 2538–2541.
14. D.A. Wong, B. Annesser, T. Birney, R. Lamond, A. Kumar, S. Johnson, et al., Incidence of contraindications to total disc arthroplasty: a retrospective review of 100 consecutive fusion patients with a specific analysis of facet arthrosis, Spine J. 7 (2007) 5–11.
15. A.R. Block, R.J. Gatchel, W.W. Deardorff, R.D. Guyer, The psychology of spine surgery, American Psychological Association, Washington, D.C, 2003.
16. R.D. Guyer, F.H. Geisler, S.L. Blumenthal, P.C. McAfee, B.B. Mullin, Effect of age on clinical and radiographic outcomes and adverse events following 1-level lumbar arthroplasty after a minimum 2-year follow-up, J. Neurosurg. Spine 8 (2008) 101–107.
17. R. Bertagnoli, J.J. Yue, R. Nanieva, A. Fenk-Mayer, D.S. Husted, R.V. Shah, et al., Lumbar total disc arthroplasty in patients older than 60 years of age: a prospective study of the ProDisc prosthesis with 2-year minimum follow-up period, J. Neurosurg. Spine 4 (2006) 85–90.

# 56

# The Role of Dynamic Stabilization and the Aging Spine

*Reginald J. Davis*

**K E Y   P O I N T S**

- The rationale behind posterior motion preservation devices is explained.
- Devices for specific clinical indications are shown.

## INTRODUCTION

Posterior dynamic stabilization of the lumbar spine is an evolving field. At the core is the concept of incremental stabilization or progressive control of motion of the spine. This contrasts with more traditional fusion techniques where stabilization entails rigid fixation with abolition of motion. These goals are achieved with surgical implantation of posteriorly placed devices, often following surgical decompression where indicated. These devices exert varying degrees of motion control at varying anatomical regions of influence, based on design.

It is a rapidly expanding field with a broad spectrum of devices, approaches, materials, and degree of imparted stabilization. Proper discussion of dynamic stabilization can only occur with organizational hierarchy, considering anatomical location, functional impact, intensity of intervention, and targeted goal of intervention. Each will be considered with relationship to the others.

## DEVICES

The devices can be largely grouped into three categories, based on anatomical location of implantation. These categories are interspinous, facet, and pedicle. These discrete anatomical insertion points allow for a targeted intervention with very specific actions and indications. There is sufficient overlap such that a broad spectrum of disease can be treated.

### Interspinous Spacers

The spinous processes and the interspinous space are the sites used with increasing frequency in treating spinal conditions. Though few conditions directly affect the spinous process itself, this anatomical location has utility in implant attachment for distraction and stabilization to a significant degree.

The rationales for interspinous devices are several. They distract the neural foramen to reduce nerve root compression. They also share load with the posterior disc, unload the facets, and assist with stability at the operated level. For the most part they are minimally invasive and easily revisable.

These devices are surgically implanted between the spinous processes or within the interlaminar space. In this location they act to control extension, unload the facets, tension the posterior annulus, as well as tension the posterior ligaments. This influence can be enhanced with surgical positioning in more flexion, or after loaded distraction. The resulting kyphosing moment can increase overall volume for neural elements.

### X-Stop (Kyphon)

X-Stop is a titanium alloy device that is designed to stop extension (Figure 56-1). The oval spacer conforms to the interspinous space, and the wings prevent lateral migration. It is minimally invasive and inserted laterally, thus preserving the supraspinous ligament. It is designed to be implanted under local anesthesia. In clinical trial, X-Stop was significantly better than non-operative treatment of lumbar spinal stenosis at 1 and 2 years post-op. The observed success rate was comparable to published reports for decompressive laminectomy, but with considerably lower morbidity.[1,5] X-Stop is currently approved by the U.S. Food and Drug Administration (FDA) for use in patients with claudication symptoms from lumbar stenosis. Patients with relief in flexion and who are otherwise comfortable sitting respond well.

### Wallis (Zimmer Spine)

The Wallis device is a PEEK interspinous spacer secured to the spinous processes using PET bands (Figure 56-2). It is designed to block extension and control flexion. Indications include isolated lumbar intervertebral instability, such as herniated discs, Modic I degenerative lesions, degenerative disc disease at a level adjacent to a previous fusion, and spinal stenosis treated without laminectomy. In long term (13 year) OUS follow-up, the device obviated the need for arthrodesis in 80% of patients.[4] The Wallis device is currently undergoing clinical evaluation and is not FDA approved.

### Diam (Medtronic)

Diam is an interspinous stabilizer composed of a silicone bumper, encased in polyester mesh, and secured with polyester sutures (Figure 56-3). It is inserted with minimal access and minimal tissue disruption. It is designed to resist extension and reduce intradiscal pressure. Indications include restoration of early segmental degeneration, correction of misalignment often seen in discectomy, and stenosis. Diam is currently undergoing clinical evaluation and is not FDA approved.

### Coflex (Paradigm)

Coflex is a titanium alloy device whose U-shaped body conforms to the interspinous and interlaminar space (Figure 56-4). It acts as a stiff spring, dynamically stabilizing extension. Lateral migration is prevented by wings compressed onto the spinous processes. Indications include lumbar stenosis, adjacent segment disease, recurrent HNP and early symptomatic disc degeneration. In OUS implantation after decompressive laminectomy in degenerative lumbar spinal stenosis, Coflex was found to be less invasive and provided similar clinical outcome in comparison with instrumented fusion.[2] Coflex is currently undergoing clinical evaluation and is not FDA approved.

### ExtenSure (NuVasive)

ExtenSure is a PEEK interspinous spacer secured by geometric conformity to the anatomy and the suturing of the supraspinous ligament (Figure 56-5). It is designed to alleviate pseudoclauditory symptoms and radicular symptoms by enlarging the central canal, lateral recess, and foramina. It also decreases or eliminates low back pain by decreasing pressure on arthritic facet joints,

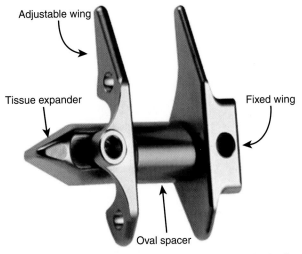

■ **FIGURE 56-1**   X-Stop device interspinous spacer (Kyphon).

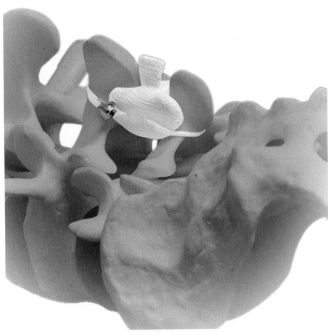

■ **FIGURE 56-3**   The Diam interspinous stabilizer (Medtronic).

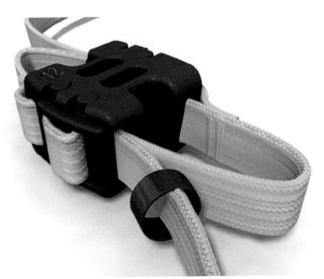

■ **FIGURE 56-2**   The Wallis device interspinous spacer (Zimmer Spine).

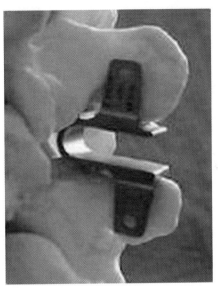

■ **FIGURE 56-4**   The Coflex device (Paradigm).

degenerative discs, or both. It also restores disc height and foraminal volume. It is indicated in moderate to severe spinal stenosis, degenerative spondylolisthesis, and mild to moderate degenerative scoliosis. ExtenSure is currently undergoing clinical evaluation and is not FDA approved.

### In-Space (Synthes)

In-Space is a laterally placed PEEK cylindrical device, secured by deployable wings (Figure 56-6). It is intended to stop segmental extension and to distract the symptomatic interspinous space. In doing so, maintenance of foraminal height, opening of the area of the spinal canal, reduction of stress on the facets, and relieving of pressure on the posterior annulus results. It is indicated in lumbar spinal stenosis, disc protrusions with discogenic low back pain, facet syndrome due to face osteoarthritis, degenerative spondylolisthesis up to grade 1, and degenerative disc disease. In-Space is not FDA approved.

### Superion (Vertiflex)

Superion is a titanium alloy interspinous device with deployable wings (Figure 56-7). It is designed for percutaneous implantation in the treatment of moderate degenerative lumbar stenosis at one or two levels. Superion is currently under clinical investigation in the United States and is not FDA approved.

### Facet Devices

The facet poses unique challenges. The anatomy and functional interrelationships are complex. The 3-D sliding synovial articulation is difficult to replicate. Physiologically, the facets have nociceptive and proprioceptive input that is vital to the proper function of the motion segment. The resulting chemical and mechanical pain generation is difficult to treat surgically. Kinematically complex, facet joints engage in coupled shear and sliding, as well as rotational load sharing, all of which can be specific to certain levels.

This results in a very complex continuum of disease. Painful inflammation, osteoarthritis, stenosis, abnormal loading, and total failure of the functional spinal unit can all originate with facet disease. These challenges are not easily overcome, addressed, or surgically treated. Facet arthroplasty, a rapidly evolving subspecialty in motion preservation, strives to address these issues in the most ergonomic manner.

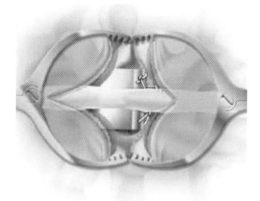

■ **FIGURE 56-5**   The ExtenSure interspinous spacer (NuVasive).

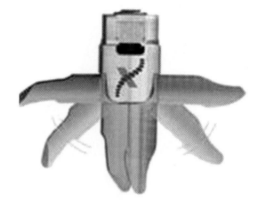

■ **FIGURE 56-7**   The Superion interspinous device (Vertiflex).

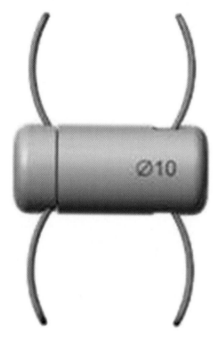

■ **FIGURE 56-6**   The In-Space device (Synthes).

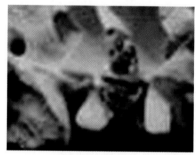

■ **FIGURE 56-8**   The Zyre interpositional arthroplasty device (Quantum Orthopedics).

multiple revision options. This concept is early technology with a paucity of clinical data. Zyre is not FDA approved.

### Fenix (Gerraspine AG)

Fenix is a cobalt chromium facet joint resurfacing device. It has superior and inferior components secured with a translaminar locking screw (Figure 56-9). It is designed to eliminate the painful components, resurface the facet joint, preserve supporting structure and anatomy, and allow or restore physiologic motion. Surgery entails removal of capsule and intraarticular cartilage, with or without decompression. Indications include significant facet disease and subarticular stenosis. Fenix has had limited clinical use and is not FDA approved.

### Anatomic Facet Replacement System (Facet Solutions)

Anatomic Facet Replacement System (AFRS) is a total facet replacement device composed of cobalt-chromium-molybdenum articular surfaces that uses conventional pedicle screw fixation (Figure 56-10). It is designed to reproduce facet anatomy and preserve or restore natural lumbar biomechanics. Surgical implantation is through a midline approach and entails total facetectomy. Indications include osteoarthritis of the facets causing stenosis, and low grade degenerative spondylolisthesis. Fixation with standard pedicle screws allows ready revision options. AFRS I is in clinical trial in the United States and is not FDA approved.

### Total Facet Arthroplasty System (Archus)

Total Facet Arthroplasty System (TFAS) is a total facet replacement device composed of cobalt-chromium articular surfaces and titanium alloy cross arm assembly (Figure 56-11). It comprises paired cephalad bearings and paired caudal housings in a "ball in cup" motion-constraining configuration. These are supported by the titanium cross arm assembly with cemented pedicle post fixation. In situ modular assembly allows for precise adjustment to individual anatomy. Proposed indications include degenerative disease of the facets, facet instability, up to grade I spondylolisthesis with neurological impairment, central or lateral spinal stenosis, at L3-L4 or L4-L5. TFAS is being clinically evaluated in the United States and is not FDA approved.

The overarching goal is reduction of pain and the return of function. The design rationales for the facet-based devices are to clinically correlate intensity of intervention to severity of disease, to allow or restore more physiological loading, to allow or restore the physiological center of rotation, and to control the range of motion of the motion segment.

The emerging technologies are thoughtfully engineered. They are well studied and modeled as the result of extensive research and analysis. The facet-based devices vary from resurfacing, through augmentation and partial replacement, to total replacement. These devices are designed to complement residual kinematics of the motion segment, or to duplicate native motion in total replacement.

### Zyre (Quantum Orthopedics)

Zyre is an interpositional arthroplasty device (Figure 56-8). It consists of a cobalt chromium intraarticular spacer, through which passes a PET cord with chromium retainers. It is minimally invasive, requires no bone resection, maintains capsular integrity, and can be implanted with or without decompression. Indications include painful degeneration of the facet with failed CMM. Advantages include minimal disruption of anatomy and

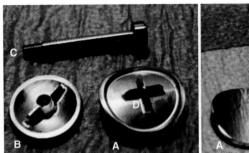

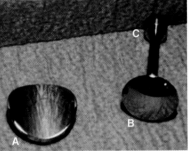

■ **FIGURE 56-9**   The Fenix facet joint resurfacing device (Getraspine AG).

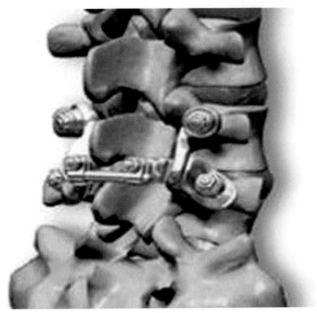

■ **FIGURE 56-10**   Anatomic Facet Replacement System (Facet Solutions).

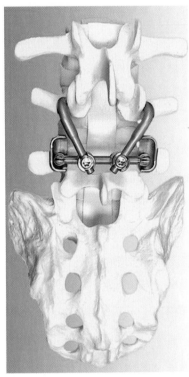

■ **FIGURE 56-11**   Total Facet Arthroplasty System (Archus).

### Total Posterior System (Impliant)

Total Posterior System (TOPS) is composed of opposing titanium plates with interlocking PCU. It is fixed to the spine with polyaxial pedicle screws (Figure 56-12). The entirety of the posterior elements is totally replaced. Motion is restored and constrained in all planes via polymeric dampening. Utilizing the same surgical technique as standard posterior fusion, it recreates the normal biomechanics of the spine, allowing full physiologic range of motion. Surgery occurs through a midline approach and laterally placed pedicle screws. Total facetectomy and removal of posterior elements is necessary. Implantation requires a precise jig assembly. Indications include moderate to severe spinal stenosis. TOPS is being clinically evaluated in the United States and is not FDA approved.

## Pedicle-Based Dynamic Rods

The pedicle-based devices offer the most secure fixation to the spine and thus the greatest opportunity to control motion. Influence is exerted on facets, posterior ligaments, and posterior disc complex. Implantation can be unloaded utilizing a neutral position of the spine, resulting in passive control of motion, or implantation can be loaded utilizing a more distracted position of the spine, resulting in more dynamic load sharing. These devices may be stand-alone or placed in conjunction with decompression or as an adjunct to fusion. There are many devices, each with unique characteristics. This results in a broad range of control exerted, and thus coverage over a wide spectrum of potential spine pathologies. All share the common goal of alleviating back and leg pain using more flexible constructs and materials to stabilize the spine while preserving anatomical structures.

### N-Hance (Synthes)

N-Hance is a flexible posterior stabilizing device that is composed of a collar of paired PCU spacers with interposed titanium ring and end caps (Figure 56-13). This unit slides over the tapered core of a 6-mm titanium rod. The construct provides elongation, compression, and angulation. N-Hance is 510K approved by the FDA as an adjunct to fusion.

### Stabilimax NZ (Applied Spine)

Stabilimax NZ is an investigational posterior stabilizing system that utilizes a dual spring configuration to confer physiologic motion parameters (Figure 56-14). It is intended to provide maximum stabilization to the spine, decreasing the abnormal motion that causes pain, while maintaining physiologic motion.

It is designed to provide stabilization of the lumbar spine in patients receiving decompression surgery for the treatment of clinically symptomatic central or lateral spinal stenosis. Stabilimax NZ is currently being clinically evaluated and is not FDA approved.

### Dynesys (Zimmer Spine)

The Dynesys Dynamic Stabilization System is a posteriorly placed pedicle-based device (Figure 56-15). It is composed of titanium alloy screws, an interposed PCU spacer, and a through-passed PET cord. During implantation of the device, the cord is placed in tension and the spacer is placed in

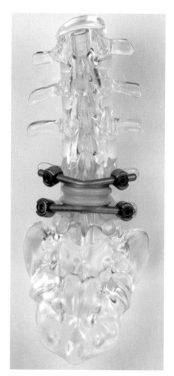

■ **FIGURE 56-12** Total Posterior System (Impliant).

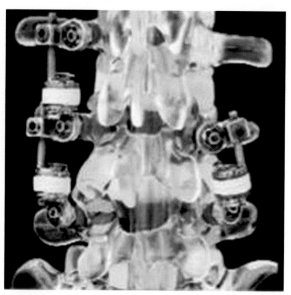

■ **FIGURE 56-14** The Stabilimax NZ investigational posterior stabilizing system (Applied Spine).

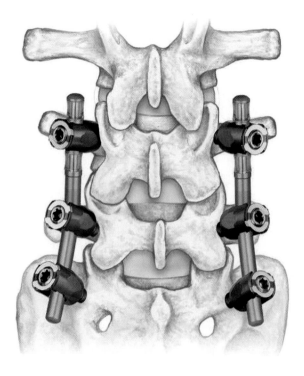

■ **FIGURE 56-13** The N-Hance flexible posterior stabilizing device (Synthes).

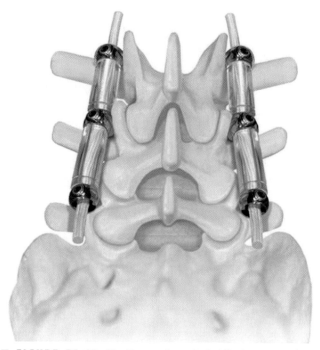

■ **FIGURE 56-15** The Dynesys Dynamic Stabilization System (Zimmer Spine).

### Dynamic TTL-Rod (Scient'x)

The Dynamic TTL-Rod is composed of titanium rods with an interposed damper (Figure 56-16). The damper is a series of washers contained within a bell housing. This configuration results in a posterior rod with micro motion of 2 mm. It is designed to stabilize the spinal segment in semirigid fashion with reduced forces at the bone screw interface. The Dynamic TTL-Rod is 510K approved as an adjunct to fusion.

### CD Horizon Legacy Peek Rod System (Medtronic)

The CD Horizon Legacy Peek Rod System is a pedicle-based, posterior rod device (Figure 56-17). It is composed of standard polyaxial pedicle screws attached to a peek rod. It is designed to provide semirigid fixation that closely replicates the natural load distribution of the lumbar spine for patients who undergo spinal fusion surgery. The CD Horizon Legacy Peek Rod System is 510K approved as an adjunct to fusion.

compression. These opposing vectors of force act through the pedicle screws to dynamically neutralize the spinal segment in flexion, extension, and at rest. The system is 510K approved as an adjunct to fusion. In prospective OUS clinical trial, dynamic neutralization proved to be a safe and effective alternative (to fusion) in the treatment of unstable lumbar conditions.[3]

Dynesys is currently in FDA panel discussion regarding approval as a nonfusion dynamic stabilization system.

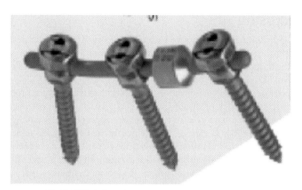

■ **FIGURE 56-16**  The Dynamic TTL-Rod (Scient'x).

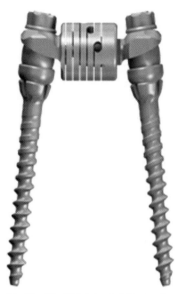

■ **FIGURE 56-18**  The DSS Spine Stabilization System (Paradigm).

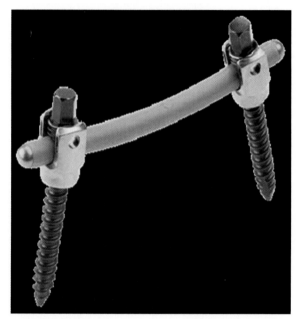

■ **FIGURE 56-17**  The CD Horizon Legacy Peek Rod System (Medtronic).

### *DSS Spine Stabilization System (Paradigm)*

The DSS Spine Stabilization System is a pedicle-based posterior coupler device (Figure 56-18). It is an entirely modular system composed of titanium monoaxial pedicle screws, upon which are placed washers and spherical spacers. This allows polyaxial orientation of the couplers. The couplers are made of titanium. The configuration of outer spiral cut housing and inner shaft with a ball-in-socket piston confers motion is all directions with stoppage within physiologic ranges. The hemispherical screw interfaces allow further polyaxial implantation. It is designed to allow physiologic motion within an overall reduced range and to restrict the neutral zone. The DSS Spine Stabilization System is 510K approved as an adjunct to fusion.

### *Dynabolt (VertiFlex)*

Dynabolt is a pedicle screw–based flexible posterior rod. It allows for full range of motion and can be delivered percutaneously. It is designed to reduce bone–screw interface stresses and to enable load sharing through the spinal column during motion. Dynabolt is 510K approved as an adjunct to fusion.

### CLINICAL APPLICATION

The aging spine demonstrates characteristic degeneration that is unique depending on anatomical location. The ligaments progress from desiccation and loss of elasticity, through inflammation, to end-stage hypertrophy and calcification. The facets suffer inflammation, capsular insufficiency,

synovial deterioration, and bony overgrowth. The metabolic and structural deterioration of bone ultimately results in osteopenia, osteoporosis, and mechanical insufficiency. These degenerative processes , individually and in combination, result in a broad spectrum of spinal conditions, which vary in severity, clinical manifestation, anatomical location, and intensity of appropriate intervention. For each of these conditions a dynamic solution can be considered. As this is still a new and evolving field, most proposed interventions are intuitive with a paucity of supporting clinical data.

### Ligament

Mild ligamentous disease, beyond simple inflammation, may result initially in ligamentous laxity. This state contributes to mild instability. In addition, thickening or buckling of specific ligaments lining the spinal canal can contribute to spinal stenosis. The interspinous spacers overall may have clinical efficacy in such cases. X-Stop has demonstrated efficacy in these patients. The dynamic rods may also be used but represent a more aggressive solution. The relative invasiveness of pedicle fixation in such cases is overkill in many instances. The facet replacement devices likewise entail more disruption of anatomy than can be recommended for otherwise mild disease.

Moderate ligamentous laxity can result in more significant instability. The abnormal motion, characterized by an increased neutral zone, can result in back pain. A greater degree of central canal stenosis can also be seen. Surgical treatment often entails direct decompression with concomitant worsening of instability. The interspinous devices could be considered in these instances, but for the most part might lack sufficient influence of translation to be effective. A more robust interlaminar device such as Coflex may be used in selected cases. The dynamic rods have much more utility in this patient population. Pedicle-based devices that control the neutral zone include DSS and Stabilimax. Following more extensive laminectomy and partial facetectomy or with greater instability, more rigid devices may be needed. Dynesys, CD Horizon Peek, and Dynamic TTL have sufficient rigidity as to be useful in up to grade 1 spondylolisthesis.

More severe ligamentous dysfunction can result in degenerative spondylolisthesis, more severe central canal stenosis, lateral or subarticular stenosis, and secondary disc failure. The stiffer pedicle-based devices could be considered here. Devices to be considered include Dynesys, Isobar, and PEEK rods. Efficacy is exceeded with greater than grade 1 spondylolisthesis, pars defect, and greater than 50% facetectomy. Fusion with traditional rigid fixation technology is then warranted.

### Facet

Mild capsular failure and intractable synovial inflammation may result in facet pain. Facet resurfacing technology, such as Zyre may be efficacious.

Moderate capsular failure and synovial dysfunction also occurs and results in significant pain and disability. Synovial cysts with lateral compression, facet overgrowth with subarticular stenosis, and degenerative subluxation of facets could be treated with facet reconstruction. Fenix and similar technologies may be indicated in such cases.

Severe facet disease results in more severe stenosis, and facet failure. This probably requires facet replacement. Applicable technologies include TFAS, Facet Solutions, and Tops.

## Canal

Moderate lumbar stenosis, beyond the mild stenosis seen with ligamentous buckling or involution, requires surgical decompression. The accompanying mild instability may be treated with interlaminar devices such as Coflex and Vertiflex.

Moderately severe stenosis with more accompanying instability may be treated with the stiffer pedicle-based devices such as Dynesys, PEEK rods, or Isobar.

## Osteopenia

Bone quality is the overarching consideration for any device implantation. Osteopenia and osteoporosis are typically contraindications to most device usage. Dynamic stabilization technologies in general have reduced forces at the bone–screw interface when compared to traditional fixation techniques. This may result in a more suitable construct for stabilization in such instances of poor bone quality.

## CONCLUSION

The aging spine is less adaptive to, and less forgiving of, less than ideally applied solutions to pathological conditions. Hence there is an even greater need for thoughtfulness of approach, broad spectrum of choice, and proper selection of technique.

Posterior dynamic stabilization of the lumbar spine offers promising solutions to a variety of challenging clinical scenarios. In most instances, inadequate clinical data exist to fully evaluate appropriateness and efficacy in specific pathological entities. Rigid clinical science is needed to support what is presently clinical intuition. Only through patient trials and physician experience will the proper use of and indication for these devices become clear. Also, further evolution of proper diagnostic techniques that specifically evaluate the dynamic elements of spine pathology will be needed to guide proper selection of technology.

## References

1. Anderson, et al., J. Neurosurg. 4 (6) (2006 Jun) 463–471.
2. S.C. Park, et al., J. Korean. Neurosurg. Soc. 46 (4) (2009 Oct) 292–299.
3. T.M. Stoll, et al., Eur. Spine J. (11 Suppl 2) (2002 Oct) S170–S178.
4. Neurosurg. Rev. 32 (3) (2009 Jul) 335–341. discussion 341–2.
5. Zucherman, et al., Eur. Spine J. 13 (1) (2004 Feb) 22–31.
6. Spine 30 (12) (2005 Jun 15) 1351–1358, 2004.

# 57

# Pedicle Screw Fixation in the Aging Spine

*Hajeer Sabet and Frank M. Phillips*

**KEY POINTS**

- When performing reconstructive spinal surgery in the elderly patient, the surgeon must consider the fragility of osteoporotic bone, the stability of the spine, and the potential failure mechanisms of any applied instrumentation.

- Increasing pedicle screw length, diameter, or both can be the first line in improving pedicle screw construct rigidity.

- Undertapping pedicle screws can achieve increased insertional torque and screw pullout strength.

- Triangulation of screws increases the overall pullout strength of the construct and provides higher resistance against loads perpendicular to the pedicle screws.

- A twofold to threefold increase in screw pullout can be achieved with the use of polymethylmethacrylate injected into the vertebral body around the screws.

## INTRODUCTION

The number of people with osteoporosis is expected to rise with the increasing longevity of the population, so spine surgeons must appreciate the impact of osteoporosis on the management of spinal disorders in the elderly. Older patients desire to remain active and are reluctant to accept disability and deformity as an inevitable consequence of aging. These patient expectations coupled with advances in spinal surgical techniques have resulted in more spinal procedures being performed on the elderly. The spinal surgeon may be required to treat direct sequelae of osteoporosis in the form of painful spinal fractures or resultant deformity, or may be required to consider osteoporosis as it relates to spinal reconstruction in the older patient. Regardless of any surgical decisions in the osteoporotic patient, the spine surgeon must ensure that the patient is being appropriately medically treated for osteoporosis.

As larger reconstructive spine surgeries are performed on older patients, the ability of the osteoporotic spine to support spinal implants must be considered. The selection of spinal instrumentation must take into account the fragility of osteoporotic bone, the stability of the spine, and the likely failure mechanisms of any applied instrumentation. The preoperative workup should include evaluation for the severity of osteoporosis, which might impact the surgeon's choice of reconstruction techniques.

Posterior instrumentation is most commonly applied to the osteoporotic spine in an effort to stabilize the spine and promote fusion after decompression of neural elements. In this situation, the anterior column is typically intact and no frank instability exists, so that posterior instrumentation alone is often adequate. Surgery primarily for deformity correction in the elderly is challenging and infrequently indicated. Posterior instrumentation may be used to correct spinal deformity; however, if the deforming forces exceed the stability of the implant–bone interface, posterior construct failure will occur.

In current clinical practice, the large majority of posterior instrumentation spinal surgeries involve pedicle screw instrumentation. In the osteoporotic spine, the weak link in the instrumentation construct is the implant–bone interface. The majority of instrumentation failures involve screw loosening and pull-out, which may lead to failure of fusion or the development of recurrent or de novo deformity. Posterior thoracolumbar instrumentation failure has been shown to correlate with bone mineral density (BMD).[1-3] Screw pull-out and also cutout through the adjacent endplate with cyclical flexion–extension loading are directly related to BMD and may occur even at physiologic loads in the osteoporotic spine.[1-3] In a biomechanical study, Soshi and colleagues[2] concluded that pedicle screw fixation should be avoided in patients with a BMD less than 0.3 g/cm$^2$.

At the time of pedicle screw insertion, the surgeon may recognize poor screw purchase in osteoporotic bone because of the low insertion torque required to advance the screw. Insertion torque not only correlates with BMD and screw pull-out, but also predicts early screw failure.[4-6] If poor screw purchase is recognized intraoperatively, the surgeon should attempt to salvage the situation rather than rely on inadequate fixation to achieve the goals of instrumentation.

## PEDICLE SCREWS IN THE OSTEOPOROTIC SPINE

### Screw Placement

The surgeon may consider increasing the length or diameter of the pedicle screw in an attempt to improve the screw purchase in bone (Table 57-1). Increasing screw length does increase screw pull-out strength, although this effect may be less pronounced in osteoporotic bone.[7,8] Use of bicortical screws in the lumbar spine is limited because of risk of vascular injury. However, in the sacrum, a bicortical screw can be placed safely and improves pull-out strength.[9,10] The inability to accurately gauge the anterior vertebral body cortex intraoperatively may affect the surgeon's ability to safely place longer screws, since screws extending beyond the anterior vertebral body may predispose to vascular injury. At the sacrum, bicortical purchase may be safely accomplished with medially directed pedicle screws with a low risk of vascular injury. Increasing screw diameter will also increase pull-out strength[7,11-13]; however, the dimensions of the pedicle being cannulated may limit the screw diameter. In the osteoporotic spine, when the screw diameter exceeds 70% of the pedicle diameter, a risk of pedicle fracture is created.[14]

Directing pedicle screws toward the stronger subchondral bone adjacent to the vertebral body endplate will improve pull-out resistance.[15,16] In the sacrum, optimal screw purchase is achieved by directing the screws toward the disc space anteriorly or through the sacral promontory.[17-19]

**TABLE 57-1  Pedicle Screw Size Relationship**

| Screw Size | 6.0 | 5.0 |
| --- | --- | --- |
| Screw outer diameter (mm) | 6.0 | 5.0 |
| Screw minor diameter (mm) | 4.8 | 3.8 |
| Tap minor diameter (mm) | 4.75 | 3.75 |

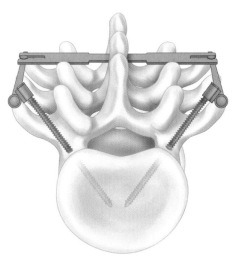

■ **FIGURE 57-1** Triangulation of pedicle screws with a cross plate. (Redrawn from P. Richard, M.D. Schlenk, M.D. Todd Stewart, et al., The biomechanics of iatrogenic spinal destabilization and implant failure, Neurosurg Focus 15(3), 2003.)

Another strategy to improve stability of the pedicle screw construct in osteoporotic bone is to distribute forces by increasing the number of fixation points to the spine by including additional levels in the construct. The advantages of this approach must be weighed against the risks and morbidity associated with the additional level surgery as well as the potential long-term consequences of a fusion spanning additional levels. The surgeon may also augment the pedicle screw construct with offset sublaminar hooks, which are well suited for use in the osteoporotic spine because they rely on the relatively unaffected cortical laminar bone for fixation.[1,20] Biomechanical studies have supported the ability of supplemental sublaminar hooks to increase the rigidity and pull-out strength of pedicle screw constructs.[21,22]

Convergence of pedicle screws with a triangulation effect can substantially increase the overall pull-out strength of the construct and provides higher resistance against loads perpendicular to the pedicle screw (Figure 57-1).[23] Triangulation of pedicle screws increased pullout strength by 143% over single pedicle screws.[23] Bilateral triangulated pedicle screws allow the screws to, in effect, hold all of the bone between the screws rather than just the bone within the threads of the individual screws. Ruland and colleagues[23] suggested that for triangulated screws to fail simultaneously, a transverse fracture through the vertebral body at the level of the tips of the pedicle screw had to occur. Kilincer and colleagues[24] demonstrated there was no biomechanical benefit to converging pedicle screws more than 60 degrees.

The ability to triangulate pedicle screws is impacted by local bony anatomy. Larger diameter pedicles at levels where the pedicles natural converge (for example L5) allow for medial angulation of the screws. Smaller diameter or deformed pedicles where pedicle morphology is more straight ahead (for example T12) are more challenging for placement of convergent screws.

## Undertapping Pedicle Screws

In osteoporotic bone, loss of fixation at the bone–screw interface is the primary mode of failure for screws. The preparation technique of the bone–implant interface is important for optimal screw purchase. Typically the path for the pedicle screw is tapped before screw placement. In osteoporotic bone, a tap with a diameter smaller than that of the pedicle screw is recommended in order to conserve cancellous bone, which is compacted around the screw heads thereby increasing screw stability. Carmouche and colleagues[25] performed a cadaveric pullout resistance study comparing tapping, undertapping, and no-tapping techniques. The authors reported that same-size tapping of lumbar and thoracic pedicle screws decreased pullout resistance when compared to undertapping or no-tapping. Kuklo and colleagues[26] reported a 93% increase in insertional torque when undertapping thoracic screws by 1 mm when compared to line-to-line tapping. Halvorson found in a cadaveric model that screw insertion technique did not affect pullout resistance with normal bone density (BMD > 1 g/cm²).[27] In osteoporotic bone, however, there was a marked benefit to undertapping by 1 mm.[27,28]

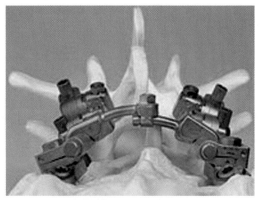

■ **FIGURE 57-2** Articulated cross-link.

## Transverse Connectors

Transverse connectors, also known as "cross-links", serve to link together and add rigidity to two screw–rod constructs (Figure 57-2). The cross-link does not directly effect fixation at the screw-bone interface, but instead augments stability of the overall construct that can indirectly facilitate fixation by minimizing micro motion. Biomechanical testing has confirmed the ability of cross-links to increase torsional and lateral stability in an unstable burst fracture model. An additive effect to stability with the application of one and then two cross-links was reported.[29] Transverse connectors had little effect on flexion-extension, lateral bending or tensile rod stress. Longer constructs such as those used to treat spinal deformity have also been tested with cross-links. Kuklo and colleagues[30] showed that in long pedicle screw–rod constructs, cross-links increased predominantly axial rotational stability, with the effect enhanced by the addition of a second cross-link (additional 15%). Location of the cross-link within the longer constructs did not significantly impact stability.

Disadvantages of cross-links include breakage[31] and hardware prominence because these are the most dorsally placed elements in the instrumentation construct. The dorsal cross-link prominence may lead to localized discomfort and at times the formation of an overlying bursa. Additionally, connectors can theoretically add to instrumentation crowding, thus reducing available bone surface area for fusion.

## Bone Cement

The bone–screw interface also may be improved by injecting polymethylmethacrylate (PMMA) bone cement into the pedicle around the pedicle screw. A twofold to threefold increase in screw pullout has not been demonstrated with the use of PMMA injected into the vertebral body through a cannulated pedicle.[2,8] Increasing the amount of PMMA injected into the pedicle has not been shown to significantly increase the pullout strength.[32] Possible risks of this technique include cement extravasation outside of the vertebra, with potential for leakage into the spinal canal or neural foramina. Other cements such as hydroxyapatite cement, calcium phosphate, and carbonated apatite have also been shown to enhance the screw–bone interface and increase pedicle screw pullout strength.[13,33,34] Moore and colleagues[33] reported that the failure modes seen with PMMA and calcium phosphate cement differed in pullout tests. With PMMA augmentation, pedicle fracture occurred at or near the junction with the vertebral body in 80% (25 of 30) of the samples. In contrast, failure of calcium phosphate augmentation occurred at the cement–screw interface in 80% (24 of 30) of the samples. In an in vivo animal model of pedicle screw augmentation, injectable calcium sulfate cement was shown to significantly improve the immediate pullout strength of pedicle screw fixation, and this effect was maintained even after the calcium sulfate cement had been absorbed completely.[35] Interestingly Kiner and colleagues[36] recently reported a biomechanical study suggesting that larger diameter pedicle screws increased construct rigidity greater than did cement augmentation. Cement augmentation of screws has been used in patients with osteoporosis and metastatic spinal tumors undergoing spinal instrumentation with acceptable clinical results and low rates of instrumentation failure.[37-39]

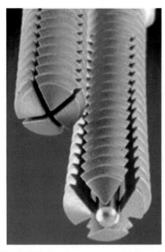

■ **FIGURE 57-3**  Biomet expandable pedicle screw.

## Expandable Screws

Recently, expandable pedicle screws have been designed that can pass through a fixed pedicle size and then expand in situ in the cancellous bone of the vertebral body to improve screw fixation. These screws are similar to those used in drywall. These allow for greater bone contact at the screw tip with no increase in pedicle insertion diameter or screw length. These screws may be particularly beneficial in the osteoporotic patient.

Various designs of expanding pedicle screws are available. In one design, the pedicle screw is cannulated to accept an expansion peg. The distal two thirds of the screw is split lengthwise by two perpendicular slots to form four anterior fins when expanded. An expansion peg (a smaller-gauge screw) is threaded into the inner core of the pedicle screw. As the expansion peg advances into the slotted portion of the screw, it spreads and opens up the slotted tip of the screw, creating fins. Withdrawal of the expansion peg collapses the fins, allowing for removal of the screw (Figure 57-3).

Ngu and colleagues[40] examined the load-to-failure strength of an expandable screw design (Omega-21, Biomet, Warsaw, Ind.). The expandable-screw pullout strength (391 N) was significantly stronger than a standard pedicle screw l (145 N) reflecting a 170% increase in pullout strength. It should be noted in this study that cemented augmented pedicle fixation had an even higher pullout resistance (599 N, or 284% increase). Cook and associates[41] found expandable screws to have an approximate 50% increase in pullout strength compared with conventional pedicle screws.

In a clinical study of 145 patients that received expandable screw fixation, 21 of these patients were osteoporotic. Of these 21 patients, 18 (86%) went on to have solid fusion, and 20 (95%) had expandable screws intact at 2 to 5 years. Expandable screw breakage occurred in 3% of all patients studied, with osteoporotic patients demonstrating a higher screw breakage rate of 5% (1/21 cases, 5/97 screws). Broken expandable screws were difficult to remove. Screw breakage most frequently occurred at the level of the prongs.

## CONCLUSION

With the aging of today's population, the spine surgeon must appreciate the effects of osteoporosis on the spine. The risk–benefit ratio of spinal surgery in the elderly osteoporotic patient must be cautiously weighed by both the surgeon and patient. The surgeon must understand the limitations of spinal instrumentation in the osteoporotic spine and should consider strategies to reduce the likelihood of construct failure.

## References

1. J.D. Coe, K.E. Warden, M.A. Herzig, Influence of bone mineral density on the fixation of thoracolumbar implants. A comparative study of transpedicular screws, laminar hooks, and spinous process wires, Spine 15 (1990) 902–907.
2. S. Soshi, R. Shiba, H. Kondo, et al., An experimental study on transpedicular screw fixation in relation to osteoporosis of the lumbar spine, Spine 16 (1991) 1335–1341.
3. M. Yamagata, H. Kitahara, S. Minami, et al., Mechanical stability of the pedicle screw fixation systems for the lumbar spine, Spine 17 (1992) S51–S54.
4. W.W. Lu, Q. Zhu, A.D. Holmes, et al., Loosening of sacral screw fixation under in vitro fatigue loading, J. Orthop. Res. 18 (2000) 808–814.
5. K. Okuyama, K. Sato, E. Abe, et al., Stability of transpedicle screwing for the osteoporotic spine. An in vitro study of the mechanical stability, Spine 18 (1993) 2240–2245.
6. T.A. Zdeblick, D.N. Kunz, M.E. Cooke, et al., Pedicle screw pullout strength. Correlation with insertional torque, Spine 18 (1993) 1673–1676.
7. D.W. Polly Jr., J.R. Orchowski, R.G. Ellenbogen, Revision pedicle screws. Bigger, longer shims—what is best? Spine 23 (1998) 1374–1379.
8. M.R. Zindrick, L.L. Wiltse, E.H. Widell, et al., A biomechanical study of intrapedicular screw fixation in the lumbosacral spine, Clin. Orthop Relat Res. 203. (1986) 99–112.
9. D.H. McCord, B.W. Cunningham, Y. Shono, et al., Biomechanical analysis of lumbosacral fixation, Spine (17 (Suppl)) (1992) S235–S243.
10. S. Mirkovic, J.J. Abitol, J. Steinman, et al., Anatomic consideration for sacral screw placement, Spine (16 (Suppl)) (1991) S289–S294.
11. R.F. McLain, T.O. McKinley, S.A. Yerby, et al., The effect of bone quality on pedicle screw loading in axial instability. A synthetic model, Spine 22 (1997) 1454–1460.
12. A.G. Brantley, J.K. Mayfield, J.B. Koeneman, et al., The effects of pedicle screw fit. An in vitro study, Spine 19 (1994) 1752–1758.
13. S.A. Yerby, E. Toh, R.F. McLain, et al., Revision of failed pedicle screws using hydroxyapatite cement. A biomechanical analysis, Spine 23 (1998) 1657–1661.
14. T. Hirano, K. Hasegawa, T. Washio, et al., Fracture risk during pedicle screw insertion in osteoporotic spine, J. Spinal Disord. 11 (1998) 493–497.
15. A.G. Hadjipavlou, C.L. Nicodemus, F.A. al-Hamdan, J.W. Simmons, M.H. Pope, Correlation of bone equivalent mineral density to pull-out resistance of triangulated pedicle screw construct, J. Spinal Disord. 10 (1) (1997) 12–19.
16. T. Lowe, M. O'Brien, D. Smith, Central and juxta-endplate vertebral body screw placement: a biomechanical analysis in a human cadaveric model, Spine 27 (4) (2002) 369–373.
17. P.A. Robertson, L.D. Plank, Pedicle screw placement at the sacrum: anatomical characterization and limitations at S1, J. Spinal Disord. 12 (3) (1999) 227–233.
18. W.W. Lu, Q. Zhu, A.D. Holmes, K.D. Luk, S. Shong, J.C. Leong, Loosening of sacral screw fixation under in vitro fatigue loading, J. Orthop. Res. 18 (5) (2000) 808–814.
19. R.A. Lehman Jr., T.R. Kuklo, P.J. Belmont Jr., R.C. Andersen, D.W. Polly Jr., Advantage of pedicle screw fixation directed into the apex of the sacral promontory over bicortical fixation: a biomechanical analysis, Spine 27 (8) (2002) 806–811. 98 (Suppl) (2003) 50–55.
20. M. Chiba, R.F. McLain, S.A. Yerby, et al., Short-segment pedicle instrumentation. Biomechanical analysis of supplemental hook fixation, Spine 21 (1996) 288–294.
21. K. Hasegawa, H.E. Takahashi, S. Uchiyama, et al., An experimental study of a combination method using a pedicle screw and laminar hook for the osteoporotic spine, Spine 22 (1997) 958–962. discussion 963.
22. A.S. Hilibrand, D.C. Moore, G.P. Graziano, The role of pediculolaminar fixation in compromised pedicle bone, Spine 21 (1996) 445–451.
23. C.M. Ruland, P.C. McAfee, K.E. Warden, et al., Triangulation of pedicular instrumentation. A biomechanical analysis, Spine 16 (Suppl. 6) (1991) S270–S276.
24. C. Kilincer, S Inceoglu, M.J. Sohn, et al., Effects of angle and laminectomy on triangulated pedicle screws. J. Clin. Neurosci. 14 (12) (2007) 1186–1191.
25. J.J. Carmouche, R.W. Molinari, T. Gerlinger, J. Devine, T. Patience, Effects of pilot hole preparation technique on pedicle screw fixation in different regions of the osteoporotic thoracic and lumbar spine, J. Neurosurg. Spine 3 (5) (2005 Nov.) 364–370.
26. T.R. Kuklo, R.A. Lehman, Jr. Effect of various tapping diameters on insertion of thoracic pedicle screws: a biomechanical analysis. Spine 28 (18): (2003) 2066–2071.
27. T.L. Halvorson, L.A. Kelley, K.A. Thomas, et al., Effects of bone mineral density on pedicle screw fixation, Spine 19 (21) (1994) 2415–2420.
28. F.M. Pfeiffer, D.L. Abernathie, D.E. Smith, A comparison of pullout strength for pedicle screws of different designs: a study using tapped and untapped pilot holes, Spine 31 (23) (2006 Nov 1) E867–E870.
29. J.C. Dick, T.A. Zdeblick, B.D. Bartel, et al., Mechanical evaluation of cross-link designs in rigid pedicle screw systems, Spine 22 (1997) 370–375.
30. T.R. Kuklo, A.E. Dmitriev, M.J. Cardoso, R.A. Lehman Jr., M. Erickson, N.W. Gill, Biomechanical contribution of transverse connectors to segmental stability following long segment instrumentation with thoracic pedicle screws, Spine 33 (15) (2008 Jul 1) E482–E487.
31. K.R. Eck, K.H. Bridwell, F.F. Ungacta, K.D. Riew, M.A. Lapp, L.G. Lenke, C. Baldus, K. Blanke, Complications and results of long adult deformity fusions down to l4, l5, and the sacrum, Spine 26 (9) (2001 May 1) E182–E192.
32. B.M. Frankel, S. D'Agostino, C. Wang, A biomechanical cadaveric analysis of polymethylmethacrylate-augmented pedicle screw fixation, J. Neurosurg. Spine 7 (1) (2007 Jul) 47–53.
33. D.C. Moore, R.S. Maitra, L.A. Farjo, et al., Restoration of pedicle screw fixation with an in situ setting calcium phosphate cement, Spine 22 (1997) 1696–1705.
34. J.C. Lotz, S.S. Hu, D.F. Chiu, et al., Carbonated apatite cement augmentation of pedicle screw fixation in the lumbar spine, Spine 22 (1997) 2716–2723.
35. X. Yi, Y. Wang, H. Lu, C. Li, T. Zhu, Augmentation of pedicle screw fixation strength using an injectable calcium sulfate cement: an in vivo study, Spine 33 (23) (2008 Nov 1) 2503–2509.
36. D.W. Kiner, C.D. Wybo, W. Sterba, Y.N. Yeni, S.W. Bartol, R. Vaidya, Biomechanical analysis of different techniques in revision spinal instrumentation: larger diameter screws versus cement augmentation, Spine 33 (24) (2008) 2618–2622.
37. P.I. Wuisman, M. Van Dijk, H. Staal, et al., Augmentation of (pedicle) screws with calcium apatite cement in patients with severe progressive osteoporotic spinal deformities: An innovative technique, Eur. Spine J. 9 (2000) 528–533.
38. J.S. Jang, S.H. Lee, C.H. Rhee, Polymethylmethacrylate-augmented screw fixation for stabilization in metastatic spinal tumors. Technical note, J. Neurosurg. 96 (2002) 131–134.
39. M.C. Chang, C.L. Liu, T.H. Chen, Polymethylmethacrylate augmentation of pedicle screw for osteoporotic spinal surgery: a novel technique, Spine 33 (10) (2008 May 1) E317–E324.
40. B.B. Ngu, S.M. Belkoff, D.E. Gelb, S. Ludwig, A biomechanical comparison of sacral pedicle screw salvage techniques, Spine 31 (6) (March 15, 2006) E166–E168.
41. S.D. Cook, J. Barbera, M. Rubi, S.L. Salkeld, T.S. Whitecloud, Lumbosacral fixation using expandable pedicle screws. an alternative in reoperation and osteoporosis, Spine J. 1 (2) (2001 Mar-Apr) 109–114.

# The Role for Biologics in the Aging Spine

## 58

*David A. Essig, Christopher P. Miller, and Jonathan N. Grauer*

---

**KEY POINTS**

- Define the current biologic options for treatment of degenerative conditions of the spine.
- Define the role for bone morphogenetic proteins (BMPs) in degenerative conditions of the spine.
- Identify bone graft substitutes and their properties.
- Discuss other potential application of biologics in the aging spine.

## INTRODUCTION

Currently, there are over 36 million people over the age of 65 years in the United States. This number is projected to increase to 71 million (nearly 20%) by 2030.[1] As the population ages there will be a similar increase in age-related diseases, such as degenerative disorders of the spine. The elderly are also living a more active lifestyle than at any other time, and thus the demand for addressing issues in this population will only increase over time. However, treating degenerative conditions of the aging spine poses particularly challenging situations to surgeons. Not only must the spinal surgeon address the spinal pathology, but these patients often have serious comorbidities that may affect the treatment options.[2,3] Therefore, patients, families, and physicians will have to weigh the additional risks of operative treatment against the benefits of reducing disabling pain and improving quality of life.

Spinal fusion is commonly considered in this population to address degeneration, deformity, and/or stabilize a decompressed segment. Although instrumentation is frequently used for initial stability, fusion is a biological event in which solid bridging bone forms between adjacent vertebrae.

Currently, iliac crest autologous bone (autograft) remains the gold standard bone graft material for achieving spinal fusion in all ages. It is an excellent choice because it is the only bone graft option that provides all of the components necessary for arthrodesis: osteoconductive matrix, osteoinductive proteins, and osteogenic cells. However, there are significant problems with using autograft including the limited supply of available bone and subjecting the patient to a secondary invasive procedure to harvest the autologous bone which is, in itself, associated with potential morbidity, such as infection, fracture, and intractable pain.[4,5] This consideration is particularly relevant for the elderly population who, because of their medical comorbidities, often have longer recovery times and more complications following surgeries of any kind. As a result, there has been significant work to develop materials to supplement or even replace iliac crest bone graft in the hope of minimizing surgical morbidities while ensuring that the treatment objectives are still achieved.

There have been few studies examining the use of biologics specifically in older patients. What has been done has focused primarily on complications as opposed to health outcomes and fusion success. Despite the limited information, older patients would intuitively seem to be an ideal target population for bone graft alternatives because of their poorer quality iliac crest bone and their higher risk for graft-associated complications. Although the roles of such biologics are still being defined, they provide an exciting adjunct or alternative treatment for spinal conditions in the aging patient population. This chapter will discuss some of these biologics designed to stimulate a successful spinal arthrodesis and their use in the elderly population.

## BONE MORPHOGENETIC PROTEINS

Bone morphogenetic proteins (BMPs), members of the transforming growth factor-beta superfamily, have gradually become better understood since their initial identification by Marshall Urist[6] in the 1960s.[7] They function by binding to the cell membrane of undifferentiated mesenchymal type of cells to promote the induction of bone formation. Although more than 12 BMPs have been identified, only a few have been explored for potential clinical use.

Two BMP molecules have been approved for use in humans. Recombinant human bone morphogenetic protein-2 (rhBMP-2) is currently approved, in conjunction with a collagen sponge and threaded intervertebral cage, for the treatment of degenerative lumbar spine disease. Recombinant human bone morphogenetic protein-7 (rhBMP-7), also referred to as osteogenic protein-1 (OP-1), currently has a humanitarian device exemption (HDE) status for posterolateral lumbar fusions in challenging fusion environments.

In a prospective, randomized trial comparing anterior lumbar interbody fusion with either rhBMP-2 implanted on a collagen sponge in a tapered fusion cage or autogenous iliac crest bone graft, there was a 94.5% fusion rate in the BMP group versus an 88.7% fusion rate in the control group, as determined radiographically.[8] Moreover, 5.9% of the subjects in the autograft control group experienced adverse events related to their bone grafting procedures, and 32% reported persistent pain at the donor site at the time of final follow-up. Back, leg, and neurologic pain scores improved in both groups to a similar extent. Nonetheless, this procedure is less commonly considered than posterior procedures in the aged population because of the increase in complication rate and recovery time associated with anterior approaches.

Posterior lumbar fusion with BMP has significant challenges including limited surface area for healing, distractive forces, and the large gap between transverse processes needing to be bridged. Furthermore, studies have demonstrated the need for a bulking agent in posterior procedures. One recent retrospective study comparing instrumented posterolateral fusion with rhBMP-2 versus iliac crest autograft demonstrated equivalent fusion masses between the two groups at 2-year follow-up.[9] Nonunion rate was 6.6% in the BMP group compared to 11.1% in the control group. No significant differences in the bulking agent used (local bone, allograft bone, demineralized bone matrix, and ceramic) were noted. Demonstrated outcomes when rhBMP-7 (OP-1) is used are comparable to those of autograft when used in uninstrumented posterolateral fusion for the treatment of degenerative spondylolisthesis.[10]

Recently Glassman and colleagues[11] reported on the utility of rhBMP-2 with an absorbable collagen sponge (ACS) compared to autograft in an elderly population (older than 60 years of age). They assessed the clinical, radiographic, and economic outcomes at 2-year follow-up for 102 patients treated by posterolateral lumbar fusion with iliac crest autograft versus rhBMP-2/ACS. They found no increased rates of complications due to the rhBMP-2

(8 of the 50 patients) in this population. In fact, there were increased perioperative complications in the autograft group (23 of the 52 patients). These complications included donor site infections, cardiac issues, pain, urinary tract infections, and neurologic deficit. Additionally, they found that the rhBMP-2 group had significantly better fusion grades on radiographic imaging and equivalent improvements in health-related quality of life outcomes for both groups.

Though BMPs provide substantial benefits in spinal arthrodesis, their use is not always without complication.[12] Potential complications include the formation of ectopic bone, hematoma and seroma formation, bone resorption and graft subsidence, antibody formation, and possible carcinogenicity. While some of the effects may be dose or carrier related, many of the applications currently considered for their use are off-label and their use has to be considered carefully. Further, the cost-to-benefit considerations remain to be elucidated.

## OTHER BONE GRAFT ALTERNATIVES

Many other potential bone graft materials have also been considered for use alone or in combination with local bone to limit morbidity associated with iliac crest autograft. Some of these alternatives include allograft, demineralized bone matrix (DBM), and synthetic materials such as ceramics. While none of these bone graft alternatives possess all three factors necessary to promote osteogenesis, their utility in specific clinical situations is being studied. No matter what substance is chosen, the local and systemic environment must be hospitable to the formation of new bone, and there must be adequate blood supply, mechanical stability, and a lack of growth-inhibiting factors (e.g., nicotine, infection).

## Allograft

Allograft bone provides an osteoconductive scaffold for new bone formation. Various allograft bone types are available. Successful use of allograft bone in spinal surgery is largely dependent on its placement. When structural allograft is implanted in the anterior column, it is associated with relatively high fusion rates, both in the cervical and the thoracolumbar regions of the spine.[13,14] However, when nonstructural allograft bone is placed under tension, as in the posterior spine, it incorporates at a slower rate than autograft and leads to lower rates of arthrodesis when used alone.[15,16]

A recent study by Anderson and associates[17] evaluated the use of morcelized femoral head allograft with and without instrumentation in the elderly. The study did not harvest autograft from any of the patients. The demonstrated successful fusion, determined by radiographs, is 68% with allograft alone and 81% with allograft plus instrumentation. Additionally, there were 15 of the 94 patients treated who required revision surgeries, a revision rate that is similar to what is seen when using autograft alone. This study demonstrated superior outcomes with allograft plus instrumentation for posterolateral fusion surgeries. However, more importantly for this review, it is one of the few studies to specifically evaluate allograft in an elderly population.

## Demineralized Bone Matrix

Demineralized bone matrix is allograft bone that has been decalcified to produce a product of collagen and noncollagenous proteins. Multiple products are available, but there are relatively limited data available regarding their efficacy, as limited regulatory requirements have been established for these minimally manipulated tissue products. Further, studies have questioned the osteoinductive nature of one product versus another, as well as lot-to-lot variability.[18,19]

There are few randomized controlled clinical trials evaluating the use of DBMs in humans. In one series, 77 patients underwent one, two, or three level noninstrumented anterior cervical discectomy and fusion procedures, using freeze-dried structural allografts filled with a DBM or autogenous iliac crest bone graft alone.[20] At a minimum of 1-year follow-up, fusion rates were 54% and 74% for the allograft/DBM and autograft groups, respectively. Despite this relatively easy fusion environment, inferior fusion rates were observed in the experimental study arm.

In contrast, another study, involving 50 subjects who received lumbar interbody fusions, reported a 96% success rate after implanting titanium mesh cages packed with a DBM and a coralline hydroxyapatite carrier.[21]

The authors performed circumferential fusions with posterior instrumentation and autograft but they did not have a control group to compare against. However, they only used the DBM anteriorly. Again, this study only used the DMB in the anterior spinal column where fusion is generally more easily achieved. This is an excellent example of how DBM could be used as a bone graft extender by eliminating the need for iliac crest bone graft (ICBG) in the anterior fusion construct.

Unfortunately, there are no studies specifically evaluating the use of DBM in the elderly. However, given the highly variable composition and ability to induce fusion between different DBM products, it is doubtful that a definitive study could be adequately performed in an elderly population that could be generalized across multiple DBM products or even across different production lots of the same product.

## Synthetic Materials (Ceramics)

Synthetic materials are being considered with increased frequency as bone graft materials. These provide an osteoconductive scaffolding and are generally used as bone graft extenders or supplements to local or iliac crest bone graft. Again, because the regulatory pathways for approval of such products are not as stringent as for other products, such as the BMPs, the studies are generally less controlled and rigorous, making the efficacy of such products more challenging to interpret.

One of the inherent disadvantages of ceramics is that they are relatively weak and brittle. When ceramics are introduced into the anterior spinal column they must be protected from the significant compressive forces by internal fixation until the graft is incorporated into the new bone growth.[13] Like allograft, ceramics are also inferior to autogenous bone when placed under tension.[22] Other biologically active materials, such as local autograft, demineralized bone matrices (DBMs), or osteoinductive growth factors, may be combined with ceramic osteoconductive matrices to form a composite graft that can then lead to increased amounts of bone formation.[23,24]

## Bone Marrow Aspirates

Autologous bone marrow represents another source of osteogenic cells and osteoinductive proteins for spinal fusion. The most significant advantage of this technique is that aspiration of bone marrow has much less morbidity than the procurement of iliac crest autograft. However, it must be used in combination with an osteoconductive matrix, bone marrow aspirate to form a composite graft. The major limitation to this technique is that unfractionated bone marrow has only moderate osteogenic potential. Even in healthy adults, it is estimated that only 1 out of every 50,000 nucleated bone marrow cells is capable of undergoing differentiation into an osteoblast.[25] Additionally, it has been shown that the number of viable bone marrow cells decreases significantly with age, which may limit utility in an elderly population.[26]

One recent study demonstrated comparable fusion rates to autograft in an instrumented posterolateral fusion study.[27] Both allograft and DBM can be combined with the osteogenic elements of bone marrow aspirate to help promote fusion. By adding bone marrow aspirate, osteogenic elements may be added to help promote fusion. Studies have shown improved fusion rates with the use of bone marrow aspirate from iliac crest when used in conjunction with autologous autograft in a bone paucity model.[28] Recently, aspirates from the vertebral bodies accessed during pedicle screw instrumentation have been shown to be an excellent source of osteogenic cells with only modest depletion with serial aspirations.[29] However, there was a reduction in the cellularity of the specimens in older individuals.

## OTHER POTENTIAL APPLICATION OF BIOLOGICS IN THE AGING SPINE

### Vertebral Body Augmentation in Vertebral Body Compression Fractures

Unique to elderly patients, vertebral compression fractures are the most common type of osteoporotic fragility fracture that can occur from low energy trauma, such as a fall from standing height or less. Although many are asymptomatic, the possible consequences of such injuries can be serious, resulting in limited ambulation, chronic pain, depression, and loss of independence. The primary goals for treatment include pain control and treatment, surgical or nonsurgical, aimed at returning the patient to full activity as quickly as possible to avoid long-term sequelae of deconditioning and muscle weakness.

Surgical options for vertebral body compression fractures include vertebroplasty and kyphoplasty to inject bone cement into the collapsed vertebrae with or without the use of an inflatable balloon to elevate the endplates prior to injecting the cement. Both procedures provide short-term improvement in pain and correction of the deformity, and long-term benefits for functional capacity and prevention of recurrent pain.[30]

A recent meta-analysis[30] comparing kyphoplasty and vertebroplasty found that both treatments resulted in significant improvements in pain and functionality compared to baseline. Compared to medical treatment there was improvement in function, but not pain. Comparing the two surgical treatments, this meta-analysis concluded that balloon kyphoplasty provided better correction of the kyphotic angle and vertebral height while also having less complications from cement extravasation and pulmonary embolism. This study concluded that balloon kyphoplasty is likely superior to traditional vertebroplasty for compression fractures refractory to conventional medical therapy; however they based their assessments on level III data because no randomized control trials were available to appropriately evaluate these treatments.[30]

Newer alternatives to the traditional polymethylmethacrylate (PMMA) bone cement used for these procedures are also being evaluated. The current cement material has a number of shortcomings including a strong exothermic polymerization reaction, which could damage surrounding tissues, lack of bioavailability and osteoconductivity, toxicity of the cement, and extremely limited resorption over time.[31,32] Thus newer cements are being developed to address some of these issues. A recent study evaluating the use of two novel variants (aluminum-free and zinc-based glass polyalkenoate cement) in an in vitro model of osteoporotic compression fractures found them to have similar material properties (injectability, radiopacity, uniaxial compression strength, and biaxial flexural modulus) to traditional cement and performed well over serial compression tests in the lab.[33]

Clinical trials for some of these new cement alternatives have begun with differing results. One study of calcium phosphate cement in balloon kyphoplasty demonstrated improvement in pain and disability outcomes, but poor resistance to flexural, tractive, and shear forces, which resulted in radiographic loss of correction.[34] The authors ultimately recommended against the routine use of this cement alternative to traditional PMMA.

The hope for future advances in cement technology is to develop materials that will accomplish the pain relief and structural correction in the short term while allowing gradual bony healing and replacement of the cement with new bone in the long run. Future research must be done for developing both the basic material science and clinical efficacy before cement alternatives are widely accepted.

## Nonfusion Applications: Addressing Disc Degeneration Directly

Much of low back pain in the aging spine is believed to be a result of disc pathology. Various studies have attempted to identify changes in disc anatomy that may play a role in the generation of back discomfort. Recent studies have demonstrated that there is an overall decrease in cellular density within the disc as well as a reduction in the production of cartilage-specific extracellular matrix components.[35] As a result, there is an overall loss of water-binding capacity and thus an alteration in the biomechanics of the disc. Despite the paucity of cells within the disc, it plays an integral role in the maintenance of matrix proteins. The reduction in cells during aging is believed to be attributable to both apoptotic and necrotic processes. A focus of recent scientific work has been to induce or augment these cells.[36] Cellular transplantation offers potential promise in the treatment of degenerative disc disease; other therapies that have been proposed are the injection of biomaterials into the disc to augment the nucleus pulposus.

However, as noted previously, these technologies are very early in their development from a clinical standpoint. Most of these technologies are only being evaluated for use early in the degenerative cascade. By the time that degeneration is more advanced, such as in the elderly population being considered here, this technology may not be applicable.

## CONCLUSION

Performing spinal surgeries in the elderly presents significant challenges to the surgeon with regard to advanced pathology and preexisting illness, which may complicate the treatment options. Iliac crest autograft has long been the gold standard treatment option for patients of all age groups because it is the only graft option that contains osteogenic cells, osteoinductive growth factors, and an osteoconductive matrix. Unfortunately, harvesting autograft also forces the patient to undergo an additional invasive procedure, which can result in significant postoperative morbidity, particularly in the elderly. The evolution of bone graft alternatives and supplements provides exciting, less morbid alternatives to the use of iliac crest autograft for spinal fusion that may be considered for use alone or in combination with local bone graft material.

The use of biologics in the elderly offers the potential to reduce complications associated with harvesting ICBG while maintaining successful fusion. A number of different types of biologics are currently available, including various recombinant growth factor signaling proteins (rhBMPs), demineralized bone matrix, and synthetic ceramics. The future of these technologies likely lies in composite grafts that use these and other biologic materials in combination to attempt to recreate and stimulate the native bone formation system. There are similar advances being made in nonfusion alternatives to surgery, such as in the treatment of vertebral compression fractures in the elderly, an increasingly common condition as the population ages and osteoporotic, fragility fractures become more prevalent. New cements used for these treatments are being developed as alternative to PMMA bone cement and will likely play an increasingly important role in the future treatment of vertebral compression fractures. Additionally, there may be a role for biologics to assist in the restoration of disc health. This may be accomplished through possible chondrocyte transplantation or through the use of BMP. This may offer the possibility of avoiding the cascade of degenerative spine disease.

As these graft alternatives continue to advance, it will be important to carefully evaluate their use in the elderly, who are the most likely to require surgery for degenerative, age-related conditions of the spine. However, regardless of how these new technologies are employed, the success of these complex surgeries will remain dependent upon the basic principles essential to achieving a solid arthodesis: proper patient selection, optimization of the biological environment and selection of the best bone graft material, preparation of the fusion bed, and maintenance of adequate biomechanical stability during bone formation.

### References

1. Federal Interagency Forum on Aging-Related Statistics. Older Americans update 2006: key indicators of well-being, In: Federal Interagency Forum on Aging-Related Statistics, U.S. Government Printing Office, Washington, DC, 2006.
2. J.M. Cloyd, F.L. Acosta Jr., C.P. Ames, Complications and outcomes of lumbar spine surgery in elderly people: a review of the literature, J. Am. Geriatr. Soc. 56–7 (2008) 1318–1327.
3. R.A. Hart, M.A. Prendergast, Spine surgery for lumbar degenerative disease in elderly and osteoporotic patients, Instr. Course Lect. 56 (2007) 257–272.
4. A.R. Gupta, N.R. Shah, T.C. Patel, Perioperative and long-term complications of iliac crest bone graft harvest for spinal surgery: a quantitative review of the literature, Int. Med. 8 (2001) 163–166.
5. J.C. Steinmann, H.N. Herkowitz, Pseudarthrosis of the spine, Clin. Orthop. Relat. Res. 284 (1992) 80–90.
6. M.R. Urist, Bone: Formation by autoinduction, Science 150 (1965) 893–899.
7. E. Carlisle, J.S. Fischgrund, Bone morphogenetic proteins for spinal fusion, Spine J. 5–6 (Suppl) (2005) 240S–249S.
8. J.K. Burkus, M.F. Gornet, C.A. Dickman, T.A. Zdeblick, Anterior lumbar interbody fusion using rhBMP-2 with tapered interbody cages, J. Spinal Disord. Tech. 15–5 (2002) 337–349.
9. S.D. Glassman, L. Carreon, M. Djurasovic, M.J. Campbell, R.M. Puno, J.R. Johnson, J.R. Dimar, Posterolateral lumbar spine fusion with INFUSE bone graft, Spine J. 7–1 (2007) 44–49.
10. J.F. Brandoff, J.S. Silber, A.R. Vaccaro, Contemporary alternatives to synthetic bone grafts for spine surgery, Am. J. Orthop. 37–8 (2008) 410–414.
11. S.D. Glassman, L.Y. Carreon, M. Djurasovic, M.J. Campbell, R.M. Puno, J.R. Johnson, J.R. Dimar, RhBMP-2 versus iliac crest bone graft for lumbar spine fusion: a randomized, controlled trial in patients over sixty years of age, Spine (Phila Pa 1976) 33–26 (2008) 2843–2849.

12. D. Benglis, M.Y. Wang, A.D. Levi, A comprehensive review of the safety profile of bone morphogenetic protein in spine surgery, Neurosurgery 62–5 (Suppl 2), 2008. ONS423-31; discussion ONS31.

13. K.M. Malloy, A.S. Hilibrand, Autograft versus allograft in degenerative cervical disease, Clin. Orthop. Relat. Res. 394 (2002) 27–38.

14. A.R. Vaccaro, K. Chiba, J.G. Heller, T. Patel, J.S. Thalgott, E. Truumees, J.S. Fischgrund, M.R. Craig, S.C. Berta, J.C. Wang, Bone grafting alternatives in spinal surgery, Spine J. 2–3 (2002) 206–215.

15. S.S. Jorgenson, T.G. Lowe, J. France, J. Sabin, A prospective analysis of autograft versus allograft in posterolateral lumbar fusion in the same patient. A minimum of 1-year follow-up in 144 patients, Spine (Phila Pa 1976) 19–18 (1994) 2048–2053.

16. P.J. Nugent, E.G. Dawson, Intertransverse process lumbar arthrodesis with allogeneic fresh-frozen bone graft, Clin. Orthop. Relat. Res. 287 (1993) 107–111.

17. T. Andersen, F.B. Christensen, B. Niedermann, P. Helmig, K. Hoy, E.S. Hansen, C. Bunger, Impact of instrumentation in lumbar spinal fusion in elderly patients, Acta Orthop. (2009) 445–450.

18. H.W. Bae, L. Zhao, L.E. Kanim, P. Wong, R.B. Delamarter, E.G. Dawson, Intervariability and intravariability of bone morphogenetic proteins in commercially available demineralized bone matrix products, Spine (Phila Pa 1976) 31-12 (2006) 1299–1306. discussion 307–8.

19. B. Peterson, P.G. Whang, R. Iglesias, J.C. Wang, J.R. Lieberman, Osteoinductivity of commercially available demineralized bone matrix. Preparations in a spine fusion model, J. Bone Joint Surg. Am. 86-A-10 (2004) 2243–2250.

20. H.S. An, J.M. Simpson, J.M. Glover, J. Stephany, Comparison between allograft plus demineralized bone matrix versus autograft in anterior cervical fusion. A prospective multicenter study, Spine (Phila Pa 1976) 20–20 (1995) 2211–2216.

21. J.S. Thalgott, J.M. Giuffre, Z. Klezl, M. Timlin, Anterior lumbar interbody fusion with titanium mesh cages, coralline hydroxyapatite, and demineralized bone matrix as part of a circumferential fusion, Spine J. 2–1 (2002) 63–69.

22. R.W. Bucholz, A. Carlton, R.E. Holmes, Hydroxyapatite and tricalcium phosphate bone graft substitutes, Orthop. Clin. North Am. 18–2 (1987) 323–334.

23. C.J. Damien, J.R. Parsons, A.B. Prewett, F. Huismans, E.C. Shors, R.E. Holmes, Effect of demineralized bone matrix on bone growth within a porous HA material: a histologic and histometric study, J. Biomater. Appl. 9–3 (1995) 275–288.

24. R.E. Kania, A. Meunier, M. Hamadouche, L. Sedel, H. Petite, Addition of fibrin sealant to ceramic promotes bone repair: long-term study in rabbit femoral defect model, J. Biomed. Mater. Res. 43–1 (1998) 38–45.

25. R.G. Burwell, The function of bone marrow in the incorporation of a bone graft, Clin. Orthop. Relat. Res. 200 (1985) 125–141.

26. G.F. Muschler, H. Nitto, C.A. Boehm, K.A. Easley, Age- and gender-related changes in the cellularity of human bone marrow and the prevalence of osteoblastic progenitors, J. Orthop. Res. 19–1 (2001) 117–125.

27. K.H. Bridwell, P.A. Anderson, S.D. Boden, A.R. Vaccaro, J.C. Wang, What's new in spine surgery, J. Bone Joint Surg Am. 90–7 (2008) 1609–1619.

28. L.J. Curylo, B. Johnstone, C.A. Petersilge, J.A. Janicki, J.U. Yoo, Augmentation of spinal arthrodesis with autologous bone marrow in a rabbit posterolateral spine fusion model, Spine (Phila Pa 1976) 24-5 (1999) 434–438. discussion 8–9.

29. R.F. McLain, C.A. Boehm, C. Rufo-Smith, G.F. Muschler, Transpedicular aspiration of osteoprogenitor cells from the vertebral body: progenitor cell concentrations affected by serial aspiration, Spine J. 9–12 (2009) 995–1002.

30. R.S. Taylor, R.J. Taylor, P. Fritzell, Balloon kyphoplasty and vertebroplasty for vertebral compression fractures: a comparative systematic review of efficacy and safety, Spine (Phila Pa 1976) 31–23 (2006) 2747–2755.

31. G. Lewis, Injectable bone cements for use in vertebroplasty and kyphoplasty: state-of-the-art review, J. Biomed. Mater. Res. B. Appl. Biomater. 76–2 (2006) 456–468.

32. G. Lewis, Properties of acrylic bone cement: state of the art review, J. Biomed. Mater. Res. 38–2 (1997) 155–182.

33. G. Lewis, M.R. Towler, D. Boyd, M.J. German, A.W. Wren, O.M. Clarkin, A. Yates, Evaluation of two novel aluminum-free, zinc-based glass polyalkenoate cements as alternatives to PMMA bone cement for use in vertebroplasty and balloon kyphoplasty, J. Mater. Sci. Mater. Med., 2009.

34. T.R. Blattert, L. Jestaedt, A. Weckbach, Suitability of a calcium phosphate cement in osteoporotic vertebral body fracture augmentation: a controlled, randomized, clinical trial of balloon kyphoplasty comparing calcium phosphate versus polymethylmethacrylate, Spine (Phila Pa 1976) 34–2 (2009) 108–114.

35. C. Hohaus, T.M. Ganey, Y. Minkus, H.J. Meisel, Cell transplantation in lumbar spine disc degeneration disease, Eur. Spine J. 4 (17 Suppl) (2008) 492–503.

36. L.M. Boyd, A.J. Carter, Injectable biomaterials and vertebral endplate treatment for repair and regeneration of the intervertebral disc, Eur. Spine J. 3 (15 Suppl) (2006) S414–S421.

# 59

# Minimally Invasive Spinal Surgery (MISS) Techniques for the Decompression of Lumbar Spinal Stenosis

*Zachary A. Smith, Farbod Asgarzadie, and Larry T. Khoo*

**K E Y   P O I N T S**

- Lumbar spinal stenosis has classically been treated via decompressive techniques, such as laminotomy, laminectomy, and foraminotomies, which are traditionally associated with a good early postoperative neurological outcome. Because the targeted population is elderly, however, perioperative and postoperative complications, such as wound infections, deep vein thrombosis, and stasis types of events, are not uncommon.

- Traditional wide bony decompressive techniques as well as their attendant musculoligamentous injury are associated with delayed instability, recurrent stenosis, and progressive back pain in a significant percentage of patients over time.

- Minimally invasive surgical techniques are associated with decreased tissue exposure and injury, thereby sparing the stabilizing soft tissue musculoligamentous and bony complexes.

- As a result, published perioperative complication rates for minimally invasive spinal surgery (MISS) decompressive techniques have been lower than traditional open decompressive rates, with equivalent 1- and 2-year neurological outcomes and efficacies. Preliminary long-term data also indicate a trend toward decreased rates of progressive axial back pain, recurrent stenotic symptoms, and delayed radiographic instability.

- New stabilizing interspinous and interfacet devices may effectively decompress vertical stenosis (i.e., neurological compression due to facet subluxation at the level of the spinal recess and foramina) without the need for excessive resection of the bony elements via classical midline approaches.

## INTRODUCTION

In elderly patients afflicted with lumbar spinal stenosis (LSS), the simple act of walking can often be rendered so painful as to be unbearable. Although standard open posterior laminectomy is well established and familiar to virtually all spine surgeons, this traditional surgical treatment of LSS is often associated with significant postoperative pain, disability, and dysfunction. With their mobility limited by the pain of recovery, these patients can also suffer from other perioperative sequelae, including deep vein thrombosis, pulmonary atelectasis, pneumonia, gastritis, ileus, pulmonary embolism, urinary tract infections, and pyelonephritis. Because LSS patients are typically elderly and frail, the morbidity of the two-edged surgical sword cuts particularly deep in them. *Primum non nocere.* Thus surgeons have increasingly employed less destructive means of achieving decompression in the hope of minimizing iatrogenic injuries.

Minimally invasive foraminotomies and discectomies have gained increasing popularity among spine surgeons for the treatment of herniated intervertebral discs. The minimally invasive microendoscopic discectomy has been particularly attractive for its small skin incision, gentle tissue dissection and excellent visualization. The technique has been shown to provide symptomatic relief equivalent to that achieved with open discectomy, with significant reductions in operative blood loss, postoperative pain, hospital stay, and narcotic usage. The evolution of minimally invasive techniques has led to safe and effective applications for the treatment of LSS. The minimally invasive percutaneous microendoscopic approach for bilateral decompression of lumbar stenosis via a unilateral approach has been described for the treatment LSS and has been shown to offer a similar short-term clinical outcome as compared to open techniques with a significant reduction in operative blood loss, postoperative stay, and use of narcotics.[1] This chapter reviews the pathophysiology of LSS; explains the rationale, indications and surgical techniques for minimally invasive LSS surgery; and presents our 4-year outcomes data.

## PATHOPHYSIOLOGY

The clinical entity of lumbar spinal stenosis is one that is familiar to almost all physicians who treat the elderly. From a pathophysiological perspective, lumbar stenosis typically results from a complex degenerative process that leads to compression of neural elements from a combination of ligamentum flavum hypertrophy, preexisting congenital narrowing (e.g., trefoil canal), intervertebral disc bulging or herniation, and facet thickening with arthropathy of the capsule soft tissues.[2-4] With the unparalleled recent advances in imaging, it has become evident that the majority of these changes and thereby the neurological compression are typically seen at the level of the interlaminar window.[2,5] These pathological changes are thus thought to be responsible for the clinical symptoms of lumbar stenosis. For these patients, the *sine qua non* feature of the history is low back and proximal leg pain that worsens with standing and walking and is alleviated by sitting and bending forward. Whether this phenomenon occurs as a result of direct neural compression or from secondary vascular ischemia of the nerve roots remains unclear. Nevertheless, this presentation of neurogenic claudication, anthropoid posture, and low back pain is becoming increasingly common as our population demographic grows older and older. Indeed, stenosis of the lumbar canal is now the most common indication for surgery of the spine for patients over the age of 65 years.[6-9] This peak incidence in the geriatric population makes the surgical treatment of spinal stenosis particularly difficult because these patients are at significantly increased surgical risk because of their often poor medical condition.

## TREATMENT OPTIONS AND GUIDELINES

The traditional treatment of lumbar stenosis usually entails an extensive resection of posterior spinal elements such as the interspinous ligaments, spinous processes, bilateral lamina, portions of the facet joints and capsule, and the ligamentum flavum. Additionally, wide muscular dissection and retraction usually are required to achieve adequate surgical visualization. These classical operations of a wide decompressive laminectomy, medial facetectomy, and foraminotomy have been used for decades with a variable degree of success.[8-11] Such extensive resection and injury of the posterior osseous and muscular complex can lead to significant iatrogenic pain, disability, and morbidity. Loss of the midline supraspinous–interspinous ligament complex can lead to a loss of flexion stability, thereby increasing the risk of delayed spinal instability.[12,13] Extensive laminectomy can also be associated with significant operative blood loss as well as prolonged postoperative pain and weakness secondary to the extensive surgical dissection and muscle detachment. Such iatrogenic injury can lead to paraspinal muscle denervation and atrophy, which may correlate with an increased incidence of "failed back syndrome" and chronic pain.[14,15] Because patients with lumbar stenosis are usually elderly and often medically frail, this delayed recovery can often result in significant morbidity. Deep venous thrombosis, pulmonary embolism, pulmonary atelectasis, pneumonia, urinary tract infections, ileus, and narcotic dependency are but some of these potentially devastating sequelae.

Whereas conservative therapy initially is a reasonable recommendation, there will inevitably be a significant proportion of patients with progressive stenotic symptoms who will ultimately require surgical intervention. In the Maine Lumbar Spine Study group, Atlas and coworkers[16] prospectively followed 97 patients over a 10-year interval. Of these, 56 were surgically treated and 41 were conservatively managed. Based on patient satisfaction assessment vehicles, 54% of surgically treated patients reported improvement versus 42% of nonsurgical patients at 10 years. In comparison, the 4-year data from the Maine Lumbar Spine Study group revealed that 70% of surgically treated patients reported a clear improvement, compared to 52% in the nonoperative group.[6] This decrease in patient satisfaction indicates that surgical benefits may not be stable over the course of time because LSS is typically a chronic and progressive disease. Hurri and colleagues,[7] in 1998, reported their longitudinal 12-year study of 75 patients with lumbar stenosis. Using the Oswestry index, their disability was scored over many years and could demonstrate no clear difference between those who were operated on versus those managed conservatively. From an extensive review of the literature, Turner concluded from his attempted meta-analysis that approximately 64% of surgically treated patients had a good outcome over a midterm period of follow-up (3 to 6 years). However, he also noted that delayed clinical progression and recurrence of stenosis symptoms was extremely common, thus reflecting the chronic degenerative nature of the underlying disease process.[13] Thus although surgical treatment appears to have a positive effect on the natural history of LSS, clinical progression and recurrence is likely. Moreover, several subgroups have been consistently identified that are particularly prone to recurrence of symptoms. These include patients with preexisting spondylolisthesis, scoliosis, prior destabilizing laminectomies, and the presence of segmental vertebral motion on flexion–extension radiographs.[17,18] According to the treatment guidelines set forth by the AANS/CNS Joint section on Disorders of the Spine and Peripheral Nerves, fusion is recommended for patients with lumbar stenosis and associated degenerative spondylolisthesis who require decompression.[19] In addition, wide decompressions leading to disruption of the facet joints has also been associated with poorer outcomes.[19] In light of these considerations, the need for a less invasive means of decompression without major disruption of the facet joints and muscular attachments as well as the option of fusion for the treatment for LSS is evident.

## SURGICAL RATIONALE

Over the past two decades, numerous surgeons have worked toward the goal of reducing the surgical morbidity of the procedure. The ideal operation for LSS would be one that could simultaneously achieve an adequate decompression of the neural elements, while at the same time minimize damage to the posterior muscular, ligamentous, and bony complex. Because the pathological changes typically are concentrated at the level of the interlaminar space, focal laminotomy was the natural first step in the evolution of surgical procedures for LSS. By sparing most of the lamina, spinous processes, and interspinous ligamentous complex, laminotomy helped to preserve the biomechanical integrity of the spine. Aryanpur and Ducker,[20] in their description of multilevel open lumbar laminotomies, reported a longitudinal good outcome rate of 79% to 85% at 2-year follow-up. As the use of the operating microscope became increasingly common among

spinal surgeons, unilateral microscopic hemilaminotomy was developed as a means of sparing the contralateral musculature as well. This procedure was characterized by unilateral multifidus retraction, ipsilateral decompression, and also contralateral microscopic decompression performed under the midline bony and ligamentous structures. For this microscopic laminotomy as described by McCulloch[21] and Young and colleagues,[22] an 80% to 95% improvement rate was reported over a 9-month follow-up period. Despite this progressive movement toward less extensive resection of the posterior bony elements, symptomatic outcomes have remained similar regardless of the aggressiveness of the surgical procedure utilized to treat LSS.[23] Indeed, in one of the only studies correlating the degree of radiographic with clinical outcome, it was observed that the satisfaction of patients with the results of surgery (e.g., Oswestry score and walking capacity) was more important in surgical outcome than the degree of decompression as seen on a postoperative CT scan.[5]

In the past decade, significant strides in microendoscopic visualization technology have been made. Accordingly, endoscopic-assisted procedures have become increasingly popular for the treatment of a wide range of spinal pathologies, including hyperhydrosis, herniated discs, tumors, and fractures. In the lumbar spine, microendoscopic-assisted discectomies (MEDs) have been used in treating herniated discs successfully for the last 5 years. The MED procedure has been particularly attractive for its small skin incision, gentle tissue dissection, excellent visualization, and ability to achieve results equivalent to those with open techniques. The microendoscopic decompressive laminotomy (MEDL) technique was thus developed as a synthesis of the unilateral hemilaminotomy, described earlier, and these MED techniques. The MEDL technique was initially validated in a series of cadaveric studies in which the equivalent bony decompressions were achieved via either an open or an endoscopic technique.[24] Since then, it has also been studied clinically with resultant good surgical outcomes, low morbidity, and a rapid postoperative functional recovery.[1] A bilateral decompression via a unilateral minimally invasive approach thus represents the next logical step in the evolution of modern surgical treatment for LSS.

## INDICATIONS FOR MISS DECOMPRESSIVE TECHNIQUES

Patients undergoing microendoscopic decompressions for LSS should meet the same selection criteria as those for open decompressive laminectomy or laminotomy. As reviewed earlier, these patients should have low back pain associated with the sine qua non description of neurogenic claudication. Because the MEDL technique is capable of decompressing the central canal, lateral recess, and the proximal part of the ipsilateral neural foramen, symptoms of radiculopathy from either foraminal stenosis or disc herniation can be successfully addressed by MEDL as well. When evidence of nerve compression is present, the MEDL should ideally be performed on the same side as these symptoms to afford maximal surgical exposure. Patients who have radicular symptoms on both sides should either be treated via a bilateral MEDL procedure or open type decompression. Similarly, a far-lateral disc herniation with coexisting central stenosis must be treated via either two MED approaches or an open technique.

Patients with evidence of LSS in addition to spondylolisthesis, deformity, or severe degenerative disc disease may benefit from a minimally invasive transforaminal interbody fusion and percutaneous posterolateral instrumentation.[19] Patients with severe spondylolisthesis or severe deformity, infection, tumor, arachnoiditis, pseudomeningocele, or cerebrospinal fluid fistula are generally not suitable candidate for MEDL. A thorough clinical and radiographic evaluation with use of dynamic flexion, extension, and lateral-bending radiographs, contrast-enhanced MRI and CT, and isotope scans should be performed to exclude these conditions. Prior surgery at the same level as the present stenotic area is also a relative contraindication. For these cases, significant epidural scarring and dense adhesions can make the MEDL technique particularly difficult with an increased risk of durotomy. However, in cases with a limited amount of decompression, a relatively intact facet complex, and little epidural scarring as shown on gadolinium-enhanced MRI, the MEDL procedure can be used to successfully achieve a repeat decompression. Redo procedures should be attempted only by surgeons who have already gained facility with the MEDL technique in a good number of simple cases. Additionally, patients undergoing redo decompression with MEDL should be clearly informed about the increased surgical risks and the possibility of conversion to an open procedure.

## Surgical Technique

After appropriate preoperative evaluation and medical clearance, the patient is brought to the operative suite where general endotracheal anesthesia is induced with adequate intravenous access and an intraarterial monitoring catheter. Local and intravenous sedation alone is generally inadequate, because the MEDL procedure requires the patient to be still for a prolonged period of time. A Foley catheter should be used for most cases. After induction, we refrain from the use of neuromuscular paralytics to better assess the nerve root during decompression. This will provide for intraoperative feedback as well as to allow for a more rapid reawakening of the patient at the end of the procedure. Because blood loss for the MEDL procedure has typically been minimal, it is important to avoid excessive fluid hydration during the case, which can often lead to cardiopulmonary complications in this population of older patients. Overall, it is crucial for the operative surgeon to have a clear working dialogue with the anesthesiologist before and during the case to clarify the nature of the procedure. This will greatly help to reduce unfortunate miscommunications and their attendant complications.

The patient is then turned into a prone position onto a radiolucent Wilson frame and Jackson table. Utmost care should be made to insure adequate padding of all pressure points, eyes, and extremities. The fluoroscopic C-arm should then be brought into the surgical field so that real-time lateral fluoroscopic images can be obtained. Ideally, this should be draped and positioned such that it can be easily swung in and out during the procedure without having to interrupt the flow of the case. The operative surgeon generally stands on the side of the approach with the C-arm and video monitors placed opposite him. However, the ultimate arrangement of the video monitor and C-arm monitor can be varied to allow for optimal ergonomic movements during the operation (Figure 59-1). Electromyographic (EMG) monitoring of motor nerve root responses can be used if desired.

Under fluoroscopic guidance with a Steinmann pin held laterally to the patient, the approximate level of the incision is marked approximately 1 to 1.5 inches off midline on the side of the approach. This incision is marked to facilitate targeting of the laminofacet junction at the spinal level to be decompressed (Figure 59-2A). A small stab incision is then made in the middle of the marked incision through which the Steinmann pin is then passed down to the medial bony facet margin. Particular care should be made to begin this approach laterally to avoid inadvertent dural penetration. The placement of the pin is then confirmed with the fluoroscope to ensure a good working trajectory (Figure 59-2B). Although we have not routinely done so, anteroposterior radiographic images can be obtained to guarantee proper pin positioning. In our early experience with minimally invasive stenosis decompression, we decompressed the ipsilateral lateral

recess before decompressing the contralateral side. For the last 4 years, we have changed our approach to contralateral decompression, a technique that has been described previously.[25] Once the guidewire has been docked on the spinolaminar junction, a skin incision is made above and below the Steinmann pin for a total length of approximately 2.5 cm. The METRx (Medtronic, Sofamor-Danek, Memphis, Tenn.) microendoscopic system's set of serial dilators (Figure 59-3) are then passed over then Steinmann pin to gently dilate the lumbar musculature and expand the lumbodorsal fascia away. Medial angulation of up to about 45 degrees is desirable at this point to ensure optimal visualization of the spinolaminar junction and ensure a proper trajectory for drilling of the anterior aspect of the lamina to the contralateral lateral recess and foramen (Figure 59-4). The 18-mm final working channel is then passed over the dilators and secured to the flexible-arm METRX retractor mounted to the table side rail. Final fluoroscopic confirmation of the working channel position is then obtained, an 18-mm working channel of adequate depth (usually 5 to 6 cm) is placed and the serial dilators are then removed. The endoscope is then attached to the tubular retractor or the operating microscope is used for the remainder of the procedure.

Bovie cautery with a long tip is then used to remove the remaining muscle and soft tissue overlying the lamina and spinolaminar junction. A long high-speed burr (e.g., AM-8, Midas Rex) is then used to core out the cancellous and deep cortical surface of the contralateral lamina, preserving the ligamentum flavum underneath and using it as a protective layer over the dura. This "intralaminar" drilling is carried out laterally to the contralateral lateral recess and foramen. Kerrison rongeurs may be used to remove the remaining laminar edge and the medial contralateral facet. After adequate contralateral bony decompression, the ligamentum flavum can be removed with use of up-angled curettes and Kerrison rongeurs.

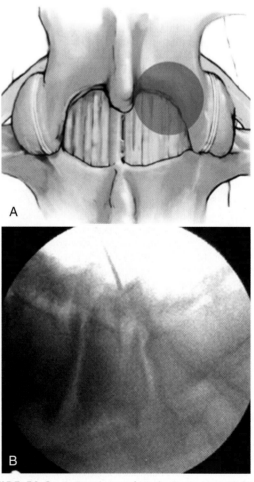

■ **FIGURE 59-2** **A,** Dorsal view of interlaminar space with highlighted spinolaminar junction target. **B,** Lateral fluoroscopic image showing percutaneous Steinmann pin placement.

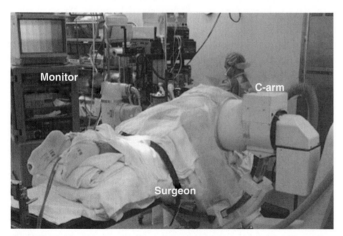

■ **FIGURE 59-1** A view of the typical operative set-up for an MEDL procedure. The patient is placed in the prone position. The C-arm is placed into the field to allow for intraoperative lateral fluoroscopy. The video monitors are placed opposite the operative side to allow easy visualization by the surgeon.

Attention is now directed toward the ipsilateral lateral recess and foramen. The tubular retractor is angled laterally toward the ipsilateral lamina-medial facet junction and drilling is carried out to thin the lamina and the medial facet complex down (Figure 59-5). With the bony edges well visualized, a small straight curette is used to scrape the inferior edge of the adjacent lamina and the medial edge of the facet complex. This exposure is then carried underneath the lamina and facet with the use of a small angled endoscopic curette (Figure 59-6 A and B). Proper placement of the curettes should be confirmed under fluoroscopy. Good dissection of the underlying flavum and dura from the bone is crucial in preventing incidental dural tears and cerebrospinal (CSF) fluid leaks. Bleeding from epidural small and edge of the flavum was controlled via long-tipped endoscopic bipolar cautery. A small angled Kerrison rongeur is then utilized to begin the laminotomy (see Figure 59-6 A to D). After adequate drilling, endoscopic Kerrison rongeurs are used to continue the removal of the lamina and medial facet. Frequent dissection with the small angled curette before biting with the Kerrison rongeur should be used to free the underlying ligament and nerve root. In this fashion, bilateral hemilaminotomies, medial facetectomies, and foraminotomies are completed (Figure 59-7).

For cases in which an ipsilateral bulging or herniated disc is present, the nerve root is retracted and the epidural veins are coagulated with bipolar cautery and dissected free over the underlying disc space. A sharp annulotomy is then made with a special endoscopic knife and a standard discectomy and internal decompression is then performed.

In cases of multiple adjacent level stenoses, the initial placement of the dilators and tubular retractor should be midway between the stenotic levels. In a patient with both L3-L4 and L4-L5 stenosis, for example, the working channel should be first docked on the L4 lamina and then swung caudad to decompress the L4-L5 level, and cephalad to subsequently decompress the L3-L4 level. For patients with a larger vertical distance between spinal segments, sharp incision of the lumbodorsal fascia and superoinferior translation of the working channel may also be needed. Figure 59-8 demonstrates the extent of multiple level decompression than can be obtained through repositioning of the working channel through a single incision. Figure 59-9 demonstrates a typical decompression achieved via MEDL for a representative case of lumbar stenosis.

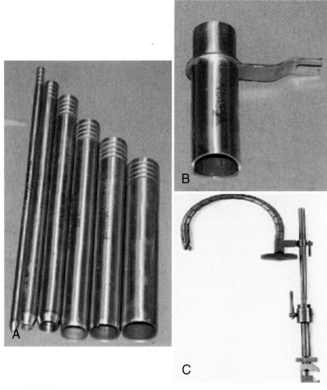

■ **FIGURE 59-3**    METRx (Medtronic Sofamor Danek, Memphis, Tenn.). Equipment Set. **A,** Sequential soft tissue dilators. **B,** 18-mm working channel with retractor arm attachment. **C,** Flexible bed-mounted retractor arm.

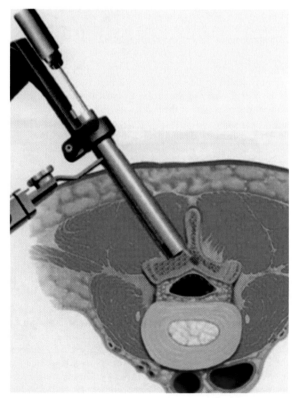

■ **FIGURE 59-4**    Medial angulation of the retractor tube ensures optimal visualization of the spinolaminar junction and facilitates a proper trajectory for drilling of the anterior aspect of the lamina to the contralateral lateral recess and foramen.

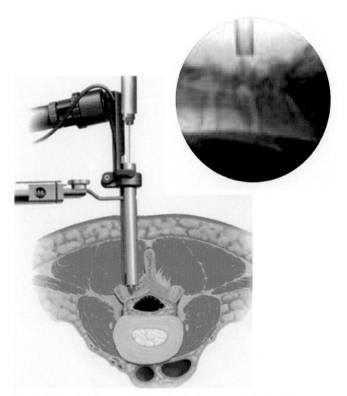

■ **FIGURE 59-5**    The tubular retractor is now angled laterally toward the ipsilateral lamina–medial facet junction.

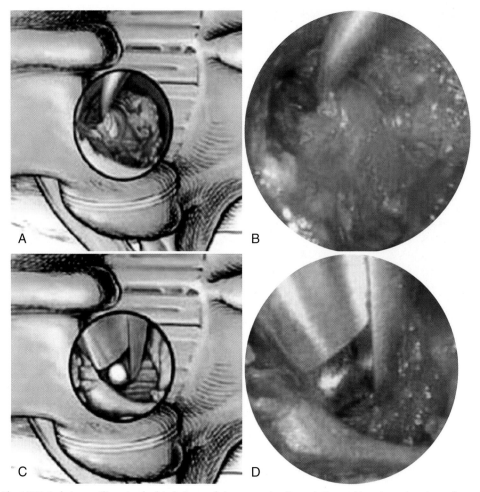

■ **FIGURE 59-6**   The MEDL technique utilizes standard techniques of decompression through the working channel under endoscopic guidance: **A,** A small angled curette is used to define the laminar edge and to mobilize the flavum. **B,** An intraoperative view through the endoscope of this maneuver is shown. **C,** Endoscopic Kerrison rongeurs are used to begin the laminotomy and decompression. **D,** An intraoperative view of the Kerrison used for the laminotomy.

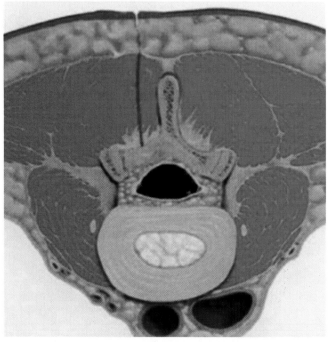

■ **FIGURE 59-7**   Bilateral hemilaminotomies, medial facetectomies, and foraminotomies are completed.

In cases in which an interbody fusion is indicated, the drill is used to remove the medial aspect of the superior articular process and expose the superior and medial aspects of the pedicle and the adjoining foramen to the level of the top margin of the disc. Coagulation and division of the inferior foraminal veins allows for about 10 to 12 mm between the exiting and traversing roots at the upper margin of the disc, allowing for thorough discectomy and interbody fusion using a single intervertebral spacer is then placed and directed just across the midline using biplanar fluoroscopy (Traxis MIS TLIF set, Abbot Spine, or Concorde Cage, Depuy Spine) (Figure 59-10). Bilateral percutaneous pedicle screws and connecting rods (Pathfinder, Abbott Spine) are placed under compression to lock the interbody fusion cage and to minimize the risk of cage migration.[26] A detailed discussion of a minimally invasive transforaminal lumbar interbody fusion is beyond the scope of this article.

After inspection of the thecal sac and nerve roots, hemostasis is obtained by bipolar cautery and gentle tamponade with thrombin-soaked Gelfoam pledgets. A single dose of intraoperative Cefazolin (Ancef) or vancomycin is typically employed during the procedure and a second dose can be given at the surgeon's discretion. The area is then copiously irrigated with lactated ringers impregnated with bacitracin antibiotics. A small piece of Gelfoam soaked with methylprednisolone (Solumedrol) was typically gently placed over the laminoforaminotomy defect. Use of epidural morphine paste or similar cocktails is reasonable if there is not evidence of dural erosion or tear. Such agents may help to reduce postoperative pain and allow for more rapid recovery and ambulation. The tubular retractor and endoscope are then removed. Because the defect is typically quite small, only a limited amount of closure need be performed and a drain is not needed. A 0-Vicryl type of reabsorbable suture is used to close the lumbodorsal fascia in a

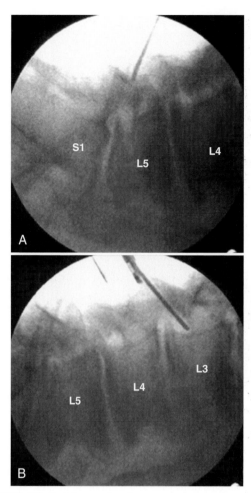

■ **FIGURE 59-8** Intraoperative fluoroscopic images demonstrate the long multilevel decompression that can be achieved through a single incision by simply angling the working channel.

figure-of-eight. Bupivacaine (Marcaine [0.25%]) is used to inject the skin edges before closure. Inverted stitches of 2-0 Vicryl suture are used to close the subcutaneous layer. A 4-0 clear Vicryl subcuticular closure is then used to carefully reapproximate the skin edges, with care taken to avoid inversion. Either Steri-Strips or Dermabond can then be used to cover the skin. Dermabond is attractive because it keeps the skin edges closely approximated for 7 to 10 days and provides a waterproof barrier. The patient can thus shower almost immediately after surgery.

For cases in which a CSF leak occurred, direct repair of the durotomy is extremely difficult because of the small size of the endoscopic procedure. Fortunately, most dural tears that occur with the microendoscopic technique are typically small as well. Thus we have typically not employed lumbar drains. Fibrin glue, fat, or muscle grafts were typically used to tamponade the dural violation. For large CSF leaks, direct repair can be attempted if specialized instruments are available for use through the endoscopic tube. A Castro-Viejo type of needle holder and long forceps are particularly useful in this regard.

## POSTOPERATIVE MANAGEMENT

The patient is awakened from anesthesia and taken to the postanesthesia recovery unit. For single-level MEDL procedures, for which an early discharge is anticipated, it is important for the surgeon to communicate preoperatively with the anesthesiologist. Long-acting inhalational and intravenous agents should be avoided to allow for rapid awakening of the patient postoperatively. Additionally, use of only short-acting muscle relaxants for initial induction will allow for better monitoring of nerve root function as well as quicker extubation of the patient after surgery.

Patients should be allowed to ambulate early on after surgery. Foley catheters, arterial lines, and unneeded intravenous lines should be removed as early as possible. Early evaluation and treatment by experienced physical therapists are important to begin the recovery and rehabilitation process. As most patients with LSS present with a limited capacity for ambulation, walking at the preoperative level should be encouraged. We typically have not used a rigid external orthosis after MEDL with or without TLIF and pedicle screw fixation, but use of a lumbar corset with metal stays or similar brace is reasonable for the patient's comfort. Depending on the level of analgesic and narcotics used preoperatively, we have generally aimed to minimize usage of postoperative pain medications. We typically employ strong nonsteroidal antiinflammatory agents in nonfusion cases (e.g., celecoxib [Celebrex], rofecoxib [Vioxx]) combined with muscle relaxants (e.g., cyclobenzaprine [Flexeril], baclofen, methocarbamol [Robaxin]). Oral narcotic medications such as hydrocodone/acetaminophen (Vicodin) and oxycodone/acetaminophen (Percocet) are used primarily on a breakthrough basis. In a comparison of MEDL with open decompression, we found that LSS patients after MEDL use significantly less narcotic medication.[1]

Patients are typically discharged when they are able to ambulate on their own and their pain on oral agents only. For patients with mild to moderate preoperative symptoms and gait limitation, discharge can frequently occur within 24 to 48 hours after surgery. For patients with long-standing severe symptoms and gait dysfunction, a course of inpatient rehabilitation may be needed to optimize their functional status before sending them home. It is important to inquire about the patient's home living situation to ensure that appropriate support and safety is available there before discharge. We routinely recommend a structured course of truncal stabilization and aerobic conditioning for these patients.

## CLINICAL OUTCOMES AND COMPLICATIONS

The results of our first 48 MEDL patients are presented here to serve as a useful guide in what to expect during clinical follow-up. As with all surgical procedures, the results of treatment with MEDL will vary directly with the patient population and selection criteria of the surgeon. Additionally, operative times, blood loss, complication rates, and postoperative length of stay will typically improve as a surgeon's facility with the MEDL procedure grows.

The patients had a mean age of 64.5 years. There was a male-to-female ratio of 3:2. The patients' clinical presentations were scored into four clinical categories: back pain, leg pain, gait limitation and distance, and urinary dysfunction. Patients who underwent fusion and patients with evidence of lumbar instability, severe deformity, spondyloptosis/severe spondylolisthesis, infection, tumor, and cauda equina syndrome were excluded from the MEDL study group. All patients had pain in their lower back, 80% reported some degree of radiating leg pain, about 96% had significant limitation in their ambulatory ability, and about 16% reported symptoms of urinary dysfunction. Before surgery, all MEDL patients demonstrated compressive central canal stenosis with or without lateral recess stenosis on MRI or CT myelogram. A historical comparative cohort of 32 patients with LSS of similar age and symptoms, and of the same gender, from the same institution treated via open laminectomies were used as a comparison.

Twenty-eight patients had a one-level procedure performed, with 20 patients having two levels done at one sitting. Overall, a total of 68 spinal segments were decompressed in the 48 patients. Typically, the choice of side for the surgical approach was that of the most clinically symptomatic side. The operative time for a single-level MEDL procedure averaged 55 minutes. The average blood loss per level decompressed was 25 ml for the MEDL group and 193 ml for the open group. No patients in the MEDL group required intraoperative or postoperative transfusions.

Our rate of dural violations and CSF leak is 4% compared to previous rates of up to 16%.[1] In our early experience with minimally invasive stenosis decompression, we decompressed the ipsilateral lateral recess before decompressing the contralateral side. We believe that this approach may in fact increase the risk of dural violations while drilling the contralateral side, since unprotected dura is exposed. With the technique described earlier and published previously,[25] the dura is entirely protected on both sides during contralateral drilling. There were no cases of neural injury

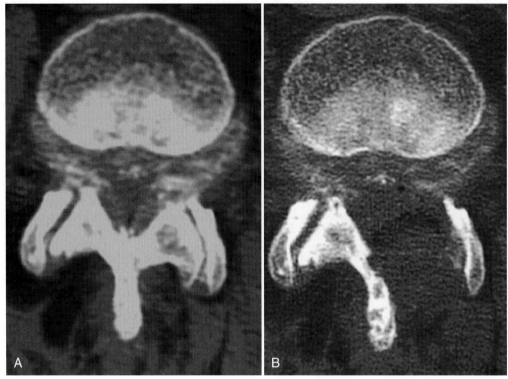

■ **FIGURE 59-9** Illustrative case of a 57-year-old man who presented with a 16-month history of neurogenic claudication type symptoms and some left-sided L5 radicular symptoms. **A,** CT myelogram shows marked L4-L5 stenosis from facet and flavum hypertrophy. **B,** Postoperative CT demonstrates the extent of decompression afforded by MEDL.

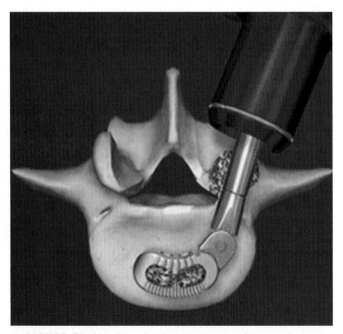

■ **FIGURE 59-10** Illustration depicting insertion of intervertebral spacer through a retractor tube.

associated with the MEDL cases, and to date there have been no cases of iatrogenic or delayed spinal instability requiring fusion.

The average length of stay for the MEDL and open surgery patients was 36 hours as compared to the significantly longer average stay of 94 hours for open surgery patients. The length of stay was often affected by postoperative problems arising from the often numerous comorbid medical conditions that these elderly patients often had. Of 48 patients with LSS initially enrolled, 4-year outcomes are available on 32 patients. All

patients reported an increase in walking endurance at 6 months that was maintained in 80% of patients at a mean of 38 months. Satisfaction of patients at 4 years was reported by 78% of the patients, with 88% reporting improvement in symptoms. Overall, the ODI scores were as follows: 46 preoperatively, 20 at 1 year, 21 at 2 years, 26 at 3 years. The SF-36 scores went from an average of 2.2 preoperatively, 3.1 at 1 year, 2.9 at 2 years, and 2.8 at 3 years.

## EMERGING TECHNOLOGIES

Although this chapter focuses primarily on direct decompressive techniques for LSS, posterior lumbar arthroplasty devices may provide symptomatic relief without direct decompression. The simplest posterior lumbar arthroplasty devices are those of interspinous distraction or blockade devices. These include the X-STOP (Saint Francis Medical, Alameda, Calif.), the Wallis System (Abbott Spine, Austin, Tex.), the Diam Device (Medtronics, Memphis, Tenn.) and the Coflex system (Paradigm Spine, New York, N.Y.) (Figure 59-11). These devices are placed between the bases of the spinous processes and provide mild distraction or blockade of the functional middle column at a given motion segment. As a result of this interposition, the volume and height of the spinal neural foramen and the lateral recess are maintained and/or slightly increased. Zucherman and colleagues[27] reported 191 patients were treated, 100 in the X-STOP group and 91 in the control group. At every follow-up visit, X-STOP patients had significantly better outcomes in each domain of the Zurich Claudication Questionnaire. At 2 years, the X-STOP patients improved by 45.4% over the mean baseline Symptom Severity score compared with 7.4% in the control group; the mean improvement in the Physical Function domain was 44.3% in the X-STOP group and −0.4% in the control group. In the X-STOP group, 73.1% patients were satisfied with their treatment compared with 35.9% of control patients.

Additionally, biomechanical cadaveric and finite modeling studies have demonstrated an increased overall stiffness of the motion segment, presumably from middle column augmentation, as well as decreases in the stresses and loading across the posterior aspect of the intervertebral disc and annu-

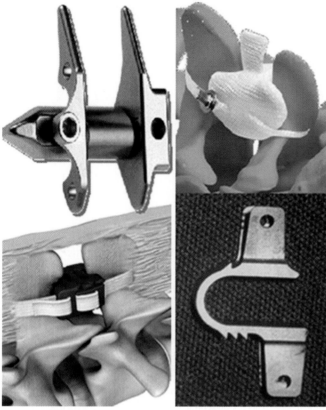

■ **FIGURE 59-11**    Interspinous devices. *Clockwise from top left*: X-Stop, Diam, Coflex, Wallis.

lus, as well as the facet joints themselves. Accordingly, several groups have reported benefits for use of interspinous devices in patients with degenerative mechanical pain without stenosis as well.[28]

## References

1. L. Khoo, R. Fessler, Microendoscopic decompressive laminotomy for the treatment of lumbar stenosis, Neurosurgery 5 (Suppl. 5) (2002) S146–S154.
2. P. Guigui, E. Barre, M. Benoist, A. Deburge, Radiologic and computed tomography image evaluation of bone regrowth after wide surgical decompression for lumbar stenosis, Spine 24 (1999) 281–289.
3. T.J. Kleeman, A.C. Hiscoe, E.E. Berg, Patient outcomes after minimally destabilizing lumbar stenosis decompression: the Port-Hole technique, Spine 25 (2000) 865–870.
4. A.C. Simotas, F.J. Dorey, K.K. Hansraj, F. Cammisa, Nonoperative treatment for lumbar spinal stenosis: clinical and outcome results and a 3-year survivorship analysis, Spine 25 (2000) 197–204.
5. A. Herno, T. Saari, O. Suomalainen, Airaksinen, The degree of decompressive relief and its relation to clinical outcome in patients undergoing surgery for lumbar spinal stenosis, Spine 24 (1999) 1010–1014.
6. S.J. Atlas, R.B. Keller, D. Robson, R.A. Deyo, D.E. Singer, Surgical and nonsurgical management of lumbar spinal stenosis: four-year outcomes from the Maine Lumbar Spine Study, Spine 25 (2000) 556–562.
7. H. Hurri, P. Slatis, K. Soini, et al., Lumbar spinal stenosis: assessment of long-term outcome 12 years after operative and conservative management, J. Spin. Dis. 11 (1998) 110–115.
8. J.N. Katz, G. Stucki, S.J. Lipson, et al., Predictors of surgical outcome in degenerative lumbar spinal stenosis, Spine 21 (1999) 2229–2233.
9. F. Postacchini, Spine update: surgical management of lumbar spinal stenosis, Spine 24 (1999) 1043–1047.
10. L.D. Herron, C. Mangelsdorf, Lumbar stenosis: results of surgical treatment, J. Spinal Disord. 4 (1991) 26–33.
11. P.L. Sanderson, P.L.R. Wood, Surgery for lumbar spinal stenosis in old people, J. Bone Joint Surg. Br. 75 (1993) 393–397.
12. R.Y.C. Tsai, R.S. Yang, R.S. Bray, Microscopic laminotomies for degenerative lumbar spinal stenosis, J. Spin. Dis. 11 (1998) 389–394.
13. G.F. Tuite, J.D. Stern, S.E. Doran, et al., Outcome after laminectomy for lumbar spinal stenosis, part I: clinical correlations, J. Neurosurg. 81 (1994) 699–706.
14. D.H. See, G.H. Kraft, Electromyography in paraspinal muscles following surgery for root compression, Arch. Phys. Med. Rehab. 56 (1975) 80–83.
15. T. Sihvonen, A. Herno, L. Paljarva, et al., Local denervation atrophy of paraspinal muscles in postoperative failed back syndrome, Spine 18 (1993) 575–581.
16. S. Atlas, B. Keller, Y. Wu, R. Deyo, D. Singer, Long-term outcomes of surgical and nonsurgical management of lumbar spinal stenosis: 8-10 year results from the Maine Lumbar Spine Study, Spine 30 (2005) 936–943.
17. A. Caputy, A. Luessenhop, Long-term evaluation of decompressive surgery for degenerative lumbar stenosis, J. Neurosurg. 77 (1992) 669–676.
18. J. Katz, S. Lipson, R. Lew, et al., Lumbar laminectomy alone or with instrumented or non-instrumented arthrodesis in degenerative lumbar spinal stenosis. Patient selection, costs, and surgical outcomes, Spine 22 (1997) 1123–1131.
19. D. Resnick, T. Choudhri, A. Dailey, et al., Guidelines for the performance of fusion procedures for degenerative disease of the lumbar spine. Part 9: fusion in patients with stenosis and spondylolisthesis, J. Neurosurg. Spine 2 (2005) 679–685.
20. J. Aryanpur, T. Ducker, Multilevel lumbar laminotomies: an alternative to laminectomy in the treatment of lumbar stenosis, Neurosurgery 26 (1990) 429–433.
21. J.A. McCulloch, Microsurgical spinal laminotomies, in: J.W. Frymoyer (Ed.), The adult spine: principles and practice, Raven Press, Ltd., New York, 1991.
22. S. Young, R. Veerapen, S.A. O'Laire, Relief of lumbar canal stenosis using multilevel subarticular fenestrations as an alternative to wide laminectomy: preliminary report, Neurosurgery 23 (5) (1988) 628–633.
23. J.A. Turner, M. Ersek, L. Herron, R. Deyo, Surgery for lumbar spinal stenosis, attempted meta-analysis of the literature, Spine 17 (1992) 1–8.
24. B.H. Guiot, L.T. Khoo, R.G. Fessler, A Minimally invasive technique for decompression of the lumbar spine, Spine 27 (4) (2002) 432–438.
25. S. Palmer, R. Turner, R. Palmer, Bilateral decompression of lumbar stenosis involving a unilateral approach with microscope and tubular retractor system, J. Neurosurg. Spine 97 (2002) 213–217.
26. R. McCaffert, L. Khoo, M. Perez-Cruet, Percutaneous pedicle screw fixation of the lumbar spine using the pathfinder system, in: M. Perez-Cruet, L. Khoo, R. Fessler (Eds.), An anatomic approach to minimally invasive spine surgery, QMP, St. Louis, 2006, pp. 599–614.
27. J.F. Zucherman, K.Y. Hsu, C.A. Hartjen, et al., A multicenter, prospective, randomized trial evaluating the X STOP interspinous process decompression system for the treatment of neurogenic intermittent claudication: two-year follow-up results, Spine 30 (12) (2005) 1351–1358.
28. J. Senegas, Mechanical supplementation by non-rigid fixation in degenerative intervertebral lumbar segments: the Wallis system, Eur. Spine J. 11 (2) (2002) S164–S169.

# 60

# Minimally Invasive Scoliosis Treatment

*Choll W. Kim, Kamshad Raiszadeh, and Steven R. Garfin*

**K E Y   P O I N T S**

- Minimally invasive spine (MIS) techniques for the treatment of scoliosis are relatively new.
- The direct lateral interbody fusion technique is a powerful method of deformity correction.
- Percutaneous pedicle screw fixation can be performed from T10 to the pelvis.
- Stenosis can be treated without laminectomy via indirect decompression.
- Endoscopic transforaminal decompression is a promising technique for treating radiculopathy due to neuroforaminal stenosis at the concavity of the scoliotic segment.

## INTRODUCTION

The degenerative cascade can occur in a variety of ways. When the disc degenerates and loses its height, shortening of the anterior spinal column occurs. In most cases, the collapse of the disc space occurs symmetrically, leading to loss of lumbar lordosis and accentuation of thoracic kyphosis. However, the disc may collapse asymmetrically, which in turn can lead to a lateral bending of the spine. When this occurs over multiple segments, a degenerative scoliosis may develop, causing imbalance in posture, often in both the coronal and the sagittal planes.[1]

The anatomic characteristics of degenerative scoliosis and idiopathic adolescent scoliosis differ significantly. Whereas scoliosis that develops in childhood is marked by significant rotation of the vertebral bodies, little rotation is appreciated in most adult degenerative scoliosis patterns. Furthermore, there is a propensity for the adult scoliosis curve to develop in the lumbar rather than the thoracic spine. This is likely due to the greater mobility of the lumbar spine, which undergoes a more clinically evident degeneration of the disc.

The treatment of scoliosis in the aging spine differs markedly from scoliosis treatment of the growing spine. The key differences are the lack of mobility of the adult spine, the presence of osteopenia and osteoporosis, the location of the curve, the curve magnitude, the need for decompression, and the frailty of older patients with their associated comorbidities. The goals of treatment differ as well. In adolescent idiopathic scoliosis, there is more concern with deformity and less with pain. In adult degenerative scoliosis symptoms are related more to pain (both back pain and nerve pain) than deformity.

As our population increases in age, the prevalence of symptomatic degenerative scoliosis will increase concomitantly. The incidence of complications is high for this type of surgery.[2] The risk of these complications increases with advanced age and other medical comorbidities. The goal of minimally invasive surgery is to decrease the soft tissue trauma associated with large midline posterior and thoracoabdominal approaches, which require take-down of the diaphragm. This chapter addresses the key indications for surgical treatment, minimally invasive strategies for scoliosis treatment, contraindications to minimally invasive surgery, and potential pitfalls of MIS treatment.

## BASIC SCIENCE OF MINIMALLY INVASIVE SPINE SURGERY

The posterior paraspinal muscles provide dynamic stability to the spinal column.[3] Numerous studies have investigated the anatomic, histologic, and radiographic properties of many of these muscles with the goal of understanding pathologic changes associated with spinal abnormalities such as chronic low back pain, disc herniation, scoliosis, and degenerative lumbar kyphosis. Paradoxically, some operations designed to treat these various spinal disorders actually disrupt these muscles and, in turn, may lead to substantial functional deficits, various pain syndromes, or both. Minimally invasive spine surgery techniques strive to minimize surgical trauma to these muscles, thereby preserving their function. Architectural studies show that the multifidus muscle stands out among all other lumbar muscles, and indeed many extremity muscles, as a most extreme example of a muscle designed to stabilize the lumbar spine against flexion. This functional design was elucidated by means of intraoperative laser diffraction and quantitative architecture measurements that demonstrated (1) an extremely large physiologic cross-sectional area, greater than that of any other lumbar spine muscle, and (2) a sarcomere length range exclusively on the ascending portion of the length–tension curve.[4] The large physiologic cross-sectional area and relatively short fibers indicate that the multifidus muscle is architecturally designed to produce large forces over a narrow range of lengths. This design allows the multifidus muscle to function more to stabilize the spine and less to provide motion of the spine. As a stabilizer, it acts to maintain optimal joint forces throughout the spine as the body assumes various positions requiring prolonged flexion (such as assembly-line work) or extension (such as standing).

## CLINICAL PRACTICE GUIDELINES

The main reason for surgical treatment of adults with scoliosis is pain. Pain can occur in several ways. First, the pain of neurogenic claudication develops with the degenerative cascade. This is exacerbated by spinal malalignment. Both lateral listhesis and anterolisthesis reduce the area of the canal. The resulting stenosis is more severe than the corresponding degree of degeneration in a well-aligned spine. If there is severe asymmetric disc collapse, the neuroforamina will close down on the side of the concavity, which in turn can cause radiculopathy.

Pain also occurs because of the degenerative arthritis that develops within the disc and facet joints. Bone-on-bone movement between motion segments can cause pain in a manner analogous to degenerative joint disease in the knee and hip. Furthermore, a malalignment will create focal areas of increased stress. Finally, postural imbalance can lead to fatigue-related muscle pain. Much as in flat back syndrome, early muscle fatigue and pain can develop as the patient tries to compensate for coronal and/or sagittal imbalance. In contrast to adolescent scoliosis, the concern for curve progression is relatively low. The pain associated with stenosis, radiculopathy, and early muscle fatigue drives surgical decision-making. It is rare to perform surgical correction of deformity in the absence of pain in adults with degenerative scoliosis.

## Endoscopic Transforaminal Decompression for Unilateral Radiculopathy

Occasionally, a patient with degenerative scoliosis will complain mainly of leg pain, with only minor back pain. In most cases, the pain is due to neuroforaminal stenosis. Traditionally, this has been treated with hemilaminectomy and foraminotomy. However, there is risk of worsening deformity due to loss of stability when excessive bony resection is necessary and when the activity of the multifidus muscle is disrupted. An extraforaminal approach has been used with good success via a Wiltse-type paramedian approach. A minimally invasive modification of this technique utilizes tubular retractors that dilate the soft tissue and minimize retraction pressures. Although this is still performed with the patient under general anesthesia, the accessibility of the neuroforamen is sufficient. However, it

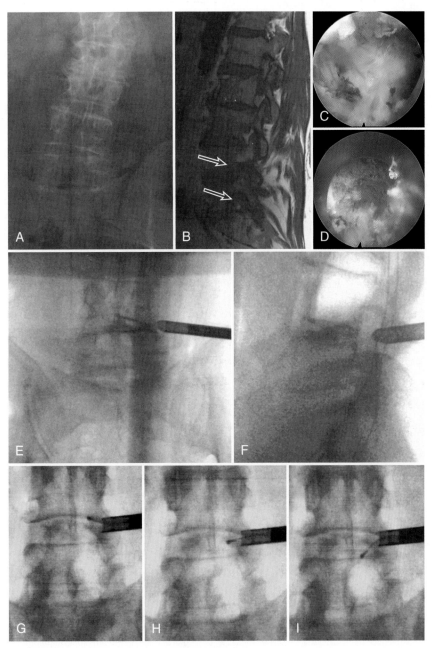

■ **FIGURE 60-1** Endoscopic Transforaminal Decompression. A 7-mm endoscopic cannula is placed at the extraforaminal opening of the affected level. A combination of bipolar probes (Ellman International, Inc., Oceanside, N.Y.), holmium side-firing lasers (Trimedyne, Inc., Irvine, Calif.), and mechanical trephines (Joimax, Inc., Campbell, Calif.) are used to release the neuroforaminal ligament, superior edge of the facet joint capsule, and lateral edge of the ligamentum flavum as it becomes confluent with the facet joint capsule. Mechanical trephines are used under fluoroscopic guidance to remove the superior edge of the superior articular process. A combination of ligamentous release with a small amount of bony resection decompresses the exiting nerve root. The angled bipolar probe is passed into the spinal canal to manually confirm adequate decompression. **A,** AP radiograph showing asymmetric disc collapse with narrowing of the left L4 and L5 neuroforamina. **B,** Left parasagittal T1-weighted MR image showing narrowing of the left L4 and L5 neuroforamina. *(open arrows)* **C,** Endoscopic view of the facet joint capsule. **D,** Endoscopic view of the semicircular removal of superior articular process using trephines. The rough cancellous bone can be seen as a superior dome in the field of view. **E,** Intraoperative AP C-arm image showing the endoscopic cannula docked at the extraforaminal opening of the left L4 neuroforamen. **F,** Intraoperative lateral C-arm image showing the endoscopic cannula docked at the extraforaminal opening of the left L4 neuroforamen. Intraoperative AP image showing the endoscopic angled probe passing through the superior (**G**), middle (**H**), and inferior (**I**) aspects of the neuroforamen. The ability to pass the probe through the neuroforamen without resistance confirms an adequate decompression.

is technically challenging to use the operating microscope because of the angle of the approach.

The endoscopic technique provides another avenue of treatment and it can be performed using local anesthesia.[5] This is advantageous for patients with significant medical comorbidities that make general anesthesia risky. Furthermore, the endoscopic technique allows a more lateral trajectory to the spine, facilitating deeper entry into the neuroforamen (Figure 60-1).

## Deformity Correction via Direct Lateral Anterior Interbody Fusion

A powerful method of deformity correction is the direct lateral interbody fusion (DLIF) technique (Figures 60-2 through 60-5). This technique was best described by Ozgur and colleagues[6] using the XLIF system (Nuvasive, San Diego, Calif.). The key feature of the technique is the ability to rest the interbody spacer along the strongest portion of the vertebra endplate, namely, the cortical rim or apophyseal ring. The

annulus inserts at this location and the cortex of the vertebral body acts as a vertical support. Because the interbody spacer is placed from the lateral position, the implant may overhang past the edge of the disc space, ensuring that the implant fully rests on the strongest portion of the endplate. If placed from an anterior or anterolateral position, the interbody spacer would enter the canal or the neuroforamen. In addition, the DLIF technique preserves the anterior longitudinal ligament. It is presumed that by keeping the integrity of this structure, the spine maintains a pivot point from which to correct an asymmetrically collapsed disc.

A comparison of interbody fusion techniques shows that the direct lateral interbody technique allows for greater deformity correction than anterior lumbar interbody fusion (ALIF), transforaminal lumbar interbody fusion (TLIF) or posterolateral fusion without interbody fusion. A radiographic comparison of various treatment groups showed that the focal Cobb angle for DLIF was two to four times that for the other treatment methods (Figure 60-6). The main drawback of this technique is approach-related nerve root irritation, which occurs in 3.4% of patients.[7]

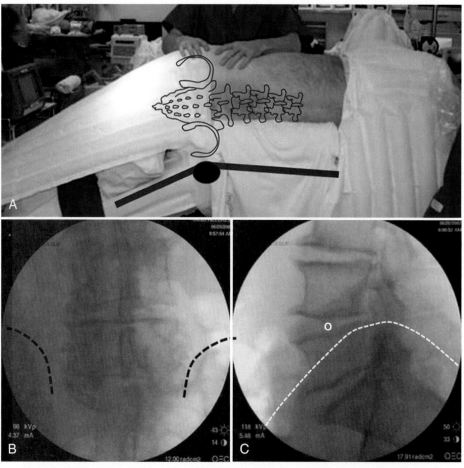

■ **FIGURE 60-2**    Lateral Positioning for Direct Lateral Interbody Fusion (DLIF). An important step in the safe application of the DLIF procedure is proper patient positioning. The patient is placed on a breaking radiolucent table. A soft support is placed at the lateral hip at the level of the iliac crest (**A**). The break in the table is placed at the same area (*black oval*). The patient is secured to the table using sticky rolls or a moldable beanbag device. Soft tape is placed at the hips (over the greater trochanters) and just below the shoulders. The hips and knees are flexed in a comfortable position at about 45 degrees. Transverse pillows are placed between the legs. A strap is then gently placed above the ankles to maintain this position. The patient must be adequately secured to the table so that the table itself can be rotated ("airplaned"), ensuring that the surgical target site is perfectly lateral relative to the floor. This is best accomplished by using the C-arm under the table flat to the floor. The table is then rolled until a perfect AP image is obtained (**B**). In most cases of degenerative scoliosis, there is some mild rotation such that the caudal vertebral body and the cephalic vertebral body cannot be in a perfect AP position simultaneously. In this instance, the caudal vertebral body is usually used as the reference level. This process is required at each level to adjust for rotational deformities between levels. The lateral image is used to target the midportion of the disc space (**C**). At L4-5, the nerve root can be at this position. In such cases, the initial dilator is targeted more anteriorly and thereafter pulled posteriorly to the disc midpoint. This allows the dilator to enter the psoas muscle anterior to the nerve root and by sweeping posteriorly creates a cuff of muscle that separates the dilator from the nerve root. The iliac crest can impede access to the L4-5 disc space (*dotted lines*). It is important to ascertain before surgery that iliac crest can be pulled out of the way by lateral bending of the patient on the operating table, as described in **A**.

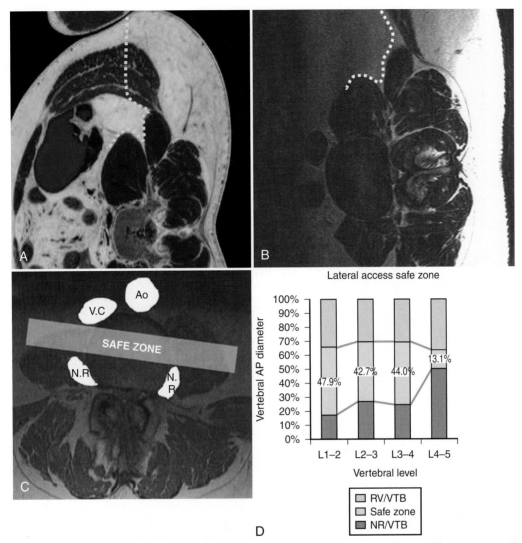

**■ FIGURE 60-3**   Direct Lateral Retroperitoneal Transpsoas Approach. The skin incision is made with the aid of the C-arm in the direct lateral position. Gentle blunt dissection is accomplished with angled Mayo scissors. The muscles of the lateral abdominal wall are entered between muscle fibers (**A**). Numerous sensory nerves are encountered, which can be swept out of the surgical corridor. The retroperitoneal space is entered by cautious, gentle spreading of the tranversus abdominis fascia, which can be thick in younger patients. Finger dissection is then used to open the potential space of the retroperitoneum. Upon entering the retroperitoneal space, the finger is immediately directed posteriorly to the inner abdominal wall as shown by the *dotted lines* (**B**). A back-and-forth motion is used to release thin reticular attachments of the retroperitoneal fat to the abdominal wall. The tip of the traverse process is used as the initial landmark. At L4-L5, the iliolumbar ligament is palpated as well as the anterior aspect of the iliacus muscle. Blunt finger dissection is further taken anteriorly over the psoas muscle, which is very soft and delicate to the touch. Care should be taken to avoid undue maceration of the fragile muscle fibers. The initial dilator is then passed down along the finger and docked gently on the surface of the psoas muscle. The initial dilator is kept in contact with the finger to facilitate safe passage of the tip through the retroperitoneal space and ensure that it does not capture any abdominal structures such as bowel or ureter. Using the C-arm, the tip of the initial dilator is positioned at the disc center and the psoas muscle entered gently using a back-and-forth twisting motion. Because the psoas muscle is soft it will not cause resistance. Neurophysiologic monitoring via free-run and triggered EMG is used to confirm that the nerve root is not in the path of the initial dilator. The safe zone for the transpsoas approach is anterior to the nerve root and posterior to the vena cava (**C**). The limits of this safe zone suddenly narrow at L4-L5 compared to the more cephalic levels (**D**).

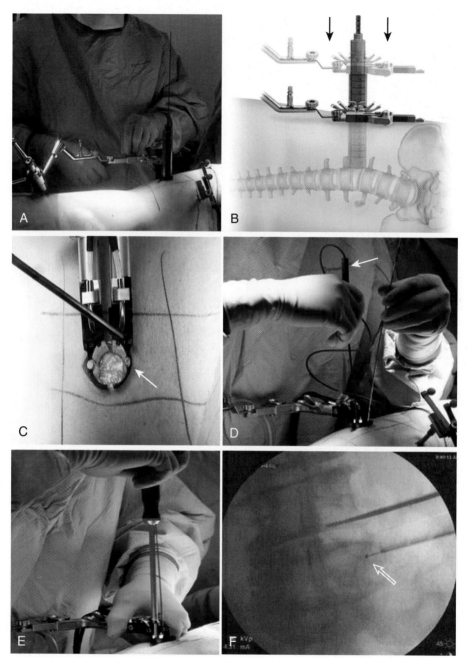

■ **FIGURE 60-4** Disc Exposure. Once the initial dilator is safely passed through the psoas muscle and positioned on the disc space, a guidewire is inserted into the disc to hold the dilators in place. Serial dilation is then performed with larger tubular rings. At each step, neurophysiologic monitoring is used to avoid the nerve root. After the final dilator, an expandable tubular retractor (**A** and **B**) is slid down using a back-and-forth motion (Medtronic Spine, Memphis, Tenn.). Thin fibers of the psoas are often found over the disc space (**C**). These fibers should be only 1 to 2 mm thick and can be swept aside with the suction tip or a Penfield 4 probe. The blades of the retractor contain slots for bone fixation screws (*white arrow,* **C**) that can be used to pass the neuromonitoring probe (NIM, Medtronic, Memphis, Tenn.) down to the bone surface (*white arrow,* **D**). The bone fixation screw is inserted through the slots in the retractor (**E**). It is best to position the bone screw immediately adjacent to the disc space (**F**). Before insertion of the bone screw, the ball-tip neuromonitoring probe (*open arrow,* **F**) is used to ensure that the bony surface is free of neural structures.

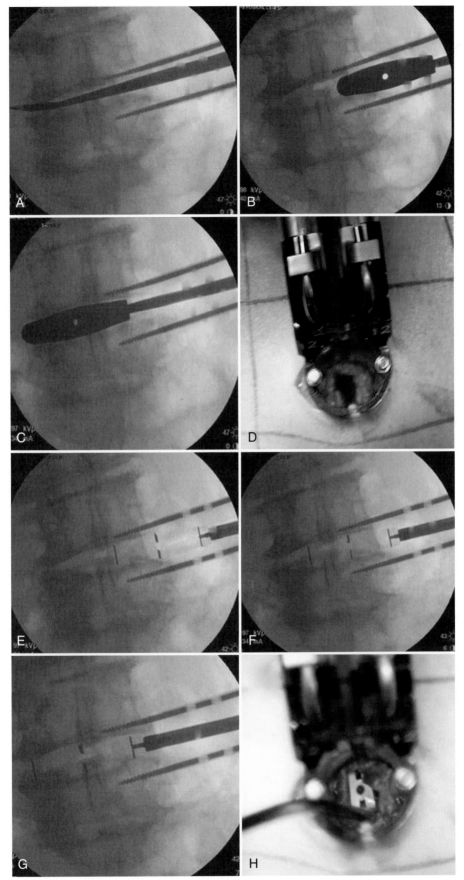

■ **FIGURE 60-5** Direct Lateral Discectomy. A key component of the DLIF discectomy is release of the contralateral annulus. This can be accomplished with a Cobb-type periosteal elevator (**A**). Using a mallet, the elevator is gently tapped until it penetrates the annulus. A palpable release can be appreciated. Although the tip of the elevator may protrude up to 1 cm past the lateral vertebral body line, no known clinical sequelae have been observed. Once a subtotal discectomy, endplate preparation, and contralateral annular release have been accomplished, smooth trials are used to dilate the disc space (**B** to **D**). The interbody device of the appropriate size is then tamped into place. Using a wide interbody spacer that rests on the lateral cortical rim of the vertebral body, a dramatic reduction and disc height restoration can be seen (**E** to **G**). The specialized retractor provides an optimal view of the surgical corridor before (**D**) and after insertion (**H**) of the interbody spacer.

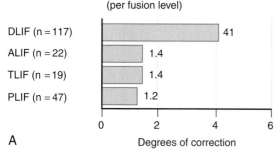

A

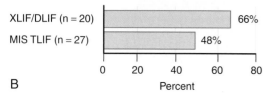

B

■ **FIGURE 60-6**  Deformity Correction using the DLIF Technique. A retrospective radiographic review comparing various fusion techniques shows the superiority of the DLIF technique for reduction of focal Cobb angle in patients with degenerative scoliosis (**A**) and reduction of spondylolisthesis (**B**).

## Minimally Invasive Posterior-Only Approaches

The most common minimally invasive posterior approach is the minimally invasive transforaminal lumbar interbody fusion (MIS TLIF). Utilizing a paramedian approach, a unilateral facetectomy may be performed on the side requiring maximum correction.[8] Interbody fusion allows for a high fusion rate and provides additional soft tissue release needed for deformity correction. The MIS TLIF strategy is particularly attractive if there is a large disc herniation, facet cyst, and/or severe stenosis requiring a direct decompression.

A key limitation is the difficulty in placing a sufficiently large interbody spacer to restore disc space height. Additionally, each level requires a separate and distinct dissection. In cases in which there are more than three levels to be corrected, this technique can be time-consuming and laborious.

## Percutaneous Pedicle Screw Fixation

Multilevel fixation with pedicle screws and rods remains one of the most significant challenges in the minimally invasive treatment of degenerative scoliosis. In contrast to open techniques, the percutaneous rods cannot be reduced into the tulip of the pedicle screws, nor can a rotation maneuver

be performed. The method of bringing the rod to the screw relies on screw extension sleeves that serve to guide the rods through each tulip and thereafter reduces the rod into the seat of the tulip so that a fixation nut can be applied (Figure 60-7). The greatest challenge occurs at the lumbosacral junction, where there is a sudden curvature due to the lordotic angle between L4 and S1 (See Figure 60-7H). Extreme care must be exercised to align the height of the tulips. With osteoporotic bone, misalignment can lead to screw pullout during the reduction maneuver. The use of bone cement injected into the pedicles immediately before screw insertion greatly improves fixation strength.[9]

## MIS Iliac Fixation

The use of iliac screws improves fusion rates at L5-S1 when the construct is long. An important technique in posterior deformity correction is insertion of iliac screws in a minimally invasive fashion.[10] By placing the insertion point of the iliac screws on the medial wall of the posterior superior iliac spine (PSIS) about 2 cm distal to the S1 screw, the tulips of the screws can be aligned so that a rod can be passed through both the S1 screw tulip and the iliac screw tulip (Figure 60-8). Meticulous attention to rod contouring is required to ensure that the construct is not under undue stress.

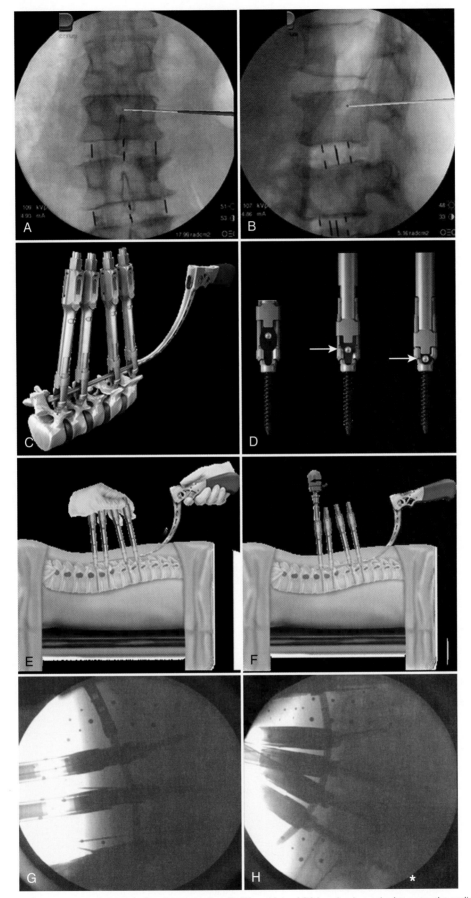

■ **FIGURE 60-7** MIS Pedicle Screw Fixation. Meticulous intraoperative AP (**A**) and lateral (**B**) imaging is required to enter the pedicle using percutaneous or mini-open techniques. A sleeve to guide rod insertion is required to facilitate passage of the rod over multiple levels (**C**, **E**). The design of the sleeve should provide a relatively large opening to simplify rod insertion and reduction of the rod down to the tulip of the pedicle screw (**D**, **F**). The depth of screw insertion should be monitored carefully using lateral C-arm imaging to avoid step-offs, which make rod reduction difficult (**G**). Careful rod contouring is also necessary, particularly if crossing the lumbosacral junction, where there is a sudden increase in lordosis (**H**). Pelvic fixation can be accomplished through a small surgical corridor that is immediately adjacent to the L5-S1 exposure (MIS pelvic screw marked by * in **H**).

## Case Studies

Minimally invasive scoliosis surgery relies on three main technologies: (1) DLIF/XLIF, (2) posterior MIS TLIF, and (3) percutaneous pedicle screw instrumentation. Using a combination of these techniques, deformities of the thoracolumbar spine spanning T10 to the pelvis can be treated. The most common and most straightforward problem is a degenerative scoliosis from L2 to L5 with back pain and neurogenic claudication (Figure 60-8). Using a lateral interbody approach, much of the stenosis can be addressed by correcting the Cobb angle and reestablishing the disc space height. In doing so, an indirect decompression can be achieved in some cases without the need for a posterior laminectomy.

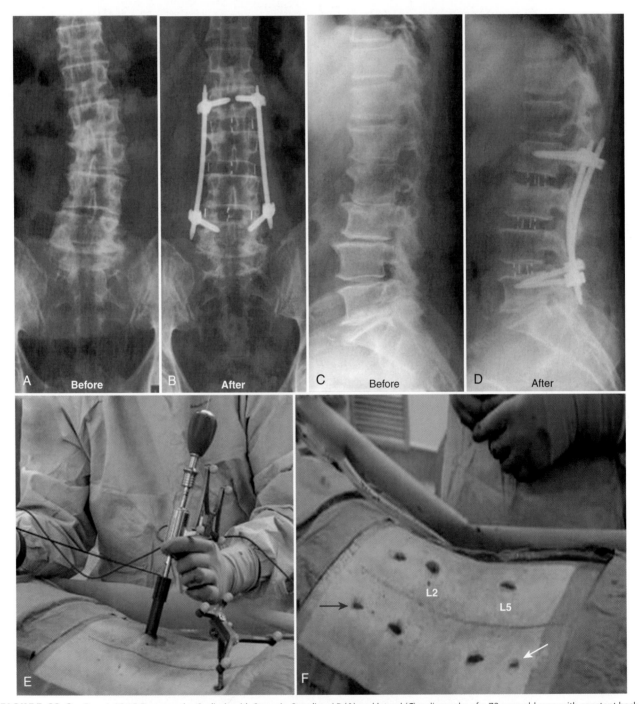

■ **FIGURE 60-8** Case 1: L2-L5 Degenerative Scoliosis with Stenosis. Standing AP (**A**) and lateral (**C**) radiographs of a 72-year-old man with constant back pain and neurogenic claudication. Patient avoided surgical treatment because of fear of intraoperative risks of traditional open surgery. Current medical problems include hypertension and mild chronic obstructive pulmonary disease. Patient underwent angioplasty 2 years ago. Surgical treatment was performed in 1 day via stage 1 direct lateral anterior interbody fusion at L2-L3, L3-L4 and L4-L5. Estimated blood loss was 50 ml, and surgical time was 127 min. The patient was repositioned and nonsegmental posterior instrumentation was performed through 18-mm percutaneous incisions. The rod was inserted through proximal stab incisions (**F,** *blue arrow*). The navigation patient reference frame was placed percutaneously on the left posterior superior iliac spine (**F,** *white arrow*). Decompression was achieved indirectly via deformity correction and disc space height restoration. No laminectomy was performed. Patient was ambulating on postoperative day 1 with resolution of leg pain. He was discharged on postoperative day 3. At 1-year postsurgery, his visual analog scale is 2-3 and his walking tolerance is 2 miles.

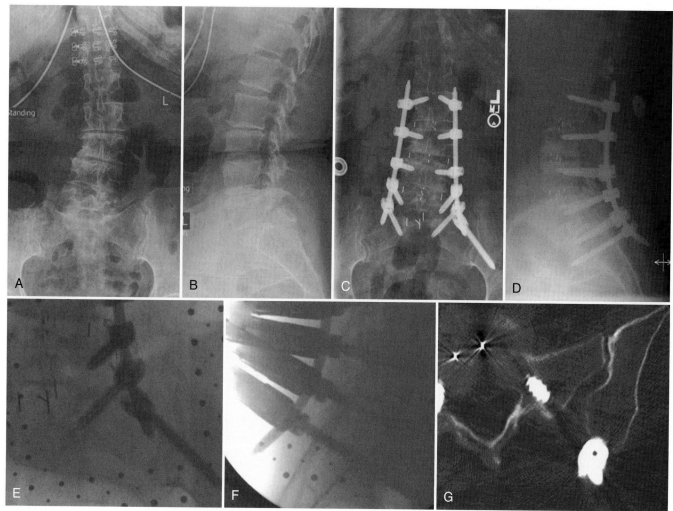

■ **FIGURE 60-9**    Case 2: L2-S1 Degenerative Scoliosis. Standing AP (**A**) and lateral (**B**) radiographs of 69-year-old woman with back pain, left posterolateral leg pain, right anterior thigh pain, and neurogenic claudication with walking and prolonged standing. Her walking tolerance was less than 100 feet, limited by worsening bilateral leg pain, left worse than right. A two-stage procedure was performed. On day 1, DLIF was performed at L2-L3, L3-L4, and L4-L5. She tolerated the procedure well with 75 ml, of estimated blood loss. Surgical time was 142 minutes. Two days later, she underwent the stage 2 procedure: left L5-S1 MIS TLIF, mini-open left iliac screw, and percutaneous pedicle screws bilaterally at L2, L3, L4, L5, and S1 (**C, D**). The rod was passed percutaneously using reduction sleeves (**E, F**). Decompression was achieved indirectly via deformity reduction and realignment. No laminectomies, except those at L5-S1 during the MIS TLIF, were performed. The iliac screw is inserted on the medial aspect of the posterior superior iliac spine about 2 cm distal to the S1 pedicle screw, such that the base of the screw tulips is aligned to accept a single rod (**E** to **G**). Estimated blood loss was 275 ml and total surgery time was 387 minutes. She was ambulatory on postoperative day 1 after stage 2 and discharged to home on postoperative day 4. She has good resolution of her leg pain and mild to moderate back pain (VAS 4-5).

In cases in which there is an oblique takeoff of L5 from the sacrum, L5-S1 fusion can be achieved using an MIS TLIF (see Figure 60-9). A novel and promising strategy for L5-S1 fusion is the use of a transsacral fixation device (Figure 60-10). Added construct stability can be achieved with additional pelvic fixation using the L5-S1 surgical corridor to expose the medial wall of the posterior-superior iliac spine (PSIS) as the entry point for the pelvic screw. This allows the tulip of the pelvic screw to align with the S1 screw so that a single rod can be used (see Figures 60-9 and 60-10).

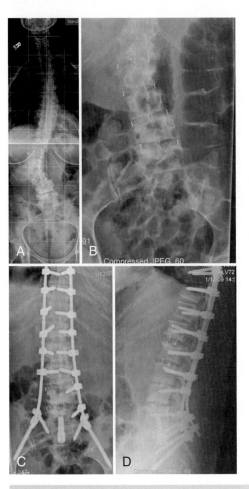

■ **FIGURE 60-10**  Case 3: T10-Pelvis Reconstruction. Standing AP (**A**) scoliosis films of a 47-year-old woman with seronegative spondyloarthropathy complaining of worsening back pain and right flank pain due to impingement of the 12th rib on the iliac crest. Radiographs from 18 months previously revealed only minimal deformity. Stage 1 DLIF was performed with marked improvement in coronal alignment (**B**). Two days later, she underwent posterior reconstruction: L5-S1 transsacral fusion, mini-open bilateral iliac screws, mini-open bilateral T10-L1 pedicle screws, and percutaneous pedicle screws bilaterally at L2-L3 with unilateral screws at L4-L5 (**C, D**). Mini-open exposures for the pedicle screws were used to expose the facet joints and posterior elements of T10-L1, which were decorticated and bone grafted. Long contoured rods were passed through proximal stab incisions and advanced through each of the rod reduction sleeves. The stage 2 procedure was tedious and difficult. Total surgical time was 9 hours, 17 minutes and estimated blood loss was 575 ml. Postoperatively, she was ambulatory on day 2 and discharged home on day 7.

## CONCLUSIONS AND DISCUSSION

The primary indication for surgical treatment is pain. The pain associated with adult degenerative scoliosis is caused by a combination of early muscle fatigue due to coronal and sagittal imbalance, spinal stenosis, radiculopathy, and facet arthropathy. Because most patients with symptomatic degenerative scoliosis are elderly, efforts to minimize the morbidity of surgical intervention is warranted. Minimally invasive techniques strive to decrease blood loss and associated fluid shifts, systemic stress responses, the need for powerful postoperative narcotic pain medications that can be poorly tolerated in the elderly patient, and disruption of muscle–tendon complexes that may provide dynamic stability needed for early ambulation and rehabilitation.

The use of minimally invasive techniques relies heavily on interbody fusion. This is the most permissive fusion environment and requires no disruption of muscle tendon complexes. This is in contrast to posterolateral fusions, which require detachment of the paraspinal muscle tendon attachment sites from the lateral aspect of the superior articular process and transverse processes. The use of interbody fusion techniques facilitates improved deformity correction by allowing an anterior release and correction of asymmetric disc height loss.

The application of MIS techniques for the treatment of scoliosis remains in evolution. The techniques remain challenging. The learning curve is exceedingly long, and only limited instrumentation is currently available. Reliance on intraoperative imaging leads to high radiation exposures for the surgical team. Future efforts must focus on improved instrumentation for rapid and accurate multilevel pedicle screw insertion. This technology must be combined with a corresponding rod insertion system that accommodates various degrees of spinal curvature as well as the sudden lordosis that occurs at the lumbosacral junction. A key aspect of this issue is the need to place the screws in line with each other such that they do not pull out during rod reduction.

## References

1. A. Ploumis, E.E. Transfledt, F. Denis, Degenerative lumbar scoliosis associated with spinal stenosis, Spine J. 7 (2007) 428–436.
2. K.J. Cho, S.I. Suk, S.R. Park, J.H. Kim, S.S. Kim, W.K. Choi, K.Y. Lee, S.R. Lee, Complications in posterior fusion and instrumentation for degenerative lumbar scoliosis, Spine (Phila Pa 1976) 32 (2007) 2232–2237.
3. N. Bogduk, J.E. Macintosh, M.J. Pearcy, A universal model of the lumbar back muscles in the upright position, Spine (Phila Pa 1976) 17 (1992) 897–913.
4. S.R. Ward, C.W. Kim, C.M. Eng, L.J. Gottschalk, A. Tomiya, S.R. Garfin, R.L. Lieber, Architectural analysis and intraoperative measurements demonstrate the unique design of the multifidus muscle for lumbar spine stability, J. Bone Joint Surg. Am. 91 (2009) 176–185.
5. A.T. Yeung, C.A. Yeung, In-vivo endoscopic visualization of patho-anatomy in painful degenerative conditions of the lumbar spine, Surg. Technol. Int. 15 (2006) 243–256.
6. B.M. Ozgur, H.E. Aryan, L. Pimenta, W.R. Taylor, Extreme lateral interbody fusion (XLIF): a novel surgical technique for anterior lumbar interbody fusion, Spine J. 6 (2006) 435–443.
7. R.Q. Knight, P. Schwaegler, D. Hanscom, J. Roh, Direct lateral lumbar interbody fusion for degenerative conditions: early complication profile, J. Spinal Disord. Tech. 22 (2009) 34–37.
8. J.D. Schwender, L.T. Holly, D.P. Rouben, K.T. Foley, Minimally invasive transforaminal lumbar interbody fusion (TLIF): technical feasibility and initial results, J. Spinal Disord. Tech. 18 (Suppl.) (2005) S1–S6.
9. D.J. Burval, R.F. McLain, R. Milks, S. Inceoglu, Primary pedicle screw augmentation in osteoporotic lumbar vertebrae: biomechanical analysis of pedicle fixation strength, Spine (Phila Pa 1976) 32 (2007) 1077–1083.
10. M.Y. Wang, S.C. Ludwig, D.G. Anderson, P.V. Mummaneni, Percutaneous iliac screw placement: description of a new minimally invasive technique, Neurosurg. Focus 25 (2008) E17.

# 61

# Lateral XLIF Fusion Techniques

*Luiz Pimenta, Etevaldo Coutinho, Jose Carlos Sauri Barraza, and Leonardo Oliveira*

**K E Y   P O I N T S**

- Appropriate patient positioning
- Retroperitoneal access
- Transpsoas access
- Disc space preparation
- Implant insertion

## INTRODUCTION

Demands of mobility and quality of life have increased in the elderly segment of society over the past decades. A rising number of elderly patients suffering from adult degenerative scoliosis may be eligible for surgical treatment.[1] The prevalence of adult scoliosis rises with age: from 4% before age 45 years, to 6% at age 59 years, to 15% in patients older than 60 years.[2]

Adult scoliosis is defined as acquired deformity in the skeletally mature patient with a Cobb angle of at least 10 degrees in the coronal plane due to asymmetric disc and facet joint degeneration. It is associated not only with severe back and/or leg pain but also with complicated surgical outcomes.[9]

All nonoperative treatments should be exhausted before considering surgical treatment. Usually, the surgical procedure is focused on two aims. The first aim is to decompress the comprised neural elements in cases of symptomatic spinal stenosis, and the second is to balance and stabilize the spine in the coronal and sagittal planes when there is imbalance.[4] Today a wide variety of approaches—anterior, posterior, or a combination—are available to achieve fusion, but all include significant operative morbidity.[5] Newer implants have improved cosmesis and correction, obtaining better results; however, the elderly patient is not a candidate for this kind of surgery because of the higher risk of complications and generally poorer bone quality in this population.[6]

The eXtreme Lateral Interbody Fusion (XLIF) approach may offer various clinical advantages over more traditional techniques for treating adult degenerative scoliosis.[7] This less invasive procedure realigns the endplates to a horizontal position through bilateral annular release, placement of a large implant across the disc space spanning the ring apophysis, and the effects of ligamentotaxis. The XLIF technique restores disc and foraminal heights, indirectly decompressing the neural elements, and promotes stabilization through an anterior intervertebral fusion stopping progression of the curve.

## INDICATIONS AND CONTRAINDICATIONS

The indications for the XLIF approach in the treatment of adult scoliosis do not differ from those for traditional techniques, except that the L5-S1 level cannot be accessed laterally.

## CLINICAL STUDY

In a larger patient series, 23 patients have 3-year follow-up (FU). Mean age is 66 years (range, 39 to 88). Three to seven levels were treated between T10 to L5. Three of these needed lateral plate fixation (Figure 61-1).

The procedures were performed without major complication in an average of 121 minutes and with <50 ml blood loss. Mean hospital stay was 40 hours. After 3-year FU, one patient (4%) presented with pseudarthrosis according to Food and Drug Administration (FDA) fusion criteria.[7] Three patients (12%) had subsidence at 6-month FU, but all were asymptomatic. Visual Analogue Scale (VAS) pain scores improved from an average of 8.1 preoperatively to 3.3 at 3-year FU. Oswestry scores improved from an average 47.8 preoperatively to 22.8 at 3-year FU. Coronal and sagittal alignments improved from average Cobb angles of 16 degrees preoperatively to 7.4 degrees at 3-year FU, and average lordosis angles of 37.8 degrees preoperatively to 48 degrees at 3-year FU. The mean preoperative Cobb angle was not high because in our earliest series we were not treating large curves. Currently, using the XLIF approach we can treat curves up to 90 degrees, with very good clinical results (Figure 61-2).

## PREOPERATIVE ASSESSMENT AND PLANNING

### Operative Technique

#### Patient Positioning

For the XLIF approach, the patient is placed and taped in a true 90-degree lateral decubitus position (Figure 62-3A), being preferable to approach from the concavity side. The table and/or patient should be laterally flexed to increase the distance between the iliac crest and the rib cage.

#### Incision and Retroperitoneal Access

The midposition of the disc of interest is identified using a Kirschner wire (K-wire) and fluoroscopy (Figure 61-3B). A small incision is created for insertion of the atraumatic tissue dilators and an expandable retractor (MaXcess, NuVasive, Inc., San Diego, Calif.), which will be the working portal. An incision posterior to this lateral marking is first made to introduce a finger into the retroperitoneal space to sweep open the space and ensure that all lateral attachments of the peritoneum are released to provide safe lateral entry (Figure 61-3C).

#### Transpsoas Access

With the retroperitoneal space identified, the finger is brought up under the lateral skin marking and an incision is made at this direct lateral location for the introduction of an initial dilator (Figure 61-3D). The finger in the retroperitoneal space is used to escort the dilator safely from the direct lateral incision to the psoas muscle. The dilator is then placed over the surface

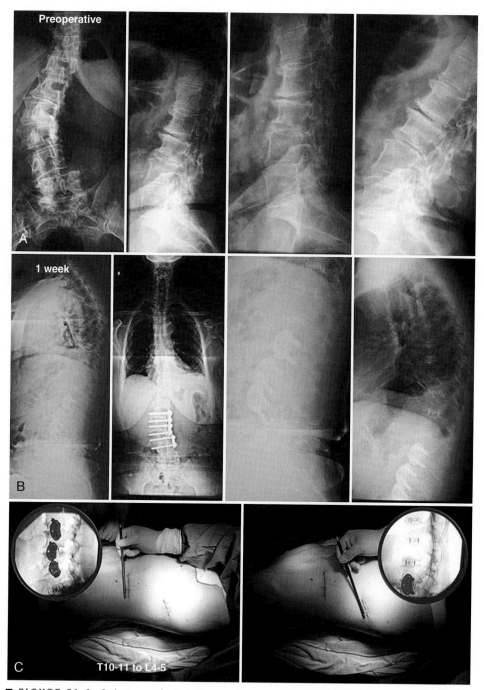

■ **FIGURE 61-1**    Patient example. **A,** A 62-year-old woman with degenerative scoliosis, back and right leg pain, neurogenic claudication, and unable to walk more than 100 m. **B,** One week after surgery, we can see improvement of the coronal balance using XLIF. **C,** Seven level surgery achieved with two small incisions.

of the psoas muscle, exactly over the disc space to be treated, confirmed by fluoroscopy. The fibers of the psoas muscle are then gently separated with the dilators until the disc is reached (Figure 61-3E). The Neuro-Vision electromyographic (EMG) monitoring system (NuVasive, Inc.) assesses the proximity of the lumbar nerve roots to the advancing dilator (Figure 61-3G). An expandable retractor (MaXcess) is advanced over the last dilator (Figure 61-3F and H).

Under direct illuminated vision, a thorough diskectomy is performed using standard instruments (Figure 61-3I). The posterior and anterior annulus are left intact. The annulotomy window is centered in the anterior lateral half of the disc space. Disc removal and release of the contralateral

annulus using a Cobb elevator (Figure 61-3J) provides the opportunity to place a long implant (Figure 61-3K) that will rest on both lateral margins of the apophyseal ring, maximizing endplate support, restoring height, and correcting imbalance alignment. Hemostasis is confirmed and no drains are required (Figure 61-3L).

## POSTOPERATIVE CARE

Patients should be encouraged to walk the same day to aid their recovery and muscle function. Postoperative pain tends to be minimal, and may be discharged after only an overnight hospital stay.

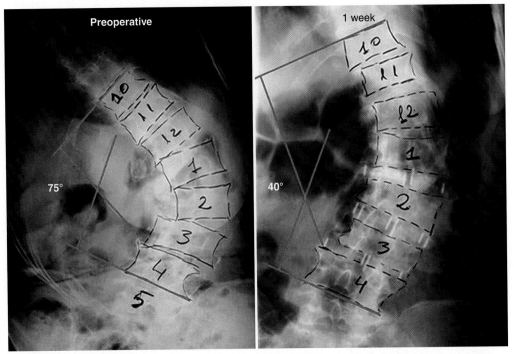

■ **FIGURE 61-2**  Patient example: An 83-year-old woman with degenerative scoliosis, pain in back and both legs, neurogenic claudication, unable to walk, huge pain even in bed. One week after surgery the subject was walking. The anteroposterior x-ray shows improvement in the correction of coronal alignment.

## COMPLICATIONS AND AVOIDANCE

In some series of adult deformity surgery, the complication rate is high, with elevated morbidity and mortality in some cases.[8] In comparison, our results demonstrate a lower level of complications due to the minimally invasive nature of the procedure. We observed minor complications in the immediate postoperative period, such as tenderness with hip flexion on the operative side and less commonly, sensory disturbance in the operative side leg. Painful dysesthesias and motor disturbance are rare, but possible. In these cases, a CT scan is recommended to rule out a psoas hematoma. If a hematoma is found, draining it improves symptoms.

In the long-term FU, subsidence was observed in some cases, already described in the results (Figure 61-4).

## CONCLUSION

The treatment for adult scoliosis differs from that for adolescent idiopathic scoliosis.[9] The most important issues are reduction of back and leg pain, and stop curve progression through fusion.[10] The complication rate has been lower than traditional surgical methods of treatment. Subsidence is the most common complication in the XLIF stand-alone technique but our experience has shown no clinical compromise in the final result. We have been successfully performing fusion using stand-alone cages through a lateral minimal invasive approach, decreasing pain, decompressing indirectly neurological structures, restoring disc height and stopping the curve progression.

This paper shows that with this less invasive procedure, good final results are obtained with low morbidity.

## References

1. F. Schwab, A. Dubey, L. Gamez, et al., Adult scoliosis: prevalence, SF-36, and nutritional parameters in an elderly volunteer population, Spine 30 (2005) 1082–1085.
2. Y. Floman, Degenerative scoliosis: indications for surgery and results, Journal of Bone and Joint Surgery-British Volume, 88-B (Suppl.) 4–5.
3. M. Aebi, The adult scoliosis, Eur. Spine J. 14 (2005) 925–948.
4. A. Ploumis, E.E. Transfledt, F. Denis, Degenerative lumbar scoliosis associated with spinal stenosis, Spine J. 7 (4) (2007 Jul-Aug) 428–436.
5. M.C. Gupta, Degenerative scoliosis options for surgical management, Orthop. Clin. N. Am. 34 (2003) 269–279.
6. C.B. Tribus, Degenerative lumbar scoliosis: evaluation and management, J. Am. Acad. Orthop. Surg. 11 (2003) 174–183.
7. B.M. Ozgur, H.E. Aryan, L. Pimenta, W.R. Taylor, Extreme Lateral Interbody Fusion (XLIF): a novel surgical technique for anterior lumbar interbody fusion, The Spine Journal 6 (2006) 435–443.
8. D.S. Bradford, B.K. Tay, S.S. Hu, Adult scoliosis: surgical indications, operative management, complications, and outcomes, Spine 24 (1999) 2617–2629.
9. H.R. Weiss, Adolescent idiopathic scoliosis (AIS)—an indication for surgery? A systematic review of the literature, Disabil. Rehabil. 30 (10) (2008) 799–807.
10. S.D. Daffner, A. Vaccaro, Adult degenerative lumbar scoliosis, Am. J. Orthop. 2 (2003) 77–82.

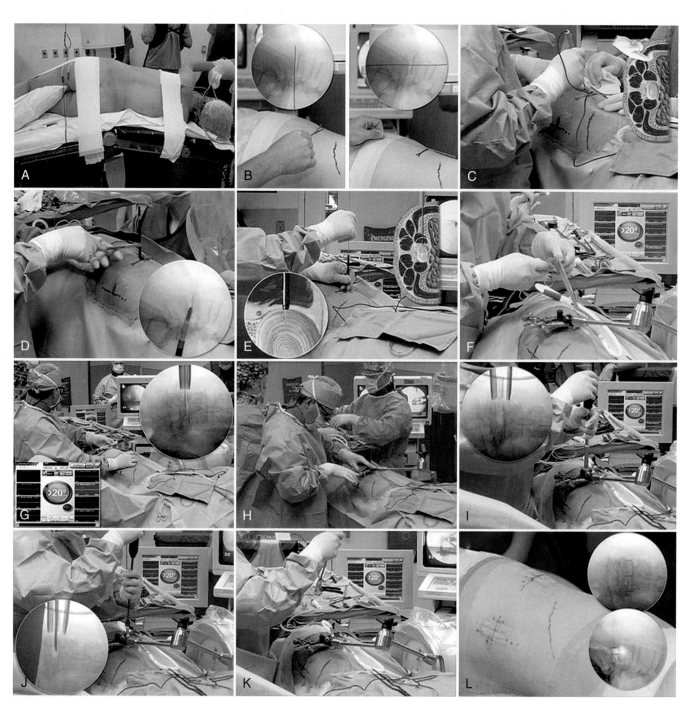

■ **FIGURE 61-3** XLIF surgical technique. **A,** Patient positioning. **B,** Index level identification. **C,** Retroperitoneal access. **D, E,** Transpsoas access. **F,** Maxcess insertion. **G,** NeuroVision Electromyographic System. **H,** Maxcess fixation. **I,** Diskectomy. **J,** Endplate preparation. **K,** Implant insertion. **L,** Surgical wound.

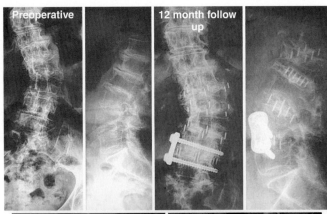

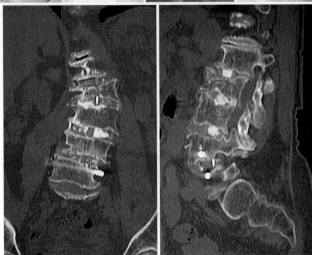

■ **FIGURE 61-4**   Patient example: An 84-year-old woman with degenerative scoliosis. Twelve months after surgery, clear evidence of fusion is seen on CT scan, despite subsidence (*red circle*). Clinical improvement after surgery was maintained.

# 62

# Pelvic Fixation of the Aging Spine

*Joseph M. Morreale, Ravi Ramachandran, Jonathan N. Grauer, and Peter G. Whang*

| K E Y   P O I N T S |
| --- |
| • Incorporation of the iliac crest into lumbosacral fusions may serve to decrease the rate of pseudarthrosis. |
| • Instrumentation that extends beyond the lumbosacral pivot point augments the stiffness of the construct. |
| • The bony fixation and pullout strength of implants progressively increase as they are placed more laterally into the pelvis (i.e., the iliac wings). |
| • Multiple screw anchors may be needed to obtain solid iliac fixation in patients with severe osteoporosis. |
| • Fully threaded screws may prevent loosening or failure by maximizing cortical purchase. |

## INTRODUCTION

Iliolumbar fixation is an important adjunctive technique that may be beneficial for the operative management of multiple conditions affecting the aging spine, including untreated idiopathic or degenerative scoliosis, sagittal plane deformities such as kyphosis or flat-back syndrome, high-grade spondylolisthesis, sacral fractures, tumors or infections requiring sacrectomy, and stenotic lesions distal to a multilevel lumbar arthrodesis. It has been well established that the biomechanical and biological conditions unique to this region make it more difficult to achieve a successful fusion. Therefore, the incorporation of

instrumentation into the pelvis is extremely valuable in many situations, because it helps to restore spinal balance and confers greater stability to the lumbosacral junction. The increasing rigidity of these constructs may also serve to enhance bone formation in complex reconstructive cases that may otherwise be prone to the development of a nonunion.

Reliable fixation to the pelvis was first achieved in the 1970s with Luque instrumentation which utilized a bar with a curved distal end that could be advanced into the iliac crest. A decade later, the Galveston method was introduced, which provided even greater fixation because it allowed for the application of contoured rods, which were inserted though the posterior superior iliac spine, in between the inner and outer tables of the pelvis, toward the sciatic notch. Nevertheless, these early systems were still found to give rise to an relatively high incidence of pseudarthrosis, ranging from 6% to 41%.[1]

Iliac screws improve on these initial approaches by taking advantage of innovations in implant design and modularity. These constructs are not only more rigid; their pull-out strength has been shown to be three times greater than that of a standard Galveston rod.[2] Given their superior biomechanical properties, it is anticipated that the use of iliac screws may reduce the risk of pseudarthrosis compared to other types of lumbosacral constructs. However, the proper placement of this instrumentation requires an intricate knowledge of pelvic anatomy in order to avoid cortical breaches through the ileum or penetration into the acetabulum.[3] Furthermore, the surgeon must also take into account the position of the screws for the purpose of contouring the rod and ensure adequate soft tissue coverage to ensure the heads will not be too prominent, which could contribute to patient discomfort.[4]

## Case Studies

### CLINICAL CASE #1—DEGENERATIVE SCOLIOSIS

A 69-year-old woman presents with complaints of severe axial low back pain that radiates into her anterior thighs in conjunction with a curvature of her thoracolumbar spine. The patient had previously been treated in a Milwaukee brace for a diagnosis of adolescent idiopathic scoliosis until skeletal maturity but had never undergone a previous spinal procedure. She feels as if her symptoms and her deformity have been worsening despite multiple conservative treatments, including physical therapy, pain medications, and a series of spinal injections. Her past medical history is notable for osteoporosis and a 30 pack-year history of smoking.

Physical examination findings include obvious thoracic and lumbar prominences upon forward flexion with some tenderness to palpation at the apices of the curves. However, her shoulders and pelvis are essentially level. She exhibits normal motor and sensory function with no long tract signs. She also has no tension signs in her lower extremities.

Posteroanterior and lateral scoliosis x-rays display a right thoracic curve from T5 to T11 and a left lumbar curve from T11 to L4, measuring 58 degrees and 67 degrees, respectively (Figure 62-1). However, her overall coronal and sagittal alignment appears to be reasonably balanced. These films demonstrate clear progression compared to previous radiographs acquired several years ago. Aside from her deformity, an MRI study of her

entire spine reveals no intraspinal abnormalities or significant compression of the neural elements.

### CLINICAL CASE #2—PATHOLOGIC FRACTURE

A 59-year-old man who initially presented with a 1-month history of axial low back pain with occasional lower extremity symptoms consistent with neurogenic claudication. The patient has a known diagnosis of colorectal cancer that was treated with multiple abdominal operations and chemotherapy. The patient is currently requiring high-dose narcotics for his pain, which is increasing in severity. His past medical history is otherwise unremarkable except for mild hypertension.

A physical examination of the patient reveals limited range of motion of the lumbar spine with diffuse tenderness to palpation. He has no apparent neurologic deficits with normal reflexes as well as negative straight leg-raising tests in both lower extremities.

Imaging studies include plain films of the lumbar spine, which demonstrate L3 and L4 vertebral body fractures (Figure 62-2). These fractures were confirmed to be burst-type injuries on a subsequent CT scan with obvious height loss, focal kyphosis, and retropulsion of fragments with approximately 25% canal compromise. An MRI study displays a large soft tissue mass extending into the epidural space at these levels, which results in significant spinal stenosis with near-obliteration of the thecal sac.

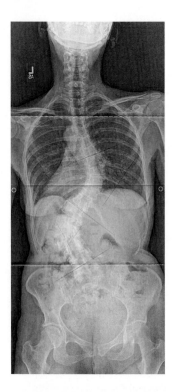

■ **FIGURE 62-1**  Posteroanterior scoliosis x-ray reveals thoracic and lumbar curves measuring 58 degrees and 67 degrees, respectively.

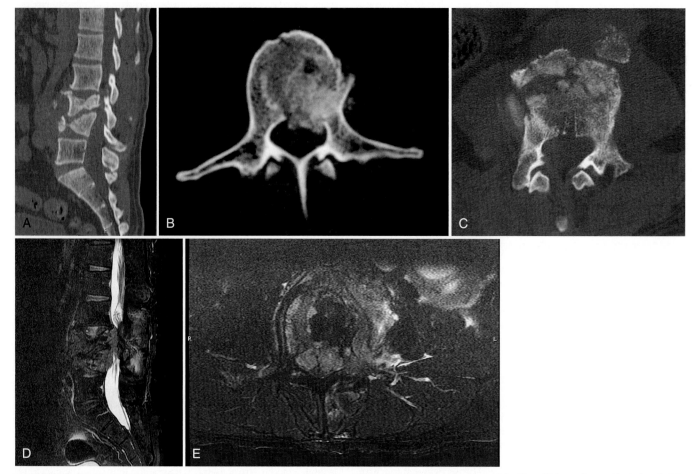

■ **FIGURE 62-2**  Sagittal (**A**) and axial (**B, C**) CT images of the lumbar spine demonstrate burst-type fractures of the L3 and L4 vertebrae with obvious height loss, focal kyphosis, and retropulsion of fragments into the spinal canal. Sagittal (**D**) and axial (**E**) views from T2-weighted MRI study confirm the presence of a large anterior epidural mass resulting in significant spinal stenosis and compression of the thecal sac.

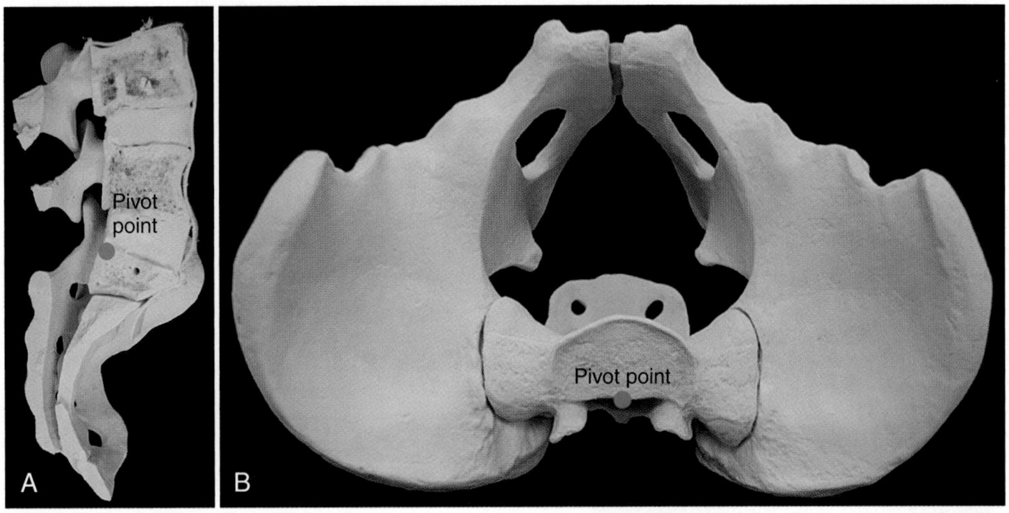

■ **FIGURE 62-3** Sagittal (**A**) and axial (**B**) cross-sectional cuts through the pelvis depicting the location of the lumbosacral pivot point (*red dot*) along the posterior aspect of the L5-S1 interspace.

## BASIC SCIENCE AND BIOMECHANICAL STUDIES

A thorough understanding of the osseous and soft tissue anatomy of the lumbosacral spine and pelvis is critical for the safe and effective insertion of iliac fixation. The sacrum is composed of five fused vertebrae and serves as a functional keystone that links two paired hemipelves posteriorly through bilateral sacroiliac articulations. Because this instrumentation is introduced into the iliac wings, which form the lateral borders of the pelvic ring, it is necessary to consider a number of different parameters such as intrailiac distance, width between the inner and outer tables, and cortical thickness. The longest intrailiac path proceeds along a line connecting the posterior superior iliac spine to the anterior inferior iliac spine, which averages approximately 141 mm in males and 129 mm in females. Similarly, the width of the iliac crest should allow for the placement of 8-mm screws in males and 6- to 7-mm implants in females; the mean cortical thickness in males and females has been shown to be 5.2 mm and 4.7 mm, respectively.[3]

In their comparison of 10 different methods of lumbosacral fixation, McCord and colleagues[5] reported that the two constructs associated with the highest loads to failure both obtained solid purchase within the iliac crests. Based on this in vitro data, the concept of the lumbosacral pivot point was elucidated, which is located at the intersection of the middle osteoligamentous column and the L5-S1 interspace (Figure 62-3). According to this paradigm, pelvic implants that extend anterior to this fulcrum increase the overall stiffness of the instrumentation because the resultant biomechanical vectors are transformed from in-line forces to cantilever bending.[6]

Three distinct zones have been designated for the purpose of categorizing sacropelvic fixation (Figure 62-4).[7] Zone 1 refers to the S1 vertebral body, Zone 2 encompasses the sacral alae and the region between S2 and the coccyx, and Zone 3 denotes the paired iliac wings. In general, the degree of stability imparted by these screws has been found to improve as they are positioned more laterally within the lumbopelvic ring (i.e., from Zone 1 to Zone 3); implants situated in Zone 3 are also better able to resist the pull-out forces that are generated by bending moments arising from the lumbosacral junction than those directed toward either Zone 1 or 2.

The use of internal fixation in the setting of osteoporosis may be particularly problematic because this instrumentation is likely to be more susceptible to loosening or failure, especially in cases involving traumatic injuries or deformity correction where it may be subjected to tremendous stresses and strains. Consequently, in these situations it may be preferable to employ longer implants that will traverse the entire length of the iliac column and engage the cortical bone superior to the acetabulum, so that they are able to withstand more significant forces.[2] Another approach that has been advocated for osteoporotic patients is the incorporation of two screws into each iliac crest. However, there are some concerns that the application of rigid

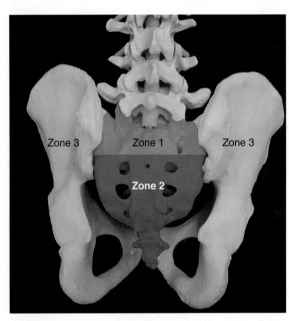

■ **FIGURE 62-4** Schematic demarcating the three zones of sacropelvic fixation: 1—S1 vertebral body; 2—the region between S2 and the coccyx as well as the sacral alae; 3—iliac wings.

iliac fixation could lead to stress shielding of an already compromised pelvis, which may predispose these individuals to insufficiency fractures.[8]

## CLINICAL PRACTICE GUIDELINES

Unfortunately there are currently no prospective, randomized, controlled clinical trials that have specifically elucidated the safety and efficacy of lumbopelvic fixation in the elderly population. Consequently, the precise indications for this surgical technique have not yet been definitively established, and there are still no validated clinical practice guidelines that may be employed to direct the management of these patients.

## CLINICAL CASE EXAMPLES: TREATMENT AND FUTURE CHALLENGES

Both of the cases presented earlier involved posterior-based spinal constructs that were reinforced with pelvic implants. The first patient with degenerative scoliosis underwent a circumferential procedure performed in a staged fashion consisting of anterior releases and interbody fusions from L2-S1 with polyetheretherketone (PEEK) cages followed by a posterior spinal arthrodesis extending from T5 to the ileum with instrumentation and autogenous bone (Figure 62-5). In the second case example, the pathologic fractures of the L3 and L4 vertebral bodies were addressed with a posterior decompression of those levels, in conjunction with an instru-

mented fusion of the motion segments between L1 and the pelvis with local and iliac crest autograft (Figure 62-6). In both of these situations the decision was made to include supplemental pelvic fixation because such extensive constructs would be expected to subject the distal screws to substantial forces that may bring about hardware failure or loosening, especially in these individuals who were suspected of having

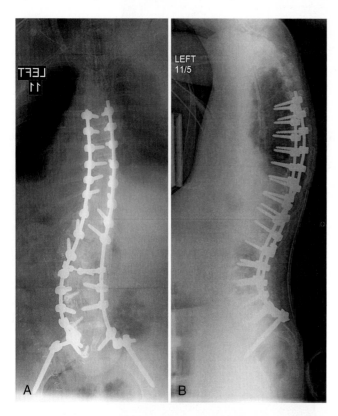

■ **FIGURE 62-5** Postoperative PA (**A**) and lateral (**B**) x-rays following a circumferential arthrodesis with extension of instrumentation into the pelvis.

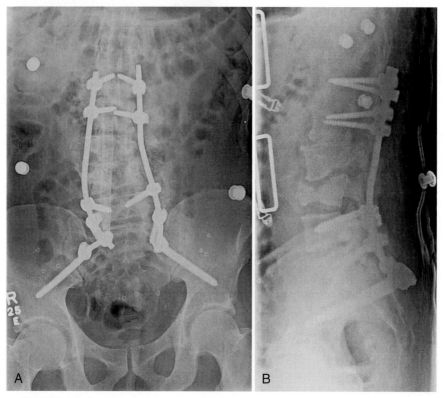

■ **FIGURE 62-6** Postoperative AP (**A**) and lateral (**B**) x-rays demonstrating a posterior lumbar construct that was augmented with iliac screws for greater stability.

osteoporosis. Thus the purpose of adding pelvic implants was to augment the rigidity of the instrumentation and create a more stable, "balanced" construct that would hopefully reduce the incidence of pseudarthrosis.

In placing pelvic screws, it may be useful to remove a portion of the posterior superior iliac spine with a Leksell rongeur or burr so that the heads may be adequately countersunk in an attempt to minimize their prominence. The probe is introduced into the window of cancellous bone and aimed between the inner and outer tables of the ileum, toward the sciatic notch (Figure 62-7). After the tract is probed for any cortical breaches, the cavity is tapped in preparation for the instrumentation; in most instances the dimensions of the iliac wing should be able to accommodate relatively large implants (i.e., 7.5 mm in diameter and up to 80 mm in length or greater). The final position of the pelvic screws should be assessed with intraoperative radiographs or fluoroscopy in AP, lateral,

and oblique views to ensure that it is entirely contained within the ileum and is not encroaching upon other critical structures, such as the hip joint (Figure 62-8).

In the future, further advances in technology may yield even stronger implants that are lower profile and easier to connect to adjoining lumbosacral instrumentation. Because of the challenges associated with the insertion of iliac screws, this approach may be well suited to the application of novel surgical navigation systems that are integrated with advanced three-dimensional imaging modalities.

## CONCLUSION

Pelvic fixation represents an effective method for enhancing the rigidity of posterior spinal fusion constructs. By obtaining secure purchase within the iliac crests, these implants confer greater stability to the axial skeleton

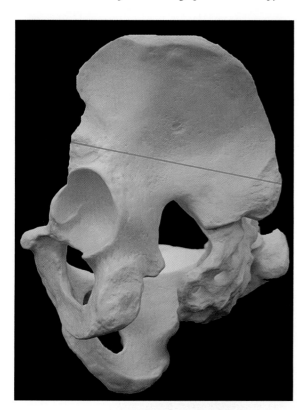

■ **FIGURE 62-7**    Lateral view of the pelvis delineating the optimal trajectory for the screw.

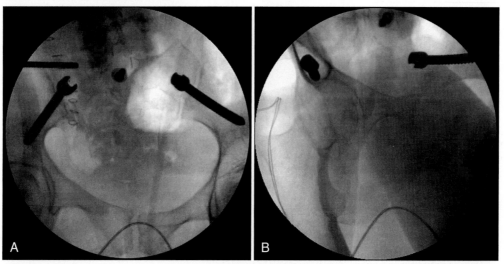

■ **FIGURE 62-8**    Anteroposterior (**A**) and oblique (**B**) fluoroscopic images are used to visualize the iliac screws during the procedure to ensure that the implants have not breached the cortical bone and are not encroaching upon the acetabulum.

and may therefore be indispensable for the treatment of patients with osteoporosis who are at greater risk for nonunion and other postoperative complications following complex spinal reconstructions.

## References

1. A. Moshirfar, F.F. Rand, P.D. Sponseller, S.J. Parazin, A.J. Khanna, K.M. Kebaish, J.T. Stinson, L.H. Riley, Pelvic fixation in spine surgery. Historical overview, indications, biomechanical relevance, and current techniques, J. Bone Joint Surg. Am. 87 (2005) 89–106.
2. R.M. Schwend, R. Sluyters, J. Najdzionek, The pylon concept of pelvic anchorage for spinal instrumentation in the human cadaver, Spine 28 (2003) 542–547.
3. T.A. Schildhauer, P. McCulloch, J.R. Chapman, F.A. Mann, Anatomic and radiographic considerations for placement of transiliac screws in lumbopelvic fixation, J. Spinal Disord. Tech. 15 (2002) 199–205.
4. N.K. Acharya, B. Bijukachhe, R.J. Kumar, V.K. Menon, Ilio-lumbar fixation—the Amrita technique, J. Spinal Disord. Tech. 21 (2008) 493–499.
5. D.H. McCord, B.W. Cunningham, Y. Shono, J.J. Myers, P.C. McAfee, Biomechanical analysis of lumbosacral fixation, Spine 17 (Suppl. 8) (1992) S235–S243.
6. E.R. Santos, M.K. Rosner, J.H. Perra, D.W. Polly, Spinopelvic fixation in deformity: a review, Neurosurg. Clin. N. Am. 18 (2007) 373–384.
7. M.F. O'Brien, Sacropelvic fixation in spinal deformity, in: R.L. DeWald (Ed.), Spinal deformities: the comprehensive text, Thieme, New York, 2003, pp. 601–614.
8. K.B. Wood, M.J. Schendel, J.W. Ogilvie, J. Braun, M.C. Major, J.R. Malcom, Effect of sacral and iliac instrumentation on strains in the pelvis: a biomechanical study, Spine 21 (1996) 1185–1191.

# 63

# Intradiscal Biologics: A Potential Minimally Invasive Cure for Symptomatic Degenerative Disc Disease?

*Rajeev K. Patel*

**K E Y   P O I N T S**

- Biological repair of injured tissues by introducing cell-based tissue replacements, genetic modifications of resident cells, or a combination thereof have been successfully applied to various tissues such as bone and cartilage.

- Application of these treatment modalities to cure symptomatic intervertebral disc degeneration is in its infancy and mostly limited to experimental studies in vitro or in animal studies.

- Attempts at gene therapy or tissue engineering demonstrate obvious potentials as well as significant shortcomings to biological cure of symptomatic degenerative disc disease.

- Knowledge gained from these attempts might be applied to cure the low back pain that often accompanies the structurally compromised intervertebral disc.

## INTRODUCTION

The development of a cell-based, biological replacement to restore, maintain, and improve the function of damaged tissues and organs has become the en vogue frontier to developing potential novel approaches to patient cures. The intervertebral disc (IVD) undergoes very extensive degenerative changes (Figure 63-1) with the various macro- and microtraumas that come with age and daily life activities. Individual differences have been demonstrated in young individuals exhibiting the disc of an elderly person and vice versa. It is generally accepted that an extremely prevalent rate and degree of asymptomatic disc degeneration exists in the general population. Therefore, differentiating normal aging from symptomatic pathological degeneration is very difficult and cannot be assessed by simply identifying the most abnormal disc on imaging (Figure 63-2). At this time, controlled provocative lumbar discography (Figure 63-3) remains our best clinical test to identify a physiologically painful structurally compromised IVD. The term "discogenic low back pain" is the term often used to indicate degenerative disc disease associated with concordant pain.

Relating recent findings regarding the molecular mechanisms in initiating or propagating degenerative alterations of the IVD will be crucial to the ultimate success in the developments of biologic strategies to cure discogenic low back pain.

## FUNCTIONAL ANATOMY OF THE INTERVERTEBRAL Disc

Intervertebral discs transmit loads from body weight and muscle activity as well as provide flexibility to the spine. The discs consist of three highly specialized structures: the endplates, the annulus fibrosus, and the nucleus pulposus The two cartilaginous endplates form the inferior and superior interface between the disc and the adjacent vertebrae, thereby enclosing the disc axially. The annulus fibrosus is made up of several lamellae consisting of parallel collagen fibers interspersed by elastin fibers. Surrounded by the annulus fibrosus is the nucleus pulposus, the gelatinous core, which consists of randomly organized collagen fibers, radially arranged elastin fibers, and a highly hydrated aggrecan-containing gel. The highly hydrated proteoglycans in the nucleus pulposus are essential to maintain the osmotic pressure and therefore have a major effect on the load-bearing properties of the disc.

It is also important to note that the intervertebral disc is a largely avascular structure. With increasing age, as growth and skeletal maturation proceed, degenerative processes begin to change the morphology and therefore the function of the disc. The most widely accepted conceptual model of spinal segmental degeneration was proposed by Kirkaldy-Willis.[1] In this model, the nucleus pulposus of degenerated discs is characterized by a decreased water and proteoglycan content leading to the loss of its gel-like appearance and hydrostatic properties. Degenerative changes of the annulus fibrosus are less obvious, but result in irregular lamellae with the collagen and elastin networks becoming more disorganized. Replacing the gel-like structure of the nucleus pulposus with fibrocartilaginous tissue results in decreased flexibility and therefore often in cleft formation with fissures. Up to 50% of the cells show signs of necrosis and some of them reveal signs of apoptosis, potentially resulting in cell loss from the disc.[2] Although there is broad consensus about these hallmarks of degeneration, the question of whether revascularization and/or reinnervation of the inner parts of the disc may occur during degeneration is still a topic of debate.[3] Although studies have described revascularization, possibly accompanied by reinnervation, of the inner parts of the IVD, it is not completely clear at

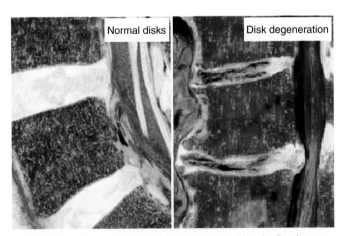

■ **FIGURE 63-1** Macroscopic pathoanatomy evident in disc degeneration compared side by side to healthy intervertebral discs.

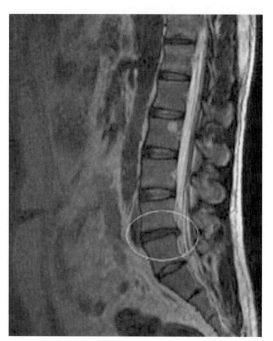

■ **FIGURE 63-2** T2-weighted sagittal MRI demonstrating segmental degenerative disc desiccation and bulging at the L4-L5 level.

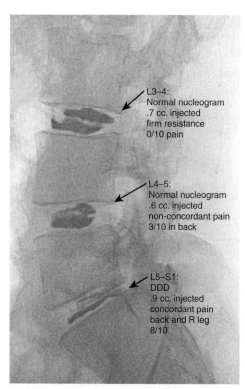

L3–4:
Normal nucleogram
.7 cc. injected
firm resistance
0/10 pain

L4–5:
Normal nucleogram
.6 cc. injected
non-concordant pain
3/10 in back

L5–S1:
DDD
.9 cc. injected
concordant pain
back and R leg
8/10

■ **FIGURE 63-3** Provocative lumbar diskography demonstrating a structurally compromised fissured L5-S1 IVD with a physiologic concordant pain elicitation under controlled pressure as well as adjacent nonphysiologic and nonpainful discs at L4-L5 and L3-L4 with intact morphologies.

which stage of degeneration these occur.[3] Clarification of this question is of special importance since the interplay between neovascularization and neo-innervation might be of crucial importance for the pain sensation caused by degenerated discs. Answers to these questions may ultimately determine the rate-limiting step to the potential of biologic cures of symptomatic degenerative disc disease.

## CAUSES OF DEGENERATIVE DISC DISEASE

Degenerative disc disease is a complex process with a multifactorial etiology. Nutritional effects, mechanical load, and genetics all likely have contributory pathologic effects on the IVD. Of these, nutrition and removal of waste products likely play a special role in realizing the potential that intradiscal biologics may ultimately hold. Insufficient nutritional supply of the cells is thought to be the major obstacle contributing to degenerative disc disease. Cells of the IVD face the precarious situation of having to maintain a huge extracellular matrix with a "fragile" supply of nutrients that is easily disturbed because the IVD is avascular and nutrition is dependent on diffusion. Because of the size of the intervertebral disc, the nutrients need to diffuse from a capillary network in the vertebral bodies, through the endplates and the disc matrix to the cells in the nucleus of the disc. The supply of nutrition becomes more restricted as the originally cartilaginous endplates become calcified as the degenerative process progresses. As glucose and oxygen is restricted because of diffusion distances, the removal of metabolic waste such as lactic acid becomes critically impaired. Measurements have demonstrated that as oxygen concentrations were very low in the nucleus and increased toward the disc surface, the lactic acid concentration showed the reverse profile. The buildup of lactic acid results in an intradiscal environment with a lowered pH. Low oxygen concentrations and acidic pH adversely affect the synthetic activity and proteoglycan synthesis rates of disc cells. This toxic environment may lead to a fall in proteoglycan content and therefore to degenerative disc disease. This suboptimal environment may lead to increased cell death and therefore reduced cell numbers in the disc.[4] Ultimately, the result of poor nutritional supply of the IVD is that very few remaining cells are confronted with the task of maintaining an extensive matrix. Unfortunately, it likely holds true that the progression of matrix degeneration becomes irreversible once the cell density falls below a minimal threshold.

## THERAPEUTIC BIOLOGIC STRATEGIES

Biologic treatments for the degenerated IVD have scarcely been utilized to regenerate or cure the painful, deteriorated disc and restore biological function. Thus far, intradiscal biologics are classified into four approaches:

1. Direct injection of a biologically active factor(s) (Figure 63-4)
2. Modification of the gene expression of resident disc cells in vivo (direct gene therapy) (Figure 63-5)
3. Supplementation with autologous implantation of in vitro cultivated and modified cells (Figure 63-6)
4. Stem-cell based gene therapies (Figure 63-7)

These applications aim for sustained delivery of biologically active substances to the disc that should drive regeneration or conserve the status quo. The nature of the respective active factor is hereby defined by our knowledge of the molecular mechanisms active in the disc during the various stages of degeneration. The applicability of the various approaches is largely dependent on our current knowledge of disc cell biology, the state of degeneration of the intervertebral disc, and potential safety issues.

### Intradiscal Injection of a "Naked" Biologically Active Factor

Percutaneous intradiscal injection would provide the most straightforward approach to delivery of an active biologic factor to the disc cells (see Figure 63-3). Although direct application of potentially beneficial factors, mostly proteins like growth factors, cytokines, or anabolic enzymes, has been used frequently in vitro, few studies have been published attempting this approach in vivo. Promising results have been reported after injecting rabbit lumbar IVD in vivo with osteogenic protein-1 (OP-1), a growth factor belonging to the Transforming Growth Factor Beta (TGF-β) superfamily of growth factors. Direct injection of this growth factor resulted in significantly increased proteoglycan synthesis and restoration of disc height that was found to be stable up to 24 weeks after injection.[5,6] Additional studies demonstrated that OP-1 injection exhibited a physiologic effect by inhibiting pain-related behavior in a rat disc degeneration model.[7,8] Subsequently, Chubinskaya and colleagues[9] documented the anticatabolic effect of intradiscal injection of

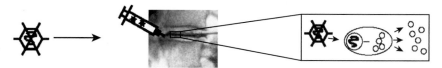

■ **FIGURE 63-4**  Intradiscal injection of a "naked" biologically active factor—done to facilitate the sustained release of an agent into the cellular matrix.

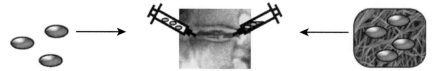

■ **FIGURE 63-5**  Modification of the gene expression of resident disc cells in vivo (direct gene therapy) utilizing a viral vector resulting in transformation and sustained expression of the active protein Z.

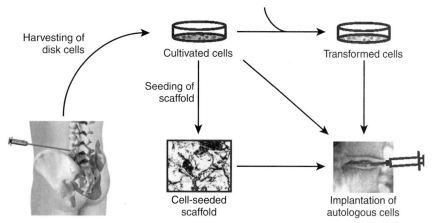

■ **FIGURE 63-6**  Supplementation with autologous implantation of in vitro cultivated and modified cells. Cultivated cells can be genetically modified in vivo before implantation (indirect gene therapy), seeded into a scaffold, or simply implanted directly.

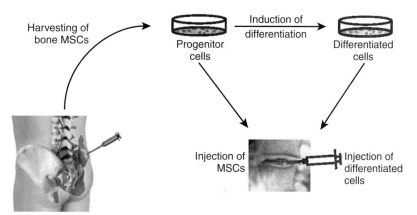

■ **FIGURE 63-7**  Stem-cell based gene therapy. Mesenchymal stem cells can be cultivated as progenitor cells and either injected directly into the disc matrix or be differentiated in vitro into a disc cell and then injected.

OP-1 in a rat model by demonstrating reduced immunostaining for aggrecanase, Matrix Metalloproteinase (MMP)-13, substance P, Tumor necrosis factor (TNF)-α, and Interleukin (IL)-1β. Because substance P is a neuropeptide linked with inflammation and pain, the aforementioned reduction in level of this noxious protein support the previously stated physiologic inhibition of pain-related behavior.[7-9] Furthermore, Miyamoto and coworkers[10] were able to demonstrate that intradiscal injection of OP-1 restored the biomechanical properties of IVDs in the rabbit model of degenerative disc disease. They reported not only that a single injection of OP-1 significantly

restored IVD height, but also that the treated discs demonstrated a higher viscous and elastic modulus due to increased proteoglycan content in the nucleus as well as increased collagen content in the nucleus and annulus. Concerns regarding the potential of ectopic bone formation in the epidural space with OP-1 therapies was addressed by Kawakami and associates.[11] They demonstrated that there was no macroscopic evidence of ectopic bone formation, no motor paresis, and no behavioral differences to motor stimuli with epidural administration of OP-1 in a rat model. The aforementioned studies demonstrate the feasibility of direct injection, yet this technique may be limited to the presence of disc cells that are still healthy, numerous, and able to respond to a biologically active agent. Taking into context the decreasing viability and synthetic activity of human disc cells during progressive degeneration, future directions for this technique may be best suited for success in the younger patient population with discogenic Low back pain (LBP) due to modestly degenerated discs in synergistic combinations with other biologically active agents.

As opposed to injecting a biologically active enzyme or growth factor, Klein and colleagues[12] published a clinical pilot study utilizing direct injection of a mixture of matrix components and aiding components known to induce proteoglycan synthesis. This solution of glucosamine and chondroitin sulfate combined with hypertonic dextrose and dimethylsulfoxide was injected into 30 patients who exhibited concordant pain on provocative lumbar discography. These patients responded well regarding reduction in a disability score and a visual analogue pain score at an average follow-up of 13 months. The authors suggested that the good outcome might be due to the combination of several components resulting in a parallel replenishing of the matrix by increased proteoglycan synthesis and induction of disc repair by simultaneous induction of multiple growth factors. This approach might prove superior to the injection of a single bioactive factor. It is conceivable that the injected matrix components are able to modulate and improve the intradiscal environment, enabling the disc cells, even in a degenerated disc, to react to the resulting secretion of growth factors and continue with the maintenance of the cellular environment. However, from this pilot study it is not clear if the injected components will be contained inside the disc in heavily degenerated discs and therefore be able to ensure a prolonged beneficial effect on the disc cells. Further controlled comparative studies are required before any therapeutic conclusions can be rendered.

Common to these injection techniques is the concern that the aforementioned demonstrated short-term effects might cease when the originally injected material has been consumed or is lost to the disc cells by diffusion. In order to provide the disc with a continuing supply of biologically active factors, it would be desirable to continuously produce the biologic of choice or include the substance in a pharmacological slow-release system as suggested for the use of growth factors.[13] Considering these data, it is conceivable that combination therapy of growth factor(s) and matrix replenishment might be the way to obtain a more sustained improvement of degenerated discs. This approach may also allow for expansion of the previously stated limitations with application of this technique to various grades of degeneration because of the requirement of a certain density of healthy disc cells.

## Gene Therapy Approaches

Prolonged supply of the discal matrix with a beneficial agent could be achieved by genetically modifying disc cells to produce a desired gene product. Because of advances in molecular genetics, techniques are readily available to insert genetic elements (DNA) into almost any type of target cell. These genetic elements usually consist of the gene encoding the desired product and a control element modulating the expression of the respective gene. Typically, two strategies can be used to achieve expression of the desired gene at the targeted site. Direct, or in vivo, gene therapy requires the direct introduction of the gene of interest into resident cells in situ (see Figure 63-4), whereas indirect, or ex vivo, gene therapy requires the removal of target cells, introduction of the gene of interest in vitro and implantation of the transformed cells (see Figure 63-5).[14] Uptake of the desired genetic material, usually in the form of pure "naked" DNA, can be optimized by application of a carrier, also called vector. Viral vectors are very efficient transporters of genetic material; they are able to enter mammalian cells, taking over DNA replication and the protein expression machinery. For the purposes of gene therapy, several engineered viruses are available that have the original viral genome removed or inactivated and, in addition, are modified to not replicate or exhibit their pathogenicity. Of interest, these viruses vary in their ability to integrate the transferred DNA into the host cell genome, their ability to invade dividing or nondividing cells, and their infection efficiency. Because of the properties of the IVD and its cells, the virus of choice needs to efficiently infect nondividing, quiescent cells. Furthermore, the low cell density inside the disc might hamper efficient infection of a sufficient fraction of the disc cells. On the other hand, the avascular and contained IVD might provide an advantageous environment to achieve high concentrations of the injected

viral vector, leading to higher efficiency of the infection process while also lessening the danger of an immune response against viral proteins.

Studies have demonstrated that adenoviral vectors are able to efficiently transform disc cells from various species. The main disadvantage of adenoviral vectors lies in the activation of innate and adaptive parts of the patient's immune system when the vector is applied in vivo. To overcome this potentially lethal complication, Lattermann and colleagues[15] recently tested an adeno-associated viral vector (AAV) for its applicability to degenerative disc disease. The authors demonstrated that AAV was able to efficiently transduce human disc cells in vitro and rabbit disc cells in vivo. Although AAV caused a humoral immune response, no significant cellular immune response, as seen with adenoviral vectors, was observed. Interestingly, despite the observed humoral immune response, significant transgene expression was observed in the preexposed animals.[15] These findings suggest that AAV might offer a valuable and safer alternative to adenoviral vectors in the future. Although the aforementioned studies suggest the feasibility of direct gene therapy using viral vectors to target disc cells, the question of the delivered gene and therefore expressed gene product remains open. Nishida and coworkers[14] published one of the initial studies to deliver an exogenous therapeutic gene in vivo using an adenoviral vector carrying the gene for TGF-b1 to modify cells of rabbit IVD. The authors found significant increases of TGF-b1 and proteoglycan production in the injected disc, suggesting the feasibility of direct gene therapy to treat intervertebral disc degeneration.[14] Lim Mineralization Protein (LMP) is another potentially beneficial gene factor that has been shown to positively affect the degenerated disc cellular matrix by increasing the disc cell production of Bone Morphogenetic Proteins (BMP) and proteoglycans in vitro.[16] In vivo studies involving the intradiscal injection of rabbit discs resulted in increased expression of the anabolic cytokines BMP-2 and BMP-7 mRNA and also led to increased production of aggrecan mRNA.[16] These data suggest that LMP-1 is also a beneficial factor that could be applied to gene therapeutics for disc degeneration. Sox9-on the other hand, does not affect the proteoglycan content of the disc cellular matrix. Sox9 is a gene transcription factor responsible for the synthesis of type II collagen, and its transfer into cells from degenerated human discs resulted in increased levels of type II collagen.[17] Injection of a Sox9-carrying adenoviral vector into traumatized rabbit discs resulted in preservation of the histologic appearance seen in healthy discs, whereas the injured control discs displayed typically recognized degenerative changes.[17] Therefore, not only increased proteoglycan production but also collagen type II production seems to be able to prevent disc degeneration in vivo, thereby offering multiple potentially therapeutic options. Although the increased production of a single gene product seems to result in the transformation of disc cells, a combination of related gene-producing factors may prove synergistic and more physiologic. In fact, Moon and coworkers[18] have already reported that the combined transfer of Transforming growth factor Beta-1 (TGF-β1), Insulin like growth factor(IGF)-1 and BMP-2 revealed the aforementioned hypothetical synergistic effect of these factors on protein synthesis by demonstrating an amplification of protein synthesis.

An opposite approach that might be a potential alternative to the use of anabolic factors to induce disc cells into the production of matrix components is the application of anticatabolic factors. Inhibition of catabolic activity would ensue in maintaining or increasing the content of the respective matrix component by slowing down its degradation without the need to force the disc cells to higher synthesis rates. Wallach and colleagues[19] recently published an in vitro study utilizing an adenoviral vector to introduce the gene encoding forTissue inhibitor of metalloproteinase (TIMP)-1 into disc cells isolated from degenerated human IVD. Gene delivery of TIMP-1 increased the proteoglycan content in the disc cell cultures, suggesting the anticatabolic approach to be a potentially promising strategy for gene therapy of degenerative disc disease.

The aforementioned index gene therapeutic approaches report results that sound promising. Despite the obvious potentials, the reality is that the application to human IVD will be challenged by the suboptimal and eventually toxic microenvironment inside the severely degenerated disc. It is questionable if the remaining compromised IVD cells in the degenerated disc will be able to produce reasonable amounts of gene-induced growth factors over extended periods of time. Furthermore, one can argue that it is unlikely that the existing starving cells are able to properly respond and produce an improved matrix even if the production of the respective gene product is achieved.

## Autologous Implantation of Cultivated, Modified Cells

Degenerated discs could be treated by supplementation of the deserted matrix with in vitro cells that have been removed, cultivated, and modified. Autologous cells are optimal because their utilization makes the potential immunological complications a moot issue. Autologous cells compatible with disc tissue have to be harvested, expanded in vitro, and subsequently implanted into the symptomatic IVD. Once the cells have been removed and cultivated in vitro, this approach allows for indirect gene therapy via genetic modification of the withdrawn cells and/or tissue engineering via seeding of the cells in supporting biomaterials before implantation into the symptomatic degenerated IVD (see Figure 63-5). The combination of these techniques potentially improves efficiency by improving cell survival or enhancing the biosynthetic activity of the implanted cells. Genetic modification of cultivated cells in vitro is technically very similar to the aforementioned approaches previously discussed. The focus in this section turns to the cultivation of disc cells and creation of suitable implants.

For several reasons, it is extremely difficult to obtain suitable and sufficient numbers of target cells from intervertebral disc tissue. Removal of nucleus pulposus cells, the obvious target cells, would require opening of the annulus fibrosus to gain access. This would almost certainly cause damage to the annulus. In addition to the very restricted accessibility, the very low cell density in degenerated discs will further complicate the acquisition of ample usable cells for successful in vitro cultivation. Therefore only a limited number of scenarios are conceivable that would allow the withdrawal of sufficient cells from the disc to perform a disc cell–based approach without further damaging the already affected disc or accelerating its degeneration. Withdrawal of herniated disc material might be one scenario that would facilitate the removal of sufficient disc cells for in vitro cultivation. However, the introduction of cells/implants after a surgical intervention on the same disc could be disputed since the outcome of microdiscectomy has been shown to be satisfactory for most patients with radiculopathy. That being said, the direct insult as well as the likely accelerated degenerative process of the surgical level post microdiscectomy predisposes that segment to discogenic LBP postoperatively. This increased risk may justify cell implantation to prevent postoperative acute and/or chronic discogenic LBP. Another potential clinical application would be the use of cell-based approaches to prevent the accelerated degeneration of discs adjacent to an interbody fusion level. Mechanical stress at segmental levels adjacent to fusion procedures is a known biomechanical issue. This is known to result in accelerated rates of degenerative disc disease and consequently discogenic low back pain at segments juxtapositioned to the fusion level (Figure 63-8). The disc material removed during the fusion procedure could be used as a source of cells to treat the adjacent disc. However, this would imply an intervention at an asymptomatic nondegenerated disc that only has the potential to degenerate in the future and is therefore rather questionable. Thus, at this time, autologous disc cell transplantation is limited to a few clinical scenarios but has the potential to prove to be a powerful approach within these limitations.

The most direct approach to support a degenerated disc by autologous cells would be injecting a suspension of ex vivo proliferated disc cells.[20] An approach to prepare autologous disc cells for subsequent transplantation into the degenerated disc is the cultivation of the disc cells in three-dimensional cultivation systems. Initial experiments by Maldonado and associates[21] demonstrated that cultivation of disc cells in three-dimensional constructs conserved the native phenotype, as demonstrated by the synthesis of matrix components similar to those observed in native discs. Since then, a wide variety of techniques have been recently applied to supply disc cells with the desired three-dimensional contructs.[22] Experimental strategies whose feasibility has been tested in vivo in animal experiments have also been undertaken. Gruber and colleagues,[23] in a study utilizing a sand rat–based model, applied autologous disc cells, expanded in routine monolayer cultures and seeded into a three-dimensional scaffold, to a hollowed cavity created in an intervertebral disc. After up to 33 weeks, no giant cell response was observed and the cells showed an appropriate morphology. In addition, no abnormality in the cell-surrounding matrix was observed, suggesting appropriate survival of the implanted cells during the analyzed time period. From their data the authors concluded that autologous disc cell implantation can be successful, although technically challenging. However, because of the immediate implantation after the seeding of the scaffold, the

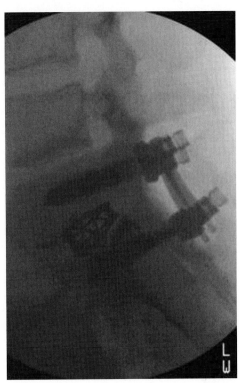

■ **FIGURE 63-8**  Lateral plain x-ray demonstrating adjacent level loss of disc height and degenerative changes at L4-L5 status post instrumented posterior lumbar interbody fusion at L5-S1.

disc cells do not have the time to synthesize appropriate amounts of matrix before encountering the adverse environment within the disc. Cultivation of the disc cells in a three-dimensional system before implantation might, therefore, improve the chances for survival in the hostile environment of the degenerated disc. Sato and coworkers[24] evaluated this approach by utilizing a nonimmunogenic atelocollagen scaffold to seed and cultivate annulus fibrosus cells. This process demonstrated an increased ability to express type II collagen mRNA and deposited more type II collagen and proteoglycan compared to cells grown in monolayers. Atelocollagen scaffolds seeded with annulus fibrosus cells have been allografted into the lacunae of recipient rabbits after laser diskectomy of the nucleus pulposus. Implantation resulted in a significant prevention of the narrowing of the intervertebral disc space up to 12 weeks postoperative compared to the nucleotomized control animals. Histological analysis also showed that the allografted cells were viable, proliferated, and produced a hyaline-like matrix in the disc tissue of the recipients. Although the rabbit model does not appropriately simulate the mechanical forces experienced by implanted disc cell in human discs, it is conceivable that cells surrounded by their own matrix might withstand mechanical forces with more success. That being said, another problem not addressed by the presented studies is the acute shortage of nutrients experienced by the cells after implantation into the degenerated disc. Considering that the nutrient supply is hardly sufficient for the original disc cells, it is questionable if the additional cells will survive for the prolonged time span likely required to provide a sustained structural improvement of the disc.

## Implantation of Mesenchymal Stem Cells

Adult mesenchymal stem cells (MSCs) are uncommitted pluripotent stem cells that are found in several tissues, such as skeletal muscle, bone marrow, synovial membranes, and the dermis.[25,26] Mesenchymal stem cells are of high plasticity and have a high capacity of multilineage differentiation. Members of the BMP family of growth factors have been used thus far to induce differentiation of mesenchymal stem cells into chondrocytes.[27] However, since BMPs are not exclusively inducing cartilage differentiation, its expression needs to be carefully timed and modulated to prevent the subsequent generation of bone structures. To overcome this problem, signal transduction and transcription factors, such as members of the Sox family as well as the Brachyury factor, that exclusively induce cartilage differentiation have been tested and demonstrated with encouraging results.[28,29] It has been found that cocultivation of MSCs with disc cells might be sufficient to induce a disc cell–like phenotype in MSCs.[30,31] Although these data originate from in vitro experiments, it might be conceivable that MSCs would also differentiate in vivo after injection into the disc. Besides the cocultivation with disc cells, cultivating of mesenchymal stem cells in three-dimensional cultivating systems appears to be sufficient to induce a nucleus pulposus–like phenotype.[32] Implantation of collagen gel–embedded mesenchymal stem cells into artificially degenerated rabbit discs resulted in preserved nuclear and annular structures, prevention of proteoglycan decrease from the nucleus pulposus, and increased disc height.[33,34] The implanted cells were shown to survive and express genetic markers typical for nucleus pulposus cells. Similar results were also found after injection of a bone-derived MSC suspension into rabbit discs and injection of gel embedded MSCs into rat coccygeal discs.[35,36]

The use of mesenchymal stem cells provides a new and exciting approach to biologically treat disc degeneration with encouraging results thus far. The comparably easy access to autologous mesenchymal stem cells allows overcoming one of the major culprits of conventional approaches. The high expandability of MSCs together with the relative ease of harvesting the cells makes this approach highly attractive. However, continued and extended studies are required to assess the structure of the newly synthesized matrix with regard to biomechanical properties and prove its value under the mechanical loads the functioning spine must bear.

## CONCLUSIONS

The mechanics of human gait confer constant and multiplanar loads to the IVD. The progressive structural alterations to the IVD that occur in continuum with spine segmental degeneration are not benign. The functions of the disc require a mechanically stable structure with a highly specialized matrix to confer the needed flexibility and physical strength to the spine. The known avascularity of the adult IVD restricts nutrient supply to diffusion and therefore poses a major challenge for the prolonged maintenance of the diskal matrix by its cellular components. The aforementioned mechanical stressors combined with the known inadequate nutrition eventually creates a toxic environment, resulting in progressive destruction of the matrix cellular structure and simultaneous extensive decay of the matrix. These properties and its alterations during degeneration define and limit the techniques applicable to biologically repair degenerated IVD and create patient cures. This might indicate that the clinical application of intradiscal biologics to regenerate the structurally compromised IVD is in the distant future. Recent studies looking at various biological approaches to maintain and improve the structurally compromised IVD provide real leads into the exciting potentials of these novel treatments. Further basic science and clinical experiments both in vivo and in vitro are required to bridge the gap between scientific potential and clinical realities.

## References

1. W.H. Kirkaldy-Willis, J.H. Wedge K. Yong-Hing et al., Pathology and pathogenesis of lumbar spondylosis and stenosis, Spine 3(4) (1978) 319–328.
2. H.E. Gruber, E.N. Hanley Jr., Analysis of aging and degeneration of the human intervertebral disc. Comparison of surgical specimens with normal controls, Spine 23 (1998) 751–757.
3. W.E. Johnson, H. Evans, J. Menage, S.M. Eisenstein, A. El Haj, S. Roberts, Immunohistochemical detection of Schwann cells in innervated and vascularized human intervertebral discs, Spine 26 (2001) 2550–2557.
4. H.A. Horner, J.P. Urban, 2001 Volvo Award Winner in basic science studies: effect of nutrient supply on the viability of cells from the nucleus pulposus of the intervertebral disc, Spine 26 (2001) 2543–2549.
5. H.S. An, E.J. Thonar, K. Masuda, Biological repair of intervertebral disc, Spine 28 (2003) S86–S92.
6. K. Masuda, Y. Imai, M. Okuma, et al., Osteogenic protein-1 injection into a degenerated disc induces the restoration of disc height and structural changes in the rabbit anular puncture, Spine 31 (7) (2006 Apr 1) 742–754.

7. H.S. An, K. Takegami, H. Kamada, C.M. Nguyen, E.J. Thonar, K. Singh, G.B. Andersson, K. Masuda, Intradiscal administration of osteogenic protein-1 increases intervertebral disc height and proteoglycan content in the nucleus pulposus in normal adolescent rabbits, Spine 30 (2005) 25–31. discussion 31–22.
8. M. Kawakami, T. Masumoto, H. Hashizume, et al., Osteogenic protein-1 inhibits degeneration and pain-related behavior induced by chronically compressed nucleus pulposus in the rat, Spine 30 (17) (2005 Sep 1) 1933–1939.
9. S. Chubinskaya, M. Kawakami, L. Rappoport, et al., Anti-catabolic effect of OP-1 in chronically compressed intervertebral discs, J. Orthop. Res. Apr. 25 (4) (2007) 517–530.
10. K. Miyamoto, K. Masuda, J.G. Kim, et al., Intradiscal injections of osteogenic protein-1 restore the viscoelastic properties of degenerated intervertebral discs, Spine J. 6 (6) (2006 Nov-Dec) 692–703.
11. M. Kawakami, H. Hashizume, T. Matsumoto, et al., Safety of epidural administration of osteogenic protein-1: behavioral and macroscopic observation, Spine 32 (13) (2007 Jun 1) 1388–1393.
12. R.G. Klein, B.C. Eek, C.W. O'Neill, et al., Biochemical injection treatment for discogenic low back pain: a pilot study, Spine J. 3 (3) (2003) 220–226.
13. K. Masuda, T.R. Oegema Jr., H.S. An, Growth factors and treatment of intervertbral disc degenration, Spine 29 (2004) 2757–2769.
14. K. Nishida, L.G. Gilbertson, P.D. Robbins, C.H. Evans, J.D. Kang, Potential applications of gene therapy to the treatment of intervertebral disc disorders, Clin. Orthop. Relat. Res. 379 (Suppl) (2000) S234–S241.
15. C. Lattermann, W.M. Oxner, X. Xiao, et al., The adeno associated viral vector as a strategy for intradiscal gene transfer in immune competent and pre-exposed rabbits, Spine 30 (2005) 497–504.
16. S.T. Yoon, J.S. Park, K.S. Kim, et al., LMP-1 upregulates intervertebral disc cell production of proteoglycans and BMPs in vitro and in vivo, Spine 29 (2004) 2603–2611.
17. R. Paul, R.C. Haydon, H. Cheng, A. Ishikawa, N. Nenadovich, W. Jiang, L. Zhou, B. Breyer, T. Feng, P. Gupta, T.C. He, F.M. Phillips, Potential use of Sox9 gene therapy for intervertebral degenerative disc disease, Spine 28 (2003) 755–763.
18. S.H. Moon, K. Nishida, L. Gilbertson, et al., Biologic response of human intervertebral disc cell to gene therapy cocktail, In: International Society for the study of the Lumber Spine (ISSLS), San Francisco, CA, 2001.
19. C.J. Wallach, S. Sobajima, Y. Watanabe, J.S. Kim, H.I. Georgescu, P. Robbins, L.G. Gilbertson, J.D. Kang, Gene transfer of the catabolic inhibitor TIMP-1 increases measured proteoglycans in cells from degenerated human intervertebral discs, Spine 28 (2003) 2331–2337.
20. T.M. Ganey, H.J. Meisel, A potential role for cell-based therapeutics in the treatment of intervertebral disc herniation, Eur. Spine J. 11 (Suppl 2) (2002) S206–S214.
21. B.A. Maldonado, T.R. Oegema Jr., Initial characterization of the metabolism of intervertebral disc cells encapsulated in microspheres, J. Orthop. Res. 10 (1992) 677–690.
22. H.E. Gruber, E.N. Hanley Jr., Recent advances in disc cell biology, Spine 28 (2003) 186–193.
23. H.E. Gruber, T.L. Johnson, K. Leslie, J.A. Ingram, D. Martin, G. Hoelscher, D. Banks, L. Phieffer, G. Coldham, E.N. Hanley Jr., Autologous intervertebral disc cell implantation: a model using Psammomys obesus, the sand rat, Spine 27 (2002) 1626–1633.
24. M. Sato, T. Asazuma, M. Ishihara, T. Kikuchi, M. Kikuchi, K. Fujikawa, An experimental study of the regeneration of the intervertebral disc with an allograft of cultured annulus fibrosus cells using a tissue-engineering method, Spine 28 (2003) 548–553.
25. P. Bianco, P. Gehron Robey, Marrow stromal stem cells, J. Clin. Invest. 105 (2000) 1663–1668.
26. P. Bianco, M. Riminucci, S. Gronthos, P.G. Robey, Bone marrow stromal stem cells: nature, biology, and potential applications, Stem Cells 19 (2001) 180–192.
27. J.M. Mason, A.S. Breitbart, M. Barcia, D. Porti, R.G. Pergolizzi, D.A. Grande, Cartilage and bone regeneration using gene-enhanced tissue engineering, Clin. Orthop. Relat. Res. 379 (Suppl) (2000) S171–S178.
28. H. Akiyama, M.C. Chaboissier, J.F. Martin, A. Schedl, B. de Crombrugghe, The transcription factor Sox9 has essential roles in successive steps of the chondrocyte differentiation pathway and is required for expression of Sox5 and Sox6, Genes. Dev. 16 (2002) 2813–2828.
29. A. Hoffmann, S. Czichos, C. Kaps, D. Bachner, H. Mayer, B.G. Kurkalli, Y. Zilberman, G. Turgeman, G. Pelled, G. Gross, D. Gazit, The T-box transcription factor Brachyury mediates cartilage development in mesenchymal stem cell line C3H10T1/2, J. Cell Sci. 115 (2002) 769–781.
30. S. Kim, C. Le Visage, K. Tateno, A. Sieber, J. Kostuik, K. Leong, Interaction of human mesenchymal stem cells with disc cells: changes in biosynthesis of extracellular matrix, Spine J. 2 (2002) 107S.
31. S.M. Richardson, R.V. Walker, S. Parker, N.P. Rhodes, J.A. Hunt, A.J. Freemont, J.A. Hoyland, Intervertebral disc cell mediated mesenchymal stem cell differentiation, Stem Cells 24 (2005) 707–716.
32. M.V. Risbud, M.W. Izzo, Cs Adams, et al., Mesenchymal stem cells respond to their microenvironment in vitro to assume nucleus pulposus-like phenotype, 2003. 30th Annual meeting: International Society for the Study of the Lumbar Spine (ISSLS), vancouver, canada.
33. D. Sakai, J. Mochida, T. Iwashina, A. Hiyama, H. Omi, M. Imai, T. Nakai, K. Ando, T. Hotta, Regenerative effects of transplanting mesenchymal stem cells embedded in atelocollagen to the degenerated intervertebral disc, Biomaterials 27 (2006) 335–345.
34. D. Sakai, J. Mochida, T. Iwashina, T. Watanabe, T. Nakai, K. Ando, T. Hotta, Differentiation of mesenchymal stem cells transplanted to a rabbit degenerative disc model: potential and limitations for stem cell therapy in disc regeneration, Spine 30 (2005) 2379–2387.
35. G. Crevensten, A.J. Walsh, D. Ananthakrishnan, et al., Intervertbral disc cell therapy for regeneration: mesenchymal stem cell implantation in rat intervertebral discs, Ann. Biomed. Eng. 32 (2004) 430–434.
36. Y.G. Zhang, X. Guo, P. Xu, et al., Bone mesenchymal stem cells transplanted into rabbit intervertebral discs can increase proteoglycans, Clin. Orthop. Relat. Res. 430 (2005) 219–226.

# PART 8

# The Future of the Aging Spine

# 64

# Endoscopic Surgical Pain Management in the Aging Spine

*Anthony T. Yeung, Christopher A. Yeung, and Christopher Meredith*

**KEY POINTS**

- The foraminal endoscopic surgical approach avoids the surgical morbidity of stripping the multifidus muscle.

- The foraminal approach is capable of intradiscal and epidural decompression under clear endoscopic visualization.

- The foraminal approach can be used to treat chronic common low back pain by denervating the nerves innervating the disc as well as the dorsal spinal column.

- Variations in foraminal normal anatomy and pathoanatomy, poorly understood by traditional surgeons, plays major role in chronic lumbar pain syndrome.

- Use of specialized miniaturized surgical tools, including the use of bipolar radiofrequency and laser, is an important and integral part of the endoscopic procedure.

## INTRODUCTION

The aging spine typically begins with disc degeneration and annular dehiscence, followed by transfer of loads from the anterior spinal column to the facets. This may produce discogenic pain and axial back pain, resulting in segmental instability with resultant deformity. If the condition becomes painful, and nonsurgical treatment is not effective, traditional surgical treatment has been limited to diskectomy and fusion. Though diskectomy has been shown to be beneficial by the SPORT[1] study, the long-term cost-effectiveness of fusion is questioned. Traditional spine surgery to treat painful degenerative disc disease such as with herniated discs, spondylolisthesis, central spinal stenosis, and neuroforaminal stenosis encompasses many different techniques. Surgical treatment, however, often results in a "failed back surgery syndrome" (FBSS) with limited success for subsequent salvage procedures. Newer minimally invasive techniques, in skilled and experienced hands, when approaching the pathology along natural muscle and tissue planes opens the door to earlier and a greater number of minimally invasive surgical options for the painful, aging spine without excessive concern about the paradoxical effects of surgery. The concept of "endoscopic surgical pain management" is addressed in this chapter, based on the senior author's (ATY) 20-year experience using his percutaneous endoscopic transforaminal surgical technique described as the YESS (Yeung Endoscopic Spine Surgery) procedure.

The YESS procedure eliminates the pain generator causing the pain syndrome, not just "masking" the pain with therapeutic injections. The approach accomplishes disc decompression by "selectively" removing degenerative nucleus, sealing and closing annular tears, decompressing spinal nerves, ablating nerves and inflammatory tissue contributing to discogenic and axial back pain, and surgically removing a wide spectrum of disc herniations. In more advanced stages, lumbar spondylolysis and isthmic and degenerative spondylolisthesis can also be addressed surgically. This brief overview provides examples of conditions that the senior author has treated endoscopically with minimal surgical morbidity, in contrast with the much more invasive traditional option. The reader is directed to the published references for more detailed information on the evolution of this new minimally invasive and innovative technique.[2-15]

Traditional surgical correction in the aging spine usually involves open decompression, fixation, and fusion techniques. The percentage of fusion surgeries for these conditions as a whole has increased dramatically in the United States over the past few decades. Between 1990 and 2001, lumbar fusion surgery increased 220%.[16] A recent article by Tosteson and colleagues,[17] examining the data from the SPORT trial, concluded that even for degenerative spondylolisthesis surgery (decompression and fusion) is not a cost-effective procedure, when examined over a 2-year period. The importance of this data is that it emphasizes the need to better identify the source of back pain and sciatica, possibly earlier treatment, and more thorough study of the complex innervations of the spine in the foramen (Figure 64-1A-C). This area, known as the "hidden zone" of MacNab, holds the answer to the effectiveness of foraminal decompression and ablation of foraminal nerves in the treatment of discogenic and facet pain. It may have an impact on health care reform that seeks to reduce the cost of care, because over 100 billion dollars a year is spent on back pain in the United States, most of it being spent on nonsurgical treatment such as physical therapy, interventional pain management, and over-the-counter and prescription drugs. We also need to reduce the need for fusion as a surgical solution for pain. This can be accomplished if we are able to not only demonstrate the efficacy and cost-effectiveness of endoscopic surgical pain management, but help establish a new subspecialty in endoscopic surgical pain management, because it requires special training to acquire proficiency.

Understanding chronic, surgically treatable back pain begins with understanding common lumbar pain. Cadaver microdissection of the nerves in the foramen reveals an extensive network of nerves arising from the spinal cord, splitting into the dorsal and ventral rami before exiting the foramen as the spinal nerve. A ramus communicans connects with the sinuvertebral nerves innervating the annulus. When there is an inflammatory response to annular tears with the development of an inflammatory membrane, the subsequent neo-neurogenesis and angiogenesis response contributes to pain that is not detected by imaging studies currently available. Better soft tissue imaging and imaging of chemical changes in the spine may help. We traditionally only grossly see the traversing and exiting spinal nerves as surgeons, and routinely fail to recognize and miss the relatively common furcal nerve, or the dorsal ramus and its medial and lateral branches that emanate from each spinal nerve. This network of nerves from the dorsal ramus contributes greatly to chronic discogenic and axial back pain not responsive to nonsurgical treatment. It is undetected by MRI or CT scan, but can be visualized endoscopically and confirmed by meticulous cadaver dissection (Figure 64-1B, C). Rational treatment calls for the appropriate and effective use of diagnostic and therapeutic diagnostic procedures such as diskography, selective nerve root blocks, foraminal

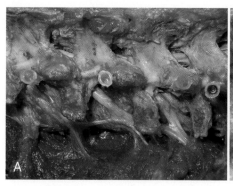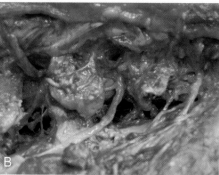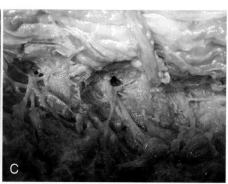

■ **FIGURE 64-1  A,** Fresh cadaver dissection of dorsal and foraminal anatomy showing the relationship of the disc annulus, spinal nerves, facets, and lamina dictating surgical access. Normal left foraminal anatomy L2-S1. Blue: hubbed needles are inserted into the disc space in the foramen accessing the posterolateral quadrant of the disk. Note the furcal nerve branch at L4-L5. The epidural space can be reached with a far lateral trajectory and/or by removing the ventral facet with trephines, lasers, or endoscopic high-speed diamond burrs. All soft tissue has been stripped from the transverse processes, including dorsal ramus innervation of the dorsal column. The intertransverse ligament covering the exiting nerves in the foramen has been stripped away. **B,** Facet innervation and the relationship of the transverse process, the interspinous ligament, and the exiting nerve in the foramen. The right exiting nerve at L3-L4 exhibits a furcal nerve branch traversing the foramen in the far lateral quadrant of the L3-L4 disc annulus. Furcal nerves are the myelinated branches of normal spinal nerves (usually the exiting nerve), commonly seen endoscopically in the foramen. When stimulated or cut, these nerves can cause dysesthesia and react like the parent spinal nerve. It does not respond like the main nerve because it is usually too small to be detected by continuous intraoperative electromyography or radicular pain reported by the patient. The endoscopic surgeon should take care to recognize and not injure these furcal nerves if they are more than 1 mm in diameter, but they cannot always be avoided. Dysesthesia, immediately postoperative or delayed, is readily treated by transforaminal epidural blocks combined with sympathetic blocks. Furcal nerves can be responsible for sciatica that is seemingly out of proportion to what is suggested by relatively normal MRI appearance, and may be part of the sciatica reported preoperatively. Note also the proximity of the intermediate and lateral branches of the dorsal ramus on the cephalic edge of the transverse process at L3. The dorsal ramus sends a medial branch that crosses the transverse process on the way to innervate the facet joint above and below the disc level. Irritation of the lateral branch, when irritated, can cause muscle spasm and an involuntary list. **C,** Dorsal ramus innovation of L3, L4, and L5 facets. The dorsal ramus emanating from the origin of the spinal nerve sends off medial, intermediate, and lateral branches to innervate the facets and the dorsal muscle column. The interspinous ligament has been removed to expose the dorsal ramus. It is found just ventral to the intertransverse ligament and can irritate the exiting nerve and its dorsal root ganglion. This poorly studied nerve can be responsible for severe chronic axial back pain associated with a degenerating disc exhibiting grade IV and V far lateral annular tears. Back pain, not just sciatica, caused by disc protrusions and annular tears can be explained by irritation of the dorsal ramus, not just the spinal nerves. Selective endoscopic diskectomy and thermal annuloplasty can reduce axial back pain and sciatica, and Intradiscal Electrothermic Therapy (IDET) cannot reach these nerves! Endoscopic rhizotomy of the branches of the dorsal ramus has shown to be a very effective means of decreasing chronic severe axial back pain.

epidural steroid blocks, facet and medial branch blocks, and sympathetic nerve blocks. Research studies, such as those by Carragee[18], that emphasize the risks and the difficulty of interpretation of diagnostic tests such as diskography without balancing the indications and usefulness of the diskography, does a disfavor to endoscopic minimally invasive surgeons who are able to look at pathoanatomy and are skilled at spinal endoscopy. This skill affords endoscopic surgeons the opportunity to treat lumbar pain and sciatica without fusion.

The politics and social-economic pressures of medicine create even more controversy as poorly qualified "experts" provide personal opinion on "standard of care" in medical-legal and insurance coverage disputes.

The information obtained from these diagnostic and therapeutic injection procedures allows the surgeon to more selectively pinpoint the pain source and to determine how to mitigate the source of pain.

## INDICATIONS AND CONTRAINDICATIONS

A widely accepted indication for foraminal endoscopic disc surgery is currently a foraminal or extraforaminal lumbar disc herniation. All sizes and types of herniations, however, are possible in the hands of a skilled and experienced endoscopic surgeon. Indications rely heavily on the skill and experience of the surgeon, as well as the patient's anatomy relative to the location of the herniation and the ability to access the herniation. Indications may also depend on injection and imaging studies to identify a painful condition of the disc. The painful condition is currently identified by preoperative diagnostic and therapeutic injections such as evocative chromodiskography, foraminal epidurography, therapeutic foraminal blocks, or selective nerve root blocks. Small disc herniations with sciatica, herniations with predominant back pain from the herniation, and annular tears that cause chemical sciatica that may be considered relative contraindications for traditional surgery because of the surgical risk-benefit ratio of the procedure, but may be an indication for foraminal endoscopic surgery. Any condition that obviously benefits from intradiscal therapy such as intradiscal debridement of diskitis is best performed percutaneous transforaminally. Contraindications are relative, dependent on percutaneous access to the

pathoanatomy and the interventionalist's experience. It is not unusual to find pathoanatomy, such as chronic granulation and inflammatory tissue in the disc or furcal nerves in the foramen, that is not apparent on preoperative imaging studies, but is clearly visualized endoscopically during foraminal endoscopic surgery.

## DESCRIPTION OF THE DEVICE

The design of the endoscope and endoscopic system is an important factor for endoscopic surgeons to consider. Techniques of endoscopic decompression vary depending on the endoscope design, the available surgical instruments, and surgical techniques practiced by the developer of the system. Not all endoscopic systems are designed for or amenable to the technique described here, but techniques and endoscopic systems continue to evolve. This chapter specifically describes the YESS transforaminal "inside-out-technique," utilizing the YESS foraminoscope (Figure 64-2) and the instruments designed for the system and technique. Not only is it important to have the necessary instruments, but specially configured cannulas are designed to expose the pathoanatomy to be surgically treated but, in the process, also protect vital anatomy such as the nerve and dura. Other systems are also evolving, so that in time, there will be similarities evolved and copied from the YESS transforaminal technique illustrated here.

## BACKGROUND OF SCIENTIFIC TESTING AND CLINICAL OUTCOMES

Peer-reviewed literature for disc herniation, first reported by Mayer and Brock[19] in 1993[3] then by Hermantin[2] in a prospective randomized study, has concluded that the results with transforaminal endoscopic (coined "arthroscopic" by Kambin[20]) diskectomy in the lumbar spine are generally similar to those with open diskectomy, but with significantly less surgical morbidity and quicker recovery (Table 64-1). The YESS technique evolved from the original Kambin technique as Yeung originally learned from Kambin. The procedure, done on an outpatient basis, utilizes local anesthesia with sedation. Patients are usually discharged an hour after surgery. Results show

PARTIAL INSTRUMENT SET FOR SELECTIVE ENDOSCOPIC DISCECTOMY (NOT TO SCALE)

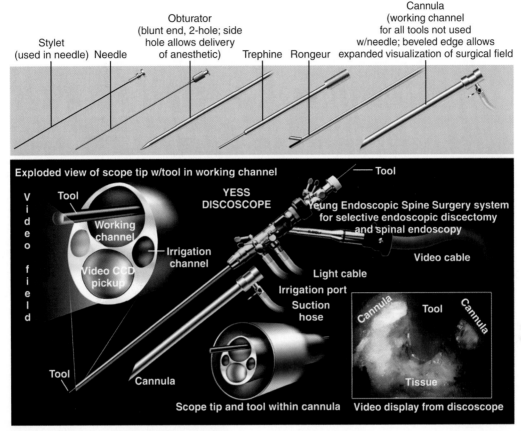

■ **FIGURE 64-2** Richard Wolf YESS Multichannel Operative Endoscope. The spinal endoscope is designed with an operative channel, multichannel irrigation for improved visualization, and a cannula system configured to enhance surgical access to pathoanatomy while protecting sensitive anatomy such as spinal nerves. *(Reprinted from Yeung CA, Hayes VM, Siddiqi FN, Yeung AT. Lumbar endoscopic posterolateral (transforaminal) approach. In Motion preservation surgery of the spine. Yue JJ, Bertagnoli R, McAfee PC, An HS (eds). Philadelphia, Saunders/Elsevier, 2008.)*

**TABLE 64-1** Microdiskectomy versus Endoscopic Diskectomy[*]

| | SURGICAL OUTCOME | |
| Level II-III Evidence | Group 1: Arthroscopic Microdiskectomy | Group 2: Microscopic Diskectomy |
| --- | --- | --- |
| Satisfactory outcome | 97% | 93% |
| "Very satisfied" | 73% | 67% |
| Disability | 27 days | 49 days |
| Narcotic use | 7 days | 25 days |
| Hospital stay | 0 day | 1 day |

From F.U. Hermantin ,T. Peters, L. Quartararo, et al. A prospective randomized study comparing the results of open discectomy with those of video-assisted arthroscopic microdiscectomy. Journal of Bone and Joint Surgery 81A ( 1999 ) 958 – 965.
[*]Sixty patients randomized, 30 per group.

that patients use less postoperative pain medication and return to work within 1 to 6 weeks. It is not unusual for individual patients to return to work in a matter of days. Long-term follow-up has demonstrated decreased recurrence (6%), less postlaminectomy syndrome, and greater patient satisfaction overall. Morganstern, a student of Yeung[21], has reported[6] that after a learning curve of approximately 70 patients utilizing the YESS technique for a wide spectrum of disc herniation types, a 90% overall good/excellent result by MacNab and modified MacNab criteria is achievable. The 90% standard was the goal established for endoscopic surgeons wishing to take up the procedure. The results for all types of herniated nucleus pulposus (HNP), through 2008, as reported in the literature are summarized in Table 64-2.

The YESS endoscopic transforaminal approach, described in this chapter, also addresses a wide spectrum of painful degenerative conditions of the lumbar spine. The results of highly selected patients for these painful conditions have been reported at national and international spine meetings, but the clinical results of endoscopic treatment contained and noncontained HNP studies were last reported in 2004. Over 3,000 cases recorded on an excel database ranging from 1- to 10-year follow-up using clinical standardized measurements such as visual analog scale (VAS), Oswestry Disability Index (ODI), SF 12 (lifestyle disability scale), and MacNab criteria are currently being collated independently for peer-reviewed publication.

The endoscopic foraminal approach, differentiated from the posterior approach, emphasizes the dilation along tissue planes without damage to normal anatomy. The foraminal approach for disc herniation utilizing the "inside-out-technique" provides easy access for central, paracentral, and subligamentous foraminal and extraforaminal disc herniations through natural tissue planes between the longissimus and psoas muscles (Figure 64-3). For foraminal and large paracentral herniations, it is easy to visualize the lateral edge of the traversing nerve (Figure 64-4) once the herniation is removed. If the fragment is large and extruded, it comes out as an intact collagenized fragment. Prodromal symptoms of disc herniation in the aging spine usually arise from annular tears, which cause recurrent back pain and sciatica before the disc herniates. The opportunity to study and treat painful annular tears endoscopically that do not heal naturally provides information on validating the theory of electrothermal therapy but also sheds light on the reasons why the usefulness of blind radiographic methods will always be limited. Identification of granulation tissue and nucleus material

**TABLE 64-2    Results of Arthroscopic Diskectomy\* versus Microdiskectomy**

| Author(s) | Number of Patients | Type of Treatment (Indications) | Mean Age (range) | Mean Follow-up (range) | Results MacNab Good/Excellent[†] |
|---|---|---|---|---|---|
| Mayer (1993) | 20 | Contained HNP Small protrusion Single | NR | NR | 80% |
| Kambin (1999) | 60 | Small protrusion Contained/extruded HNP | NR | NR | 97% |
| Yeung (2000) | 500 | All patient groups | 42 25-69 | NR | 86% |
| Lew/Mehalic (2001) | 49 | Far lateral HNP | NR | NR | 85% |
| Yeung (2001) | 307 | HNP—all types All patient groups | NR 18-72 | 23 NR | 84% |
| Tsou/Yeung (2002) | 219 | HNP with neurologic deficit | NR | NR | 93% |
| Ruetten (2005) | 463 | All HNP | NR | NR | 81% |
| Choi/Lee (2007) | 41 | Extraforaminal HNP | 58.7 32-74 | 34.1 NR | 92% |
| Ruetten (2008) | 178 | All HNP | 43 20-68 | NR 1-24 mo | 82% |
| Hoogland (2008) | 262 | Recurrent HNP | NR | NR | 86% |

\*Term coined by Kambin; later used generically to denote endoscopic foraminal diskectomy. ( P. Kambin, Arthroscopic microdiskectomy. Mt Sinai J Med 58(2) (1991) 159-64).
[†]MacNab criteria: Good—occasional back or leg pain not interfering with normal work or recreation; Excellent—no pain, no restriction of activity.

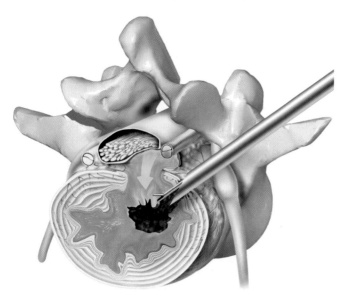

■ **FIGURE 64-3** Basic "Inside-Out-Technique" for Endoscopic Disc Decompression. Uniportal technique for selective endoscopic diskectomy. After introduction of a beveled cannula, endoscopic microrongeurs are used for visualized fragmentectomy. This is followed by use of specialized hinged rongeurs and straight and flexible shavers to remove the soft nucleus from the annular herniation defect. *(Reprinted from Yeung CA, Hayes VM, Siddiqi FN, Yeung AT. Lumbar endoscopic posterolateral (transforaminal) approach. In Motion preservation surgery of the spine. Yue JJ, Bertagnoli R, McAfee PC, An HS (eds). Philadelphia, Saunders/Elsevier, 2008.)*

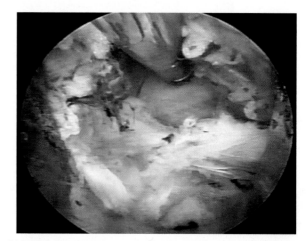

■ **FIGURE 64-4** Traversing Nerve after Removal of a Extruded Foraminal HNP. Indigo carmine dye stains the degenerative nucleus blue, helping the surgeon to selectively remove not only the extruded, sequestered disc herniation, but also the loose degenerative disc material, which could become the source of a recurrent herniation. Here, the decompressed traversing nerve is clearly visualized to confirm complete decompression of the herniation. Intraoperative or postoperative CT scan or MRI is not needed to confirm complete decompression of the spinal nerve when visual confirmation confirms successful removal of the herniation. The real-time extraction of the herniation fragment, followed by direct visualization of the decompressed nerve, confirmed by the conscious patient providing immediate feedback reporting immediate relief of leg pain, precludes the need for traditional evidence based medicine calling for a double-blind, randomized study to validate the selective endoscopic diskectomy technique or any visualized endoscopic technique designed to address the pathoanatomy.

in the annular layers (Figure 64-5A) provides a good prognosis for those tears treated with thermal annuloplasty. The nucleus material that weakens the annulus must be removed before the annulus is cauterized to close the tear. Using a biportal approach and a 70-degree scope, cauterization and confirmation of successful thermal annuloplasty under direct endoscopic visualization provide confirmation that the tear is closed and sealed (Figure 64-5B).

The technique for endoscopic foraminoplasty in more advanced disc degeneration and foraminal narrowing is associated with central and foraminal stenosis, not only for lateral recess stenosis but also for foraminal

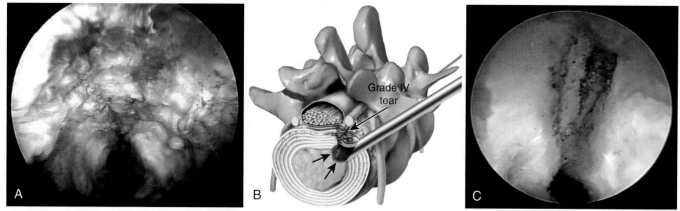

■ **FIGURE 64-5** Endoscopic Thermal Annuloplasty of Annular Tears. **A,** Painful annular tear identified endoscopically after intraoperative chromo-diskography confirms the presence of a grade IV annular tear with disc tissue embedded in the annular fibers. Tears that don't heal have imbedded disc material preventing the tear from healing naturally. The nucleus material must be removed from the annular layers before the results of thermal annuloplasty is predictable. This is the reason the surgical results of IDET is not predictable. Selective endoscopic diskectomy removes degenerative disc material as well as the nucleus embedded in the annulus. Endoscopic thermal annuloplasty follows. Tears vary in size, location, and type. One or two quadrant posterior and posterolateral tears in patients with 20% to 25% remaining annular thickness have good long-term results following endoscopic thermal annuloplasty. More extensive tears will also heal, but can tear again. Painful annular tears are best diagnosed with Evocative Chromo-Discography and confirmed by endoscopic visualization of the tear. Diskography performed by the surgeon evokes the pain, while the indigo carmine dye helps locate the tear. Granulation and inflammatory tissue are often found adjacent to the tear, and visual documentation of tear closure provides evidence of endoscopic thermal annuloplasty in the treatment of painful annular tears as a source of pain in the aging spine. **B,** Illustration of selective endoscopic diskectomy and thermal annuloplasty technique for a grade IV Tear. **C,** Grade III-IV annular tear cauterized and closed with bipolar radiofrequency thermal annuloplasty as viewed through a 70-degree scope. The prognosis for this tear is good because the tear is completely closed, and 20% to 24% of the annulus is still preserved after closing the tear.

decompression of the ventral facet in tall discs to gain "inside-out" access to sequestered herniations in the epidural space. A foraminoplasty cannula exposes the ventral aspect of the superior facet for endoscopic decompression (Figure 64-6A), which helps strip the capsule and define the undersurface of the facet to be removed with trephines and burrs (Figure 64-6B). Degenerative spondylolisthesis is often associated with disc protrusions and lateral stenosis, whereas sciatica from isthmic spondylolisthesis, due to the mechanical compression of the axilla and subarticular recess (Figure 64-6C), is effectively treated by endoscopic foraminal decompression in selected patients. These patients usually improve temporarily with foraminal diagnostic and therapeutic injections. Endoscopic decompression of the foramen can provide enough relief that the patient will avoid fusion. Failed back surgery syndrome (FBSS) patients with lateral recess stenosis and recurrent disc herniation also respond well. When the support is shifted posteriorly to the facet joints, synovitis and facet cysts may form. These cysts may impinge on the spinal nerves. Pedunculated cysts are sometimes visualized endoscopically, especially if the cyst wall is stained by indigo carmine or is visualized in the course of a diskectomy for chronic sciatica (Figure 64-7). Degenerative and isthmic spondylolisthesis (Figure 64-8A-D) can also be treated endoscopically with proper interventional injection workup. Impingement from the disc or superior facet of the inferior vertebra can be sorted out with diagnostic and therapeutic injections. If evocative diskography evokes concordant back pain and/or sciatica, and foraminal epiduralgrams and therapeutic injections provide information of the pathoanatomy, then careful preoperative planning will provide information on the likely outcome of foraminal decompression.

## CLINICAL PRESENTATION AND EVALUATION

The clinical presentation and evaluation for endoscopic decompression are the same as for the techniques used for traditional transcanal surgery. FBSS patients, however, represent a large and diverse group of spine surgery patients who have previously undergone spine surgery to treat back pain, yet they continue to suffer from back pain and sciatica after one or more spine surgeries. FBSS can be the result of an initial failure to recognize all of the pain generators, failure of the initial surgery (inadequate disc removal), recurrence of the original pathology (recurrent disc herniation), or progression of the underlying condition (lumbar spondylosis and facet arthrosis). The endoscopic applications outlined in this chapter are applicable to all of these conditions and often obviate the need for large instrumented fusions

or implants such as spinal cord stimulators. Preoperative evaluation incorporates correlation of the findings on imaging studies such as MRI, CT scan, diskography, and CT/diskography.

## OPERATIVE TECHNIQUE(S)

### Anesthesia

The procedure is carried out in an operating room. Local anesthesia using 0.5% to 1% lidocaine, supported by an anesthesiologist using fentanyl and midazolam (Versed), is all the anesthesia needed. Some surgeons and anesthesiologists are more comfortable with general anesthesia, and it is an acceptable standard of care to use general anesthesia, but there is greater chance of nerve injury from anatomic variations of the position of the exiting nerve and with anomalous nerves in the foramen, such as the furcal nerves. The patient's ability to feel pain during the procedure provides an additional safety factor for foraminal surgery.

### Position

The prone position is preferred because it provides a more intuitive for the surgeon and lends greater flexibility when using a biportal approach working inside the disc space. The biportal approach provides greater visual control of the flexible shavers and larger surgical instruments. A six-step protocol in standardizing optimal needle and instrument placement is extensively published, and not within the scope of this chapter.

### Procedure

The procedure and technique described are those preferred by the author. In every instance, diskography is an integral part of the technique. The diagnostic value of the subjective provocative response is valuable for confirming the disc as the source of the pain. Not only is evocative Chromo-Discography a clinical confirmatory test that links the suspected painful disc to the patient's subjective pain complaints, but the blue staining of the degenerated nucleus pulposus and annular defects, using the vital dye indigo carmine in 10% concentration, visually identifies normal and degenerative portions of the disc and annulus in contained or uncontained herniations. Contiguous disc fragments in the epidural space, disc tissue embedded in the annular defects, and herniation tracts are stained by the dye for targeted

## ENDOSCOPIC FORAMINAL-PLASTY

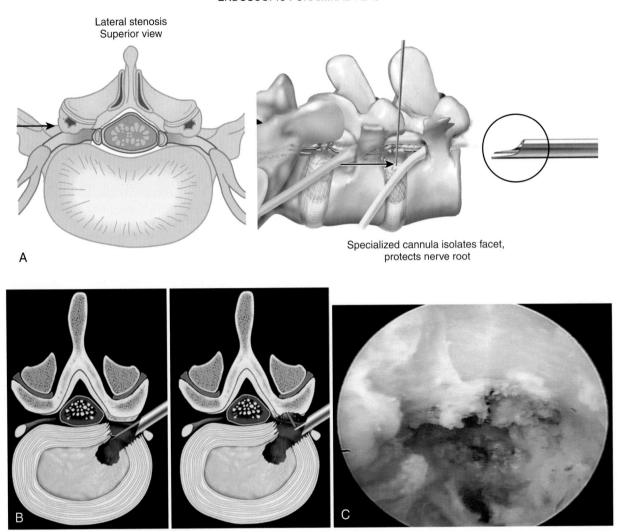

■ **FIGURE 64-6    A,** Endoscopic foraminal decompression. In more advanced aging, foraminal stenosis and osteophytosis can cause impingement of the spinal nerves. A specially configured cannula is placed under the facet for foraminal decompression. A side-firing laser is useful to strip the capsule from the facet; then a trephine and high-speed diamond burr are used to decompress the ventral portion of the facet to enlarge the foramen and elevate the foraminal window to gain access to the epidural space. The exiting nerve is then followed into the epidural space to decompress the axilla between the traversing and the exiting nerve. Decompression continues until the lateral edge of the traversing nerve is visualized or until fat is seen in the foramen. **B,** Foraminal decompression may be performed in conjunction with disc decompression or as a stand-alone procedure. Here, the illustration demonstrates the use of the holmium:yttrium-aluminum-garnet side-firing laser to strip the capsule from the ventral facet. More extensive decompression may be further performed with trephines, endoscopic Kerrison rongeurs, high-speed endoscopic burrs, or rasps. **C,** Decompressed exiting nerve for lateral recess stenosis. A high-speed diamond burr was used to complete the superior facet decompression to free the exiting nerve by stripping the facet capsule and removing 4 mm from the ventral surface of superior facet.

removal. Nonionic Isovue 300 contrast is used for radiographic visualization of the injectate. It is mixed with indigo carmine in a 10:1 ratio. In a nondegenerated disc, the roentgenographic contrast permeates the nucleus pulposus and forms a compact oval or bilobular nucleogram. There is no dye penetration into the substance of the normal impermeable annular collagen layers. Therefore the absence of an annulogram represents a normal annulus. In degenerated conditions, clefts, crevices, tears, and migrated fragments of nucleus will be filled with contrast both inside the disc and along the herniation tract.

A syringe is attached to the needle via an extension tube and the surgeon correlates the patient's response to the application of the injectate. Manual pressure, graded light, moderate, and high, is accurate enough to correlate the patient's response to the injection, thereby correctly used here the pain generated by the diskography process with the volume and pressure of the manual injection. This must also be correlated with the diskogram pattern. The literature promotes the use of a transducer to record the intradiscal pressures during the diskogram process. Surgeons who perform their own diskography, however, rapidly learn to correlate the findings with the

endoscopic pathoanatomy and become more proficient at patient selection. For patients with ambiguous clinical complaints, a preoperative diskography may help clarify the nature of the spinal problem. However, intraoperative diskography has the advantage of outlining the disc herniation as identified on the preoperative MRI study and assists the surgeon in removal of the disc. Ultimately the herniated disc material is extracted under endoscopic visualization.

The endoscopic approach uses a posterolateral approach, located typically 10 to 12 cm from the midline of the spine in a 160- to 180-pound patient, and uses an access cannula with 6- to 7-mm inner diameter and 7- to 8-mm outer diameter. It allows for the use of foramimal endoscopes with 2.8-, 3.1-, and 4.0-mm working channels that provide excellent, clear visualization of and access to the foraminal structures containing the disc and annulus, the epidural space, and ventral surface of the facet joint, including the pedicle and vertebral body. A combination of trephines, Kerrison rongeurs, high-speed drills, articulating graspers, flexible pituitary graspers, and various laser delivery systems can be used to ablate nerves, enlarge the neural foramen, remove facet and foraminal osteophytes, and decompress the spinal canal compressing neural structures without any destruction of the posterior spinal structures. Foraminal decompression is capable of treating a treating a wide variety of the pathologies discussed here. Its application potential in the elderly is virtually limitless, as it allows for outpatient and minimally invasive treatment of many spine disorders currently managed with either large, open surgeries or pain medications alone. The emergence of foraminal spinal endoscopy offers a bridge for treating many spinal ailments in patients who might not fare well with large open surgeries yet need something more than pain management.

## POSTOPERATIVE CARE

A postoperative lumbar corset will make the patient feel more comfortable. Before removal of the access cannula, routine use of depomedrol 80 mg delivered with 0.5% bupivacaine (Marcaine) (1-2 ml) will provide immediate postoperative analgesia; there have been no instances of infection from the use of steroids. The patient should be instructed to avoid bending, lifting, and twisting for 4 to 6 weeks to allow the annulus to heal and to reduce the incidence of recurrent disc herniation from the foraminal access portal and from an annular defect produced by the disc herniation. Physical therapy is not required but can be considered on an individual basis. Patients are instructed to use their pain as a guide to activity after the 6-week period.

## COMPLICATIONS AND AVOIDANCE

The risk of serious complications or injury is low—approximately 1% or less in the authors' experience. As with any surgery, there are the usual risks of infection, nerve injury, dural tears, bleeding, and scar tissue formation. Transient dysesthesia, the most common postoperative complaint, occurs in approximately 5% to 15% of cases and is almost always transient. Its cause remains incompletely understood, but a detailed study of foraminal anatomy reveals an extensive network of nerves that can be surgically irritated, even with the most careful use of surgical instruments. Dysesthesia may also be related to nerve recovery, operating adjacent to the dorsal root ganglion of the exiting nerve, or a small hematoma adjacent to the ganglion of the exiting nerve, because it can occur days or even weeks after surgery. There are also anomalous nerve fibers in the annular tissue, which may be furcal nerves or

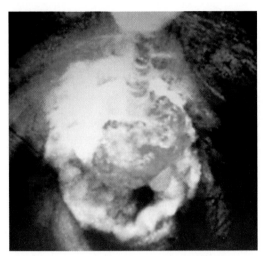

■ **FIGURE 64-7**  Pedunculated Synovial Cysts. Pedunculated cysts may be difficult to see on MRI because they may vary in size and are sometimes seen incidentally during foraminal surgery. It does not have to be located adjacent to the facet joint, because the cyst may be medial or lateral to the joint. Here the cyst, accompanied by a plexus of blood vessels, is found in the foramen compressing the exiting nerve. Usually a cyst is suspected from the finding of a bright signal adjacent to the facet capsule.

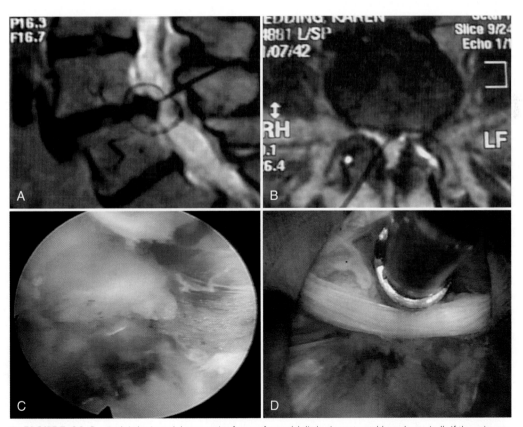

■ **FIGURE 64-8**  Both isthmic and degenerative forms of spondylolisthesis are treatable endoscopically if the pain generator can be demonstrated to come from the disc or foramen. **A,** Lateral MRI demonstrates a degenerative spondylolisthesis with a disc protrusion contributing to central stenosis. The disc can be decompressed endoscopically, but the risk of instability with further slippage is increased. **B,** There is foraminal stenosis causing sciatica. This patient had right sciatica, not left; good relief was obtained with a foraminal epidural block on the right. **C,** Endoscopic foraminoplasty identified impingement of the exiting nerve by the tip of the superior facet of the inferior vertebra. **D,** A furcal nerve was found in the foramen, possibly also contributing to the patient's sciatica. His sciatica resolved following foraminal endoscopic decompression.

## ADVANTAGES AND DISADVANTAGES

The visualization of conjoined nerves, furcal nerve branches, and anomalous anatomy such as sympathetic nerves may shed light on why current imaging studies cannot fully explain the reason(s) that some patients with identical imaging studies have debilitating pain and others do not. The advantages of endoscopic visualization of dorsal and foraminal pathoanatomy provide greater opportunity for surgical treatment. When the degenerative process creates conditions that are demonstrated to produce pain, ablation of nerves responsible for pain is a viable surgical procedure that causes very little surgical morbidity as compared to the traditional techniques such as fusion. These variations in normal anatomy and anomalous nerves in the foramen also present a new set of surgical risks to the endoscopic surgeon. Irritation or surgical injury to these sensitive nerves, often unavoidable, is considered a risk that is fortunately very small compared with the benefit of pain relief.

nerves growing into an inflammatory membrane in the area of the foramen that is not the traversing or exiting nerve. It could show up in the surgical specimen without permanent effect on the patient, but may cause temporary dysesthesia. Using blunt techniques to dilate the annular fibers has limited surgical morbidity and the excisional biopsy of tissues (anomalous nerves) caused by neo-neurogenesis and angiogenesis from the surgical specimen, but dysesthesia cannot be avoided completely, because it has occurred even when there were no adverse intraoperative events and in cases in which the continuous electromyography (EMG) and somatosensory evoked potentials (SEP) did not show any nerve irritation. The symptoms are sometimes so minimal that most endoscopic surgeons do not report it as a "complication." The more severe dysesthetic symptoms are similar to a variant of complex regional pain syndrome, but usually less severe, and without the skin changes. Postoperative dysesthesia is treated with transforaminal epidurals, sympathetic blocks, and the off-label use of pregabalin 150 mg/day or gabapentin titrated to as much as 1800 to 3200 mg/day. Gabapentin is approved by the U.S. Food and Drug Administration (FDA) for postherpetic neuralgia, but is effective in the treatment of neuropathic pain. The close proximity of sympathetic nerves and their role in disc innervation is still poorly understood, but treatment of dysesthesia by blocking the sympathetic trunk has produced dramatic results, especially when provided early in the course of postoperative dysesthesia.

Avoidance of complications is enhanced by the ability to visualize normal and pathoanatomy clearly, as well as through the use of local anesthesia and conscious sedation rather than general or spinal anesthesia. Adopting the "inside-out-technique" will give the surgeon more leeway in planning the surgical approach, since direct targeting to the herniation based on imaging studies may provide some "surprises" when visualization is not as clear as anticipated because of bleeding, and the herniation turns out to be more than a simple herniation not appreciated by the imaging study. Staying inside the disc space or returning to the disc space when visualization is obscured to reorient the surgeon is an important factor to consider. In experienced hands, some surgeons have safely utilized general anesthesia when circumstances make it safer for the patient. With use of a local anesthetic, the patient usually remains comfortable during the entire procedure, with the exception of periods such as during Evocative Chromo-Discography annular fenestration, or when instruments are manipulated past the exiting nerve. Local anesthesia of 0.50% lidocaine permits generous use of this diluted anesthetic for pain control but allows the patient to feel pain when the nerve root is manipulated. Nerves can also be adherent to the annulus or nucleus. Pain experienced by the patient is very helpful to the surgeon when probing or operating in the foramen, as it permits documentation or release of these adhesions before removing the herniation.

## CONCLUSIONS AND DISCUSSION

In summary, endoscopic posterolateral lumbar diskectomy and foraminal decompression provides a visualized method for minimal access to the disc and epidural space that avoids surgical morbidity to the dorsal muscle column. This endoscopic approach also allows for the visualization of foraminal and intradiscal pathology that is not appreciated by the traditional approach. Inflammation pays a major role in pain production.

The correlation of these conditions and findings with pain generation may open the door to a better understanding of the degenerative process causing lumbar disc herniations, and our concept of surgical intervention that encourages patient selection for earlier intervention may evolve as well. Following foraminal diskectomy and decompression, the traversing nerve, exiting nerve, axilla, and epidural space are all able to be probed and visualized. It is not always necessary to directly visualize all structures if there is good indirect evidence that the painful structure is being appropriately addressed; an example is decompression of a central disc herniation by visualizing the annulus and annular tears with an intradiscal view of the annulus. Patients can also provide confirmation that their leg pain is gone when undergoing surgery under conscious sedation. A closer study of posterior column and facet innervation will also open the door for endoscopic nerve ablation techniques that can be used for axial back pain.

In this area of health care reform, identifying the pain generator early, and treating it with a minimally invasive technique with surgical pain management, may lead to cost savings by decreasing our dependence on drug usage for chronic pain, and large expensive destructive surgery spine surgery such as fusion. Any technology to help surgeons attain proficiency through surgical training simulators or improved imaging capability, preoperatively or intraoperatively, should be part of the equation in health care reform.

## References

1. J.N. Weinstein, T.D. Tosteson, J.D. Lurie, A.N. Tosteson, B. Hanscom, J.S. Skinner, et al., Surgical vs nonoperative treatment for lumbar disc herniation: the Spine Patient Outcomes Research Trial (SPORT): a randomized trial, JAMA 296 (2006) 2441–2450.
2. F.U. Hermantin, T. Peters, L. Quartararo, P. Kambin, A prospective, randomized study comparing the results of open discectomy with those of video-assisted arthroscopic microdiscectomy, Journal of Bone and Joint Surgery 81A (1999) 958–965.
3. A.T. Yeung, Minimally invasive disc surgery with the Yeung Endoscopic Spine System (YESS), Surg. Technol. Int. VIII (2000) 267–277.
4. A.T. Yeung, P.M. Tsou, Posterolateral endoscopic excision for lumbar disc herniation: surgical technique, outcome, and complications in 307 consecutive cases, Spine 27 (2002) 722–731.
5. P.M. Tsou, A.T. Yeung, Transforaminal endoscopic decompression for radiculopathy secondary to intra-canal non-contained lumbar disc herniations: outcome and technique, Spine J. 2 (2002) 41–48.
6. A.T. Yeung, C.A. Yeung, Advances in endoscopic disc and spine surgery: foraminal approach, Surg. Technol. Int. XI (2003) 253–261.
7. P.M. Tsou, C.A. Yeung, A.T. Yeung, "Selective endoscopic discectomy™ and thermal annuloplasty for chronic lumbar discogenic pain: a minimal access visualized intradiscal procedure", Spine J. 2 (2004) 563–574.
8. A.T. Yeung, M.H. Savitz, L.T. Khoo, et al., Complications of minimally invasive spinal procedures and surgery Part IV: percutaneous and intradiscal techniques, in: A.R. Vacarro, J.J. Regan, A.H. Crawford (Eds.), Complications of pediatric and adult spinal surgery, Marcel Dekker, New York, 2004, pp. 547–571.
9. A.T. Yeung, C.A. Yeung, Percutaneous foraminal surgery: the YESS technique, in: D. Kim, R. Fessler, J. Regan (Eds.), Endoscopic spine surgery and instrumentation, Thieme, New York, 2005.
10. A.T. Yeung, C.A. Yeung, In vivo endoscopic visualization of patho-anatomy in painful degenerative conditions of the lumbar spine, Surg. Technol. Int. XV (2006) 243–256.
11. A.T. Yeung, C.A. Yeung, Microtherapy in low back pain, in: H.M. Mayer (Ed.), Minimally invasive spine surgery, second ed., Springer Verlag, Berlin Heidelberg, 2006, pp. 267–277.
12. C. Kauffman, C.A. Yeung, A.T. Yeung, Percutaneous lumbar surgery, in: Rothman Simeone, H.N. Herkowitz, S.R. Garfin, F.J. Eismont, G.R. Bell, M.D. Balderston (Eds.), The spine, 5th edition, Elsevier/ Mosby Saunders, Philadelphia, 2006.
13. A.T. Yeung, Incorporating adjunctive minimally invasive surgical technologies in endoscopic foraminal surgery: one surgeon's experience with endoscopic treatment of painful degenerative conditions of the lumbar spine, SAS J. 2007.
14. A.T. Yeung, C.A. Yeung, Minimally invasive techniques in the management of lumbar disc herniation, Orthop. Clin. North Am. 38 (3) (2007) 363–372.
15. A. Yeung, C.A. Yeung, Arthroscopic lumbar discectomy, in: advanced reconstruction: spine, American Academy of Orthopedic surgeon publication, Chicago, Illinois Publication Project 2009 (in Press)
16. B.I. Martin, S.K. Mirza, B.A. Comstock, et al., Reoperation rates following lumbar spine surgery and the influence of spinal fusion procedures, Spine 32 (3) (2007) 382–387.
17. A.N.A. Tosteson, J.D. Lurie, T.D. Tosteson, et al., Surgical treatment of spinal stenosis with and without degenerative spondylolisthesis, Annals of Internal Medicine 149 (12) (2008) 845–854.
18. E.J. Caragee, Is Lumbar discography a determinate of discogenic low back: Provocative discography reconsidered: current Pain and Headache Reports 4 (2007) 301–308
19. H.M. Mayer, M. Brock, Percutaneous endoscopic lumbar discectomy (PELD), Neurosurg Rev 16 (2) (1993) 115–120.
20. P. Kambin, Nass, Arthroscopic Microdiscectomy, Spine Journal 3 (Suppl. 3) (2003) 60S–64S. (Review).
21. P.M. Tsou, A.T. Yeung, Transforaminal endoscopic decompression for radiculopathy secondary to intracanal noncontained lumbar disc herniations: outcome and technique, Spine Journal 2 (1) (2002) 41–48.
22. P. Kambin, Arthroscopic microdiskectomy, Mt Sinai J Med 58 (2) (1991) 159–164

# 65

# Dorsal Endoscopic Rhizotomy for Chronic Nondiscogenic Axial Low Back Pain

*Anthony T. Yeung, Yinggang Zheng, and Christopher A. Yeung*

### KEY POINTS

- The dorsal ramus branches off the origin of the spinal nerve and sends off medial, intermediate, and lateral branches to innervate the facet joint and the tissues surrounding the facet.
- The medial branch, going to the facet joint at the level of the transverse process and one level below, is usually protected by periosteal tissue or an osseous tunnel as it crosses the transverse process to innervate the facet joint of two spinal segments.
- Dorsal endoscopic rhizotomy is more surgically effective than percutaneous electrode radiofrequency for ablation of the nerves innervating the dorsal column.
- Visualization of the medial, intermediate, and lateral branches of the dorsal ramus provides direct surgical confirmation of nerve ablation.
- The results of a prospective nonrandomized study concluded that endoscopic rhizotomy is a safe and effective technique to treat chronic, facet-mediated axial back pain.

## INTRODUCTION

Traditional treatment of low back pain from an aging spine encompasses many techniques. When surgery is contemplated, diskectomy, laminectomy, and fusion are the most common surgical procedures utilized. Diskectomy, the most common surgical procedure for sciatica and back pain, may exacerbate the back pain, especially when there is concomitant spinal instability. Chronic back pain may therefore be a consequence following surgical diskectomy. Natural progression of the degenerative process also results in lumbar spondylosis, facet arthrosis, spinal stenosis, and spondylolisthesis in the time line of an aging spine, which may also be the source of pain generation. The costs of surgical procedures to correct these conditions vary widely, depending on the surgical procedures chosen and implemented by the surgeon. Fusion, the traditional procedure for back pain, is usually recommended with caution because of its surgical morbidity and high cost. Failed back surgery syndrome (FBSS), with a paucity of effective salvage procedures, then result when surgical treatment fails. One recent study by Katz[1] estimated that the annual costs associated with all treatments of back pain in the United States are over $100 billion. This cost estimate does not even consider the difficult-to-calculate economic loss due to loss of productivity from disabling low back pain. Back surgeries to relieve back pain, however, continue to steadily increase in the United States, partly because of expansion of surgical techniques and implants used to facilitate fusion. Hazard[2] documented an increase in these numbers from 300,413 in 1994 to 392,948 in 2000. Though the majority of these surgeries are successful in relieving back pain, a significant percentage is not. Some studies estimate that, at best, only 60% of these surgeries are successful.[3,4] These data, along with the data reported in the Spine Outcomes Research Trial (SPORT),[5] demonstrate that although most spine surgeries are cost-effective, even the 2-year results for degenerative spondylolisthesis, the premier indication for one-level fusion, is questioned. With good patient selection, accurate diagnostic criteria, and a low cost, a minimally invasive surgical option, addressing just the innervation of the facet-mediated pain generator, may be a viable minimally invasive procedure to be considered before the definitive surgical fusion or joint replacement option is considered.

The Yeung Endoscopic Spine Surgery (YESS) decompressive approach, described in Chapter 64, details a transforaminal endoscopic approach that utilizes a minimally invasive surgical technique enabling disc and foraminal decompression as well as ablation of painful nerves and removal of chemical mediators in the disc, annulus, and foramen. Presumed primary sensory nerves innervating the disc and facet can be ablated, and pathologic conditions causing inflammation (and, therefore, pain) are addressed. The technique, expanded to target denervation of the branches of the dorsal ramus responsible for facet mediated pain, is the subject of this chapter.

Lumbar spondylolysis, facet arthrosis, spondylolisthesis, both isthmic and degenerative, that may also be associated with spinal stenosis, are traditionally treated with open decompression, dynamic stabilization, or fusion. A recent article by Weinstein et al,[5] examining the data from the SPORT trial, concluded that degenerative spondylolisthesis surgery (decompression and fusion) is not a cost-effective procedure when examined over a 2-year period. These data highlight the need to better evaluate back pain patients with more specific diagnostic procedures, such as evocative diskography, selective nerve root blocks, foraminal epidural steroids, and facet and medial branch blocks. The information obtained from these procedures in experienced hands allows the surgeon to more selectively choose who might benefit from surgical intervention. Many of the pain generators can also be addressed earlier in the disease process if surgery does not cause significant paradoxical effect on the aging spine. In this chapter we outline a technique for performing endoscopic medial, intermediate, and lateral branch rhizotomy arising from the dorsal ramus, a sensory branch from the origin of the main spinal nerve, that we have termed, dorsal endoscopic rhizotomy.

The endoscopic applications outlined in this chapter are therefore applicable to all painful conditions arising from the facet joint complex.

## INDICATIONS AND CONTRAINDICATIONS

Endoscopic rhizotomy has been performed successfully, and remains effective at over 3-year follow-up in most patients in our pilot study. It is appropriate for the following conditions causing axial back pain.

### Ideal Indications

Patients who will most likely benefit from selective endoscopic rhizotomy include the following:

1. Axial back pain solely from arthropathy of the lumbar facet joints without leg pain: The diagnostic imaging of these patients may present with

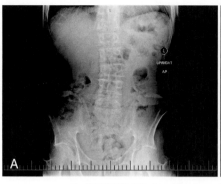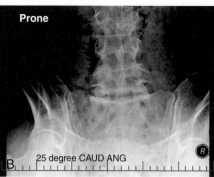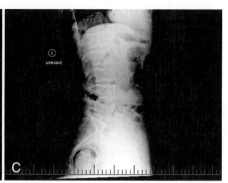

■ **FIGURE 65-1a, 1b, 1c**     Ideal patient with single level facet arthrosis and chronic, non-debilitating axial back pain.

narrowing disc space, but the discogenic contribution to back pain is thought to be a minor contributor. These patients are usually not debilitated, but the patients' pain significantly affects their activities of daily living (Figure 65-1A-C).
2. Axial back pain mostly from facet arthrosis with very mild buttock and thigh pain: Pain is approximately 90% in the back and 10% in the leg.
3. Subacute and chronic axial back pain following a posttraumatic injury to the facet joints refractory to nonsurgical treatment.
4. Axial back pain from adjacent disc level of fusion demonstrating spondylosis and facet arthrosis causing pain without disc segment instability.
5. All of the previously mentioned patients should have more than 80% pain relief after controlled diagnostic and therapeutic medial branch block (MBB).

## Relative Indications

Patients in the following categories should expect only partial relief of axial back pain from dorsal ramus rhizotomy:

1. Axial back pain associated with mild buttock pain and leg pain: In general, back pain is about 50% to 80% and leg pain is 20% to 50%, with pain coming from the facet as well as the disc.
2. Axial back pain from facet is 50% with leg pain 50% in general: Patients received previous benefit from medial branch block, plus transforaminal epidural block. The patient has a strong desire for relief of axial back pain more permanently with a minimally invasive procedure, while intermittent sciatica is tolerable.
3. Patient has axial back pain, 40% to 50%, and leg pain, 50% to 60%, with stenosis and instability indicated for surgical decompression and fusion, but the patient elects a less invasive staged procedure or whose medical condition does not allow for higher-risk surgical procedure. The patient would be satisfied to have a decreased pain level and partially improve the quality of life, in addition to reduced pain medication dose. These patients, indicated for fusion, should not have high expectation with dorsal endoscopic rhizotomy.
4. FBSS without pseudarthrosis and gross deformity presenting with axial back pain only and responding well to MBB.
5. Patient associated with mild and stable spondylolisthesis, but presenting with axial back pain of facet origin.
6. All of the previously mentioned categories of patients should have 50% to 80% pain relief after MBB before dorsal endoscopic rhizotomy. This group of patients should be very realistic about the anticipated pain relief.

## Patients with Poor Indications for Dorsal Ramus Rhizotomy

Patients with lumbosacral radiculopathy whose debilitating leg pain is greater than back pain:

1. Multiple-level disc disease with confirmed severe concordant discogenic pain by evocative diskography, and minimal relief with medial branch blocks

2. Significant motion segment instability or hypermobility
3. Pseudarthrosis following failed fusion
4. FBSS with more leg pain than back pain without known etiology
5. Patients with multiple debilitating painful conditions: severe multilevel stenosis including foraminal stenosis associated with scoliosis without good response to MBB
6. SI joint dysfunction
7. Severe osteoporosis, particularly with vertebral compression fracture
8. Severe depression, fibromyalgia, rheumatoid arthritis, and ankylosing spondylitis as well as autoimmune diseases
9. Drug dependency
10. Psychosocial problems and pending litigation
11. No benefit from MBB

Patients initially benefiting from dorsal endoscopic rhizotomy, who have recrudescence of some of their back pain, may have pain from progression of vertical load forces shifting to the facets, such as progressive degenerative scoliosis. These patients will have relief for 2 to 3 years before the effect of rhizotomy fails. Spinal pain, however, may also come from multiple causes and multiple anatomic structures in the spine. Certain conditions such as anomalous nerves in the foramen may not be detectable using currently available technology, but may be visualized endoscopically. For a structure to be implicated, it needs to be shown to be a source of pain from reliable diagnostic techniques. Endoscopic examination of the foramen during foraminal surgery, discussed in Chapter 64 on foraminal surgery for painful conditions of the lumbar spine, identifies some of these nerve structures and anomalies. The known structures responsible for pain in the spine include, but are not limited to, the vertebral bodies, intervertebral discs, nerve roots, facet joints, ligaments, muscles, and sacroiliac joints. Postlaminectomy syndrome (FBSS) following operative procedures may affect these structures, and, except for recurrent disc herniation or lateral recess stenosis, may not be surgically correctable. Contraindications for facet rhizotomy are pain syndromes not involving the facet joint in some way. Neural blockade or nerve block therapy, however, is a validated procedure that, when performed properly, can implicate the facet joint as responsible for spinal pain in up to 40% of patients with low back pain.[7] Patients with this condition usually have moderate to severe back pain that does not have a strong radicular component. Pain is aggravated by hyperextension of the spine, and may present with tenderness to palpation at the level of the suspected facet joint. Patient selection, therefore, depends more on the patient's response to proper administration of medial branch blocks rather than facet injections, because the procedure targets the nerve innervating the facet joint. Although x-ray, CT scan, and MRI findings of degenerative disc disease, lumbar spondylosis, and facet arthrosis are helpful in concluding that the facet is involved in axial back pain, the success of surgical ablation of the branches of the dorsal ramus is dependent on clear interpretation and effective resolution of axial back pain from medial branch blocks. Adding low-dose steroids (methylprednisolone [Depo-Medrol]) to longer-acting anesthetic agents such as 0.5% bupivacaine provides long enough relief of axial back pain to help make a clinical decision on the projected effectiveness of endoscopic rhizotomy. Patient selection for the procedure for the prospective study begun in 2006 was indicated for patients receiving at least 50% back pain relief, but the pilot study demonstrated endoscopic rhizotomy is most successful for those reporting 80% to 90% relief of their axial back pain following a medial branch block.

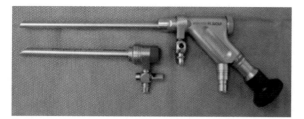

■ **FIGURE 65-2** Yeung Endoscopic Spine System (YESS) rhizotomy scope and cannula.

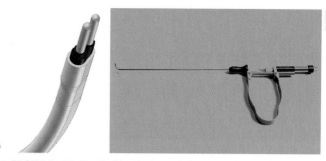

■ **FIGURE 65-3** Flexible Bipolar Radiofrequency Probes. *Left:* Probes designed for small nerve transection. (1.5- to 2-mm gap). *Right:* Standard Ellman Triggerflex (Elliquence, Inc.).

Contraindications are relative, since there may be limitations on the effects of nerve denervation. In patients with multiple or nonspecific pain generators such as myofascial pain syndrome, sacral iliac joint pain, or those with a soft tissue source of pain where no nerve root pathology exists, have less satisfactory results, even if there is a facet-component. Therefore, including these patients who also have facet-mediated pain may serve as relative contraindications. However, if the patient understands that the relief they get from facet rhizotomy is limited to the facet joint, then a satisfactory result can be obtained. The effect of facet denervation in the pain management literature cites pain relief lasting only 6 months to 1 year.[8,9] This is because current techniques of radiofrequency lesioning may not be complete. Dorsal endoscopic rhizotomy, however, was able to attain pain relief for this time frame more effectively, because the surgeon is able to confirm adequate ablation of a visualized nerve branch or the consistent location at least of the medial branch. Patients who fail to get relief from radiofrequency ablation have been shown to get significantly more relief following dorsal endoscopic rhizotomy. These patients may be offered dorsal endoscopic rhizotomy cautiously, because we assume that failure may be due to poor patient selection rather that technique failure. An ongoing continued review of A. Yeung's 2006 prospective pilot study (presentation made at the International Society for Minimally Invasive spine surgery in January 2007. Information not published.) reveals a majority of patients still experiencing continued relief since the inception of the study (up to 3 years). Because of multiple pain sources in patients with an aging spine, results of endoscopic rhizotomy are less predictable in patients who were only partially relieved of back pain obtained from the diagnostic blocks. Each injection should be individually evaluated for clinical efficacy. In patients with only very temporary pain relief, another trial block may be considered. Patients unable to stop taking their anticoagulants for stroke, transient ischemic attacks, and thrombophlebitis are at greater risk for surgical morbidity. These patients are operated on with caution, risking complications from bleeding at the surgical site. However, the ability to cauterize a small wound to control bleeding may make the contraindication a relative one.

## DESCRIPTION OF THE DEVICE

A YESS (Yeung Endoscopic Spine System) rhizotomy endoscope was developed with the Richard Wolf Surgical Instrument Company (Vernon Hills, Ill.) specifically for dorsal ramus rhizotomy. The length of the scope is designed to allow the endoscope to rest on the fluid adapter with a focal length that will keep the transverse process and the nerves in focus (Figure 65-2). The endoscope has two cannula configurations, a standard round cannula with a flat opening and a cannula with a beveled opening to allow flexible curved bipolar radiofrequency electrodes and side-firing lasers to exit the wall of the cannula for tissue coagulation and resection (Figure 65-3). Straight and side-firing lasers, in addition to two types of radiofrequency electrodes, are recommended because it is a more aggressive surgical tool for stripping the periosteum and soft tissue envelope that may shield the medial branch.

## BACKGROUND OF SCIENTIFIC TESTING AND CLINICAL OUTCOMES

Radiofrequency has been extensively used for ablation of the medial branch in treating facet joint pain for years. It has been reported that most patients only benefited from short term relief of pain.[8,9] It is also observed that recurrent axial pain from the same lesioned facet may be due to reinnervation by regrowth of nerves. For this assumption, repeat radiofrequency for

recurrence is common. Finding the exact location of the medial branch, however, is not only essential to ablate the nerve, but in our study, the medial branch was sometimes found to be buried in a periosteal tunnel up to several millimeters thick. Blind, even perfectly placed, thin wire electrodes may not be able to adequately ablate the nerve. Efforts have been made to improve the radiofrequency technique by needle position, making multiple lesions and using larger needles.[10] To continue this effort, the senior author (ATY) embarked on an endoscopic surgical technique in 2005 using the FDA-approved Vertebris 3.1-mm spine endoscope spine system for foraminal lumbar surgery. In the YESS system, bipolar radiofrequency flex probe and Ho:YAG laser are important surgical tools for tissue ablation and thermomodulation. It has been reported that percutaneous laser medial branch rhizotomy provided better and longer-lasting results than radiofrequency lesioning,[8,9] and this reasoning is confirmed by using the same tools in selective endoscopic rhizotomy. Derby and Lee[10] reported in 2006 that a more aggressive ablative process gives better results than traditional percutaneous techniques utilizing two needle electrodes during lumbar facet rhizotomy in an experimental model. The literature also supports multiple ablations with radiofrequency because it provided better results than a single lesion. A prospective study was initiated by the senior author in March 2006 before Dr. Linqiu Zhou reported his work on cryotherapy for dorsal ramus syndrome at the 19th International Intradiscal Therapy Meeting in April 2006. Dr Zhou was involved in the Chinese study of over 2630 patients that utilized a cryotherapy technique targeting the dorsal ramus to relieve pain from chronic muscle spasm, and upper lumbar back pain. The paper presented by Dr. Zhou and colleagues, titled "The Spinal Dorsal Ramus and Low Back Pain," presented evidence that anatomic dissections of the dorsal ramus at L1 and L2 extended two to three segmental levels below L2.[11]

A prospective, nonrandomized study was initiated by the senior author to determine whether the dorsal ramus, particularly the medial branch, could be visualized endoscopically, and whether endoscopic rhizotomy of the medial branch and visualized intermediate and lateral branches of the dorsal ramus would produce better results than conventional rhizotomy techniques. The pilot study of 50 consecutive patients was initiated in March, 2006, and was first reported at the 25th International Jubilee Course on Percutaneus Endoscopic Spine Surgery and Complementary Techniques at Zurich, Switzerland in January, 2007.[6] Inclusion criteria were lumbar degenerative conditions that resulted in facet pain from the aging spine or postoperative facet-mediated pain (Table 65-1). We primarily targeted the medial branch in the osseous tunnel with an endoscope and attempted to ablate it under visual control. This resulted in excellent axial pain relief in the vast majority of patients receiving endoscopic rhizotomy. There were no complications. When the nerve branch was traced to the dorsal ramus, it resulted in fenestration of the intertransverse ligament, bleeding, and painful feedback from the patient during the ablation process. Twitching muscles could also be felt by the surgeon. Temporary ache and mild dysesthesia were reported by the patients, but no patient was worse. Ultimately, 90% (45/50) of the patients still had relief at 6 months follow-up. Only five patients had recurrence of their back pain at 6 months. Aggressive ablation of the dorsal ramus or inadvertent penetration of the probe and cannula deep to the intertransverse ligament sometimes caused bleeding and temporary dysesthesia, This led to the use of indigo carmine dye to help guide the surgeon to stay dorsal to the ligament in pursuing the nerve. We

**TABLE 65-1   Inclusion Criteria of Pilot Study on Selective Endoscopic Rhizotomy**

**Pilot Study Inclusion Criteria: Endoscopic Medial Branch and Dorsal Ramus Rhizotomy**

- Mri evidence of facet arthrosis
- Failed or not satisfied with nonsurgical pain management
- At least 50% relief with medial branch blocks
- No psycho-social or litigation problems
- No workman's comp
- Includes patients with increased back pain subsequent to discectomy

**TABLE 65-2   Results of Prospective Nonrandomized Study**

**Prospective Non randomized Pilot Study**

Method:
Endoscopic medial branch And D.R.Rhizotomy
- 50 consecutive patients
- 2-9 month follow-up
- VAS
- Oswestry

Preliminary Early Results
- 45/50 (90%) still had relief at 6 month follow-up and were satisfied
- Ave VAS 6.2 to 2.5
- Ave Oswestry 48 to 28

therefore conclude that ablation of the dorsal ramus is not needed, even if potentially more effective in relieving back pain, because it may cause unacceptable unforeseen complications by ablation near the dorsal root ganglion. VAS and Oswestry scores were tabulated. VAS decreased from 6.2 to 2.5 and Oswestry from 48 to 28; 90% of patients had continued improvement at 6 months follow-up (Table 65-2). The extended study continues, and recent review of patient data by an independent reviewer and co-author (Y. Zheng) further confirmed the previous study results. In carefully selected ideal patients, satisfactory results were achieved in more than 90% patients without complications. These encouraging data and satisfactory feedback from patients motivated the authors to introduce this new minimally invasive endoscopic surgical technique.

## CLINICAL PRESENTATION AND EVALUATION

Patients who complain of chronic axial back pain are evaluated with x-rays and MRI or CT scan. A history is taken to rule out nonfacet sources of chronic back pain. After informed consent is discussed with the patient, the goals and expected results of selective endoscopic rhizotomy are understood, the patient is offered this surgery as an alternative to nonsurgical pain management or, sometimes, traditional surgical management consisting of decompression and stabilization.

## OPERATIVE TECHNIQUE

### Anesthesia

Surgery can be performed under local or monitored anesthetic care (MAC), obviating the need for general anesthesia. Most patients are sedated with fentanyl and midazolam (Versed), but some anesthesiologists choose to use propofol since the procedure is short and the patient is comfortable after the surgical site is anesthetized with 0.5% bupivacaine (Marcaine) with epinephrine.

Its application potential in the elderly is virtually limitless, especially since it allows for the outpatient and minimally invasive treatment of chronic back pain currently managed with either large, open surgeries or strictly with pain management and pain medications.

## Position

The patient is placed prone with the lumbar spine placed on a kyphotic frame with the back parallel to the floor. Reducing lumbar lordosis for the purpose of surgical access to the transverse process helps to prevent inadvertent penetration of surgical instruments into the foramen where the irritation of the dorsal root ganglion and exiting spinal nerve can cause surgical morbidity.

## Procedure

The procedure begins with needles placed on the transverse process just lateral to the facet in the muscle interval between the multifidus and longissimus muscle (Wiltse's paramedian approach). Isovue 300, mixed with 10% indigo carmine dye, is injected into the interval to help the surgeon identify the tissue plane endoscopically. Indigo carmine dye is used to mark the tissue planes and the level of the transverse process dorsal to the intertransverse ligament. At times dye can be seen leaking to the facet joint capsule or to the foramen, at times even outlining the location of the dorsal ramus if there is a breach of the foraminal ligament leading to the foramen. The endoscope is then inserted through the cannula and docked on the transverse process (Figure 65-4). The medial branch of the dorsal ramus is first targeted (Figure 65-5). It is not always visualized because the nerve is protected by a soft tissue envelope. However, when the nerve is identified crossing the transverse process, it is transected under direct vision, as is the lateral branch. A modification of the technique begins with wagging the blunt obturator to develop the tissue plane between the multifidus and longissimus muscle. This facilitates visualization of the lateral branch of the dorsal ramus, cephalad to the edge of the transverse process (Figure 65-6). If the nerve is not identified, all the soft tissues are stripped to the periosteum of the transverse process adjacent to the lateral facet, especially to the cephalad edge of the transverse process. In the first 50 patients of the prospective study, the nerves at the base of the transverse process were mainly targeted, while looking primarily for the medial branch. The intermediate and lateral branch was targeted when visualized. With the wagging maneuver, the intermediate and lateral branch was visualized more easily. After 100 patients, continued surgical experience and greater surgeon experience allowed for more aggressive dissection along the tissue plane between the multifidus and longissimus muscles to actively look for multiple lateral branches to ablate, sometimes following the branches to the dorsal ramus. Care, however, is taken to stay dorsal to the intertransverse ligament to avoid irritation of the exiting spinal nerve and the dorsal root ganglion in the foramen. Our cadaver dissections provided even more anatomic information on the complexity of facet innervation, especially from L3 cephalad (Figure 65-7). This finding, plus some anatomic dissections with demonstrating caudal connections of the dorsal ramus with segments below (Figure 65-8), provides evidence that rhizotomies of the dorsal ramus above the level of imaging involvement may have a role in the treatment of axial facet mediated pain. We do not, however, recommend routine ablation of the dorsal ramus because it is very benign to ablate the branches of the dorsal ramus at the involved spinal segment, and the risk of neuroma and spinal nerve injury is lessened significantly.

The medial branch of the dorsal ramus was more difficult to identify than the lateral or intermediate branches because it may be buried in thick periosteum or capsular tissue, but ablation of soft tissue to cortical bone assured ablation of the medial branch. The Ho:YAG laser (Trimedyne, Inc., Santa Ana, CA) was found to be the most effective surgical tool for ablation through thick collagenous tissue. If the procedure is modified to develop the plane between the multifidus and longissimus muscles, much like a dissection using Wiltse's approach to the transverse process for pedicle screw placement. It is easier to visualize the intermediate and lateral branches. The literature contains illustrations of the anatomy of the dorsal ramus and its branches at the transverse process (see Figure 65-4).

## POSTOPERATIVE CARE

The patient is sent home if his insurance allows endoscopic rhizotomy as an outpatient procedure; otherwise the surgery is performed in a hospital and the patient is admitted for overnight observation until the patient opts to go home. There is no postoperative treatment plan specific to rhizotomy. The patient is returned to his or her normal or desired activity level.

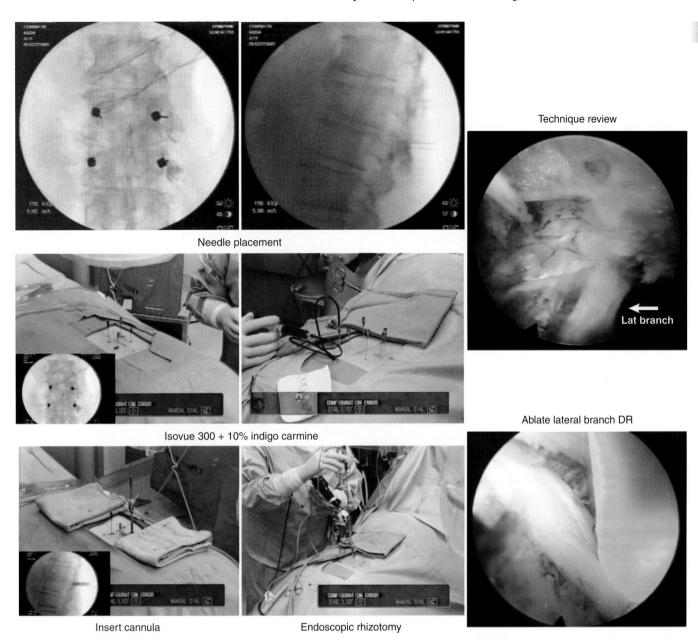

Technique review

Lat branch

Needle placement

Isovue 300 + 10% indigo carmine

Ablate lateral branch DR

Insert cannula                    Endoscopic rhizotomy

■ **FIGURE 65-4**    Selective endoscopic rhizotomy surgical technique.

## ADVANTAGES AND DISADVANTAGES

A visualized nerve ablation is more effective than the traditional blind percutaneous technique. The ability to ablate the medial branch will eliminate facet pain, and ablating the selected lateral branch that innervates the longissimus muscle and lateral soft tissues helps to decrease paravertebral muscle spasm. Because the lateral branches are multisegmental, ablation of the lateral branch has met with no clinically adverse symptoms. With the procedure being a new technique, the disadvantage may currently come from the limited availability of surgeon training and surgical equipment.

## COMPLICATIONS AND AVOIDANCE

Rarely, transient dysesthesia may result, especially when there was inadvertent penetration of the intertransverse ligament or if the patient felt pain during the ablative procedure. Ablation of the lateral branch may cause the muscles to twitch, but the patient should have no pain. Staying dorsal to the intertransverse ligament avoids the possibility of exiting and foraminal nerve injury. The use of indigo carmine dye helps the surgeon stay dorsal to the foramen. Avoiding ablation of the dorsal ramus may remove risk of neuroma formation or irritation of anomalous nerves such as furcal nerves and autonomic nerves in the foramen described in Chapter 64.

## CONCLUSIONS AND DISCUSSION

Endoscopic ablation of the medial branches, along with a selected lateral branch of the dorsal ramus, is effective in relief of chronic axial back pain from facet joint and may decrease the need and consideration of fusion as a surgical means of relieving chronic axial back pain (Figure 65-9, Box 65-1). It is certainly more cost-effective in the short term compared to fusion. A large-scale and long-term follow-up is needed to observe whether the technique can decrease the trend toward more fusion procedures in managing axial back pain in the aging spine. Endoscopic rhizotomy offers a bridge for treating many spinal ailments in patients who might not fare well with large open surgeries yet need something more than conventional pain management. To understand selective endoscopic rhizotomy, the detailed surgical anatomy of the dorsal lumbar rami and its significance for dorsal rhizotomy is reviewed.

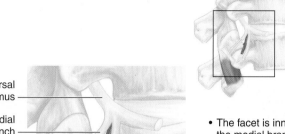

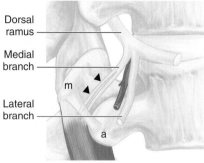

- The facet is innervated by the medial branch of the dorsal ramus at its own level and to the level below.
- Traditional denervation ablates only the medial branch in the osseous tunnel.
- **Lateral branch to dorsal column may contribute to chronic back pain.**
  **–Longissimus muscle**
  **–Soft tissue lateral to multifidus**

■ **FIGURE 65-5**    Anatomy of the medial branch of the dorsal ramus.

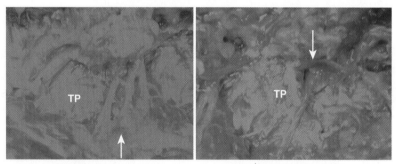

Lateral branches

Dorsal ramus ventral to intertransverse ligament

Medial branch stripped off transverse process

■ **FIGURE 65-6**    Location of the lateral branch of the dorsal ramus in relation to the transverse process.

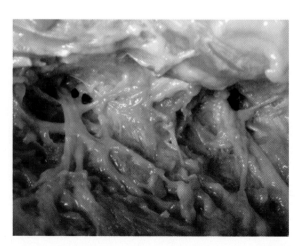

■ **FIGURE 65-7**    Cadaver dissection of the dorsal ramus and its branches in relation to the transverse process.

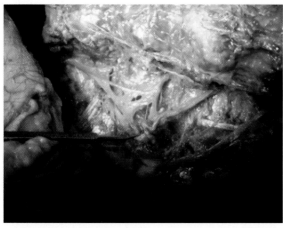

■ **FIGURE 65-8** The dorsal ramus is shown to connect through the a plexus via the gray communicans that connects with nerves that innervate the disc, then also sends branches to one or two segments caudally. This explains how discogenic pain may also cause axial back pain.

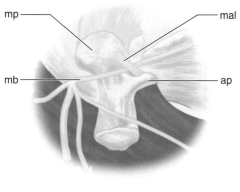

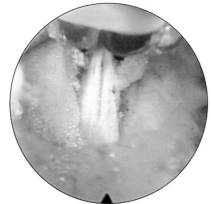

Lateral branch of dorsal ramus

■ **FIGURE 65-9** Lateral branch of dorsal ramus.

## Anatomy of the Lumbar Dorsal Ramus

There are five pairs of lumbar spinal nerves (Figure 65-10). Centrally, the spinal nerve consists of ventral and dorsal roots. The ventral root comes from the anterior horn of the spinal cord and the dorsal root comes from the posterior horn of the spinal cord. The dorsal root has a dorsal ganglion after leaving the spinal cord and before joining the ventral root. The ganglion contains the cell bodies of the sensory fibers in the dorsal root. The ganglion lies within the dural sleeve of the nerve root and occupies the upper and medial part of the intervertebral foramen. The ventral and dorsal roots join together laterally become the spinal nerve

in the intervertebral foramen. After leaving the spinal canal just outside the foramen, the spinal nerve divides into a larger ventral ramus innervating the lower extremities and a smaller dorsal ramus innervating the zygapophyseal joint, back muscles, and ligaments.

### L1 to L4 Dorsal Rami

Bogduk described the lumbar dorsal rami in detail from his anatomical dissection of cadavers.[10] (Bogduk 1980) The L1 to L4 dorsal rami project at almost a right angle to the spinal nerve. The main stem is only about 5 mm long. It runs dorsocaudally through the intertransverse space, deep to the intertransversarii mediales. They are divided into three branches: medial, lateral, and intermediate.

The medial branch (MB) passes dorsally and caudally toward the superior border of the root of the subadjacent transverse process. From there it continues dorsally and caudally lying inside the groove formed by the junction of the root of the transverse process with the base of the superior articular process. In this region, the nerve is bound to the periosteum by a layer of connective tissue, which coats the facet joint and transverse process. The MB continuously courses caudally. At the caudal border of the facet joint, the MB turns medially through a groove between the mamillary process and accessory process, covered and held by the mamillo-accessory ligament. After passing this groove, the MB runs medially and caudally across the vertebral lamina. It lies deep to the multifidus and also sends off articular branches to the facet joint and interspinous process. MB sends off proximal zygapophysial nerve (PZN) and distal zygapophyseal nerve (DZN). PZN innervates the cephalaic facet joint from its caudal side upward, and DZN innervates the caudal facet joint from cephalad side downward. Ultimately MB enters the multifidus muscle via its deep surface.

The lateral branch (LB) crosses the subadjacent transverse process and courses laterally, caudally, the and dorsally through the iliocostalis lumborum. The L1-L3 branches pierce the dorsal layer of thoracolumbar fascia and become cutaneous. L3 LB is bound down to the iliac crest. L4 LB remains entirely intramuscular.

The intermediate branch (IMB) runs dorsally and caudally distributing to the longissimus thoracis muscle. IMB also has intersegmental communicating loops.

### L5 Dorsal Ramus

The L5 dorsal ramus is longer than the L1-L4 dorsal rami. It courses the superior border of the ala of the sacrum, lying in the groove formed by the junction of the ala and the superior articular process of the sacrum. It divides into medial and intermediate branches, lacking a lateral branch. The medial branch curves medially around the caudal aspect of the lumbosacral facet joint and ends in the multifidus muscles. The intermediate branch innervates the longissimus thoracis and communicates with the S1 dorsal ramus. Ablation of the branches of the dorsal ramus, with its complex innervation, may provide axial back pain relief beyond the level surgically ablated. Care is taken when the dorsal ramus is ablated because partial ablation of a large nerve may result in dysesthesia or the formation of a neuroma. No patient, however, considered themselves as worse, even if the procedure did not provide the anticipated or desired pain relief.

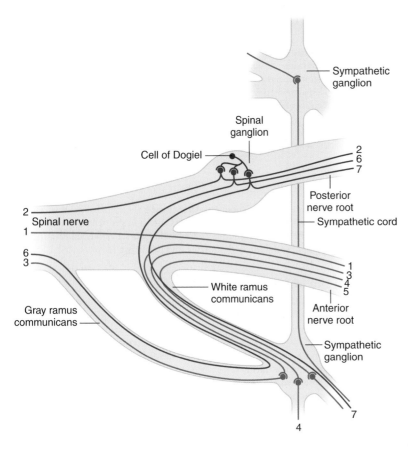

■ **FIGURE 65-10** Connections with the spinal nerves. Communications are established between the sympathetic and spinal nerves through what are known as the gray and white rami communicantes. The gray rami convey sympathetic fibers into the spinal nerves and the white rami transmit spinal fibers into the sympathetic. Each spinal nerve receives a gray ramus communicans from the sympathetic trunk, but white rami are not supplied by all the spinal nerves. The gray ramus commuincans connects the spinal nerve with sympathetic and autonomic nerves in a complex innervation of the disc and posterior elements.. Chronic back pain from an aging spine most likely involves not just the spinal nerve, but its autonomic connections.

# References

1. J.N. Katz, Lumbar disc disorders and low-back pain: socioeconomic factors and consequences, J. Bone Joint. Surg. Am. 88 (Suppl 2) (2006) 21–24.
2. R.G. Hazard, Failed back surgery syndrome: surgical and nonsurgical approaches, Clin. Orthop. Relat. Res. 443 (2006) 228–232.
3. B.I. Martin, S.K. Mirza, B.A. Comstock, et al., Reoperation rates following lumbar spine surgery and the influence of spinal fusion procedures, Spine 32 (3) (2007) 382–387.
4. B.K. Weir, G.A. Jacobs, Reoperation rate following lumbar discectomy. An analysis of 662 lumbar discectomies, Spine 5 (4) (1980) 366–370.
5. J.N. Weinstein, T.D. Tosteson, J.D. Lurie, Tosteson An, B. Hanscom, J.S. Skinner, et al., Surgical vs nonoperative treatment for lumbar disc herniation: the Spine Patient Outcomes Research Trial (SPORT): a randomized trial, JAMA 296 (2006) 2441–2450.
6. A.T. Yeung, Endoscopic medial branch and dorsal ramus rhizotomy for chronic axial back pain: a pilot study, International 25th Jubilee Course on Percutaneus Endoscopic Spine Surgery and Complementary Techniques. Zurich, Switzerland. January 24-25, 2007.
7. S. Datta, M. Lee, F.J. Falco, D.A. Bryce, S.M. Hayek, Systematic assessment of diagnostic accuracy and therapeutic utility of lumbar facet joint interventions, Pain Physician. 12 (2) (2009) 437–460.
8. K. Iwatsuki, T. Yoshimine, K. Awazu, Alternative denervation using laser irradiation in lumbar facet syndrome, Lasers Surg. Med. 39 (3) (2007) 225–229.
9. Kantha Sri. Lumbar facet joint denervation by laser thermo-coagulation. 18th International Intradiscal Therapy Society Meeting May 25-28, 2005, San Diego, CA.
10. R. Derby, C.H. Lee, The efficacy of a two needle electrode technique in percutaneous radio-frequency rhizotomy: An investigational laboratory study in an animal model, Pain Physician. 9 (3) (2006) 207–213.
11. Linqiu Zhou, Carson D. Schneck, Zhenhai Shao. The spinal dorsal ramus and low back pain. Presented at the 19th Annual Meeting of International Intradiscal Therapy Society. Phoenix, AZ. Apr. 5-9, 2006.
12. N. Bogduk, A.S. Wilson, W. Tynan, The human lumbar dorsal rami, J. Anat. 134 (1982) 383–397.

# 66

# Economics of Spine Care

*Stephen H. Hochschuler and Donna D. Ohnmeiss*

## INTRODUCTION

Health care has changed much in recent years, and will likely continue to do so. While some amazing advancements have been made in fields ranging from diagnostic imaging to new pharmaceuticals, as well as new surgical interventions, numerous challenges have arisen with respect to cost and access. Regardless of the economic and political discussions of health care, there is certainty that amid the changing current climate, the population is aging. The first of the baby boomers are entering their 60s and will soon become part of the Medicare population. This will greatly increase the number of older patients who will expect high-quality care. In this chapter, the authors will provide an overview of the economics affecting health care, current challenges, and how these topics fit into providing spine care to an aging population.

## OVERVIEW OF THE ECONOMY AND HEALTHCARE

The year 2008 ended with great economic changes and challenges to be addressed by the incoming Obama administration in 2009. The biggest names in the financial world, such as Lehman Brothers, Merrill Lynch, Bear Stearns, Wells Fargo, AIG, and Citibank were plummeting into ruin. Icons of American industry such as GM, Ford, Chrysler, and others such as Circuit City, were facing complete failure. These financial problems swept the globe in a wave of uncertainty. Many turned to the federal government for bailout support. The government chose an avenue of giving large companies billions of dollars in bailouts and stimulus packages to try to avert a total meltdown of the economy. It is proposed that saving these large businesses as well as creating jobs through highway improvement and other shovel-ready projects will increase confidence in the financial system and let people feel confident enough to spend money to fuel the economic recovery. This is a somewhat confusing issue, however, because a large part of the problem was based on too much credit without enough savings and now, in the short term, the government hopes to change the present course of recession with more spending. How well this course of action works will not be determined for several years. On an individual level, millions have lost their savings for retirement, and millions have lost their jobs, leading to the loss of homes and even access to health insurance.

Health care represents some of the best and worst in the United States. Great advances continue to be made in imaging and other diagnostic procedures, implants are continually patented and developed, and widespread use of the Internet has produced a much more educated patient than in years ago. However, problems with our health care system include the many uninsured (due to lack of availability, lack of affordability, and persons opting to not pay for insurance although they can afford it), workers becoming uninsured through layoffs or illness, workers with insurance having requests for treatment denied by insurers, escalating costs, decreasing physician reimbursements, lack of access, frivolous medical-related lawsuits, unnecessary procedures being prescribed, and inadequate quality assessment and feedback systems. With respect to costs, new terms, such as "medical foreclosure" and "medical bankruptcy" have been added to our vocabulary in recent years.

The amount of resources consumed by health care continues to grow rapidly, well ahead of the pace of inflation. In 2007, the estimated spending was $2.2 trillion and was expected to rise to $4.3 trillion by 2017.[1]

At that time, it is estimated that health care spending will represent 19.5% of the gross domestic product. The paradox lies in what Americans are getting for their health care dollars. While the United States spends more on health care than any other country, in 2004, it ranked twenty-third in life expectancy for men and twenty-fifth for women.[2] Approximately 20% of Americans between the ages of 18 and 64 years do not have health insurance.[3] Among the working population in this age group, the average premium for workplace-based health insurance rose more than 115% from 1999 to 2008, burdening both employees and employers.[4] One of the problems for this group is insurance being linked to employment. If someone loses his or her job, he also loses his access to affordable insurance coverage. Many in this group also feel that even if they have insurance, once a health problem arises, they are often denied coverage for treatment.

On the other hand, insurers struggle with escalating costs charged for newly developed drugs and implants, as well as the potential for add-on technologies to be used during an operation or a course of treatment. They also are accountable for meeting the demands of their investors to consistently produce a competitive profit margin. The Internet has helped greatly in educating patients about various health-related conditions and potential treatment options. However, the Internet, along with direct-to-consumer marketing, has produced patients with greater demands for their health care providers to prescribe particular medications and perform various procedures that the consumers may not otherwise ask for.

The concept of competitive effectiveness is at present (April 2009) a topic being addressed in Washington as a solution for rising health care costs. Although on the surface the concept is irrefutable, there is much concern that when Washington makes these decisions without significant physician and patient input and then adds cost-effectiveness, health care rationing, such as is seen in Canada and England, might well result.

One possible scenario to address the 47 million uninsured as well as revamping health care insurance might be a government-sponsored program to subsidize health savings accounts (HSAs). This would make the patient the source of purchasing health care and, just as with purchasing a car, the consumer would purchase what is needed based on comparative analysis of different procedures, providers, and implants. Pay-for-performance, which insurers are proposing, would be carried out in HSA scenario to the individual and not capricious treatment decisions made by the insurance companies. In addition, such a system would afford patients the much-sought after portability.

Other areas of health care have changed drastically during the past several years. There is much less trust in the FDA's ability to adequately monitor the safety of food, medications, and medical devices; use and promotion of products off-label has come to merit investigation by the FBI and other federal agencies; concern has arisen over the financial relationships between industry and physicians; and, for many years, physicians have felt obligated to practice defensive medicine to help ward off exorbitant malpractice lawsuits.

## OVERVIEW OF SPINE CARE

Spine care is far from immune from the challenges health care is facing. Guyer described this paradox in spine care with the excitement of numerous new devices and treatments contrasted with financial challenges.[5] As previously mentioned, there is a problem with the physician–medical manufacturer relationship. As the health care market became more competitive, spine companies looked to new ways of improving and marketing products. At the same time, declining reimbursements led physicians to look for other avenues of revenue. This led to companies teaming with surgeon-consultants to design new implants. The companies provide the engineering expertise and the surgeons provide expertise in knowing what types of devices are needed and what designs are most feasible for use. Unfortunately, some companies and surgeons elected to abuse this productive collaboration and instead turn it into an unethical practice of payment for use of certain products and payments for services that were never rendered. This has resulted in a declining interaction between industry and physicians, reduced funding to support research and education, public disclosure of financial relationships and investigations, and arrests for inappropriate payments to physicians as well as for off-label promotion by physicians and corporate employees. Groups such as Advamed have emerged, and continue to refine guidelines for interaction between industry and physicians. Others have suggested banning any relationship or support from industry to physicians or organizations. This drastic a measure would undoubtedly have severely detrimental effects on research as well as new product development.

Although back pain is a multibillion-dollar problem annually in the United States, there is surprisingly little solicitation for federal grants to support research in this area. Ultimately, without corporate support, back pain research and education would be severely limited, a step that cannot be beneficial by any measure.

## BACK PAIN IN A CHANGING POPULATION

The increasing percentage of the population that is over 60 years will impact spine care. Much of the focus in the past has been on younger patients, in whom the majority of back pain has been related to herniated discs and painful disc degeneration. In many publications dealing with the treatment of painful spinal conditions, the mean age has been in the 40s. With the influx of baby boomers into the Medicare population, the dominant needs in spine care will likely shift. Their needs will be oriented toward stenosis, osteoporotic spinal fractures, and degenerative scoliosis. One should remember some of the characteristics of this generation as well. They generally want to be active and demand quality service. A few steps have already been taken toward designing surgical interventions for older patients. In recent years, implants such as interspinous devices have been introduced and they continue to evolve. Osteoporotic fractures are now treated with procedures such as kyphoplasty and vertebroplasty. It is likely that we will continue to see increased focus on the development of therapies for those 50 to 60 years old and older that are often minimally invasive and focused on return to activity.

There has been great enthusiasm for the movement away from traditional spinal fusion toward motion-preserving technologies. Singh et al projected that by 2010, 47.9% of the spine market will be arthroplasty devices.[6] This was estimated to be approximately $2.18 billion.

It is to be noted that the medical spine market does not necessarily follow the traditional pattern of economics, with respect to the pricing of devices varying with supply and demand. One example of this was described by Lieberman who applied it to pedicle screws.[7] While the basic design of the pedicle screw and rod systems changed little from 1900 to 2000, their prices rose from $135 to $160 to $225 to $700. The continual increase was not attributed to increasing development or manufacturing costs, but rather to what the market would bear. As noted by Hochschuler on this topic, with many new technology items such as computers, time and competition drive the prices lower if there are no significant enhancements of the product.[6] However, what was seen with pedicle screws is that the number of companies offering screw and rod systems increased through the years, but the prices increased rather than decreased.

One item that is often discussed is the cost-effectiveness of spinal surgery. Unfortunately, there have been very few studies investigating this topic. However, in the few studies that do exist, spine surgery has been found to be in line with other commonly accepted surgeries. One of the strategies employed to address the cost-effectiveness of spinal surgery has been to compare various procedures to well-accepted surgical procedures. Polly et al reviewed the SF-36 results reported in 11 different fusion studies and

compared them, based on cost per unit of change in the physical component scores of the SF-36, to results reported from total hip replacement, total knee replacement, and carotid artery bypass surgery.[8] Their analysis found that fusion was more cost-effective than bypass surgery, similar to knee replacement, and less cost-effective than hip replacement. However, it should be noted that 9 of the 11 fusion studies included in the analysis were based on IDE trials. This may have somewhat skewed the results, due to the rigorous patient selection criteria employed in most trials. Also, the surgical protocol in such studies does not allow the use of multiple bone graft types, off-label use of bone graft or implants, or the decision to use additional items such as anterior lumbar plates, "door stop" screws with anterior graft or cages, or other items. This restriction of implants may have lowered the costs of fusion in the IDE trials compared to typical use patterns. Another study investigated the cost-effectiveness of spinal decompression by comparing it to total hip replacement.[8] The authors found decompression to be 50% more cost-effective than hip replacement. Some of this may be attributable to the lack of implants used in spinal decompression.

As advances have been made in spinal surgery, one item of debate has been the use of bone morphogenic protein (BMP) to enhance spinal fusion. While this material has been attributed to producing a high fusion rate, its cost has been the source of concern. One study analyzing this issue found that the operative cost of using BMP was greater; however, over time BMP became cost-neutral due to the reduced costs of future care associated with iliac crest donor site pain and subsequent costs related to a higher rate of pseudarthrosis in fusion surgeries performed not using BMP.[9]

As interest in spine surgery has moved away from fusion to motion-preserving technologies, the concern about costs has moved into this arena as well. One such intervention is total disc replacement (TDR). While this technology holds the promise of reducing pain and allowing motion of the operated segment, questions about the costs related to its use have arisen. Guyer et al reported the results of a cost-effectiveness model comparing the operative costs and treatment costs through a 24-month postoperative period.[10] TDR was compared to ALIF with BMP and cages, ALIF with iliac crest autograft, and PLIF using autograft and pedicle screw fixation. The cost model suggests that operative costs, as well as costs throughout the follow-up, were significantly less in the TDR group compared to each of the fusion procedures. Also comparing the costs of TDR to fusion, Patel et al reviewed hospital costs related to single-level TLIF, circumferential fusion, ALIF alone, and TDR.[11] They found the total hospital costs of TDR were significantly less than any of the three fusion groups. The cost of TDR was similar to TLIF and ALIF, if the cost associated with using BMP in these fusion procedures was not included. Levin et al also reported that single-level TDR was related to significantly lower hospital charges compared to circumferential fusion.[12] However, they found no significant difference in the charges for two-level procedures.

The evaluation of TDR in Switzerland is perhaps a predictor of the future on a global basis for the evaluation of new spinal implants. The Swiss government required a national registry of all TDR procedures. From the data collected, a decision would be made concerning the reimbursement for use of the device. The early data from that registry have recently been published.[13] The authors referred to this process as following the "health technology assessment" principle of "coverage with evidence development." Prospective data for 427 patients were analyzed. Pain scores, quality of life, and medication usage all improved significantly. The rate of complications occurring with the surgery and/or initial hospital stay was 3.9% for single-level cases and 8.6% for two-level procedures. Rehospitalization and revisions occurred in 3.1% of single-level cases and 1.4% of two-level cases. The authors concluded that TDR appeared to be a relatively safe and effective procedure, at least in the short-term. But what may be more important about this study is that it creates a comprehensive model to evaluate new technologies. The use of such registries may help to address many concerns that arise in IDE trials and individual studies with respect to how generalizable are study results to broad-scale use. It also provides the collection of data for a large number of subjects so that the occurrence of complications can be identified more quickly than in relatively small studies.

The lumbar spine has generally received much more attention than the cervical region. However, there are many patients with significant neck pain and related cost of treatment. With the aging population, the number of cervical problems related to degenerative spinal conditions is likely to increase.

In analyzing surgery for cervical spine disease, Patil et al found that the number of procedures doubled in the years from 1990 to 2000.[14] During that time, the patient age and number of comorbidities increased; however, mortality and length of hospital stay decreased. Inflation-adjusted costs of cervical surgery increased 48% during the decade, to surpass $2 billion.

The many recent and emerging advances in spine care contribute to this being a very exciting time for spine care providers. Alternatives to spinal fusion using the patient's own iliac crest for graft material have been realized in the form of BMP and other fusion materials. Even more exciting has been the development of total disc replacements for the lumbar and cervical spine. Designs of dynamic stabilization devices are numerous. Total facet replacements are being evaluated. The arena of minimally invasive spine surgery is growing rapidly. However, who pays for all of these advances? Which patients are most likely to benefit from expensive treatment options and which can achieve good results with less expensive interventions?

The costs related to back pain were reported to range between $100 and $200 billion a year in the United States.[15] Much of this cost was due to patients missing work. The same authors reported that, annually, less than 5% of patients use 75% of the total cost of back pain. Another high cost area for back pain is surgical implants. This was reported to be $2.5 billion in 2003.

One component of back pain costs that is not often addressed is the cost related to time off work. Ekman et al reported that costs related to loss of productivity were about 84% of the total societal costs of back pain.[16] These data suggest that one means of reducing the overall costs of back pain is incorporating strategies to keep back pain patients at work as long as possible and to return them to work as soon as possible after back pain–related absence.

## Osteoporosis

Osteoporosis is a major concomitant factor in aging patients with back pain. It is estimated that 55% of Americans, or 44 million persons, who are at least 50 years of age have either osteoporosis or osteopenia.[17] The costs related to this disease were estimated to be $19 billion in 2005, and were expected to rise to $25.3 billion by 2025. Although not all of these costs can be attributed to spinal fractures in the elderly, these account for a significant part of the costs in the osteoporotic population. In addition, new fixation techniques designed to be employed in the elderly spine with osteoporosis are being developed.

## COMPENSATION

With the government's emphasis on cost reduction, rising costs need to be addressed. Part of cost-cutting to date has included decreasing compensation to surgeons. Data over the last 10 years show that hospital income has increased 18%, spinal device companies' income has increased 154%, while the spine surgeon's payment has decreased 30%. However, there not only needs to be more appropriate dollar reconciliation of the entities, but plaintiff attorneys' involvement in the system and malpractice settlements need to be addressed, as well as the whole adjudication process. In addition, insurance companies need to redesign products to help reduce costs and make portability possible or a one-payer government system will evolve.

## MEDICAL TOURISM

One issue that has arisen in recent years is medical tourism. There are many web pages that offer highly discounted medical services with the added allure of foreign travel. While some patients feel that this may be their only option for some expensive procedures for which they do not have insurance or for which their insurance denies coverage, it is a system that has yet to be fully tested. Many questions arise, such as how can they be assured that they are traveling to a quality facility? Will patients receive quality implants including tissue transplanted from others? What happens if a complication arises? What if the patient dies overseas? How will complications that arise after return to the United States be treated and paid for? Also of concern is can America compete fairly in this arena? In many countries offering medical tourism packages, the cost of health care delivery is heavily subsidized by the government, which helps drive the cost down. Also, in those countries,

the need to pay malpractice and similar insurances by physicians, clinics, hospitals, and manufacturers does not exist. This also contributes significantly to the ability to charge less for medical care.

## COST-EFFECTIVENESS

While the concept of assessing treatments based on cost-effectiveness certainly has merit and appears to be relatively straightforward, such studies are extremely difficult to perform in the United States, due to HIPAA and the lack of any comprehensive data-capture system to assess all costs, not just the hospitalization costs related to a single surgical event. There is no way for researchers to have access to complete patient records. A surgeon can access the costs incurred at his/her center and possibly the operative costs at the hospital where the surgery was performed. However, one cannot get access to costs related to treatment provided outside of these entities. Such costs would be any services provided off-campus such as physical therapy, chiropractic, medication, pain management, and in some cases, reoperation. In addition, care providers do not have access to the indirect costs such as disability payments made to a patient due to their back pain. All these are important in determining the true cost-effectiveness of an intervention. These difficulties, coupled with the wide variety of procedures and implants used, make detailed cost analysis very difficult. If such studies are performed, they will likely be criticized by those who disagree with the results due to all of the potential problems with getting reliable full datasets for patients.

There have been a few cost-effectiveness studies performed for spinal surgery. From the SPORT (Spine Patient Outcomes Research Trial) study, the cost-effectiveness of decompression and decompression with fusion were compared to nonoperative treatment for lumbar spinal stenosis.[18] Based on the cost per quality-adjusted life-year (QALY) over a 2-year follow-up, the authors reported that the economic value of spinal surgery for this group compares favorably with other health-related interventions.

Considering the rapidly expanding number of treatment options and additional items that may be used, the cost-effectiveness calculation becomes even more complicated. For example, consider the cost-effectiveness of anterior lumbar fusion. The simplest procedure may use a femoral ring allograft and a graft extender. The cost of this simple procedure is greatly reduced compared to cages packed with BMP, use of an anterior plate, and the use of interoperative neural monitoring. Can it be shown that any or all of the additional costs associated with the latter procedure result in a proportionally better outcome? To date, there are too few outcome data available to address questions such as these, but they are relevant to the tune of several thousand dollars difference in the cost of a single-level ALIF. Unfortunately, while there may be sound biomechanical or litigious reasons for many of the implants used in spine surgery, there are currently no clinical data available to demonstrate the benefits of many such interventions. As with many things, the key likely does not lie in a simplistic dichotomy, either beneficial or not beneficial. The real answer more likely lies in the need to determine which combinations of implants and services are needed in which subgroups of patients. Those with multiple risk factors for failures or with unusually shaped anatomy may merit the use of more expensive constructs, while such costs cannot be justified in simple cases.

## WHERE TO GO FROM HERE

As previously mentioned, there is a movement going on in general to shift from the current practice of medicine to one employing evidence-based guidelines and cost-effectiveness to determine care. While this approach appears logical, there are several potential shortcomings. These include lack of rigorous research, inability to collect comprehensive cost data, and decisions made by bureaucrats in Washington without appropriate input from physicians or patients.

Care providers have been reluctant to embrace treatment based solely on evidence-based– and cost-effectiveness–based information. It is essential to allow doctors the freedom to use their education and experience gained from many years of practice. However, just as with residency training, accountability with, perhaps, peer review might prove efficacious. The all-important relationship of physician with industry needs clarification with appropriate compensation. No one wishes for businessmen or engineers to design new implants in isolation. In no other field other than those receiving bailout support has any professional organization agreed with a government or Advamed mandate as to hourly consulting fees. If this is to be accepted in medicine, the authors suggest that a cap be applied to apply to Wall Street executives, lawyers, accountants, etc.

In closing, no doubt there are changes on the horizon in spine medicine. If health care is allowed to expand undeterred, our country will be bankrupt. Hard decisions need to be made. It is in our common interest to involve all factions, which must include patients and doctors, with transparency and full disclosure as to the goals and consequences of various scenarios.

## References

1. S. Keehan, A. Sisko, C. Truffer, et al., Health spending projections through 2017: the baby-boom generation is coming to Medicare, Health Affairs 27 (2008) w145–w155.
2. National Center for Health Statistics: Health, United States, 2008, Hyattsville, MD, 2009.
3. Centers for Disease Control: Early release of selected estimates based on data from the 2007 national health interview survey, June, 2008.
4. Employee health benefits: 2008 annual survey. In: The Henry J. Kaiser Family Foundation 1-8, 2008.
5. R.D. Guyer, The paradox in medicine today: exciting technology and economic challenges, Spine J. 8 (2008) 279–285.
6. K. Singh, A.R. Vaccaro, T.J. Albert, Assessing the potential impact of total disc arthroplasty on surgeon practice patterns in North America, Spine J. 4 (2004) 195S–201S.
7. I.H. Lieberman, Disc bulge bubble: spine economics 101, Spine J. 4 (2004) 609–613.
8. D.W. Polly, S.D. Glassman, J.D. Schwender, et al., SF-36 PCS benefit-cost ratio of lumbar fusion comparison to other surgical interventions: a thought experiment, Spine 32 (2007) S20–26.
9. S.J. Ackerman, M.S. Mafilios, D.W. Polly, Economic evaluation of bone morphogenetic protein versus autogenous iliac crest bone graft in single-level anterior lumbar fusion: an evidence-based modeling approach, Spine 27 (2002) S94–99.
10. R.D. Guyer, S.G. Tromanhauser, J.J. Regan, An economic model of one-level lumbar arthroplasty versus fusion, Spine J. 7 (2007) 558–562.
11. V.V. Patel, S. Estes, E.M. Lindley, E. Burger, Lumbar spinal fusion versus anterior lumbar disc replacement: the financial implications, J. Spinal Disord. Tech. 21 (2008) 473–476.
12. D.A. Levin, J.A. Bendo, M. Quirno, et al., Comparative charge analysis of one- and two-level lumbar total disc arthroplasty versus circumferential lumbar fusion, Spine 32 (2007) 2905–2909.
13. E. Schluessmann, P. Diel, E. Aghayev, et al., SWISSspine: a nationwide registry for health technology assessment of lumbar disc prostheses, Eur. Spine J. 2009.
14. P.G. Patil, D.A. Turner, R. Pietrobon, National trends in surgical procedures for degenerative cervical spine disease: 1990-2000, Neurosurgery 57 (2005) 753–758.
15. J.N. Katz, Lumbar disc disorders and low-back pain: socioeconomic factors and consequences, J. Bone Joint Surg. Am. 88 (Suppl. 2) (2006) 21–24.
16. M. Ekman, O. Johnell, L. Lidgren, The economic cost of low back pain in Sweden in 2001, Acta Orthop. 76 (2005) 275–284.
17. National Osteoporosis Foundation: Fast facts, http://www.nof.org/osteoporosis/disease facts.htm. Accessed February 17, 2010.
18. A.N. Tosteson, J.S. Skinner, T.D. Tosteson, et al., The cost effectiveness of surgical versus nonoperative treatment for lumbar disc herniation over two years: evidence from the Spine Patient Outcomes Research Trial (SPORT), Spine 33 (2008) 2108–2115.

# 67

# Micro- and Nanotechnology and the Aging Spine

*Lisa A. Ferrara*

## INTRODUCTION

In the United States by the year 2000, approximately 20% of all Americans were older than 65. Twelve percent were older than 85. With an aging population, a higher proportion of the elderly seek orthopedic treatment, due to the prevalence of musculoskeletal complaints. Currently, 25% of orthopedic patients are 65 and older. The Census Bureau projects that the 65 and older population will double from 33 million to 65 million by 2030, while the younger age groups will remain the same. Physicians will be faced with a greater number of individuals who are experiencing intellectual failure, immobility, instability, incontinence, insomnia, degenerative musculoskeletal disorders, and iatrogenic problems.

The aging process presents a cascade of events that affect the health of the musculoskeletal system, in particular, the human spine. The maximum bone mineral density of an individual is reached between the ages of 18 to 20 years of age. As aging progresses, muscle size and strength begin to decrease, by as early as age 25. Accompanying these changes are reductions in hormone levels for both men and women, contributing to a decline in bone density and muscular strength. As we age, the musculoskeletal system experiences degenerative changes resulting in fibrosis, stiffening, and shrinkage of the soft tissue; bone loss; joint changes; and tissue desiccation due to a reduction in proteoglycans and a change in collagen type (i.e., intervertebral disc).[10] With respect to the aging spine, this fibrosis and stiffening reduces the osmotic properties of the disc and the ability of the disc to obtain and/or maintain vital nutrients while eliminating noxious wastes. Disc desiccation initiates a cascade of progressive degenerative events leading to loss of disc height, degenerative facets, and compression of the neural structures resulting in pain. The degenerative process continues as the discs of the spine undergo these arthritic bony changes, resulting in altered loading patterns on the spine, further enhancing the patient's pain and neurological deficits.

As a result, the elder population suffers from a variety of degenerative disorders afflicting the spine, such as osteoporosis, degenerative disc disease, compromised facet joints, spondylotic myelopathies, and stenosis, all resulting in pain and loss of motion. However, the longer life expectancies and increased levels of activity at a much later stage in life place greater demands on the spine and musculoskeletal system. Over the last decade, there has been a surge in orthopedic implant development and spinal arthroplasty devices to preserve or restore long-term joint motion.

As the overall life expectancy continues to increase worldwide, the need for improved medical care increases and is expected to continue as the baby boom generation crosses into the senior phase of their lives. With continued development of novel medical technologies and a changing health care environment, microinvasive technological advancements in medicine continue to progress, especially within the orthopedic and neurosurgical arena, where a new generation of medicine is evolving.

Smart technology or "smart systems" are terms used to define systems that are capable of imitating human intelligence. A smart system with respect to medical devices is a system that can automatically sense and respond to a changing environment once implanted into the human body. Smart technologies employ smart microsensors that can sense minuscule changes in pH, chemistry, stress, strain, pressures, and temperatures; smart materials that change their properties in response to a particular stimulus; microelectromechanical technologies that can sense and respond at the cellular level; and nanoelectromechanical technologies that behave at the molecular level.

With respect to the aging spine, the ability to sense adverse changes in vivo and manipulate cells and molecules presents the possibility of promising treatments for debilitating diseases and musculoskeletal disorders. Smart materials that have the ability to repair and reorganize human tissue and eventually allow for an engineered material and scaffold to be substituted by newly regenerated tissue provide an attractive solution for implant and tissue longevity. Such novel materials should be capable of nonlinear responses to imitate the mechanics of living tissue. Smart biosensors and tooling can lend to improved surgical techniques and patient outcomes. The incorporation of micro- or nanotechnology into spinal implants and surgical tooling can enhance surgical accuracy; provide precision cutting techniques for microsurgery with minuscule tissue damage; manipulate cellular and subcellular structures; develop genetic engineering clinical strategies; monitor and respond to tissue-targeting feedback; and create biosensors that can provide the surgeon with real-time, continuous biofeedback with respect to implant performance during the lifespan of the applied treatment. Smart materials with preprogrammed porosities can function as biological sieves for implantable drug delivery systems, controlled differentiated tissue growth, and disease barriers. Finally, ultra-small tweezers that are of nanosize allow for manipulation of molecules to change the course of a disease.

The areas in which such interventions may become clinically applicable in the aging spine include nuclear regeneration and replacement technologies, neural regeneration, localized delivery of pharmaceuticals such as bone morphogenetic proteins for localized and controlled bone growth, delivery of antibiotics and pain medications for long-term steady-state delivery, and monitoring of implant lifespan. Nucleus regeneration may involve the employment of semipermeable membranes that allow specific cells or humoral agents to pass into a disc space that spur and nurture the regeneration process. Neural regeneration techniques must not only overcome the humoral stimulation barriers required to induce regeneration, they must overcome physical barriers and the complexity of the nervous system involving complex synaptic connections that are poorly understood. MEMS/NEMS and polymer technologies can be utilized to create textured surfaces that facilitate neural growth, while grids and tubes that can be electrically stimulated can be used for orienting neuronal growth.

## SPINAL ETIOLOGIES[12,13,21]

### Degenerative Disc and Congenital Disorders

The normal aging process results in degenerative disorders due to normal wear and tear of the joints and soft tissues. Although the process of aging results in disc desiccation, facet degeneration, osteophyte formation, and a cascade of mechanical and chemical events that lead to degenerative conditions that cause pain and neurological changes, the ability of the body to heal the tissues still occurs, although at a slower rate with progressive aging.

**Arthritis** affects approximately 80% of people over the age of 55 in the United States.[1,12] It is often triggered by injury, a weakened immune system, and/or hereditary factors. Symptoms include inflammation, joint pain, and progressive deterioration of joint surfaces over time which may result in anatomical changes of the joint surface, and edema inside the joint accompanied by tissue debris. This condition demonstrates mechanical instability in the joint related to the wearing away of the cartilage that is responsible for friction-free motion of the joint. The debris causes an inflammatory response that can induce bone overgrowth and osteophyte formation that eventually interferes with joint mobility. Rheumatoid arthritis is a progressive form of arthritis that can be painfully destructive and may cause the interior joint tissues to swell and thicken, resulting in joint disintegration and eventual significant deformity.

**Osteophytes** or bone spurs are visible indications of a changing mechanical environment and are often found in areas affected by arthritis such as the disc or joint spaces where cartilage has deteriorated. The formation of osteophytes is the body's attempt to halt the motion of the arthritic joint and deal with the degenerative process, but often causes impingement on the surrounding nerve roots.

Ankylosing spondylitis is a chronic hereditable disease characterized by progressive inflammation of the spine with early sacroiliac joint involvement, followed by hardening of the anulus fibrosus and surrounding connective tissue and arthritic changes in the facet joints.[5;6] The disease eventually results in a loss of segmental mobility and "stiffening" of the spinal tissues.

## Spinal Stenosis

Spinal stenosis is a disorder causing narrowing of the spinal canal or the neuroforamen through which nerves exit the spinal column, thereby placing pressure on the spinal cord. It occurs in all areas of the spine, however, most often in the lumbar and cervical areas. Lumbar spinal stenosis-related symptoms include pain, weakness, or numbness in the legs, calves, or buttocks, and are exacerbated when walking short distances and reduced when sitting, bending forward, or lying down. Cervical spinal stenosis demonstrates similar symptoms in the shoulders, arms, and legs, in addition to fine motor skill and balance disturbances. Treatment for spinal stenosis includes drug therapy such as nonsteroidal antiinflammatory drugs to reduce swelling and pain, and analgesics to relieve pain. Further conservative approaches to pain involve corticosteroid injections (epidural steroids) to reduce swelling and treat acute pain. Certain medical conditions may confound the diagnosis and affect treatment choices. Diabetes-related peripheral vascular disease and diabetic neuropathy or polyradiculopathy may superficially mimic the neurogenic claudication of spinal stenosis, causing pain and neurological deficits to the patient.

## Osteoporosis

Osteoporosis is defined as the loss of bone mass and density due to a loss of calcium exchange, which significantly compromises the strength of the vertebral body.[1] It is often detected during the later stages of bone loss and will weaken the mechanical integrity of the spinal column. Deformities may develop as the vertebral segments lose a great deal of the cancellous structure, and eventually lead to compression and crush fracture resulting in a kyphotic posture. Loss of bone strength may cause spontaneous fractures to occur, in which the patient's own body weight alone may cause vertebrae to collapse leading to compressed nerves.

## Spinal Deformity (Scoliosis, Kyphosis)

Scoliosis, kyphosis, and sagittal imbalance are spinal deformities that are degenerative in nature in the older spine. Scoliosis is a three-dimensional deformity that affects the coronal, sagittal, and axial planes. Kyphosis causes sagittal imbalance and is identified as a degenerative curvature that affects the sagittal plane. Lumbar deformities can be classified as idiopathic with superimposed degenerative changes and de novo degenerative scoliosis, in

which the deformity starts at age 40 or greater, resulting from osteoporosis and/or age-related degenerative disc changes. These deformities are characterized by the location of their curvatures (i.e., thoracic, lumbar, or thoracolumbar) and can be biplanar in nature. Treatment for such pathology often results in a fusion with rigid instrumentation for curvature correction. Currently, trapezoidal mesh cages with bone morphogenic protein (BMP) are used to provide the anterior column support and improved curve correction with BMP to ensure fusion incorporation. However, this is a surgically-invasive approach requiring significant rigid stabilization implants, and is subject to early failure if the surrounding bone integrity is suboptimal or compromised, as that of the older spine.

## Spinal Tumors

These are rare in occurrence. The physician is interested in determining the cause of the tumor, whether there is a past history of cancer, and relieving associated pain. If the patient's primary condition is breast or lung cancer, it is possible for the cancer to metastasize to the spine. Tumors can occur in anyone without a history of disease. Fortunately not all spinal tumors are malignant.

The foregoing are just a few of the spinal etiologies that can be associated with the aging spine. Currently, there are conservative and surgical treatment options for these disorders. However, the conservative treatments do not address the individual's long-term pain and well-being, while the surgical options provide immediate treatment and address the pathology, but are much more invasive and short-lived with respect to the patient's lifespan and quality of life.

## NANOMEDICINE AND THE AGING SPINE

Bionanotechnology is the merging of biology with nanotechnology (performs at the molecular level) by incorporating fabricated nanostructured materials and electronics into a living biological environment with functions that will diagnose and respond therapeutically. This term also applies to biomicrotechnology, which incorporates microstructured materials (performs at the cellular level) and electronics into a living environment. The application of these technologies in a clinical environment has been termed nanomedicine. Microelectromechanical systems (MEMS) and nanoelectromechanical systems (NEMS) are microsized systems capable of performing biological tasks at the cellular or molecular level and are deemed "smart technologies." The specific application of micro or nanobiotechnology to develop micro/nanosized medical devices will revolutionize medicine with the potential to regenerate tissue, restore mobility, and increase the longevity of spinal implantation, as well as improve the quality of life and activity levels for the aging population.

## Drug Delivery Therapies[7,19]

Over the last few decades, considerable advances have been made toward drug delivery technologies. However, considerable challenges still exist. The continuous release of therapeutic agents over extended time periods following a preprogrammed temporal profile, local delivery of the drug at a constant rate to the diseased microenvironment to overcome systemic toxicity, improved ease of administration, increased patient compliance, minimized risk of side effects, reduced hospital stay, and independent application all pose significant challenges to the effectiveness of the delivered pharmaceutical. Injected or ingested drugs follow first-order kinetics with high blood levels of the drug immediately after initial dosing, followed by an exponential decay in blood concentration. The rapid rise in the drug can lead to toxicity, and the efficacy of the drug is diminished as the drug levels fall exponentially. A continuous drug release profile in a controlled manner for maintaining blood levels is an optimal release design. Currently, most controlled drug delivery systems are transdermal and subcutaneous in nature, with current research, focused on the development of implantable systems that will deliver therapeutic agents in a steady state manner, well underway. The treatment of certain diseases such as osteoporosis and arthritis that require the chronic administration of drugs could benefit from the presence of implantable devices. These devices have the capabilities to provide localized continuous delivery to the physiological site. The benefits of implantable drug delivery systems include the reduction of side effects with improved feedback in a manner that mimics the physiological release profiles of the immune system.

Micro and nanoengineered delivery devices have the potential to improve drug delivery. Numerous materials that were once injected are now capable of being inhaled or swallowed through novel nanodelivery devices, thus improving patient compliance. However, the issues with fluctuating blood levels and drug maintenance still exist. Therefore, a variety of microfabricated devices such as microparticles, microneedles, microchips, nanoporous membranes, and micropumps have been employed in the development of drug delivery systems for the goal of long-term implantation. In essence, this is analogous to the behavior of the immune system. MEMS and NEMS have provided an alternative to current means of drug delivery. The technology allows for systems to be employed that will ease application of the drug and reduce the pain of delivery for injectable drugs. Microneedles of accurate, repeatable micron dimensions have been precisely designed in arrays with reproducible lumen dimensions that pierce tissue allowing for delivery of the drug in a localized manner, yet are small enough to avoid pain and significant tissue damage (Figure 67-1). Human nerves are insensitive to micro- or nanoscale needles, making microneedle arrays for drug delivery ideal for the elderly patient with fragile skin. Implantable nano-channeled needles for drug delivery can provide improvement of control and optimization of pharmocodynamics, by maintaining prolonged steady state of the drug performance and reducing the blood level fluctuation potential and toxicity risks associated with conventional drug delivery. The drug release rates can be accurately modeled and predicted due to the reproducibility of the microneedles.[7] Eventually, these systems will be externally controlled by telemetric means where a small drug delivery "chip" is implanted directly to the diseased site and the chemical environment monitored and pharmaceutical agents delivered in response to a change in the chemistry, thus serving both as a diagnostic tool and therapeutic agent for diseased tissue.

Nanopore technology has been implemented in the development of microfabricated nanoporous membranes that are biologically, thermally, chemically, and mechanically stable once implanted into tissue and are also ideal for drug delivery systems and molecular sieves. These membranes are ideal biological sieves that have uniform pore size and very low thickness, making them ideally suited for drug delivery due to the ability of the membranes to have controlled diffusion and sustained release. The pore size, pore length, and pore density can all be highly controlled and serve as ideal diffusion barriers. A drug reservoir can also be fitted to the device for sustained delivery to the tissues.[7,19]

## Micro- and Nanoscale Smart Polymer Technologies

There are numerous types of smart polymers or polymers that exhibit a sharp phase transition from hydrophilic to hydrophobic in response to an environmental stimulus such as pH, temperature, pressure, or strain. Numerous applications exist for these smart polymers or stimuli-responsive polymers, such as drug delivery and drug targeting systems, biodetectors,

biosensors, and artificial muscles. Smart polymers are macromolecules capable of undergoing rapid, reversible phase transitions from a hydrophilic to a hydrophobic phase and are thermodynamic systems that undergo a phase transition for a certain range of parameters such as pressure, temperature, and pH.[8,15-18,20] Furthermore, there are protein-based polymers that will adhere to surrounding tissue or behave as a barrier to scar tissue, as well as polymers that are electroactive in nature whose properties change drastically upon change of stimulus. Additionally, polymers that respond differently to changing mechanical properties such as strain rates have numerous potential uses in the musculoskeletal system in terms of replacement devices or shock absorbers in the human joints. Aging often results in degenerative joints that have less efficient shock-absorbing behavior, which is further amplified in the spine, where each intervertebral disc serves as a shock absorber to spinal motion. Fast strain rates imposed on these types of polymers would elicit a stiffening response, whereas slow strain rates would elicit a greater elastic zone with greater deformation. Finally, the physical state of a smart polymer coating on the surface of another material can switch from hydrophobic to hydrophilic, where in the hydrophobic state, the surfaces have been found to adhere to proteins and cells and can be patterned after human cells. In the hydrophilic state, these proteins would be released. Such a technology can be incorporated into applications toward engineering human tissue, such as an intervertebral disc or cancellous bone and can provide adhesive or barrier functions to the surrounding tissues.

## Nanocoatings

With the advent of spine arthroplasty implants for motion preservation, adherence of the implant to the surrounding bony interface is often challenging for long-term fixation. Biocompatible thermal spray coatings such as titanium plasma sprays and hydroxyapatite coatings (HA) are the conventional means for improving an implant's fixation to the surrounding bone environment by promoting osseointegration at the interface. The HA coatings are generally 50 to 75 μm thick, and have a mean roughness of 7.5 to 9.5 μm, with a porosity of 1% to 10%, and a bond strength between 20 and 30 MPa. Titanium powders are generally sprayed and exhibit thickness of 350 μm to 600 μm, with a mean roughness of 30 μm and a porosity of 15% to 40%, with a bond strength of 25 MPa.[4,14,14] However, the wide range in porosity and thickness can have limiting effects with respect to osseointegration.

Nanocoatings or nanostructured thermal spray coatings exhibit enhanced mechanical performance when compared to the conventional biomedical thermal spray coatings used on orthopedic implants, due to the uniformity and consistency in porous replication. Further characteristics such as higher wear resistance, higher bond strength with the substrate, higher resistance to delamination, higher toughness, and higher plasticity have also been observed with nanostructured coatings.[4,9] These structures have been used extensively in the dental arena and tend to have a higher affinity for osteoblast proliferation and uniform bone formation at the interfaces. Improvement of these qualities using nanostructured technologies can lead

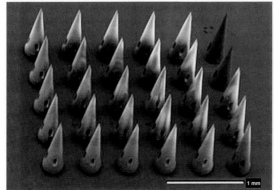
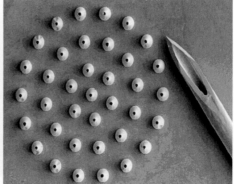

■ **FIGURE 67-1**   Microscope image shows an array of hollow microneedles that are approximately 1000 microns tall next to a hypodermic needle typical of those now used to inject drugs and vaccines. *(Images from Google image, Microneedles. From Mark Prausnitz, Georgia Tech's School of Chemical and Biomolecular Engineering.)*

to improved fixation of implants at the bone interface and the potential to increase the implant's lifespan within compromised or osteoporotic bone of the aging spine.

## Biosensors and Biochips

Although the exact pathomechanism by which a degenerative intervertebral disc leads to neural inflammation and pain has not been determined, modern techniques of chemical analysis can be implemented to identify biochemical markers that participate in the degenerative cascade, and possibly with the onset of pain. Clinical studies have shown that both the anulus fibrosus and nucleus pulposus cells of the intervertebral disc express factors such as neurotrophins NGF and BDNF that may influence and enhance innervation and pain in the degenerated disc. Expression of such markers as oncogenes Trk-A and Trk-B by the cells of the nondegenerated and degenerated disc suggests an autocrine role for neurotrophins in the regulation of disc cell biology. Additionally, several cytokines have been implicated in the process of IVD degeneration and herniation, with the investigations predominantly focused on interleukin 1 (IL-1) and tumor necrosis factor-alpha (TNF-α) as possible markers involved in the pathogenesis of IVD degeneration.

Chemical markers are macromolecules present in the membranes and fluids in the vicinity of the pathology. The ability to identify degenerative markers could lead to treatment strategies that could diagnose early spinal degeneration and provide treatments at an early stage, when the tissue is capable of healing and reversal of the disease is possible. Microfabricated biosensors can detect and target particular disease-related molecules and proteins. The current methods for protein detection involve labeling procedures that are time-consuming; also, proteins must be in high concentrations for detection, at a point that may not be reversible with respect to tissue healing. Implantable microsized biosensors provide a favorable approach that allows for real-time analysis in minuscule dosages to shorten the detection time and treatment options for the patient. Cantilever-based biosensors for diagnostics have become a promising tool for detection of biomolecular interactions with greater accuracy than conventional methods (Figure 67-2). A nanocantilever and/or microcantilever are devices that can act as physical, chemical, or biological sensors by detecting changes in cantilever bending or vibrational frequency. It is the miniaturized counterpart of a diving board that moves up and down at a regular interval, thus translating molecular or protein recognition into a mechanical motion, at either the nano- or microscale. The mechanical motion can be detected by an optical or piezoresistive readout detector system and, therefore, molecules adsorbed on a microcantilever can cause vibrational frequency changes and deflection

of the microcantilever. Biomolecules that are immobilized on the surface of the cantilever beam relay a surface stress to a readout system. If this surface stress is disrupted by a variation in molecular mass or when a specific mass of a molecule is adsorbed on its surface, such as that of a diseased molecule, the readout will reflect the change and the diseased molecule can be detected at a very early time point and at small manageable dosages for successful treatment. Using a cantilever based on the detection of changes in vibrational frequency, the viscosity, density, and flow rate also can be measured and monitored.[2]

Biochips or Lab-on-a-chip (Figure 67-3)[3] are microfluidic devices that can conduct several laboratory functions and fluid analyses at rapid speeds designed with microchannels smaller than a single cell, with large surface-area-to-volume ratio where liquids follow a laminar flow pathway. "Lab-on-a-chip" indicates generally the scaling of single or multiple lab processes down to chip-format. Conventional lab work conducted on patients' blood samples are used to detect disease-related biochemical changes, and often take as long as one to two weeks to obtain diagnostic results. The biochip can conduct a continuous analysis on minuscule amounts of blood within seconds in multiple iterations, and provide more than just a snapshot of information. In doing so, earlier detection of degenerative disease is possible.

Early detection of diseased molecules can lead to earlier treatment of the degenerative processes related to the aging spine, with the potential to halt or reverse the progression of the disease. The degenerative cascade may start with disc degeneration and desiccation, resulting in height loss, facet hypertrophy, and the bony abnormalities that accompany the degenerative cascade, including osteoporosis. If detected early, the cascade could be interrupted and the progression halted.

## THE POTENTIAL FOR MICRO/NANOTECHNOLOGY IN THE AGING SPINE

The advancement of micro and nanotechnologies discussed in this section presents novel opportunities for increasing the lifespan and improving the quality of life for the aging population. Micro/nanotechnology has the potential to change the future of medicine and patient care. The areas of concentration for micro/nanomedicine are: (1) therapeutic delivery systems with the potential to deliver gene and pharmaceutical targeting specific cellular pathways, (2) development of novel biomaterials and tissue engineering to guide tissue regeneration, and (3) biosensors and biochips for diagnostic monitoring and therapeutic responses. For the aging patient with the degenerative spine, micro/nanomedicine provide the potential of reversing osteoporosis through nanomanipulation of molecules, gene therapy, localized

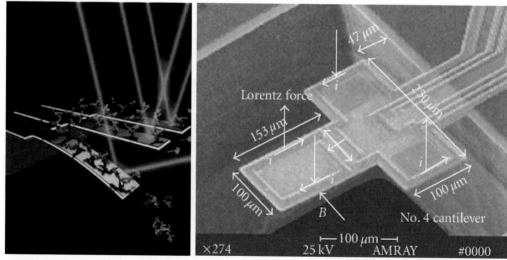

■ **FIGURE 67-2**   NEMS piezoresistive cantilever structures fabricated as cancer detection systems or to detect molecular changes in living tissue or fluids. The right image shows actual multiplanar cantilever detection systems. (*Left image from* http://www.eurekalert.org/features/doe/2001-10/drnl-cm061802.phpen. *Right image from Li X, Yu H, Gan X, Xiaoyuan X, Pengcheng X, Jungang L, Liu M, and Yongxiang L: Integrated NEMS/MEMS resonant cantilevers for ultrasensitive biological detection, ed 2 Journal of Sensors (637734): 1-9, 2009.*)

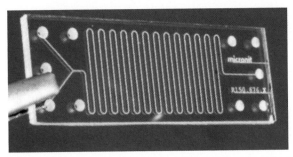

**■ Figure 67-3** Example of the Lab-on-a-chip concept, in which blood can be repeatedly sampled in minuscule amounts and the data accurately transmitted remotely.

drug delivery, and the development of nano- and microscaffolds that are osteoinductive and osteoconductive and can regenerate bone tissue. Biosensors and biochips will not only diagnose degenerative disorders of the spine, but provide the possibility of treating degenerative etiologies detected early in the cascade, to avoid the eventual fusion alternative, which has numerous challenges in the compromised spine of the aging individual.

## References

1. http://www.spineuniverse.com/displayarticle.php/article65.html. Accessed February 17, 2010.
2. http://www.azonano.com/details.asp?ArticleID=1927. Accessed February 17, 2010.
3. http://en.wikipedia.org/wiki/Lab-on-a-chip. Accessed February 17, 2010.
4. P. Bansal, N.P. Padture, A. Vasiliev, Improved interfacial mechanical properties of Al2O3-13wt% TiO2 Plasma-sprayed coatings derived from nanocrystalline powders, Acta Materialia. 51 (2003) 2959.
5. E. Benzel, L. Ferrara, S. Roy, et al., Biomaterials and implantable devices: discoveries in the spine surgery arena, Clin. Neurosurg. 49 (2002) 209–225.
6. E. Benzel, L. Ferrara, S. Roy, A. Fleischman, Micromachines in spine surgery, Spine 15 (29) (2004) 6–601.
7. T. Desai, S. Bhatia, Therapeutic micro/nano technology, Springer, 2006.
8. I.Y. Galaev, B. Mattiasson, 'Smart' polymers and what they could do in biotechnology and medicine, Trends Biotechnol. 17 (1999) 335–340.
9. M. Gell, Development and implementation of plasma sprayed nanostructured ceramic coatings, Surface and Coatings Technology 48 (2001) 146–147.
10. B.H. Guiot, R.G. Fessler, Molecular biology of degenerative disc disease, Neurosurgery 47 (2000) 1034–1040.
11. X. Li, H. Yu, X. Gan, X. Xiaoyuan, X. Pengcheng, L. Jungang, M. Liu, L. Yongxiang, Integrated NEMS/MEMS resonant cantilevers for ultrasensitive biological detection, J. Sensors (637734) (2009) 1–9.
12. Millenium Research Group: US markets for spinal implants, 2006, 5413, 2006.
13. C.A. Niosi, T.R. Oxland, Degenerative mechanics of the lumbar spine, Spine J. 4 (202S) (2004) 208S.
14. C.J. Oosterbos, A.I. Rahmy, A.J. Tonino, Hydroxyapatite coated hip prosthesis followed up for 5 years, Int. Orthop. 25 (2001) 17–21.
15. N.A. Peppas, P. Bures, W. Leobandung, et al., Hydrogels in pharmaceutical formulations, Eur. J. Pharm. Biopharm. 50 (2000) 27–46.
16. N.A. Peppas, K.B. Keys, M. Torres-Lugo, et al., Poly(ethylene glycol)-containing hydrogels in drug delivery, J. Control. Release 62 (1999) 81–87.
17. N.A. Peppas, J.J. Sahlin, Hydrogels as mucoadhesive and bioadhesive materials: a review, Biomaterials 17 (1996) 1553–1561.
18. N.A. Peppas, K.M. Wood, J.O. Blanchette, Hydrogels for oral delivery of therapeutic proteins, Expert Opin. Biol. Ther. 4 (2004) 881–887.
19. D.E. Resiner, Bionanotechnology; global prospects, CRC Press, 2008.
20. K.E. Uhrich, S.M. Cannizzaro, R.S. Langer, et al., Polymeric systems for controlled drug release, Chem. Rev. 99 (1999) 3181–3198.
21. A. White, M. Panjabi, Clinical biomechanics of the spine, ed 2. J.B. Lippincott Company, Philadelphia, 1978.

# 68

# Guided Lumbar Interbody Fusion

*Ali Araghi*

**KEY POINTS**

- Guided lumbar interbody fusion (GLIF) technique is a curvilinear minimally invasive approach to the lateral spine, leveraging all adherent benefits of lateral procedures with the patient in the prone position.

- Allows for a circumferential fusion without repositioning the patient. This minimizes procedural time and allows simultaneous access to the posterior and anterior columns, enabling the surgeon to perform circumferential releases prior to placement of structural anterior column support.

- Delivers a large implant with a large amount of bone graft directly across the anterior column engaging the apophyseal rings for maximum support.

- Allows for direct visualization through the ARC Portal System, via the hinged lids, allowing the surgeon to easily confirm anatomy, to inspect disc preparation and to ensure safe implantation of the interbody spacer.

- Provides an alternative approach where other conventional access methods may be difficult, to better accommodate patient pathologies.

## INTRODUCTION

Interbody lumbar fusion techniques have become increasingly popular because of improved rates of fusion, restoration of disc and foraminal height, and promotion of lordosis.[1] Accessing the anterior column of the lumbar spine lowers the incidence of pseudoarthrosis and recreates the patient's normal sagittal alignment.[2] Late results of alleviating these effects through posterior fixation techniques alone show a significant loss of disc height at the injured segment and kyphotic deformation,[3] necessitating access to the anterior column of the spine for interbody fusion. Conventional methods for accessing the anterior spine use an anterior retroperitoneal approach known as an anterior lumbar interbody fusion (ALIF), whereby a surgeon must mobilize the great vessels, sympathetic plexus, and ureter. This approach is associated with considerable surgical trauma, and higher rates of morbidity. As a result, most of these techniques typically require the presence of an experienced general or vascular surgeon, due to the risk of serious complications.[2]

Gaining popularity are techniques that access the anterior lumbar spine from a lateral retroperitoneal approach with the patient positioned in a lateral decubitus position. These procedures allow access to the anterior spine with little risk of injuring the peritoneum or great vessels, reducing the surgical risks compared to a standard ALIF operation. Since 1973, similar retroperitoneal approaches were documented to access the lumbar spine for performing lumbar sympathectomies and, starting in 1997 and 1998, Rosenthal et al. and McAfee et al., respectively, reported on minimally invasive anterior retroperitoneal approaches to the spine for anterior lumbar fusion. Early results show these alternative lateral approaches to the lumbar spine to be safe and effective for anterior fusion of the first through the fifth lumbar vertebrae.[2]

The guided lumbar interbody fusion (GLIF) technique is a lateral retroperitoneal approach whereby the lateral spine is accessed through a curvilinear portal with the patient in the prone position. Accessing the lateral spine while maintaining the patient in a prone position offers many advantages over similar lateral retroperitoneal approaches and conventional ALIF techniques. First and foremost, this procedure allows the addition of posterior fixation without having either to break the sterile field to rotate the patient mid-surgery or to stage a series of surgeries. This reduces the surgical time required for a full circumferential fusion procedure (otherwise known as a 360), which directly relates to decreased anesthesia time and costs for the patient, surgeon, and hospital.

## INDICATIONS/CONTRAINDICATIONS

Surgical indications for spinal fusion include discogenic pain, segmental spinal instability, progressive degenerative scoliosis, symptomatic spondylolisthesis, postsurgical pseudarthrosis, discitis, stenosis, degenerative disc disease, and lumbar vertebral fractures that may be alleviated with a lateral transpsoas approach.

Contraindications include systemic infection, osteoporosis, significant comorbidities, degenerative spondylolisthesis grade 3 or higher, and bilateral retroperitoneal scarring.

Additionally, the GLIF technique should be considered for revision surgery on patients with significant scar tissue from previous anterior or posterior approaches to the spine.

## DESCRIPTION OF THE DEVICE

At the center of the GLIF technique is the ARC Portal System, a curvilinear lighted retractor system with a hinged top (Figure 68-1). This instrument is delivered over sequential dilators to the disc space, and the hinged top can be opened to gain direct visualization of key surgical landmarks during disc preparation. The device has proximal and distal stabilization capabilities to prevent portal migration during the procedure. In addition to the ARC Portal System, the GLIF technique utilizes specialized instrumentation to efficiently prepare the disc space for implant delivery.

## BACKGROUND OF SCIENTIFIC TESTING / CLINICAL OUTCOMES

Bergey and Regan report, in a study conducted on 28 patients between 1996 and 2003, that early results show the lateral endoscopic transpsoas approach to the lumbar spine to be a safe, minimally invasive method for anterior fusion of the first through the fifth lumbar vertebrae. Their study indicates a risk of groin/thigh paresthesias and/or pain, but they report that these symptoms have proven to be transient. Of the 28 cases, eight patients experienced the transient groin/thigh numbness and/or pain; six patients experienced a small peritoneal perforation due to blunt dissection, with no bowel injuries; and two patients were converted to a mini-open lateral approach. Their report concludes that "this approach can be successfully combined with percutaneous pedicle screw fixation to provide a minimally invasive approach for circumferential fusions."[4]

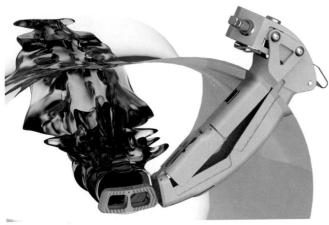

**■ FIGURE 68-1**   The retracted ARC Portal System against a representative lumbar spine.

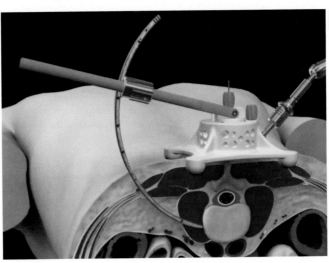

**■ FIGURE 68-2**   The Calibrated Introducer delivering the Initial Dilator.

More recently, an extreme lateral interbody fusion technique (XLIF) has been adopted, with positive results. Pimenta indicates, in a study conducted to evaluate the XLIF technique for fixating lumbar degenerative scoliosis, that the transpsoas lateral approach has lower morbidity, does not require the use of endoscopes, avoids risks associated with anterior approaches, and avoids the invasion of the posterior spinal canal. Analyzing a consecutive series of 80 patients, Pimenta found the transpsoas approach to be a safe, reproducible, minimally invasive technique able to reconstruct sagittal balance, correct degenerative scoliosis, avoid the potential risks to the anterior approach, and promote rapid recovery.[5]

Wright reports similar results in a study of his first 10 patients to undergo the XLIF technique at Washington University. He reports the ability to perform a full discectomy, restore disc and foraminal height, as well as to achieve indirect canal decompression from L1 to L5. There were no vascular, visceral, or neurological complications. Nine out of ten patients ambulated on the day of surgery and were discharged on postoperative day one. One-year radiographic follow-up showed evidence of fusion. Additionally, the study indicated minimal narcotic requirement. Complications included three of 10 patients having transient pain with hip flexion that resolved by 6 weeks. His paper compared patients over 300 lb to those less than 300 lb, and found the surgical corridor to remain essentially the same length with no difference in outcomes, OR times, or blood loss. Hence, among one of the advantages of this technique he cited was that it is particularly useful in obese patients in whom anterior or posterior approaches would be more difficult.[6]

## CLINICAL PRESENTATION AND EVALUATION

This technology is novel and is currently in the alpha phase of release. At the time this chapter was published, only a few devices had been implanted using this technique. There have been no surgical complications to date, and follow-up data are presently being collected for better clinical evaluation.

## OPERATIVE TECHNIQUE

Proper patient positioning and delivery of the initial dilator are integral to the success of a GLIF technique. To facilitate proper trajectory of the instrumentation, the Calibrated Introducer was developed to repeatedly and reliably deliver the instruments to the surgical site (Figure 68-2).

The patient is positioned on the operating table in the prone position, and lateral fluoroscopy is used to locate the proper operative level. The Calibrated Introducer is placed along the midline of the patient's back, directly above the operative level, and then secured with a Table Fixation Arm. The Calibrated Introducer is adjusted to locate the posterior one third of the operative disc space, which in turn identifies the axis of rotation for the curvilinear trajectory. Dilator 1 is attached to the Calibrated Introducer swing arm (centered on the identified axis of rotation) and rotated until the distal tip of Dilator 1 touches the patient's skin. At this location, a 4 cm transverse

incision is made through the patient's skin and fascia. A finger is used to palpate through the subcutaneous tissue into the retroperitoneal space, and can be used to sweep the peritoneum anteriorly and identify either the psoas muscle or the anterior tops of the transverse processes.

Using the surgeon's finger as a guide, Dilator 1 is advanced along the calibrated trajectory and delivered into the retroperitoneal space, through the psoas muscle, and up to the annular wall of the desired location. Throughout this step and the following sequential dilaution procedure, standard neuromonitoring technology can be utilized to ensure safe delivery of the dilators around the nervous structures. Proper dilator placement is confirmed with lateral fluoroscopy, then anterior-posterior fluoroscopy. A guidewire is delivered through the cannula of Dilator 1 into the vertebral disc and then Dilator 1 is impacted into the intervertebral disc space, approximately 3 to 4 cm or to the midline. At this point, fluoroscopy can be used to verify final placement of the initial dilator. The guidewire and Calibrated Introducer can then be removed. Dilator 1 implanted into the intervertebral disc space provides a fixed trajectory to the surgical site for the following access instrumentation.

Sequential dilation is performed using Dilator 2 and Dilator 3 to retract the soft tissue through the retroperitoneal space and psoas muscle in preparation for the delivery of the access portal. The ARC Portal is delivered over Dilator 3 and gently manipulated until the instrument is fully seated against the lateral wall of the anterior spinal column (Figure 68-3). Throughout the procedure, anterior-posterior fluoroscopy is used to confirm instrument placement and trajectory. Final placement of the device is maintained using a Table Fixation Arm. An Anterior Awl that retracts from the ARC Portal is deployed into the intervertebral disc space to establish distal fixation to the spine, and the dilators are removed.

The hinged top of the ARC Portal is then opened using a toeing wrench to expose the operative site (Figure 68-4). Direct visualization is used to identify local anatomy and prepare the operative corridor for the subsequent disc-preparatory and implant insertion steps/operations. The distal perimeter of the ARC Portal can be explored using standard neuromonitoring equipment. Penfield dissectors or elevators can be used to isolate and tuck residual tissue behind the edges of the portal. Bipolar electrocautery can also be used, if necessary, to further prepare for disc visualization. A Posterior Tang, which extends into the intervertebral disc space and attaches to the ARC Portal, is assembled using the Posterior Tang Guide to complete the protected working zone within the intervertebral disc space between the Anterior Awl and Posterior Tang.

Specialized instrumentation is used to efficiently clean the disc space through the ARC Portal. The lateral annulus and disc nucleus are removed using an adapted annulotomy knife, annulus punch, and a series of curved pituitary rongeurs. Specialized osteotomes, Cobb elevators, curettes and rasps may be used to remove cartilaginous material from the endplates and release the contralateral annulus. Alternatively the Rotating Actuator with auxiliary Shaver Blades and Rotating Distractor attachments can be used to clear the disc space (Figure 68-5). The Shaver Blade and Rotating Distractor attachments can be used as a guide to determine an appropriate Implant Trial size used in the following step.

After the disc space has been sufficiently cleared, Implant Trials are used to determine the appropriate size of the implant with respect to height and foot print size. The GLIF system offers a range of footprint sizes: lengths, heights, and lordotic angles. Anterior-posterior fluoroscopy is used to verify placement of the Implant Trial. An implant is attached to the Impacting Inserter, and the interior channels of the implant are filled with graft material. The Impacting Inserter and implant are delivered through the ARC Portal into the disc space (Figure 68-6). Ideal implant placement is centered across the disc space, resting on both lateral edges of the disc on an anterior-posterior projection. On a lateral view, the implant should ideally be placed between the anterior third and middle of the disc space. Placement of the implant is confirmed by both anterior-posterior fluoroscopy and lateral fluoroscopy. The ARC Portal can be collapsed and all instruments are then removed.

## POSTOPERATIVE CARE

Radiographic follow-up until fusion has occurred is prudent. Postoperative bracing is predicated on the patient's bone quality, the degree of instability present preoperatively, the choice of additional fixation, and intraoperative variables, as well as surgeon choice.

## COMPLICATIONS AND AVOIDANCE

The GLIF technique is a curvilinear access to the lumbar spine with the patient in the prone position, affecting the anatomic areas between the following borders: the 12th rib and diaphragm in the cephalad direction; the erector spinae, abdominal and oblique muscles posteriorly; the peritoneum, aorta, and vena cava anteriorly; and the iliac crest in the caudal direction. This window of anatomic landmarks confines the fascia, peritoneal fat, spinal plexus, and various traversing nerves. The following analysis reviews surgical techniques and anatomic precautionary areas that may be encountered with the GLIF technique.

Dissecting from the skin to the retroperitoneal space should be approached in a muscle-splitting approach. Mayer describes a blunt, muscle-splitting approach in which each muscular layer (external oblique, internal oblique, transverse abdominal muscles) is dissected in the direction of its fiber orientation. Care is taken to preserve the iliohypogastric and ilio-inguinal nerves, which occasionally cross the surgical field at the level of L4-L5 between the layers of the internal oblique and transverse abdominal muscles.[7]

The major drawback in a lateral retroperitoneal approach is traversing past the large psoas muscle, which covers the spine along its lateral aspect. Additionally, the psoas muscle has various nerves bordering and traversing through its confines, including the genitofemoral nerve and spinal plexus. The psoas muscle acts as a stabilizer for the lumbar spine, like guy wires

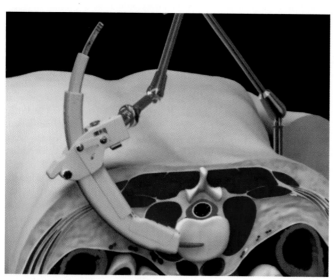

■ **FIGURE 68-3** The ARC Portal delivery over sequential dilators.

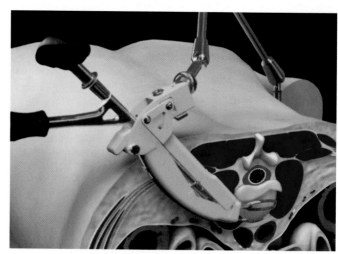

■ **FIGURE 68-5** The Rotating Actuator delivered through the ARC Portal. The Proximal T-Handle is used to actuate the attached shaver bit, which is delivered into the intervertebral disc space.

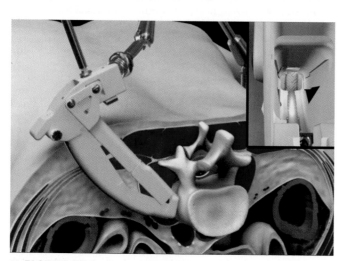

■ **FIGURE 68-4** A retracted ARC Portal System, with inset view showing an exposed annulus view down the ARC Portal.

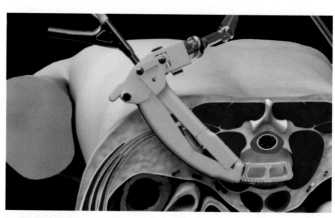

■ **FIGURE 68-6** Delivery of an implant through the ARC Portal using the Impacting Inserter.

stabilizing a ship's mast, during activities such as lifting, by using compressive loading and bilateral activation.[8] Thus, preserving the psoas muscle function can be related to better spinal stability and protection.

Regarding direction of approach, Bergey reports that a "left-sided approach to the surgery is preferred to a right-sided approach because it is easier to dissect the aorta off the spine than to dissect around the more friable inferior vena cava." Bergey concludes in his study that the advantage of a lateral transpsoas approach over a standard anterior transperitoneal approach is in the ease of access to the upper lumbar spine (L1-L4), a place where anterior techniques are frequently complicated by the location of the great vessels. As the indications of minimally invasive lateral approaches expand to treatment of coronal plane deformities, other factors play a larger role. The concave side of such curves usually allows convergence to one point and minimizes the number of incisions needed to approach more than one level. However, the disc is being approached from the collapsed side, and it will take more work to access the disc. Once the annulotomy is made from the side of the collapse, theoretically it should allow the maximal release and optimize the correction.

Bergey expressed concern about a 30% incidence of transient groin/thigh pain, these symptoms being consistent with the cutaneous innervation of the genitofemoral nerve. As a result, Bergey recommends staying in the anterior one third of the psoas muscle to avoid nerve root injury. Visualization and protection of the genitofemoral nerve should avoid permanent paresthesias in the anterior thigh.[2] The genitofemoral nerve mainly branches from the L1 and L2 nerve root, travels through the psoas major muscle anteriorly, and descends along with the abdominal surface of the psoas major. Moro et al. report that the level where the genitofemoral nerve passes through the psoas major muscle ranges from the cranial third of the L3 vertebral body to the caudal third of the L4 vertebral body. [9] It then descends on the surface of the psoas muscle, normally under the cover of the peritoneum, and divides into the genital and femoral branches. The genital branch passes outward on the psoas major and pierces the fascia transversalis or passes through the internal abdominal ring. It then descends along the back part of the spermatic cord to the scrotum, and supplies, in the male, the cremaster muscle. In the female, it accompanies and ends in the round ligament. The femoral branch of the genitofemoral nerve descends on the external iliac artery, sending a few branches to it and, after passing beneath the Poupart ligament to the thigh, supplies the skin of the anterior aspect of the thigh about midway between the pelvis and knee.[2] Moro states that the risk of injuring the genitofemoral nerve increases when splitting the psoas major muscle at lower levels. However, there are reports of having succeeded in remitting the symptoms without a serious problem. [9]

Moro's anatomic study of the lumbar plexus with respect to retroperitoneal endoscopic surgery clarifies the safety zone of the psoas major muscle during retroperitoneal endoscopic surgery using cadavers. Lumbar spines were removed from embalmed cadavers, and from L1-L5, each specimen was cut in parallel with the lumbar disc space and the lumbar vertebra at the cranial third and caudal third of each lumbar vertebral body. The distribution and relationship of the lumbar plexus and nerve roots was analyzed using computer images. Moro reports, from the results of the study, that the safety zone may be at L2-L3 and above, due to the presence of the genitofemoral nerve between the cranial third of the L3 vertebral body and L4-L5. If the possibility of damaging the genitofemoral nerve is not considered, the safety zone should be at L4-L5 and above. Moro recommends starting from the abdominal edge of the vertebra when spreading the psoas major muscle at L2-L3 and below, because nerves are not located in the abdominal surface of the vertebra. Because the lumbar plexus and nerve roots were wholly contained within the psoas major muscle, one can safely split between the psoas major muscle and vertebral body to protect the nerves (retract posteriorly). Moro continues, stating that the method for retracting the psoas muscle anteriorly and reaching to the lateral surface of the vertebral body may be useful; however, according to the present study, it is the danger zone where the lumbar plexus and nerve roots are located in the center of the vertebral body and dorsally. Additionally, at the L5-S1 level, there are the L4 nerve root, L5 nerve root, femoral nerve, and obturator nerve between the psoas major muscle and the lumbar quadratus muscle. Therefore, those nerve tissues must be checked and protected with the endoscope or the alternative transperitoneal approach should be considered. [9]

---

### ADVANTAGES/DISADVANTAGES OF GLIF

- Advantages
  1. Access allows addition of posterior fixation and posterior releases without rotating patient, to reduce procedural time, anesthesia, and blood loss, which can also help in driving down costs
  2. Delivers an implant directly across anterior column, engaging the apophyseal ring without requiring drastic repositioning
  3. Allows for a larger implant to be delivered with a larger amount of bone graft
  4. Protects / avoids mobilization of the great vessels
  5. Retroperitoneal approach decreases incidence of injuring the peritoneum
  6. Preserves the spine's natural stabilization elements:
     ○ Anterior longitudinal ligament
     ○ Posterior longitudinal ligament
     ○ Posterior elements (facets / lamina)
  7. Allows direct visualization, via hinged portal, allowing the surgeon to easily confirm anatomy and ensure soft tissue and nerves are protected
  8. Provides alternative approach for revision procedures
- Disadvantages
  1. Initial trajectory is defined using blind dilator techniques, although neurostimulation can be used
  2. A learning curve is associated with new procedures

---

Intraoperative neurologic surveillance may also provide added benefit in avoiding the exiting nerve roots, especially at L4-L5, where the L3 nerve root can cross the disc space and may be at risk if the approach is in the anterior one half of the psoas muscle.[2] Peloza validates the use of an electrically elicited electromyography (EMG) monitoring system for nerve avoidance during a posterolateral approach to the spine. Electrically elicited EMG monitoring works by initiating an electrical impulse that causes nearby nerves to depolarize, which generates a muscle contraction in the corresponding myotome(s). These impulses can be detected using peripheral EMG electrodes. Peloza uses adhesive EMG surface electrodes applied to the patient's legs, providing EMG monitoring of the myotomes associated with the spinal levels of interest: vastus medialis for L2-L4, tibialis anterior for L4-L5; biceps femoris for L5-S2; medial gastrocnemius for S1-S2. Peloza concludes that such a system could assist the spine surgeon in safely accessing the intervertebral disc space for minimally invasive lumbar interbody procedures.[10]

### CONCLUSION/DISCUSSION

Published literature indicates that the lateral transpsoas retroperitoneal approach to the spine can be a safe, minimally invasive method for accessing the anterior lumbar spine. Early results show low rates of morbidity, few serious complications, successful rates of fusion, minimal narcotic requirements, and no difference in surgical outcomes comparing obese to nonobese cases. Results from studies of XLIF, which is most analogous to the GLIF technique, state that the surgical corridor for obese patients and nonobese patients is essentially the same, thus making this technique easier on obese patients in whom anterior or posterior approaches would be more difficult. The data suggest that a lateral access to the lumbar spine is most preferable at the lower levels between L2 and L5; above L2 presents challenges associated with the ureter and renal artery and below L5 can be more easily approached with a transperitoneal approach because those levels do not require mobilization of the great vessels, as they are below the vessel bifurcation.

The most significant complications associated with transpsoas approaches are groin/thigh pain related to disruption of the genitofemoral nerve or peritoneal perforation while establishing exposure to the spinal column and damaging the exiting nerve roots / lumbar plexus. However, symptoms related to interference of the genitofemoral nerve seem to be transient and are reported to remit in 6 weeks. As with any surgical procedure there should be a "bailout" plan; in this case it would be to convert to mini-open in the case of encountering scar tissue from previous surgeries or any other unforeseen complication. These less conventional lateral approaches to the spine have a steep learning curve and hands-on training in a laboratory is recommended.

Published articles indicate a left-sided approach to the surgery is preferred because it is easier to dissect the aorta off the spine than to dissect around the more fragile vena cava. The literature reinforcs the necessity of correct patient positioning and accurately finding the location of the incision. Diligently positioning the patient and locating the incision will aid in a smoother operation and procedure, as reorienting surgical portals can often be cumbersome. The access instrumentation and technique should be constructed to promote ideal "muscle-splitting" techniques compared to muscle-sacrificing techniques. Handling of the psoas muscle should be done with care, as the area in and around the muscle indicates the most significant area for injury. The literature shows that it is optimal for the anterior one third of the psoas muscle to be carefully dissected and, optionally, aided by the use of intraoperative neurologic surveillance. Postoperative prescription of bracing for up to 3 months may also be considered.

## References

1. M.P. Steinmetz, D.K. Resnick, Use of a ventral cervical retractor system for minimal access transforaminal lumbar interbody fusion: technical case report, Operative Neurosurgery 60 (2) (2007) E175–E176.
2. D.L. Bergey, A.T. Villavicencio, T. Goldstein, J.J. Regan, Endoscopic lateral transpsoas approach to the lumbar spine, Spine 29 (15) (2004) 1681–1688.
3. A. Olinger, U. Hildebrandt, W. Mutschler, M.D. Menger, First clinical experience with an endoscopic retroperitoneal approach for anterior fusion of lumbar spine fractures from levels T12 to L5, Surg. Endosc. 13 (1999) 1215–1219.
4. D. Bergey, J. Regan, Lateral endoscopic transpsoas spinal fusion: review of technique and clinical outcomes in a consecutive series, Spine J. 3 (5) (2003) S166.
5. L. Pimenta, R. Diaz, F. Phillips, F. Bellera, F. Vigna, M. Da Silva, XLIF: 90 degrees, minimally invasive surgical technique to treatment lumbar degenerative scoliosis in adults: clinical and radiological results in a 15 months follow-up study, Minimally Invasive and Reconstructive Spine Department at Santa Rita Hospital World Spine III Interdisciplinay Congress in Spine Care Meeting, Rio Janeiro, Brazil, 2005.
6. N.M. Wright, XLIF: the first 10 patients at Washington University, Washington University School of Medicine. St. Louis, Missouri World Spine III, Rio de Jinero, Brazil, (Sep 2005).
7. M.H. Mayer, A new microsurgical technique for minmally invasive anterior lumbar interbody fusion, Spine 22 (6) (1997) 691–699.
8. P.L. Santaguida, S.M. McGill, The psoas major muscle: a three dimensional geometric study, J. Biomech 28 (3) (1995) 339–345.
9. T. Moro, S.I. Kikuchi, S.I. Konno, H. Yaginuma, An anatomic study of the lumbar plexus with respect to retroperitoneal endoscopic surgery, Spine 28 (5) (2003) 423–428.
10. J. Peloza, Validation of neurophysiological monitoring of posterolateral approach to the spine via discogram procedure, 9th International Meeting on Advanced Spine Techniques, Center for Spine Care, Dallas, Texas, 2002.

# Laser and Ozone Spinal Decompression

# 69

*James J. Yue and David A. Essig*

**KEY POINTS**

- Define the postulated etiologies of mechanical and radicular pain.
- Define the theory of laser disc decompression.
- Define the role for laser disc decompression.
- Define the postulated mechanism of action of ozone-oxygen chemodiscolysis.
- Define the role of ozone-oxygen chemodiscolysis.

## INTRODUCTION

Low back pain is one of the most frequent chief complaints in medical practices. Approximately 80% of the populations of Western countries will suffer from at least one episode of low back pain in their life. Pain is often characterized as either radicular or postural. While radicular pain is often due to an offending disc herniation, the etiology of low back pain is poorly understood. Proposed pathogenesis includes both mechanical and inflammatory mechanisms, including deformation of the annulus, stimulation of the nociceptive components of the spinal root, ischemia, venous stasis, prostaglandins, and cell-mediated immune response.[1] Various surgical procedures have been utilized to address the treatment of low back pain. These include both motion-sparing and fusion interventions. While these procedures have excellent short-term effects, they have been linked to longer-term complications including recurrent disc herniation, postoperative scarring, and adjacent motion segment disease. As a result, less invasive procedures have been developed. Two such procedures, laser spinal decompression and ozone chemodiscolysis, have shown significant promise.

## LASER DECOMPRESSION

Peter Choy and David Asher were the first to use laser energy to evaporate disc material in 1986. Their initial results were poor, but subsequent studies have had good to excellent outcomes in upto 80% of patients.[2] While various different lasers have been described, most of them use approximately 1200 joules per disc in a pulsatile manner. The principles of treatment are based on the hypothesis that the intervertebral disc functions as a closed hydraulic system. Thus, an increase in water content within the disc increases the pressure, as a result of the inelastic annulus fibrosus. The energy from the laser seeks to evaporate intradiscal material to decrease intradiscal pressure. Furthermore, the energy is hypothesized to denature and renature proteins, causing irreversible changes to the structure of the disc and its ability to rehydrate.[3]

As a result of the laser's energy, the biomechanical properties of the disc are also affected. Experiments have shown that there is a negative correlation between laser energy and disc stiffness. While there is a decrease in intradiscal pressure, there is an overall increase in disc circumference and height as a result of the decrease in disc stiffness. The duration of these biomechanical changes has also been shown to be a function of laser energy. High-energy lasers have been shown to maintain disc height reductions on radiographs and MRI at 12 weeks of follow-up in animal studies.[3]

There is significant debate as to the type of laser most suitable for percutaneous laser decompression. Optical analysis of the properties of degenerative discs and the lasers used in clinical practice has revealed that the wavelength of the Ho:YAG laser provides the highest absorption rate (83% at 2060 nm wavelength). $CO_2$ lasers have also been found to be the most effective at ablating disc material in vitro.[3] No matter what type of laser is chosen, a temperature of 100° C must be attained within the nucleus pulposus for the treatment to be affective. It is important that this heat be confined to the nucleus so as to avoid the potential for destruction of the vertebral endplates, possibly causing a sterile spondylodiscitis, which has been reported in animal models. Clinical complications that have been reported include discitis, vertebral osteomyelitis, worsening of low back pain, and failure of the percutaneous probe requiring surgical decompression. Overall, the complication rate is believed to be around 0.5%.[2]

While there is significant debate with regard to the optimum amount of energy that should be delivered to ablate the nucleus pulposus to reduce intradiscal pressure, indications for the procedure are confined to contained disc herniations. Patients with extruded disc herniations, sequestered herniations, narrowed intervertebral spaces, vertebral abnormalities, or those patients experiencing severe neurologic symptoms should be excluded from receiving treatment.[4] Although there is a lack of randomized controlled trials regarding percutaneous laser disc decompression, observational studies have shown positive evidence in support of the technique. These studies have shown an average relief of 72% at 1 year, with sample sizes of at least 50 patients. A systematic review of the literature revealed Level II-2 evidence for short- and long-term relief with a Grade 1C strong recommendation.[4]

## OZONE CHEMODISCOLYSIS

The concept of chemodiscolysis or chemonucleolysis first gained popularity with chymopapain approximately 40 years ago. However, it fell out of favor as a result of reports of serious neurologic complications in addition to reports of anaphylaxis. Recently, there has been resurgence in the popularity of chemodiscolysis using an oxygen-ozone mixture delivered percutaneously. This technique is based on the principle that pain is generated by mechanical pressure as well as by radicular and periganglionic inflammation.[1] Herniated discs are believed to cause pain through an autoimmune reaction as well as through the triggering of cytokine release. An oxygen-ozone mixture is believed to achieve its effect not only through chemodiscolysis, but also through an antiinflammatory effect similar to a corticosteroid. Postulated mechanisms of action of $O_2$-$O_3$ gas include improved oxygenation to reduce tissue hypoxia, inhibition of proteases, release of immunosuppressive cytokines, and disc dehydration through rupture of water molecules.

The approach is similar to other percutaneous disc techniques. Using CT guidance, a needle is inserted via a paravertebral approach into the center of the disc. A mixture of oxygen and ozone gas is injected into the disc and the foraminal spaces. In a recent study of 2900 patients who were treated with this method, good results with regard to the VAS score were achieved in 85% of patients, with no neurologic or infectious complications reported.[5] Furthermore, a recent randomized study contrasting intraforaminal steroid and local anesthetic injections with oxygen-ozone injection demonstrated that oxygen-ozone was more effective at 6 months than steroid injections.[6]

## CONCLUSION

Although percutaneous laser disc decompression and oxygen-ozone chemo-discolysis are exciting new technologies, there is a lack of prospective data concerning their effectiveness compared to other interventional procedures. To date, studies have been unable to show an advantage over standard lumbar discectomy.[7] Furthermore, while specific exclusion criteria exist, including sequestered or extruded disc herniations as well as severe neurologic dysfunction, the specific patient that could best benefit is not well defined. It is unclear whether these treatments offer a temporizing solution or a cure for discogenic and radicular pain. Also, will these minimally invasive techniques bias future operative procedures? Further studies will hopefully delineate the appropriate clinical scenarios for these techniques as well as their long-term results.

## References

1. C. Andreula, M. Muto, M. Leonardi, Interventional spinal procedures, Eur. J. Radiol. 50 (2) (2004) 112–119.
2. V. Singh, R. Derby, Percutaneous lumbar disc decompression, Pain Physician 9 (2) (2006) 139–146.
3. B. Schenk, P.A. Brouwer, M.A. van Buchem, Experimental basis of percutaneous laser disc decompression (PLDD): a review of literature, Lasers Med. Sci. 21 (4) (2006) 245–249.
4. V. Singh, et al., Percutaneous lumbar laser disc decompression: a systematic review of current evidence, Pain Physician 12 (3) (2009) 573–588.
5. M. Muto, et al., Low back pain and sciatica: treatment with intradiscal-intraforaminal O(2)-O(3) injection: our experience, Radiol. Med. 113 (5) (2008) 695–706.
6. M. Gallucci, et al., Sciatica: treatment with intradiscal and intraforaminal injections of steroid and oxygen-ozone versus steroid only, Radiology 242 (3) (2007) 907–913.
7. J.N. Gibson, G. Waddell, Surgical interventions for lumbar disc prolapse: updated Cochrane Review, Spine 32 (16) (2007) 1735–1747.

# 70

# The Biochemistry of Spinal Implants: Short- and Long-Term Considerations

*Shawn Hermenau, Anne Prewett, and Ravi Ramachandran*

## KEY POINTS

- Biocompatibility of a material is directly related to the host's response to an implanted object. It is multifactorial in nature and may include implant material, size, shape, location of implant, and duration of implantation.

- Release of biomaterial from an implant may have local and systemic effects. Local or systemic toxicity, mutagenesis, carcinogenesis, and hypersensitivity reactions are all examples of biologic response to implanted materials.

- Major metals used today all have relatively safe biologic profiles and are relatively inert, but biologic responses have been documented and are well described.

- Polymers and hydrogels are new and emerging fields of implants with minimal biologic effects.

- Bone grafting material can be classified into several groups based on desired effects. These materials are typically inert and can be used safely.

## HISTORICAL BACKGROUND

In 1892, Sir William Aruthnot Lane began to fix tibia fractures with ordinary steel (Figure 70-1). He was successful in treating a large number of patients, but noted that the steel plates he used became corroded after time. Fortunately, and unbeknown to him, the rust that formed acted as a pseudo-insulator (oxide layer), and prevented further degradation and, likely, failure of the plate. If he had used a dissimilar metal, this layer would not have formed and a severe electrolyte reaction would have ensued, leading to the destruction of the metal and inflammation of the tissues. Though metals had previously been implanted in patients, it was with this advancement that the use of metal implants for fracture stabilization became a practical procedure.[1]

The use of implantable material is not new in orthopedics. For centuries, the use of biomaterials has enabled us to heal patients as well as to learn more about material properties and the body's response to these materials. This learning process has produced the arsenal of safe materials used today. The "safety" of a material is in part determined by its biocompatibility.

Biocompatibility, or the clinical success of a biomaterial, is directly dependent upon the response of the host tissue to perturbation brought about by the foreign material. Biocompatibility is very dependent on the site of implantation, the function and size of the implant, and the duration of implantation. An unintentional consequence of implanting objects into a host is the solubility of implanted material and its dissemination into bodily tissue. This dissemination may be local or throughout the body at distant sites, with little or no effect or with potentially life-threatening effects.

This chapter will review the major implantable materials in orthopedics and biologic or tissue responses that may occur. The section is broken down into metals, polymers, hydrogels and biologics.

## Tissue Response to Biomaterials

The biocompatibility of a material is directly related to the tissue response generated by the material. These are time-dependent processes and can be viewed in two different but interconnected ways: first, the bulk properties of a material, and, second, the physiochemical surface properties of the material, both of which contribute to the initial incorporation and long-term survival of biologic prostheses (Table 70-1).

The bulk properties of a material can mimic those that they are intended to replace or augment. Material designs are targeted for the optimization of function with specific prostheses — wear, strength, and modulus of elasticity. Typically, the bulk materials may have low and unintended systemic distribution in the body over time and may be responsible for potential negative effects such as hypersensitivity or carcinogenicity.

The surface physiochemical or biochemical properties of a material directly relate to incorporation of implants and are more crucial to the short-term success or biocompatibility of a material or implant. The effects of material surface biochemistry are seen in protein adsorption and mediation of cell attachment in the implant assimilation.

Tissue response to implanted biomaterials typically follows a predictable pattern. First, tissue injury and blood-material interaction occurs in the wound bed. During this phase, a hydration shell is formed around the implant. This stage is crucial to determining which proteins and molecules and, hence, cells will adhere to the prosthesis during later stages of incorporation. Hours after implantation, the material becomes covered with proteins from the extracellular matrix, marking the second stage of implantation. The third stage may occur from minutes to days after implantation and is marked by the arrival of cells that adhere to the material surface. Cell adherence through integrins is mediated by earlier protein precursors and adsorption. Intercellular protein adsorption occurs, and further cell-mediated changes are seen on the material surface. Enrichment of surface proteins (Vroman effect) may mediate cell adherence and subsequent incorporation of the device into a specific biologic tissue. This final stage may take days (biodegradable suture), months (bioabsorbable implants), or years (total disc replacement), depending upon the implanted material and clinical goals. Adverse responses can occur throughout the assimilation process. Blood clots, fibrous capsule formation, or foreign body giant cell formation may result as a consequence of exaggerated or prolonged stimulation of the immune system.

## METALS

Current implantable metal alloys with wide use in orthopedics are 316L stainless steel, cobalt-chromium alloys, titanium alloys, and tantalum (Table 70-2). In general, metals are used routinely for weight-bearing or load-bearing implants such as plates, nails, stems, and screws. Though biocompatibility is good with metals, there are issues of concern. Corrosion, metallic toxicity, hypersensitivity, genotoxicity, and carcinogenesis all have been described in the literature with the use of metallic implants.

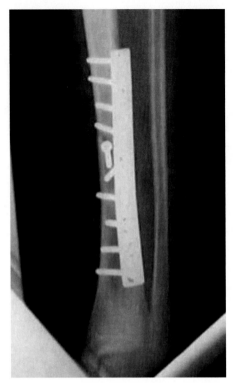

■ **FIGURE 70-1**  Tibial plating with an example of metallic implant.

**TABLE 70-1**  **Common Tissue-Implant Interactions**

| Implant-Tissue Reaction | Consequence |
| --- | --- |
| Toxic | Tissue necrosis |
| Biologically inert—smooth surface | Implant is encapsulated without bonding |
| Biologically inert—porous surface | Tissue grows into pores and forms mechanical bonds |
| Bioactive | Tissue forms interfacial bond with implant (bioactive fixation) |
| Dissolution of implant | Implant resorption and replacement with soft tissue or bone |

## Metal Types

### Titanium

Although titanium has excellent heat and corrosion resistance capabilities, it is difficult to form and machine into desired shapes. Also, its extreme chemical reactivity with air, combined with other factors, has caused the cost of titanium components to be very high. It is used in aerospace applications where weight and temperature resistance are very important, and in military applications, where it provides extreme corrosion resistance and durability. Titanium is also used in biomedical applications such as prosthetics and implants, due to its biologic inertness.

Pure titanium and titanium alloys are used in the making of orthopedic implants such as total disc replacements, stems, nails, and plates. There are several titanium alloys that have been developed. The most commonly used alloy is Ti-6Al-4V. Ti-6Al-4V is composed of titanium, aluminum (6%), and vanadium (4%). These alloys have high corrosion resistance compared to stainless steel and Co-Cr. A passive oxide coat ($TiO_2$) forms on titanium and its alloys, which protects the metal further from corrosion and enhances the metal's biocompatibility profile.

These materials are classified as biologically inert biomaterials or bioinert. As such, they remain essentially unchanged when implanted into patients. The human body is able to recognize these materials as foreign, and tries to isolate them by encasing them in fibrous tissues. However, they do not elicit any adverse reactions and are generally well tolerated. Furthermore, they do not induce allergic reactions such as those observed with stainless steel and cobalt-chrome implants, which have some nickel in their composition and may elicit a nickel hypersensitivity reaction in surrounding tissues.

Titanium and its alloys possess suitable mechanical properties to be used in orthopedics, such as strength, bending strength, and fatigue resistance. Other specific properties that make it a desirable biomaterial are density and elastic modulus. In terms of density, it has a significantly lower density than other metallic biomaterials, implying that these implants will be lighter than similar items fabricated out of stainless steel or cobalt-chrome alloys. Having a lower elastic modulus compared to the other metals is desirable, as the metal tends to behave more like bone itself, which is desirable from a biomechanical perspective. This implies that the bone hosting the biomaterial is less likely to atrophy and resorb.

As a clinical benefit, the scatter associated with titanium is far less than with other metals and makes future imaging studies better. These are not ferromagnetic metals and are safe to use in MRI magnets.

### Cobalt-Chrome

The main components of cobalt-chrome alloys are cobalt, chromium, molybdenum, and some nickel. Cobalt alloys are combined with chromium and molybdenum to increase the metal's corrosion resistance. Cobalt-chrome alloy was the first alloy that was introduced in dentistry in the 1930s, and since then, has proved its clinical effectiveness as a biomaterial.

The components of Co-Cr are elemental, as noted above, and therefore must be classified as more biologically favorable in principle, as elements that have no function in the human body. For essential elements, the body has diverse ways of decomposition and utilization. There appears to be certain threshold values, below which no interaction takes place.

Ores of cobalt are accompanied by nickel. Complete separation of the elements is never possible. The relevant standards stipulate a maximum nickel content of 0.1%. Concentrations of greater than 0.1% have to be declared. Alloys with less than 0.1% of nickel can be designated as nickel-free. In standard cobalt-chrome implants, the release of nickel will amount to approximately 0.00003 mg/cm$^2$ (0.03 µg/cm$^2$) in the first week and constantly decline thereafter. If one compares this to the daily uptake in food, i.e., approximately 0.19 to 0.90 mg, (190 to 900 µg), toxicological or allergic stress appears very improbable.

### Stainless Steel (316L)

The composition of stainless steel has varying percentages of iron, chromium, nickel, molybdenum, and carbon. The most common stainless steel alloy in orthopedic implants is SS 316L. The designation 316L by the ATSG is broken down as follows: the 300 series represents the austenitic family (crystalline structure) of steel, and the L means that the carbon content of the stainless steel is below 0.03%; this will reduce the sensitization effect, precipitation of chromium carbides at grain boundaries, due to the high temperatures produced by welding. The effect of these precipitates can weaken the material by increased corrosion at the grain boundaries. Stainless steel is chemically treated with nitric oxide to form a passive oxide layer, to further increase its corrosion resistance.

Stainless steel is a strong material, with better ductile properties than all the other implantable materials. It has fallen out of favor in the United States, but worldwide is still the most commonly used metal implant. The decrease in U.S. utilization is due to the superior strength, corrosion resistance, and mechanical properties of titanium and cobalt-chrome. Additionally, the biocompatibility profile of stainless steel is less favorable than the other metals, with more reports of hypersensitivity reactions because of its higher nickel content.

### Tantalum

Tantalum is a gray, heavy, and very hard metal. When pure, it is ductile and can be drawn into fine wire, which is used as a filament for evaporating metals such as aluminum. Tantalum is almost completely immune to chemical attack at temperatures below 150° C, and is attacked only by hydrofluoric

**TABLE 70-2    Relative Metallic Properties**

| Characteristic | 316L Stainless Steel | Cobalt Chrome | Titanium | Tantalum |
|---|---|---|---|---|
| Stiffness | Medium | High | Low | Low |
| Strength | Medium | Medium | High | High |
| Corrosion resistance | Low | Medium | High | High |
| Biocompatibility | Low | Medium | High | High |

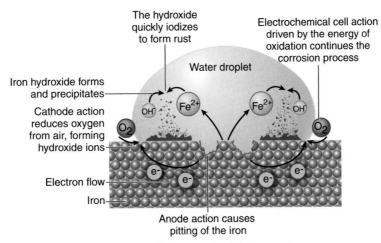

■ **FIGURE 70-2**    Example of pitting corrosion.

acid, acidic solutions containing the fluoride ion, and free sulfur trioxide. At high temperatures, tantalum becomes much more reactive. Tantalum is used to make a variety of alloys with desirable properties such as high melting point, high strength, and good ductility. Tantalum readily forms oxides and is most stable as +5 tantalum pentoxide. Elemental tantalum unites strength and corrosion resistance with excellent biocompatibility. Tantalum is the metal used in the construction of Trabecular Metal (Zimmer). The cellular structure of Trabecular Metal resembles bone and approximates its physical and mechanical properties more closely than any other prosthetic material. Its unique, highly porous, trabecular configuration is conducive to bone formation, enabling rapid and extensive tissue infiltration and strong attachment.

## Corrosion

Most fluids in the human body are of similar chloride content and pH to sea water (20 g/L and 7.4); therefore many metals used in orthopedic implants have been those most resistant to corrosion in sea water. Corrosion is, simply, the dissolution of metallic ions in aqueous solution. Electrochemical cells are produced in the body when these metallic implants are used and equilibria of metallic ions in solution are achieved within body fluids over time (Figure 70-2).

Generally three types of corrosion exist with the use of metallic implants and include (1) galvanic, (2) crevice or pitting, and (3) fretting corrosion. Galvanic corrosion is corrosion due to the use of dissimilar metals in contact with one another or electrochemical dissolution. Pitting corrosion is a form of localized corrosion that leads to the creation of small holes or defects in the metal (Figure 70-3). The driving power for pitting corrosion is the lack of oxygen around a small area. This area becomes anodic while the area with excess of oxygen becomes cathodic, leading to very localized galvanic corrosion. The corrosion penetrates the mass of the metal, with limited diffusion of ions, further increasing the localized lack of oxygen. The mechanism of pitting corrosion is probably the same as crevice corrosion. Finally, fretting corrosion, as defined by the ASM Handbook on Fatigue and Fracture, is: "A special wear process that occurs at the contact area between two materials under load and subject to minute relative

motion by vibration or some other force." The relative small motion causes mechanical wear and material transfer at the surface of the metals, followed by oxidation of that debris and the freshly exposed surface. This debris then acts as an additional abrasive product that is often harder than the original metal and perpetuates the process.

## Distribution of Metal in Body Fluids

A prosthetic device constitutes a pool of trace elements or alloy in the body, which, when mobilized by corrosion, dissolution, and wear, are distributed in local tissue or potentially at sites distant to the original site of implantation. Metallic particles can be found in local tissues such as articular joint capsules, muscle, and regional lymph nodes, or at distant tissues such as abdominal paraaortic lymph nodes, liver, spleen, and pancreas. Studies have looked at distribution of metal ions in body fluids following prosthetic joint implantation. Only slight increased levels of Co and Cr in serum and urine have been noted in patients 2.5 years after implantation of the prosthesis.[1] Another paper reported increased deposition of metallic particles in the liver, spleen, and abdominal paraaortic lymph nodes, in a postmortem study. Larger metallic burdens were seen in patients with failed total joint replacements. In most of the patients evaluated in the postmortem study, the concentration of metallic particles in the liver and spleen was low, and no toxic effects were apparent on histological exam of the surrounding tissue.[2]

Animal studies have shown that nickel, cobalt, or molybdenum introduced into tissue is quickly transported and eliminated in the urine within a relatively short time. Chromium is not eliminated as quickly and can accumulate in tissues and red blood cells. The hexavalent Cr often will be reduced to trivalent Cr and become cell-associated, therefore accumulating in the body.

## Mutagenesis

Metallic particles disseminated throughout the body are feared to have potentially deleterious effects. Some early studies were published raising the question of biomaterials being responsible for mutagenesis at distant

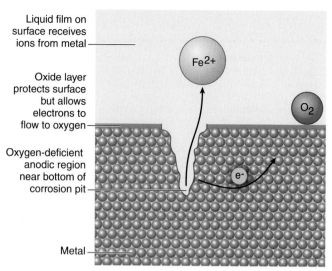

Liquid film on surface receives ions from metal

Oxide layer protects surface but allows electrons to flow to oxygen

Oxygen-deficient anodic region near bottom of corrosion pit

Metal

■ **FIGURE 70-3** Example of electrochemical cell around metallic implant.

sites in the body. Mutagenesis, or genotoxicity, is the disruption of DNA resulting in the production of aberrant proteins that lead to cellular or tissue dysfunction. Genotoxicity or mutagenesis can serve as an indicator for the potential carcinogenicity of a material. A paper in 2003 looked at potential mutagenesis of cobalt-chrome and titanium implants. The conclusion was that neither material showed evidence of mutagenesis in bacterial assay and mammalian cell assays. Although, by itself, this is not enough evidence to be able to state that these implants are not mutagenic or genotoxic, in combination with the reports of cancer (next section) in patients with Co-Cr or titanium implants, it appears to be supported clinically.

## Carcinogenicity

Although local and systemic deposits of metallic ions have been demonstrated in patients with implanted metal, the associative relationship of these toxic effects has yet to be established. Concentration-related connections between orthopedic implants and malignant degeneration have been questioned and potential case reports have been published. The International Agency for Research on Cancer concluded that implanted foreign bodies of metallic titanium, cobalt-chromium, and stainless steel appear not to be directly carcinogenic in humans.

There is sufficient evidence in experimental animals for the carcinogenicity of implants of cobalt, nickel, and nickel alloy powder containing approximately 66% to 67% nickel, 13% to 16% chromium and 7% iron. This noted, there is inadequate evidence in experimental animals to establish the carcinogenicity of orthopedic-type implant materials of chromium metal, stainless steel, titanium metal, or titanium-based alloys.

There is inadequate evidence in humans for the carcinogenicity of metallic implants and metallic foreign bodies, although numerous case reports and small power studies have been published and controversy has been generated. Out of the large number of patients with orthopedic implants, a total of 35 cases have been reported of malignant neoplasms arising from the bone or the soft tissue in the region of an implant. Fourteen cohort studies of patients following total knee or total hip replacement from six countries were performed to investigate cancer incidence in these populations. One study showed a small increase in overall cancer incidence, while the remaining studies showed overall decreases. Four of these studies suggested a possible increased risk for specific cancers, including Hodgkin disease, non-Hodgkin lymphoma, leukemia, and kidney cancer. However, results of several other studies were not consistent with this observation. Additionally, two case-control studies, one including cases with soft-tissue sarcoma and the other including lymphoma and leukemia, were carried out in the United States. These studies failed to establish a causal effect. Most of the studies did not have information on possible confounding variables such as immunosuppressive therapy or

rheumatoid arthritis for the lymphomas and analgesic drugs for kidney cancer. The follow-up in most of the studies may have been too short to evaluate cancer occurring many years after exposure. A total of 23 cases of sarcomas, 23 cases of carcinomas, and 7 cases of brain tumors have been reported at the site of metallic foreign bodies, mainly bullets and shrapnel fragments.

## Hypersensitivity

The first report of hypersensitivity with a metallic orthopedic implant was in 1966 by Foussereau and Laugier. They reported on a patient with an eczematous dermatitis and associated this hypersensitivity reaction with nickel. Since then, a growing body of literature has described metal hypersensitivity reactions to stainless steel, cobalt-chromium, and, to a lesser degree, titanium implants. Though well documented, these metal hypersensitivity reactions remain unpredictable and poorly understood events relative to orthopedic implants.

The prevalence of metal hypersensitivity in the general population is approximately 10% to 15%. Metals known to cause reactions are nickel, beryllium, cobalt, chromium, and to a far lesser extent, titanium and tantalum. Nickel is the most common sensitizer, with a prevalence of approximately 14%. Cross-reactivity between nickel and cobalt exists. In patients with metal prostheses, the prevalence of metal hypersensitivity is approximately 25%, and in patients with failed prostheses, the prevalence reaches 60%. It is unclear whether the failure is a result of hypersensitivity or whether increased degradation products in the body due to the implant failure result in increased hypersensitivity reactions.

Dermal contact and ingestion of metals is known to result in an immune response causing hives, eczema, redness, and itching. Resultant metallic degradation products may sensitize the body and generate similar effects. A temporal association between implantation and clinical manifestations of these symptoms has been shown. Implant-related hypersensitivity reactions are typically cell-mediated reactions (type IV delayed-type hypersensitivity).

Implant degradative products from corrosion or mechanical wear will react and bind to proteins in tissue and form organometallic complexes. It is these complexes that become antigens, sensitize T cells, and eventually result in a T-cell–mediated immune response. T cell release of cytokines, including IL-3, granulocyte-macrophage colony stimulating factor, INF-α, and TNF-β, then leads to the activation and infiltration of macrophages responsible for the immune response seen in these delayed-type hypersensitivity reactions.

Clinically, the immunologic response within the periprosthetic area may include vasculitis, fibrosis, muscle necrosis, osteolysis, and metallosis. This cascade of events may result in mechanical failure of the device or inability of the implant to be integrated into the biologic system, and may mandate removal of the biomaterial. Removal of a device that has served its function and can be safely removed should be considered, as this may alleviate some of the symptoms for the patients.

Though hypersensitivity reactions to orthopedic implants are not common, more frustrating is the lack of predictability for avoiding this complication. No evidence exists to support the use of routine allergy testing or skin testing of metals in patients undergoing implantation of a metallic device. In the event of temporally related skin symptoms and metallic implantation, skin sensitivity testing should be considered. Until more studies are conducted to better define the role of delayed-type and humoral immune hypersensitivity reactions in patients with metallic implants, the risk to patients should be considered minimal.

## POLYMERS

### Introduction

Synthetic polymers are occupying a growing role in implant construction. They accord numerous advantages including radiolucency and elasticity. While the vast majority are biologically inert, their wear and degradation processes and properties reflect on their suitability as implants. The following sections will outline the principal polymers used in disc arthroplasty, in fusion, and as bioabsorbable interbody spacers.

## UHMWPE

The polymer with which spine surgeons have had the most experience and the longest-reaching data is ultra high molecular weight polyethylene (UHMWPE). The material is composed of extremely long chains, with molecular weights numbering in the millions. The longer chain serves to transfer load effectively to the polymer backbone, resulting in a very tough material. UHMWPE is highly resistant to corrosive chemicals, exhibits low moisture absorption, has a low coefficient of friction, and is both self-lubricating and resistant to abrasion.

Total disc arthroplasty's CHARITÉ Artificial Disc has been implanted since the 1980s. The implant consists of two metallic endplates that articulate with a central UHMWPE disc. Modern manifestations of this design, still incorporating the UHMWPE articulation, include the Synthes Pro-Disc-C, the Cervitech PCM, the LDR Spine Mobi-C, the Aesculap AG Activ-C, and the DePuy Spine Discover.

## PEEK

Polyether ether ketone (PEEK) is an organic polymer thermoplastic. Molecularly, it consists of phenylene rings that are linked via oxygen bridges. There have been no reports of biologic adverse response/reaction with this material. The plastic is used either alone or with a carbon fiber reinforcement. It is a member of the polyaryletherketone family, which includes several other polymers with applications in spine surgery.

The first utilization of PEEK was in spinal cages in the 1990s, by AcroMed. An advantage of the polymer in this function is its radiolucency, which facilitates radiographic assessment of fusion in vivo. The majority of current implants employing PEEK are cervical and lumbar spinal cages. Examples include Zimmer Spine's BAK Vista radiolucent Interbody Fusion System, Surgicraft's STALIF anterior lumbar fusion cage, Scient'x's CC interbody fusion cage, Depuy Spine's OCELOT Stackable Cage System, and the Nubac Disc Arthroplasty Device.

Recent studies with PEEK cages attempt to accelerate fusion by incorporating hydroxyapatite, 40% β-tricalcium phosphate/60% hydroxyapatite, or rhBMP-2. Possible applications for the material in posterior dynamic stabilization, interspinous process decompression systems, posterior rods, and total disc replacement are also being explored.

## PLA and PGA

Bioabsorbable devices in the spine are composed of polymers known as alpha-polyesters or poly-(alpha-hydroxy) acids. These include polylactic acid (PLA) and polyglycolic acid (PGA). PLA is based on a lactic acid monomer, while PGA is based on a glycolic acid monomer. Both substances safely degrade completely in vivo and are used in bioabsorbable interbody spacers.

Advantages of bioabsorbable polymers over metals in spine surgery include the avoidance of imaging artifact on postoperative radiographs and a modulus of elasticity closer to that of native bone, lessening stress-shielding. As the implant is ultimately resorbed, complications such as implant erosion and migration may be avoided. Disadvantages of the use of bioabsorbable polymers are an initial strength that cannot match their metal counterparts and the possibility of generating an inflammatory response with breakdown products.

## Implant Performance and Failure

The reaction of the implants and the materials that compose them with the body is largely a result of the processes of wear, degradation, and oxidation. In the following section, we will discuss the theoretical and observed complications specific to polymer implants.

## UHMWPE

Given our relatively short experience with the application of UHMWPE in spine surgery, most relevant in vivo clinical data come from retrieval studies of the CHARITÉ Artificial Disc. Some data have also been published on the ProDisc-L. Both implants are constructed with a UHMWPE insert. Relevant wear data concerning other materials are largely a product of lab studies. Decades of experience from total hip and knee arthroplasty have demonstrated that UHMWPE wear particles have the ability to cause implant failure through macrophage-mediated aseptic osteolysis. Similar complications have been observed in spine surgery. Osteolysis has been observed around certain total disc replacement designs, including the CHARITÉ implant. The particle load and resulting inflammatory response in the periprosthetic area is reported to be proportional to that observed in total hip arthroplasty.

CHARITÉ components, retrieved for intractable pain and/or facet degeneration, frequently displayed one-sided wear patterns. The dome of the components typically exhibited burnishing, and the rim showed evidence of plastic deformation, burnishing, and fracture, thought to be produced by impingement. Similar patterns are described in the ProDisc-L and Prodisc-C.

In addition to impingement, rim damage observed in polyethylene total disc replacement retrievals has also been associated with postirradiation oxidation. Analysis of explanted CHARITÉ cores has shown that the exposed rim experiences severe oxidation after 10 or more years. The central dome is protected from in vivo oxidation due to contact with the metallic endplates.

The end product of UHMWPE wear is the creation of wear debris and ensuing aseptic loosening. The biology of aseptic loosening has been extensively studied and described in the hip and knee total joint arthroplasty literature. The cellular response to UHMWPE consists primarily of giant cells and macrophages. The magnitude of the response is directly related to the volume of debris. The role of these cells is to detect, phagocytose, and degrade any foreign material. In the process, these cells release chemical messengers, including cytokines and other mediators of the inflammatory process. As a result, a foreign-body granulomatous response is initiated. Macrophages fuse, forming giant cells to wall off the foreign material. Osteoclasts are activated by the cytokines IL-1b, IL-6, IL-8, PGE2, and TNF-α. Osteolysis is postulated to be the product of both osteoclastic and macrophage– and giant-cell–mediated bone resorption.

## PEEK

Theoretical implant complications of PEEK cages are the same as those observed with metal devices. These include subsidence, wear, debris production, and fracture. Wear debris has been identified in periprosthetic biopsies, but no evidence of an inflammatory reaction to the particles has been described. In vitro and in vivo studies suggest that PEEK particles appear to be harmless to the spinal cord.

Examination of systemic, intramuscular, and intracutaneous toxicity of PEEK has revealed no adverse side effects. There do not appear to be issues with sensitization or gene toxicity. Extensive in vitro testing with fibroblast, macrophage, and osteoblast cell lines shows no cytotoxicity, immunogenesis, or genotoxicity of PEEK.

## PLA and PGA

Alpha polyesters are degraded by hydrolysis. The process releases their respective monomers, which are then incorporated into normal cellular physiologic processes. Lactic acid is produced from PLA, and glycolic acid from PGA. Lactic acid eventually ends up in the citric acid cycle, while glycolic acid can be excreted in urine. The rate of degradation is based both on factors inherent to the implant and polymer, including molecular weight, crystallinity, and porosity, and other local factors including vascularity and loading conditions.

As the implant begins to degrade and fragment, particle removal via a foreign-body reaction begins. The rate of degradation is associated with the degree of inflammatory response, synovitis, and even activation of the complement cascade. PLA has the slower rate of degradation, while PGA has the faster. As a result, PLA degradation has been associated with a foreign-body reaction as late as 143 weeks after implantation, while a foreign-body response reaction to PGA has been seen as early as 3 to 6 weeks after implantation. As a result of this inflammatory response, complications such as sterile sinus tract formation, synovitis, hypertrophic fibrous encapsulation, and osteolysis have been described.

## HYDROGELS

## Synthetic Hydrogels

Synthetic polymers exhibit low toxicity, and have been used in medical applications for a period of more than 60 years. Many polymer systems have been employed, including polyacrylonitrile, polyamides, polyethylene, polymethylmethacrylate, polytetrafluoroethylene, polyurethanes, and silicones. Products made from these polymers have been used as bone and tissue replacements, as drug delivery devices, and have been variously employed in nearly all medical disciplines, including heart surgery, orthopedic surgery, ophthalmology, gynecology, and plastic surgery with remarkable success. Synthetic polymers are also utilized in topical applications and as coatings for stents and other implants.

As a result of their synthesis, hydrophobic polymers generally contain minute amounts of residual impurities, such as monomers, degradation products, stabilizers, catalysts, and solvents. Regardless of the purity of the polymer, there is the potential for small quantities of these impurities to migrate into the recipient of products devised from these polymer systems. These impurities are very difficult to remove completely from the polymers, and they can migrate over long time periods from the polymers into the surrounding tissue.

Water-insoluble, hydrophilic polymers that absorb large quantities of water relative to their initial weight are called hydrogels. Through the absorption of water or surrounding media, hydrogels expand in both weight and volume and can be viewed to some extent as "solidified water." Synthetic hydrogels may have several important advantages as biomaterials, when compared with the classic hydrophobic polymers.

Hydrogels are typically permeable to aqueous solutes, thereby permitting the removal of water-soluble impurities by simple aqueous extraction. As hydrogels are principally composed of water, they are highly biocompatible and exhibit reduced potential to invoke an inflammatory process. The potential for fibrosis and encapsulation is diminished with hydrogel implants relative to traditional hydrophobic synthetic polymer implants. As a result, hydrogels show low adherence to tissues, making them excellent candidate materials for adhesion barriers. Hydrogels also exhibit low friction relative to surrounding tissue. The higher the water content of the hydrogel, the lower the friction.

Protein and lipids can be deposited on the surface of hydrophobic polymers due to denaturation. Cell adhesion proteins are frequently denatured in this fashion and can lead to cellular attachment and fibrosis. Hydrogels, due to their high water content, are resistant to lipid and cell attachment and spreading. As a result, hydrogels often exhibit low adhesion of platelets and other thrombotic cellular elements.

Hydrogels are permeable to water and to small molecular weight water-soluble substances. Part of the water in the swollen hydrogel is available as free water, which provides a diffusion path through the polymer's structure for molecules up to a certain size. At the same time, the polymer network acts as a barrier for larger molecules and for cells, bacteria, and viruses.

One of the first hydrogels used widely was Ivalon. Composed of polyvinylalcohol cross-linked with formaldehyde or glutaraldehyde, the material was hard in the dry state, and soft and pliable in the swollen state. The material found uses as an implantable device and was used variously as a repair material for anorectal reconstruction, breast augmentation, middle ear tympanoplasty, and orthopedic surgery. Complications related to loss of tensile strength and a tendency to become brittle over long-term surgical implantation limited its use.

The potential of synthetic hydrogels as biomaterials was first recognized by Wichterle and Lim in the 1950s. Hydrogels based on hydroxyethylmethacrylate (HEMA), sparingly cross-linked by diesters of diglycols (mono-, di-, tri-, and tetra-) and methacrylic acid were tested on animals mid-century and later developed for soft contact lenses. They later were tested for use as an implant material for reconstructive, plastic, ophthalmic, thoracic, orthopedic, and general surgery; and for drug delivery. Covalently cross-linked polyHEMA is very stable chemically and thermally, and is resistant to enzymatic degradation. This polymer is extensively used in the soft contact lens industry, either as pure poly(HEMA) or in various copolymers, such as PolyHEMA and Polyvinylalcohol. In addition, both polyHEMA and PVA are resistant to degradation due to the carbon-carbon backbone, which is chemically very stable. Polymers such as polyamides, polyesters, and polyurethanes lack the C-C backbone yet have found a wide application as medical hydrogels. Although their in vivo stability cannot match the stability of polymers with the C-C backbone, they have been found to be stable in tissue for over 1 year, with no loss of mass or mechanical properties. Their widest application in medicine today is found in hydrophilic coatings on stents and catheters, wound and burn dressings, and controlled drug release formulations.

## Hydrolyzed Pan Hydrogels – Development and History

The last group of synthetic hydrogels is the HPANs. It is a family of thermoplastic hydrogels, based on acrylic multiblock copolymers. HPAN copolymers form hydrogels using phase separation and formation of crystalline clusters, which cause physical cross-linking. HPAN copolymers are formed by a partial controlled hydrolysis of polyacrylonitrile (PAN). Their formation requires just a simple chemical reaction (hydrolysis) and they contain no monomers, cross-linkers, catalysts, or other toxic residuals.

HPAN hydrogels belong to a family of hydrogels based on partial hydrolysis of PAN, generally called HPANs (hydrolysed PANs). First generation of HPANs was developed in the Institute of Macromolecular Chemistry of the Czechoslovak Academy of Sciences in the Czech Republic, and its synthesis, composition, and properties were described in a number of papers. These materials were found to be highly biocompatible and were used in contact lenses and orthopedic implants.

Additional HPAN advantages as compared to other hydrogels are:

(1) Mechanical strength even at high water content: HPAN hydrogels are comparable in elasticity and tensile strength to tissues with a similar water content, such as cornea, vitreous body, cartilage, and nucleus pulposus of the intervertebral disc. These materials are particularly resistant to tear propagation. HPAN is probably stronger and more resistant to mechanical damage than any other current synthetic hydrogel of the same liquid content.

(2) As for other hydrogels, HPAN hydrogels are permeable to water-soluble compounds. The maximum size of these molecules (permeation limit) can be controlled by the water content of the hydrogel. Molecules smaller than the permeation limit (drugs, nutrients, metabolites, salts, gases) can be transported through the hydrogel using either diffusion or hydraulic flow mechanisms. At its maximum water content, HPAN can pass solutes of molecular weight up to 100,000 Daltons. Highly-hydrated HPAN has also very high hydraulic permeability similar to cartilages and comparable tissues.

## BIOLOGICS

### Bone Graft

Bone graft is required to fill voids to achieve fusion of motion segments and to unite fractured bones. The ideal bone graft, considered the gold standard to which all others are compared, is autogenous bone graft or autograft. The ideal bone graft substitute should be osteogenic, biocompatible, bioabsorbable, able to provide structural support, easy to use clinically, and cost-effective.

The normal host response to autograft is divided into several phases. As mentioned earlier, with any "foreign" object implanted into the body there is hemorrhage and inflammation, and next, invasion by vascular elements from the periphery that bring in precursor cells to osteoblasts and osteoblasts themselves. The rim of osteoblasts deposits new bone on the outer edges of the graft and remodeling begins. This stage may take weeks to months, depending on the type of graft, and is completed after the graft is fully incorporated into the host tissue in a seamless fashion.

The bone grafts and their substitutes are divided according to their properties of osteoconduction, osteoinduction, osteogenesis, or a combination of these. Osteogenic refers to a material that produces bone-forming cells that directly lay down new bone in an area. Osteoinductive refers to a material that can stimulate the differentiation of stem cells into osteogenic cells. Osteoconductive materials are those that provide a porous scaffold to support the formation of new bone. In addition, there are materials that provide more than one of the above characteristics and are considered combination materials (Table 70-3).

Osteoconduction refers to the process in which the three-dimensional structure of a substance is conducive to the ongrowth and ingrowth of new bone. Osteoconductive bone graft substitutes are commercially available and vary in chemical composition, structure, and resorption rates. Understanding the basics of each type and the reason to use a specific one of them will assist with surgical success. The Table 70-3 groups these materials into classes and describes some of their basic properties.

**TABLE 70-3** Bone Grafting

| Bone Graft Family | Description | Classes |
|---|---|---|
| Osteoconductive | Provides structure or scaffold to support bone formation | Ca-Phosphate, ceramics, synthetic polymers, bioactive glass, allograft |
| Osteoinductive | Induces differentiation of cells and new bone growth | BMP, demineralized bone matrix |
| Osteogenesis | Provides stem cells with osteogenic potential that directly form new bone | Bone marrow aspirate |
| Combined | Combinations of above | Autograft |

BMP or bone morphogenic protein is an osteogenic substance that has significant potential for increasing union rates in orthopedic surgery, but which is a source of significant controversy. Infuse (Medtronic), or rHBMP-2, has had tremendous results in demonstrating efficacy of bone production and increasing fusion rates. This product appears to have a great application in high-risk patients undergoing lumbar fusion. These indications for its use are very specific and should be limited to this small set of patients. Recently, the FDA notified health care professionals of life-threatening complications associated with the recombinant human bone morphogenic protein (rhBMP) when it is used in the cervical spine. The agency had received 38 reports of complications during the previous 4 years, associated with its use in cervical spine fusions, for which it is not approved. The complications included swelling of neck and throat tissue, which resulted in compression of the airway and/or neurological structures in the neck. Some reports describe difficulty swallowing, breathing, or speaking. NASS and AANS have all come out with statements recommending that surgeons not use BMP off-label in the cervical spine.

## SUMMARY

Biocompatibility of a biomaterial is directly dependent upon the response of the host tissue. Factors that influence this response are the site of implantation, the function and size of the implant, and the duration of implantation. An unintentional consequence of implanting objects into a host is the solubility of implanted material and its dissemination into bodily tissue. This dissemination may be local or throughout the body at distant sites, with little or no effect or with potentially life-threatening effects.

Metals used today (titanium, Co-Cr, and stainless steel 316L) have generally good biologic profiles and are considered safe to implant. Hypersensitivity reactions may occur and are most likely with nickel exposure. No good screening tests are available to determine who may experience an exaggerated immune response with metal implantation. Corrosion is another large part of a metal's biocompatibility profile and plays a part in a potential hypersensitivity reaction which in itself can lead to mechanical failure of the implant.

Plastic compounds are a growing area of research and have been safely used in orthopedic surgery. They accord numerous advantages, including radiolucency and elasticity. While the vast majority are biologically inert, the material's wear and degradation processes and properties reflect on their suitability as implants.

Biologic implants such as bone graft are usually biologically inert or biocompatible. Different bone grafts are divided based on the materials' ability to stimulate bone production directly, induce the growth of bone from host tissue, or be a scaffold to facilitate the ingrowth of bone produced by the host. It is crucial when using these products that specific goals or indications are used, in order to achieve successful surgical outcomes.

## References

1. M. Rang, The story of orthopaedics, Saunders Publishing Philadelphia, 2000.
2. J.M. Anderson, et al., Foreign body reaction to biomaterials, Sem Immunology 20 (2008) 86–100.
3. C.G. Lewis, et al., Metal carcinogenesis in total arthoplasty, Clin. Orthop. 329S (1996) S264–S268.
4. J.A. Disegi, et al., Stainless steel in bone surgery, Injury 31 (2000) S-D2–6.
5. American Society for Testing and Materials, Handbook.
6. F.W. Sunderman, et al., Cobalt, chromium, and nickel concentrations in body fluids of patients with porous-coated knee or hip prostheses, J. Ortho. Research. 7 (1989) 307–315.
7. R.M. Urban, et al., Dissemination of wear particles to the liver, spleen, and abdominal lymph nodes of patients with hip or knee replacement, J. Bone Joint Surg. 82-A (4) (2000) 457–477.
8. A. Katzer, et al., In vitro toxicity and mutagenicity of CoCrMo and Ti6Al wear particles, Toxicology 190 (2003) 145–154.
9. International Agency for Research on Cancer, Surgical implants and other foreign bodies, IARC Monographs on the Evaluation of Carcinogenic Risks to Humans 74, 1999.
10. N. Hallab, et al., Metal sensitivity in patients with orthopaedic implants, J. Bone Joint Surg 83-A (3) (2001) 428–436.
11. S.M. Kurtz, et al., The clinical performance of UHMWPE in the spine, in: S.M. Kurtz (Ed.), Ultra-high molecular weight polyethylene in total joint replacement and medical devices, Academic Press, , 2009.
12. E. Ingham, J. Fisher, Biological reactions to wear debris in total joint replacement, Inst. Mech. Eng. 214 (1) (2000) 21–37.
13. S.M. Kurtz, J.N. Devin, PEEK Biomaterials in trauma, orthopaedic, and surgical implants, Biomaterials 28 (32) (2007) 4845–4869.
14. W.J. Ciccone, et al., Bioabsorbable implants in orthopaedics: new developments and clinical applications, JAAOS 9 (5) (2001) 280–288.
15. D.J. Hak, The use of osteoconductive bone graft substitutes in orthopaedic trauma, JAAOS Vol. 15 (9) (2007) 525–536.
16. Electrochemical Corrosion. http://www.chem1.com/acad/webtext/elchem/ec7.html. Accessed February 18, 2010.